Family
Medical
Companion

Family
Medical
Companion

ISBN 1 85534 334 7

Printed and bound by Firmin-Didot (France),
Group Herissey. No d'impression : 35402.

Contents

Medical Terms

A

abdomen the region of the body which lies below the THORAX, being divided from it by the DIAPHRAGM, and above the PELVIS. The abdominal cavity contains the DIGESTIVE ORGANS (e.g. the STOMACH and INTESTINES), the EXCRETORY ORGANS (BLADDER and KIDNEYS) and, in females, the REPRODUCTIVE ORGANS (WOMB and OVARIES).

ablation the surgical removal (i.e. by cutting) of any part of the body.

abortifacient one of a number of drugs used to bring about an induced ABORTION.

abortion the removal of an embryo or foetus from the womb, either by natural expulsion or by human intervention, before it is considered to be viable at the 24th week of pregnancy. An abortion may be SPONTANEOUS, and this is commonest during the first three months of pregnancy and is thought to be most often associated with abnormalities in the foetus. Or an abortion may be INDUCED, when it is also known as THERAPEUTIC, or TERMINATION OF PREGNANCY, and is carried out for medical or social reasons.

Unless the mother's life is at risk, UK legislation requires a therapeutic abortion to be carried out before 24 weeks' gestation. A THREATENED ABORTION occurs when the foetus is alive but there is bleeding from the UTERUS and/or pain. If the foetus has died the abortion is referred to as INEVITABLE. An INCOMPLETE ABORTION describes the situation where some of the foetal material is left behind in the uterus.

HABITUAL ABORTION is where a woman loses each foetus in three consecutive pregnancies before the 20th week. The foetus weighs less than 500 grams and an abnormality in the uterus is one of the reasons why this occurs.

ABO system a blood group classification. *See* BLOOD GROUPS.

abrasion a superficial injury caused by the mechanical rubbing off of the skin surface or outer layer of a mucous membrane. Also known as a GRAZE.

abruptio placentae bleeding from the PLACENTA after the 28th week of PREGNANCY which may result in the placenta becoming completely or partially detached from the wall of the UTERUS.

abscess a collection of pus at a localized site anywhere in the body resulting from an infection caused by bacteria. Treatment is by the surgical opening of the abscess and by the administration of ANTIBIOTICS.

abscission the surgical removal of tissue by cutting.

acardia the condition which describes the congenital absence of the heart. It may arise where there are SIAMESE TWINS, in which case one heart is responsible for the circulation of both infants.

acetone a chemical substance which is formed in the body when normal metabolism is upset, as during prolonged bouts of vomiting, starvation, DIABETES MELLITUS, and sometimes as a result of severe fevers, particularly in children. The acetone is excreted in the urine and in the breath, and in diabetes may be a forewarning of coma.

acetylcholine an important organic chemical substance present in the body, which is known as a NEUROTRANSMITTER and is involved in the transmission of electrical impulses along nerves.

achalasia means failure to relax and usually refers to a condition called achalasia of the cardia. It describes the situation where the muscle fibres surrounding the opening of the OESOPHAGUS (gullet) into the stomach do not relax properly, and hinder the passage of swallowed food.

Achilles tendon this is a large, thick tendon present in the lower leg which attaches the calf muscles to the heel bone enabling this to be moved. It is prone to damage during the playing of energetic sports.

achondroplasia this is the commonest cause of DWARFISM in which the long bones of the limbs are abnormally short. It is inherited as a dominant characteristic which affects both sexes.

acidosis describes a condition in which the acidity of the blood and body fluids rises to an abnormally high level due to a failure in the mechanisms which regulate the acid/base balance in the body. It is commonly caused by a faulty metabolism of fat, as in DIABETES MELLITUS or during starvation and excessive vomiting.

It may also have a respiratory origin e.g. during drowning when a higher than normal level of carbon dioxide is retained in the body. It also occurs as a result of kidney failure (renal acidosis), when too much sulphuric and phosphoric acids are retained within the body or an excess of bicarbonate is excreted.

acne a disorder of the skin, the commonest of which is *acne vulgaris* in adolescents, characterized by the presence of pustules and blackheads.

SEBACEOUS GLANDS in the skin become overactive (due to hormonal influence) and there is a greater production of SEBUM and proliferation of bacteria which cause infection. The hair follicles become blocked and pustules form which eventually turn black. The condition usually resolves with time but can be eased with creams and sometimes antibiotics. Other forms of acne also occur. *See* ROSACEA.

acoustic descriptive of anything relating to the sense of hearing or sound.

acquired a condition or malady that is not CONGENITAL but arises after birth.

action potential *see* **nerve impulse**.

acupuncture a method of traditional healing practised in China which involves the insertion of fine needles at various points beneath the skin. The needles are moved by rotation or electric current and the system has been proved to be effective in the relief of symptoms, sometimes being employed as an alternative to ANAESTHESIA.

acute a disease or condition which is short-lived, and which starts rapidly with severe symptoms.

adactyly describes the absence of fingers or toes (digits).

Adam's apple a projection of the thyroid cartilage of the LARYNX which is visible beneath the skin of the throat.

addiction a broadly-used term which describes a state of physical and psychological dependence upon a substance or drug.

Addison's disease a disease caused by the failure of the ADRENAL GLANDS to secrete certain substances (the adrenocortical hormones), because the adrenal cortex has been damaged. This damage commonly used to be caused by tuberculosis but now, it may more often result from disturbances in the immune system. The symptoms of the disease are low blood pressure (hypotension), wasting, weakness, and dark pigmentation of the skin. A complete cure can be effected by replacing the deficient hormones with hormone replacement therapy.

adenitis refers to inflammation of one or more glands.

adenoidectomy the removal, by surgery, of the ADENOIDS.

adenoids a clump of lymphoid tissue situated at the back of the nose (in the nasopharynx). The adenoids may become swollen as a result of persistent throat infections, and may obstruct breathing through the nose.

adhesion this refers to the joining together of two surfaces which should normally be separate, and results from severe inflammation. Bands of fibrous tissue are formed which join the structures together. Adhesions may form within a joint which is damaged and inflamed, or following abdominal surgery when they may form between loops of the intestine, etc. Adhesions at a joint restrict its movement, a condition known as ankylosis, and can sometimes be resolved by manipulation. Adhesions within the abdomen or involving the lungs (resulting from PLEURISY) may require surgery to separate the fibrous bands.

adipose tissue a type of loose, fibrous, connective tissue containing a mass of fat cells. Excess food is laid down and stored within the fat cells and adipose tissue is found beneath the skin and around the kidneys. It provides a reserve energy store and also has an insulating function.

adjuvant therapy a type of drug therapy used in the management of certain cancers following on from radiotherapy, or surgical removal of a primary tumour. The aim is to destroy secondary tumours where there is a risk of these occurring and it is sometimes used in the treatment of breast cancer.

adrenal glands each of the two kidneys within the body bears an adrenal gland upon its upper surface. The adrenal glands, also known as suprarenal glands, are important ENDOCRINE organs, producing HORMONES that regulate various body functions. Each adrenal gland has two parts, an outer cortex and an inner medulla which secrete a variety of hormones. Two of the most important ones are ADRENALINE and CORTISONE.

adrenaline a very important hormone produced by the medulla of the adrenal glands which, when released, prepares the body for 'fright, flight or fight' by increasing the depth and rate of respiration, raising the heartbeat rate and improving muscle performance.

It also has an inhibitive effect on the processes of digestion and excretion. It can be used medically in a variety of ways, for instance in the treatment of bronchial asthma, where it relaxes the airways. It may be applied to wounds to check bleeding, as it constricts blood vessels in the skin, and also to stimulate the heart when there is cardiac arrest. Adrenaline is also known as epinephrine. *See* ADDISON'S DISEASE.

adrenocorticotrophic hormone (*or* **ACTH**) is an important substance produced and stored by the anterior PITUITARY GLAND. It regulates the release of corticosteroid hormones from the adrenal glands and is used medically, by injection, to test their function. It is also used in the treatment of asthma and rheumatic disorders.

adult respiratory distress syndrome (*or* **ARDS**) describes the condition of severe respiratory failure brought about by a number of different disorders. There is a lack of oxygen in the blood, which exhibits itself by imparting a blue tinge to the skin, and rapid breathing and pulse rate. The syndrome may be caused by physical damage to the lungs, by infection or by an adverse reaction following surgery or transfusion. It is often fatal.

aetiology (*or* **etiology**) the scientific study of the causes of disease.

afterbirth a mass of tissue consisting of the placenta, umbilical cord and membranes, which is detached and expelled from the womb during the third stage of labour following a birth.

afterpains pains caused by uterine contractions following a birth, which help to restore the uterus to its normal size. They may also indicate that a piece of placenta has been retained which the womb is trying to expel.

agoraphobia an abnormal fear of public places or open spaces.

AIDS this refers to *A*cquired *I*mmune *D*eficiency *S*yndrome, which was first recognized in Los Angeles in the USA in 1981. The causal agent was identified in 1983 as being the human immunodeficiency virus, known as HIV, a ribonucleic acid (RNA) RETROVIRUS. The virus has been found in blood, other body fluids, semen and cervical secretions and is mainly transmitted by sexual activity.

The HIV virus affects the T-LYMPHOCYTES of the immune system, and leaves the patient increasingly unable to resist certain infections and tumours which are particularly associated with AIDS. Although they may take a long time to develop, these infections eventually prove to be fatal and at the present time there is no known cure for AIDS.

air embolism a bubble of air in a blood vessel which interferes with the outward flow of blood from the right ventricle of the heart. The air may enter the circulation after an injury, surgery or infusion into a vein. The symptoms are chest pain and breathlessness, leading to acute heart failure.

air passages these are all the openings and passages through which air enters and is taken into the lungs. These are the nose, pharynx (throat), larynx, trachea (windpipe) and bronchial tubes. Air entering via this route has dust particles removed, and is warmed and moistened before entering the lungs.

albinism an inherited disorder in which there is a lack of pigmentation in the skin, hair and eyes. The pigment involved is melanin.

albino an individual affected by albinism, who typically has pink skin and eyes and white hair. The pink colour is imparted by blood in the blood vessels in the skin which, in a normal person, is masked by the presence of the pigment melanin. Albino people additionally suffer from poor eyesight and have increased sensitivity to sunlight, tending to burn easily.

alimentary canal the whole of the passage along which food is passed, starting at the mouth and ending at the anus.

alkalosis an abnormal rise in the alkalinity (a decrease in pH) of the blood and body fluids due to a failure or swamping of the mechanisms which regulate the acid-base balance in the body. It may arise through acid loss following prolonged vomiting, or occur in a patient who has been treated for a gastric ulcer with a large amount of alkalis.

Respiratory alkalosis may arise if breathing is too deep for the amount of physical exertion being undertaken. The symptoms of alkalosis include muscular cramps and fatigue.

allantois a structure which develops early in the life of an embryo and grows out from the hindgut, becoming attached to the wall of the womb. It later develops into the placenta and umbilical cord.

allele one of several forms of a GENE at a given place on the CHROMOSOME. They are usually present on different chromosomes and are responsible for certain characteristics of the PHENOTYPE. It is the dominance of one allele over another that determines the phenotype of the individual.

allergen any substance, usually a protein, which causes a hypersensitive (allergic) reaction in a person who is exposed to the allergen. There are a great variety of allergens which cause reactions in different tissues and body functions. The respiratory system and skin are often affected.

allergy a state of hypersensitivity in an affected individual to a particular allergen, which produces a characteristic response whenever the person is exposed to the substance. In an unaffected person, antibodies present in the bloodstream destroy their particular antigens (ALLERGENS). However, in an affected individual this reaction causes some cell damage and there is a release of substances such as histamine and bradykinin, which cause the allergic reaction. Examples of allergies are dermatitis, hay fever, asthma and the severe response known as ANAPHYLAXIS.

alopecia *see* **baldness**.

alpha fetoprotein a type of protein formed in the liver and gut of the foetus and which is detectable in the amniotic fluid and maternal blood. It is normally present in small amounts in the AMNIOTIC FLUID but when the foetus has a neural tube defect (SPINA BIFIDA or ANENCEPHALY), this level rises higher during the first six months of pregnancy. It can be detected by a maternal blood test at about the 16th week of pregnancy, and confirmed by AMNIOCENTESIS. If a foetus has DOWN'S SYNDROME, the level of alpha fetoprotein may be abnormally low. Alpha fetoprotein is also produced by some adult tissues if there is an abnormality present such as a type of liver cancer known as HEPATOMA.

alternative medicine the name describes all forms of healing other than western-orientated medical practice and includes acupuncture, homeopathy, osteopathy, naturopathy, faith healing and herbal remedies.

altitude sickness (*or* **mountain sickness**) This condition affects individuals (usually mountaineers) who are exposed to high altitudes to which they are unaccustomed. At high altitudes (4500m above sea level) there is a lack of oxygen and reduced atmospheric pressure. This causes a person to breathe more deeply and rapidly (hyperventilate) with a consequent lowering of CO_2 levels in the blood. Symptoms of altitude sickness are nausea, headache, exhaustion and anxiety. In severe cases there may be pulmonary OEDEMA in which excess fluid collects in the lungs, and this requires urgent medical treatment at a lower altitude.

alveolus (*plural* **alveoli**) a small sac or cavity which in numbers forms the alveolar sacs at the end of the BRONCHIOLES in the lungs. Each alveolus is fed by a rich blood supply via capillaries (*see* CAPILLARY) and is lined with a moist membrane where oxygen and carbon dioxide, the respiratory gases, are exchanged. The alveolar sacs provide an enormous surface area for efficient respiration.

Alzheimer's disease the commonest cause of dementia afflicting those in middle or old age, and a degenerative disease of the cerebral cortex for which there is no cure. Symptoms include progressive loss of memory and speech, and paralysis. The cause is not understood but is the subject of ongoing research.

amenorrhoea an absence of MENSTRUATION, which is normal before puberty, during PREGNANCY, and while breast-feeding is being carried out and following the MENOPAUSE. Primary amenorrhoea describes the situation where the menstrual periods do not begin at puberty. This occurs if there is a chromosome abnormality (such as TURNER'S SYNDROME) or if some reproductive organs are absent. It can also occur where there is a failure or imbalance in the secretion of hormones. In secondary amenorrhoea, the menstrual periods stop when they would normally be expected to be present. There are a variety of causes including hormone deficiency, disorders of the HYPOTHALAMUS, psychological and environmental stresses, during starvation, ANOREXIA nervosa or depression.

amines naturally-occurring compounds found in the body which have an important role in a variety of functions. They are derived from AMINO ACIDS and ammonia and include such substances as ADRENALINE and HISTAMINE.

amino acids the end products of the digestion of PROTEIN foods and the building blocks from which all the protein components of the body are built up. They all contain an acidic carboxyl group (-COOH) and an amino group ($-NH_2$) which are both bonded to the same central carbon atom. Some can be manufactured within the body whereas others, the ESSENTIAL AMINO ACIDS, must be derived from protein sources in the diet.

amnesia loss of memory which may be partial or total. *Anterograde* amnesia is the loss of memory of recent events following a trauma of some kind. *Retrograde* amnesia is the inability to remember events that preceded a trauma. Other types of amnesia are *post-traumatic* and *hysterical* and more than one kind may be experienced by an individual.

amniocentesis a procedure carried out to sample the amniotic fluid surrounding a foetus in order to test it in the laboratory. A fine needle is inserted through the abdominal wall of the mother and the amniotic sac is pierced so that a small quantity of fluid can be drawn off. The amniotic fluid contains ALPHA FETOPROTEIN and cells from the embryo, and various disorders such as Down's syndrome and spina bifida can be detected. It is usually carried out between the 16th and 20th week of pregnancy if a foetal abnormality is suspected.

amnion a fibrous, tough membranous sac which lines the womb and encloses the foetus floating within it surrounded by amniotic fluid. A caul is a piece of the amnion.

amnioscopy the procedure by which an instrument (an endoscope) is inserted either by means of an incision through the mother's abdominal wall or through her cervix, in order to view the foetus. An amnioscope is used if the procedure is carried out abdominally and a fetoscope if through the cervix.

amniotic cavity the cavity, filled with fluid, which is enclosed by the amnion and surrounds the foetus.

amniotic liquid the liquid within the amniotic cavity, which is clear and composed mainly of water containing foetal cells, lipids and urine from the foetus. At first it is produced by the amnion but its volume is supplemented by urine from the kidneys of the foetus. It is circulated by being swallowed by the foetus and excreted by the kidneys back into the cavity, and has an important protective function. The amniotic fluid ('waters') is released when the membranes rupture during labour.

amniotomy this refers to the artificial rupture of membranes, or ARM, which is carried out surgically by means of an instrument called an amnihook. The amnion is ruptured in order to induce the onset of labour.

amphetamines a group of drugs that are chemically similar to adrenaline and have a stimulating effect on the central nervous system. They act on the SYMPATHETIC NERVOUS SYSTEM and produce feelings of mental alertness and wellbeing, eliminating tiredness. However, they are highly addictive and dangerous and their medical use (mainly in the treatment of hyperkinetic syndrome, a mental disorder in children) is very strictly controlled.

ampicillin a type of semi-synthetic penicillin used to treat various infections and usually given by mouth or by injection.

ampoule a small plastic or glass bubble which is sterile and sealed, usually containing one dose of a drug to be administered by injection.

amputation the surgical removal of any body part, but generally a limb.

anabolic (steroids) refers to the effect of enhancing tissue growth by promoting the build-up of protein e.g. to enhance muscle bulk. Anabolic steroids are synthetic male sex hormones (which mimic ANDROGEN), and are used medically to aid

weight gain after wasting illnesses and to promote growth in children with certain types of dwarfism. They may also be used in the treatment of osteoporosis. Anabolic steroids should not be taken by healthy people as they have serious side effects, especially after prolonged use, and have been misused by athletes.

anaemia a decrease in the ability of the blood to carry oxygen due to a reduction in the number of red blood cells or in the amount of haemoglobin which they contain. Haemoglobin is the pigment within the red blood cells which binds to oxygen. There are a number of different types of anaemia and a variety of reasons for it, and treatment depends upon the underlying cause.

anaesthesia a loss of sensation or feeling in the whole or part of the body, usually relating to the administration of ANAESTHETIC drugs so that surgery can be performed.

anaesthetic a substance which, when administered, produces a loss of sensation in the whole (general anaesthetic) or part (local anaesthetic) of the body. General anaesthetics result in a loss of consciousness and usually a combination of drugs are used to achieve an optimum effect. These act to depress the activity of the CENTRAL NERVOUS SYSTEM, have an ANALGESIC effect and relax muscles, enabling surgical procedures to be carried out with no awareness on the part of the patient. Local anaesthetics block the transmission of nerve impulses in the area where they are applied so that no pain is felt. Commonly used ones are cocaine and lignocaine. They are used for minor surgical procedures and in dentistry.

anaesthetist a doctor who is medically specialized in the administration of anaesthetics.

analgesia a state of reduced reaction to pain, but without loss of consciousness. It may be due to drugs (*see* ANALGESICS) or it may happen accidentally should nerves become diseased or damaged.

analgesics drugs or substances which relieve pain, varying in potency from mild, such as paracetamol and aspirin, to very strong e.g. pethidine and morphine.

anaphylaxis a response exhibited by a hypersensitive individual when confronted with a particular ANTIGEN. It results from the release of histamine in body tissues following the antigen-antibody reaction within cells. An allergic reaction is an example of mild anaphylaxis. Anaphylactic shock is a much rarer and more serious condition, which can follow the injection of drugs or vaccines, or a bee sting, to which the individual is hypersensitive. Its onset is immediate and results from a widespread release of histamine in the body. The symptoms include severe breathing difficulties, swelling (OEDEMA), a fall in blood pressure, acute URTICARIA and heart failure. Death may follow if the individual is not soon treated with adrenaline by injection.

anaplasia the condition in which cells and tissues become less differentiated and distinctive and revert to a more primitive form. This state is typical in tumours which are malignant and growing very rapidly.

anastomosis in surgery, this refers to the artificial joining together of two or more tubes which are normally separate e.g. between parts of the intestine or blood vessels. In anatomy, this is the area of communication between the end branches of adjacent blood vessels.

anatomy the scientific study of the body structure of man and animals.

androgen one of a group of hormones which is responsible for the development of the sex organs and also the secondary sexual characteristics in the male. Androgens are steroid HORMONES and the best-known example is TESTOSTERONE. They are mainly secreted by the TESTES in the male but are also produced by the adrenal cortex and by the ovaries of females, in small amounts.

anencephaly a failure in the development of a foetus resulting in the absence of the cerebral hemispheres of the brain and some skull bones. If the pregnancy goes to term the infant dies soon after birth, but spontaneous abortion occurs in about 50% of affected pregnancies. Anencephaly is often associated with SPINA BIFIDA and is the most common developmental defect of the central nervous system. Anencephaly can be detected during the pregnancy by measuring the amount of ALPHA FETOPROTEIN present. *See also* AMNIOCENTESIS.

aneuploidy this describes the condition in which an abnormal number of chromosomes are present in the cells of an affected individual. The number of chromosomes is either more or less than the normal exact multiple of the HAPLOID number (half the full complement) and is characteristic of DOWN'S SYNDROME and TURNER'S SYNDROME. *See* EUPLOID.

aneurysm a balloon-like swelling of the wall of an artery which occurs when it becomes weakened or damaged in some way. There may be a congenital weakness in the muscular wall of the artery involved, as is often the case within the brain. Damage may also be the result of infection, particularly SYPHILIS, or degenerative conditions

e.g. ATHEROMA. There is a danger within the brain that an aneurysm may rupture causing a SUBARACHNOID HAEMORRHAGE or cerebral haemorrhage. The surgical treatment of aneurysms has greatly advanced and is very successful in many cases.

angina pectoris a suffocating, choking pain which is felt in the chest. The pain is felt or brought on by exercise and relieved by rest, and occurs when the blood supply to the heart muscle is inadequate. During exercise the demand for blood (supplied by the coronary arteries) is increased and if the supply is insufficient, because the arteries are damaged, chest pain results. The coronary arteries may be damaged by ATHEROMA, the most common cause. Angina pectoris is usually first treated with drugs but if the condition worsens, coronary-artery bypass surgery (ANGIOPLASTY) may need to be performed.

angiocardiography an X-ray examination technique of the activity of the heart involving the injecting of a radio-opaque substance. The X-ray film obtained is called an angiocardiogram.

angiography an examination technique of blood vessels using X-rays, made possible by first injecting a radio-opaque substance. If the blood vessels being examined are arteries, it is called arteriography and if veins, venography or phlebography.

angioma a clump of distended blood vessels pushing onto the surface of the brain. It may cause epilepsy and occasionally a vessel may burst to cause a SUBARACHNOID HAEMORRHAGE.

angioneurotic oedema a short-lived painless swelling which may result from infection, allergic reaction to drugs or food, stress, or it can be hereditary.

angioplasty a surgical method used to widen or reopen a narrowed or blocked blood vessel or heart valve. A balloon is inserted and then inflated to clear the obstruction.

angitis (*or* **vasculitis**) this describes the condition where there is inflammation of the walls of small blood vessels, usually in patches.

anorexia means a loss of appetite. *Anorexia nervosa* is a psychological disorder which is commonly associated with young female individuals. The person has a false and distorted image of herself as fat and a fear or phobia relating to obesity, and becomes unable to eat. The person may take laxatives and induce vomiting, as well as starving herself, in order to lose weight. Accompanying symptoms include AMENORRHOEA, low blood pressure, ANAEMIA and a risk of sudden death from heart damage. Treatment consists of psychotherapy, along with persuasion to eat.

anoxia the condition when the body tissues do not receive sufficient oxygen. It may be due to high altitudes (and thus lower atmospheric pressure), a lack of red blood cells, or a disease such as PNEUMONIA which limits the amount of oxygen reaching the lung surfaces and therefore reduces that available for transfer to the blood.

antacids substances which neutralize acidity, usually hydrochloric acid in the digestive juices of the stomach. An example is sodium bicarbonate.

antagonistic action an action in which systems or processes act against each other so that the activity of one reduces that of the other. Two muscles may operate in this way, the contraction of one necessitating the relaxation of the other, as in the movement of a limb. In addition, hormones and drugs act antagonistically, the release of one limiting the effect of the other.

antenatal before birth. Pregnant women attend antenatal clinics, which monitor the health of both mothers and their unborn babies.

anthrax a serious infectious disease of cattle and sheep, which can be transmitted to man and is caused by a bacillus, *B. anthracis*. The spores of the bacillus remain viable for many years and are resistant to destruction. People can be infected by handling contaminated skins, fleeces and bones and the spores may either be inhaled or enter through a cut in the skin. The danger is increased if the infected skins are dry, so that spores and dust are inhaled. The disease takes two forms in man, either affecting the lungs (if the spores are inhaled) causing pneumonia (*Wool sorter's disease*), or the skin (if infected through a cut), known as malignant pustule, a severe ulceration. The disease is now rare in the UK, but can be fatal, although it is usually successfully treated with large doses of PENICILLIN and tetracycline ANTIBIOTIC drugs.

antibiotic a substance, derived from a microorganism, which kills or inhibits the multiplication of other microorganisms, usually bacteria or fungi. Well-known examples are penicillin and streptomycin.

antibodies protein substances of the GLOBULIN type which are produced by the lymphoid tissue and circulate in the blood. They react with their corresponding ANTIGENS and neutralize them, rendering them harmless. Antibodies are produced against a wide variety of antigens and these reactions are responsible for IMMUNITY and ALLERGY.

anticholinergic side effects the effects that may be experienced when taking anticholinergic drugs. The drugs compete with the NEUROTRANSMITTER ACETYLCHOLINE at the synapses of nerves, resulting in side effects such as dry mouth, nausea, vomiting, retention of urine, constipation and impaired vision.

anticoagulants drugs or substances which delay or tend to prevent blood clotting, examples of which are warfarin and heparin. These are used in the treatment of EMBOLISM and THROMBOSIS to disperse blood clots in vessels.

anticonvulsants drugs which are used to reduce the severity of epileptic fits (convulsions) or to prevent them from occurring.

antidepressants drugs which are administered in order to alleviate the symptoms of depression.

antidote a substance which counteracts the effect of a particular poison.

antiemetic a drug taken to prevent vomiting, such as are used for travel sickness (*see* MOTION SICKNESS) and VERTIGO.

antigens any substances which cause the formation by the body of ANTIBODIES to neutralize their effect. Antigens are often protein substances, regarded as 'foreign' and 'invading' by the body, and elicit the production of antibodies against them. *See* ALLERGEN, ALLERGY and ANAPHYLAXIS.

antihistamines drugs which counteract the effects of histamine release in the body. They are widely used to treat allergic reactions of various sorts, particularly to relieve skin conditions. Those taken by mouth have a sedative effect and so care must be taken while they are being used.

anti-inflammatory anything which reduces inflammation. Typical anti-inflammatory drugs are the antihistamines, non-steroidal anti-inflammatory drugs (NSAID types, used especially in the treatment of rheumatic disease) and glucocorticoids.

antimetabolites a group of drugs used particularly in the treatment of certain cancers which mimic substances (metabolites) present in the cells. The antimetabolites combine with enzymes which would otherwise use the metabolites for cell growth. Hence they reduce the growth of cancer cells but also have attendant side effects which can be severe.

antiperistalsis *see* **peristalsis**.

antiseptics substances which prevent the growth of disease-causing microorganisms, such as bacteria, and which are applied to the skin to prevent infection and to cleanse wounds. Examples are iodine and crystal violet.

antiserum a serum, usually prepared from horses,

which contains a high concentration of antibody against a particular antigen. It is injected to give immunity against a particular disease or toxin.

anuria a failure of the kidneys to produce urine which may result from a number of disorders which cause a prolonged drop in blood pressure. Anuria is typical of increasing URAEMIA and HAEMODIALYSIS may be necessary.

anus the opening of the alimentary canal at the opposite end from the mouth, through which faeces are voided. The anus is at the lower end of the bowel and its opening is controlled by two muscles, the internal and external sphincters.

anxiety *see* **neurosis**.

aorta the major large artery of the body, which arises from the left ventricle of the heart and which carries blood to all areas. The other arteries of the body are all derived from the aorta.

aortic stenosis a narrowing of the opening of the aortic valve, resulting in the obstruction of the flow of blood from the left ventricle to the aorta. A common cause of this is calcium deposits formed on the valve associated with ATHEROMA, or damage caused by previous RHEUMATIC FEVER. Also, the condition may arise congenitally. The effect is that the left ventricle muscle has to work harder in order to try to maintain the blood flow, and becomes thicker as a result. The symptoms of aortic stenosis include ANGINA PECTORIS and breathlessness. The condition is treated surgically by valve replacement.

apgar score a method of assessing the health of an infant immediately after birth, carried out at one minute and five minutes after delivery. The breathing, muscle tone, response to stimuli, heartbeat rate and skin colour are assessed and each awarded a maximum of two points. Further detailed monitoring of progress follows if a low score is achieved.

aphasia speechlessness caused by disease or injury to those parts of the brain which govern the activities involved in speech-making. It is caused by THROMBOSIS, EMBOLISM or HAEMORRHAGE of a blood vessel within the brain, as in a STROKE, or by a TUMOUR. It may be temporary if the blood supply is not permanently damaged, but often the power of speech continues to be impaired and is associated with other intellectual disorders.

aphonia loss of the voice, which may be caused by disease or damage to the LARYNX or mouth, or to nerves controlling throat muscles, or may result from HYSTERIA.

aplasia a complete or partial failure in the correct development of an organ or tissue.

apnoea a temporary halt in breathing which may result from a number of different causes. Apnoea is quite common in newborn infants and can be registered by an apnoea monitor which sounds an alarm if the baby ceases to breathe.

apocrine the term for sweat glands that occur in hairy parts of the body. The odours associated with sweating are due to bacterial action on the sweat produced. *See also* PERSPIRATION.

appendicectomy (*or* **appendectomy**) the surgical operation to remove the vermiform APPENDIX.

appendicitis inflammation of the vermiform APPENDIX, which, in its acute form, is the most common abdominal emergency in the western world, usually requiring treatment by APPENDICECTOMY. It is most common in young people during their first 20 years, and the symptoms include abdominal pain which may move about, appetite loss, sickness and diarrhoea. If not treated the appendix can become the site of an ABSCESS, or become gangrenous, which eventually may result in PERITONITIS. This arises because infected material spreads from the burst appendix into the peritoneal cavity. Appendicectomy at an early stage is highly successful and normally results in a complete cure.

appendix a blind-ended tube which is an appendage of various organs within the body. It normally refers to the vermiform appendix, which is about 9 to 10 cm long, and projects from the CAECUM (a pouch) of the large intestine. It has no known function and can become the site of infection, probably as the result of obstruction. *See* APPENDICECTOMY and APPENDICITIS.

areola means a small space and usually refers to the brown-coloured, pigmented ring around the nipple of the breast.

arm strictly, this refers to the section of the upper limb between the elbow and the shoulder, but is usually used to describe the whole limb.

arrhythmia any disturbance in the normal rhythm of heartbeat. The built-in pacemaker of the heart is the sinoatrial node situated in the wall of the right atrium, which itself is regulated by the AUTONOMIC NERVOUS SYSTEM. The electrical impulses produced by the pacemaker control the rate and rhythm of heartbeat. Arryhthmias occur when these electrical impulses are disturbed, and there are various different types, including EXTRASYSTOLE (ectopic beats), ectopic tachycardias, heart block and FIBRILLATION. Most heart diseases cause arrhythmias but they may also arise for no obvious cause.

arteriectomy the surgical removal of a part or the whole of an artery.

arteriogram the recording of an arterial pulse which appears as a trace in wave form. It may be recorded on an oscilloscope screen or on a paper strip by various methods.

arteriography the X-ray examination of an artery following the injection of a radio-opaque substance.

arteriole a small branch of an artery leading to a capillary.

arterioplasty surgery to reconstruct an artery, which is carried out especially in the treatment of ANEURYSMS.

arteriosclerosis a vague term used to describe several degenerative conditions affecting the arteries. *See* ATHEROMA and ATHEROSCLEROSIS.

arteritis inflammation of an artery.

artery a blood vessel which carries blood away from the heart. Oxygenated (bright red) blood is carried by the arteries to all parts of the body. However, the pulmonary arteries carry dark, unoxygenated blood from the heart to the lungs. An artery has thick, elastic walls, which are able to expand and contract, and contain smooth muscle fibres. This smooth muscle is under the control of the SYMPATHETIC NERVOUS SYSTEM.

arthritis inflammation of the joints or spine, the symptoms of which are pain and swelling, restriction of movement, redness and warmth of the skin. There are many different causes of arthritis including OSTEOARTHRITIS, RHEUMATOID ARTHRITIS, TUBERCULOSIS and RHEUMATIC FEVER.

arthropathy any joint disorder or disease.

arthroplasty the operation to repair a diseased joint by constructing a new one, often involving the insertion of artificial materials.

artificial insemination SEMEN collected from a donor is inserted by means of an instrument into the vagina of a woman in the hope that she will conceive. The semen may be from her husband or partner (AIH) or from an anonymous donor (AID) and is introduced near the time of ovulation. Usually AIH is used if the partner is impotent and AID if he is sterile.

artificial respiration an emergency procedure carried out when normal respiration has ceased, in order to artificially ventilate the lungs, usually referred to as 'artificial respiration'. In hospital, where a seriously ill person is unable to breathe unaided, artificial respiration is achieved by means of a machine known as a ventilator.

asbestosis a disease of the lungs, which is a form of pneumoconiosis caused by the inhalation of asbestos dust. Asbestos has been used in many industries and the dust causes scarring of the lungs.

There is a serious risk of MESOTHELIOMA or cancer of the lung and those working with asbestos have to adhere to strict health and safety procedures.

asepsis a state of complete absence of harmful pathogenic microorganisms achieved by various sterilization techniques. This is the optimum state in which operations are carried out.

asphyxia the state of suffocation during which breathing eventually stops and oxygen fails to reach tissues and organs. It occurs as a result of drowning, strangulation and breathing in poisonous fumes.

Also, it can result from obstruction of the air passages, either by a foreign body lodged at the opening (e.g. a piece of food) or by swelling due to a wound or infection. In the state of asphyxia, the heartbeat rate rises and the person gasps for breath, and there is a rise in blood pressure and blueness in the skin. Eventually a state of paralysis ensues, followed by death. However, if asphyxia is due to the inhalation of narcotic fumes there is no struggle and the person may die peacefully during sleep.

aspiration the process of removing fluid or gases from cavities in the body by means of suction. The instrument used is called an aspirator and various types exist depending upon site of use.

aspirin a type of drug in widespread use which is correctly called acetylsalicylic acid. It is used to relieve mild pain e.g. headache, neuralgia and that associated with rheumatoid arthritis. It is also used to combat fever, and is also helpful in the prevention of CORONARY THROMBOSIS. In susceptible individuals it may cause irritation and bleeding of the stomach lining and is not normally given to children under the age of 12 years. High doses will cause dizziness and possibly mental confusion.

asthma a condition characterized by breathing difficulties caused by narrowing of the airways (bronchi, *see* BRONCHUS) of the lung.

It is a distressing condition, with breathlessness and a paroxysmal wheezing cough, and the extent to which the bronchi narrow varies considerably. Asthma may occur at any age but usually begins in early childhood, and is a hypersensitive response which can be brought on by exposure to a variety of ALLERGENS, exercise, stress or infections. An asthma sufferer may have other hypersensitive conditions, such as eczema and hay fever, and it may be prevalent within a family. It may or may not be possible for a person to avoid the allergen(s) responsible for an asthma attack. Treatment involves the use of drugs to dilate the airways (bronchodilators), and also inhaled corticosteroids.

astigmatism a defect in vision which results in sight being blurred and distorted. It is caused by abnormal curvature of the CORNEA, and possibly also at the LENS, of the EYE, so that not all the light entering is focused on the retina. Treatment is by wearing glasses with special cylindrical lenses, which produce the opposite distortion and cancel out that of the eye itself.

astringent a substance that causes cells to contract by losing proteins from their surface. They cause localized contraction of blood vessels and are applied to minor wounds of the skin, and are used in mouthwashes and eyedrops.

ataxia a loss of coordination in the limbs, due to a disorder of the CENTRAL NERVOUS SYSTEM. There may be a disease of the sensory nerves (sensory ataxia) or of the CEREBELLUM (cerebellar ataxia). An ataxic person produces clumsy movements and lacks fine control. *See* FRIEDREICH'S ATAXIA and LOCOMOTOR ATAXIA.

atheroma a degenerative condition of the arteries. The inner and middle coats of the arterial walls become scarred and fatty deposits (CHOLESTEROL) are built up at these sites. The blood circulation is impaired and it may lead to such problems as ANGINA PECTORIS, STROKE and heart attack. The condition is associated with the western lifestyle, i.e. lack of exercise, smoking, obesity and too high an intake of animal fats.

atherosclerosis similar to ATHEROMA, being a degenerative disease of the arteries, associated with fatty deposits on the inner walls, leading to reduced blood flow.

athlete's foot a fungal infection of the skin particularly occurring between the toes and often due to ringworm.

atrium (*plural* **atria**) one of the two thin-walled upper chambers of the heart, which receive blood from major veins. The right atrium receives (deoxygenated) blood from the venae cavae and the left atrium is supplied with (oxygenated) blood from the pulmonary vein. (Atria also refers to various other chambers in the body.)

atrophy wasting of a body part, due to lack of use, malnutrition, or as a result of ageing. The ovaries of women atrophy after the menopause and muscular atrophy accompanies certain diseases. *See* POLIOMYELITIS.

aural relating to the ear.

auricle the external flap of the ear, known as the pinna. Also, an ear-shaped appendage of the ATRIUM of the heart.

autism a severe mental disorder of childhood in which there is a failure in emotional development and an inability to communicate. There are accompanying behavioural problems and autism may be caused by brain damage and genetic factors. Autistic individuals exhibit stereotyped patterns of behaviour and may or may not be intellectually impaired. They require intensive and prolonged education in order to progress.

autoantibody an antibody produced by the body against one of its own tissues, which is a feature of AUTOIMMUNE DISEASE.

autoclave equipment used to sterilize surgical equipment and dressings, etc., by means of steam at high pressure. It is one of the most important methods of sterilization.

autograft a graft of skin or tissue taken from one part of a person's body and transferred to another region. Since the graft is 'self' it is not rejected by the body's immune system.

autoimmune disease one of a number of conditions resulting from the production of antibodies by the body which attack its own tissues. For reasons which are not understood the immune system loses the ability to distinguish between 'self' and 'non-self'. Autoimmune disease is currently thought to be the cause of a number of disorders, including acquired haemolytic anaemia (*see* HAEMOLYSIS), PERNICIOUS ANAEMIA, RHEUMATOID ARTHRITIS, RHEUMATIC FEVER and DIABETES MELLITUS.

autoimmunity a failure of the immune system in which the body develops antibodies that attack components or substances belonging to itself. *See* AUTOANTIBODY and AUTOIMMUNE DISEASE.

autonomic nervous system the part of the nervous system which controls body functions that are not under conscious control, e.g., the heartbeat and other smooth muscles and glands. It is divided into the SYMPATHETIC and PARASYMPATHETIC NERVOUS SYSTEMS.

autopsy (*or* **post mortem**) the examination and dissection of a body after death.

aversion therapy a type of psychological conditioning, which links an unpleasant stimulus to the undesirable behaviour that needs to be eliminated. An example is the use of a drug which induces vomiting in an alcoholic person each time he or she takes a drink. The unpleasant association induces the person to give up alcoholic drink. Electric shock is also commonly used in aversion therapy, which is a method of treatment for such conditions as sexual perversion, compulsive behaviour (e.g. gambling) and drug addicton.

axon *see* **neuron**.

B

Babinski reflex a reflex response of the foot (*see* PLANTAR REFLEX). When the sole is stroked the big toe turns up and the others fan out. This is normal for infants up to two years but abnormal thereafter.

bacillus (*plural* **bacilli**) a term for any bacterium that is rod-shaped. Also a genus of Gram-positive (*see* GRAM'S STAIN) bacteria that includes *B. anthracis*, the cause of anthrax.

backache pain in the back which may vary in intensity, sharpness and cause. Much back pain is due to mechanical/structural problems, including fractures, muscle strain or pressure on a nerve. Other causes include tumours, bone disease such as OSTEOPOROSIS, referred pain from an ulcer, and inflammation e.g. SPONDYLITIS. Treatment is varied and may be surgical, heat treatment, ultrasound, medications etc.

backbone *see* **spinal column.**

bacteria (*singular* **bacterium**) single-cell organisms that underpin all life-sustaining processes. GRAM'S STAIN is a test used to distinguish between the two types (Gram-positive and Gram-negative). They are also identified by shape: spiral, (spirilli), rod-like (bacilli), spherical (cocci), comma-shaped (vibrid) and spirochaetal (that are corkscrew-like). Bacteria are the key agents in the chemical cycles of carbon, oxygen, nitrogen and sulphur. Some are responsible for disease in plants and animals e.g. tuberculosis, typhoid, syphilis and cholera.

bactericide something that kills bacteria, used especially when referring to drugs and antiseptics.

bacteriology the study of bacteria.

bacteriophage a virus that attacks a BACTERIUM. The phage replicates in the host which is ultimately destroyed as new phages are released. Each phage is specific to a certain bacterium and uses are found in genetic engineering in cloning and certain manufacturing processes.

baldness the gradual depletion of hair on the head which is to a great extent hereditary. Baldness is a symptom of some diseases, e.g. SYPHILIS, MYXOEDEMA and anaemia, and *alopecia* is a patchy baldness of the scalp that can affect other areas of the body. Baldness is often preceded (for several years) by SEBORRHOEIC ECZEMA which causes hair follicles to lose their capacity to produce hair in the natural cycle of replacement.

ballottement the technique whereby a floating structure in the body can be gently pushed so that it rebounds, as with a foetus.

balsam one of several resinous substances, in the main derived from evergreens, that contain BENZOIC ACID, e.g. Friar's balsam and balsam of tolu. They are used to alleviate colds and may be applied to abrasions.

bandage a material pad or strip wrapped around a part of the body to hold a dressing in place, immobilize a limb or maintain pressure on a compress. There are several types including crepe, domette (used in orthopaedics), elastic (for support), tubular (for easy application and maintenance of light pressure) and PLASTER OF PARIS bandages which are used as splints.

barbiturate drugs that are derived from barbituric acid and which have anaesthetic, hypnotic or sedative effects. Barbiturates reduce blood pressure and temperature and depress the central nervous system and respiration. TRANQUILLIZERS are replacing barbiturates to lessen drug abuse.

barium sulphate a heavy chemical powder used in X-ray examinations. Due to its opaque (to X-rays) nature, it forms a shadow in whatever cavity it lies. It is used for the examination of the stomach and intestines and can be used to trace a meal through the bowels.

barrier cream a cream, lotion or ointment put onto the skin to provide protection against irritants, allergens, sunlight, etc. Water-repellent silicones are frequently used.

basal ganglion GREY MATTER at the base of the CEREBRUM, which is involved in the subconscious control of voluntary movement.

base pairing linking of the two strands of a DNA molecule between the bases of the constituent NUCLEOTIDES. The bases differ in structure: adenine and guanine being purines; thymine, cytosine and uracil being pyrimidines, and a purine bonds to a pyrimidine e.g. A - T, C - G. The particular nature of the base pairing produces a highly structured DNA that can be replicated precisely (ensuring accurate transmission of genetic information from parent to daughter cell).

BCG vaccine Bacillus Calmette-Guérin vaccine, named after the two French bacteriologists and first introduced in France in 1908. It is used as a vaccine against TUBERCULOSIS, usually administered intradermally, and complications are rare. A pre-vaccination test is applied to all save the newborn and vaccination is given to those showing a negative result. Vaccination is usually given to: schoolchildren aged 10 to 14; children of Asian origin, because tuberculosis has a high incidence in this ethnic group; health workers and others.

bed sores (*or* **pressure sores** *or* **decubitus ulcers**) sore and ulcerated skin caused by constant pressure on an area of the body. Bedridden, particularly unconscious patients, are at risk and their position has to be changed to relieve the prone areas: heels, buttocks, elbows, lower back etc. The best action is preventative, because healing may be slowed by reduced blood supply.

behaviour therapy the treatment of behavioural disorders through the use of psychotherapy. Existing responses or patterns of behaviour are replaced through the use of therapies such as AVERSION THERAPY.

Bell's palsy a paralysis of the facial muscles on either or both sides of the face caused by infection/inflammation, when it may be temporary. Permanent paralysis may result from a basal skull fracture, stroke, etc. The paralysis results in an inability to open and close the eye, smile and close the mouth on the side affected.

B endorphin a painkiller released by the PITUITARY in response to pain and stress.

bends (*or* **compressed air illness** *or* **Caisson disease**) workers operating in high pressure in diving bells or at depth underwater may suffer if surfacing too rapidly. Pain in the joints (the bends), headache and dizziness (decompression sickness) and paralysis may be caused by the formation of nitrogen bubbles in the blood, which then accumulate in different parts of the body. Death may occur. The symptoms can be relieved by increasing the atmospheric pressure on the sufferer, causing the nitrogen to redissolve.

Benedict's test a test for glucose and reducing sugars. It consists of a solution of copper sulphate, sodium carbonate and sodium citrate to which the sample is added. The resulting solution is boiled and sugar is indicated by a rust-coloured precipitate. The test is used to detect sugar in urine if DIABETES is suspected.

benign used most frequently with reference to tumours, meaning not harmful.

benzene hexachloride a rapidly acting insecticide.

benzhexol (*or* **benzhexol hydrochloride**, *or* **trihexyphenidyl hydrochloride**) a drug prescribed in the treatment of PARKINSON'S DISEASE.

benzocaine used in various forms, a local anaesthetic for relief of painful skin conditions including those within the mouth.

benzodiazepines a group of drugs that act as tranquillizers (e.g. diazepam), hypnotics (flurazepam) and anticonvulsants, depending upon the duration of action.

benzoic acid an antiseptic used to preserve certain pharmaceutical preparations and foodstuffs. It is also used in treating fungal infections of the skin, and urinary tract infections.

benzoin a resin used in the preparation of compounds which are inhaled in the treatment of colds, bronchitis (e.g. Friar's BALSAM), etc.

benzothiadiazines DIURETIC compounds taken orally, which reduce the reabsorption of chloride and sodium ions in the renal tubules of the KIDNEY. A secondary effect is a lowering of the blood pressure and a primary use is to relieve OEDEMA in heart failure.

benzoyl peroxide a bactericidal agent used as a bleach in the food industry and also as a treatment for ACNE.

beri beri a disease causing inflammation of the nerves, due to a dietary lack of vitamin B₁ (thiamine), which results in fever, paralysis and palpitations and can occasionally precipitate heart failure. Beri beri is most prevalent in southeast Asia, China and Japan and is due to the removal of rice husks in processing.

beta blocker drugs used to treat ANGINA, reduce high blood pressure and manage abnormal heart rhythms. Certain receptors of nerves in the SYMPATHETIC NERVOUS SYSTEM are blocked, reducing heart activity. A notable side effect is constriction of bronchial passages which may adversely affect some patients.

biceps a muscle that is said to have two heads e.g. the biceps of the upper arm (*biceps brachii*) and the biceps on the back of the thigh (*biceps femoris*).

bifurcation the branching of, for example, a blood vessel into two. Also the TRACHEA where it forms two bronchi (*see* BRONCHUS).

biguanides substances, taken orally, that reduce

blood sugar level and are used in the treatment of *diabetes mellitus*. The result is that glucose production in the liver is reduced.

bile a viscous, bitter fluid produced by the LIVER and stored in the GALL BLADDER, a small organ near the liver. It is an alkaline solution of bile salts, pigments (*see* BILIRUBIN), some mineral salts and CHOLESTEROL, which aids in fat digestion and absorption of nutrients. Discharge of bile into the intestine is increased after food and of the amount secreted each day (up to one litre), most is reabsorbed with the food, passing back into the blood to circulate back to the liver. If the flow of bile into the intestine is restricted, it stays in the blood, resulting in jaundice.

bile duct a duct that carries BILE from the liver. The main duct is the hepatic which joins the cystic duct from the GALL BLADDER to form the common bile duct which drains into the small INTESTINE.

bilirubin one of the two important BILE pigments, formed primarily from the breakdown of HAEMOGLOBIN from red blood cells. Bilirubin is orange-yellow in colour while its oxidized form biliverdin is green. The majority of bile produced daily is eventually excreted and confers colour to the stools.

bioassay the determination of a drug's activity or potency by comparing its effects on a living organism with that of a reference sample of known strength. In the absence of other methods, bioassay is used in determining the strength of biological materials e.g. hormones.

bioavailability the term used to describe the amount of a drug that becomes available at its target, after administration and having followed a particular route. The amount may be low for drugs administered by mouth since food affects bioavailability through the alteration of the rate of absorption. Components of food, e.g. calcium, may act as a chelating agent (restricting the amount of the drug that is free), also reducing the absorption of a drug.

biochemistry the study of the chemistry of biological processes and substances in living organisms. Such studies contribute to the overall understanding of cell metabolism, diseases and their effects.

biofeedback the provision of information to a subject about his or her autonomic physiological responses (e.g. blood pressure, heart rate) by means of electronic instrumentation. The subject becomes able, through responding to the generated signals, to control the function in question (this is called *operant conditioning*). It is

uncertain how this is achieved, although it can be effective in regulating, for example, hypertension.

biopsy an adjunct to diagnosis, which involves removing a small sample of living tissue from the body for examination under the microscope. The technique is particularly important in differentiating between benign and malignant tumours. A biopsy can be undertaken with a hollow needle inserted into the relevant organ.

biotin one of a number of vitamins in the B-complex that are synthesized by bacteria in the intestine. It also occurs in liver, meat, eggs, vegetables, milk and cereals. A biotin deficiency can occur only if large amounts of egg white are ingested, because a constituent, avidin, binds to the biotin. Serious deficiency results in dermatitis, muscle pains, anorexia and changes in heart activity.

birthmark (*or* **naevus**) an agglomeration of dilated blood vessels creating a malformation of the skin, and is present at birth. These may occur as a large port-wine stain which can now be treated by laser, or a strawberry mark which commonly fades in early life. *See also* MOLE.

bismuth a metal of which various salts are used in medicine. It occurs in treatments for diarrhoea, haemorrhoids and externally in the management of skin conditions.

bladder a sac of fibrous and muscular tissue that contains secretions and which can increase and decrease in capacity. Discharge of the contents is through a narrow opening. *See* GALL BLADDER and URINARY ORGANS.

blastocyst a spherical mass of cells that forms an early stage in human development and occurs at the time of implantation in the uterus wall.

blindness being unable to see, a condition which may vary from a total lack of light perception (total blindness) through degrees of visual impairment. The commonest causes of blindness are GLAUCOMA, senile CATARACT, vitamin A deficiency (night blindness) and DIABETES MELLITUS.

blood a suspension of red blood cells (or corpuscles) called erythrocytes, white blood cells (leucocytes) and platelets (small disc-shaped cells involved in blood clotting) in a liquid medium, blood PLASMA. The circulation of blood through the body provides a mechanism for transporting substances. Its functions include:

1) carrying oxygenated blood from the heart to all tissues via the arteries while the veins return deoxygenated blood to the heart.

2) carrying essential nutrients, e.g. glucose, fats and amino acids to all parts of the body.

3) removing the waste products of metabolism— ammonia and carbon dioxide, to the liver where urea is formed and then transported by the blood to the kidneys for excretion.

4) carrying important molecules, e.g. hormones, to their target cells.

The red blood cells, produced in the bone marrow, are haemoglobin-containing discs while the white varieties vary in shape and are produced in the marrow and lymphoid tissue. The plasma comprises water, proteins and electrolytes and forms approximately half the blood volume.

blood bank a unit in which blood is collected, processed and stored, prior to its use in transfusions.

blood clot a hard mass of blood platelets, trapped red blood cells and fibrin. After tissue damage, blood vessels in the area are constricted and a plug forms to seal the damaged are. The plug formation is initiated by an ENZYME released by the damaged blood vessels and platelets.

blood count (*or* **complete blood count** *or* **CBC**) a count of the numbers of red and white blood cells per unit volume of blood. The count may be performed manually using a microscope, or electronically.

blood groups the division and classification of people into one of four main groups, based upon the presence of ANTIGENS on the surface of the red blood cells (corpuscles). The classifying reaction depends upon the SERUM of one person's blood agglutinating (clumping together) the red blood cells of someone else. The antigens, known as agglutinogens react with antibodies (agglutinins) in the serum. There are two agglutinogens termed A and B and two agglutinins called anti-A and anti-B. This gives rise to four groups: corpuscles with no agglutinogens, group O; with A; with B and with both A and B (hence blood group AB). The agglutinin groups match those of the agglutinogens, thus a person of blood group B has anti-A serum in their blood. It is vital that blood groups are matched for transfusion because incompatibility will produce blood clotting.

The Rhesus factor is another antigen (named after the Rhesus monkey, which has a similar antigen), those with it being Rh-positive and those without Rh-negative. About 85% of people are Rh-positive. If a Rh-negative person receives Rh-positive blood, or if a Rh-positive foetus is exposed to antibodies to the factor in the blood of the Rh-negative mother, then HAEMOLYSIS occurs in the foetus and newborn child. This may cause the stillbirth of the child, or jaundice after birth. Testing of pregnant women is thus essential.

blood poisoning *see* **septicaemia**.

blood pressure the pressure of the blood on the heart and blood vessels in the system of circulation. Also the pressure that has to be applied to an artery to stop the pulse beyond the pressure point.

Blood pressure peaks at a heartbeat (SYSTOLE) and falls in between (DIASTOLE). The systolic pressure in young adults is equivalent to approximately 120mm mercury (and 70mm in diastole). The pressure also depends upon the hardness and thickness of vessel walls and blood pressure tends to increase with age as arteries thicken and harden.

A temporary rise in blood pressure may be precipitated by exposure to cold; a permanent rise by kidney disease and other disorders. A lower blood pressure can be induced by a hot bath or be caused by exhaustion. The instrument used to measure blood pressure is the SPHYGMOMANOMETER.

blood sugar glucose concentration in the blood for which the typical value is 3.5 to 5.5 mmol/l (millimoles per litre). *See also* HYPOGLYCAEMIA and HYPERGLYCAEMIA.

blood transfusion the replacement of blood lost due to injury, surgery, etc. A patient may receive whole blood or a component e.g. packed red cells (red blood cells separated from the PLASMA, used to counteract anaemia and restore HAEMOGLOBIN levels). Blood from donors is matched to the recipient for BLOOD GROUP and haemoglobin. Donor blood can be stored for three weeks before use if kept just a few degrees above freezing, after which the platelets, leucocytes and some red blood cells become non-viable. Plasma and serum are also transfused and, in the dried form, plasma can be stored for up to five years.

blood vessel the veins and arteries and their smaller branchings, venules and arterioles, through which blood is carried to and from the heart.

blue baby the condition whereby an infant is born with CYANOSIS due to a congenital malformation of the heart. The result is that blue (i.e. deoxygenated) blood does not go through the lungs to be oxygenated but is pumped around the body. Surgery can usually be performed to correct the condition.

boil (*or* **furuncle**) a skin infection in a hair follicle or gland that produces inflammation and pus. The infection is often due to the bacterium *Staphylococcus*, but healing is generally quick upon release of the pus or administration of antibiotics. Frequent occurrence of boils is usually investigated to ensure the patient is not suffering from DIABETES MELLITUS.

bolus a chewed lump of food ready for swallowing.

bonding the creation of a link between an infant and its parents, particularly the mother. Factors such as eye to eye contact, soothing noises, etc., are part of the process.

bone the hard connective tissue that with CARTILAGE forms the skeleton. Bone has a matrix of COLLAGEN fibres with bone salts (crystalline calcium phosphate or hydroxyapatite, in which are the bone cells, OSTEOBLASTS and OSTEOCYTES). The bone cells form the matrix.

There are two types of bone: compact or dense, forming the shafts of long bones; and spongy or cancellous, which occurs on the inside and at the ends of long bones, and also forms the short bones. Compact bone is a hard tube covered by the periosteum (a membrane) and enclosing the marrow and contains very fine canals (*see* HAVERSIAN CANALS) around which the bone is structured in circular plates *See also* BONE DISEASES, BONE MARROW.

bone diseases *see* **osteomyelitis, osteochondritis, osteosarcoma** and **achondroplasia.**

bone marrow a soft tissue found in the spaces of bones. In young animals all bone marrow, the red marrow, produces blood cells. In older animals the marrow in long bones is replaced by yellow marrow which contains a large amount of fat and does not produce blood cells. In mature animals the red marrow occurs in the ribs, sternum, vertebrae and the ends of the long bones (e.g. the femur [the thigh bone]). The red marrow contains MYELOID tissue, with ERYTHROBLASTS, from which red blood cells develop. LEUCOCYTES also form from the myeloid tissue and themselves give rise to other cell types.

botulism the most dangerous type of food poisoning, caused by the anaerobic bacterium *Clostridium botulinum*. The bacterium is found in oxygen-free environments e.g. in contaminated food in bottles or tins. During growth it releases a toxin of which one component attacks the nervous system. It has a very small lethal dose and symptoms commence with a dry mouth, constipation and blurred vision and worsen to muscle weakness. Death is caused by paralysis of the muscles involved in respiration.

bovine spongiform encephalopathy (*or* **BSE**) a disease of cattle that proves fatal and which is similar to scrapies in sheep and CREUTZFELDT-JAKOB DISEASE in humans.

bow legs (*or* **genu varum**) a deformity in which the legs curve outwards producing a gap between the knees when standing. Small children may exhibit this to some degree but continuance into adult life or its later formation is due to abnormal growth of the EPIPHYSIS. It can be corrected by surgery.

brachial adjective meaning 'of the upper arm', hence brachial artery etc.

brachycardia slowness of the heartbeat and pulse to below sixty per minute.

bradykinesia the condition in which there is abnormally slow movement of the body and limbs and slowness of speech, as may be caused by PARKINSON'S DISEASE.

bradykinin a polypeptide derived from plasma proteins, which causes smooth muscle to contract. It is also a powerful dilator of veins and arteries.

brain the part of the CENTRAL NERVOUS SYSTEM contained within the cranium. Vertebrates have a highly complex brain, which is connected via the spinal cord to the remainder of the nervous system. The brain interprets information received from sense organs and emits signals to control muscles. The brain comprises distinct areas: the CEREBRUM, CEREBELLUM, PONS, MEDULLA OBLONGATA and mid-brain or MESENCEPHALON. GREY MATTER and WHITE MATTER make up the brain, in different arrangements, and a dense network of blood vessels supplies the grey matter and both blood vessels and nerve cells are supported by a fibrous network, the NEUROGLIA.

The average female brain weighs 1.25kg, and the male 1.4kg and the maximum size occurs around the age of 20, whereupon it decreases gradually. Three membranes (the MENINGES) separate the brain from the skull and between each pair is a fluid-filled space to cushion the brain. There are twelve nerves connected to the brain, mainly in the region of the brainstem, and four arteries carrying blood to the brain. Two veins drain the central portion and many small veins open into venous SINUSES, which connect with the internal jugular vein.

brain diseases many brain diseases are indicated by some impairment of a facility e.g. a loss of sensation or an alteration in behaviour. *See* APHASIA, CONCUSSION, EPILEPSY, HYDROCEPHALUS and MENINGITIS.

brainstem death (*or* **brain death**) a complete and continuous absence of the vital reflexes controlled by centres in the brainstem (breathing, pupillary responses, etc.). Tests are performed by independent doctors and repeated after an interval, before death is formally confirmed. At this point, organs may be removed for transplant, providing suitable permission has been obtained.

breast the MAMMARY GLAND which produces milk. Each breast has a number of compartments with lobules surrounded by fatty tissue and muscle fibres. Milk formed in the lobules gathers in branching tubes or ducts that together form lactiferous ducts. Near the nipple the ducts form ampullae (small 'reservoirs'), from which the ducts discharge through the nipple.

breast cancer a CARCINOMA or SARCOMA which is the commonest cancer in women. Incidence is low in countries where breast-feeding persists and animal fat intake in the diet is low. The first sign may be a lump in the breast or armpit (the latter being due to spread to the lymph nodes). A localized tumour may be removed surgically and in addition, radio, chemo- and hormone therapy can form part of the treatment.

breast screening procedures adopted to detect breast cancer as early as possible. In addition to self-examination, there are many formal programmes of screening.

breathlessness is caused fundamentally by any condition that depletes blood oxygen resulting in excessive and/or laboured breathing to gain more air. The causes are numerous, ranging from lung diseases or conditions (PNEUMONIA, EMPHYSEMA, BRONCHITIS) to heart conditions and obesity. In children, narrowing of the air passages is a cause, as is ASTHMA.

breech presentation the position of a baby in the uterus whereby it would be delivered buttocks first, instead of the usual head-first delivery. The baby, and possibly the mother, may be at risk in such cases.

brittle bone disease *see* **osteogenesis imperfecta**.

bronchiole very fine tubes occurring as branches of the bronchi (*see* BRONCHUS). The bronchioles end in alveoli (*see* ALVEOLUS) where carbon dioxide and oxygen are exchanged.

bronchitis occurring in two forms, acute and chronic, bronchitis is the inflammation of the bronchi. Bacteria or viruses cause the acute form, which is typified by the symptoms of the common cold initially, but develops with painful coughing, wheezing, throat and chest pains and the production of purulent (pus-containing) mucus. If the infection spreads to the BRONCHIOLES (bronchiolitis) the consequences are even more serious, as the body is deprived of oxygen. Antibiotics and EXPECTORANTS can relieve the symptoms.

Chronic bronchitis is identified by an excessive production of mucus and may be due to recurrence of the acute form. It is a common cause of death among the elderly and there are several parameters of direct consequence to its cause: excessive smoking of cigarettes; cold, damp climate; obesity; respiratory infections. Damage to the bronchi and other complications may occur giving rise to constant breathlessness. Bronchodilator drugs are ineffective in treatment of the chronic form.

bronchodilator drugs used to relax the SMOOTH MUSCLE of the bronchioles, thus increasing their diameter and the air supply to the lungs. They are used in the treatment of ASTHMA.

bronchus (*plural* **bronchi**) air passages supported by rings of cartilage. Two bronchi branch off from the TRACHEA and these split into further bronchi. The two main bronchi branch to form five lobar bronchi, then twenty segmental bronchi and so on.

brown fat *see* **adipose tissue**.

brucellosis a disease of farm animals (pigs, cattle, goats) caused by a species of a Gram-negative bacillus, *Brucella* (*see* GRAM'S STAIN). It may be passed to man through contact with an infected animal or by drinking contaminated, untreated milk. In cattle the disease causes contagious abortion but in man it is characterized by fever, sweats, joint pains, backache and headache. The use of antibiotics and sulphonamides over a period of time is usually effective and although brucellosis itself is rarely fatal, it may have serious complications e.g. MENINGITIS or PNEUMONIA.

bruises injuries of, and leakage of blood into, the subcutaneous tissues, but without an open wound. In the simplest case minute vessels rupture and blood occupies the skin in the immediate area. A larger injury may be accompanied by swelling. A bruise begins as blue/black in colour, followed by brown and yellow as the blood pigment is reabsorbed.

buccal generally pertaining to the mouth, specifically the inside of the cheek or the gum next to the cheek.

bulimia an insatiable craving for food. *Bulimia nervosa* is an overwhelming desire to eat a lot of food followed by misuse of laxatives or induced vomiting to avoid weight gain. Although there is no attempt to hide the condition, it is psychological in origin, and the sufferers have a fear of obesity. There are many similarities with anorexia nervosa but there is little success in treatment.

burns burns and scalds show similar symptoms and require similar treatment, the former being caused by dry heat, the latter by moist heat. Burns may also be due to electric currents or chemicals. Formerly burns were categorized by degrees (a system developed by Dupuytres, a French surgeon) but are now either superficial, where sufficient tissue remains to ensure skin regrows, or deep where grafting will be necessary.

Severe injuries can prove dangerous because of shock due to fluid loss at the burn. For minor burns and scalds, treatment involves holding the affected area under cold water. In more severe cases, antiseptic dressings are normally applied and in very severe cases, hospitalization is required. Morphine is usually administered to combat the pain. If the burns exceed 9%, then a TRANSFUSION is required.

C

caecum an expanded, blind-ended sac at the start of the large intestine between the small intestine and colon. The small intestine and vermiform appendix open into the caecum.

Caesarian section a surgical operation to deliver a baby by means of an incision through the abdomen and uterus. It is performed when there is a risk to the health of the baby or the mother through normal delivery, either as a planned or as an emergency procedure.

caesium 137 a radioactive substance produced artificially from caesium, which is used in RADIOTHERAPY.

caffeine a substance obtained from coffee and tea, which has a stimulating effect on the central nervous system. It is used as a component of medicines given to relieve headache and also has DIURETIC properties. In addition, it acts as a cardiac stimulant and has a beneficial effect in the treatment of certain forms of asthma.

calamine zinc carbonate, which is a mild astringent and is a component of lotions used to relieve itchy, painful skin conditions such as eczema, urticaria and sunburn.

calciferol a form of VITAMIN D which is manufactured in the skin in the presence of sunlight or derived from certain foods e.g. liver and fish oils. Its main role is in calcium metabolism, enabling calcium to be absorbed from the gut and laid down in bone. A deficiency of vitamin D leads to the bone disease OSTEOMALACIA and also RICKETS.

calcification the deposition of calcium salts, which is normal in the formation of bone, but may occur at other sites in the body. See OSSIFICATION.

calcium a metallic element which is essential for normal growth and functioning of body processes. It is an important component of bones and teeth and has a role in vital metabolic processes e.g. muscle contraction, passage of nerve impulses and blood clotting. Its concentration in the blood is regulated by various THYROID HORMONES. Calcium is an essential element in a normal healthy diet and is found in dairy products such as milk and cheese.

calcium-channel blockers (or calcium antagonists) drugs which inhibit the movement of calcium ions into smooth muscle and cardiac muscle cells. Their effect is to relax the muscle and reduce the strength of contraction and to cause vasodilation. They are used in the treatment of high blood pressure and angina.

callus material which forms around the end of a broken bone, containing bone-forming cells, cartilage and connective tissue. Eventually this tissue becomes calcified.

calorie a term applied to a unit of energy which is the heat required to raise the temperature of one gram of water by one degree centigrade.

cancer a widely-used term describing any form of malignant tumour. Characteristically, there is an uncontrolled and abnormal growth of cancer cells, which invade surrounding tissues and destroy them. Cancer cells may spread throughout the body via the bloodstream or lymphatic system, a process known as METASTASIS, and set up secondary growths elsewhere. There are known to be a number of different causes of cancer, including cigarette smoking, radiation, ultraviolet light, some viruses and possibly the presence of cancer GENES (oncogenes). Treatment depends upon the site of the cancer but involves radiotherapy, chemotherapy and surgery, and survival rates in affected people are showing encouraging improvements.

candidiasis those infections caused by Candida (a yeast-like fungus), such as THRUSH and VAGINITIS.

cannula a hollow tube which is used to draw off fluid from a body cavity. It fits tightly round a solid core, with a sharp pointed end (known as a trocar) which aids insertion. Once the cannula is correctly situated, the trocar is withdrawn so that fluid can run through the tube.

capillary a fine blood vessel, which communicates with an ARTERIOLE or VENULE. Capillaries form networks in most tissues and have walls which are only one cell thick. There is a constant exchange of substances (oxygen, carbon dioxide, nutrients, etc.) between the capillaries, arterioles and venules supplying the needs of the surrounding tissues.

capsule a sheath of connective tissue or membrane surrounding an organ. The adrenal gland, kidney and spleen are all housed within a capsule. A JOINT capsule is a fibrous tissue sheath surrounding various joints. A capsule is also used to describe a small, gelatinous pouch containing a drug, which can be swallowed.

carbaryl an insecticide substance which is especially used in preparations for the elimination of head lice.

carbohydrates organic compounds which include sugars and starch and contain carbon, hydrogen and oxygen. They are the most important source of energy available to the body and are an essential part of the diet. They are eventually broken down in the body to the simple sugar, glucose, which can be used by cells in numerous metabolic processes.

carbolic acid phenol derived from coal tar, the forerunner of modern antiseptics. A strong disinfectant, it is used in lotions and ointments such as CALAMINE lotion, but is highly poisonous if ingested.

carbon dioxide (*or* **carbonic acid**) a gas formed in the tissues as a result of metabolic processes within the body. Medically, carbon dioxide is used combined with oxygen during anaesthesia. At very low temperatures (-75°C) carbon dioxide forms a snow-like solid known as 'dry ice'. This is used on the skin to freeze a localized area and also in the treatment of warts.

carbon monoxide (CO) an odourless and colourless gas which is highly dangerous when inhaled, leading to carbon monoxide poisoning. In the blood it has a very great affinity for oxygen and converts haemoglobin into carboxyhaemoglobin. The tissues of the body are quickly deprived of oxygen because there is no free haemoglobin left to pick it up in the lungs. Carbon monoxide is present in coal gas fumes and vehicle exhaust emissions.

The symptoms of poisoning include giddiness, flushing of the skin (due to carboxyhaemoglobin in the blood, which is bright red), nausea, headache, raised respiratory and pulse rate and eventual coma, respiratory failure and death. An affected person must be taken into the fresh air and given oxygen and artificial respiration if required.

carcinogen any substance which causes damage to tissue cells likely to result in cancer. Various substances are known to be *carcinogenic* including tobacco smoke, asbestos and ionizing radiation.

carcinoma a cancer of the EPITHELIUM, i.e. the tissue that lines the body's internal organs and skin.

cardiac arrest the failure and stopping of the pumping action of the heart. There is a loss of consciousness and breathing and the pulse ceases. Death follows very rapidly unless the heartbeat can be restored. Methods of achieving this include external CARDIAC MASSAGE, artificial respiration, DEFIBRILLATION and direct cardiac massage.

cardiac cycle the whole sequence of events which produces a heartbeat, which normally takes place in less than one second. The atria (*see* ATRIUM) contract together and force the blood into the ventricles (DIASTOLE). These then also contract (SYSTOLE) and blood exits the heart and is pumped around the body. As the ventricles are contracting the atria relax and fill up with blood once again.

cardiac massage a means of restoring the heartbeat if this activity has suddenly ceased. Direct cardiac massage, which is only feasible if the person is in hospital, involves massaging the heart by hand through an incision in the chest wall. Another method, used in conjunction with artificial respiration, is by rhythmic compression of the chest wall while the person is laid on his or her back. The heel of the hand is placed on the chest in the lower region of the breastbone, and firmly compressed between 60 and 80 times a minute, alternating with mouth-to-mouth resuscitation.

cardiac muscle specialized muscle unique to the heart, consisting of branching, elongated fibres possessing the ability to contract and relax continuously.

cardiac pacemaker *see* **pacemaker** and **sinoatrial node**.

cardiology the area of medicine concerned with the study of the structure, function and diseases of the heart and circulatory system.

cardiomyopathy any disease or disorder of the heart muscle which may arise from a number of different causes, including viral infections, congenital abnormalities and chronic alcoholism.

cardiopulmonary bypass an artificial mechanism for maintaining the body's circulation while the heart is intentionally stopped in order to carry out cardiac surgery. A 'heart-lung' machine carries out the functions of heart and lungs until surgery is completed.

cardiovascular system the heart and the whole of the circulatory system, which is divided into the *systemic* (arteries and veins of the body) and *pulmonary* (arteries and veins of the lungs). The cardiovascular system is responsible for the transport of oxygen and nutrients to the tissues, and removing waste products and carbon dioxide from them, taking these to the organs from which they are eventually eliminated.

carotid artery one of two large arteries in the neck which branch and provide the blood supply to the head and neck. The paired common carotid arteries arise from the AORTA on the left side of the heart and from the innominate artery on the right. These continue up on either side of the neck and branch into the internal and external carotids.

carotid body a small area of specialized reddish-coloured tissue situated one on either side of the neck, where the common carotid artery branches to form the internal and external carotids. It is sensitive to chemical changes in the blood, containing chemoreceptors, which respond to oxygen, carbon dioxide and hydrogen levels. If the oxygen level falls, impulses are transmitted to the respiratory centres in the brain, resulting in an increase in the rate of respiration and heartbeat.

carpus (*plural* **carpi**) latin for wrist, consisting of eight small bones which articulate with the ULNA and RADIUS of the forearm on one side and with the *metacarpals* (bones of the hand) on the other.

cartilage a type of firm connective tissue, which is pliable and forms part of the skeleton. There are three different kinds, hyaline cartilage, fibrocartilage and elastic cartilage. *Hyaline* cartilage is found at the joints of movable bones and in the trachea, nose and bronchi, and as costal cartilage joining the ribs to the breastbone. *Fibrocartilage*, which consists of cartilage and connective tissue, is found in the intervertebral discs of the spinal column and in tendons. *Elastic* cartilage is found in the external part of the ear (pinna).

casein a type of protein found in milk which is curdled in the stomach by the action of the enzyme, rennin. Casein is the main protein in cheese and is used medically in preparations for the treatment of malnutrition.

catabolism the biochemical processes within the body (metabolism) are divided into two different sorts — those that build up or produce (synthesize) substances, known as anabolism, and those which break down material (lysis), known as catabolism. In catabolism, more complex materials are broken down into simpler ones with a release of energy, as occurs during the digestion of food.

catalepsy a mental disorder in which the person enters a trance-like state. The body becomes rigid like a statue and the limbs, if moved, stay in the position in which they are placed. There is no sense of recognition or sensation and there is a loss of voluntary control. The vital body functions are shut down to a minimum level necessary for life and, in fact, may be so low as to resemble death. The condition is brought on by severe mental trauma, either as a result of a sudden shock or by a more prolonged depression. It may last for minutes or hours or, rarely, for several days.

cataract a condition in which the lens of the eye becomes opaque, resulting in a blurring of vision. It may arise from a number of different causes, including injury to the eye, as a congenital condition (e.g. DOWN'S SYNDROME) or as a result of certain diseases such as DIABETES. However, the commonest cause is advancing age, during which changes naturally take place in the lens involving the protein components. This is known as senile cataract. Cataract is treated by surgical removal of the whole or part of the affected lens.

catatonia when a patient becomes statue-like, remaining rigid. It is a symptom of mental disease and often a feature of catatonic SCHIZOPHRENIA. Treatment involves tranquillizers and possibly intravenous barbiturates.

catheter a fine flexible tube which is passed into various organs of the body, either for diagnostic purposes or to administer some kind of treatment. One of the commonest kinds is a urethral catheter inserted into the bladder to clear an obstruction, draw off urine or wash out this organ.

caul a piece of membrane (part of the amnion) which sometimes partly covers a newborn baby.

cauterize the application of a heated instrument known as a cautery to destroy living tissue or to stop a haemorrhage. It is used in the treatment of warts and other small growths on the skin.

cavernous sinus one of a pair of cavities located on either side of the sphenoid bone behind the eye sockets at the base of the skull. Venous blood drains into it from the brain, part of the cheek, eye and nose, and leaves through the facial veins and internal jugular.

cell the basic building block of all life and the smallest structural unit in the body. Human body cells vary in size and function and number several billion. Each cell consists of a cell body surrounded by a membrane. The cell body consists of a substance known as cytoplasm, containing various organelles, and also a nucleus. The nucleus contains the CHROMOSOMES, composed of the genetic material, the DNA. Most human body cells contain 46 chromosomes (23 pairs), half being derived from the individual's father and half from the mother. Cells are able to make exact copies of themselves by a process known as MITOSIS, and a full complement of chromosomes is received by each daughter cell. However, the human sex cells (sperm and ova) differ in always containing half the number of chromosomes. At fertilization, a sperm and ovum combine and a complete set of chromosomes is received by the new embryo. *See* MITOSIS and MEIOSIS.

central nervous system the brain and the spinal cord, which receives and integrates all the nervous information from the peripheral nervous system.

cephalosporins a group of semi-synthetic antibiotics derived from a mould called *Cephalosporium*. They are effective against a broad spectrum of microorganisms and are used to treat a variety of infections. They are sometimes able to destroy organisms which have become resistant to penicillin.

cerebellum the largest part of the hindbrain consisting of a pair of joined hemispheres. It has an outer grey cortex, which is a much folded layer of grey matter, and an inner core of white matter. The cerebellum coordinates the activity of various groups of voluntary muscles and maintains posture and balance.

cerebral cortex the outer layer of grey matter of the cerebral hemispheres of the CEREBRUM. It is highly folded and contains many millions of nerve cells, and makes up about 40% of the brain by weight. The cerebral cortex controls intellectual processes, such as thought, perception, memory and intellect, and is also involved in the senses of sight, touch and hearing. It also controls the voluntary movement of muscles and is connected with all the different parts of the body.

cerebral palsy an abnormality of the brain which usually occurs before or during birth. It may arise as a development defect in the foetus due to genetic factors, or by a (viral) infection during pregnancy. A lack of oxygen during a difficult labour or other trauma to the infant can result in cerebral palsy. After birth, the condition can result from haemolytic disease of the newborn, or infection of the brain e.g. MENINGITIS. It can also be caused by cerebral thrombosis or trauma. The condition is characterized by spastic paralysis of the limbs, the severity of which is variable. Also, there may be involuntary writhing movements called athetosis, and balance and posture are also affected. There is often mental subnormality and speech impairment and sometimes EPILEPSY.

Treatment may involve surgery but also physiotherapy, speech and occupational therapy, and special education.

cerebrospinal fluid a clear, colourless fluid with a similar composition to LYMPH. It fills the ventricles and cavities in the CENTRAL NERVOUS SYSTEM and bathes all the surfaces of the brain and spinal cord. The brain floats in it and it has a protective function, acting as a shock absorber helping to prevent mechanical injury to the central nervous system. The cerebrospinal fluid is secreted by the choroid plexuses in the ventricles of the brain and it contains some white blood cells (but no red), salts, glucose and enzymes. It is reabsorbed by veins back into the bloodstream.

cerebrum the largest and most highly developed part of the brain consisting of a pair of cerebral hemispheres, divided from each other by a longitudinal fissure. The cerebral hemispheres are covered by the CEREBRAL CORTEX, below which lies white matter in which the BASAL GANGLIA are situated. The cerebrum controls complex intellectual activities and also all the voluntary responses of the body.

cervical relating to the neck but often used in connection with the neck of the womb (uterus).

cervical cancer cancer of the neck or cervix of the womb, which is one of the most common cancers affecting women. In the precancerous stage, readily detectable changes occur in the cells lining the surface of the cervix. These can be identified by means of a CERVICAL SMEAR test and, if treated at this stage, the prevention and cure rates of the cancer are very high. Early cancer is treated by CRYOSURGERY, DIATHERMY, laser treatment and electrocoagulation. The sexual behaviour of a woman influences her risk of contracting cervical cancer. Early sexual intercourse and numerous different partners are now recognized to increase the risk.

cervical smear a simple test, involving scraping off some cells from the cervix and examining them microscopically. The test is carried out every three years to detect early indications of cancer and is a form of preventative medicine.

cervix a neck-like structure, especially the cervix uteri ,or neck of the womb. It is partly above and partly within the vagina projecting into it and linking it with the cavity of the uterus via the cervical canal.

chemoreceptor a cell or number of cells that detect the presence of specific chemical compounds. In the presence of the chemical an electrical impulse is sent along a specialized sensory nerve to the brain, where the information is received and decoded. Chemoreceptors are present in the nose and taste buds. *See also* CAROTID BODY.

chemotherapy the treatment of disease by the administration of chemical substances or drugs. It includes the treatment of infectious diseases with antibiotics and other types of drug. Also, the treatment and control of various tropical diseases and, especially in recent years, many different forms of cancer with ANTIMETABOLITE drugs.

chest the chest or thorax is the upper part of the body cavity, separated from the lower abdomen by the DIAPHRAGM. The chest cavity is enclosed within the rib cage. The thoracic skeleton consists of the ribs and costal cartilages attached to the sternum (breastbone) at the front. At the back, the ribs join the thoracic vertebrae of the spine. The thorax contains the lungs, heart and oesophagus and above it lies the neck and head.

chicken pox a highly infectious disease which mainly affects children and is caused by the *Varicella zoster* virus. There is an incubation period of two to three weeks and then usually a child becomes slightly feverish and unwell. Within 24 hours an itchy rash appears on the skin, which consists of fluid-filled blisters. Eventually these form scabs, which fall off after about one week. The treatment consists of the application of calamine lotion to reduce the itching, and isolation from other children.

The disease is uncommon in adults as a childhood attack gives lifelong immunity and most children are exposed to chicken pox at some stage. However, the virus may remain within the system and become active later as shingles (*Herpes zoster*).

chilblain a round, itchy inflammation of the skin, which usually occurs on the toes or fingers during cold weather, and is caused by a localized deficiency in the circulation. Chilblains may sometimes be an indication of poor health or inadequate clothing and nutrition. Keeping the feet and hands warm, paying attention to the diet and exercise to improve the circulation help to prevent chilblains.

chiropody the branch of medicine concerned with the health of the foot including its normal structure and development, diseases and their treatment. The medical practitioner is termed a chiropodist.

chiropractor a person who practises chiropractic, which is a system of manipulation, mainly of the vertebrae of the spine, to relieve stress on nerves which might be causing pain.

chloral hydrate a type of sedative drug which is given mainly to elderly people and children. Within half an hour of being taken by mouth (usually as a syrup), it induces sleep and its effects last for about eight hours. It is useful when used sparingly, but harmful in large doses causing toxic effects and addiction.

chlorhexidine (*or* **hibitane**) chlorhexidine is an antiseptic substance, which is used in preparations to cleanse the skin. It is also used in LOZENGES for mild infections of the mouth and throat. Dilute solutions are effective as mouthwash.

chloroform a volatile and colourless liquid which is a compound of carbon, hydrogen and chlorine ($CHCl_3$). It was once widely in use as a general anaesthetic but it affects the rhythm of the heart and also causes liver damage. Hence, it is little used today, except in very low concentrations as a preservative and in some LINIMENTS.

choking violent coughing and interference in breathing, caused by an obstruction in the airway in the region of the larynx. The obstruction is usually a piece of food and if it is large there is a danger of suffocation. If the coughing fails to dislodge the obstruction it is necessary to use other methods to aid a choking person. A child can be held upside down by the legs and struck firmly on the back, as this results in the object being dislodged more easily. With adults it may be necessary to use the HEIMLICH'S MANOEUVRE in order to force the obstruction out.

cholera an infection of the small intestine, caused by the BACTERIUM *Vibrio cholerae*. It varies in degree from very mild cases to extremely severe illness and death. The disease originated in Asia but spread widely last century, when there were great cholera epidemics in Britain and elsewhere. During epidemics of cholera, the death rate is over 50% and these occur in conditions of poor sanitation and overcrowding. The disease is spread through contamination of drinking water by faeces of those affected by the disease, and also by flies landing on infected material and then crawling on food.

Epidemics are rare in conditions of good sanitation but when cholera is detected, extreme attention has to be paid to hygiene, including treatment and scrupulous disposal of the body waste of the infected person. The incubation period for cholera is one to five days and then a person suffers from severe vomiting and diarrhoea (known as 'cholera diarrhoea' or 'rice water stools'). This results in severe dehydration and death may follow within 24 hours. Treatment involves bed rest and the taking by mouth of salt solutions, or these may need to be given intravenously. Tetracycline or other sulphonamide drugs are given to kill the bacteria. The death rate is low (5%) in those given proper and prompt treatment but the risk is greater in children and the elderly. Vaccination against cholera can be given but it is only effective for about six months.

cholesterol a fatty insoluble molecule (sterol), which is widely found in the body and is synthesized from saturated fatty acids in the liver. Cholesterol is an important substance in the body, being a component of cell membranes and a precursor in the production of steroid hormones (sex hormones) and bile salts. An elevated level of blood cholesterol is associated with ATHEROMA, which may result in high blood pressure and coronary thrombosis, and this is seen in the disease DIABETES MELLITUS. There appears to be a relationship between the high consumption of saturated animal fats (which contain cholesterol) in the western diet and the greater incidence of coronary heart disease among, for example, Western Europeans and North Americans. It is generally recommended that people in these countries should reduce their consumption of saturated fat and look for alternatives in the form of unsaturated fats which are found in vegetable oils.

choline an organic compound which is a constituent of some important substances in the body such as phospholipids, lecithin and ACETYCHOLINE. It is sometimes classed as part of the vitamin B complex but this essential compound can also be synthesized by the body.

choluria bile in the urine, which occurs when there is an elevated level of bile in the blood. This may result from the condition known as obstructive JAUNDICE, when the bile ducts become obstructed so that bile manufactured in the liver fails to reach the intestine. The urine is dark-coloured and contains bile salts and pigments.

chorea a disorder of the nervous system characterized by the involuntary, jerky movements of the muscles, mainly of the face, shoulders and hips. *Sydenham's chorea* or *St Vitus' dance* is a disease that mainly affects children and is associated with acute rheumatism. About one third of affected children develop rheumatism elsewhere in the body, often involving the heart, and the disease is more common in girls than in boys. If the heart is affected there may be problems in later life but treatment consists of rest and the giving of mild sedatives. The condition usually recovers over a period of a few months. *Huntington's chorea* is an inherited condition, which does not appear until after the age of 40 and is accompanied by dementia. *Senile chorea* afflicts some elderly people but there is no dementia. *See also* RHEUMATIC FEVER.

chorion one of two foetal membranes completely surrounding the embryo and forming the placenta.

chorionic gonadotrophic hormone a hormone produced during pregnancy by the placenta, large amounts of which are present in the urine of a pregnant woman. The presence of this hormone is the basis of most pregnancy tests. Also known as human chorionic gonadotrophin (HCG), it is given by injection to treat cases of delayed puberty and, with another hormone called follicle-stimulating hormone, women who are sterile, owing to a failure in ovulation. It is also used to treat premenstrual tension.

choroid plexus an extensive network of blood vessels present in the ventricles of the brain and responsible for the production of the CEREBROSPINAL FLUID.

chromosomes the rod-like structures present in the nucleus of every body cell, which carry the genetic information or genes. Each human body cell contains 23 pairs of chromosomes (apart from the sperm and ova), half derived from the mother and half from the father. Each chromosome consists of a coiled double filament (double helix) of DNA with genes carrying the genetic information arranged linearly along its length. The genes determine all the characteristics of each individual. Twenty-two of the pairs of chromosomes are the same in males and females. The 23rd pair are the sex chromosomes, males have one X and one Y, whereas females have two X chromosomes. *See* CELL and SEX-LINKED INHERITANCE.

chyme the partly digested food which passes from the stomach into the intestine. It is produced by the mechanical movements of the stomach and the acid secretions present in the gastric juice.

cilia fine hair-like projections, especially found lining the epithelium of the upper respiratory tract. These beat and help to maintain the flow of air and remove and trap particles of dust.

circulation of the blood the basic circulation is as follows: all the blood from the body returns to the heart via the veins, eventually entering the right atrium through the inferior and superior venae cavae. This contracts and forces the blood into the right ventricle and from there it is driven to the lungs via the pulmonary artery. In the lungs, oxygen is taken up and carbon dioxide is released. The blood then passes into the pulmonary veins and is returned to the left atrium of the heart. Blood is forced from the left atrium into the left ventricle and from there into the aorta. The aorta branches, giving off the various arteries which carry the blood to all the different parts of the body. The blood eventually enters the fine network of arterioles and capillaries and supplies all the tissues and organs with oxygen and nutrients. It passes into the venules and veins, eventually returning to the right atrium through the vena cavae to complete the cycle.

circumcision a surgical removal of the foreskin (or prepuce) of the penis in males and part or all of the external genitalia (CLITORIS, labia minora, labia majora) in females. In females and usually in males, the procedure is carried out for religious reasons. Male circumcision may be required in the medical conditions known as PHIMOSIS and PARAPHIMOSIS. Female circumcision is damaging and not beneficial to a woman's health.

cirrhosis a disease of the liver in which fibrous tissue resembling scar tissue is produced as a result of damage and death to the cells. The liver becomes yellow-coloured and nodular in appearance. There are various types of the disease, including alcoholic cirrhosis and postnecrotic cirrhosis, caused by viral hepatitis. The cause of the cirrhosis is not always found (cryptogenic cirrhosis) but the progress of the condition can be halted if this can be identified and removed. This is particularly applicable in alcoholic cirrhosis, where the consumption of alcohol has to cease.

clavicle the collar bone, forming a part of the shoulder girdle of the skeleton. It is the most commonly fractured bone in the body.

cleft palate a developmental defect in which a fissure is left in the midline of the palate as the two sides fail to fuse. It may also involve the lip (HARE LIP) and the condition can be corrected by surgery.

clitoris a small organ present in females, situated where the labial folds meet below the pubic bone. It contains erectile tissue which enlarges and hardens during sexual stimulation.

clone a group of cells that are derived from one cell (by asexual division) and are genetically identical.

clostridium a group of bacteria which are present in the intestine of man and animals. Some species are responsible for serious diseases such as botulism, tetanus and gas GANGRENE.

clot the term applied to a semi-solid lump of blood or other fluid in the body. A blood clot consists of a fine network of FIBRIN in which blood corpuscles are caught. *See* COAGULATION.

coagulation (of the blood) the natural process in which blood is converted from a liquid to a semi-solid state to arrest bleeding (haemorrhage). A substance known as prothrombin and calcium are normally present in the blood, and the enzyme thromboplastin is present in the platelets (*see* BLOOD). When bleeding occurs, thromboplastin is released and prothrombin and calcium are converted by the enzyme into THROMBIN. A soluble protein called fibrinogen is always present in the blood and is converted by thrombin into FIBRIN, which is the final stage in the coagulation process. A fibrous meshwork or clot is produced, consisting of fibrin and blood cells, which seals off the damaged blood vessel. In normal healthy conditions, thromboplastin is not released and so a clot cannot form. The coagulation or clotting time is the time taken for blood to clot and is normally between three and eight minutes.

coagulation factors these are substances present in plasma which are involved in the process of blood coagulation. They are designated by a set of Roman numerals, e.g. Factor VIII, and lack of any of them means that the blood is unable to clot. *See* HAEMOPHILIA.

cobalt-60 an artificial radioisotope, which emits gamma radiation and is used in RADIOTHERAPY.

cocaine an alkaloid substance derived from the leaves of the coca plant, which is used as a local anaesthetic in nose, throat, ear and eye surgery. It has a stimulating effect on the central nervous system when absorbed, in which fatigue and breathlessness (caused by exertion) disappear. However, it is highly addictive and damaging to the body if it is used often and hence it is very strictly controlled. It is also one of the drugs given for pain relief in cases of terminal cancer.

coccyx the end of the backbone, which consists of four fused and reduced vertebrae which correspond to the tail of other mammals. The coccyx is surrounded by muscle and joins with the SACRUM, a further group of fused vertebrae which is part of the PELVIS.

cochlea a spiral-shaped organ resembling a snail shell, forming a part of the inner ear, and concerned with hearing. It consists of three fluid-filled canals, with receptors which detect pressure changes caused by sound waves. Nerve impulses are sent to the brain, where the information is received and decoded.

codeine a substance derived from morphine, which is used for pain relief and to suppress a cough.

cod liver oil oil derived from the pressed fresh liver of cod, which is a rich source of vitamins D and A, and is used as a dietary supplement.

coeliac disease also known as gluten enteropathy, this is a wasting disease of childhood in which the intestines are unable to absorb fat. The intestinal lining is damaged due to a sensitivity to the protein gluten, which is found in wheat and rye flour. An excess of fat is excreted and the child fails to grow and thrive. Successful treatment is by adhering strictly to a gluten-free diet throughout life.

cofactor some ENZYMES can only work if their particular cofactor is present. Cofactors may be inorganic (e.g. metal ions) or non-protein organic substances (e.g. coenzymes), and they may activate their enzyme or actually take part in the reaction itself.

cold (*or* **common cold**) widespread and mild infection of the upper respiratory tract, caused by a virus. There is inflammation of the mucous membranes and symptoms include feverishness, coughing, sneezing, runny nose, sore throat, headache and sometimes face ache due to catarrh in the sinuses. The disease is spread by coughing and sneezing and treatment is by means of bed rest and the taking of mild ANALGESICS.

cold sore *see* **herpes**.

colectomy surgical removal of the colon.

colic spasmodic, severe abdominal pain which occurs in waves with brief interludes in between. Intestinal colic is usually the result of the presence of some indigestible food which causes the contraction of the intestinal muscles. Infantile colic, common in young babies, is due to wind associated with feeding. An attack of colic is generally not serious but can result in a twisting of the bowel which must receive immediate medical attention. Colic-type pain may also be caused by an obstruction in the bowel such as a tumour, which again requires early medical treatment.

colitis inflammation of the colon, the symptoms of which include abdominal pain and diarrhoea, sometimes blood-stained. *Ulcerative colitis* tends to affect young adults and tends to occur periodically over a number of years. There is abdominal discomfort, fever, frequent watery diarrhoea containing mucus and blood, and anaemia. The condition can be fatal but usually there is a gradual recovery. Treatment is by means of bed rest, drug treatment with corticosteroids and iron supplements, and a bland, low-roughage

diet. Colitis may be due to infections caused by the organism *Entamoeba histolytica* (amoebic colitis) and by bacteria (infective colitis). It may also occur in CROHN'S DISEASE.

collagen a protein substance that is widely found in large amounts in the body in connective tissue, tendons, skin, cartilage, bone and ligaments. It plays a major part in conferring tensile strength to various body structures.

collar bone *see* **clavicle**.

colon the main part of the large intestine, which removes water and salts from the undigested food passed into it from the small intestine. When water has been extracted the remains of the food (faeces) are passed on to the rectum.

colostomy a surgical operation to produce an artificial opening of the colon through the abdominal wall. The colostomy may only be temporary, as part of the management of a patient's condition e.g. to treat an obstruction in the colon or rectum. However, if the rectum or part of the colon has been removed because of cancer the colostomy is permanent and functions as the anus.

colostrum the first fluid produced by the mammary glands of the breasts after birth. It is a fairly clear fluid containing antibodies, serum and white blood cells and is produced during the first two or three days prior to the production of milk.

colour blindness a general term for a number of conditions in which there is a failure to distinguish certain colours. It is more prevalent in males than in females and is usually inherited. The most common form is Daltonism, in which reds and greens are confused. This is a sex-linked disorder, the recessive gene responsible being carried on the X chromosome and hence more likely to be present in males. The cause of colour blindness is thought to be a failure in the operation of the CONES, the light-sensitive cells in the RETINA of the eye which detect colours.

coma a state of deep unconsciousness from which a person cannot be roused. There may be an absence of pupillary and corneal reflexes and no movements of withdrawal when painful stimuli are applied. It may be accompanied by deep, noisy breathing and strong heart action and can be caused by a number of different conditions. These include apoplexy, high fever, brain injury, diabetes mellitus, carbon monoxide poisoning and drug overdose. A comatose person may eventually die, but can recover, depending upon the nature of the coma and its cause.

commensal a term applied to any organism (usually

a microorganism) which lives in or on the body of another organism without causing either benefit or harm. Examples in man are bacteria living in the gut or on the skin.

comminuted fracture a serious injury to a bone in which more than one break occurs, accompanied by splintering and damage to the surrounding tissues. It usually results from a crushing force, with damage to nerves, muscles and blood vessels, and the bone is difficult to set.

commissure a joining or connection of two similar structure, on either side of a midline. It is usually applied to bundles of nerve fibres connecting the right and left side of the brain and spinal cord.

compress a pad soaked in hot or cold water, wrung out and applied to an inflamed or painful part of the body. A hot compress is called a fomentation.

computerized tomography a diagnostic technique in radiology whereby 'slices' of the body are recorded using a special X-ray scanner known as a CT scanner. The information is integrated by computer to give an image in cross-section of the tissue under investigation. The technique is used for investigations of the brain, for example if a tumour, haematoma or abscess is present. Whole body scans may be required for a number of conditions, but are particularly useful when malignancy is present, supplying information about the position and outline of a tumour and the extent of spread of cancer.

concretions hard, stony masses of various sizes formed within the body. Examples are gallstones and kidney stones, and they are usually composed of mineral salts. Also known as calculi (*single* **calculus**).

concussion a loss of consciousness caused by a blow to the head. The sudden knock to the head causes a compression wave which momentarily interrupts the blood supply to the brain. The unconsciousness may last for seconds or hours and when the person comes round there may be some headache and irritability, which can last for some time. A mild case of concussion may not involve complete loss of consciousness but be marked by giddiness, confusion and headache. In all cases, the person needs to rest and remain under observation.

condyle a rounded knob which is found at the ends of some bones e.g. on the femur and humerus, and which articulates with an adjacent bone.

cone a type of photoreceptor (light-sensitive cell) found in the RETINA of the eye, which detects colour. Cones contain the pigment retinene and the protein opsin and there are three different types, which react to light of differing wavelengths (blue, green and red).

congenital diseases or conditions that are present at birth.

conjunctivitis inflammation of the mucous membrane (conjunctiva) that lines the inside of the eyelid and covers the front of the eye. The eyes become pink and watery and the condition is usually caused by an infection which may be bacterial or viral or the microorganism *Chlamydia* may be responsible. Treatment depends upon cause but a number of drugs are used often in the form of eyedrops.

connective tissue supporting or packing tissue within the body which holds or separates other tissues and organs. It consists of a ground material composed of substances called mucopoly-saccharides. In this, certain fibres such as yellow elastic, white collagenous and reticular fibres are embedded along with a variety of other cells, e.g MAST CELLS, MACROPHAGES, fibroblasts and fat cells. The constituents vary in proportions in different kinds of connective tissue to produce a number of distinct types. Examples are adipose (fatty) tissue, cartilage, bone, tendons and ligaments.

constipation the condition in which the bowels are opened too infrequently and the faeces become dry, hard and difficult and painful to pass. The frequency of normal bowel opening varies between people but when constipation becomes a problem, it is usually a result of inattention to this habit or to the diet. To correct the condition a change of lifestyle may be needed, including taking more exercise, fluid and roughage in the diet. Laxatives and enemas are also used to alleviate the condition. Constipation is also a symptom of the more serious condition of blockage of the bowel (by a tumour), but this is less common.

contraception prevention of conception. Pregnancy can be prevented by *barrier methods*, in which there is a physical barrier to prevent the sperm from entering the cervix. These comprise the condom (sheath) and diaphragm (cap). As well as being a contraceptive, the sheath reduces the risk of either partner contracting a sexually transmitted disease, including HIV infection. Non-barrier methods do not interpose this physical barrier and include the INTRAUTERINE CONTRACEPTIVE DEVICE (coil) and oral contraceptives (the Pill), which are hormonal preparations. Depot preparations are also hormonal drugs that are given by injection, planted under the skin (subcutaneous implants) and released from intravaginal rings, and have a long-lasting effect.

Sterilization of either a man or woman provides a means of permanent contraception. It is also possible to give a high dose of oral contraceptives within 72 hours of unprotected intercourse, but this is usually regarded as an emergency method. The rhythm method of contraception involves restricting sexual intercourse to certain days of a woman's monthly cycle when conception is least likely to occur.

controlled drugs those drugs which, in the UK, are subject to the restrictions of the Misuse of Drugs Act 1971. They are classified into three categories: Class A includes LSD, morphine, cocaine and pethidine, Class B includes cannabis, amphetamines and barbiturates and Class C comprises amphetamine-related drugs and some others.

convulsions (*or* **fits**) involuntary, alternate, rapid, muscular contractions and relaxations throwing the body and limbs into contortions. They are caused by a disturbance of brain function and in adults usually result from epilepsy. In babies and young children they occur quite commonly but, although alarming, are generally not serious. Causes include a high fever due to infection, brain diseases, such as meningitis, and breath-holding, which is quite common in infants and very young children. Convulsions are thought to be more common in the very young because the nervous system is immature. Unless they are caused by the presence of disease or infection which requires to be treated, they are rarely life-threatening.

corn (*and* **bunion**) a small, localized portion of hardened, thickened skin, occurring on or between the toes, which is cone-shaped. The point of the cone, known as 'the eye', points inwards and causes pain. It is caused by pressure from poorly-fitting shoes. A bunion is found over the joint at the base of the largest toe and is also caused by tight-fitting footwear. With a bunion, the joint between the toe and the first metatarsal bone becomes swollen and forms a lump beneath the thickened skin, due to bending caused by the shoe. A hammer toe is similar but involves the second toe, which becomes bent at the joint to resemble a hammer, because shoes or boots are too tight or pointed.

cornea the outermost, exposed layer of the EYE, which is transparent and lies over the iris and lens. It refracts light entering the eye, directing the rays to the lens, and thus acting as a coarse focus. It is a layer of connective tissue which has no blood supply of its own but is supplied with nutrients from fluid within the eye (the aqueous humour). It is highly sensitive to pain, and presence or absence of response if the cornea is touched is used as an indicator of a person's condition, for example in a comatose patient.

corneal graft (*or* **keratoplasty**) a surgical procedure to replace a damaged or diseased cornea with one from a donor. Sometimes only the outer layers of the cornea are replaced (lamellar keratoplasty) or the whole structure may be involved (penetrating keratoplasty).

coronary angioplasty *see* **angioplasty**.

coronary arteries the arteries that supply blood to the heart and which arise from the AORTA.

coronary artery disease any abnormal condition that affects the arteries of the heart. The commonest disease is coronary ATHEROSCLEROSIS, which is more prevalent in those populations with high fat, saturated fat, refined carbohydrates etc. in their diet. ANGINA is a common symptom of such diseases.

coronary bypass graft a surgical operation which is carried out when one or more of the coronary arteries have become narrowed by disease (ATHEROMA). A section of vein from a leg is grafted in to bypass the obstruction and this major operation is usually successful and greatly improves a person's quality of life.

coronary thrombosis a sudden blockage of one of the coronary arteries by a blood clot or thrombus, which interrupts the blood supply to the heart. The victim collapses with severe and agonizing chest pain, often accompanied by vomiting and nausea. The skin becomes pale and clammy, the temperature rises and there is difficulty in breathing. Coronary thrombosis generally results from ATHEROMA, and the part of the heart muscle which has its blood supply disrupted dies, a condition known as MYOCARDIAL INFARCTION. Treatment consists of giving strong pain-relieving drugs such as morphine. Also specialist care in a coronary care unit is usually required to deal with ARRHYTHMIA, heart failure and CARDIAC ARREST, which are the potentially fatal results of coronary thrombosis.

corpus luteum the tissue that forms within the ovary after a Graafian follicle (the structure which contains the egg) ruptures and releases an ovum at the time of OVULATION. It consists of a mass of cells containing yellow, fatty substances, and secretes the hormone PROGESTERONE which prepares the womb to receive a fertilized egg. If the egg is not fertilized and no implantation of an embryo takes place, the corpus luteum degenerates. However, if a pregnancy ensues, the corpus luteum expands and secretes progesterone until this function is taken over by the placenta at the fourth month.

cortex the outer part of an organ situated beneath its enclosing capsules or outer membrane. Examples are the adrenal cortex of the adrenal glands, renal cortex of the kidneys and cerebral cortex of the brain. *Compare* MEDULLA.

corticosteroids any steroid hormone manufactured by the adrenal cortex, of which there are two main types. Glucocorticosteroids such as cortisol and cortisone are required by the body mainly for glucose metabolism and for responding to stress. Mineralocorticosteroids, e.g. aldosterone, regulate the salt and water balance. Both groups are manufactured synthetically and used in the treatment of various disorders. Glucocorticosteroids are potent anti-inflammatory agents and are used in the treatment of conditions where inflammation is involved.

cortisone a glucocorticosteroid hormone produced by the adrenal cortex. It is used medically to treat deficiency of corticosteroid hormones. Deficiency occurs in ADDISON'S DISEASE and if the adrenal glands have had to be surgically removed for some reason. Its use is restricted because it causes severe side effects including damage to the muscle and bone, eye changes, stomach ulcers and bleeding, as well as nervous and hormonal disturbances.

costal cartilage a type of cartilage connecting a rib to the sternum (breastbone).

cot death *see* **sudden infant death syndrome**.

cradlecap a form of seborrhoea or dermatitis of the scalp which affects young babies and responds to an ointment containing white soft paraffin, salicylic acid and sulphur.

cramp prolonged and painful spasmodic muscular contraction, which often occurs in the limbs but can affect certain internal organs (*see* COLIC and GASTRALGIA). Cramp may result from a salt imbalance, as in heat cramp. Working in high temperatures causes excessive sweating and consequent loss of salt. It can be corrected and prevented by an increase of the salt intake. Occupational cramp results from continual repetitive use of particular muscles, e.g. writer's cramp. Night cramp occurs during sleep and is especially common among elderly people, diabetics and pregnant women. The cause is not known.

cranial nerves twelve pairs of nerves which arise directly from the brain, each with dorsal and ventral branches known as *roots*. Each root remains separate and is assigned a roman numeral as well as a name. Some cranial nerves are mainly sensory while others are largely motor and they leave the skull through separate apertures. The cranial and spinal nerves are an important part of the *peripheral nervous system* which comprises all parts lying outside the brain and spinal cord.

cranium the part of the skull that encloses the brain, formed from eight fused and flattened bones that are joined by immovable suture JOINTS.

crepitus the grating sound heard when the ends of fractured bones rub together, and also from the joints of those suffering from arthritis. It also occurs in *chondromalacia patellae,* which is a roughening of the inner surface of the kneecap which produces the grating sound and pain. Crepitus also denotes the sound heard by means of a STETHOSCOPE from an inflamed lung when there is fluid in the alveoli.

cretinism a syndrome caused by lack of thyroid hormone, which is present before birth and is also called *congenital hyperthyroidism.* It is characterized by dwarfism, mental retardation and coarseness of skin and hair. Early diagnosis and treatment with thyroid extract (thyroxine) is vital as this greatly improves a child's intellectual and other abilities. In the UK, blood serum from newborn babies is tested for thyroxine level in order to detect this condition.

Creutzfeldt-Jakob disease (*or* **CJD** *or* **spongiform encephalopathy**) a fatal disease of the brain thought to be caused by a SLOW VIRUS. There is a spongy degeneration of the brain and rapid progressive dementia. The disease usually strikes in middle and early old age and is usually fatal within a year. Similar diseases in animals are bovine spongiform encephalopathy (BSE) in cattle and scrapie in sheep, which, it is alleged by some scientists, may be transmittable to man. Recently there has been alarm that some adults treated in childhood for dwarfism with extracts of pituitary glands obtained from corpses, may be at risk of contracting Creutzfeldt-Jakob disease. It is alleged that some of the pituitary glands obtained may have been infected with the virus and that the disease has been passed on and has already caused some deaths.

Crohn's disease (*or* **ileitis**) this is a condition in which there is inflammation of part of the ILEUM, in the lower part of the small intestine. This leads to ulceration and thickening, with symptoms of pain, diarrhoea and weight loss. Although the cause of Crohn's disease is not known there is thought to be a genetic link, as the condition can occur in families.

croup a group of diseases characterized by a swelling, partial obstruction and inflammation of the entrance to the larynx, occurring in young children. The breathing is harsh and strained, producing a typical crowing sound, accompanied by coughing and feverishness. Diphtheria used to be the most common cause of croup but it now usually results from a viral infection of the respiratory tract (LARYNGOTRACHEOBRONCHITIS). The condition is relieved by inhaling steam (a soothing preparation such as tincture of benzoin is sometimes added to the hot water) and also by mild sedatives and/or painkillers. Rarely, the obstruction becomes dangerous and completely blocks the larynx, in which case emergency TRACHEOSTOMY or nasotracheal INTUBATION may be required. Usually, the symptoms of croup subside and the child recovers, but then he or she may have a tendency towards attacks on future occasions.

cryosurgery the use of extreme cold to perform surgical procedures, usually on localized areas to remove unwanted tissue. The advantages are that there is little or no bleeding or sensation of pain, and scarring is very much reduced. An instrument called a cryoprobe is used, the fine tip of which is cooled by means of a coolant substance contained within the probe. The coolants used are carbon dioxide, nitrous oxide gas and liquid nitrogen. Cryosurgery is used for the removal of cataracts and warts and to destroy some bone tumours.

culture a population of bacteria, viruses and other microorganisms or cells grown in the laboratory on a nutrient base known as a *culture medium*.

curare an extract from the bark of certain South American trees which relaxes and paralyses voluntary muscle. The pure alkaloid substance obtained from the bark is known as d-tubocurarine chloride and it is used as a muscle relaxant in anaesthesia.

Cushing's syndrome a metabolic disorder, which results from excessive amounts of CORTICOSTEROIDS in the body, due to an inability to regulate cortisol or adrenocorticotropic hormone (ACTH). The commonest cause is a tumour of the PITUITARY GLAND (producing secretion of ACTH) or a malignancy elsewhere e.g. in the lung or adrenal gland requiring extensive therapy with corticosteroid drugs. Symptoms include obesity, reddening of face and neck, growth of body and facial hair, OSTEOPOROSIS, high blood pressure and possible mental disturbances.

cuticle another name for the outer layer of the skin or EPIDERMIS. It refers to the outer layer of flattened cells covering a hair.

cyanide poisoning poisoning with any of the salts of hydrocyanic acid, which paralyses every part of the nervous system and is usually fatal within minutes. The person rapidly becomes unconscious and this is followed by convulsions and death. The antidotes are amyl nitrite, sodium thiosulphate and cobalt edetate, which may save life if quickly administered.

cyanocobalamin *see* **vitamin B**$_{12}$.

cyanosis a blue appearance of the skin, due to insufficient oxygen within the blood. It is first noticeable on the lips, tips of the ears, cheeks and nails and occurs in heart failure, lung diseases and asphyxia, and in 'blue babies', who have congenital heart defects.

cystic fibrosis (*or* **CF**) a genetic disease, the defective gene responsible for it being located on human chromosome no. 7. The disease affects all the mucus-secreting glands of the lungs, pancreas, mouth and gastrointestinal tract and also the sweat glands of the skin. A thick mucus is produced which affects the production of pancreatic enzymes and causes the bronchi to widen (bronchiectasis) and become clogged. Respiratory infections are common and the sweat contains abnormally high levels of sodium and chloride. The stools also contain a lot of mucus and have a foul smell. The disease is incurable and cannot be diagnosed by antenatal tests.

However, the outlook for affected children has greatly improved and treatment consists of physiotherapy to relieve bronchial congestion, taking pancreatic enzyme tablets, vitamins and prompt treatment of respiratory infections when these occur.

cystitis inflammation of the bladder, normally caused by bacterial infection, the causal organism usually being *E. coli*. It is marked by the need to pass urine frequently, accompanied by a burning sensation. There may be cramp-like pains in the lower abdomen, with dark strong urine which contains blood. The condition is common in females and is usually not serious, but there is a danger that the infection may spread to the kidneys.

Treatment is by means of antibiotics and also by drinking a lot of fluid, possibly with the addition of bicarbonate of soda. The prevalence of the condition in females is due to the fact that the urethra is much shorter in women than in men, and the bacteria (which are present and harmless in the bowel) are more likely to gain access to both to the urinary tract and the vagina.

cysts small, usually benign, tumours containing fluid (or soft secretions) within a membranous sac. Examples are wens, caused by blockage of sebaceous glands in the skin, cysts in the breasts, caused by blocked milk ducts, and ovarian cysts, which may be large and contain a clear, thick liquid. *Dermoid cysts* are congenital and occur at sites in the body where embryonic clefts have closed up before birth. These may contain fatty substances, hair, skin, fragments of bone and even teeth. *Hydatid cysts* are a stage in the life cycle of certain parasites (tapeworm) and may be found in man, especially in the liver.

cytomegaloviruses a number of viruses belonging to the *Herpes* group which give infected cells a swollen appearance. They cause severe effects in those whose immune system is disrupted and are responsible for a serious disease of newborn babies, called cytomegalic disease. The virus is transmitted to the baby before or during birth and can cause jaundice, enlargement of the liver and spleen and mental retardation.

cytoplasm the jelly-like substance within the cell wall which surrounds the nucleus and contains a number of organelles.

cytotoxic a substance which damages or destroys cells. Cytotoxic drugs are used in the treatment of various forms of cancer and act by inhibiting cell division. However, they also damage normal cells and hence their use has to be carefully regulated in each individual patient. Cytotoxic drugs may be used in combination with RADIOTHERAPY or on their own.

D

dead space the volume of air, primarily in the TRACHEA and bronchi, that does not take part in the oxygen/carbon dioxide exchange. In each breath taken into the lungs, this proportion does not contribute directly to the respiratory process.

deafness a partial or complete loss of hearing. The deafness may be temporary or permanent, conductive or sensory, congenital or acquired. Congenital hearing loss is not a common cause. In many cases, the loss is due to a problem in the cochlea, the auditory nerve or the brain-nerve deafness. This is a common condition in the elderly although no particular cause can be identified. Other causes include exposure to industrial noise or explosions.

Conductive hearing loss is due to poor transmission of sound waves to the inner ear, possibly due to OTITIS, which can cause middle ear inflammation and perforation of the eardrum. This latter condition can be treated by surgery or the use of a hearing aid.

decidua the soft epithelial tissue that forms a lining to the uterus during pregnancy and which is shed at birth.

defibrillation the application of a large electric shock to the chest wall of a patient whose heart is fibrillating (*see* FIBRILLATION). The delivery of a direct electric countershock hopefully allows the pacemaker to set up the correct rhythm again.

degeneration the deterioration over time of body tissues or an organ resulting in a lessening of its function. The changes may be structural or chemical and there are a number of types: fatty, FIBROID, calcareous (as with CONCRETIONS), mucoid and so on. Degeneration may be due to ageing, heredity or poor nutrition. Poisons such as alcohol also contribute to degeneration, as with CIRRHOSIS.

dehydration the removal of water. More specifically, the loss of water from the body through diuresis, sweating, etc., or a reduction in water content due to a low intake. Essential body electrolytes (such as sodium chloride and potassium) are disrupted and after the first symptom, thirst, irritability and confusion follow.

delirium a mental disorder typified by confusion, agitation, fear, anxiety, illusions and sometimes hallucinations. The causal cerebral dysfunction may be due to deficient nutrition, stress, toxic poisoning or mental shock.

delirium tremens (*or* **DTs**)a form of DELIRIUM due often to partial or total withdrawal of alcohol after a period of excessive intake. Symptoms are varied and include insomnia, agitation, confusion and fever, often with vivid hallucinations. The treatment involves lessening and removing the dependence on alcohol, accompanied by sedation with drugs such as BENZODIAZEPINES.

delta waves one of the four types of brain waves and the slowest of the four. Delta waves are associated with deep sleep. If delta waves are seen in the *electroencephalogram* of a waking adult, brain damage is indicated e.g. as with epileptics and around brain tumours.

deltoid the muscle, triangular in shape, that covers the shoulder and is attached to the collar bone, shoulder blade and humerus. It enables the arm to be raised from the side.

dementia a mental disorder typified by confusion, disorientation, memory loss, personality changes and a lessening of intellectual capacity. Dementia occurs in several forms: SENILE DEMENTIA, ALZHEIMER'S DISEASE and multi-infarct dementia. The causes are various and include vascular disease, brain tumour, SUBDURAL HAEMATOMA, HYDROCEPHALUS and hyperthyroidism.

demyelination the process whereby the myelin sheath surrounding a nerve fibre is destroyed, resulting in impaired nerve function. This is associated with MULTIPLE SCLEROSIS but can also happen after a nerve has been injured.

denaturation the disruption, usually by heat, of the weak bonds that hold a protein together. Extremes of temperature are fatal to most animals because the ENZYMES (which are proteins) that perform essential catalytic functions in life-sustaining biochemical processes are irreversibly denatured.

dendrite one of numerous thin branching extensions of a nerve cell. The dendrites are at the 'receiving end' of the nerve cell (neuron) and they form a network which increases the area for receiving impulses from the terminals of axons of other neurons at the SYNAPSE.

dentine the material which forms the bulk of a tooth, lying between the pulp cavity and the enamel. It is similar to bone in composition but contains blood capillaries, nerve fibres and extensions of odontoblasts (cells producing the dentine).

depilation the removal of hair from the body, whether temporarily by shaving or use of chemicals, or permanently by electrolysis. The latter method destroys the hair follicles.

depot with reference to a drug, being injected or implanted for slow absorption into the circulation.

depressant a drug which is used to reduce the functioning of a system of the body e.g. a respiratory depressant. Drugs such as opiates, general anaesthetics, etc., are depressants.

depression a mental state of extreme sadness dominated by pessimism, in which normal behaviour patterns (sleep, appetite, etc.) are disturbed. Causes are varied: upsetting events, loss, etc., and treatment involves the use of therapy and drugs. *See also* MANIC DEPRESSIVE PSYCHOSIS.

dermatitis an inflammation of the skin which is similar in many respects to, and often interchanged with, ECZEMA. It is characterized by erythema (redness due to dilatation of capillaries near the surface), pain and PRURITIS. Several forms of dermatitis can be identified. Contact dermatitis is caused by the skin coming into contact with a substance to which the skin is sensitive. A large range of compounds and materials may cause such a reaction. Treatment usually involves the use of a corticosteroid. Light dermatitis manifests itself as a reddening and blistering of skin exposed to sunlight. This occurs on hands, face and neck during the summer months. Some individuals become sensitized by drugs or perfumes in cosmetics, while others have an innate sensitivity. Erythroderma or exfoliative dermatitis involves patches of reddened skin which thicken and peel off. It is often associated with other skin conditions e.g. PSORIASIS. Corticosteroids form a central part of the treatment in this case.

desensitization the technique whereby an individual builds up resistance to an allergen by taking gradually increasing doses of the allergen over a period of time. Also in the treatment of phobias, where a patient is gradually faced with the thing that is feared and concurrently learns to relax and reduce anxiety.

detached retina when the retina becomes detached from the choroid (a layer of the eyeball with blood vessels and pigment that absorbs excess light, preventing blurred vision). The detachment may be due to tumour or inflammation, or to the leaking of vitreous humour through holes in the retina to fill the space between retina and choroid, thus disrupting the fine attachments. The condition can be corrected by surgery, whereby heat binds the retina and choroid together using scar tissue.

diabetes insipidus a rare condition which is completely different from DIABETES MELLITUS and is characterized by excessive thirst (*see* POLYDIPSIA) and POLYURIA. It is due to a lack of the antidiuretic hormone or the inability of the kidney to respond to the hormone.

diabetes mellitus a complex metabolic disorder involving carbohydrate, fat and protein. It results in an accumulation of sugar in the blood and urine and is due to a lack of INSULIN produced by the pancreas, so that sugars are not broken down to release energy. Fats are thus used as an alternative energy source. Symptoms include thirst, POLYURIA and loss of weight, and the use of fats can produce KETOSIS and KETONURIA. In its severest form, convulsions are followed by a diabetic coma.

Treatment relies upon dietary control, with doses of insulin or drugs. Long-term effects include thickening of the arteries, and in some cases the eyes, kidneys, nervous system, skin and circulation may be affected. *See also* HYPOGLYCAEMIA and HYPERGLYCAEMIA.

diagnosis the process whereby a particular disease or condition is identified after consideration of the relevant parameters, viz. symptoms, physical manifestations, results from laboratory tests and so on. In many instances the diagnosis requires greater skills than does the treatment.

dialysis the use of a semipermeable membrane to separate large and small molecules by selective diffusion. Starch and proteins are large molecules while salts, glucose and amino acids are small molecules. If a mixture of large and small molecules is separated from distilled water by a semi-permeable membrane, the smaller molecules diffuse into the water which is itself replenished. This principle is the basis of the artificial kidney which, because a patient's blood is processed, is known as HAEMODIALYSIS.

diaphragm a membrane of muscle and tendon that separates the thoracic and abdominal cavities. It is covered by a SEROUS MEMBRANE and attached at the lower ribs, breastbone and backbone. The diaphragm is important in breathing, when it bulges up to its resting position during exhalation. It flattens during inhalation and in so doing it reduces pressure in the thoracic cavity and helps to draw air into the lungs.

Also, a rubber bowl-shaped cap used as a contraceptive with spermicidal cream. It fits inside the VAGINA, over the neck of the UTERUS.

diaphysis the central part or shaft of a long bone.

diarrhoea increased frequency and looseness of bowel movement, involving the passage of unusually soft faeces. Diarrhoea can be caused by food poisoning, COLITIS, IRRITABLE BOWEL SYNDROME, DYSENTERY, etc. A severe case will result in the loss of water and salts which must be replaced and antidiarrhoeal drugs are used in certain circumstances.

diastase (amylases) ENZYMES that break down starch into sugar. Specifically, diastase is the part of malt containing amylase. Diastase is used to help in the digestion of starch in some digestive disorders.

diastasis the separation of a growing bone from the shaft.

diastole the point at which the heart relaxes between contractions, when the ventricles fill with blood. This usually lasts about half a second, at the end of which the ventricles are about three-quarters full.

diathermy the use of high-frequency non-lethal electric currents to produce heat in a part of the body. The heat generated increases blood flow and is used for the relief of deep-seated pain such as NEURITIS, SCIATICA and particularly painful rheumatic conditions. The use of currents in this way can be adopted to cauterize tissues and small blood vessels (the latter because the blood coagulates on contact with the heated element).

dietetics the study and application of the science of nutrition to all aspects of food and feeding for individuals and groups in health and disease.

digestion the process of breaking down food into substances that can be absorbed and used by the body. Digestion begins with the chewing and grinding of food, at which point it is mixed with saliva to commence the process of breakdown. Most digestion occurs in the stomach and small intestine. In the stomach the food is subject to gastric juice which contains pepsins to break down proteins and hydrochloric acid. The food is mixed and becomes totally soluble before passing into the small intestine as CHYME, where it is acted upon by pancreatic juice, bile, bacteria and succus entericus (intestinal juices).

Water is absorbed in the intestine in a very short time, while the bulk of the food may take several hours. The chyme forms chyle due to the action of bile and pancreatic juice. Fats are removed from this in emulsion form into the lymph vessels (*see* LACTEAL) and then into the blood. Sugars, salts and amino acids move directly into the small blood vessels in the intestine and the whole process is promoted by microfolding of the intestine wall producing finger-like projections (villi). The food passes down the intestine due to muscle contractions of the intestine wall and ultimately the residue and waste are excreted.

digitalis a powder derived from the leaf of the wild foxglove (*Digitalis purpurea*), which finds use in cases of heart disease. It acts in two ways; strengthening each heartbeat and increasing each pause (DIASTOLE), so that the damaged heart muscle has longer to rest. It also has a diuretic effect. Digitalis poisoning may occur with prolonged use or an overdose. Symptoms include vomiting, nausea, blurred vision, irregular heartbeat and possible breathing difficulties and unconsciousness.

dilatation and curettage (*or* **D & C**) the technique whereby the cervix is opened using DILATORS and then the lining is scraped using a curette. Such sampling is performed for the removal of incomplete abortions and tumours, to diagnose disease of the uterus or to correct bleeding, etc.

dilator an instrument employed to increase the opening of an orifice. Also, a muscle that increases the diameter of a vessel, or organ. The same term is applied to drugs that achieve a similar effect.

dipeptide a compound comprising two amino acids joined by a peptide bond (a characteristic chemical linkage where the amino group — NH_2 — of one amino acid is joined to the carboxyl group —COOH—of another).

diphtheria a serious, infectious disease caused by the bacterium *Corynebacterium diphtheriae*, commonest in children. The infection causes a membranous lining on the throat which can interfere with breathing and eating. The toxin produced by the bacterium damages heart tissue and the central nervous system and it can be fatal if not treated. The infection is countered by injection of the antitoxin with penicillin or erythromycin taken to kill the bacterium. Diphtheria can be immunized against.

diplegia paralysis on both sides of the body.

diplopia double vision. It is caused by dysfunction in the muscles that move the eyeballs such that rays of light fall in different places on the two retinae. The condition can be due to a nervous disease, intoxication or certain diseases such as diphtheria.

disc a flattened circular structure, such as the cartilage between vertebrae.

disinfection the process of killing PATHOGENIC organisms (not spores) to prevent the spread of infection. Different compounds are used, appropriate to the surface being disinfected.

dislocation injuries to joints such that bones are displaced from their normal, respective positions. Associated effects include bruising of the surrounding tissues and tearing of the ligaments that hold the bones together. Most dislocations are simple rather than compound (the latter being where the bone punctures the skin), and acquired rather than CONGENITAL. Immediate treatment involves the application of a splint or bandage to render the joint stable and immobile. Repositioning the bone (REDUCTION) requires skill, after which the limb must be fixed to avoid a repetition. Even after some time, care is necessary when using the limb.

diuresis an increase in urine production due to disease, drugs, hormone imbalance or increased fluid intake.

diuretic a substance that increases urine formation and excretion, and which may work specifically within the kidney e.g. by prevention of sodium and therefore water reabsorption, or outside the kidney.

diverticulitis the inflammation of diverticula (*see* DIVERTICULUM) in the large intestine. During the condition, there are cramp-like pains in the left side of the abdomen, possibly with constipation and fever. Treatment normally involves complete rest with no solid food, and antibiotics.

diverticulosis the condition in which there are DIVERTICULA in the large intestine, occurring primarily in the lower colon. They are caused by the muscles of the bowel forcing the bowel out through weak points in the wall. It is thought that it may be related to diet, but symptoms are not always produced.

diverticulum (*plural* **diverticula**) in general, a pouch extending from a main cavity. Specifically applied to the intestine, a sac-like protrusion through the wall, many of which usually develop later in life. The formation of diverticula is DIVERTICULOSIS and their inflammation is known as DIVERTICULITIS.

DNA (*or* **deoxyribonucleic acid**) a nucleic acid, and the primary constituent of CHROMOSOMES. It transmits genetic information from parents to offspring in the form of GENES. It is a very large molecule comprising two twisted nucleotide chains, which can store enormous amounts of information in a stable but not rigid way, i.e. parental traits and characteristics are passed on but evolutionary changes are allowed to occur.

donor a person who donates part of his or her body for use in other people. Blood is the most common donation but many tissues and organs are now used, including kidneys, livers, hearts, skin, corneas, bone marrow etc. Organ donations occur when the donor has been certified as brainstem dead. *See* BRAINSTEM DEAD.

donor insemination *see* **artificial insemination**

dopa an amino acid compound formed from tyrosine (an amino acid synthesized in the body), which is a precursor of DOPAMINE and NORADRENALINE (norepinephrine in America). A drug form, levodopa or l-dopa, is used to treat PARKINSON'S DISEASE, as it can increase the concentration of dopamine in the basal ganglia.

dopamine a catecholamine derived from DOPA and an intermediate in the synthesis of NORADRENALINE. (Catecholamines comprise benzene, hydroxyl groups and an amine group and are physiologically important in the functioning of the nervous system, mainly as NEUROTRANSMITTERS). It is found mainly in the basal ganglia of the brain and a deficiency is typical in PARKINSON'S DISEASE.

dosage the overall amount of a drug administered, determined by size, frequency and number of doses and taking into account the patient's age, weight and possible allergic reactions. Modern techniques enable controlled dosage using transdermals (drugs absorbed from a plaster on the skin) and implantable devices. The latter are polymeric substances containing the drug and placed just beneath the skin, which deliver the correct dose at any predetermined rate.

Down's syndrome (formerly called mongolism) a syndrome created by a CONGENITAL CHROMOSOME disorder which occurs as an extra chromosome 21, producing 47 in each body cell. Characteristic facial features are produced — a shorter, broader face with slanted eyes (similar to the Mongolian races, hence the term mongolism). It also results in a shorter stature, weak muscles and the possibility of heart defects and respiratory problems. The syndrome also confers mental retardation.

Down's syndrome occurs once in approximately 600 to 700 live births and although individuals may live beyond middle age, life expectancy is reduced and many die in infancy. The incidence increases with the age of the mother from 0.04% of children to women under 30 to 3% to women at 45. It is therefore likely that above 35 an AMNIOCENTESIS test would be made.

Drosophila a fruit fly that is used a great deal in genetic research because they breed easily and quickly and have just four pairs of chromosomes that are visible under the microscope. It is used to study linkage (when two or more GENES occur on the same CHROMOSOME and their respective characteristics are thus inherited together) and cytogenetics (inheritance related to all structure and function).

drug binding when a drug is attached to a protein, fat or component of tissues.

drug clearance is defined as the volume of blood which in one minute is completely cleared of a drug.

drug interactions when a patient is prescribed several drugs, there is the possibility for interactions between some or all of the medications. There are several ways in which the interaction may occur e.g. one drug displacing another at the site of action thus affecting its effectiveness; as alteration in the rate of destruction of one drug by another (by altering the activity of liver enzymes); prevention of absorption.

drug metabolism the process by which a drug is altered by the body into a metabolite (i.e. necessary for metabolic action), which may be the active agent and the process which ultimately results in the removal of the drug and thus determines the length of time over which it is active.

Dublin-Johnson syndrome a rare, chronic and hereditary condition in which there is an excess of BILIRUBIN in the blood, leading to gall bladder disorders, jaundice and abnormal pigmentation of the liver.

duct a narrow tube-like structure joining a gland with an organ or the body surface, through which a secretion passes e.g. sweat ducts opening onto the skin.

ductless gland a gland which releases the secretion directly into the blood for transport around the body, e.g. the pituitary and thyroid. Some glands, such as the PANCREAS, operate as ductless glands (for INSULIN), but secrete a digestive juice via ducts into the small intestine.

ductus arteriosus when a foetus is in the uterus, the lungs do not function and the foetal blood bypasses the lungs by means of the ductus

arteriosus which takes blood from the pulmonary artery to the aorta. The vessel stops functioning soon after birth.

duodenal ulcer the commonest type of PEPTIC ULCER. Duodenal ulcers may occur after the age of 20 and are more common in men. The cause is open to debate but probably results from an abrasion or break in the duodenum lining which is then exacerbated by gastric juice. Smoking seems to be a contributory but not causal factor.

The ulcer manifests itself as an upper abdominal pain roughly two hours after a meal that also occurs during the night. Food (e.g. milk) relieves the symptom and a regime of frequent meals and milky snacks, with little or no fried food and spices and a minimum of strong tea and coffee is usually adopted. Recent drug treatments enable the acid secretion to be reduced, thus allowing the ulcer to heal. Surgery is required only if there is no response to treatment, if the PYLORUS is obstructed or if the ulcer becomes perforated. The latter is treated as an emergency.

duodenum the first part of the small intestine where food (CHYME) from the stomach is subject to action by BILE and pancreatic enzymes. The duodenum also secretes a hormone secretion that contributes to the breakdown of fats, proteins and carbohydrates. In the duodenum, the acid conditions pertaining from the stomach are neutralized and rendered alkaline for the intestinal enzymes to operate.

dura mater *see* **meninges** and **brain**.

dwarfism an abnormal underdevelopment of the body manifested by small stature. There are several causes including incorrect functioning of the PITUITARY or THYROID gland. Pituitary dwarfism produces a small but correctly proportioned body and if diagnosed sufficiently early, treatment with growth hormone can help. A defect in the thyroid gland may result in CRETINISM or in the activity of digestive organs and their secretions. RICKETS may also be responsible for dwarfism.

dysarthria poorly articulated speech which sounds weak or slurred due to impairment of the control of muscles that effect speech. The cause may be damage in the brain or to the muscles themselves. Dysarthria occurs with strokes, multiple sclerosis, cerebral palsy and so on.

dysentery an infection and ulceration of the lower part of the bowels that causes severe diarrhoea with the passage of mucus and blood. There are two forms of dysentery caused by different organisms. Amoebic dysentery is due to *Entamoeba histolytica* which is spread via infected food or water and occurs mainly in the tropics and sub-tropics. The appearance of symptoms may be delayed but in addition to diarrhoea there is indigestion, anaemia and weight loss. Drugs are used in treatment.

Bacillary dysentery is caused by the bacterium *Shigella* and spreads by contact with a carrier or contaminated food. Symptoms appear from one to six days after infection and include diarrhoea, cramp, nausea and fever and the severity of the attack varies. Antibiotics may be given to kill the bacteria but recovery usually occurs within one to two weeks.

dyslexia a disorder that renders reading or learning to read difficult. There is usually an associated problem in writing and spelling correctly. A very small number of children are affected severely and boys are more prone than girls by a factor of three.

dyspepsia (*or* **indigestion**) after eating there may be discomfort in the upper abdomen/lower chest with heartburn, nausea and flatulence accompanying a feeling of fullness. The causes are numerous and include GALLSTONES, PEPTIC ULCER, HIATUS HERNIA and diseases of the liver or pancreas.

dysphasia a general term for an impairment of speech whether it is manifested as a difficulty in understanding language or in self-expression. There is a range of conditions with varying degrees of severity. *Global aphasia* is a total inability to communicate, however some individuals partially understand what is said to them. *Dysphasia* is when thoughts can be expressed up to a point. *Non-fluent dysphasia* represents poor self-expression but good understanding while the reverse is called *fluent dysphasia.* The condition may be due to a stroke or other brain damage and can be temporary or permanent.

E

ear the sense organ used for detection of sound and maintenance of balance. It comprises three parts, the external or outer, middle and inner ear, the first two acting to collect sound waves and transmit them to the inner ear, where the hearing and balance mechanisms are situated.

The outer ear (*auricle* or *pinna*) is a cartilage and skin structure which is not actually essential to hearing in man. The middle ear is an air-filled cavity that is linked to the PHARYNX via the EUSTACHIAN TUBE. Within the middle ear are the ear (or auditory) ossicles, three bones called the *incus, malleus* and *stapes* (anvil, hammer and stirrup respectively). Two small muscles control the bones and the associated nerve (the chorda tympani). The ossicles bridge the middle ear, connecting the eardrum with the inner ear and in so doing convert sound (air waves) into mechanical movements which then impinge upon the fluid of the inner ear.

The inner ear lies within the temporal bone of the skull and contains the apparatus for hearing and balance. The COCHLEA is responsible for hearing and balance is maintained by the semi-circular canals. The latter are made up of three loops positioned mutually at right angles and in each is the fluid endolymph. When the head is moved the fluid moves accordingly and sensory cells produce impulses that are transmitted to the brain.

earache pain in the ear may be due directly to inflammation of the middle ear but is often referred pain from other conditions e.g., infections of the nose or larynx or tooth decay.

eating disorders *see* **anorexia** and **bulimia.**

ECG *see* **electrocardiogram.**

echocardiography the use of ULTRASOUND to study the heart and its movements.

echography (*or* **ultrasonography**) the use of sound waves (ULTRASOUND) to create an image of the deeper structures of the body, based upon the differences in reflection of the sound by various parts of the body.

eclampsia (of pregnancy) convulsions that occur during pregnancy, usually at the later stages or during delivery. Although the cause is not known the start of convulsions may be associated with cerebral OEDEMA or a sudden rise in blood pressure. Kidney function is usually badly affected. The condition is often preceded for days or weeks by symptoms such as headache, dizziness and vomiting, and seizures follow. The fits differ in severity and duration and in the one in twelve fatalities, there may be a cerebral haemorrhage or pneumonia, or the breathing may gradually fade. The condition requires immediate treatment as it threatens both mother and baby. Treatment is by drugs and reduction of outside stimuli, and a CAESARIAN SECTION is undertaken.

ectopic referring to something or some event that is not in its usual place or occurring at its usual time e.g. an ectopic pregnancy is one that is outside the uterus.

eczema an inflammation of the skin that causes itching, a red rash and often small blisters that weep and become encrusted. This may be followed by the skin thickening and then peeling off in scales. There are several types of eczema, *atopic* being one of the most common. (Atopic is the hereditary tendency to form allergic reactions due to an antibody in the skin.) A form of atopic eczema is infantile eczema, which starts at three or four months and it is often the case that eczema, hay fever and asthma is found in the family history. However, many children improve markedly as they approach the age of ten or eleven. The treatment for such conditions usually involves the use of HYDROCORTISONE or other steroid creams and ointments.

EEG *see* **electroencephalogram.**

ejaculation the emission of semen from the penis via the urethra. It is a reflex action produced during copulation or masturbation and the sensation associated with it is called orgasm.

elbow the joint at which the arm bends and the arm and forearm meet. It is the articulation of the humerus, ulna and radius which allows backward/forward movement of the radius and ulna and a rotation of the radius on the ulna. Ligaments hold the joint and it is covered front and back by strong muscles.

electrocardiogram (*or* **ECG**) a record of the changes in the heart's electrical potential, on an instrument called an electrocardiograph. The subject is connected to the equipment by leads on the chest and legs or arms. A normal trace has one wave for the activity of the atria and others relating to the ventricular beat. Abnormal heart activity is often indicated in the trace and it therefore forms a useful diagnostic aid.

electroconvulsive therapy a somewhat drastic treatment for severe DEPRESSION and sometimes SCHIZOPHRENIA. An electric current is passed through the brain, producing a convulsion. The convulsion is controlled by administering an anaesthetic and a muscle relaxant. There is no memory of the shock and there may be temporary amnesia, with headache and confusion — symptoms that usually dissipate within a few hours. It is a treatment that is used much less than was the case and even then it is considered suitable for only very carefully chosen patients.

electroencephalogram (*or* **EEG**) a record of the brain's electrical activity measured on an electroencephalograph. Electrodes on the scalp record the charge of electric potential — or brain waves. There are four main types of waves: alpha, beta, theta and delta. Alpha waves, with a frequency of ten per second, occur when awake and delta waves (seven or less per second) occur in sleeping adults. The occurrence of delta waves in wakeful adults indicates brain damage or cerebral tumours.

electrolytes *sensu stricto* – a compound that dissolves in water to produce a solution containing ions that is able to conduct an electrical charge. In the body, electrolytes occur in the blood plasma, all fluid and interstitial fluid and normal concentrations are imperative for normal metabolic activity. Some diseases alter the electrolyte balance, either through vomiting or diarrhoea or because the kidney is malfunctioning. The correct balance can be restored through oral or intravenous dosage or by DIALYSIS.

elephantiasis a dramatic and debilitating enlargement of skin and underlying connective tissue due to inflammation of the skin, subcutaneous tissue and the blocking of lymph vessels, preventing drainage. Inflammation and blocking of vessels is due to parasitic worms — filariae which are carried to man by mosquitoes. The parts of the body most commonly affected are the legs, scrotum and breasts, in some cases to enormous proportions. The associated muscles of a limb may degenerate due to the abnormal pressure on them, and eventually overall health suffers. Prevention is the key, by eradication of the mosquitoes, but some relief is gained by using certain drugs early in the history of the disease.

emaciation particularly severe leanness caused by lack of nourishment or disease. It tends to be associated with diseases such as tuberculosis or diseases producing diarrhoea over a long period of time.

embolectomy the surgical, and often emergency, removal of an EMBOLUS or clot to clear an arterial obstruction.

embolism the state in which a small blood vessel is blocked by an EMBOLUS, or fragment of material, which the circulatory system has carried through larger vessels. This plug may be fragments of a clot, a mass of bacteria, air bubbles that have entered the system during an operation or a fragment of tumour. The blockage leads usually to the destruction of that part of the organ supplied by the vessel. The most common case is a pulmonary embolism. Treatment utilizes an anticoagulant drug such as warfarin or heparin, EMBOLECTOMY or streptokinase. The latter is an enzyme capable of dissolving blood clots.

embolus material carried by the blood which then lodges elsewhere in the body (*see* EMBOLISM). The material may be a blood clot, fat, air, a piece of tumour etc.

embryo the stage of development from two weeks, when the fertilized ovum is implanted in the uterus, to two months.

embryology the study of the embryo, its growth and development from fertilization to birth.

embryo transfer (*see also* IN VITRO FERTILIZATION) the fertilization of an ovum by sperm and its development into an early embryo, outside the mother, and its subsequent implantation in the mother's uterus. Such procedures result in what is popularly termed a 'test-tube baby'.

emesis is the medical term for vomit.

emetics a substance that causes vomiting. Direct emetics, such as mustard in water, copper sulphate, alum or a lot of salty water, irritate the stomach, while indirect emetics such as apomorphine and ipecacuanha act on the centre of the brain that controls the act of vomiting. Tickling the throat is also classed as an emetic (indirect). Emetics tend to be used little nowadays, but great care must be exercised if their use is advocated.

emollients substances that soften or soothe the skin whether in the form of a powder, oil or preparation, often used in the treatment of eczema. Examples are olive oil, glycerin and French chalk.

emphysema refers, in the main, to an abnormal condition of the lungs where the walls are overinflated and distended and changes in their structure occur. This destruction of parts of the walls produces large air-filled spaces which do not contribute to the respiratory process. Acute cases of emphysema may be caused by whooping cough or bronchopneumonia, and chronic cases often accompany chronic bronchitis which itself is due in great part to smoking. Emphysema is also developed after tuberculosis when the lungs are stretched until the fibres of the alveolar walls are destroyed. Similarly in old age, the alveolar membrane may collapse producing large air sacs, with decreased surface area.

encephalins PEPTIDES that act as NEUROTRANSMITTERS. Two have been identified, both acting as analgesics when their release controls pain. They are found in the brain and in nerve cells of the spinal cord.

encephalitis inflammation of the brain. It is usually a viral infection and sometimes occurs as a complication of some common infectious diseases, e.g. measles or chicken-pox. There are several forms of the disease including *Encephalitis lethargica* (sleepy sickness or epidemic encephalitis), which attacks and causes swelling in the basal ganglia, cerebrum and brainstem which may result in tissue destruction; Japanese encephalitis, which is caused by a virus carried by mosquitoes and tick-borne encephalitis, which occurs in Europe and Siberia. In most cases there is no readily available treatment other than reducing pressure on the brain to relieve symptoms.

encephalography any technique used to record brain structure or activity e.g. EEG.

encephaloid the term given to a form of cancer that superficially resembles brain tissue.

encephalomyelitis inflammation of the brain and spinal cord, typified by headaches, fever, stiff neck and back pain, with vomiting. Depending upon the extent of the inflammation and the patient's condition, encephalomyelitis may cause paralysis, personality changes, coma or death.

encephalopathy any disease affecting the brain or an abnormal condition of the brain's structure and function. It refers in particular to degenerative and chronic conditions such as Wernicke's encephalopathy, which is caused by a THIAMINE deficiency and associated with alcoholism.

endemic the term used to describe, for example, a disease that is indigenous to a certain area.

endocarditis inflammation of the ENDOCARDIUM, heart valves and muscle, caused by a bacterium, virus or rheumatic fever. Those at greatest risk are patients with some damage to the endocardium from a CONGENITAL deformity or alteration of the immune system by drugs. Patients suffer fever, heart failure and/or EMBOLISM. Large doses of an antibiotic are used in treatment and surgery may prove necessary to repair heart valves that become damaged. If not treated the condition is fatal.

endocardium a fine membrane lining the heart, which forms a continuous membrane with the lining of veins and arteries. At the cavities of the heart it forms cusps on the valves and its surface is very smooth to facilitate blood flow.

endocrine glands DUCTLESS GLANDS that produce HORMONES for secretion directly into the bloodstream (or lymph). Some organs e.g. the PANCREAS also release secretions via a DUCT. In addition to the pancreas the major endocrine glands are the THYROID, PITUITARY, PARATHYROID, OVARY and TESTIS. Imbalances in the secretions of endocrine glands produce a variety of diseases.

endocrinology the study of the ENDOCRINE GLANDS, the hormones secreted by the glands and the treatment of any problems.

endogenous referring to within the body, whether growing within, or originating from within or due to internal causes.

endometriosis the occurrence of ENDOMETRIUM in other parts of the body e.g. within the muscle of the uterus, in the ovary, FALLOPIAN TUBES, PERITONEUM and possibly the bowel. Because of the nature of tissue, it acts in a way similar to that of the uterus lining and causes pelvic pain, bleeding and painful menstruation. The condition occurs between puberty and the menopause and ceases during pregnancy. The treatment required may include total hysterectomy, but occasionally the administration of a steroid hormone will alleviate the symptoms.

endometritis inflammation of the ENDOMETRIUM caused commonly by bacteria, but it can also be due to a virus, parasite or foreign body. It is associated with fever and abdominal pain and occurs most after abortion or childbirth or in women with an INTRAUTERINE CONTRACEPTIVE DEVICE.

endometrium the womb's mucous membrane lining that changes in structure during the menstrual cycle, becoming thicker with an increased blood supply later in the cycle. This is in readiness for receiving an embryo but if this does not happen, the endometrium breaks down and most is lost in menstruation.

endorphins a group of compounds, PEPTIDES that occur in the brain and have pain-relieving qualities similar to morphine. They are derived from a substance in the PITUITARY and are involved in endocrine control. In addition to their opiate effects, they are involved in urine output, depression of respiration, sexual activity and learning. *See also* ENCEPHALINS.

endoscope the general term for an instrument used to inspect the interior of a body cavity or organ, e.g. the gastroscope is for viewing the stomach. The instrument is fitted with lenses and a light source and is usually inserted through a natural opening, although an incision can be used.

enema the procedure of putting fluid into the rectum for purposes of cleansing or therapy. An evacuant enema removes faeces and consists of soap in water or olive oil while a barium enema is given to permit an X-ray of the colon to be taken. The compound barium sulphate is opaque to X-rays. The insertion of drugs into the rectum is a therapeutic enema.

engagement the stage in a pregnancy when the presenting part of the foetus which is usually the head, descends into the pelvis of the mother.

enteral the term meaning relating to the intestine.

enteral feeding the procedure of feeding a patient who is very ill through a tube via the nose, to the stomach. Through the tube is given a liquid, low-waste food and there are a number of proprietary brands, some containing whole protein, some amino acids. This is a particularly useful technique when a patient suffers tissue damage with an ensuing reduction of muscle and plasma proteins after a major operation, burns, renal failure, etc.

enteric fevers *see* **typhoid fever** and **paratyphoid fever**.

enteritis inflammation of the intestine, due usually to a viral or bacterial infection, causing diarrhoea.

enterovirus a virus that enters the body via the gut where it multiplies and from where they attack the central nervous system. Examples are POLIOMYELITIS and the Coxsackie viruses (the cause of severe throat infections, MENINGITIS, and inflammation of heart tissue, some muscles and the brain).

enzyme any protein molecule that acts as a catalyst in the biochemical processes of the body. They are essential to life and are highly specific, acting on certain substrates at a set temperature and pH. Examples are the digestive enzymes amylase, lipase and trypsin. Enzymes act by providing active sites (one or more for each enzyme) to which substrate molecules bind, forming a short-lived intermediate. The rate of reaction is increased, and after the product is formed, the active site is freed. Enzymes are easily rendered inactive by heat and some chemicals. The names of most enzymes end in *-ase*, and this is added onto the name of the substrate, thus a peptidase breaks down peptides. Enzymes are vital for the normal functioning of the body and their lack or inactivity can produce metabolic disorders.

epidemic a disease that affects a large proportion of the population at the same time. Usually an infectious disease that occurs suddenly and spreads rapidly, e.g. today there are influenza epidemics.

epidemiology the study of epidemic disease. It involves aspects such as occurrence and distribution, causes, control and prevention. Included are the obvious epidemics such as cholera and smallpox and also those either associated with more recent times (e.g. related to diet, lifestyle, etc.) or those about which much more is now known. Thus, the link between smoking and cancer, diet and coronary disease are also included.

epidermis the outer layer of the skin, which comprises four layers and lies over the dermis. The top three layers are continually renewed as cells from the innermost germinative layer (called *the Malpighian layer* or *stratum germinativum*) are pushed outwards. The topmost layer (*stratum corneum*) is made up of dead cells where the CYTOPLASM has been replaced by KERATIN. This layer is thickest on the palms and the soles of the feet.

epidural anaesthesia anaesthesia in the region of the pelvis, abdomen or genitals produced by local anaesthetic injected into the epidural space of the spinal column (the epidural space is that space between the vertebral canal and the dura mater of the spinal cord).

epiglottis situated at the base of the tongue, a thin piece of cartilage enclosed in MUCOUS MEMBRANE that covers the LARYNX. It prevents food from passing into the larynx and TRACHEA when swallowing. The epiglottis resembles a leaf in shape.

epiglottitis inflammation of the mucous membrane of the EPIGLOTTIS. Swelling of the tissues may obstruct the airway and swift action may be necessary, i.e. a TRACHEOSTOMY, to avoid a fatality. The other symptoms of epiglottitis are sore throat, fever and a croup-like cough and it occurs mainly in children, usually during the winter.

epilepsy a neurological disorder involving convulsions, seizures and loss of consciousness. There are many possible causes or associations of epilepsy, including cerebral trauma, brain tumour, cerebral haemorrhage and metabolic imbalances, as in HYPOGLYCAEMIA. Usually an epileptic attack occurs without warning, with complete unconsciousness and some muscle contraction and spasms. Some drugs are used in treatment, although little can be done during the fit itself.

epiphysis the softer end of a long bone that is separated from the shaft by a plate (the epiphyseal plate) of cartilage. It develops separately from the shaft but when the bone stops growing it disappears as the head and shaft fuse. Separation of the epiphysis is a serious fracture because the growing bone may be affected.

episiotomy the process of making an incision in the PERINEUM to enlarge a woman's vaginal opening to facilitate delivery of a child. The technique is used to prevent tearing of the perineum.

epithelioma an epithelial (*see* EPITHELIUM) tumour used formerly to describe any carcinoma.

epithelium (*plural* **epithelia**) tissue made up of cells packed closely together and bound by connective material. It covers the outer surface of the body and lines vessels and organs in the body. One surface is fixed to a basement membrane and the other is free and it provides a barrier against injury, microorganisms and some fluid loss. There are various types of epithelium in single and multiple (or stratified) layers and differing shapes, *viz.* cuboidal, squamous (like flat pads) and columnar. The shape suits the function, thus the skin is formed from stratified squamous (and KERATINIZED) epithelium, while columnar epithelia, which can secrete solutions and absorb nutrients, line the intestines and stomach.

Epstein Barr virus the virus, similar to the herpes virus, that causes infectious mononucleosis (GLANDULAR FEVER) and is implicated in HEPATITIS.

erection the condition whereby erectile tissue in the penis (and to some degree the clitoris) is engorged with blood, making it swell and become hard. It is due primarily to sexual arousal, although it does occur during sleep, due to physical stimulation, and it also occurs in young boys. It is a prerequisite of vaginal penetration for emission of semen.

eruption an outbreak, or rash upon the skin usually

in the form of a red and raised area, possibly with fluid-containing vesicles or scales/crusts. It may be associated with a disease such as measles or chickenpox, a drug reaction or a physical or short-lived occurrence e.g. nettlerash.

erysipelas an infectious disease, caused by *streptococcus pyogenes*. It produces an inflammation of the skin with associated redness. Large areas of the body may be affected and other symptoms may include vesicles, fever and pain, with a feeling of heat and a tingling sensation. In addition to being isolated, patients are given penicillin.

erythema an inflammation or redness of the skin in which the tissues are congested with blood. The condition may be accompanied by pain or itching. There are numerous causes, some bacterial/viral and others physical e.g. mild sunburn.

erythroblast cells occurring in the red bone marrow that develop into red blood cells (called ERYTHROCYTES). The cells begin colourless but accumulate HAEMOGLOBIN and in mammals the nucleus is lost.

erythrocyte the red blood cell that is made in the bone marrow and occurs as a red disc, concave on both sides, full of HAEMOGLOBIN. These cells are responsible for carrying oxygen to tissues and carbon dioxide away. The latter is removed in the form of the bicarbonate ion (HCO_3^-), in exchange for a chloride ion (Cl^-). There are approximately five million erythrocytes in one millilitre of blood and they are active for about 120 days before being absorbed by MACROPHAGES.

erythromycin an antibiotic used for bacterial and mycoplasmic infections. It is similar to penicillin in its activity and can be taken for infections that penicillin cannot be used to treat.

escherichia a group of Gram-negative (*see* GRAM'S STAIN) rod-shaped bacteria (*E. coli*) normally found in the intestines and common in water, milk, etc. *E. coli* is a common cause of infections of the urinary tract.

essential amino acid of the twenty amino acids required by the body, a number are termed essential, because they must be in the diet, as they cannot be synthesized in the body. The essential ones are: isoleucine, leucine, lysine, methionine, phenylalanine, threonine, tryptophan and valine. In addition, infants require arginine and histidine. A lack leads to protein deficiency, but they are available in meat, cheese and eggs, and all eight would be obtained if the diet contained corn and beans.

essential fatty acid there are three polyunsaturated

acids in this category which cannot be produced in the body — arachidonic, linoleic and linolenic. These compounds are found in vegetable and fish oils and are vital in metabolism and proper functioning. A deficiency may cause such symptoms as allergic conditions, skin disorders, poor hair and nails and so on.

essential hypertension high blood pressure with no identifiable cause. Arteriosclerosis is a complication of, and often associated with, hypertension. Other complications include cerebral haemorrhage, heart failure and kidney failure. There are now several drugs that reduce blood pressure, including betablockers and methyldopa. Lifestyle is an important factor for some sufferers: excessive weight should be lost, excess salt intake avoided and strain of all types lessened.

etiology *see* **aetiology**.

eugenics the study of how the inherited characteristics of the human population can be improved by genetics or selective/controlled breeding.

euploid term meaning with a chromosome number that is an exact multiple of the normal (haploid) number.

eustachian tube tubes, one on each side, that connect the middle ear to the PHARYNX. The short (about 35 to 40mm) tube is fine at the centre and wider at both ends and is lined with mucous membrane. It is normally closed but opens to equalize air pressure on either side of the eardrum. It was named after the 16th-century Italian anatomist Eustachio.

euthanasia intentionally hastening the death of someone who is suffering from a disease that is painful, incurable and inevitably fatal. The patient and/or their relatives consent to this, whether it is achieved by administering a lethal drug or by withholding treatment.

Ewing's sarcoma a malignant bone cancer that develops from the marrow in the pelvis or long bones. It occurs in young adults and children and soon spreads around the body. It is uncommon but very malignant although recent use of anticancer drugs has prolonged the life expectancy of sufferers. The cancer was named after the American pathologist James Ewing, who determined that it was different from OSTEOSARCOMA.

excision in general terms, cutting out. More specifically the removal of, for example, a gland or tumour from the body.

excoriation injury of the surface of the skin (or other part of the body) caused by the abrasion or scratching of the area.

excreta waste material discharged from the body. The term is often used specifically to denote faeces.

excretion the removal of all waste material from the body, including urine and faeces, the loss of water and salts through sweat glands and the elimination of carbon dioxide and water vapour from the lungs.

exogenous originating outside the body. It can also refer to an organ of the body.

expectorants a group of drugs that are taken to help in the removal of secretions from the lungs, bronchi and trachea. The drugs work in one of several ways or can be used to combine their effects. Some dry up excess mucus and sputum while others render these secretions less viscous, to promote their removal. There are other varieties that work in still different ways.

extrapyramidal side effects are those caused by drugs that interfere with this system of nerves and pathways that connect the basal ganglia, cerebral cortex, cerebellum, thalamus (*see individual entries*) and spinal neurones, which are involved mainly with reflex muscular movements.

extrasystole (*or* **ectopic beat**) a heartbeat that is outside the normal rhythm of the heart and is due to an impulse generated outside the SINOATRIAL NODE. It may go unnoticed or it may seem that the heart has missed a beat. Extrasystoles are common in healthy people, but they may result from heart disease, or nicotine from smoking, or caffeine from excessive intake of tea and coffee. Drugs can be taken to suppress these irregular beats.

eye the complicated organ of sight. Each eye is roughly spherical and contained within the bony ORBIT in the skull. The outer layer is fibrous and comprises the opaque SCLERA and transparent CORNEA. The middle layer is vascular and is made up of the *choroid* (the blood supply for the outer half of the retina), *ciliary body* (which secretes aqueous humour) and the IRIS. The inner layer is sensory, the RETINA. Between the cornea and the LENS is a chamber filled with aqueous humour and behind the lens is a much larger cavity with vitreous humour. Light enters the eye through the cornea and thence via the aqueous humour to the lens, which focuses the light onto the retina. The latter contains CONE and ROD cells, which are sensitive to light and impulses are sent to the visual cortex of the brain via the optic nerve.

F

face the front-facing part of the head which extends from the chin to the forehead. There are fourteen bones in the skull, supporting the face, and numerous fine muscles are responsible for movements around the eyes, nose and mouth producing expression. These are under the control of the seventh cranial nerve, which is a mixed sensory and motor nerve known as the FACIAL NERVE.

facial nerve the cranial nerve, which has a number of branches and supplies the muscles which control facial expression. It also has branches to the middle ear, taste buds, salivary glands and lacrimal glands. Some branches are motor and others sensory in function.

facial paralysis paralysis of the facial nerve, which leads to a loss of function in the muscles of the face, producing a lack of expression in the affected side. It occurs in the condition known as *Bell's palsy,* in which there may also be a loss of taste and inability to close the eye. The condition is often temporary, if caused by inflammation which recovers in time. However, if the nerve itself is damaged by injury or if the person has suffered a stroke, the condition is likely to be permanent.

factor VIII this is one of the COAGULATION FACTORS normally present in the blood and is known as antihaemophilic factor. If the factor is deficient in males it results in HAEMOPHILIA.

faeces the end waste product of digestion, which is formed in the colon and discharged from the bowels via the ANUS. Also known as stools, it consists of undigested food (chiefly cellulose), bacteria, mucus and other secretions, water and bile pigments which are responsible for the colour. The condition and colour of the faeces are indicators of general health e.g. pale stools are produced in JAUNDICE and COELIAC DISEASE and black stools often indicate the presence of digested blood.

fainting (*or* **syncope**) this is a temporary and brief loss of consciousness caused by a sudden drop in the blood supply to the brain. It can occur in perfectly healthy people, brought about by prolonged standing or emotional shock. It may also result from an infection, during pregnancy, from severe pain or loss of blood through injury. Fainting is often preceded by giddiness, blurred vision, sweating and ringing in the ears. Recovery is usually complete, producing no lasting ill-effects, although this depends upon the underlying cause.

Fallopian tubes a pair of tubes, one of which leads from each ovary to the womb. At the ovary, the tube is expanded to form a funnel with finger-like projections, known as fimbriae, surrounding the opening. This funnel does not communicate directly with the ovary but is open to the abdominal cavity. However, when an egg is released from the ovary the fimbriae move and waft it into the Fallopian tube. The tube is about 10 to 12cm long and leads directly into the womb at the lower end through a narrow opening.

false rib *see* **rib**.

farmer's lung an allergic condition caused by sensitivity to inhaled dust and fungal spores that are found in mouldy hay or straw. It is a form of allergic alveolitis (inflammation of the ALVEOLI of the lungs) characterized by increasing breathlessness. The condition may be treated by CORTICOSTEROID drugs but can only be cured by avoidance of the allergen.

fascioliasis a disease of the liver and bile ducts caused by the organism *Fasciola hepatica* or liver fluke. Human beings and animals are hosts to the adult flukes and the eggs of the parasite are passed out in faeces. These are taken up by a certain species of snail which forms an intermediate host for the parasite, from which the larval stages are deposited on vegetation, especially wild watercress. Human beings are then infected, especially by eating wild watercress, which should always be avoided.

Symptoms include fever, loss of appetite, indigestion, nausea and vomiting, diarrhoea, abdominal pain, severe sweating and coughing. In severe cases the liver may be damaged and there may be jaundice and even death. Chemotherapy is required to kill the flukes, the principal drugs being chloroquine and bithionol.

fat *see* **adipose tissue.**

fatigue physical or mental tiredness following a prolonged period of hard work. Muscle fatigue resulting from hard exercise is caused by a build, up of *lactic acid.* Lactic acid is produced in muscles (as an end product of the breakdown of GLYCOGEN to produce energy), and builds up when there is an insufficient supply of oxygen. The muscle is unable to work properly until a period of rest and restored oxygen supply enables the lactic acid to be removed.

fatty acids a group of organic compounds each consisting of a long, straight hydrocarbon chain and a terminal carboxylic acid (COOH) group. The length of the chain varies from one to nearly thirty carbon atoms and the chains may be *saturated* or *unsaturated.* Some fatty acids can be synthesized within the body but others, the ESSENTIAL FATTY ACIDS, must be obtained from food. Fatty acids have three major roles within the body.

(1) They are components of glycolipids (lipids containing carbohydrate) and phospholipids (lipids containing phosphate). These are of major importance in the structure of tissues and organs.

(2) Fatty acids are important constituents of triglycerides (lipids which have three fatty acid molecules joined to a glycerol molecule). They are stored in the cytoplasm of many cells and are broken down when required to yield energy. They are the form in which the body stores fat.

(3) Derivatives of fatty acids function as hormones and intracellular messengers.

favism an inherited disorder which takes the form of severe haemolytic ANAEMIA (destruction of red blood cells) brought on by eating broad beans. A person having this disorder is sensitive to a chemical present in the beans and also to certain drugs, particularly some antimalarial drugs. It is caused by the lack of a certain enzyme, glucose 6-phosphate dehydrogenase, which plays an important role in glucose metabolism. The defective gene responsible is passed on as a SEX-LINKED dominant characteristic and appears to persist in populations where it occurs, because it also confers increased resistance to malaria. Favism is found in African-Americans, Yemenite Jews in Israel and in some people living in the Mediterranean region and in Iran.

febrile having a fever.

femoral describing the femur or area of the thigh e.g. femoral artery, vein, nerve and canal.

femur the thigh bone, which is the long bone extending from the hip to the knee and is the strongest bone in the body. It is the weight-bearing bone of the body and fractures are common in old people who have lost bone mass. It articulates with the pelvic girdle at the upper end, forming the hip joint and at the lower end with the patella (kneecap) and tibia to form the knee joint.

fertilization the fusion of SPERMATOZOON) and OVUM to form a *zygote* which then undergoes cell division to become an embryo. Fertilization in humans takes place high up in the FALLOPIAN TUBE near the ovary and the fertilized egg travels down and becomes implanted in the womb.

fever an elevation of body temperature above the normal which accompanies many diseases and infections. The cause of fever is the production by the body of endogenous pyrogen which acts on the thermo-regulatory centre in the hypothalamus of the brain. This responds by promoting mechanisms which increase heat generation and lessen heat loss, leading to a rise in temperature. Fever is the main factor in many infections caused by bacteria or viruses and results from toxins produced by the growth of these organisms. Examples of these *primary* or *specific* fevers are diphtheria, scarlet fever and typhoid fever. An *intermittent fever* describes a fluctuating body temperature, which commonly accompanies MALARIA, in which the temperature sometimes returns to normal. In a *remittent fever* there is also a fluctuating body temperature but this does not return to normal. In a *relapsing fever*, caused by bacteria of the genus *Borella*, transmitted by ticks or lice, there is a recurrent fever every three to ten days following the first attack which lasts for about one week.

Treatment of fever depends upon the underlying cause. However, it may be necessary to reduce the temperature by direct methods such as sponging the body with tepid water, or by giving drugs such as ASPIRIN. As well as a rise in body temperature, symptoms of fever include headache, shivering, nausea, diarrhoea or constipation. Above 105°F (40.6°C), there may be delirium or convulsions, especially in young children.

fibreoptic endoscopy a method of viewing internal structures such as the digestive tract and tracheo-bronchial tree using fibreoptics. Fibreoptics uses illumination from a cold light source which is passed down a bundle of quartz fibres. The instruments used are highly flexible compared to the older form of endoscope and can be employed to illuminate structures which were formerly inaccessible. Using fibreoptic endoscopy, direct procedures can be carried out, such as BIOPSY and polypectomy (surgical removal of a POLYP).

fibrillation the rapid non-synchronized contraction or tremor of muscles, in which individual bundles of fibres contract independently. It applies especially to heart muscle and disrupts the normal beating so that the affected part is unable to pump blood. Two types of fibrillation may occur, depending upon which muscle is affected. Atrial fibrillation, often resulting from ATHEROSCLEROSIS or rheumatic heart disease, affects the muscles of the atria and is a common type of arrhythmia. The heartbeat and pulse are very irregular and cardiac output is maintained by the contraction of the ventricles alone. With ventricular fibrillation the heart stops pumping blood so that this, in effect, is cardiac arrest. The patient requires immediate emergency resuscitation or death ensues within minutes.

fibrin the end product of the process of blood COAGULATION, comprising threads of insoluble protein formed from a soluble precursor, FIBRINOGEN, by the activity of the enzyme thrombin. Fibrin forms a network which is the basis of a blood clot. *See* COAGULATION.

fibrinogen a COAGULATION FACTOR present in the blood, which is a soluble protein and the precursor of FIBRIN. *See* COAGULATION.

fibrocystic disease of the pancreas *see* **cystic fibrosis**.

fibroid a type of benign tumour found in the womb (uterus), composed of fibrous and muscular tissue and varying in size from 1 or 2mm to a mass weighing several pounds. They more commonly occur in childless women and those over the age of 35. Fibroids may present no problems but alternatively can be the cause of pain, heavy and irregular menstrual bleeding, urine retention or frequency of MICTURITION and sterility. Fibroids can be removed surgically but often the complete removal of the womb (HYSTERECTOMY) is carried out.

fibroma a benign tumour composed of fibrous tissue.

fibrosarcoma a malignant tumour of connective tissue particularly found in the limbs and especially the legs.

ibrosis the formation of thickened connective or scar tissue, usually as a result of injury or inflammation. This may affect the lining of the ALVEOLI of the lungs (pulmonary interstitial fibrosis) and causes breathlessness. *See also* CYSTIC FIBROSIS.

fibrositis inflammation of fibrous connective tissue, muscles and muscle sheaths, particularly in the back, legs and arms, causing pain and stiffness.

fibrous tissue a tissue type which occurs abundantly throughout the body. *White fibrous tissue* consists of collagen fibres, a protein with a high tensile strength and unyielding structure, that forms ligaments, sinews and scar tissue, and occurs in the skin. *Yellow fibrous tissue* is composed of the fibres of another protein, elastin. It is very elastic and occurs in ligaments which are subjected to frequent stretching, such as those in the back of the neck. It also occurs in arterial walls and in the walls of the alveoli (*see* ALVEOLUS), and in the dermis layer of the skin.

fibula the outer, thin, long bone which articulates with the larger tibia in the lower leg.

fissure a natural cleft or groove or abnormal break in the skin or mucous membrane e.g. an anal fissure.

fistula an abnormal opening between two hollow organs or between such an organ or gland and the exterior. These may arise during development so that a baby may be born with a fistula. Alternatively, they can be produced by injury or infection, or as a complication following surgery. A common example is an anal fistula, which may develop if an abscess present in the rectum bursts and produces a communication through the surface of the skin. An operation is normally required to correct a fistula, but healing is further complicated in the case of an anal fistula because of the passage of waste material through the bowels.

fit any sudden convulsive attack; a general term which is applied to an epileptic seizure, convulsion or bout of coughing.

flap a section of tissue, usually skin, which is excised from the underlying tissues except for one thin strip (pedicle), which is left for blood and nervous supply. The flap is used to repair an injury at another site in the body, the free part being sutured into place. After about three weeks, when the healing process is well underway, the remaining strip is detached and sewn into place. Flaps are commonly used in plastic surgery and also following amputation of a limb. *See* SKIN GRAFTING.

flat foot an absence of the arch of the foot so that the inner edge lies flat on the ground. It may occur in children in whom the ligaments of the foot are soft, or in older, obese adults or those who stand for long periods. Treatment is by means of exercises, built-up footwear and, in extreme cases, surgery.

flatulence a build-up of gas in the stomach or bowels which is released through the mouth or anus.

flexion bending of a joint, or the term may also be applied to an abnormal shape in a body organ.

flexor any muscle that causes a limb or other body part to bend.

flutter an abnormal disturbance of heartbeat rhythm, which may affect the atria or ventricles but is less severe than FIBRILLATION. The causes are the same as those of fibrillation and the treatment is also similar.

flux an excessive and abnormal flow from any of the natural openings of the body e.g. alvine flux, which is diarrhoea.

foetus an unborn child after the eighth week of development.

follicle any small sac, cavity or secretory gland. Examples are hair follicles and the Graafian follicles of the ovaries in and from which eggs mature and are released.

fontanelle openings in the skull of newborn and young infants in whom the bone is not wholly formed and the sutures are incompletely fused. The largest of these is the *anterior fontanelle* on the top of the head, which is about 2.5cm square at birth.

The fontanelles gradually close as bone is formed and are completely covered by the age of 18 months. If a baby is unwell, for example with a fever, the fontanelle becomes tense. If an infant is suffering from diarrhoea and possibly dehydrated, the fontanelle is abnormally depressed.

food poisoning an illness of the digestive system caused by eating food contaminated by certain bacteria, viruses or chemical poisons (insecticides) and metallic elements such as mercury or lead. Symptoms include vomiting, diarrhoea, nausea and abdominal pain and these may arise very quickly and usually within 24 hours. Bacteria are the usual cause of food poisoning and proliferate rapidly producing toxins which cause the symptoms of the illness. Those involved include members of the genera *Salmonella, Staphylococcus, Campylobacter* and also *Clostridium botulinum*, the causal organism of botulism. Food poisoning may be fatal, the old and the young being especially at risk.

foot the part of the lower limb below the ankle made up of eleven small bones and having a structure similar to that of the hand. The *talus*, which

articulates with the leg bones and the *calcaneus*, which forms the heel, are the largest of these.

foramen a hole or opening which usually refers to those which occur in some bones. For example, the *foramen magnum* is a large hole at the base of the skull (in the *occipital bone*) through which the spinal cord passes out from the brain.

forceps surgical instruments, of which there are many different types, which are used as pincers.

foreskin the PREPUCE, which is a fold of skin growing over the end (glans) of the penis.

fossa a natural hollow or depression on the surface or within the body. Examples include the fossae within the skull, which house different parts of the brain, and the cubital fossa, a hollow at the front of the elbow joint.

fovea any small depression, often referring to the one which occurs in the RETINA of the EYE in which a large number of the light-sensitive cells called CONES are situated. It is the site of greatest visual acuity, being the region in which the image is focused when the eyes are fixed on an object.

fracture any break in a bone, which may be complete or incomplete. In a *simple fracture* (or *closed fracture*) the skin remains more or less intact but in a *compound fracture* (or *open fracture*) there is an open wound connecting the bone with the surface. This type of fracture is more serious as it provides a greater risk of infection and more blood loss. If a bone which is already diseased suffers a fracture (such as often occurs in older women who have OSTEOPOROSIS), this is known as a *pathological fracture*. A *fatigue fracture* occurs in a bone which suffers recurrent, persistent stress, e.g. the *March fracture* sometimes seen in the second toe of soldiers after long marches.

A GREENSTICK FRACTURE only occurs in young children whose bones are still soft and tend to bend. The fracture occurs on the opposite side from the causal force. A *complicated fracture* involves damage to surrounding soft tissue including nerves and blood vessels. A *depressed fracture* refers only to the skull when a piece of bone is forced inwards and may damage the brain. *See also* COMMINUTED FRACTURE.

freckles small, brown spots occurring on the skin, especially in people with red hair or with a fair complexion. They often occur after exposure to the sun as a result of an increased production of the skin pigment, melanin.

Freudian treatment involves helping a person to recover and talk about buried memories os sexual trauma. *See* FREUD'S THEORY.

Freud's theory a theory devised by Sigmund Freud (1856-1939) which states that psychological disorders result from previous trauma of a sexual nature, which the person did not come to terms with adequately at the time and the memory of which has been repressed.

Friedreich's ataxia an inherited disorder caused by degeneration of nerve cells in the brain and spinal cord. It appears in children, usually in adolescence, and the symptoms include unsteadiness during walking and a loss of the knee-jerk reflex, leading progressively to tremors, speech impairment and curvature of the spine. The symptoms are increasingly disabling and may be accompanied by heart disease. *See also* ATAXIA.

frontal lobe the anterior part of the *cerebral hemisphere* of the CEREBRUM of the brain, extending back to a region called the central sulcus, which is a deep cleft on the upper, outer surface.

frostbite damage to the skin and underlying tissues caused by extreme cold and especially affecting the 'extremities', i.e. fingers, toes, nose and cheeks. The affected parts become white and numb and may develop blisters. The skin hardens and gradually turns black, and if the frostbite is fairly superficial, this eventually peels off exposing tender red skin underneath. However, in severe cases, deeper layers of tissue become frozen and are destroyed and amputation may be necessary, especially where infection has set in. *See* GANGRENE.

frozen shoulder painful stiffness of the shoulder joint, which limits movement and is more common in older people between the ages of 50 and 70. It may result from injury but often there is no apparent cause. Treatment involves exercises and sometimes injections of corticosteroid drugs, and usually there is a gradual recovery.

fumigation the use of vapours from strong chemicals to bring about disinfection or disinfestation of clothing, rooms or buildings.

fundus the enlarged base of an organ farthest away from its opening, or a point in the RETINA of the EYE opposite the pupil.

fungal diseases diseases or infections caused by fungi.

G

gait the way in which a person walks, including speed, rhythm, etc.

galactorrhoea flow of milk from the breast, not associated with childbirth or nursing. It may be a symptom of a tumour in the pituitary gland.

gall another term for BILE.

gall bladder a sac-like organ situated on the underside of the liver which stores and concentrates BILE. It is approximately 8cm long and 2.5cm at its widest and its volume is a little over 30cm³. When fats are digested, the gall bladder contracts, sending bile into the DUODENUM through the common bile duct. GALLSTONES, the most common gall bladder disease, may form in certain circumstances.

gallstones stones of varying composition, that form in the GALL BLADDER. Their formation seems to be due to a change in bile composition rendering cholesterol less soluble. Stones may also form around a foreign body. There are three types of stone: cholesterol, pigment and mixed, the latter being the most common. Calcium salts are usually found in varying proportions. Although gallstones may be present for years without symptoms, they can cause severe pain and may pass into the common bile duct to cause, by the resulting obstruction, jaundice.

gamete a mature germ or sexual cell, male or female, that can participate in fertilization e.g. OVUM and SPERMATOZOON.

gamma globulin (or immune gamma globulin) a concentrated form of the antibody part of human blood, used for immunization against certain infectious diseases e.g. measles, poliomyelitis, hepatitis A, etc. It is of no use when the disease is diagnosed but can prevent or modify it if given before.

ganglion (plural ganglia) 1. a mass of nervous tissue containing nerve cells and SYNAPSES. Chains of ganglia are situated on each side of the spinal cord while others are sited near to or in the appropriate organs. Within the central nervous system some well-defined masses of nerve cells are called ganglia e.g. basal ganglia (see BASAL GANGLION).

2. a benign swelling that often forms in the sheath of a tendon and is fluid-filled. It occurs particularly at the wrist, and may disappear quite suddenly.

gangrene death of tissue due to loss of blood supply or bacterial infection. There are two types of gangrene, dry and moist. Dry gangrene is caused purely by loss of blood supply and is a late stage complication of DIABETES MELLITUS in which ATHEROSCLEROSIS is present. The affected part becomes cold and turns brown and black and there is an obvious line between living and dead tissue. In time the gangrenous part drops off.

Moist gangrene is the more common type and is due to bacterial infection which leads to putrefaction and issuing of fluids from the tissue, accompanied by an obnoxious smell. The patient may suffer from fever and ultimately die of blood poisoning. See also GAS GANGRENE.

gas gangrene a form of GANGRENE that occurs when wounds are infected with soil bacteria of the genus Clostridium. The bacterium produces toxins that cause decay and putrefaction with the generation of gas. The gas spreads into muscles and connective tissue, causing swelling, pain, fever and possibly toxic delirium, and if untreated the condition quickly leads to death. Some of these bacteria are anaerobic (exist without air or oxygen), hence surgery, oxidizing agents and penicillin can all be used in treatment.

gastralgia term meaning pain in the stomach.

gastrectomy the surgical removal of, usually, part of the stomach. This may be performed for stomach cancer, severe peptic ulcers or to stop haemorrhaging.

gastric anything relating to the stomach.

gastric glands glands that are situated in the MUCOUS MEMBRANE of the stomach and secrete GASTRIC JUICE. The glands are the cardiac, pyloric and fundic.

gastric juice the secretion from the GASTRIC GLANDS in the stomach. The main constituents are hydrochloric acid, rennin, mucin and pepsinogen, the latter forming pepsin in the acid conditions.

The acidity (which is around pH 1 to 1.5) also destroys unwanted bacteria.

gastric ulcer an erosion of the stomach MUCOSA caused by such agents as acid and bile. It may penetrate the muscle and perforate the stomach wall (*see* PERFORATION). Typical symptoms include burning pain, belching and possibly nausea when the stomach is empty or soon after eating. Relief may be found with antacid compounds, but surgery may be necessary.

gastritis inflammation of the stomach lining (MUCOSA). It may be due to bacteria or excessive alcohol intake.

gastroenteritis inflammation of both the stomach and intestines, leading to vomiting and diarrhoea. It is most commonly due to viral or bacterial infection and fluid loss can be serious in children.

gastroenterology the study of diseases that affect the gastrointestinal tract, including the pancreas, gall bladder and bile duct, in addition to the stomach and intestines.

gastroenterostomy an operation undertaken to reroute food from the stomach to enable an obstruction to be relieved. It consists of making an opening in the stomach and the nearby small intestine and joining the two together. It is often performed with a gastrectomy.

gastroscope a flexible instrument comprising fibreoptics or a miniature video camera that permits internal visual examination of the stomach. It is possible to see all areas of the stomach and take specimens using special tools. The tube is introduced via the mouth and oesophagus.

gastrostomy the creation, usually by surgery, of an opening into the stomach from the outside. This permits food to be given to a patient who cannot swallow due to oesophageal cancer, post-oesophageal surgery or who may be unconscious for a long time.

gauze a material with open weave that is used for bandages and dressings.

gavage forced feeding. Adopted when a patient is too weak to feed himself or herself or when an insane person refuses food. A stomach tube or naso-gastric tube is used.

gene the fundamental unit of genetic material found at a specific location on a CHROMOSOME. It is chemically complex and responsible for the transmission of information between older and younger generations. Each gene contributes to a particular trait or characteristic. There are more than 100,000 genes in man and gene size varies with the characteristic e.g. the gene that codes for the hormone INSULIN is 1700 BASE PAIRS long.

There are several types of gene, depending upon their function and in addition genes are said to be dominant or recessive. A dominant characteristic is one that occurs whenever the gene is present while the effect of a recessive gene (say a disease) requires that the gene be on both members of the chromosome pair i.e. it must be HOMOZYGOUS. *See also* SEX-LINKED DISORDERS.

genetic code specific information carried by DNA molecules that controls the particular AMINO ACIDS and their positions in every protein and thus all the proteins synthesized within a cell. Because there are just four nucleotides a unit of three bases becomes the smallest unit that can produce codes for all 20 amino acids. The transfer of information from gene to protein is based upon three consecutive nucleotides called *codons*. A change in the genetic code results in an amino acid being inserted incorrectly in a protein, resulting in a mutation.

genetic counselling the provision of advice to families about the nature and likelihood of inherited disorders and the options available in terms of prevention and management. With modern techniques of antenatal diagnosis it is possible to determine at an early stage of a pregnancy whether a child will be abnormal.

genetic engineering (*or* **recombinant DNA technology**) the artificial modification of an organism's genetic make-up. More specifically, for example, the insertion of GENES from a human cell which are inserted into a bacterium where they perform their usual function. Thus it is possible to produce, on a commercial scale, hormones such as INSULIN and GROWTH HORMONE by utilizing a bacterium with a human gene. The organism often used is *Escherichia coli*. The process has other applications, including production of monoclonal antibodies.

genetic fingerprinting the technique that utilizes an individual's DNA to identify that person. DNA can be extracted from body tissues and used in settling issues of a child's maternity or paternity. In forensic medicine samples of blood, etc., at the scene of a crime are taken to match a suspect to the criminal.

genetics the study of heredity and variation in individuals and the means whereby characteristics are passed from parent to offspring. The classical aspects of the subject were expounded by Mendel, an Austrian monk, in the early 19th century. Now there are several subdisciplines, including population genetics and molecular genetics.

genetic screening the procedure whereby

individuals are tested to determine whether their gene make-up suggests they carry a particular disease or condition. If it is shown that someone carries a genetically linked disease then decisions can be taken regarding future children. *See also* SEX-LINKED DISORDERS.

genital the term describing anything relating to reproduction or the reproductive organs.

genitalia the male or female reproductive organs, often referring to the external parts only.

genito-urinary medicine the subdiscipline concerned with all aspects of sexually transmitted diseases.

genito-urinary tract (**urogenital** in US) the genital and urinary organs and associated structures: kidneys, ureter, bladder, urethra and genitalia.

geriatrics the subdiscipline of medicine that deals with all aspects of diseases and conditions that affected the aged.

German measles (*or* **rubella**) a highly infectious viral disease occurring mainly in childhood, which is mild in effect. Spread occurs through close contact with infected individuals and there is an incubation period of two to three weeks. The symptoms include headache, shivering and sore throat, with a slight fever. There is some swelling of the neck and soon after the onset a rash of pink spots appears, initially on the face and/or neck, and subsequently spreading over the body. The rash disappears in roughly one week but the condition remains infectious for three or four more days.

    Immunity is usually conferred by the infection and although it is a mild disease it is important because an attack during the early stages of pregnancy may cause foetal abnormalities. Girls are therefore immunized around the age of 12 or 13.

germs microorganisms. The term is used particularly for microorganisms that are PATHOGENIC.

gestation the length of time from fertilization of the ovum to birth. *See also* PREGNANCY.

giardiasis the disease caused by the parasite *Giardia lamblia* which inhabits the small intestine. Although usually harmless, it may cause diarrhoea. It is contracted from untreated drinking water but is readily treated with medication.

giddiness *see* **vertigo.**

gingivitis inflammation of the gums.

gland an organ or group of cells that secretes a specific substance or substances. ENDOCRINE GLANDS secrete directly into the blood while *exocrine* glands secrete onto an epithelial surface

via a duct. Some glands produce fluids, e.g. milk from the mammary glands and saliva from the sublingual gland. The THYROID gland is an endocrine gland releasing hormones into the bloodstream. A further system of glands, the lymphatic glands, occur throughout the body in association with the lymphatic vessels. *See* LYMPH.

glandular fever (*or* **infectious mononucleosis**) an infectious viral disease caused by the Epstein Barr virus. It produces a sore throat and swelling in neck lymph nodes (also those in the armpits and groin). Other symptoms include headache, fever and a loss of appetite. The liver may be affected and the SPLEEN may become enlarged or even ruptured, which requires surgery. The disease is diagnosed by the large number of MONOCYTES in the blood and although complications tend to be rare, total recovery may take many weeks.

glaucoma a condition which results in loss of vision due to high pressure in the EYE, although there is usually no associated disease of the eye. There are several types of glaucoma which occur at differing rates but all are characterized by high intra-ocular pressure (due to the outflow of AQUEOUS HUMOUR being restricted) which damages nerve fibres in the RETINA and optic nerve. Treatment involves reduction of the pressure with drops and tablets (to reduce production of aqueous humour) and if necessary surgery is undertaken to create another outlet for the aqueous humour.

gleet discharge due to chronic GONORRHOEA.

glia (*or* **neuroglia** *or* **glial cells**) CENTRAL NERVOUS SYSTEM connective tissue composed of a variety of cells. The *macroglia* are divided into astrocytes, which surround brain capillaries, and oligodendrocytes which form MYELIN sheaths. The *microglia* perform a mainly scavenging function. Glial cells are present in ten to fifty times the number of neurons in the nervous system.

globulin a group of globular proteins that occur widely in milk, blood, eggs and plants. There are four types in blood SERUM: a₁, a₂, b, and g. The alpha and beta types are carrier proteins like haemoglobin, and gamma globulins include the IMMUNOGLOBULINS involved in the immune response.

glottis the opening between the VOCAL CORDS. Also used for the part of the LARYNX involved with sound production.

glucagon a hormone important in maintaining the level of the body's blood sugar. It works antagonistically with INSULIN, increasing the supply of blood sugar through the breakdown of

GLYCOGEN to glucose in the liver. Glucagon is produced by the ISLETS OF LANGERHANS when blood sugar level is low.

glue ear (*or* **secretory otitis media**) a form of OTITIS, common in children, which occurs as an inflammation of the middle ear, with the production of a persistent sticky fluid. It can cause deafness and may be associated with enlarged adenoids. In treatment of the condition the adenoids may be removed and GROMMETS inserted.

gluteal the term given to the buttocks or the muscles forming them.

gluteus one of the three muscles of each buttock. The *gluteus maximus* shapes the buttock and extends the thigh, the *gluteus medius* and *minimus* abduct (move the limb away from the body) the thigh while the former also rotates it.

glycogen sometimes called animal starch, is a carbohydrate (polysaccharide) stored mainly in the liver. It acts as an energy store which is liberated upon hydrolysis. *See* GLUCAGON.

glycosuria the presence of sugar (glucose) in the urine which is usually due to DIABETES MELLITUS.

goitre swelling of the neck due to THYROID GLAND enlargement. The thyroid tries to counter the dietary lack of iodine necessary to produce thyroid hormone, by increasing the output, thereby becoming larger. The endemic or simple goitre is due to this cause. Other types are caused by HYPERPLASIA and autoimmune diseases, for example when antibodies are produced against antigens in the thyroid gland.

gold salts (*or* **gold compound**) chemicals containing gold that are used in minute quantities to treat RHEUMATOID ARTHRITIS. They are given by injection into muscles and because side effects may include skin reactions, blood disorders, mouth ulcers and inflammation of the kidneys, very careful control is kept on the dosage.

gonads the reproductive organs that produce the GAMETES and some hormones. In the male and female the gonads are the testes and ovaries respectively.

gonadotrophin (*or* **gonadotrophic hormone**) hormones secreted by the anterior PITUITARY GLAND. Follicle-stimulating hormone (FSH) is produced by males and females, as is luteinizing hormone (LH); interstitial cell-stimulating hormone (ICSH) in males. FSH controls, directly or indirectly, growth of the ova and sperm, while LH/ICSH stimulates reproductive activity in the GONADS.

gonorrhoea the most common VENEREAL DISEASE, which is spread primarily by sexual intercourse but may be contracted through contact with infected discharge on clothing, towels etc. The causative agent is the bacterium *Neisseria gonorrhoeae* and it affects the mucous membrane of the vagina, or in the male, the urethra. Symptoms develop approximately one week after infection and include pain on urinating with a discharge of pus. Inflammation of nearby organs may occur (testicle, prostate in men; uterus, Fallopian tubes and ovaries in women) and prolonged inflammation of the urethra may lead to formation of fibrous tissue causing STRICTURE. Joints may also be affected and later complications include ENDOCARDITIS, arthritis and CONJUNCTIVITIS.

If a baby is born to a woman with the disease, the baby's eyes may become infected, until recently a major cause of blindness (called *ophthalmia neonatorum*). Treatment is usually very effective through the administration of penicillin, sulphonamides or tetracycline.

gout a disorder caused by an imbalance of URIC ACID in the body. Uric acid is normally excreted by the kidneys but sufferers of gout have an excess in their bloodstream, which is deposited in joints as salts (urates) of the acid. This causes inflammation of the affected joints and painful gouty arthritis with destruction of the joints. The kidneys may also be damaged, with formation of stones. Deposits of the salts (called *tophi*) may reach the stage where they prohibit further use of the joints, causing hands and feet to be set in a particular position. Treatment of gout is through drugs that increase the excretion of the urate salts or slow their formation.

Graafian follicle *see* **follicle**.

graft the removal of some tissue or an organ from one person for application to or implantation into the same person or another individual. For example, a skin graft involves taking healthy skin from one area of the body to heal damaged skin, and a kidney (or renal) graft (or transplant) is the removal of the organ from one person (usually a recently dead individual) to another. Numerous types of graft are now feasible, including skin, bone, cornea, cartilage, nerves and blood vessels, and whole organs such as kidney, heart and lung.

Gram's stain a technique described by H. C. J. Gram, the Danish bacteriologist, in 1884, which involves using a stain to differentiate between certain bacteria. Bacteria on a microscope slide are first stained with a violet dye and iodine, then rinsed in ethanol to decolourize and a second red stain added. *Gram-positive* bacteria keep the first stain and appear violet when examined under the microscope, while *Gram-negative* forms lose the first but take up the second stain, thus appearing red. The difference in staining is due to the structure of the bacteria cell walls.

grand mal a convulsive epileptic fit involving involuntary muscular contractions and lack of respiration. The latter produces bluish skin and lips (CYANOSIS) during the *tonic* phase. Convulsive movements follow and often the tongue is bitten and bladder control is lost (the *clonic* phase). Upon awakening the patient has no recall of the event.

granulocyte *see* **leucocyte**.

granulocytosis is when the blood has an abnormally high number of granulocytes. *See* LEUCOCYTE.

Graves' disease a disorder typified by thyroid gland overactivity (*see* HYPERTHYROIDISM), an enlargement of the gland, and protruding eyes. It is due to antibody production and is probably an autoimmune response (*see* AUTOIMMUNE DISEASE). Patients commonly exhibit excess metabolism (because thyroid hormones control the body's metabolism); nervousness, tremor, hyperactivity, rapid heart rate, an intolerance of heat, breathlessness and so on. Treatment may follow one of three courses; drugs to control the thyroid's production of hormones; surgery to remove part of the thyroid; or radioactive iodine therapy.

gravid another term for pregnant.

greenstick fracture a fracture occurring in bones with some flexibility (and therefore in children) where the bone is not broken right across but just on the outer arc of the bend.

grey matter a part of the CENTRAL NERVOUS SYSTEM comprising the central part of the spinal cord and the cerebral cortex and outer layer of the cerebellum in the brain. It is brown-grey in colour and is the coordination point between the nerves of the central nervous system. It is composed of nerve cell bodies, DENDRITES, SYNAPSES, glial cells (supporting cells, *see* GLIA) and blood vessels.

groin the area where the abdomen joins the thighs.

grommet a small tube with a lip at either end that is inserted into the eardrum to permit fluid to drain from the middle ear. It is used in the treatment of secretory otitis media (GLUE EAR).

growing pains pains similar to rheumatism that occur in the joints and muscles of children. They are usually insignificant and may be due to fatigue or bad posture but must be dealt with in case the cause is more serious e.g. bone disease, or rheumatic fever.

growth hormone (*or* **somatotrophin** *or* **FH**) a HORMONE produced and stored by the anterior PITUITARY GLAND that controls protein synthesis in muscles and the growth of long bones in legs and arms. Low levels result in DWARFISM in children and overproduction produces gigantism.

Guillain-Barré syndrome a condition of the nervous system whereby the myelin sheath that surrounds the nerve fibres is destroyed, resulting in the rapid onset of muscle weakness and paralysis. It is thought that this may be a disorder of the immune system that can develop from a mild infection.

gullet another term for the OESOPHAGUS.

gynaecology the subdiscipline of medicine that deals with diseases of women, particularly concerning sexual and reproduction function and diseases of reproductive organs.

gynaecomastia the abnormal enlargement of breasts in men which may be due to drugs, hormone imbalance or testicular or pituitary cancer.

H

haem a compound containing iron, composed of a pigment which is known as a *porphyrin,* which confers colour. It combines with a protein called globin in the blood to form HAEMOGLOBIN. The prefix *haem* also indicates anything relating to blood.

haemangioma a benign tumour of the blood vessels. It may be visible on the skin as a type of NAEVUS (birthmark) e.g. a *strawberry haemangioma.*

haemarthrosis bleeding into a joint which causes swelling and pain and may be the result of injury or disease. It can be a symptom of HAEMOPHILIA.

haematemesis vomiting of blood which may occur for a number of different reasons. Common causes are ulcers, either gastric or duodenal, or gastritis, especially when this is caused by irritants or poisons such as alcohol. Also blood may be swallowed and subsequently vomited as a result of a nosebleed.

haematinic a substance which increases the amount of haemoglobin in the blood e.g. ferrous sulphate. Haematinic drugs are often prescribed during pregnancy.

haematocoele leakage of blood into a cavity causing a swelling. A haematocoele usually forms as a result of an injury due to the rupture of blood vessels and the leaking of blood into a natural body cavity.

haematology the scientific study of blood and its diseases.

haematoma a collection of blood forming a firm swelling — a bruise. It may occur as a result of injury or a clotting disorder of the blood, or if blood vessels are diseased.

haematuria the presence of blood in the urine which may have come from the kidneys, ureter, bladder or urethra. It indicates the presence of inflammation or disease such as a stone in the bladder or kidney.

haemodialysis the use of an *artificial kidney* to remove waste products from a person's blood using the principle of DIALYSIS. It is carried out when a person's kidneys have ceased to function and involves passing blood from an artery into the dialyser on one side of a semi-permeable membrane. On the other side of the membrane, a solution of electrolytes of similar composition to the blood is circulated. Water and waste products pass through the membrane into this solution while cells and proteins are retained within the blood. The purified blood is then returned to the patient's body through a vein.

haemoglobin the respiratory substance contained within the red blood cells, which contains a pigment responsible for the red colour of blood. It consists of the pigment HAEM and the protein globin and is responsible for the transport of oxygen around the body. Oxygen is picked up in the lungs by arterial blood and transported to the tissues, where it is released. This (venous) blood is then returned to the lungs to repeat the process, *See* OXYHAEMOGLOBIN.

haemoglobinopathy any of a number of inherited diseases in which there is an abnormality in the formation of haemoglobin. Examples are THALASSAEMIA and SICKLE-CELL ANAEMIA.

haemoglobinuria the presence of haemoglobin in the urine caused by disintegration of red blood cells, conferring a dark red or brown colour. It can sometimes result from strenuous exercise or after exposure to cold in some people. It is also caused by the ingestion of poisons such as arsenic, and is a symptom of some infections, particularly *blackwater fever*, a severe and sometimes fatal form of MALARIA.

haemolysis the destruction (lysis) of red blood cells which may result from infection or poisoning, or as an antibody response.

haemolytic disease of the newborn a serious disease affecting foetuses and newborn babies which is characterized by HAEMOLYSIS leading to anaemia and severe jaundice. In severe cases the foetus may die due to heart failure and OEDEMA (termed *hydrops foetalis*). The usual cause is incompatibility between the blood of the mother and that of the foetus. Generally the foetus has Rh-positive red blood cells (i.e. they contain the rhesus factor) while that of the mother is Rh-negative. The mother produces antibodies to the Rh factor present in the foetal blood and these are passed to the foetus in the placental circulation. This then produces the haemolysis of the foetal red blood cells.

The incidence of the disease has been greatly reduced by giving a Rh-negative mother an injection of anti-D immunoglobulin, following the birth of a Rh-positive baby. This prevents the formation of the antibodies which would harm a subsequent baby and is also given to Rh-negative women following miscarriages or abortions.

haemophilia a hereditary disorder of blood coagulation in which the blood clots very slowly. It is a sex-linked recessive condition carried on the X chromosome and hence it affects males, with females being the carriers. There are two types of haemophilia due to a deficiency of either one of two COAGULATION FACTORS in the blood. Haemophilia A is caused by deficiency of factor VIII and haemophilia B by deficiency of factor IX, called *Christmas factor*. The severity of the disease depends upon how much less of the coagulation factor than normal is present in the blood. The symptoms of haemophilia are prolonged bleeding from wounds and bleeding into joints, muscles and other tissues. In the past, the outlook for haemophiliacs was poor with few surviving into adult life. However, now the condition can be treated by injections or transfusions of plasma containing the missing coagulation factor and, with care, a sufferer can hope to lead a much more normal life. *See* SEX-LINKED DISORDERS.

haemopoiesis formation of blood cells (particularly *erythrocytes*, the red blood cells) and platelets, which takes place in the bone marrow in adults but in a foetus it occurs in the liver and spleen.

haemorrhage bleeding — a flow of blood from a ruptured blood vessel which may occur externally or internally. A haemorrhage is classified according to the type of vessels involved: *Arterial H* — bright red blood spurts in pulses from an artery. *Venous H* — a darker-coloured steady flow from a vein. *Capillary L* — blood oozes from torn capillaries at the surface of a wound. In addition, a haemorrhage may be *primary*, i.e. it occurs at the moment of injury. It is classed as *reactionary* when it occurs within 24 hours of an injury and results from a rise in blood pressure. Thirdly, a *secondary haemorrhage* occurs after a week or ten days as a result of infection (sepsis). Haemorrhage from a major artery is the most serious kind, as

large quantities of blood are quickly lost and death can occur within minutes. Haemorrhages at specific sites within the body are designated by special names e.g. *haematuria* (from the kidney or urinary tract), *haemoptysis* (from the lungs) and *haematemesis* (from the stomach).

haemorrhoids (*or* **piles**) varicose and inflamed veins around the lower end of the bowel situated in the wall of the anus. They are classified as internal, external or mixed, depending upon whether they appear beyond the anus. They are commonly caused by constipation or diarrhoea, especially in middle and older age, and may be exacerbated by a sedentary lifestyle. They may also occur as a result of childbearing. The symptoms of haemorrhoids are bleeding and pain, and treatment is by means of creams, injections and suppositories. Attention to diet (to treat constipation) and regular exercise are important, but in severe cases, surgery to remove the haemorrhoids may be necessary.

haemostasis the natural process to arrest bleeding, involving blood coagulation and contraction of a ruptured blood vessel. The term is also applied to a number of surgical procedures designed to arrest bleeding such as the use of ligatures and DIATHERMY. A haemostatic substance stops or prevents haemorrhage e.g. phytomenadone.

haemothorax a leakage of blood into the pleural cavity of the chest, usually as a result of injury.

hair a thread-like outgrowth from the epidermis layer of the skin, which is a dead structure consisting of KERATINIZED cells. The part above the skin has three layers, an outer CUTICLE, a CORTEX containing pigment which confers colour, and an inner core. The lower end of the hair (*root*) lies within the skin and is expanded to form the *bulb*, which contains dividing cells that are continuously pushed upwards. This is contained within a tubular structure known as the *hair follicle*. A small *erector pili* muscle attached to the hair follicle in the DERMIS of the skin operates to erect the hair.

halitosis 'bad breath', which may arise for a number of reasons, including the type of food recently eaten, disease of the teeth or infections of the throat, nose or lungs.

hallucination a false perception of something that is not there, which may involve any of the senses of sight, hearing, smell, taste and touch. They may be caused by a psychological illness e.g. SCHIZOPHRENIA or damage to the brain, and also by certain drugs. They can also be a symptom of fever and deprivation, such as lack of sleep.

hallucinogen a substance or drug which causes HALLUCINATIONS e.g. mescaline or lysergic acid diethylamide.

hammer toe a deformity affecting a toe, usually the second, caused by a permanent bending (flexion) of the middle joint. It is usually caused by pressure from footwear and often a painful bunion develops on the surface. If all the toes are affected, the condition is known as a *claw foot*. Protective pads and strapping, corrective footwear and sometimes surgery, are used to alleviate the condition.

hamstring any of four tendons at the back of the knee which are attached to the *hamstring muscles* and anchor these to the TIBIA and FIBULA. The hamstring muscles are responsible for the bending of the knee joint.

hand the extremity of the upper limb below the wrist, which has a highly complex structure and an 'opposable' thumb, which is unique to man. The human hand is highly developed in terms of structure, nervous supply and function and communicates with a large area on the surface of the brain. It is capable of performing numerous functions with a high degree of precision. When there is brain damage and paralysis, the uses of the hand tend to be lost early and more permanently, compared to movements in the leg and face. The skeletal structure of the hand consists of eight small *carpal* bones in the wrist, five *metacarpal* bones in the region of the palm and three *phalanges* in each finger.

haploid the description for a cell nucleus or organism with half the normal number of chromosomes. This is the case with GAMETES and is important at fertilization to ensure the *diploid* chromosome number is restored.

hare lip a congenital developmental deformity which results in the presence of a cleft in the upper lip. It is brought about by a failure in the fusion of three blocks of embryonic tissue and is often associated with a CLEFT PALATE.

Hartmann's solution a solution of salts which is given to replace lost fluid in cases of dehydration, acidosis and after HAEMORRHAGE while awaiting cross-matched blood for transfusion.

Haversian canal one of numerous small channels or cylindrical tubes which run through compact bone (the outer layer of bones) and contain blood vessels and nerves. They form part of the *Haversian system*, consisting of the canals surrounded by concentric, alternate layers of bone *lamellae* and *lacunae* or spaces, which house bone cells. These form cylindrical units in the compact bone and the lacunae are linked up by minute channels called *caniculi*.

hay fever an allergic reaction to pollen, e.g. that of grasses, trees and many other plants, which affects numerous individuals. The symptoms are a blocked and runny nose, sneezing and watering eyes due to the release of histamine. Treatment is by means of antihistamine drugs and, if the allergen can be identified, *desensitization* may be successful. This involves injecting or exposing the individual to controlled and gradually increasing doses of the allergen until antibodies are built up.

headache pain felt within the head which is thought to be caused by dilation of intracranial arteries or pressure upon them. Common causes are stress, tiredness, feverishness accompanying an infection such as a cold, an excess of close work involving the eyes, dyspepsia, rheumatic diseases, high blood pressure and uraemia. Headache may indicate the presence of disease or disorder in the brain e.g. an infection such as MENINGITIS, TUMOUR or ANEURYSM, the result of injury and concussion.

heart the hollow, muscular organ which acts as a pump and is responsible for the circulation of the blood. The heart is cone-shaped with the point downwards and is situated between the lungs and slightly to the left of the midline. The heart projects forwards and lies beneath the fifth rib. The wall consists mainly of CARDIAC MUSCLE lined on the inside by a membrane known as the ENDOCARDIUM. An external membrane known as the PERICARDIUM surrounds the heart. A SEPTUM divides the heart into right and left halves, each of which is further divided into an upper chamber known as an ATRIUM and a lower one called a VENTRICLE. Four valves control the direction of blood flow at each outlet, comprising the aortic, pulmonary, tricuspid and mitral (bicuspid). These valves prevent backflow once the blood has been forced from one chamber into the next. *See* CIRCULATION OF THE BLOOD.

heart attack *see* **cardiac arrest**.

heart block a condition describing a failure in the conduction of electrical impulses from the natural pacemaker (the SINOATRIAL NODE) through the heart, which can lead to slowing of the pumping action.

There are three types: in first degree (partial or incomplete) heart block there is a delay in conduction between atria (*see* ATRIUM) and VENTRICLES but this does not cause slowing. In second degree heart block, there is intermittent slowing because not all the impulses are conducted between atria and ventricles. In third-degree (or complete) heart block there is no electrical conduction, the heartbeats are slow and the ventricles beat at their own intrinsic slow rhythm. This causes blackouts (*see* STOKES-ADAMS SYNDROME) and can lead to heart failure.

Heart block is more common in elderly people where degenerative changes have occurred. However, it may also be CONGENITAL or result from other forms of heart disease such as MYOCARDITIS, CORONARY THROMBOSIS, CARDIOMYOPATHY and VALVE DISEASE. For second- and third-degree heart block, treatment involves the use of an artificial pacemaker.

heartburn a burning pain or discomfort felt in the region of the heart and often rising upwards to the throat. It is caused by regurgitation of the stomach contents, the burning being caused by the acid in gastric juice or by OESOPHAGITIS. It is relieved by taking antacid tablets or alkaline substances such as sodium bicarbonate.

heat exhaustion exhaustion and collapse due to overheating of the body and loss of fluid following unaccustomed or prolonged exposure to excessive heat. It is more common in hot climates and results from excessive sweating leading to loss of fluids and salts and disturbance of the electrolyte balance in body fluids. In the mildest form, which is *heat collapse*, blood pressure and pulse rate fall, accompanied by fatigue and light-headedness, and there may be muscular cramps. Treatment involves taking drinks of salt solution, or these may be given intravenously and avoidance by gradual acclimatization to the heat, especially if hard physical work is to be carried out.

heatstroke (*or* **heat hyperpyrexia**) a severe condition following exposure of the body to excessive heat, characterized by a rise in temperature and failure of sweating and temperature regulation. There is a loss of consciousness, followed by coma and death, which can occur rapidly. The body must be cooled by sponging and salt solutions given either by mouth or intravenously.

heel the part of the foot behind the ankle joint formed by the *calcaneus* or heel bone.

Heimlich's manoeuvre a procedure to dislodge a foreign body which is blocking the larynx, causing CHOKING. The person carrying out the procedure encircles the patient from behind with his or her arms. A fist is made with one hand slightly above the patient's navel and below the ribs. With the free hand, the fist is thrust firmly into the abdomen with a rapid upward push which may need to be repeated several times. As a result of this, the foreign particle is expelled through or into the patient's mouth.

Henle's loop *see* **kidney**.

heparin an anticoagulant substance naturally present in the body, produced by liver and some white blood cells and in some other sites. It acts by inhibiting and neutralizing the action of the enzyme thrombin (*see* BLOOD COAGULATION) and is a polysaccharide (carbohydrate) containing sulphur and amino groups. It is used medically to prevent blood coagulation in patients with thrombosis and also in blood collected for sampling.

hepatectomy surgical removal of the whole or part of the liver.

hepatic vein one of the veins which drains blood from the liver leading to the inferior vena cava.

hepatitis inflammation of the liver due to the presence of toxic substances or infection caused by viruses. *Acute hepatitis* produces abdominal pain, jaundice, itching, nausea and fever. *Chronic hepatitis* has a similar range of symptoms which may persist for years and lead eventually to CIRRHOSIS. Alcohol abuse is a common cause of hepatitis, which may also result as a side effect from a number of drug treatments or from overdose. Many virus infections can cause hepatitis, such as HIV and GLANDULAR FEVER.

However, the so-called hepatic viruses are designated A, B, C, D, and E. Hepatitis A causes *infectious hepatitis* (epidemic hepatitis). It is transmitted by eating food contaminated by a person who has the virus, and is common in conditions of poor hygiene and sanitation. Hepatitis E acts in a similar way and both produce symptoms of fever, sickness and jaundice. Recovery is usually complete unless the symptoms are acute, and immunity from a future attack is conferred. *Serum hepatitis* is caused by viruses B, C and D, the route of infection being blood or blood products. Serum hepatitis is most common where infected needles have been used among drug addicts. The infection may also be passed on by tattooing needles and also through sexual intercourse with an infected individual. The mortality rate is 5-20%, but many patients make a gradual recovery from the illness, which is characterized by fever, chills, fatigue, headaches and jaundice. All these viruses may persist in the blood for a long time and if B is involved, the condition is known as *chronic type-B hepatitis*. Cancer (hepatocellular carcinoma) is common in populations where the B virus is prevalent. Various drugs are used to combat viral hepatitis, including interferon.

hepatoma a malignant tumour of the liver which is rare in Western countries except among those with CIRRHOSIS. It is common in parts of the Far East and Africa and a suspected cause is the *aflatoxin* or poison produced by a fungus which contaminates stored peanuts and cereals. The cancer often produces alpha fetoprotein, which is detectable in the blood and is an indicator of the presence of the malignancy.

heredity the principle applied to the passing on of all bodily characteristic, from parents to offspring. *See* GENETICS.

hermaphrodite an individual possessing both male and female sex organs or in whom ovarian and testicular cells are present in the gonads (*ovotestis*). This condition is extremely rare and the individual is usually sterile with reduced SECONDARY SEXUAL CHARACTERISTICS.

hernia the protrusion of a part or whole of an organ from out of its normal position within the body cavity. Most commonly, a hernia involves part of the bowel. A *congenital hernia* is present at birth, a common one being an *umbilical hernia* in which abdominal organs protrude into the umbilical cord. This is due to a failure during foetal development and can be corrected by surgery. An *acquired hernia* occurs after birth, a common example being an *inguinal hernia* in which part of the bowel bulges through a weak part of the abdominal wall (known as the inguinal canal). Another common type is a *hiatus hernia*, in which the stomach passes through the hiatus (a hole allowing passage of the oesophagus) from the abdomen into the chest cavity. A *reducible hernia* is freely movable and can be returned by manipulation into its rightful place. An *irreducible hernia* describes the opposite situation and an *incarcerated hernia* is one which has become swollen and fixed in its position. An *obstructed hernia* is one involving the bowel. The contents of the hernia are unable to pass further down and are held up and obstructed.

The most dangerous situation is a *strangulated hernia* in which the blood supply has been cut off due to the protrusion itself. This becomes painful and eventually gangrenous and requires immediate surgery as it is life-threatening. Strenuous physical activity can lead to the production of a hernia which usually develops gradually. Although short-term measures are employed to control a hernia or reduce its size, the usual treatment is by means of surgery to return and retain the protrusion in its proper place. *See* HERNIOPLASTY.

hernioplasty the surgical operation to repair a hernia.

heroin a white crystalline powder, also known as dimorphine hydrochloride, which is derived from morphine. It is a very potent analgesic (painkiller), but is highly addictive and dangerous.

herpes infectious inflammation of the skin and mucous membranes, characterized by the development of small blisters, and caused by a number of different *Herpes* viruses. The *Herpes simplex* virus, types I and II, are the cause of cold sores which usually affect the lips, mouth and face. The virus is usually acquired in childhood and once present persists for life. It can be contracted without causing any symptoms but tends to flare up from time to time producing the cold sores.

Herpes simplex is also the cause of genital herpes, in which the blisters affect the genital region. *Herpes zoster,* or shingles, is produced by a virus which causes chicken pox in children. The virus affects the course of a nerve, producing severe pain and small yellowish blisters on the skin. Often the affected areas are the abdomen, back, face and chest and although the disease subsides after about three weeks, the blisters form scabs which eventually drop off and the pain can persist for months. This is known as *post-herpetic neuralgia* and pain-relieving drugs are needed to help relieve the condition. Other herpes viruses are the CYTOMEGALOVIRUS and EPSTEIN BARR virus.

heterosexual describes sexual behaviour between individuals of opposite sexes.

heterozygous the situation in which each member (ALLELE) of a pair of genes determining a certain characteristic is dissimilar. Usually one is dominant and this is the form exhibited in the individual's body, but either type can be passed on in the gametes (sex cells). *Compare* HOMOZYGOUS.

hexachlorophane an antiseptic, disinfectant substance similar to phenol, the use of which is now limited in soaps and creams as it may produce toxic effects when absorbed through the skin.

hiatus hernia *see* **hernia.**

hindbrain the part of the brain which consists of the MEDULLA OBLONGATA, PONS and CEREBELLUM.

hip the region on either side of the body where the FEMUR (thigh bone) articulates with the PELVIS.

hip joint a ball-and-socket joint made up of the

head of the FEMUR, which rests inside a deep, cup-shaped cavity (the acetabulum) in the hip bone. The hip bone (or innominate bone) is itself made up of three fused bones, the PUBIS, ISCHIUM and ILIUM, which form part of the PELVIS.

hirsutism the growth of dark, coarse hair on the body of a female, on the face, chest, abdomen and upper back. This is either due to a greater sensitivity of hair follicles to a normal level of male hormones (androgens) producing hair of a more masculine type, or, there may be an excessive production of androgens responsible for the growth of the hair. The condition may be the result of an underlying disorder such as an ADRENAL tumour but there is a wide normal variation in the amount of body hair present in individuals and between females of different races.

histamine a substance derived from histidine, which is an amino acid. It is widely found throughout all the body tissues and is responsible for the dilation of blood vessels (arterioles and capillaries) and the contraction of smooth muscle, including that of the bronchi of the lungs. Histamine is released in great quantities in allergic conditions and ANAPHYLAXIS. *See also* ALLERGY.

histology the scientific study of tissues, involving such techniques as light and electron microscopy and the use of dyes and stains.

HIV the human immunodeficiency virus, responsible for the condition known as AIDS. The virus affects and destroys a group of lymphocytes (T-lymphocytes) which are part of the body's natural defences (the IMMUNE SYSTEM).

hives a common name for **urticaria** (or nettle rash).

HLA antigens these are the human leucocyte antigens. There are four genes responsible for their production (A, B, C, D), which are located on chromosome six which make up the HLA system. One GENE or set of genes is inherited from each parent and produce, the HLA antigens on the surfaces of cells throughout the body. These antigens are the means by which the IMMUNE SYSTEM recognizes 'self' and rejects 'non-self' and this is very important in organ transplantation. The closer the match of HLAs between donor and recipient, the greater the chances of success. If two individual share identical HLA types, they are described as being *histocompatible.*

Hodgkin's disease a malignant disease of unknown cause affecting the lymphatic system, in which there is a gradual and increasing enlargement of lymph glands and nodes throughout the body. The accompanying symptoms include loss of weight, sweating, anaemia and a characteristic type of fever (known as Pel-Ebstein fever). The person becomes gradually weaker and the glands may attain a very large size. The outlook is good, especially if the disease is detected early, and treatment is by means of surgery, radiotherapy and chemotherapy (with a combination of drugs), one or more of these being employed.

holistic relating to 'wholeness'. A holistic approach to patient care does not just concentrate on the physical disease or condition but takes note of all the factors in that person's life.

homeopathy a system of medicine devised by Samuel Hahnemann (1755–1843), which is part of ALTERNATIVE MEDICINE in the UK. It is based on the premise that 'like cures like' and so a patient is given minute quantities of compounds that can, in themselves, produce symptoms of the disease or malady being treated.

homosexual describes sexual behaviour between individuals of the same sex. The adjective is usually now applied to males, lesbian being the corresponding term for females.

homozygous the situation in which each member (ALLELE) of a pair of genes determining a certain characteristic is the same. Hence only one form of the GENE can be passed on in the gametes (sex cells) to the offspring. Genes which are normally recessive can be expressed in the body of a person who is homozygous for that particular characteristic, for example, ALBINISM. *Compare* HETEROZYGOUS.

hormone a naturally produced chemical substance produced by the body, which acts as a messenger. A hormone is produced by cells or glands in one part of the body and passes into the bloodstream. When it reaches another specific site, its 'target organ', it causes a reaction there, modifying the structure or function of cells, perhaps by causing the release of another hormone. Hormones are secreted by the ENDOCRINE GLANDS and examples are the sex hormones, e.g. TESTOSTERONE secreted by the testes, and oestradiol and PROGESTERONE secreted by the ovaries.

housemaid's knee a painful condition resulting from a swelling of the bursa (fluid-filled fibrous sac) in front of the kneecap. It is brought about by too much kneeling.

HRT *see* **menopause**.

human chorionic gonadotrophin a hormone secreted by the PLACENTA during early pregnancy under the influence of which the CORPUS LUTEUM of the OVARY produces OESTROGEN, PROGESTERONE and relaxin. These are essential for the maintenance of pregnancy. Pregnancy can be detected early on by a laboratory procedure which tests for the presence of human chorionic gonadotrophin in the urine.

human leucocyte antigen *see* **HLA antigens.**

human T-cell lymphocytotrophic virus (*or* **HTLV**) a group of viruses including the AIDS (HIV) virus, which is HTLV III. These viruses are responsible for LYMPHOMAS.

humerus the bone of the upper arm which articulates with the shoulder blade (SCAPULA) of the PECTORAL GIRDLE and the ULNA and RADIUS at the elbow.

humour a natural fluid in the body, the best-known examples being the aqueous and vitreous humours of the EYE.

Huntington's chorea *see* **chorea.**

hydrocephalus an abnormal collection of cerebrospinal fluid within the skull which causes, in babies and children, a great increase in the size of the head. Hydrocephalus results either from an excessive production of fluid or from a defect in the mechanism for its reabsorption, or from a blockage in its circulation. The cause may be CONGENITAL, and it often accompanies SPINA BIFIDA in babies, or infection (meningitis) or the presence of a TUMOUR. Hydrocephalus causes pressure on the brain, with drowsiness, irritability and mental subnormality in children. Treatment involves surgery to redirect the fluid but is not always successful. About 50% of children survive if the progress of the condition is halted and one third of these go on to enjoy a normal life with little or no physical or mental impairment.

hydrocortisone a STEROID glucocorticoid hormone, produced and released by the cortex of the ADRENAL GLANDS (a CORTICOSTEROID). It is closely related to cortisone, being released in response to stress and playing a significant part in carbohydrate metabolism. Medically it has a number of uses, especially in the treatment of ADDISON'S DISEASE and inflammatory, allergic and rheumatic conditions e.g. eczema and rheumatoid arthritis. Hydrocortisone is contained in ointments in creams or given by mouth or injection, depending upon the condition under treatment. Prolonged use may cause side effects including peptic ulcers, stunting of growth in children, CUSHING'S SYNDROME and damage to bone and muscle tissue.

hydroxocobalamin this is a cobalt-containing (cobalamin) substance used in the treatment of

vitamin B$_{12}$ deficiencies, such as pernicious ANAEMIA.

hymen a thin membrane that covers the lower end of the VAGINA at birth, which usually tears to some extent before a girl reaches puberty.

hyperadrenalism a condition in which the adrenal glands are overactive, producing the symptoms of CUSHING'S SYNDROME.

hyperalgesia an extreme sensitivity to pain.

hypercalcaemia a high blood calcium level often associated with bone tumours such as hyper-parathyroidism (*see* PARATHYROID) and OSTEOPOROSIS. Symptoms include anorexia, muscle pain and weakness.

hyperglycaemia the presence of excess sugar (glucose) in the blood, as in DIABETES MELLITUS, caused by insufficient INSULIN to cope with carbohydrate intake. The condition can lead to a diabetic coma.

hyperkalaemia a high blood potassium level often seen with kidney failure of which the signs are diarrhoea, nausea and muscle weakness.

hyperlipidaemia (*or* **hyperlipaemia**) the presence of an excess concentration of fat in the blood. An excess of CHOLESTEROL in the blood may lead to CORONARY ARTERY DISEASE and ATHEROMA. An excess of triglycerides may lead to pancreatitis.

hyperplasia increased growth in size and number of the normal cells of a tissue so that the affected part enlarges e.g. the breasts during pregnancy. *Compare* HYPERTROPHY and NEOPLASM.

hypersensitivity abnormal allergic response to an ANTIGEN to which the person has previously been exposed. Hypersensitive responses vary from quite mild such as hay fever to very severe and life-threatening e.g. ANAPHYLACTIC SHOCK. *See also* ALLERGY.

hypertension high blood pressure (in the arteries). *Essential* hypertension may be due to an unknown cause, or kidney disease or endocrine diseases. *Malignant* hypertension will prove fatal if not treated. It may be a condition itself or an end stage of essential hypertension. It tends to occur in a younger age group and there is high diastolic blood pressure (*see* DIASTOLE) and kidney failure. Previously a rapidly fatal condition, antihypertensive drugs have revolutionized treatment and given sufferers a near-normal life.

hyperthermia extremely high and abnormal body temperature, i.e. a fever. Also, a method of treatment of certain diseases by artificially inducing a state of fever, achieved by a variety of techniques.

hyperthyroidism excessive activity of the thyroid

gland — an overactive thyroid. It may be caused by increased growth of the gland, by the presence of a tumour, or due to GRAVES DISEASE.

hypertrophy increase in size of an organ due to enlargement of its cells (rather than in their number) often in response to a greater demand for work. An example is the increase in size of the remaining kidney if the other is removed for some reason. *Compare* HYPERPLASIA.

hyperventilation breathing at an abnormally rapid rate when at rest, which may be a response to stress and, if not checked, results in unconsciousness because the concentration of carbon dioxide in the blood falls. If the carbon dioxide level in the blood is abnormally high, due to impaired gas exchange in the lungs, e.g. in such cconditions as pulmonary OEDEMA and pneumonia, hyperventilation may occur. *See also* HYPOVENTILATION.

hypnosis a state of altered attention resembling sleep in which the mind is more receptive to recall of memories of past events and to suggestion. The person who induces this state in another is known as a *hypnotist*. One of the ways of inducing hypnosis is to ask the patient to fix his or her eyes on a given point or source of light and then rhythmically repeat soothing words in a low voice. Some people appear to be more easily *hypnotized* than others and there are three merging levels of hypnosis, *light, medium* and *deep*. Hypnosis is a useful form of treatment in psychiatry and also in pain relief e.g. during labour and dental repair. It is also used in the treatment of asthma and alcoholism.

hypnotics substances or drugs that induce sleep e.g. BARBITURATES and *chloral hydrate*.

hypocalcaemia a low blood calcium level possibly resulting from kidney failure, pancreatitis, vitamin D deficiency or hypoparathyroidism, and producing heart ARRHYTHMIAS, TETANY and reduction of the sense of touch (lips, tongue, feet and hands).

hypochondria an abnormal preoccupation by an individual with the state of his or her health. In its severest form the person wrongly believes that he or she is suffering from a number of illnesses and is extremely anxious and depressed. Treatment is by means of psychotherapy and antidepressant drugs but the condition tends to be difficult to cure.

hypodermic beneath the skin. The term is usually used in reference to injections given by means of a *hypodermic syringe*.

hypoglycaemia a lack of sugar in the blood, which occurs in starvation, and also with DIABETES MELLITUS, when too much insulin has been given and insufficient carbohydrates have been eaten. The symptoms include weakness, sweating, light-headedness and tremors and can lead to coma. The symptoms are alleviated by taking in glucose either by mouth, or injection in the case of hypoglycaemic coma.

hypokalaemia a low blood potassium level producing weakness and abnormal ECG, which may be caused by ADRENAL tumour, starvation, treatment of diabetic acidosis or diabetic therapy.

hypoplasia underdevelopment of a tissue or organ such as can occur in the teeth due to illness or starvation (dental hypoplasia). It is marked by lines of brown enamel across the teeth.

hypothalamus an area of the forebrain in the floor of the third ventricle, having the thalamus above and pituitary gland below. It contains centres controlling vital processes, e.g. fat and carbohydrate metabolism, thirst and water regulation, hunger and eating, thermal regulation and sexual function. It also plays a part in the emotions and in the regulation of sleep. It controls the sympathetic and parasympathetic nervous systems and secretions from the pituitary gland.

hypothermia describes the bodily state when the core temperature falls below 35°C, due to prolonged exposure to cold. At first, shivering occurs and the heart works harder to increase the flow of blood around the body. However, eventually shivering ceases and, with increasing chilling, the function of the body organs becomes disturbed and cardiac output falls. The tissues require less oxygen as their functions start to fail, but eventually the heart is unable to supply even this reduced demand. The symptoms of hypothermia are fatigue and confusion, followed by unconsciousness and death. Elderly people are particularly at risk through inadequate heating in the home.

Occasionally, a state of artificial hypothermia is induced during surgery to reduce the oxygen requirements of the tissues and enable the circulation to be briefly halted.

hypoventilation an abnormally slow rate of shallow breathing, which may result from injury or the effects of drugs on the respiratory centre in the brain. The effect is to increase the amount of carbon dioxide in the blood and lessen that of oxygen. Eventually this leads to death due to a lack of oxygen supply to cells and tissues.

hysterectomy the surgical removal of the womb either by means of an abdominal incision or through the VAGINA. It is commonly carried out if fibroids are present or if the womb is cancerous, and also if there is excessive bleeding.

hysteria a type of neurosis which is difficult to define and in which a range of symptoms may occur. These include paralysis, seizures and spasms of limbs, swelling of joints, mental disorders and amnesia. The person is vulnerable to suggestion. Two types are recognized, *conversion hysteria*, which is characterized by physical symptoms and *dissociative hysteria*, in which marked mental changes occur. *Mass hysteria* affects a group, especially those gathered together under conditions of emotional excitement. A number of people may suffer from giddiness, vomiting and fainting which runs through the whole crowd. Recovery occurs when those affected are separated from the others under calmer conditions. Treatment for hysteria is by means of psychotherapy, especially involving suggestion.

I

ichthyosis a generally hereditary skin condition in which the skin is very dry and looks cracked, producing a resemblance to fish scales. There is particular medication to take but vitamin A may help. The treatment is thus external and involves special baths and the application of ointments.

idiopathic the term given to a disease indicating that its cause is not known.

idiot savant someone who although suffering severe mental retardation is able to perform unusual and often astonishing mental feats or who exhibits remarkable musical ability e.g. feats of memory, complex mental mathematical manipulations or the ability to commit to memory previously unheard music and then play it.

ileectomy removal by surgery of all or part of the ILEUM.

ileitis inflammation of the ILEUM with pain, bowel irregularity and loss of weight. The intestine may become thickened and if the tract becomes blocked, surgery is required immediately. The specific cause is not known but it may occur in association with tuberculosis, bacterial infection (by *Yersinia enterocolitica*), Crohn's disease (chronic inflammation of the bowel) and typhoid.

ileostomy a surgical procedure in which an opening is made in the abdominal wall, to which the ileum is joined. This creates an artificial anus through which the waste contents of the intestines are collected in a special bag. This procedure is undertaken to allow the COLON to heal after surgery or colitis, or in association with other surgery in treating cancer of the rectum.

ileum the lower part of the small intestine between the JEJUNUM and the CAECUM.

ileus an obstruction of the intestine (often the ILEUM) which may be mechanical due to worms or a gallstone from the gall bladder, or it can be due to loss of the natural movement of the intestines (peristalsis). This latter condition may be caused by surgery, injury to the spine or PERITONITIS.

iliac arteries those arteries supplying blood to the lower limbs and pelvic region.

ilium the largest of the bones that form each half of the pelvic girdle. It has a flattened wing-like part fastening to the SACRUM by means of ligaments.

immune the state of being protected against an infection by the presence of antibodies specific to the organism concerned.

immunity the way in which the body resists infection due to the presence of ANTIBODIES and white blood cells. Antibodies are generated in response to the presence of ANTIGENS of a disease. There are several types of immunity: *active immunity* is when the body produces antibodies and continues to be able to do so, during the course of a disease whether occurring naturally (also called *acquired immunity*) or by deliberate stimulation. *Passive immunity* is short-lived and due to the injection of ready-made antibodies from someone who is already immune.

immunization producing immunity to disease by artificial means. Injection of an antiserum will produce temporary passive immunity. Active immunity is produced by making the body generate its own antibodies and this is done by the use of treated antigens (vaccination or INOCULATION). VACCINE is used for immunization and it may be treated live bacteria or viruses or dead organisms or their products.

immunoglobulins a group of high molecular weight proteins that act as ANTIBODIES and are present in the SERUM and secretions. Designated Ig, there are five groups each with different functions identified by a particular letter.

Immunoglobulin A (Ig A) is most common and occurs in all secretions of the body. It is the main antibody in the MUCOUS MEMBRANE of the intestines, bronchi, saliva and tears. It defends the body against microorganisms by combining with a protein in the mucosa.

Ig D is found in the serum in small amounts but increases during allergic reactions.

Ig E is found primarily in the lungs, skin and mucous membrane cells and is an anaphylactic antibody (*see* ANAPHYLAXIS).

Ig G is synthesized to combat bacteria and viruses in the body.

Ig M (or macroglobulin) has a very high molecular weight (about five or six times that of the others) and is the first produced by the body when antigens occur. It is also the main antibody in blood group incompatibilities.

immunology the study of immunity, the immune system of the body and all aspects of the body's defence mechanisms.

immunosuppression the use of drugs (immunosuppressives) that affect the body's immune system and lower its resistance to disease. These drugs are used in transplant surgery to maintain the survival of the transplanted organ, and to treat autoimmune diseases. The condition may also be produced as a side effect e.g. after chemotherapy treatment for cancer. In all instances, there is an increased risk of infection.

immunotherapy the largely experimental technique of developing the body's IMMUNITY to a disease by administering drugs or gradually increasing doses of the appropriate allergens, thereby modifying the immune response. The most widely studied disease is cancer, where this forms an auxiliary treatment to drug therapy.

impaction a descriptive term for things being locked or wedged together; or stuck in position. For example a wisdom tooth is impacted when it cannot erupt normally because of other tissues blocking it. Also, impacted faeces form a block in the colon or rectum and an impacted fracture is where the adjacent ends are locked together.

impetigo a staphylococcal and infectious skin disease found primarily in children. It spreads quickly over the body, starting as a red patch which forms pustules that join to create crusted yellowish sores. It is easily spread by contact or through towels, etc., and must be treated quickly, otherwise it may continue on an individual for months. Treatment with antibiotics is usually effective.

implant a drug, tissue or artificial object inserted or grafted into the skin or an organ. Drugs are often inserted into the skin for controlled release and in radiotherapy, treatment of prostate tumours, or head/neck cancers can include embedding a capsule of radioactive material in the tissue. A surgical implant covers a tissue graft e.g. a blood vessel, insertion of a pacemaker or a hip prosthesis.

implantation 1. the placing of an IMPLANT. 2. the attachment of the BLASTOCYST to the uterus wall during the very early stages of embryo development.

impotence when a man is unable to have sexual intercourse through lack of penile ERECTION, or less commonly to ejaculate having gained an erection. The cause may be *organic* and due to a condition or disease (DIABETES or endocrine gland disorder) or more commonly *psychogenic*, i.e. due to psychological or emotional problems such as anxiety, fear or guilt.

incision a surgical cut into tissue or organ, or the act of making the cut.

incisor the tooth with a chisel edge to it, used for biting. They form the four front teeth in each jaw.

incontinence an inability to control bowel movements or passage of urine. Urinary incontinence may be due to a LESION in the brain or spinal cord, injury to the sphincter, or damage to the nerves of the bladder. Stress incontinence occurs during coughing or straining and is common in women due to weakening of muscles through childbirth. There are other categories of incontinence, depending on the cause or the frequency of urine passage and the stimulus causing urination.

incubation 1. the time between a person being exposed to an infection and the appearance of symptoms. Incubation periods for diseases tend to be quite constant, some commoner ones being; measles, 10 to 15 days; German measles, 14 to 21; chicken pox, 14 to 21; mumps, 18 to 21; and whooping cough, 7 to 10. 2. the time taken to start and grow microorganisms in culture media. 3. the process of caring for a premature baby in an incubator.

incubator 1. the transparent box-like container in which premature babies are kept in controlled, infection-free conditions. 2. a heated container for growth of bacterial cultures in laboratories.

indigestion *see* **dyspepsia**.

induction the commencement of labour by artificial means, either by administering drugs to produce uterine contractions, or by AMNIOTOMY.

In anaesthesia, it is the process prior to the required state of anaesthesia and includes premedication with a sedative.

infant a child from birth to 12 months.

infant mortality (*or* **infant mortality rate**) a statistical measure of infant deaths, calculated as the number of deaths of infants under one year, per 1000 live births (in any given year). The figure is regarded as a measure of social conditions in a country rather than a guide to the medical services.

infarction the formation of an *infarct* or dead area of tissue in an organ or vessel due to the obstruction of the artery supplying blood. The obstruction may be caused by a blood clot or an EMBOLUS.

infection when PATHOGENS invade the body causing disease. Bacteria, viruses, fungi, etc and are all included and they enter the body, multiply and after the INCUBATION period symptoms appear. The organisms reach the body in many ways: airborne droplets, direct contact, sexual intercourse, by VECTORS, from contaminated food or drink etc.

infertility when a couple are unable to produce offspring naturally. Female infertility may be because of irregular or no ovulation, blocked FALLOPIAN TUBES or ENDOMETRIOSIS; while a low sperm count or other deficiency in the spermatozoa can lead to male infertility. Treatment can include drug therapy, surgery, or more recently the technique of *in vitro* fertilization.

infestation when animal parasites occur on the skin, in the hair or within the body (e.g. parasitic worms).

inflammation the response of the body's tissues to injury, which involves pain, redness, heat and swelling (*acute* inflammation). The first sign when the tissues are infected or injured physically or chemically is a dilation of blood vessels in the affected area, increasing blood flow, resulting in heat and redness. The circulation then slows a little and white blood cells migrate into the tissues, producing the swelling. The white blood cells engulf invading bacteria, dead tissue and foreign particles. After this either the white blood cells migrate back to the circulation, or there is the production and discharge of pus, as healing commences. *Chronic* inflammation is when repair is not complete and there is formation of scar tissue.

influenza a highly infectious disease caused by virus that affects the respiratory tract. Symptoms include headache, weakness and fever, appetite loss and general aches and pains. Sometimes there is the complication of a lung infection, which requires immediate treatment. There are three main strains of influenza virus, designated A, B and C. The viruses quickly produce new strains, which is why an attack of one is unlikely to provide protection against a later bout of the disease. Epidemics occur periodically and in Britain virus A is responsible for the majority of outbreaks.

ingestion the process of chewing and swallowing food and fluid, which then goes into the stomach. Also, the means whereby a *phagocyte* (a cell that can surround and break down cell debris, foreign particles and microorganisms) takes in particles.

inhalants substances taken into the body by INHALATION. The substances can be in several forms: inhaling the steam of a hot solution; as a pressurized aerosol of droplets of particles; or as a non-pressurized passive inhaler, where powdered medication is drawn into the body by inhaling deeply. Sufferers of asthma use inhalers to deliver drugs to the bronchi (bronchodilator drugs) for relief from attacks.

inhalation 1. (*or* **inspiration**) the act of drawing air into the lungs. 2. the medication breathed in, whether in gas or vapour of particulate form, to ensure contact with and/or treatment of conditions of the throat, bronchi or lungs.

injection the means whereby a liquid (often a drug) is introduced into the body using a syringe when it would otherwise be destroyed by digestive processes. The location of the injection depends upon the speed with which the drug is to be absorbed and the target site. Thus injections may go into the skin (*intradermal*), beneath the skin (*subcutaneous*, as with INSULIN). For slow absorption an *intramuscular* injection would be used, and *intravenous* for fast delivery.

inner ear *see* **ear**.

innervation the nerves serving a particular organ, tissue or area of the body which carries MOTOR impulses to the target and sensory impulses away from it and towards the brain.

inoculation the process whereby a small quantity of material is introduced into the body to produce or increase immunity to the disease related to the injected material. *See* IMMUNIZATION and VACCINATION.

in-patient someone admitted to a hospital for a stay to undergo treatment or investigation.

insemination injection of semen into the vagina whether by sexual intercourse or artificial means. *See* ARTIFICIAL INSEMINATION.

insomnia being unable to remain asleep or to fall asleep in the first instance, resulting in debilitating tiredness. It may be caused by a painful condition but is more likely to be due to anxiety.

insulin a pancreatic hormone produced in the ISLETS OF LANGERHANS that initiates uptake of glucose by body cells and thereby controls the level of glucose in the blood. It works by stimulating proteins on cell surfaces within muscles and other tissues to take up the glucose for their activity. A lack of hormone results in the sugar derived from food being excreted in the urine — the condition

DIABETES MELLITUS. For such cases, insulin can be administered by injection.

intercostal the term given to nerves, muscles, etc. that are situated between the ribs.

interferon glycoproteins released from cells infected with a virus which restrict, or *interfere* with, the growth of viruses. They also limit the growth of cells, hence their use in cancer treatment (which is as yet of indeterminate value). There are three human interferons: a from white blood cells, b from connective tissue and g from lymphocytes (*see* INTERLEUKINS). Sufficient quantities of interferon can now be produced by GENETIC ENGINEERING.

interleukins one of several cytokines (molecules secreted by a cell to regulate other cells nearby — *see* INTERFERON) that act between LEUCOCYTES. There are eight interleukins currently recognized and some are involved in functions such as the recognition of ANTIGENS, enhancing the action of MACROPHAGES and the production of other cytokines e.g. interleukin 2 promotes the production of g-interferon and is used in the treatment of MELANOMA.

intervertebral disc fibrous cartilaginous discs that connect adjacent vertebrae and permit rotational and bending movements. The discs make up approximately 25% of the backbone length and they act as shock absorbers providing cushioning for the brain and spinal cord. With age the discs lose their effectiveness and may be displaced.

intestinal flora the bacteria usually found in the intestine, some of which synthesize vitamin K. An acidic surrounding is produced by the bacteria and this helps lessen infection by pathogens unable to withstand the acidic conditions.

intestine the part of the ALIMENTARY CANAL or tract between stomach and anus where final digestion and absorption of food matter occur, in addition to the absorption of water and production of faeces. The intestine is divided into the small intestine comprising DUODENUM, ILEUM and JEJUNUM, and the large intestine made up of the CAECUM, vermiform APPENDIX, COLON and RECTUM. The length of the intestine in man is about 9 metres.

intolerance when a patient is unable to metabolize a drug. There is usually an associated adverse reaction.

intoxication being poisoned by drugs, alcohol or other toxic substances.

intracranial term meaning within the skull and applied to diseases, structures etc.

intracranial pressure the pressure within the cranium, more specifically the pressure as maintained by all tissues: brain, blood, cerebrospinal fluid, etc. An increase in the pressure can occur through injury, haemorrhage or tumour, and treatment will be necessary.

intramuscular term meaning within a muscle, as with an intramuscular injection.

intrauterine contraceptive device (*or* **IUD**) a plastic or metal device, often in the shape of a coil about 25mm long, that is placed in the uterus. The device probably prevents conception by interfering with potential implantation of the embryo. There are sometimes side effects e.g. back pain and heavy menstrual bleeding, but it is a reasonably effective method.

intravenous term meaning relating to the inside of a vein, hence intravenous injections are made into a vein, and blood transfusions are intravenous.

intubation the insertion of a tube into the body through a natural opening. It is commonly, though not exclusively, used to keep an airway open by insertion into the mouth or nose into the larynx. The same technique may be adopted to enable an anaesthetic gas or oxygen to be delivered.

intumescence swelling of an organ.

intussusception an eventual obstruction of the bowel caused by one part of the bowel slipping inside another part beneath it, much as a telescope closes up. The commonest sufferers are young children and the symptoms include pain, vomiting and the passage of a jelly-like blood-stained mucus. If the condition does not right itself corrective treatment is essential either by a barium enema or surgery.

invasion when bacteria enter the body; but more commonly used to describe the process whereby malignant cancer cells move into nearby normal and deeper tissues and gain access to the blood vessels.

in vitro referring to a biological or biochemical reaction or process that occurs literally 'in glassware', i.e. in a test-tube or a similar piece of laboratory apparatus.

in vitro fertilization (*or* **IVF**) the process of fertilizing an OVUM outside the body. The technique is used when a woman has blocked FALLOPIAN TUBES or when there is some other reason for sperm and ovum not uniting. The woman produces several ova (due to hormone therapy treatment), which are removed by laparoscopy (*see* LAPAROSCOPE). These are mixed with sperm and incubated in culture medium until the ova are fertilized and at the BLASTOCYST stage these are implanted in the mother's uterus. The first successful live birth utilizing this technique was in 1978 and the phrase 'test-tube baby' was coined.

in vivo referring to biological processes that occur in a living organism.

involuntary muscle one of two types of muscle not under voluntary or conscious control, such as the blood vessels, stomach and intestines. The heart muscle is slightly different (*see* CARDIAC MUSCLE).

involution the process whereby an organ decreases in size e.g. the return of the uterus to its normal size after childbirth. Also applied to degeneration of organs in old age, i.e. atrophy.

iridectomy the surgical removal of part of the IRIS, often undertaken to correct the blockage of aqueous humour (*see* EYE), associated with GLAUCOMA. It may also be necessary for removal of a foreign body or as part of CATARACT surgery.

iridotomy an incision into the IRIS.

iris the part of the EYE that controls the amount of light to enter. It is in effect a muscular disc and to reduce the amount of light entering, circular muscles contract. To increase the aperture in dim light, radiating muscles contract. The varying sized hole is the PUPIL. The iris can be seen through the CORNEA, which is transparent and, is the coloured part of the eye, this latter feature is due to pigment cells containing melanin (blue is little; brown is more).

irradiation the use in treatment of any form of radiating energy, i.e. electromagnetic radiation in the form of X-rays, a, b or g radiation, also heat and light. Some radiations are used in diagnosis or cancer treatments, others for relief of pain (heat treatment), etc.

irrigation the washing out of a wound or body cavity with a flow of water or other fluid.

irritable bowel syndrome (*or* **IBS**) a condition caused by abnormal muscular contractions (or increased motility) in the COLON, producing effects in the large and small intestines. Symptoms include pain in the abdomen which changes location, disturbed bowel movements with diarrhoea then normal movements or constipation, heartburn and a bloated feeling due to wind. The specific cause is unknown and no disease is present, hence treatment is limited to relief of anxiety or stress (which may be a contributory factor), some drug therapy to reduce muscle activity and careful choice of diet, to include a high fibre content.

irritant a general term encompassing any agent that causes irritation of a tissue e.g. nettle stings, chemicals and gases.

ischaemic relating to a decrease in blood supply to a part of the body or an organ, caused by a blockage or narrowing of the blood vessels. It is often associated with pain.

ischium one of the three bones that comprise each half of the PELVIS. It is the most posterior and it supports the weight of the body when sitting.

islets of Langerhans clusters of cells within the PANCREAS which are the ENDOCRINE part of the gland. There are three types of cells termed alpha, beta and delta, the first two producing GLUCAGON and INSULIN respectively, both vital hormones in the regulation of blood sugar levels. The third hormone produced is somatostatin (also released by the HYPOTHALAMUS), which works antagonistically against growth hormone by blocking its release by the pituitary gland. The islets were named after Paul Langerhans, a German pathologist.

isolation the process whereby a patient with an infectious disease is kept apart from non-infected people. This often includes people who may have contracted the disease but who have yet to show any symptoms. Isolation may also be necessary to ensure a patient does not come into contact with irritating environmental factors.

In *surgery*, when a structure or organ is kept apart from all around it through the use of instruments.

isometric literally 'equal measurement'. Isometric exercises are undertaken to build up muscle strength by increasing tension in the muscles without contraction e.g. by pushing against something that cannot move.

isotopes atoms that differ from other atoms of the same element due to a different number of neutrons in the nucleus. Isotopes have the same number of protons and therefore the same atomic number, but a different mass number (total number of protons and neutrons). Radioactive isotopes decay into other elements or isotopes through the emission of alpha, beta or gamma radiation, and some radioactive isotopes can be produced in the laboratory. RADIOTHERAPY uses such isotopes in the treatment of cancer.

itching a skin condition or sensation prompting scratching to obtain relief. The causes are numerous and include mechanical irritation e.g. by clothing or lice, skin diseases or conditions such as ECZEMA, allergies, etc.

J

jaundice a condition characterized by the unusual presence of bile pigment (BILIRUBIN) in the blood. The BILE produced in the liver passes into the blood instead of the intestines and because of this there is a yellowing of the skin and the whites of the eyes.

There are several types of jaundice: *obstructive*, due to bile not reaching the intestine due to an obstruction e.g. a GALLSTONE; *haemolytic*, where red blood cells are destroyed by HAEMOLYSIS; *hepatocellular*, due to a liver disease such as HEPATITIS, which results in the liver being unable to use the bilirubin. *Neonatal jaundice* is quite common in newborn infants, when the liver is physiologically immature but it usually lasts only a few days. The infant can be exposed to blue light which converts bilirubin to biliverdin, another (harmless) bile pigment.

jaw a term for the bones that carry the teeth and associated soft tissues. More specifically, they are the upper jaw (*maxilla*) and the lower jaw (*mandible*). The maxillae are fixed, while the mandible (which is one bone after the age of about 12 months) hinges on part of the temporal bone, in front of the ear.

jejunum the part of the small intestine lying before the ILEUM and after the DUODENUM. Its main function is the absorption of digested food and its lining has numerous finger-like projections (villi) that increase the surface area for absorption. The villi are longer in the jejunum than elsewhere in the small intestine.

joints connections between bones (and cartilages). Joints can be divided upon their structure and the degree to which they permit movement. *Fibrous* joints are fixed by fibrous tissue binding bones together e.g. the bones of the skull. *Cartilaginous* joints are slightly movable. These have discs of cartilage between bones so that only limited movement is permitted over one joint but over several adjacent joints, considerable flexure is achieved, as with the spine. The final category is *synovial* joints, which can move freely. Each synovial joint comprises the bones, cartilage over the ends, then a *capsule* (sheath of fibrous tissue), from which the ligaments form, and a SYNOVIAL MEMBRANE, with synovial fluid to lubricate the joint.

This type of joint then occurs in two forms: hinge joints allowing planar movement (e.g. the knee) and ball-and-socket joints permitting all-round movement (e.g. the hip). Joints are subject to various conditions and diseases including SYNOVITIS, epiphysitis (inflammation of the EPIPHYSIS), GOUT, RHEUMATISM and dislocations.

jugular a general term for structures in the neck.

jugular vein any of the veins in the neck, particularly the anterior, internal and external. The anterior jugular vein is an offshoot of the external jugular and runs down the front of the neck. The external jugular itself drains the scalp, face and neck while the larger internal jugular drains the face, neck and brain and is sited vertically down the side of the neck.

K

kala-azar *see* **leishmaniasis.**

kaolin (*or* **china clay**) a white powder form of aluminium silicate used in cases of skin irritation. It is also an adsorbent taken internally to treat DIARRHOEA.

Kaposi's sarcoma a condition involving malignant skin tumours which form from the blood vessels. Purple lumps, due to the tumours, form on the feet and ankles, spreading to arms and hands. The disease is common in Africa but less so in western countries, although it is associated with AIDS. Radiotherapy is the primary treatment but chemotherapy may also be required.

keloid (*or* **cheloid**) scar tissue which forms due to the growth of fibrous tissue over a burn or injury, creating a hard, often raised patch with ragged edges.

keratin a fibrous, sulphur-rich protein made up of coiled polypeptide chains. It occurs in hair, fingernails and the surface layer of the skin.

keratosis a condition of the skin whereby there is a thickening and overgrowth of the horny layer (or *stratum corneum*) of the SKIN. The condition is usually induced by excessive sunlight and can occur as scales and patchy skin pigmentation (*actinic keratosis*) or as yellow/brown warts (*seborrhoeic keratosis*). It is essential to avoid overexposing skin to sunlight if the condition is to be prevented or treated.

Kernig's sign the inability of someone with MENINGITIS to straighten his or her legs at the knee when the thighs are at right angles to be body. It is symptomatic of the disease.

ketoacidosis acidosis resulting from a disorder in the metabolism of carbohydrates which produces a build-up of KETONES in the body. It is mainly a complication of DIABETES MELLITUS and produces a fruity smell on the breath, also symptoms such as nausea, vomiting, dehydration, shortness of breath, weight loss and coma, if untreated.

ketogenesis the normal production of KETONES in the body, due to metabolism of fats. Excess production leads to KETOSIS.

ketone an organic compound that contains a carbonyl group (C=O) within the compound. Ketones can be detected in the body when fat is metabolized for energy when food intake is insufficient.

ketone body one of several compounds (e.g. acetoacetic acid) produced by the liver due to metabolism of fat deposits. These compounds normally provide energy, via KETOGENESIS, for the body's peripheral tissues. In abnormal conditions, when carbohydrate supply is reduced, ketogenesis produces excess ketone bodies in the blood (KETOSIS), which may then appear in the urine (KETONURIA).

ketonuria (*or* **acetonuria** *or* **ketoaciduria**) the presence of ketone bodies (*see* KETONE and KETONE BODY) in the urine due to starvation or DIABETES MELLITUS, causing excessive KETOGENESIS and KETOSIS.

ketosis the build-up of ketones in the body and bloodstream due to a lack of carbohydrates for metabolism, or failure to use fully available carbohydrates, resulting in fat breakdown (*see* KETOGENESIS and KETONURIA). It is induced by starvation, DIABETES MELLITUS or any condition in which fats are metabolized quickly and excessively.

kidney one of two glands/organs that remove nitrogenous wastes, mainly UREA, from the blood and also adjust the concentrations of various salts. The kidney measures approximately 10cm long, 6cm wide and 4cm thick, and is positioned at the back of the abdomen, below the diaphragm. Blood is supplied to the kidney by the renal artery and leaves via the renal vein. Each kidney is held in place by fat and connective tissue and comprises an inner medulla and outer cortex. The kidneys produce and eliminate URINE by a complex process of filtration and reabsorption. The 'active' parts are the nephrons which filter blood under pressure, reabsorbing water and other substances. A nephron comprises a renal tubule and blood vessels. The tubule expands into a cup shape (*Bowman's capsule*) that contains a knot of capillaries (the *glomerulus*) and the latter bring the water, urea, salts, etc. Filtrate passes from the glomerulus through three areas of the tubule (proximal convoluted tubule; the loop of Henle, distal convoluted tube, which together form a shape resembling a hairpin) leaving as urine.

kinin one of a group of polypeptides that lower blood pressure through dilation of the blood vessels and cause SMOOTH MUSCLE to contract. They are associated with inflammation, causing local increases in the permeability of tissue capillaries. In addition they play some part in the allergic response and ANAPHYLAXIS. Kinins do not normally occur in the blood but form under these conditions or when the tissue is damaged (*see also* BRADYKININS).

Klinefelter's syndrome a genetic imbalance in males in which there are 47 rather than 46 CHROMOSOMES, the extra one being an X chromosome producing a genetic make-up of XXY instead of the usual XY. The physical manifestations are small testes which atrophy, resulting in a lack of sperm production, enlargement of the breasts, long thin legs and little or no facial or body hair. There may be associated mental retardation and pulmonary disease.

knee the joint connecting the thigh to the lower leg, formed by the femur, tibia and kneecap (PATELLA). It is a hinge type of synovial JOINT with very strong ligaments binding the bones together. Although the knee is a strong joint, it is complex and injuries can be serious.

knee jerk *see* **reflex action**.

knock-knee (*or* **genu valgum**) an abnormal curvature of the legs such that when the knees are touching, the ankles are spaced apart. When walking, the knees knock and severe cases can lead to stress on the joints in the legs, with arthritis. Surgery may be performed to correct the condition, which in the past was commonly due to RICKETS but is now due mainly to poor muscles.

Korsakoff's syndrome a neurological disorder described by the Russian neuropsychiatrist Sergei Korsakoff (1854-1900), characterized by short-term memory loss, disorientation and confabulation (the invention and detailed description of events, situations and experiences to cover gaps in the memory). The condition is caused primarily by alcoholism and a deficiency of thiamine (vital in converting carbohydrate to glucose).

kwashiorkor a type of malnutrition seen especially among children in Africa. It is due to a deficiency in dietary protein and foods normally eaten for energy. It occurs when a child is weaned from the breast onto an adult diet that is inadequate such that the child cannot eat enough to get sufficient protein. The result is appetite loss, diarrhoea, OEDEMA, anaemia, and other conditions due to, for example, VITAMIN deficiencies. Initially the condition responds well to first-class protein, but it is less straightforward with more prolonged cases.

kyphosis an abnormal outward curvature of the spine, causing the back to be hunched. There is an increased curvature of the spine, which may be caused by weak musculature or bad posture (mobile kyphosis) or it may be due to collapsed vertebrae (fixed kyphosis), as in OSTEOPOROSIS of the aged.

L

labia (*singular* **labium**) meaning lips, as in the folds of skin enclosing the VULVA (the *labia majora* and *minora*).

labial pertaining to the lips. Also, the tooth surface next to the lips.

labour the process of giving birth from dilatation of the CERVIX to expulsion of the afterbirth. It usually commences naturally although some labours are induced (*see* INDUCTION). The cervix expands and at the same time the muscles of the uterus wall contract, pushing part of the AMNION down into the opening. The amnion ruptures releasing the 'waters' but these two events do not necessarily occur at the same time. The second stage is the actual delivery of the child which passes through the bony girdle of the pelvis, via the VAGINA to the outside. Initially the head appears at the cervix and the uterine contractions strengthen. These contractions are augmented by abdominal muscular contractions when the baby is in the vagina. When the baby's head is clear, the whole body is helped out and the umbilical cord severed. The final stage, accomplished by some contractions, is expulsion of the PLACENTA and membranes.

On average, labour lasts 12 hours (less for subsequent pregnancies) and in the second stage an EPISIOTOMY may be necessary to facilitate the emergence of the head. In most cases, the baby lies head down at delivery although some are delivered feet or buttocks first (BREECH PRESENTATION). Other complications tend to be rare and maternal mortality is very low in the west.

labyrinth part of the inner ear (*see* EAR) consisting of canals, ducts and cavities forming the organs of hearing and balance. There are two parts: the *membranous labyrinth*, comprising the semicircular canals and associated structures and the central cavity of the cochlea, and the *bony labyrinth*, a system of canals filled with perilymph and surrounding the other parts.

laceration a wound with jagged edges.

lacrimal relating to tears.

lacrimal gland one of a pair of glands situated above and to the side of each eye that secrete saline and slightly alkaline tears that moisten the conjunctiva (the mucous membrane lining the inside of the eyelid). The glands comprise part of the *lacrimal apparatus*, the remainder being the lacrimal ducts (or canaliculi), through which the tears drain to the lacrimal sacs and the nasal cavity.

lactase the enzyme that acts on milk sugar (LACTOSE) to produce glucose and galactose.

lactation the process of milk secretion by the MAMMARY GLANDS in the breast, which begins at the end of pregnancy. COLOSTRUM is produced and secreted before the milk. Lactation is controlled by hormones and stops when the baby ceases to be breast-fed.

lacteal vessels forming part of the lymphatic system. They occur as projections with a closed end extending into villi (*see* VILLUS) in the small intestine and take up digested fats as a milky fluid called chyle.

lactose milk sugar found only in mammalian milk and produced by the MAMMARY GLANDS. It is made up of one molecule of glucose and one molecule of galactose. People with a low level of activity of the enzyme LACTASE, or none at all, cannot absorb lactose, a condition called lactose intolerance.

lacuna (*plural* **lacunae**) an anatomical term meaning a small depression, cavity or pit, especially in compact bone.

laminectomy the surgical procedure in which access is gained to the spinal cord by the removal of the arch of one or more vertebrae. It is adopted when a tumour is to be removed, or a slipped disc is to be treated.

lancet a surgical knife that is small and pointed and sharp on both edges.

lanugo fine, downy hair that covers the foetus between the fifth and ninth months. It is lost in the ninth month and is thus seen only on babies born prematurely.

laparoscope a type of ENDOSCOPE with a light source and a means of viewing the object, that is inserted into the abdominal cavity through a small incision. This allows a surgeon to view the organs in the cavity, and a laparoscope is also used to enable some minor operations to be performed using instruments inserted through a second incision.

laparoscopy the use of a LAPAROSCOPE to examine the organs in the abdominal cavity. Carbon dioxide is injected into the cavity to expand it before the laparoscope is inserted. In addition to being used purely for observation, a laparoscopy is also useful for taking a biopsy, for sterilizations and for collecting ova for IN VITRO FERTILIZATION.

laparotomy a general term for any incision into the abdominal cavity. Types of laparotomy include COLOSTOMY and APPENDICECTOM.

large intestine *see* **intestine**.

laryngectomy surgical excision of all or part of the LARYNX. This procedure is adopted for cancer of the larynx.

laryngitis inflammation of the mucous membrane that lines the LARYNX and vocal cords. It is due to viral infection in the main, but also to bacteria, chemical irritants, heavy smoking or excessive use of the voice. *Acute* laryngitis accompanies infections of the upper respiratory tract and the symptoms include pain, a cough and difficulty in swallowing. *Chronic* laryngitis may be due to recurrence of the acute form, but is often attributable to excessive smoking, worsened by alcohol. Changes occurring in the vocal cords are more permanent and the symptoms are as for the acute form, but longer-lasting.

laryngoscope a type of endoscope used to examine the larynx.

laryngotracheobronchitis an acute inflammation of the major parts of the respiratory tract, causing shortness of breath, a croup-like cough and hoarseness. It occurs usually through viral infection and particularly in young children where there may be some obstruction of the LARYNX (*see also* CROUP). The main airways, bronchi, become coated with fluid generated by the inflamed tissues, resulting in the shortness of breath. Treatment is through inhalations, antibiotics if appropriate, and if the obstruction is serious, hospitalization may be necessary for INTUBATION, TRACHEOSTOMY, etc.

larynx part of the air passage connecting the PHARYNX with the TRACHEA and also the organ producing vocal sounds. It is situated high up in the front of the neck and is constructed of cartilages with ligaments and muscles. The ligaments bind together the cartilages and one pair of these form the VOCAL CORDS. The larynx is lined with mucous membrane and in all is about 5cm long.

laser (*L*ight *A*mplification by *S*timulated *E*mission of *R*adiation) a device that produces a powerful and narrow beam of light where the light is of one wavelength in phase. This produces a beam of high-energy light which can be used in surgery. Different lasers can be used for different procedures, for example the argon laser heats and coagulates tissues because haemoglobin absorbs the energy — this is therefore used to seal bleeding vessels. The carbon-dioxide laser is used to make incisions because water in cells absorbs the energy, thus destroying the cells. Lasers are also used in retina surgery, and in the removal of birthmarks.

Lassa fever a highly contagious viral infection first reported from Lassa in Nigeria. It takes 3-21 days to incubate and results in fever and headache, acute muscular pains, sore throat and some difficulty in swallowing. Death often occurs due to heart or kidney failure and pregnant women show a high mortality rate. Little can be done because it is a viral infection but treatment with plasma from patients who have recovered may help.

laudanum a NARCOTIC ANALGESIC prepared from opium, used widely in the past.

laughing gas the common name for NITROUS OXIDE.

laxative a substance that is taken to evacuate the bowel or to soften stools. Typical laxatives include castor oil, senna, and its derivatives. *See also* PURGATIVE.

Legionnaire's disease a bacterial infection and a form of pneumonia caused by *Legionella pneumophila*. It produces an illness similar to influenza with symptoms appearing after a 2–10 day incubation period. Fever, chills, head- and muscular aches may progress to PLEURISY and chest pains. Antibiotic treatment is usually effective e.g. erythromycin.

The disease was named after an outbreak in America in 1976 at the American Legion convention. The bacterium is found in nature, particularly in water, and static water provides ideal conditions for multiplication. Inhalation of an aerosol of water is the likeliest way of becoming infected and air-conditioning cooling towers are a particular source of infected water. It is vital that infected systems be cleaned and chlorinated.

leishmaniasis a common tropical and sub-tropical disease (in Africa, Asia, South America and the Mediterranean) caused by the parasitic protozoa

Leishmania, which are transmitted by the bites of sandflies. Depending upon the region, it affects people of differing ages and there are two forms, *visceral* and *cutaneous*; in the former, internal organs are affected while in the latter it affects the skin but also the mucous membranes.

Visceral leishmaniasis results in fever, enlargement of the glands, liver and SPLEEN and roughly three quarters of untreated cases result in fatalities. Cutaneous leishmaniasis produces skin ulcers that go by various names, and may include the nose and throat. The drug commonly used is a salt of sodium that contains antimony.

lens the part of the eye that focuses incoming light onto the RETINA. It is composed of a fibrous protein, crystallin, and is enclosed in a thin capsule.

leprosy a serious disease caused by the bacterium *Mycobacterium leprae* that attacks the skin, nerves and mucous membranes and has an incubation period of several years. There are two forms of the disease, *tuberculoid* and *lepromatous*, depending upon the resistance of the host (the former occurs in those with a higher degree of immunity). The tuberculoid form produces discoloured patches of skin with some numbness but is generally benign and often heals untreated.

Lepromatous leprosy is a much more serious and progressively destructive form of the disease, creating lumps in the skin, thickening of skin and nerves, inflammation of the iris and numbness of the skin, with muscle weakness and paralysis. The more serious cases show deformity and considerable disfigurement and sometimes blindness. There is also an intermediate form with symptoms of both types (indeterminate leprosy).

Although many millions of people are affected, drugs therapy is quite effective, providing a combination of antibiotics is used (because the bacterium develops resistance to one of the sulphone drugs commonly used).

leptomeningitis inflammation of two of the three MENINGES surrounding the brain and spinal cord. Specifically, the inner two (pia mater and arachnoid) are affected.

leptospirosis an acute infectious disease caused by bacteria in the genus *Leptospira*. The disease varies from the mild form of an influenza type of illness to the more serious cases involving fever, liver disease and therefore jaundice, and possibly kidney disease or meningitis. In such cases there may be fatalities. The organism occurs in the urine of rats and dogs and this renders workers on farms, sewage works, etc., more susceptible, but it can be contracted by bathing or immersion in contaminated water e.g. canals. Antibiotics can be given but must be administered at an early stage to be effective.

One particular species, *L. icterohaemorrhagiae*, which is transmitted by rats, is responsible for the type called Weil's disease.

lesbian *see* **homosexual**.

lesion a wound or injury to body tissues. Also an area of tissue which because of damage due to disease or wounding does not function fully. Thus primary lesions include tumours and ulcers, and from primary lesions secondaries may form.

lethargy the state of being inactive mentally and physically and one that approaches the unconscious. The cause may be psychological or physical. The lethargy associated with the aftermath of glandular fever is well-known but it may also be due to ANAEMIA, DIABETES MELLITUS or MALNUTRITION, amongst others.

leucocyte (*or* **leukocyte**) a white blood cell, so called because it contains no HAEMOGLOBIN. It also differs from red blood cells in having a nucleus. Leucocytes are formed in the bone marrow, spleen, thymus and lymph nodes and there are three types: granulocytes, comprising 70% of all white blood cells, lymphocytes (25%) and monocytes (5%). Granulocytes help combat bacterial and viral infection and may be involved in allergies. LYMPHOCYTES destroy foreign bodies, either directly or through production of antibodies, and MONOCYTES ingest bacteria and foreign bodies by the process called *phagocytosis* (engulfing microorganisms and cell debris to remove them from the body). In disease, immature forms of leucocytes may appear in the blood (ultimately forming both red and white blood cells).

leucocytosis except for pregnancy, menstruation and during exercise, an abnormal and temporary increase in the number of white blood cells in the blood. It usually accompanies bacterial but not viral infections, because the body's defence mechanism is fighting the bacteria by producing leucocytes. A blood sample may thus form a useful diagnostic tool for a condition which has not yet manifested any physical symptoms.

leucopenia a fall in the number of LEUCOCYTES (white blood cells) in the blood.

leucorrhoea a discharge of white- or yellow-coloured mucus from the vagina. It may be a normal condition (physiological discharge), increasing before and after menstruation, but a large discharge probably indicates an infection somewhere in the genital tract. A common cause is the infection called THRUSH but it may also be due to GONORRHOEA, in which case the treatment will differ.

leukaemia a cancerous disease in which there is an uncontrolled proliferation of LEUCOCYTES in the bone marrow. The cells fail to mature to adult cells and thus cannot function as part of the defence mechanism against infections. This leads to anaemia, bleeding and easy bruising, with enlargement of the spleen, liver and lymph nodes. Acute leukaemia has a sudden onset and development while the chronic form may take years to develop the same symptoms.

The cause of leukaemia is unknown, although it has been attributed to viruses, exposure to toxic chemicals or ionizing radiations. In addition to the acute and chronic forms, it is further classified by the predominant white blood cells, thus acute lymphoblastic leukaemia, acute myeloblastic leukaemia (myeloblast is an early form of granulocytes, *see* LEUCOCYTE), chronic lymphatic leukaemia. The treatment involves radiotherapy, chemotherapy and bone-marrow transplants and although there is no cure, the outlook has improved over recent years. The survival or remission rate varies with the type of leukaemia.

libido the sexual drive, often associated with psychiatric illnesses. Lack of libido may be due to illness or a lack of sex hormones due to an endocrine disorder.

Librium a minor tranquillizer used in the treatment of anxiety. It is taken orally and relaxes muscles, although there are side effects such as nausea and skin reactions.

lice (*singular* **louse**) insects parasitic on man. Lice are wingless and attach themselves to hair or clothing by means of their legs and claws. They suck blood, are particularly resistant to crushing and have to be removed using special shampoos and combs. *See also* PEDICULOSIS.

ligament bands of fibrous connective tissue composed chiefly of COLLAGEN, that join bones together, restricting movement and preventing dislocation. Ligaments strengthen joints and most joints are surrounded by a capsular ligament. Also, a layer of SEROUS MEMBRANE e.g. the PERITONEUM that supports or links organs.

ligation the procedure of tying off a duct or blood vessel to prevent flow during surgery, etc. The application of a LIGATURE.

ligature material for tying firmly around a blood vessel or duct to stop bleeding or prevent flow. The material may be wire, silk, catgut, etc.

lightening a sensation experienced by many pregnant women, normally towards the last month of the pregnancy, whereby the foetus settles lower in the pelvis. This lessens the pressure on the diaphragm and breathing becomes easier.

light reflex the mechanism whereby the PUPIL of the EYE opens in response to direct light or consensual pupillary stimulation (i.e. stimulation of one pupil with light results in a response from the other pupil).

lignocaine a commonly used local anaesthetic. It is given by injection for minor surgery and dental treatment and it can be applied directly to the eyes, throat, etc., because it is absorbed directly through mucous membranes. It is also used in the treatment of some disorders in heart rhythm.

limb an appendage of the body. Also a branch of an internal organ.

linctus a medicine, particularly to treat coughs, that is thick and syrup-like.

lingual term meaning relating to the tongue, or something close to the tongue e.g. lingual nerve, or the lingual surface of a tooth.

liniment a creamy/oily substance for rubbing onto the skin to alleviate irritation or pain. Many of the compounds are poisonous, containing substances such as camphor, turpentine and even belladonna.

linkage two or more GENES are said to be linked together if they occur close to each other on the same CHROMOSOME. The genes are thus likely to be inherited together as will be characteristics that they represent. This is because the linked genes are more likely to be together in nuclei formed as a result of meiosis (the chromosomal division that produces the GAMETES).

lint a cotton fabric (formerly linen) used for surgical dressings which has one fluffy side and one smooth, the latter being placed against the skin.

lipolysis the breakdown of lipids into FATTY ACIDS via the action of the enzyme lipase.

lipoma a benign tumour made up of fat cells which can occur in the fibrous tissues of the body, often beneath the skin. The only problem associated with such structures may be their size and position.

liposarcoma a malignant tumour of fat cells which is very rare, particularly under the age of 30. It occurs in the buttocks or thighs.

liposome a spherical droplet of microscopic size comprising fatty membranes around an aqueous vesicle. Liposomes are created in the laboratory by adding an aqueous solution to a phospholipid gel (phospholipids are compounds containing FATTY ACIDS and a phosphate group). Liposomes bear some resemblance to living cell components and are studied on this basis. Additionally, they can be introduced into living cells and are used to transport toxic drugs to a specific treatment site. The liposomes retain the drug while in the blood and on passing through the chosen organ the membrane is melted by selectively heating the organ and the drug is released. This technique is used for certain forms of cancer.

listeriosis an infectious disease caused when the Gram-positive (*see* GRAM'S STAIN) bacterium *Listeria monocytogenes*, which attacks animals, is contracted by man through eating infected products. It produces symptoms similar to influenza or it may cause MENINGITIS or ENCEPHALITIS. The old and frail are more susceptible, as are the newborn. It may terminate a pregnancy or damage the foetus if contracted during a pregnancy. Antibiotics such as penicillin provide an effective treatment.

Little's disease CEREBRAL PALSY on both sides of the body but where the legs are affected more than the arms.

liver a very important organ of the body, with many functions critical in regulating metabolic processes. It is also the largest gland in the body weighing around 1.4kg. It occupies the top right-hand part of the abdominal cavity and is made up of four lobes. It is fastened to the abdominal wall by ligaments and sits beneath the DIAPHRAGM, and upon the right kidney, large intestine, DUODENUM and stomach.

There are two blood vessels supplying the liver: the hepatic artery delivers oxygenated blood, while the hepatic portal vein conveys digested food from the stomach. Among its functions, the liver converts excess glucose to GLYCOGEN for storage as a food reserve; excess amounts of AMINO ACIDS are converted to urea for excretion by the kidneys; BILE is produced for storage in the GALL BLADDER and LIPOLYSIS occurs; some poisons are broken down (detoxified), hence the beneficial effect of the hepatic portal vein carrying blood to the liver rather than it going around the body first.

The liver also synthesizes blood-clotting substances such as FIBRINOGEN and prothrombin and the anticoagulant HEPARIN; it breaks down red blood cells at the end of their life and processes the haemoglobin for iron, which is stored; vitamin A is synthesized and stored and it also stores vitamins B12, D, E and K. In the embryo it forms red blood cells. Such is the chemical and biochemical activity of the liver that significant heat energy is generated and this organ is a major contributor of heat to the body.

lobe certain organs are divided by fissures into large divisions, which are called lobes, e.g. the brain, liver and lungs.

lobectomy the removal of a lobe of an organ e.g. lung or brain. A lobe of a lung may be removed for cancer or other disease.

lobotomy in general, cutting a lobe. More specifically, a neurosurgical operation rarely performed now, which involved severing the nerve fibres in the frontal lobe of the brain. It was performed to reduce severe depression or emotional conditions but produced serious side effects such as epilepsy and personality changes. Modern techniques permit the production of small LESIONS in specific areas and side effects are rare.

lobule a small lobe. Also, a division of an organ that is smaller than a lobe e.g. the lobules of the liver.

lochia the material discharged through the vagina from the uterus after childbirth, which takes a few weeks. Initially it consists mainly of blood, then it becomes more mucus but with some blood and then a whitish mixture of cell fragments and microbes.

lockjaw *see* **tetanus**.

locomotor ataxia an unsteady gait which is one symptom of TABES DORSALIS, a form of SYPHILIS. The organism destroys sensory nerves producing further symptoms such as pains in the legs and body, loss of bladder control and blurred vision due to optic nerve damage.

loin that area of the back between the lower ribs and the pelvis.

lumbago pain of any sort in the lower back. It can be muscular, skeletal or neurological in origin. A severe and sudden case may be due to a strained muscle or slipped disc and the latter is usually the cause of lumbago with SCIATICA.

lumbar a general term for anything relating to the LOINS e.g. lumbar vertebrae.

lumbar puncture the procedure whereby a hollow needle is inserted into the spinal canal in the lumbar region (usually between the third and fourth lumbar vertebrae) to obtain a sample of cerebrospinal fluid. The fluid is used in diagnosis of diseases of the nervous system, or to introduce drugs, anaesthetics, etc.

lumbar vertebrae numbering five, the lumbar vertebrae are between the SACRUM and the thoracic vertebrae at the lowest part of the back. These vertebrae are not fused and have strong attachment points (processes) for the muscles of the lower back.

lumpectomy the surgical removal of a tumour with the tissue immediately around it but leaving intact the bulk of the tissue and the lymph nodes. This applies particularly to breast cancer when the procedure is often followed by radiotherapy and is undertaken for patients with a small tumour (less than 2cm) and no metastases (*see* METASTASIS) to nearby lymph nodes or organs elsewhere in the body.

lungs the sac-like, paired organs of respiration situated with their base on the DIAPHRAGM and the top projecting into the neck. Each lung consists of fibrous, elastic sacs that are convoluted to provide a large surface area for gaseous exchange. Air enters the body through the windpipe or TRACHEA, which branches into two bronchi (*see* BRONCHUS), one to each lung. Further branching then occurs, into numerous BRONCHIOLES. The bronchioles divide further and then end in alveoli (*see* ALVEOLUS) which are tiny sac-like structures where the gaseous exchange occurs. The exchange of oxygen and carbon dioxide occurs between the many blood capillaries on one side of the membrane and the air on the other. The lungs are served by the pulmonary arteries and pulmonary veins.

The *total lung capacity* of an adult male is five to six litres although only about half a litre (500ml) is exchanged in normal breathing (called the *tidal volume*).

lupus erythematosus (*or* **LE**) a skin disease of the lupus group. The cause of the condition is as yet unknown, although it is thought to be an autoimmune disorder. It is characterized by raised reddened patches on the skin of the face, neck, ears, arms and scalp, which may cause scarring. About 10% of LE sufferers go on to develop SYSTEMIC LUPUS ERYTHEMATOSUS (SLE).

Lyme disease an arthritic disease with rashes, fever and possibly carditis (inflammation of the heart) and ENCEPHALITIS. It is caused by a spirochaete (a type of BACTERIUM) that is transmitted by tick bite. Symptoms may not appear until some time after the bite but antibiotics can be used in treatment.

lymph a colourless, watery fluid that surrounds the body tissues and circulates in the lymphatic system. It is derived from blood and is similar to plasma comprising 95% water, with protein, sugar, salts and LYMPHOCYTES. The lymph is circulated by muscular action and it passes through LYMPH NODES, which act as filters, and is eventually returned to the blood via the thoracic duct (one of the two main vessels of the lymphatic system).

lymphadenectomy removal of LYMPH NODES when, for example, a node has become cancerous due to it draining the area around an organ with a malignancy.

lymphadenitis inflammation of the LYMPH NODES, which become enlarged, hard and tender. The neck lymph nodes are commonly affected in association with another inflammatory condition.

lymphadenoma *see* **Hodgkin's disease**.

lymphangiography the technique of injecting a radio-opaque substance into the lymphatic system to render it visible on an X-ray, used primarily in investigating the spread of cancer.

lymphatic gland *see* **gland**.

lymphatics (*or* **lymphatic system**) the network of vessels, valves, nodes, etc., that carry lymph from the tissues to the bloodstream and help maintain the internal fluid environment of the body. Lymph drains into capillaries and larger vessels, passing through nodes and going eventually into two large vessels (the thoracic duct and right lymphatic duct), which return it to the bloodstream by means of the innominate veins.

lymph nodes small oval structures that occur at various points in the LYMPHATICS. They are found grouped in several parts of the body, including the neck, groin and armpit and their main functions are to remove foreign particles and produce LYMPHOCYTES, important in the IMMUNE response.

lymphocyte a type of white blood cell (LEUCOCYTE) produced in the bone marrow and also present in the SPLEEN, THYMUS GLAND and lymph nodes, which forms a vital component of the immune system. There are two types: B cells and T cells. B cells produce antibodies and search out and bind with particular antigens. T cells circulate through the thymus gland, where they differentiate. When they contact an antigen, large numbers of T cells are generated which secrete chemical compounds to assist the B cells in destroying e.g. bacteria.

lymphocytosis when the blood contains an increased number of lymphocytes, as during many diseases or lymphocytic LEUKAEMIA.

lymphoedema the build-up of LYMPH in soft tissues, causing swelling. It may be due to obstruction of the vessels by parasites, tumour or inflammation. A secondary form of lymphoedema may occur after removal of lymph vessels in surgery, or by blocking. The condition occurs most in the legs and treatment comprises use of elastic bandages and DIURETIC drugs.

lymphography *see* **lymphangiography**.

lymphoid tissues tissues that are involved in the formation of lymph, lymphocytes and antibodies, such as the spleen, thymus and lymph nodes.

lymphoma a tumour, usually malignant, of the lymph nodes. Often several lymph nodes become enlarged and subsequent symptoms include fever, anaemia, weakness and weight loss. If much of the lymphoid tissue is involved, there may be enlargement of the liver and spleen. Life expectancy is often very low, although treatment with drugs often produces a marked response. Radiotherapy may be used for localized varieties. *See also* HODGKIN'S DISEASE.

lymphosarcoma a tumour of the lymphatics resulting in enlargement of the glands, spleen and liver. In general, an older term applied to lymphomas other than HODGKIN'S DISEASE.

lysis the destruction of cells by antibodies called *lysins*, thus haemolysis is the break-up of red blood cells by haemolysin. Also, more generally, the destruction of cells or tissues due to breakdown of the cell membranes.

lysozyme an enzyme present in tears, in nasal secretions and on the skin, that has an antibacterial action (by breaking the cell wall of the bacterium). Lysozyme also occurs in the white of eggs.

M

macrocephaly an abnormal enlargement of the head when compared with the rest of the body. *See* MICROCEPHALY, HYDROCEPHALUS.

macrocyte a red blood cell (erythrocyte) which is abnormally large. Macrocytes are characteristic of PERNICIOUS ANAEMIA.

macrocytosis the condition in which abnormally large red blood cells (erythrocytes) are present in the blood. It is characteristic of macrocytic anaemias such as those caused by the deficiency of vitamin B_{12} (*see* CYANOCOBALAMIN and PERNICIOUS ANAEMIA) and folic acid. Macrocytes are also produced in those anaemias in which there is an increased rate of production of erythrocytes.

macrophage a large scavenger cell (PHAGOCYTE), numbers of which are found in various tissues and organs, including the LIVER, SPLEEN, BONE MARROW, LYMPH NODES, CONNECTIVE TISSUE and the *microglia* of the CENTRAL NERVOUS SYSTEM. They remove foreign bodies such as bacteria from blood and tissues. *Fixed macrophages* remain in one place in the connective tissue, *free microphages* are able to migrate between cells and gather at sites of infection to remove bacteria and other foreign material.

macula a small area or spot of tissue that is distinct from the surrounding region e.g. the *yellow spot* in the retina of the eye.

macules spots of small pigmented areas in the skin, which may be thickened. They appear as a result of pregnancy, sunburn, eczema or psoriasis, and may be symptomatic of other diseases such as syphilis and those affecting internal organs.

malabsorption syndrome a group of diseases in which there is a reduction in the normal absorption of digested food materials in the small intestine. The food materials involved are commonly fats, vitamins, minerals, amino acids and iron. The diseases include COELIAC DISEASE, PANCREATITIS, CYSTIC FIBROSIS, SPRUE and STAGNANT LOOP SYNDROME, and also surgical removal of a part of the small intestine.

malaria an infectious disease caused by the presence of minute parasitic organisms of the genus *Plasmodium* in the blood. The disease is characterized by recurrent bouts of fever and anaemia, the interval between the attacks depending upon the species. The parasite is transmitted to man by the *Anopheles* mosquito, (common in sub-tropical and tropical regions) being present in the salivary glands and passed into the bloodstream of a person when the insect bites. Similarly, the parasite is ingested by the mosquito when it takes a blood meal from an infected person. Efforts to control malaria have centred on destruction of the mosquito and its breeding sites. Once injected into the blood, the organisms concentrate in the liver where they multiply and then re-enter the bloodstream destroying red blood cells. This releases the parasites causing shivering, fever, sweating and anaemia. The process is then repeated, with hours or days between attacks. Drugs are used both to prevent infection, although they may not be totally effective, and to cure the disease once present.

malignant a term used in several ways but commonly referring to a tumour that proliferates rapidly and destroys surrounding healthy tissue, and which can spread via the lymphatic and blood system to other parts of the body. The term is also applied to a more serious form of a disease than the usual one which is life-threatening, such as *malignant smallpox* and malignant HYPERTENSION.

malnutrition a condition caused either by an unbalanced diet, i.e. too much of one type of food at the expense of others, or by an inadequate food intake (*subnutrition*) which can lead to starvation. The condition may also arise due to internal dysfunction e.g. MALABSORPTION or other *metabolic* disturbance within the body.

malposition (*and* **malpresentation**) the situation in which the head of an unborn baby before and near delivery is not in the usual (occipitoanterior) position. In *malposition* the baby is head down but a wider part of the skull is presented to the pelvic opening due to the angle of the head. In *malpresentation* the baby is not head down. Both these conditions prolong and complicate labour and, in the latter case especially, are likely to require delivery by CAESARIAN SECTION.

mammary gland a gland present in the female breast which produces milk after childbirth.

mammography a special X-ray technique used to determine the structure of the breast and useful in the early detection of tumours and in distinguishing between benign and malignant tumours.

mammoplasty plastic surgery of the breasts to decrease or increase size and other shape.

mania a form of mental illness characterized by great excitement and euphoria which then gives way to irritability as in MANIC DEPRESSIVE PSYCHOSIS.

manic depressive psychosis a form of severe mental illness in which there are alternating bouts of MANIA and great depression. During the manic phase, the person may be incoherent in thought and speech and outrageous and sometimes violent in behaviour. Drug treatment is required for both phases of the illness and there seems to be an inherited tendency towards acquiring it. Drugs are also helpful in reducing the frequency of attacks between which the person is normally quite well.

mantoux test a test for the presence of a measure of immunity to tuberculosis. A protein called *tuberculin*, extracted from the tubercle bacilli (bacteria), is injected in a small quantity beneath the skin of the forearm. If an inflamed patch appears within 18–24 hours it indicates that a measure of immunity is present and that the person has been exposed to tuberculosis. The size of the reaction indicates the severity of the original tuberculosis infection, although it does not mean that the person is actively suffering from the disease at that time.

marasmus a wasting condition in infants usually due to defective feeding. The child has a low body weight (less than 75% of normal) and lacks skin fat, and is pale and apathetic. Various disorders and diseases can bring this about, including prolonged vomiting and diarrhoea, organ disease e.g. of the heart, kidneys and lungs, infections and parasitic diseases and MALABSORPTION. Treatment depends upon the cause but the provision and gradual increase of nourishment and fluids is always of primary importance.

Marfan's syndrome an inherited disease of the connective tissue which produces defects in the skeleton, heart and eyes. The affected person is abnormally tall and thin, having spindly, elongated fingers and toes (arachnodactyly),

spine and chest deformities and weak ligaments. Heart defects include a hole in the septum separating the right and left atrium (*atrial septal defect*) and narrowing of the AORTA (coarction of the aorta). The lenses of the eyes are partially dislocated.

mastalgia pain in the breast.

mast cell a large cell, many of which are found in loose connective tissue. The cytoplasm contains numerous granules with chemicals important in the body including histamine, serotonin, heparin and the antibody immunoglobulin E. All are important in allergic and inflammatory responses.

mastectomy surgical removal of the breast, usually performed because of the presence of a tumour. Mastectomy may be *simple,* leaving the skin (and possibly the nipple) so that an artificial breast (prosthesis) can be inserted, or it may be *radical,* in which case the whole breast, pectoral muscles and lymph nodes beneath the armpit are all removed, generally performed because a cancer has spread.

mastication chewing of food in the mouth, the first stage in the digestive process.

mastitis inflammation of the breast, usually caused by bacterial infection during breast-feeding, the organisms responsible gaining access through cracked nipples. *Cystic mastitis* does not involve inflammation, but the presence of cysts (thought to be caused by hormonal factors) causes the breast(s) to be lumpy.

mastoidectomy surgical removal of the inflamed cells in the MASTOID PROCESS of the temporal bone of the skull, which is situated behind the ear, when these have become infected. *See* MASTOIDITIS.

mastoiditis inflammation of the mastoid cells and mastoid antrum, usually caused by bacterial infection, which spreads from the middle ear. Treatment is by means of antibiotic drugs and sometimes surgery. *See* MASTOID PROCESS and MASTOIDECTOMY.

mastoid process a breast-like projection of the temporal bone of the skull, which contains numerous air spaces (mastoid cells) and is situated behind the ear. It provides a point of attachment for some of the neck muscles and communicates with the middle ear through an air-filled channel called the *mastoid antrum. See* MASTOIDITIS.

measles an extremely infectious disease of children caused by a virus and characterized by the presence of a rash. It occurs in epidemics every two or three years. After an incubation period of 10–15 days the initial symptoms are those of a cold with coughing, sneezing and high fever. It is at this stage that the disease is most infectious and spreads from one child to another in airborne droplets before measles has been diagnosed. This is the main factor responsible for the epidemic nature of the disease. Small red spots with a white centre (known as *Koplik spots*) may appear in the mouth on the inside of the cheeks. Then a characteristic rash develops on the skin, spreading from behind the ears and across the face and also affecting other areas. The small red spots may be grouped together in patches and the child's fever is usually at its height while these are developing. The spots and fever gradually decline and no marks are left upon the skin, most children making a good recovery. However, complications can occur, particularly pneumonia and middle-ear infections, which can result in deafness. A vaccine now available has reduced the incidence and severity of measles in the UK.

meatus a passage or opening, e.g. the *external auditory meatus* linking the *pinna* of the outer ear to the eardrum.

meconium the first stools of a newborn baby, which are dark green and slimy and contain bile pigments, mucus and debris from cells and passed during the first two days after birth.

media the middle layer of a tissue or organ. Usually it is applied to the middle layer of the wall of a vein or artery comprising alternating sheaths of smooth muscle and elastic fibres.

mediastinum the space in the chest cavity between the two lungs which contains the heart, aorta, oesophagus, trachea, thymus gland and phrenic nerves.

medication any substance introduced into or on the body for the purposes of medical treatment e.g. drugs and medicated dressings.

medulla refers to the inner portion of a tissue or organ when there are two distinct parts. Examples include the adrenal medulla and the medulla of the kidneys. *Compare* CORTEX.

medulla oblongata the lowest part of the brainstem which extends through the FORAMEN *magnum* to become the upper part of the spinal cord. It contains important centres which govern respiration, circulation, swallowing and salivation.

megaloblast an abnormally large form of any of the cells that go on to produce erythrocytes (red blood cells). In certain forms of anaemia (megaloblastic anaemias) they are found in the bone marrow and their presence is due to a deficiency of vitamin B_{12} or of folic acid. They indicate a failure in the

maturation process of erythrocytes which results in anaemia.

megaloblastic anaemia a blood disorder in which there are a large number of large but immature red blood cells. It is usually found when there is a vitamin B_{12} deficiency or PERNICIOUS ANAEMIA.

megalomania a form of insanity in which a person suffers from delusions of grandeur about his or her greatness and power. It can accompany certain mental illnesses such as schizophrenia.

meiosis a type of cell division which occurs in the maturation process of the gametes (sperm and ova) so that the sex cells eventually contain only half the number of chromosomes of the parent cells from which they are derived. The daughter cells also have genetic variation from the parent cells, brought about by a process known as 'crossing over' which occurs during meiosis. When sperm and ovum fuse at fertilization, the full chromosome number is restored in a unique combination in the embryo. There are two phases of division in meiosis each of which is divided into four stages, namely *prophase, metaphase, anaphase* and *telophase.*

melanin a dark brown pigment found in the skin and hair and also in the choroid layer of the eye. Melanin is contained and produced within cells known as *melanocytes* in the dermis layer of the skin. When the skin is exposed to hot sunshine, more melanin is produced giving a 'suntan'. In dark-skinned races more melanin is produced by greater activity of the melanocytes and it helps to protect the skin from harmful ultraviolet radiation.

melanoma an extremely malignant tumour of the melanocytes, the cells in the skin which produce melanin. Melanomas are also found, although less commonly, in the mucous membranes and in the eye. There is a link between the occurrence of melanoma of the skin and exposure to harmful ultraviolet light during sunbathing. A highly malignant form can also arise from the pigmented cells of moles. Melanoma can be successfully treated by surgery if it is superficial and caught at an early stage. However, it commonly spreads, especially to the liver and lymph nodes, in which case the outlook is poor. The incidence of malignant melanoma is increasing and has attracted much attention in connection with the formation of holes in the ozone layer, which screens the earth from harmful UV radiation. Most experts recommend that people should cover exposed skin, use sunscreen creams and avoid the sun at the hottest part of the day.

membrane a thin composite layer of lipoprotein surrounding an individual cell or a thin layer of tissue surrounding an organ, lining a cavity or tube or separating tissues and organs within the body.

memory the function of the brain which enables past events to be stored and remembered. It is a highly complex function, which probably involves many areas of the brain including the temporal lobes. Memory involves three stages, comprising registration, storage and recall (of information). Information is committed either to the short-term or the long-term memory. Most forgetfulness involves the retrieval of information, and memory of a particular item is improved if the context in which it was registered and stored can be recreated. This technique is used by the police when trying to gain information from witnesses in the field of reconstruction of a crime.

Ménière's disease a disease first described by the Frenchman, Prosper Ménière in 1861, which affects the inner ear, causing deafness and TINNITUS (ringing in the ears), vertigo, vomiting and sweating. The disease is most common in middle-aged men, with severe attacks of vertigo followed by vomiting. The time interval between attacks varies from one week to several months, but the deafness gradually becomes more pronounced. The symptoms are caused by an over-accumulation of fluid in the labyrinths of the inner ears, but the reason for this is not known. Treatment is by a variety of drugs and surgery, neither of which are completely successful.

meninges the three connective tissue membranes which surround the spinal cord and brain. The outermost layer (meninx) is called the *dura mater,* which is fibrous, tough and inelastic, and also called the *pachymeninx*, closely lining the inside of the skull and helping to protect the brain. It is thicker than the middle layer, the *arachnoid mater*, which surrounds the brain. The innermost layer, the *pia mater*, is thin and delicate and lines the brain. Cerebrospinal fluid circulates between it and the arachnoid mater and both these inner layers are richly supplied with blood vessels which supply the surface of the brain and skull. These two inner membranes are sometimes collectively called the *pia-arachnoid* or *leptomeninges.*

meningioma a slow-growing tumour affecting the MENINGES of the brain or spinal cord, which exerts pressure on the underlying nervous tissue. It may cause paraplegia if present in the spinal cord or other losses of sensation. In the brain it causes increasing neurological disability. A meningioma can be present for many years without being detected. The usual treatment is surgical removal if the tumour is accessible. Malignant meningiomas, known as *meningeal sarcomas*, can invade surrounding tissues. These are treated by means of surgery and also radiotherapy.

meningitis inflammation of the meninges (membranes) of the brain (*cerebral meningitis*) or spinal cord (*spinal meningitis*), or the disease may affect both regions. Meningitis may affect the *dura mater* membrane, in which case it is known as *pachymeningitis*, although this is relatively uncommon. It often results as a secondary infection due to the presence of disease elsewhere, as in the case of *tuberculous meningitis* and *syphilitic meningitis*. Meningitis which affects the other two membranes (the *pia-arachnoid* membranes) is known as *leptomeningitis*. This is more common and may be either a primary or secondary infection. Meningitis is also classified according to its causal organism and may be either viral or bacterial. *Viral meningitis* is fairly mild and as it does not respond to drugs, treatment is by means of bed rest until recovery takes place. *Bacterial meningitis* is much more common and is caused by the organisms responsible for tuberculosis, pneumonia and syphilis. Also, the *meningococcus* type of bacteria causes one of the commonest forms of the disease, *meningococcal meningitis*. The symptoms are a severe headache, sensitivity to light and sound, muscle rigidity especially affecting the neck, KERNIG'S SIGN, vomiting, paralysis, coma and death. These are caused by inflammation of the meninges and by a rise in INTRACRANIAL PRESSURE. One of the features of meningitis is that there is a change in the constituents and appearance of the cerebrospinal fluid, and the infective organism can usually be isolated from it and identified. The onset of the symptoms can be very rapid and death can also follow swiftly. Treatment is by means of antibiotic drugs and sulphonamides.

menopause (*or* **climacteric**) this is the time in a woman's life when the ovaries no longer release an egg cell every month and menstruation ceases. The woman is normally no longer able to bear a child and the age at which the menopause occurs is usually between 45 and 55. The menopause may be marked by a gradual decline in menstruation or in its frequency, or it may cease abruptly. There is a disturbance in the balance of sex hormones and this causes a number of physical symptoms including palpitations, hot flushes, sweats, vaginal dryness, loss of libido and depression. In the long term, there is a gradual loss of bone (OSTEOPOROSIS) in postmenopausal women, which leads to greater risk of fractures, especially of the femur in the elderly. All these symptoms are relieved by HRT (hormone replacement therapy) involving oestrogen and progesterone, which is now generally recognized to be of great benefit.

menorrhagia when menstruation is unusally long or heavy, which may result in anaemia.

menstrual cycle and menstruation the cyclical nature of the reproductive life of a sexually mature female. One OVUM develops and matures within a GRAAFIAN FOLLICLE in one of the ovaries. When mature, the follicle ruptures to release the egg which passes down the FALLOPIAN TUBE to the uterus. The ruptured follicle becomes a temporary ENDOCRINE GLAND called the CORPUS LUTEUM, which secretes the HORMONE, PROGESTERONE. Under the influence of progesterone the uterus wall (ENDOMETRIUM) thickens and its blood supply increases in readiness for the implantation of a fertilized egg. If the egg is not fertilized and there is no pregnancy, the thickened endometrium is shed, along with a flow of blood through the vagina (menstruation). The usual age at which menstruation starts is 12–15 but it can be as early as 10, or as late as 20. The duration varies and can be anything from 2–8 days, the whole cycle usually occupying about 29–30 days.

mercaptopurine a type of ANTIMETABOLITE, CYTOTOXIC drug which prevents the proliferation of malignant cancer cells and is used in the treatment of certain kinds of LEUKAEMIA, and Crohn's disease (a disease of the digestive tract).

mesencephalon otherwise known as the mid-brain, which connects the PONS and CEREBELLUM with the *cerebral hemispheres*.

mesentery a double layer of the peritoneal membrane (PERITONEUM) which is attached to the back wall of the abdomen. It supports a number of abdominal organs including the stomach, small intestine, spleen and pancreas and contains associated nerves, lymph and blood vessels.

mesothelioma a malignant tumour of the PLEURA of the chest cavity and also of the PERICARDIUM or PERITONEUM. It is usually associated with exposure to asbestos dust but may arise independently with no known cause. Most mesotheliomas are in sites which render them inoperable, and chemotherapy and radiotherapy are used but often with limited success.

metabolism the sum of all the physical and chemical changes within cells and tissues that maintain life and growth. The breakdown processes which occur are known as *catabolic* (*catabolism*), and those which build materials up are called *anabolic* (*anabolism*). The term may also be applied to describe one particular set of changes e.g. *protein metabolism*. *Basal metabolism* is the minimum amount of energy required to maintain the body's vital processes e.g. heartbeat and respiration and is usually assessed by means of various measurements taken while a person is at rest.

metacarpal bone one of the five bones of the middle of the hand, between the PHALANGES of the fingers and the CARPAL bones of the wrist, forming the *metacarpus*. The heads of the metacarpal bones form the knuckles. *See* HAND.

metaplasia an abnormal change which has taken place within a tissue e.g. *myeloid metaplasia*, where elements of bone marrow develop within the spleen and liver. Also, *squamous metaplasia*, which involves a change in the EPITHELIUM lining the BRONCHI of the lungs.

metastasis the process by which a malignant tumour spreads to a distant part of the body, and also refers to the secondary growth that results from this. The spread is accomplished by means of three routes: the blood circulation, lymphatic system and across body cavities.

metatarsal bone one of the five bones in the foot lying between the toes and the TARSAL bones of the ankle, together forming the *metatarsus*. The metatarsal bones are equivalent to the METACARPAL BONES in the hand.

methadone a strong ANALGESIC and narcotic drug resembling morphine which is used in pain relief and as a cough suppressant. Additionally, it is used as a heroin substitute in the treatment of addiction.

methyldopa a drug that is used to reduce high blood pressure, especially in pregnancy.

metritis inflammation of the womb.

MHC major histocompatibility complex — a group of genes located on chromosome 6 which code for the HLA ANTIGENS.

microbiology the scientific study of microorganisms, i.e. those that are too small to be studied with the naked eye. They include viruses and bacteria, some of which are major causes of disease in man and animals.

microcephaly the condition in which there is abnormal smallness of the head compared to the rest of the body. *See* MACROCEPHALY.

microsurgery surgery performed with the aid of an operating microscope using high-precision miniaturized instruments. It is routine for some operations on the eye, larynx and ear and increasingly in areas inaccessible to normal surgery e.g. parts of the brain and spinal cord. Microsurgery is also performed in the rejoining of severed limbs, fingers, toes, etc., where very fine suturing of minute blood vessels and nerves is required.

microwave therapy the use of very short wavelength electromagnetic waves in the procedure known as DIATHERMY.

micturition the act of urination.

middle ear *see* **ear**.

midwifery the profession devoted to the care of mothers during pregnancy and childbirth and of mothers and babies during the period after delivery. A member of the profession is known as a *midwife*.

migraine a very severe throbbing headache, usually on one side of the head, which is often accompanied by disturbances in vision, nausea and vomiting. Migraine is a common condition and seems to be triggered by any one or several of a number of factors. These include anxiety, fatigue, watching television or video screens, loud noises, flickering lights (e.g. strobe lights) and certain foods, such as cheese and chocolate or alcoholic drinks. The cause is unknown but thought to involve constriction followed by dilation of blood vessels in the brain and an outpouring of fluid into surrounding tissues. The attack can last up to 24 hours and treatment is by means of bed rest in a darkened, quiet room and pain-relieving drugs.

miscarriage *see* **abortion**.

mitobronitol a type of drug used in the treatment of leukaemia which prevents the growth of cancer cells.

mitochondrion a tiny rod-like structure, numbers of which are present in the CYTOPLASM of every CELL. *Mitochondria* contain enzymes and ATP involved in cell METABOLISM.

mitosis the type of cell division undergone by most body cells by means of which growth and repair of tissues can take place. Mitosis involves the division of a single cell to produce two genetically identical daughter cells each with the full number of chromosomes. *Compare* MEIOSIS.

mitral incompetence (or **mitral regurgitation**) this is the condition in which the MITRAL VALVE of the heart is defective and allows blood to leak back from the left ventricle into the left atrium. It is often caused by rheumatic fever, as a congenital defect or as a result of a heart attack. The left ventricle is forced to work harder and enlarges, but eventually may be unable to cope and this can result in left-sided heart failure. Other symptoms include atrial FIBRILLATION, breathlessness and embolism. Drug treatment and/or surgery to replace the defective valve may be required (*mitral prosthesis*). *See* MITRAL STENOSIS *and* HEART.

mitral stenosis the condition in which the opening between the left atrium and left ventricle is narrowed due to scarring and adhesion of the MITRAL VALVE. This scarring is often caused by rheumatic fever and the symptoms are similar to those of MITRAL INCOMPETENCE, accompanied also by a *diastolic murmur*. It is treated surgically by widening the stenosis (mitral VALVOTOMY) or by valve replacement — *mitral prosthesis*.

mitral valve (formerly known as the *bicuspid valve*) this is located between the atrium and ventricle of the left side of the heart, attached to the walls at the opening between the two. It has two cusps or flaps and normally allows blood to pass into the ventricle from the atrium, but prevents any backflow.

MMR vaccine a recently introduced vaccine (1988) which protects against MEASLES, MUMPS and RUBELLA (German measles) and is normally given to children during their second year.

mole a dark-coloured pigmented spot in the skin which is usually brown. It may be flat or raised and may have hair protruding from it. Some types can become malignant, *see* MELANOMA.

monocyte the largest type of white blood cell (leucocyte) with a kidney-shaped nucleus found in the blood and lymph. It ingests foreign bodies such as bacteria and tissue particles.

mononucleosis *see* **glandular fever**.

monozygotic twins (*or* **identical twins**) these are children who are derived from a single fertilized egg.

morbidity the state of being diseased, the *morbidity rate* being expressed as the number of cases of a disease occurring within a particular number of the population.

moribund dying.

morning sickness vomiting and nausea, most common during the first three months of pregnancy.

morphine a narcotic and very strong analgesic drug which is an alkaloid derived from opium. It is used for the relief of severe pain but tolerance and dependence may occur. *See* ADDICTION.

motion sickness (*or* **travel sickness**) produces

symptoms of vomiting, nausea and headache caused by travel via car, boat or aeroplane. The symptoms are caused by overstimulation of the balance mechanism in the inner ear through numerous changes in position and an inability to rapidly adjust to them. Although unpleasant, the symptoms are generally not serious and a number of drugs are used to alleviate the condition or to try to prevent its onset.

motor nerve a nerve containing motor neurone fibres which carries electrical impulses outwards from the central nervous system to a muscle or gland to bring about a response there.

motor neurone one of the units or fibres of a MOTOR NERVE. An *upper motor neurone* is contained entirely within the central nervous system having its cell body in the brain and its *axon* (a long process) extending into the spinal cord where it SYNAPSES with other neurones. A *lower motor neurone* has its cell body in the spinal cord or brainstem and an axon that runs outwards via a spinal or cranial MOTOR NERVE to an effector muscle or gland, *see* NERVE.

motorneurone disease a disease of unknown cause which most commonly occurs in middle age and is a degenerative condition affecting elements of the central nervous system (i.e. the corticospinal fibres, motor nuclei in the brain stem and the cells of the anterior horn of the spinal cord). It causes increasing paralysis involving nerves and muscles and is ultimately fatal.

mouth the opening which forms the beginning of the alimentary canal and in which food enters the digestive process. The entrance is guarded by the lips, behind which lie the upper and lower sets of teeth embedded in the jaw. The roof of the mouth is called the palate, the front part being hard and immobile while behind lies the mobile soft palate. The tongue is situated behind the lower teeth and SALIVARY GLANDS which are present secrete saliva into the mouth through small ducts. Saliva contains the enzyme ptyalin, which begins the breakdown of starch while the chewing action of the teeth and manipulation with the tongue reduces the food to a more manageable size so that it can be swallowed.

mucosa another term for MUCOUS MEMBRANE.

mucous membrane a moist membrane which lines many tubes and cavities within the body and is lubricated with MUCUS. The structure of a mucous membrane varies according to its site and they are found, for example, lining the mouth, respiratory, urinary and digestive tracts. Each has a surface EPITHELIUM, a layer containing various cells and glands which secrete mucus. Beneath this lie connective tissue and muscle layers, the *laminae propria* and *muscularis mucosa* respectively, the whole forming a pliable layer.

mucus a slimy substance secreted by MUCOUS MEMBRANES as a lubricant, and composed mainly of glycoproteins of which the chief one is *mucin*. It is a clear viscous fluid which may contain enzymes and has a protective function. It is normally present in small amounts but the quantity increases if inflammation and/or infection is present.

multiple births twins, triplets, quadruplets, quintuplets and sextuplets born to one mother. While naturally-occurring twins are relatively common, other multiple births are normally rare. Their incidence has increased with the advent of *fertility drugs*, although often some of the infants do not survive.

multiple sclerosis (*or* **MS**) a disease of the brain and spinal cord which affects the MYELIN sheaths of nerves and disrupts their function. It usually affects people below the age of 40 and its cause is unknown, but is the subject of much research. The disease is characterized by the presence of patches of hardened (sclerotic) connective tissue irregularly scattered through the brain and spinal cord. At first the fatty part of the nerve sheaths breaks down and is absorbed, leaving bare nerve fibres, and then connective tissue is laid down. Symptoms depend upon the site of the patches in the central nervous system and the disease is characterized by periods of progression and remission. However, they include unsteady gait and apparent clumsiness, tremor of the limbs, involuntary eye movements, speech disorders, bladder dysfunction and paralysis. The disease can progress very slowly but generally there is a tendency for the paralysis to become more marked.

mumps an infectious disease of childhood usually occurring in those between the ages of 5 and 15, and caused by a virus which produces inflammation of the *parotid salivary glands*. The incubation period is 2–3 weeks, followed by symptoms including feverishness, headache, sore throat and vomiting, before or along with a swelling of the parotid gland on one side of the face. The swelling may be confined to one side or spread to the other side of the face and also may go on to include the *submaxillary* and *sublingual salivary glands* beneath the jaw. Generally after a few days the swelling subsides and the child recovers but remains infectious until the glands have returned to normal. The infection may spread to the pancreas and, in 15–30% of males, to the testicles. In adult men this infection can cause sterility. More rarely, inflammation in females can affect the ovaries and breasts, and MENINGITIS is another occasional complication, especially in adults. A protective vaccine is now available, see MMR.

Münchausen's syndrome a rare mental disorder in which a person tries to obtain hospital treatment for a non-existent illness. The person is adept at simulating symptoms and may self-induce these or cause self-inflicted injury to add authenticity. The person may end up having unnecessary treatment and operations and is resistant to psychotherapy.

murmur a characteristic sound which can be heard using a STETHOSCOPE, caused by uneven blood flow through the heart or blood vessels when these are diseased or damaged. Heart murmurs can also be present in normal individuals, especially children, without indicating disease. Murmurs are classified as *diastolic* (when the ventricles are relaxed and filling with blood) or *systolic* (when they are contracting).

muscle the contractile tissue of the body which produces movements of various structures both internally and externally. There are three types of muscle: 1. *striated* or *voluntary muscle* which has a striped appearance when viewed under a microscope and is attached to the skeleton. It is called 'voluntary' because it is under the control of the will and produces movements, for example, in the limbs. 2. *smooth* or *involuntary muscle* which has a plain appearance when viewed microscopically and is not under conscious control but is supplied by the autonomic nervous system. Examples are the muscles which supply the digestive and respiratory tracts. 3. *cardiac muscle*, the specialized muscle of the walls of the heart, which is composed of a network of branching, elongated fibres which rejoin and interlock, each having a nucleus. It has a somewhat striated appearance and where there are junctions between fibres, irregular transverse bands occur, known as *intercalated discs*. This muscle is involuntary and contracts and expands rhythmically throughout a person's life. However, rate of heartbeat is affected by activity within the vagus nerve.

muscle cramp *see* cramp.

muscle relaxants substances or drugs which cause muscles to relax. They are mainly used in anaesthesia to produce relaxation or paralysis of muscles while surgery is being carried out e.g. tubocurarine and gallamine. Others are administered to counteract muscular spasms, which are a feature of spastic conditions such as PARKINSON'S DISEASE e.g. diazepam.

muscular dystrophy (*or myopathy*) this is any of a group of diseases which involve wasting of muscles and in which a hereditary factor is involved. The disease is classified according to the groups of muscles which it affects and the age of the person involved. The disease usually appears in childhood and causes muscle fibres to degenerate and to be replaced by fatty and fibrous tissue. The affected muscles eventually lose all power of contraction causing great disability and affected children are prone to chest and other infections which may prove fatal in their weakened state. The cause of the disease is not entirely understood but the commonest form, *Duchenne muscular dystrophy*, is sex-linked and recessive. Hence, it nearly always affects boys, with the mother as a carrier, and appears in very early childhood. *See also* SEX-LINKED DISORDERS.

mutagen any substance or agent which increases the rate of mutation in body cells, examples being various chemicals, viruses and radiation. Mutagens increase the number rather than the range of mutations beyond that which might be expected.

mutation a change which takes place in the DNA, (the genetic material) of the CHROMOSOMES of a cell, which is normally a rare event. The change may involve the structure or number of whole chromosomes or take place at one GENE site. Mutations are caused by faulty replication of the cell's genetic material at cell division. If normal body (*somatic*) cells are involved there may be a growth of altered cells or a tumour, or these may be attacked and destroyed by the immune system. In any event, this type of mutation cannot be passed on — if the sex cells (ova or sperm) are involved in the mutation, the alteration may be passed on to the offspring producing a changed characteristic.

mutism the refusal or inability to speak, which may result from brain damage or psychological factors. Speechlessness is most common in those who have been born deaf (deaf-mutism).

myalgia pain in a muscle.

myalgic encephalomyelitis (*or ME*) a disorder characterized by muscular pain, fatigue, general depression and loss of memory and concentration. The cause is not understood, but seems to follow on from viral infections such as influenza, hence it is also called post-viral fatigue syndrome. Recovery may be prolonged and there is no specific treatment.

myasthenia gravis a serious and chronic condition of uncertain cause which may be an autoimmune disease. It is more common among young people, especially women (men tend to be affected over 40). Rest and avoidance of unnecessary exertion is essential to conserve muscle strength as there is a reduction in the ability of the neurotransmitter, ACETYLCHOLINE, to effect muscle contraction. There is a weakening which affects skeletal muscles and those for breathing and swallowing, etc. However, there is little wasting of the muscles themselves. It seems the body produces antibodies which interfere with the acetylcholine receptors in the muscle, and that the THYMUS GLAND may be the original source of these receptors. Surgical removal of the thymus gland is one treatment. Other treatment is by means of drugs, e.g. Pyridodstigmine, which inhibit the activity of the enzyme *cholinesterase*, which destroys excess acetylcholine. Other *immunosuppressive* drugs are used to suppress production of the antibodies which interfere with the receptors.

mycosis any disease which is caused by fungi, e.g. thrush and ringworm.

myelin a sheath of phospholipid and protein that surrounds the axons of some NEURONS. It is formed by specialized cells known as *Schwann cells*, each of which encloses the axon in concentric folds of its cell membrane. These folds then condense to form myelin, the neuron then being described as *myelinated*. Schwann cells produce myelin at regular intervals along the length of the axon and electrical impulses pass more rapidly along myelinated nerve fibres than along non-myelinated ones.

myelitis 1. any inflammatory condition of the spinal cord such as often occurs in MULTIPLE SCLEROSIS. 2. bone marrow inflammation. *See* OSTEOMYELITIS.

myelofibrosis a disease, the cause of which is unknown, in which FIBROSIS takes place within the bone marrow, and many immature red and white blood cells appear in the circulation because of the resultant anaemia. There is an enlargement of the SPLEEN, and blood-producing (myeloid) tissue is abnormally found both here and in the liver.

myelography a specialized X-ray technique involving the injection of a radio-opaque dye into the central canal of the spinal cord in order to distinguish the presence of disease. The X-rays are called *myelograms*.

myeloid means like or relating to bone marrow or, like a *myelocyte*. This is a cell which is an immature type of granulocyte responsible for the production of white blood cells.

myeloma a malignant disease of the bone marrow in which tumours are present in more than one bone at the same time. The bones may show 'holes' when X-rayed due to typical deposits, and certain abnormal proteins may be present in the blood and urine. Treatment is by chemotherapy and radiotherapy. *Myelomatosis* is the production of myeloma, which is usually fatal.

myocardial infarction *see* **coronary thrombosis**.

myocarditis inflammation of the muscle in the wall of the heart.

myocardium the middle of the three layers of the HEART wall, which is the thick, muscular area. The outer layer is the *epicardium* (forming part of the *pericardium*) and the inner the *endocardium*.

myoglobin an iron-containing pigment which is similar to HAEMOGLOBIN, and occurs in muscle cells. It binds oxygen from haemoglobin and releases it in the muscle cells.

myoma a benign tumour in muscle, often in the WOMB.

myomectomy surgical removal of FIBROIDS from the muscular wall of the WOMB (UTERUS).

myometrium the muscular tissue of the WOMB, composed of smooth muscle and surrounding the ENDOMETRIUM. Its contractions are influenced by the presence of certain hormones and are especially strong during LABOUR.

myopathy *see* **muscular dystrophy**.

myopia short-sightedness, corrected by wearing spectacles with concave lenses.

myxoedema a disease caused by underactivity of the thyroid gland (HYPOTHYROIDISM). There is a characteristic development of a dry, coarse skin and swelling of subcutaneous tissue. There is intellectual impairment, with slow speech and mental dullness, lethargy, muscle pain, weight gain and constipation. The hair thins and there may be increased sensitivity to cold. As the symptoms are caused by the deficiency of thyroid hormones, treatment consists of giving THYROXINE in suitable amounts.

N

naevus *see* **birthmark**.

nail the horny structure at the end of a finger or toe. It is formed of keratin, which is derived from the epidermis (superficial layer of the skin made up from an outer dead part and a living cellular part beneath). The *body* is the part of the nail showing, while the *root* is beneath the skin. The pale crescent is called the *lunula.*

narcolepsy a condition whereby a person has a tendency to fall asleep a few times per day for several minutes or hours. The attacks may occur when in quiet surroundings or may be induced by laughter and the person may be woken easily. It is thought that it may be an immune-related disease and lasts for life. Drugs (amphetamine type) may be taken to ensure attacks do not occur at certain times but regular doses are considered ill-advised in view of possible mental effects.

narcosis a state induced by narcotic drugs in which a person is completely unconscious or nearly so but can respond a little to stimuli. It is due to the depressant action of the drugs on the body.

narcotic a drug that leads to a stupor and complete loss of awareness. In particular, opiates derived from morphine or produced synthetically produce various conditions: deep sleep, euphoria, mood changes and mental confusion. In addition, respiration and the cough reflex are depressed and muscle spasms may be produced. Because of the dependence resulting from the use of morphine-like compounds, they have largely been replaced as sleeping drugs.

nasal cavity one of two cavities in the nose, divided by a SEPTUM, which lie between the roof of the mouth and the floor of the cranium.

nasogastric tube a small-diameter tube passed through the nose into the stomach for purposes of introducing food or drugs or removing fluid (ASPIRATION).

nausea a feeling of being about to vomit. It may be due to motion sickness, early pregnancy, pain, food poisoning or a virus.

nebula a slight opacity or scar of the cornea that does not obstruct vision but may create a haziness.

Also ,an oily substance that is applied in a fine spray.

nebulizer a device for producing a fine spray. Many inhaled drugs are administered in this way, and it is an effective method of delivering a concentrated form of medication e.g. bronchodilators.

necropsy an autopsy (post mortem) which results in little disfigurement.

necrosis death of tissue in a localized area or organ, caused by disease, injury or loss of blood supply.

neomycin an antibiotic, usually applied as a cream, which is effective against a wide spectrum of bacteria. Its main use is as a skin treatment.

neonatal term meaning relating to the first 28 days of life.

neoplasm a new and abnormal growth of cells, i.e. a tumour, which may be benign or malignant.

nephrectomy surgical removal of all (*radical*) or part (*partial*) of the kidney. It may be necessary to remove a tumour (in which case the surrounding fat and adrenal gland will probably also be removed) or to drain an ABSCESS.

nephritis inflammation of the KIDNEY, which may be due to one of several causes. Types of nephritis include glomerulonephritis (when the glomerulus is affected), acute nephritis, hereditary nephritis, etc.

nephron *see* **kidney**.

nephrotic syndrome a disorder of the kidneys in which the blood pressure is raised and there is excess protein in the urine and low levels of albumin in the blood. Nephrotic syndrome is usually secondary to another condition e.g. DIABETES MELLITUS, LEUKAEMIA or SYSTEMIC LUPUS ERYTHEMATOSUS.

nerve a bundle of nerve fibres comprising NEURONS and glial (supporting) cells (*see* GLIA), all contained in a fibrous sheath, the perineurium. Motor nerves carry (efferent) impulses in motor neurons from the brain (or spinal cord) to muscles or glands and a sensory nerve carries (afferent) impulses in sensory neurons from sensory organs to the brain or spinal cord. Most large nerves are mixed nerves containing both motor and sensory nerves.

nerve block (*or* **conduction anaesthesia**) the technique of blocking sensory nerves sending pain impulses to the brain, thus creating anaesthesia in that part of the body. It is achieved by injecting the tissue around a nerve with local anaesthetic (e.g. LIGNOCAINE) to permit minor operations.

nerve impulse the transmission of information along a nerve fibre by electrical activity which has its basis in the formation of chemical substances and the generation of the *action potential*. This is a change in electrical potential across the cell membrane (between inside and outside) of an axon (nerve cell) as an impulse moves along. It is a temporary and localized occurrence caused by a stimulus which travels down the axon and the voltage is caused by sodium ions (Na$^+$) entering the axon and changing the potential across the cell membrane from -65mV to +45mV (millivolts). When the stimulus has passed the membrane is restored to its resting potential. When a stimulus is continually received several hundred pulses travel along the nerve per second.

nerve injury nerves may be injured by being severed. Pressure may damage a nerve directly or push it against a bone. Damage to a sensory nerve results in a lack of or lessening in sensation, while paralysis of muscles will result from damage to the associated motor nerve.

nervous system the complete system of tissues and cells, including NERVES, NEURONS, SYNAPSES and receptors (a special cell sensitive to a particular stimulus which then sends an impulse through the nervous system). The nervous system operates through the transmission of impulses (*see* NERVE IMPULSE) that are conducted rapidly to and from muscles, organs etc. It consists of the central nervous system (brain and spinal cord) and the peripheral nervous system which includes the cranial and spinal nerves. *See* AUTONOMIC NERVOUS SYSTEM.

neuralgia strictly, pain in some part or the whole of a nerve (without any physical change in the nerve), but used more widely to encompass pain following the course of a nerve or its branches, whatever the cause. Neuralgia often occurs at the same time each day and is frequently felt as an agonizing pain. It occurs in several forms and is named accordingly, e.g. SCIATICA, trigeminal neuralgia (affecting the face, *see* TRIGEMINAL NERVE) and intercostal neuralgia (affecting the ribs). Treatment often involves the application of ointments, and the taking of painkilling drugs. If such treatments do not bring relief, it is possible

to freeze the nerve or destroy part of it by surgery.

neuritis inflammation of a nerve or nerves which may be due to inflammation from nearby tissues, or a more general condition in which the nerve fibres degenerate. This latter condition (*polyneuritis*) is due to a systemic poison such as alcohol or long-term exposure to solvents such as naphtha.

neuroendocrine system one of a number of dual, control systems regulating bodily functions through the action of nerves and hormones.

neuroglia the fine web of tissues that support nerve fibres. *See* GLIA.

neurohormone a hormone that is secreted by the nerve endings of specialized nerve cells (i.e. neurosecretory cells) and not by an endocrine gland. They are secreted into the bloodstream or directly into the target tissue. Included are NORADRENALINE and VASOPRESSIN (produced in the HYPOTHALAMUS and secreted by the pituitary gland, active in the control of water reabsorption in the kidneys).

neuroleptic any drug that induces neurolepsis, i.e. reduced activity, some indifference to the surroundings and possibly sleep. They are used to quieten disturbed patients suffering from delirium, brain damage or behavioural disturbances.

neurology the subdiscipline of medicine that involves the study of the brain, spinal cord and peripheral nerves, their diseases and conditions and the treatment of those conditions.

neuromuscular blockade the blocking of impulses at the NEUROMUSCULAR JUNCTION to paralyse a part of the body for surgery. *See also* NERVE BLOCK.

neuromuscular junction the area of membrane between a muscle cell and a motor NEURON forming a SYNAPSE between the two. Nerve impulses travel down the neuron and each releases ACETYLCHOLINE, which depolarizes the enlarged end of the neuron (the motor end plate) slightly. These small depolarizations are totalled until a threshold of -50mV is reached, and this results in the production of an ACTION POTENTIAL that crosses the synapse into the muscle fibre, producing a muscle contraction.

neuron a nerve cell, vital in the transmission of impulses. Each cell has an enlarged portion (the cell body) from which extends the long, thin axon for carrying impulses away. Shorter, more numerous dendrites receive impulses. The transmission of impulses is faster in axons that are covered in a sheath of MYELIN.

neuropathy any disease that affects the peripheral

nerves, whether singly (mononeuropathy) or more generally (polyneuropathy). The symptoms depend upon the type and the nerves affected.

neurosis (*plural* **neuroses**) a mental disorder, but one where the patient retains a grasp on reality (unlike PSYCHOSIS). Neuroses may be due to depression, phobia, hysteria or hypochondria. Anxiety is the commonest version, although this does respond to treatment. In practice, the boundary between neurosis and psychosis is vague.

neurosurgery surgical treatment of the brain, spinal cord or nerves, including dealing with head injuries, intracranial pressure, haemorrhages, infections and the treatment of tumours.

neurotic someone afflicted with a neurosis. More generally, a nervous person who acts on emotions more than reason.

neurotransmitter one of several chemical substances released in minute quantities by axon tips into the SYNAPSE to enable a nerve impulse to cross. It diffuses across the space and may depolarize the opposite membrane allowing the production of an action potential (*see* NERVE IMPULSE). Outside the central nervous system ACETYLCHOLINE is a major neurotransmitter, and NORADRENALINE is released in the SYMPATHETIC NERVOUS SYSTEM. Acetylcholine and noradrenaline also operate within the central nervous system, as does DOPAMINE, amongst others.

neutropenia a fall in the number of neutrophils (a type of granulocyte or white blood cell) in the blood, resulting from bone-marrow tumours, acute leukaemia, and other conditions.

nifedipine a drug used in the treatment of ANGINA and high blood pressure.

night blindness (*or* **nyctalopia**) poor vision in dim light or at night due to a deficiency within the cells responsible for such vision (*see* ROD). The cause may be a lack of VITAMIN A in the diet or a congenital defect.

nitrous oxide (formerly called laughing gas) a colourless gas used for anaesthesia over short periods. Longer effects require its use with oxygen and it may be used as a 'carrier' for stronger anaesthetics.

non-steroidal anti-inflammatory drugs (*or* **NSAID**) a large group of drugs used to relieve pain, and also inhibit inflammation. They are used for conditions such as rheumatoid arthritis, sprains, etc., and include aspirin. The main side effect is gastric ulcer or haemorrhage but the synthesis of new compounds has led to some with milder side effects.

noradrenaline (**norepinephrine** in US) a NEUROTRANSMITTER of the SYMPATHETIC NERVOUS SYSTEM, secreted by nerve endings and also the adrenal glands. It is similar to ADRENALINE in structure and function. It increases blood pressure by constricting the vessel, slows the heartbeat and increases breathing both in rate and depth.

nose the olfactory organ, and also a pathway for air entering the body, by which route it is warmed, filtered and moistened before passing into the lungs. The 'external' nose leads to the NASAL CAVITY, which has a mucous membrane with olfactory cells.

notifiable diseases diseases that must be reported to the health authorities to enable rapid control and monitoring to be undertaken. The list varies between countries but in the UK includes acute poliomyelitis, AIDS, cholera, dysentery, food poisoning, measles, meningitis, rabies, rubella, scarlet fever, smallpox, tetanus, typhoid fever, viral hepatitis and whooping cough.

nuclear magnetic resonance an analytical technique based upon the absorption of electromagnetic radiation over specific frequencies for those nuclei that spin about their own axes. The result is a change in orientation of the nuclei and certain elements are particularly susceptible (hydrogen, fluorine and phosphorus). The technique has been developed into a medical imaging tool which can create an image of soft tissues in any part of the body.

nucleic acid a linear molecule that occurs in two forms: DNA (deoxyribonucleic acid) and RNA (ribonucleic acid), composed of four NUCLEOTIDES. DNA is the major part of CHROMOSOMES in the cell nucleus while RNA is found outside the nucleus and is involved in protein synthesis.

nucleotide the basic molecular building block of the nucleic acids RNA and DNA. A nucleotide comprises a five-carbon sugar molecule with a phosphate group and an organic base. The organic base can be a *purine* e.g. adenine and guanine or a *pyrimidine* e.g. cytosine and thymine, as in DNA. In RNA uracil replaces thymine.

nucleus (*plural* **nuclei**) the large organelle (a membrane-bounded cell constituent) that contains the DNA. Unless it is dividing, a nucleolus with RNA is present. During cell division the DNA, which is normally dispersed with protein (as chromatin), forms visible CHROMOSOMES.

O

obesity the accumulation of excess fat in the body, mainly in the subcutaneous tissues, generally caused by eating more food than is necessary to produce the required energy for each day's activity. The effects of obesity are serious, being associated with increased mortality or cause of illness from cardiovascular disease, diabetes, gallbladder complaints, hernia and many other conditions. Treatment involves a low-energy diet but more drastic measures (e.g. stapling of the stomach and wiring of the jaws) may be necessary.

obstetrics the subdiscipline of medicine that deals with pregnancy and childbirth and the period immediately after birth; midwifery.

occipital bone a bone of the SKULL which is shaped like a saucer and forms the back of the cranium and part of its base. Arising from the base of thin bone are two occipital condyles that articulate with the first cervical vertebrae (the atlas) of the spinal column.

occlusion the closing or blocking of an organ or duct. In dentistry it is the way the teeth meet when the jaws are closed.

occult a term meaning not easily seen, not visible to the naked eye.

occupational diseases (*or* **industrial diseases**) diseases, specific to a particular occupation, to which workers in that occupation are prone. There are many lung conditions including: PNEUMOCONIOSIS (from coal mining), SILICOSIS (mining, stone dressing, etc.), ASBESTOSIS and FARMER'S LUNG (from fungal spores). In addition, there are dangers from excessive noise, irritant chemicals, occupations resulting in musculoskeletal disorders, decompression sickness (*see also* BENDS) radiation and infections from either animals or humans.

occupational therapy the treatment of both psychiatric and physical conditions by encouraging patients to undertake activities to enable them use what skills they have and to achieve some independence and self-confidence. The activities may vary enormously from craft and woodwork to social and community activities.

oculomotor nerve either of a pair of cranial nerves which are involved in eye movements including movement of the eyeball, and alterations in the size of the pupil and lens.

oedema an accumulation of fluid in the body, possibly beneath the skin or in cavities or organs. With an injury the swelling may be localized or more general, as in cases of kidney or heart failure. Fluid can collect in the chest cavity, abdomen or lung (PULMONARY OEDEMA). The causes are numerous, e.g. CIRRHOSIS of the liver, heart or kidney failure, starvation, acute NEPHRITIS, allergies or drugs. To alleviate the symptom, the root cause has to be removed. Subcutaneous oedema commonly occurs in women before menstruation, as swollen legs or ankles, but does subside if the legs are rested in a raised position.

oesophagoscope an instrument for inspecting the oesophagus. It has a light source and can be used to open the tube if narrowed, remove material for biopsy or remove an obstruction.

oesophagus the first part of the ALIMENTARY CANAL lying between the PHARYNX and stomach. The mucous membrane lining produces secretions to lubricate food as it passes and the movement of the food to the stomach is achieved by waves of muscular movement called *peristalsis.*

oestradiol the major female sex hormone. It is produced by the ovary and is responsible for development of the breasts, sexual characteristics and premenstrual uterine changes.

oestrogen one of a group of STEROID hormones secreted mainly by the ovaries and to a lesser extent by the adrenal cortex and placenta. (The testes also produce small amounts.) Oestrogens control the female secondary sexual characteristics, i.e. enlargement of the breasts, change in the profile of the pelvic girdle, pubic hair growth and deposition of body fat. High levels are produced at ovulation and with PROGESTERONE they regulate the female reproductive cycle.

Naturally occurring oestrogens include OESTRADIOL, oestriol and oestrone. Synthetic varieties are used in the contraceptive pill and to treat gynaecological disorders.

olfaction the sense of smell. *See* NOSE.

olfactory nerve one of a pair of sensory nerves for smell. It is the first cranial nerve and comprises many fine threads connecting receptors in the mucous membrane of the olfactory area, which pass through holes in the skull, fuse to form one fibre and then pass back to the brain.

oncogene any GENE directly involved in cancer, whether in viruses or in the individual.

oncogenic any factor or substance that causes cancer. This may be an organism, a chemical or some environmental condition. Some viruses are oncogenic and have the result of making a normal cell become a cancer cell.

oncology the subdiscipline of medicine concerned with the study and treatment of tumours, including medical, surgical aspects and their treatment with radiation.

oocyte a cell in the OVARY that undergoes MEIOSIS to produce an OVUM, the female reproductive cell. A newborn female already has primary oocytes, of which only a small number survive to puberty, and even then only a fraction will be ovulated. *See* OVULATION.

operculum a lid, plug or flap. A term used in several areas of medicine e.g. it is a plug of mucus blocking the cervix in a pregnant woman; it is also used in neurology and dentistry.

ophthalmology the branch of medicine dealing with the structure of the eye, its function, associated diseases and treatment.

ophthalmoplegia paralysis of the muscles serving the EYE, which may be internal (affecting the iris and ciliary muscle) or external (those muscles moving the eye itself).

ophthalmoscope an instrument, with a light source, used to examine the interior of the EYE. Some focus a fine beam of light into the eye and the point upon which it falls can be seen, while others form an image of the inside of the eye which can be studied.

opiate one of several drugs, derived from opium and including morphine and codeine. They act by depressing the central nervous system, thus relieving pain and suppressing coughing. Morphine and heroin, its synthetic derivative, are narcotics.

opium a milky liquid extracted from the unripe seed capsules of the poppy, *Papaver somniferum*, which has almost 10% of anhydrous morphine. Opium is a NARCOTIC and ANALGESIC.

opportunistic an infection that is contracted by someone with a lower resistance than usual. This may be due to drugs or another disease, such as DIABETES MELLITUS, cancer or AIDS. In normal circumstances, in a healthy person the infecting organism would not cause the disease.

optic atrophy a deterioration and wasting of the optic disc due to degeneration of fibres in the optic nerve. It may accompany numerous conditions, including DIABETES, ARTERIOSCLEROSIS or GLAUCOMA, or may be due to a congenital defect, inflammation or injury, or toxic poisoning from alcohol, lead, etc.

optic chiasma (*or* **optic commissure**) the cross-shaped structure formed from a crossing over of the optic nerves running back from the eyeballs to meet beneath the brain in the midline.

orchidectomy removal of one or both (castration) testes, usually to treat a malignant growth.

orchidopexy the operation performed to bring an undescended testis into the scrotum. It is undertaken well before puberty to ensure normal development subsequently.

organ any distinct and recognizable unit within the body that is composed of two or more types of tissue and that is responsible for a particular function or functions. Examples are the liver, kidney, heart and brain.

orgasm the climax of sexual arousal which in men coincides with ejaculation and comprises a series of involuntary muscle contractions. In women there are irregular contractions of the vagina walls.

orthodontics a part of dentistry dealing with development of the teeth and the treatment of (or prevention of) any disorders.

orthopaedics the subdiscipline of medicine concerned with the study of the skeletal system and the joints, muscles etc. It also covers the treatment of bone damage or disease whether CONGENITAL or acquired.

orthopnoea a severe difficulty in breathing that is so bad that a patient cannot lie and has to sleep in a sitting position. It usually only occurs with serious conditions of the heart and lungs.

osmosis the process whereby solvent molecules (usually water) from one part of the body move through a semi-permeable membrane to another part with a higher concentration of molecules. Cell membranes function as semi-permeable membranes and osmosis is very important in regulating water content in living systems.

ossicle the term for a small bone, often applied to those of the middle ear, the auditory ossicles (*see*

EAR), which transmit sound to the inner ear from the eardrum.

ossification (*or* **osteogenesis**) bone formation, which occurs in several stages via special cells called OSTEOBLASTS. COLLAGEN fibres form a network in connective tissue and then a cement of polysaccharide is laid down. Finally, calcium salts are distributed among the cement as tiny crystals. The osteoblasts are enclosed as bone cells (OSTEOCYTES).

osteitis inflammation of bone, caused by damage, infection or bodily disorder. Symptoms include swelling, tenderness, a dull aching sort of pain and redness over the affected area.

osteoarthritis a form of ARTHRITIS involving joint cartilage with accompanying changes in the associated bone. It usually involves the loss of cartilage and the development of OSTEOPHYTES at the bone margins. The function of the joint (most often the thumb, knee and hip) is affected and it becomes painful. The condition may be due to overuse, and affects those past middle age. It also may complicate other joint diseases. Treatment usually involves administering ANALGESICS, possibly anti-inflammatory drugs and the use of corrective or replacement surgery.

osteoblast a specialized cell responsible for the formation of bone.

osteochondritis inflammation of bone and cartilage.

osteochondrosis a disease affecting the OSSIFICATION centres of bone in children. It begins with degeneration and NECROSIS but it regenerates and calcifies again.

osteocyte a bone cell formed from an osteoblast that is no longer active and has become embedded in the matrix of the bone.

osteogenesis imperfecta (*or* **brittle bone disease**) a hereditary disease which results in the bones being unusually fragile and brittle. It may have associated symptoms, namely transparent teeth, unusually mobile joints, dwarfism, etc. It may be due to a disorder involving COLLAGEN, but there is little that can be done in treatment.

osteomalacia a softening of the bones, and the adult equivalent of rickets, which is due to a lack of VITAMIN D. This vitamin is obtained from the diet and is produced on exposure to sunlight, and it is necessary for the uptake of calcium from food.

osteomyelitis bone-marrow inflammation caused by infection. This may happen after a compound fracture or during bone surgery. It produces pain, swelling and fever and high doses of antibiotics are necessary.

osteophyte bony projections that occur near joints or intervertebral discs where cartilage has degenerated or been destroyed (*see* OSTEOARTHRITIS). Osteophytes may in any case occur with increasing age, with or without loss of cartilage.

osteoporosis a loss of bone tissue due to it being resorbed, resulting in bones that become brittle and likely to fracture. It is common in menopausal women and results from long-term steroid therapy. It is also a feature of CUSHING's SYNDROME. Hormone replacement therapy is a treatment available to women.

osteosarcoma the commonest and most malignant bone tumour that is found most in older children. The femur is usually affected but metastases are common (*see* METASTASIS). It produces pain and swelling and although amputation used to be the standard treatment, surgery is now possible, with replacement of the diseased bone and associated chemotherapy and/or radiotherapy. It remains, nevertheless, a serious cancer with a relatively poor survival rate.

osteosclerosis a condition in which the density of bone tissue increases abnormally. It is due to tumour, infection or poor blood supply, and may be due to an abnormality involving osteoclasts, cells that resorb calcified bone.

otitis inflammation of the ear. This may take several forms, depending upon the exact location, which produce diverse symptoms e.g. inflammation of the inner ear (*otitis interna*), affects balance, causing vertigo and vomiting while *otitis media* is usually a bacterial infection of the middle ear resulting in severe pain, and a fever requiring immediate antibiotic treatment. *Secretory otitis media* is otherwise known as GLUE EAR.

otology the subdiscipline of medicine concerned with the ear, its disorders and diseases and their treatment.

otosclerosis the hereditary condition in which there is overgrowth of bone in the inner ear which restricts and then stops sound being conducted to the inner EAR from the middle ear. The person affected becomes progressively more deaf, often beginning with TINNITUS, but surgery is effective.

ovarian cyst a sac filled with fluid that develops in the ovary. Most are benign but their size may cause swelling and pressure on other organs. For those cysts that do become malignant, it is possible that its discovery comes too late to allow successful treatment. ULTRASOUND scanning can be adopted to detect tumours at an early stage.

ovariotomy literally, cutting into an ovary, but more

generally used for surgical removal of an ovary or an ovarian tumour.

ovary the reproductive organ of females which produces eggs (ova) and hormones (mainly OESTROGEN and PROGESTERONE). There are two ovaries, each the size of an almond, on either side of the uterus, and each contains numerous Graafian FOLLICLES in which the eggs develop. At OVULATION an egg is released from a follicle. The follicles secrete oestrogen and progesterone, which regulate the menstrual cycle and the uterus during pregnancy.

ovulation the release of an egg from an OVARY (i.e. from a mature Graafian follicle), which then moves down the FALLOPIAN TUBE to the uterus.

Ovulation is brought about by secretion of *luteinizing hormone* secreted by the anterior PITUITARY GLAND.

ovum (*plural* **ova**) the mature, unfertilized female reproductive cell, which is roughly spherical, with an outer membrane and a single nucleus.

oxygenator a machine for oxygenating blood outside the body. It is used during heart surgery and the patient's blood is pumped through the machine.

oxytocin a hormone from the PITUITARY GLAND that causes the uterus to contract during LABOUR and prompts lactation due to contraction of muscle fibres in the milk ducts of the breasts.

P

pacemaker the part of the heart that regulates the beat — the SINOATRIAL NODE. Also, in patients with a HEART BLOCK, a device inserted into the body to maintain a normal heart rate. There are different types of pacemaker, some being permanent, others temporary; some stimulate the beat while others are activated only when the natural rate of the heart falls below a certain level.

paediatrics the branch of medicine that deals with children.

paedophilia an abnormal sexual attraction to children.

Paget's disease (of bone) otherwise known as *osteitis deformans*. A chronic bone disease, particularly of the long bones, skull and spine, which results in the bones becoming thickened, disorganized and also soft, causing them to bend. The cause is unknown and, although there is also no cure, good results are being obtained with CALCITONIN. The main symptom is pain.

palate the roof of the mouth which separates the cavity of the mouth below from that of the nose above. It consists of the *hard* and *soft* palate. The hard palate is located at the front of the mouth and is a bony plate covered by mucous membrane. The soft palate is a muscular layer that is also covered by mucous membrane. The movable soft palate is important in the production of sounds and speech.

palliative a medicine or treatment that is given to effect some relief from symptoms, if only temporarily, but does not cure the ailment. This is often the case in the treatment of cancer.

pallor an abnormal paleness of skin because of a reduced blood flow, or a lack of the normal pigments. It may be due directly to ANAEMIA or SHOCK, to spending an excessive amount of time indoors.

palpation examination of the surface of the body by carefully feeling with hands and fingertips. It is often possible to distinguish between solid lumps or swelling and cystic swellings.

palpitation when the heart beats noticeably or irregularly and the person becomes aware of it.

The heartbeat is not normally noticed but with fear, emotion or exercise it may be felt, unpleasantly so. Palpitations may also be due to neuroses, ARRHYTHMIA or heart disease, and a common cause is too much tea, coffee, alcohol or smoking. Where an excess is the cause (tea, coffee, etc.), this can be eliminated. For disease-associated palpitations, drugs can be used for control.

palsy the term used formerly for paralysis and retained for the names of some conditions.

pancreas a gland with both ENDOCRINE and exocrine functions. It is located between the DUODENUM and SPLEEN, behind the stomach, and is about 15cm long. There are two types of cells producing secretions. The first are the *acini,* which produce pancreatic juice which goes to the intestine via a system of ducts. This contains an alkaline mixture of salt and enzymes — trypsin and chymotrypsin to digest proteins, amylase to break down starch and lipase to aid digestion of fats. The second cell types are in the ISLETS OF LANGERHANS and these produce two hormones, INSULIN and GLUCAGON, secreted directly into the blood for control of sugar levels. *See also* DIABETES MELLITUS, HYPOGLYCAEMIA and HYPERGLYCAEMIA.

pancreatectomy surgical removal of the PANCREAS (or part of it) to deal with tumours or chronic PANCREATITIS. After *total* or *subtotal* pancreatectomy (where all or almost all is removed) the pancreatic secretions to aid digestion and control blood sugar have to be administered.

pancreatitis inflammation of the PANCREAS, occurring in several forms, but often associated with gallstones or alcoholism. Any bout of the condition that interferes with the function of the pancreas may lead to the development of DIABETES and MALABSORPTION.

pandemic an epidemic that is so widely spread that it affects large numbers of people in a country or countries.

Papanicolaou test (*or* **Pap test**) another name for a CERVICAL SMEAR.

papilla any small protuberance such as the papillae on the tongue.

papilloma usually benign growths on the skin surface or mucous membrane e.g. WARTS.

paracentesis the procedure of tapping or taking off (excess) fluid from the body by means of a hollow needle or CANNULA.

paracetamol a drug that has analgesic effects and also reduces fever. It is taken for mild pain (headache, etc.). It may cause digestive problems. Excessive doses can produce liver failure, causing progressive NECROSIS in a matter of days and very large doses are fatal. In the early stages of poisoning the stomach can be washed out and drugs administered to protect the liver.

parainfluenza viruses a group of viruses that cause respiratory tract infections with usually mild influenza-like symptoms. Infants and young children affected most. There are four types of the virus, virulent at different times of the year.

paralysis muscle weakness or total loss of muscle movement, which varies depending upon the causal disease and its effect on the brain. Various descriptive terms are used to qualify the parts of the body affected, thus hemiplegia affects one side of the body (*see also* DIPLEGIA, PARAPLEGIA, QUADRIPLEGIA). Paralysis is really a symptom of another condition or disease e.g. brain disease such as a cerebral haemorrhage or THROMBOSIS causing hemiplegia, disease or injury of the spinal cord leading to paraplegia, or POLIOMYELITIS (infantile paralysis). In addition there is the paralysis associated with MOTORNEURONE DISEASE.

paramedical a term for professions working closely with medics e.g. nurses, radiographers and dietitians.

paranoia an abnormal mental condition typified by delusions associated with a certain, complicated system which usually involves feelings of persecution or grandeur. The complex web of delusion may develop with time, and with some logic, so that it may appear plausible and the person seems normal in other aspects and behaviour, save for that involving the delusions.

paraphimosis constriction of the penis due to retraction of an abnormally tight foreskin which contracts on the penis behind the glans, and cannot be easily moved. Swelling and pain may be caused and usually circumcision is necessary to prevent a recurrence.

paraplegia PARALYSIS of the legs. It may be caused by injury or disease of the spinal cord and often bladder and rectum are also affected.

parasite any organism that obtains its nutrients by living in or on the body of another organism (the *host*). The extent to which the host is damaged by the parasite ranges from virtually no effect to, in extreme cases, death. Parasites in humans include worms, viruses, fungi, etc.

parasympathetic nervous system one of the two parts of the AUTONOMIC NERVOUS SYSTEM that acts antagonistically with the SYMPATHETIC NERVOUS SYSTEM. The parasympathetic nerves originate from the brain and lower portion of the spinal cord (sacral region). The AXONS of this system tend to be longer than sympathetic nerves and SYNAPSES with other neurons are close to the target organ. The parasympathetic system contracts the bladder, decreases heart rate, stimulates the sex organs, promotes digestion, etc.

parathyroidectomy surgical removal of the PARATHYROID GLANDS, usually in treatment of hyperparathyroidism (hyperactivity of one or all of the glands).

parathyroid glands four small glands located behind or within the thyroid gland, that control the metabolism of calcium and phosphorus (as phosphate) in the body. The hormone responsible, parathormone (or simply parathyroid hormone) is produced and released by the glands. A deficiency of the hormone leads to lower levels of calcium in the blood, with a relative increase in phosphorus. This produces tetany, a condition involving muscular spasms, which can be treated by injection. This is also known as *hypoparathyroidism* and is often due to removal or injury of the glands during thyroidectomy. If the hormone is at high levels calcium is transferred from bones to the blood, causing weakness and susceptibility to breaks.

paratyphoid fever a bacterial infection caused by *Salmonella paratyphi A, B* or *C*. Symptoms resemble those of typhoid fever and include diarrhoea, a rash and mild fever. It can be treated with antibiotics and temporary immunity against the *A* and *B* form is gained by vaccination with TAB vaccine.

parenteral nutrition provision of food by any means other than by the mouth. For patients with burns, renal failure, etc., or after major surgery, this mode of feeding may be necessary and is accomplished intravenously. Protein, fat and carbohydrate can all be delivered as special solutions containing all the essential compounds. The main hazard of such a system is the risk of infection and reactions to the solutions introduced e.g. HYPERGLYCAEMIA, can result.

Parkinson's disease a progressive condition

occurring in mid to late life which results in a rigidity of muscles affecting the voice and face, rather than those in the limbs. A tremor also develops possibly in one hand initially and then spreading to other limbs and it appears most pronounced when sitting. The disease is usually due to a deficiency in the NEUROTRANSMITTER dopamine, due to degeneration of the basal ganglia of the brain (*see* BASAL GANGLION). There is no cure available, but a number of drugs are able, to varying degrees, to control the condition.

parotid gland one of a pair of salivary glands situated in front of each ear and opening inside on the cheek near the second last molar of the upper jaw.

parotitis inflammation of the PAROTID GLAND, which as epidemic or infectious parotitis is called MUMPS.

paroxysm a sudden attack. A term used especially about convulsions.

parturition *see* **labour**.

pasteurization the sterilization of food by heating it to a certain temperature. This destroys potentially harmful bacteria, thus milk is heated to 62°–65°C for 30 minutes, followed by rapid cooling. Infections avoided by this process include tuberculosis and typhoid, scarlet fever, diphtheria and food poisoning.

patch test a test undertaken to identify the substances causing a person's allergy. Different allergens are placed in very small amounts on the skin. A red flare with swelling will develop if the person is allergic. This commonly happens within 15 minutes but may take up to 72 hours.

patella the kneecap. An almost flat bone, shaped somewhat like an oyster shell, that lies in front of the knee in the tendon of the thigh muscle.

patellar reflex *see* **reflex action**.

pathogen the term applied to an organism that causes disease. Most pathogens affecting humans are bacteria and viruses.

pathology the study of the causes, characteristics and effects of disease on the body by examining samples of body fluids and products whether from a living patient or at autopsy.

pectoral the descriptive term for anything relating to the chest.

pectoral girdle (*or* **shoulder girdle**) the skeletal structure to which the bones of the upper limbs are attached. It is composed of two shoulder blades (SCAPULAE) and two collar bones (CLAVICLES) attached to the vertebral column and breastbone (STERNUM) respectively.

pedicle a narrow roll of skin by which a piece of skin for grafting is attached. It is used when it is not possible to place an independent graft on the site, perhaps because of poor blood supply. Also, the term for a narrow neck of tissue connecting a tumour to its tissue of origin.

pediculosis a deficiency disease caused by a lack of nicotinic acid, part of the VITAMIN B complex. It occurs when the diet is based on maize (rather than wheat) with an associated lack of first-class protein (meat and milk). The reason is that although maize contains nicotinic acid it is in an unusable form and also it does not contain the amino acid tryptophan, which the body can use to produce nicotinic acid. The symptoms are dermatitis, diarrhoea and depression.

pelvic girdle (*or* **hip girdle**) the skeletal structure to which the bones of the lower limbs are attached. It is made up of the two hip bones, each comprising the ilium, pubis and ischium, fused together.

pelvic inflammatory disease (*or* **PID**) an acute or chronic infection of the UTERUS, ovaries or FALLOPIAN TUBES. It is due to infection elsewhere e.g. the appendix, which spreads, or an infection carried by the blood. It produces severe abdominal pain which usually responds to antibiotics but surgery may sometimes be necessary to remove diseased tissue.

pelvis the skeletal structure formed by the hip bones, sacrum and coccyx, which connects with the spine and legs. The female pelvis is shallower and the ilia are wider apart and there are certain angular differences from the male, all of which relate to childbearing. The pelvis is a point of contact for the muscles of the legs and it partially envelops the BLADDER and RECTUM. In males it also includes the PROSTATE GLAND and seminal vesicles, while in females it contains the womb and ovaries.

penicillin the antibiotic derived from the mould *Penicillium notatum*, which grows naturally on decaying fruit, bread or cheese. The genus used for production of the drug is *P. chrysogenum*. Penicillin is active against a large range of bacteria and it is non-toxic. It is usually given by injection but can be taken orally. There are many semi-synthetic penicillins acting in different ways including Ampicillin and Propicillin. Some patients are allergic to penicillin but there tend to be very few serious side effects.

penis the male organ through which the URETHRA passes, carrying urine or semen. It is made up of tissue that is filled with blood during sexual arousal, producing an erection, which enables penetration of the vagina and ejaculation of semen. The glans is the end part, normally covered by the FORESKIN (prepuce).

peptic ulcer an ulcer in the stomach (GASTRIC ULCER), oesophagus, duodenum (DUODENAL ULCER) or JEJUNUM. It is caused by a break in the mucosal lining due to the action of acid and pepsin (an enzyme active in protein breakdown) either because of their high concentrations or due to other factors affecting the mucosal protective mechanisms.

peptide an organic compound made up of two or more amino acids and collectively named by the number of amino acids. A dipeptide therefore contains two, and a polypeptide many.

percussion the diagnostic aid which involves tapping parts of the body (particularly on back and chest) with the fingers to produce a vibration and note-like sound. The sound produced gives an indication of abnormal enlargement of organs, and the presence of fluid in the lungs.

perforation when a hole forms in a hollow organ, tissue or tube e.g. the stomach, eardrum etc. In particular, it is a serious development of an ulcer in the stomach or bowels because on perforation the intestine contents, with bacteria, enter the peritoneal cavity (*see* PERITONEUM) causing PERITONITIS. This is accompanied by severe pain and shock and usually corrective surgery is required.

pericarditis inflammation of the PERICARDIUM. It may be due to URAEMIA, cancer or viral infection, and produces fever, chest pain and possible accumulation of fluid.

pericardium the smooth membrane surrounding the heart. The outer *fibrous* part covers the heart and is connected to the large vessels coming out of the heart. The inner *serous* part is a closed SEROUS MEMBRANE attached both to the fibrous pericardium and the heart wall. Some fluid in the resulting sac enables smooth movement as the heart beats.

perinatal mortality foetal deaths after week 28 of pregnancy and newborn deaths during the first week or two of life. The main causes of perinatal mortality are brain injuries during birth, congenital defects and lack of oxygen in the final stages of pregnancy (called *antepartum anoxia*). Perinatal *deaths* are due to complications involving the placenta, congenital defects and birth asphyxia.

perineum the area of the body between anus and urethral opening.

periodontal descriptive term relating to the tissues surrounding the teeth.

peripheral nervous system those parts of the nervous system excluding the central nervous system (brain and spinal cord). It comprises the afferent (sensory) and efferent (motor) cells, which include 12 pairs of cranial nerves and 31 pairs of spinal nerves. The motor nervous system then comprises the somatic nervous system, carrying impulses to the skeletal muscles, and the autonomic nervous system, which is further divided into the sympathetic and the parasympathetic nervous system (*see individual entries*).

peripheral neuritis inflammation of the nerves of the peripheral system.

peritoneum the SEROUS MEMBRANE that lines the abdominal cavity. That lining the abdomen walls is the *parietal* peritoneum, while the *visceral* peritoneum covers the organs. The folds of peritoneum from one organ to another are given special names e.g. MESENTERY. Both are continuous and form a closed sac at the back of the abdomen in the male, while in the female there is an opening from the Fallopian tube on either side.

peritonitis inflammation of the peritoneum. It may be caused by a primary infection due to bacteria in the bloodstream (e.g. tuberculous peritonitis), resulting in pain and swelling, fever and weight loss. Secondary infection results from entry into the abdominal cavity of bacteria and irritants (e.g. digestive juices) from a perforated or ruptured organ e.g. duodenum or stomach. This produces severe pain and shock and surgery is often necessary.

pernicious anaemia a type of ANAEMIA due to VITAMIN B12 deficiency which results from dietary lack or the failure to produce the substance that enables B12 to be absorbed from the bowel. This in turn results in a lack of red blood cell production and MEGALOBLASTS in the bone marrow. The condition is easily treated by regular injections of the vitamin.

perspiration (*or* sweat) the excretion from millions of tiny sweat glands in the skin. Sweat that evaporates from the skin immediately is *insensible*, while that forming drops is *sensible perspiration*. Sweat is produced in two types of sweat glands. The *eccrine* glands are found mainly on the soles of the feet and palms of the hands. The *apocrine* glands are in the armpits, around the anus and genitalia and sweat is produced in response to stimuli such as fear and sexual arousal. The major function of sweating, however, is the regulation of body temperature.

Perthes' disease a hip condition in children between the ages of four and ten, which is self-healing. Due to OSTEOCHONDROSIS of the EPIPHYSIS of the femur, a limp is developed with associated pain. Rest is essential, as is immobilizing traction, until the pain subsides and then a special splint is fitted to permit walking until the condition is fully healed.

pertussis *see* **whooping cough**.

pessary an instrument that fits into the vagina to treat a PROLAPSE. Also, a soft solid that is shaped for insertion into the vagina and contains drugs for some gynaecological disorder (also used for inducing labour).

pethidine a drug with ANALGESIC and mild sedative action for relief of moderate pain. It may be given by mouth or injection but side effects include nausea, dizziness and dry mouth, and prolonged use may create dependence.

petit mal the lesser type of epileptic seizure, which is IDIOPATHIC. It consists of brief periods (seconds) of unconsciousness, when the eyes stare blankly but posture is maintained. Children suffering frequently may have learning difficulties but the condition may disappear in adult life.

phaeochromocytoma a small vascular tumour (usually benign) of the inner part of the ADRENAL GLAND. It causes uncontrolled secretion of adrenaline and noradrenaline, producing increased heart rate, palpitations, high blood pressure, sweating and weight loss, and there may be heart failure.

phagocytosis *see* **leucocyte**.

phalanges (*singular* **phalanx**) the bones of the digits (fingers and toes), which number fourteen in each hand and foot. The thumb and big toe comprise two, while all the other digits have three phalanges.

phallus penis, or a penis-like object. Also, the term used for the embryonic penis before the final development of the urethral duct.

phantom limb the feeling that a limb or part of a limb is still attached to the body after it has been amputated. This is probably due to stimulation of the severed nerves and usually wears off with time.

pharmaceutical relating to pharmacy or drugs.

pharmacist a trained, qualified and registered person who is authorized to keep and dispense medicines.

pharmacology the branch of medicine concerning the preparation, properties, uses and effects of drugs.

pharmacy the preparation of drugs (and their dispensing), or the place where this function is undertaken.

pharyngectomy surgical excision of part of the pharynx.

pharyngitis inflammation of the PHARYNX and therefore throat, commonly due to a virus, and resulting in a sore throat. It is often associated with TONSILLITIS.

pharynx the region extending from the beginning of the oesophagus up to the base of the skull, at the cavity into which nose and mouth open. It is muscular, with a mucous membrane, and acts as the route for both food (to the oesophagus) and air (to the larynx). The EUSTACHIAN TUBES open from the upper part of the pharynx.

phenobarbitone a very widely-used BARBITURATE. It can be given orally or by injection and is taken as an anticonvulsant in epilepsy, and to treat insomnia or anxiety. It may produce drowsiness and some skin reactions and continued use should be avoided, lest dependence ensue.

phenotype the detectable, observable characteristics of an individual that are determined by the interaction of his or her GENES (genotype) and the environment in which he or she develops. The expression of the dominant gene masks the presence of a recessive one, as only the expressed gene affects the phenotype.

phenylketonuria a genetic disorder that results in the deficiency of an ENZYME that converts phenylalanine, an ESSENTIAL AMINO ACID, to tyrosine. Children can be severely mentally retarded by an excess of phenylalanine in the blood damaging the nervous system. The responsible gene is recessive, therefore the condition occurs only if both parents are carriers. However, there is a test for newborn infants (the Guthrie test) that ensures the condition can be detected and the diet can be modified to avoid phenylalanine and thus any brain damage.

phial a small glass bottle-like receptacle for storing medicines.

phimosis a condition in which the edge of the FORESKIN is narrowed and cannot be drawn back over the glans of the PENIS. To avoid inflammation and an exacerbation of the problem, circumcision may be necessary.

phlebectomy removal of a vein, or part of a vein, sometimes undertaken in the treatment of VARICOSE VEINS.

phlebitis inflammation of a vein. This commonly occurs as a complication of VARICOSE VEINS, producing pain and a hot feeling around the vein, with possible THROMBOSIS development. Drugs and elastic support are used in treatment.

phlebothrombosis the obstruction of a vein by a blood clot, common in the deep veins of the leg (in particular the calf) and resulting from heart failure, pregnancy, injury and surgery, which may change the clotting factors in the blood. The affected leg may swell and there is the danger that the clot may move, creating a PULMONARY EMBOLISM. Large clots may be removed surgically, otherwise the treatment involves anticoagulant drugs and exercise.

phlebotomy the opening of a vein, or its puncture, to remove blood or to infuse fluids.

phlegm a general term (non-medical) for sputum, mucus.

phobia an anxiety disorder and irrational fear of certain objects, animals, situations, events, etc. Avoiding the situation can lead to significant disruption, restriction of normal life or even suffering. There is a variety of phobias, including animal, specific and social phobias, and treatment involves behaviour therapy.

phonation the production of speech sounds.

photophobia an atypical sensitivity to light. Exposure produces discomfort and actions to evade the light source. The condition may be associated with medications, or migraine, meningitis, etc.

phrenic nerve the nerve to the muscles of the DIAPHRAGM, arising from the third, fourth and fifth cervical spinal nerves.

physical concerning the body as opposed to the mind.

physician a registered medical practitioner who deals with non-surgical practice.

physiology the study of the functions of and processes within the body and its various organs.

physiotherapy the use of physical methods to help healing. It may involve exercise, massage and manipulation, heat treatment and the use of light and ultraviolet radiation, etc.

pia mater *see* **brain** and **meninges**.

pica an abnormal desire to eat non-food substances such as soap, chalk, glue, clay, etc. The disorder may arise during early childhood or in mental illness. Although it also occurs during pregnancy, the desire is more often for unusual foods and an excess of ordinary foods.

pigment an organic colouring agent e.g. the blood pigment HAEMOGLOBIN, BILE pigments, rhodopsin (found in the RODS of the RETINA) and MELANIN.

piles *see* **haemorrhoids**.

pilus a hair or structure like a hair.

pimples (*or* **papules**) small swellings on the skin that are inflamed and may contain pus. The cause is often infection of a pore that is blocked with fatty secretions from the SEBACEOUS GLANDS. On the face, the condition is called ACNE.

pituitary gland (*or* **hypophysis**) a small, but very important, endocrine gland at the base of the HYPOTHALAMUS. It has two lobes, the anterior *adenohypophysis* and the posterior *neurohypophysis*. The pituitary secretes hormones that control many functions and is itself controlled by hormonal secretions from the hypothalamus. The neurohypophysis stores and releases peptide hormones produced in the hypothalamus, namely OXYTOCIN and VASOPRESSIN. The adenohypophysis secretes GROWTH HORMONE, GONADOTROPHIN, prolactin (involved in stimulating lactation), ACTH and THYROID-stimulating hormones.

placebo an inactive substance, taken as medication, that nevertheless may help to relieve a condition. The change occurs because the patient expects some treatment (even if nothing need, in reality, be done) and an improvement reflects the expectations of the patient.

New drugs are tested in trials against placebos when the effect of the drug is measured against the placebo response, which happens even when there is no active ingredient in the placebo.

placenta the organ attaching the embryo to the UTERUS. It is a temporary feature comprising maternal and embryonic tissues and it allows oxygen and nutrients to pass from the mother's blood to the embryo's blood. There is, however, no direct contact of blood supplies. The embryo also receives salt, glucose, amino acids, some peptides and antibodies, fats and vitamins. Waste molecules from the embryo are removed by diffusion into the maternal circulation. It also stores GLYCOGEN for conversion to glucose if required and secretes hormones to regulate the pregnancy. It is expelled after birth.

placenta praevia when the placenta is situated in the bottom part of the uterus, next to or over the cervix. In the later stages of pregnancy, there may be placental separation causing bleeding, which will require attention. In the more extreme cases, a Caesarian section will be necessary for delivery.

plague any epidemic disease that results in a high death rate. Specifically, the bubonic plague, transmitted to man from infected rats by the rat flea. After an incubation period of two to six days the symptoms occur as headache, weakness, fever, aches in the limbs and delirium. The lymph nodes (especially in the groin) swell and become painful (buboes; hence *bubo*nic) and may burst, releasing pus. In other cases, the infective fluid may not be released, and there may be subcutaneous haemorrhaging with creation of black patches (gangrenous) on the skin, leaching to ulcers (hence the old term — *black* death). If the bacteria enter the blood (septicaemic plague) death follows rapidly, but the most serious is pneumonic plague, when the lungs are affected.

Preventive actions are very important in such cases, particularly to eliminate the carriers. However, the disease can be treated effectively with antibiotics and sulphonamides.

plantar descriptive term meaning relating to the sole of the foot.

plaque a surface layer on teeth formed from bacteria and food debris and later, calcium salts.

plasma a light-coloured fluid component of BLOOD, in which the various cells are suspended. It contains inorganic salts with protein and some trace substances. One protein present is FIBRINOGEN.

plaster of Paris a type of calcium sulphate (gypsum) used to make plaster models in dentistry and plaster casts in orthopaedics. When mixed with water it sets firmly and in the preparation of a splint for fractures, bandages impregnated with the plaster are used. These are easily applied and moulded to the shape of the limb.

plastic surgery a branch of surgery that deals with the repair or rebuilding of damaged, deformed or missing parts of the body. *Cosmetic* plastic surgery is merely for the improvement of appearance but most is to repair burns, accident damage or congenital defects.

platelet (*or* **thrombocyte**) a disc-like structure in the blood, involved in the halting of bleeding.

pleura the SEROUS MEMBRANE that covers the lungs (*visceral*) and the inside of the chest wall (*parietal*). The membranes have a smooth surface, which is moistened to allow them to slide over each other.

pleural cavity the small space between the PLEURA, which slide over each other when breathing in and out. Should gas or fluid enter the cavity due to infection or injury the space increases and may hinder breathing.

pleurectomy removal, by surgery, of part of the PLEURA to overcome PNEUMOTHORAX or to excise diseased areas.

pleurisy (*or* **pleuritis**) inflammation of the PLEURA resulting in pain from deep breathing, and a resulting shortness of breath. There is a typical frictional rub heard through a stethoscope. Pleurisy is often due to PNEUMONIA in the adjacent lung and is always associated with disease in the lung, diaphragm, chest wall or abdomen, e.g. TUBERCULOSIS, ABSCESSes or bronchial carcinoma.

plexus a network formed from intersecting nerves and/or blood vessels, or lymphatic vessels.

pneumoconiosis a general term for a chronic form of lung disease caused by inhaling dust while working. Most of the cases are anthracosis (coal miner's pneumoconiosis), SILICOSIS and asbestosis.

pneumonectomy the surgical removal of a lung performed mainly for cancer but also for tuberculosis.

pneumonia a bacterial infection of the lungs resulting in inflammation and filling of the ALVEOLI with pus and fluid. As a result the lung becomes solid and air cannot enter. The symptoms vary, depending upon how much of the lung is unavailable for respiration, but commonly there will be chest pain, coughing, breathlessness, fever and possibly CYANOSIS. Pneumonia may be caused by several bacteria, viruses or fungi, but bacterial infection is commonest. Bronchopneumonia affects the bronchi and bronchioles, lobar pneumonia the whole lobes of the lung(s). Antibiotic treatment is usually effective, although it helps to know which is the infecting organism, to provide the most specific treatment. *See also* VIRAL PNEUMONIA.

pneumonitis inflammation of the lungs by chemical or physical agents.

pneumothorax air in the PLEURAL CAVITY, which enters via a wound in the chest wall or lung. When this happens, the lung collapses, but if the air is absorbed from the pleural cavity the lung reinflates.

pock a small eruption on the skin, which may contain pus, typical of chicken-pox and smallpox.

poliomyelitis (*or* **infantile paralysis** *or* **polio**) an infectious disease, caused by a virus, which attacks the central nervous system. The virus is taken in by mouth, passes through the digestive system and excreted with the faeces. Hands may be contaminated, leading to further spread. The incubation period is 7–12 days and there are several types of condition, depending upon the severity of the attack. In some cases the symptoms resemble a stomach upset or influenza; in others there is in addition some stiffness of muscles. Paralytic poliomyelitis is less common, resulting in muscle weakness and paralysis, while the most serious cases involve breathing when the diaphragm and related muscles are affected (bulbar poliomyelitis). Treatment of the disease involves relief of the symptoms, including bed rest, and for the bulbar form, a respirator may be required.

Immunization is highly effective and the disease has almost been eradicated in most countries. However, booster doses are advisable when visiting countries with a high incidence of the disease.

polydactyly the condition in which there are extra fingers or toes.

polydipsia an intense thirst, abnormally so. It is a characteristic symptom of DIABETES MELLITUS and certain other diseases.

polyp a growth from a mucous membrane and attached to it by a stalk. Most are benign but may cause obstructions or infections. They commonly occur in the sinuses, nose, or possibly the bladder or bowels. Their removal is usually relatively straightforward, unless a more extensive operation proves necessary to reach the affected organ.

polyuria the passing of a larger than normal quantity of urine which is also usually pale in colour. It may be due merely to a large fluid intake, or to a condition such as DIABETES, or a kidney disorder.

pons tissue that joins parts of an organ e.g. the *pons Varolii*, a part of the brainstem, links various parts of the brain including the medulla oblongata and thalamus.

pore a small opening, e.g. sweat pores.

porphyria a group of disorders that are hereditary in which there is increased production of porphyrins (natural pigments as found in e.g. haemoglobin) leading to abdominal pain, sensitivity to light and neuropathy (disease of the peripheral nerves).

portal vein a vein within the hepatic portal system that carries blood to the liver from other abdominal organs (stomach, spleen, intestine, etc.). It is atypical in that it does not take blood directly to the heart but ends in a capillary network.

posseting the term for the normal habit of some quite healthy babies to regurgitate small amounts of a recently-taken meal.

post mortem *see* **autopsy** and **necropsy**.

postpartum the term meaning relating to the first few days after birth.

poultice (*or* **fomentation**) hot, moist material applied to the body to soften the skin, soothe irritations, ease pain or increase the circulation locally.

pox pus-filled pimples, as in chicken-pox or smallpox. Also, the small pit-like depressions that are scars of smallpox.

precancerous any condition that is not malignant but will become so if left untreated.

pre-eclampsia the development of high blood pressure in pregnancy, sometimes with OEDEMA, which unless treated may result in ECLAMPSIA.

pregnancy the period of time, lasting approximately 280 days from the first day of the last menstrual period, during which a woman carries a developing foetus. Signs of a pregnancy include cessation of menstruation, increase in size of the breasts, MORNING SICKNESS, and later in the pregnancy the obvious sign of enlargement of the abdomen. A foetal heartbeat and movements also follow later. Many of these changes are hormone-controlled, by progesterone (from the OVARY and PLACENTA).

pregnancy test various tests are used to check for pregnancy, most based on the presence of CHORIONIC GONADOTROPHIC HORMONE in the urine.

premature birth a birth occurring before the end of the normal full term. The definition refers to babies weighing less than 2° kilograms. In many cases the cause is unknown but in some it may be due to PRE-ECLAMPSIA, kidney or heart disease or multiple pregnancy. Premature babies often require incubator care.

premedication drugs given to a patient before an operation in which an anaesthetic will be used. It is usually a sedative and a drug to reduce secretions of the lungs which could be inhaled otherwise.

premenstrual tension *or* **syndrome** (*or* **PMT** *or* **PMS**) the occurrence for up to ten days before menstruation, of such symptoms as headache, nervousness and irritability, emotional disturbance, depression and fatigue, with other physical manifestations such as swelling of legs and breasts, and constipation. The condition usually disappears soon after menstruation begins. The cause is not known, although the hormone PROGESTERONE is probably involved in some way.

premolar two teeth between the canines and molars on each side of the jaw.

prenatal diagnosis *see* **amniocentesis**.

prepuce *see* **foreskin**.

presentation the point, during LABOUR, at which some part of the foetus lies at the mouth of the womb. In the majority of cases the head presents, but *see* BREECH PRESENTATION.

pressure sores *see* **bed sores**.

prickly heat (*or* **heat rash** *or* **miliaria**) an itchy rash due to small red spots, which are minute vesicles caused by the blocking of sweat or sebaceous glands in the skin. Scratching may produce infection but the condition itself is not serious.

prima gravida the technical term for a woman in her first pregnancy.

progesterone a steroid hormone that is vital in pregnancy. It is produced by the CORPUS LUTEUM of the OVARY when the lining of the uterus is prepared for the implanting of an egg cell. Progesterone is secreted under the control of other hormones (prolactin from the anterior PITUITARY, and luteinizing hormone, also from the pituitary, which stimulates ovulation and formation of the corpus luteum) until the placenta adopts this role later in the pregnancy. The function of progesterone is to maintain the uterus and ensure no further eggs are produced. Small amounts of this hormone are also produced by the testes.

prognosis a forecast of the likely outcome of a disease, based upon the patient's condition and the course of the disease in other patients at other times.

prolapse a moving down of an organ or tissue from its normal position due to the supporting tissues weakening. This may happen to the lower end of the bowel (in children) or the uterus and vagina in women who have sustained some sort of injury during childbirth. In the latter case prolapse may result in the uterus itself showing on the outside. Surgery can shorten the supporting ligaments and narrow the vaginal opening.

prolapsed intervertebral disc (*or* **slipped disc**) the intervertebral disc provides cushioning for the brain and spinal cord and is composed of an outer fibrous layer over a pulpy centre. A slipped disc is caused by the inner layer being pushed through the fibrous layer to impinge upon nerves, causing pain (commonly lumbago or sciatica). The prolapse usually occurs during sudden twisting or bending of the backbone and is more likely to occur during middle age. Treatment involves bed rest on a flat, firm surface, probably with manipulation and physiotherapy at a later stage. If absolutely necessary, the disc can be removed, but this is now less common.

prone lying face downwards.

prophylactic some treatment or action that is taken to avoid disease or a condition e.g. taking a medication to prevent angina.

proprietary name the trade name given to a drug by the company manufacturing it.

prostaglandin (*or* **PG**) a group of compounds derived from essential fatty acids that act in a way that is similar to hormones. They are found in most body tissues (but especially semen) where they are released as local regulators (in the uterus, brain, lungs, etc.). A number have been identified, two of which act antagonistically on blood vessels. PGE causing dilation, PGF constriction. Certain prostaglandins cause uterine contraction in labour, and others are involved in the body's defence mechanisms.

prostatectomy surgical excision of the PROSTATE GLAND, performed to relieve urine retention caused by enlargement of the prostate. It is also done to counter poor flow of urine or frequent urination. The operation can be undertaken from several approaches: via the urethra, from the bladder, or from the PERINEUM (for a BIOPSY).

prostate gland a gland in the male reproductive system which is located below the bladder, opening into the URETHRA. Upon ejaculation, it secretes an alkaline fluid into the semen which aids sperm motility. In older men, the gland may become enlarged, causing problems with urination (*see* PROSTATECTOMY).

prostatitis inflammation of the PROSTATE GLAND due to bacterial infection. The symptoms tend to be similar to a urinary infection although in the chronic form obstructions may form, necessitating PROSTATECTOMY.

prostheses (*singular* **prosthesis**) artificial devices fitted to the body, ranging from dentures to hearing aids, pacemakers and artificial limbs.

protein a large group of organic compounds containing carbon, hydrogen, oxygen, sulphur and nitrogen, with individual molecules built up of AMINO ACIDS in long polypeptide chains. Globular protein includes ENZYMES, ANTIBODIES, carrier proteins (e.g. HAEMOGLOBIN) and some HORMONES. Fibrous proteins have elasticity and strength and are found in muscle, connective tissue and also chromosomes.

Proteins are thus vital to the body and are synthesized from their constituent amino acids, which are obtained from digestion of dietary protein.

proteinuria the condition in which protein (usually albumin) is found in the urine. It is important because it may signify heart or kidney disease. Proteinuria may also occur with fever, severe anaemia and intake of certain drugs or poisons.

pruritus another term for itching, of whatever origin.

psittacosis a bacterial infection of parrots and budgerigars that can be transmitted to man. It causes headache, shivering, nosebleeds, fever and lung problems. It is treatable with antibiotics.

psoriasis a chronic skin disease for which the cause is unknown and the treatment is palliative. The affected skin appears as itchy, scaly red areas, starting usually around the elbows and knees. It often runs in families and may be associated with anxiety, commencing usually in childhood or adolescence. Treatment involves the use of ointments and creams, with some drugs and vitamin A.

psychedelic drugs drugs that affect the mind and consciousness, and which are often hallucinogens.

psychiatrist a qualified physician who deals with mental disorders including emotional and behavioural problems.

psychiatry the study of mental disorders, their diagnosis, treatment/management and prevention.

psychoanalysis a method of treating mental ill-health by uncovering repressed fears, and dealing with them in the conscious mind. This school of psychology began with Sigmund Freud.

psychogeriatrics the branch of psychiatry dealing with mental ill-health in old people.

psychology the study of the mind, its working and resulting behaviour patterns. There are many schools of psychology, including experimental (laboratory experiments to study topics such as learning), PSYCHOANALYSIS, ethology (study of animal behaviour in the natural environment) and behaviourism.

psychopathic when a person has a mental disorder resulting in antisocial behaviour with little or no guilt for any such acts committed. In addition, psychopaths do not show any ability for showing affection, sympathy or love to others and punishment does not deter a repeat of any criminal act.

psychosis a very serious state of mental ill-health, essentially insanity. The sufferer loses touch with reality and may suffer delusions and hallucinations. Schizophrenia and manic depressive psychosis are two important psychoses.

psychosomatic the term meaning relating to both mind and body and used most often for illnesses and conditions that result from the effects of excessive emotional stress upon the body. Numerous physical ailments can be triggered in this way, from nausea, abdominal pains, ulcer and asthma to dizziness, insomnia and ARRHYTHMIA. The causes of the stress may be even more numerous but essentially fall into categories such as personal/marital; occupational; social. Although psychological treatment may help, attention to the physical symptoms is more effective.

psychotherapy the treatment of mental disorders, or the mental part of an ailment by psychological means, i.e. by concentrating upon and working through the mind. There are several approaches to this method of treatment including group therapy, psychoanalysis, and behavioural therapy.

psychotropic drugs drugs that affect the mind and its moods e.g. antidepressants, sedatives and stimulants.

puberty the changes that occur in boys and girls around the age of 10 to 14, which signify the beginnings of sexual maturity and the subsequent functioning of reproductive organs. It is apparent through the appearance of secondary sexual characteristics, such as a deepening of the voice in boys and growth of breasts in girls. In addition, girls commence menstruation and in boys the size of testicles increases. In both sexes body shape changes noticeably and body hair grows. The changes are initiated by PITUITARY GLAND hormones acting on the ovaries and testes.

pubis one of three bones, and the most anterior, that makes up each half of the pelvic girdle.

puerperal fever an infection, now rare in developed countries, which occurs within two or three days of childbirth when a mother is susceptible to disease. Because the body's resources are low and the genital tract after childbirth provides ready access for bacteria, it is essential that clean conditions are maintained to avoid infection. A mild infection of the genital tract may cause fever, high temperature and pulse. Inflammation, and possibly PERITONITIS may result from infection of local lymph and blood vessels, while access to the general circulation can cause septicaemia. Serious cases are, however, rare. Preventative measures are vital, but infections respond to antibiotic treatment.

pulmonary relating to the lungs.

pulmonary embolism a condition involving the blocking of the pulmonary artery or a branch of it by an EMBOLUS (usually a blood clot). The clot usually originates from PHLEBOTHROMBOSIS of the leg. The seriousness of the attack relates to the size of the clot. Large pulmonary emboli can be immediately fatal. Smaller ones may cause death of parts of the lung, PLEURISY and coughing up of blood. Anticoagulant drugs are used in minor cases, streptokinase may be used to dissolve the clot, or immediate surgery may be necessary. Several embolisms may produce PULMONARY HYPERTENSION.

pulmonary hypertension an increase in blood pressure in the pulmonary artery due to increased resistance to the flow of blood. The cause is usually disease of the lung (such as BRONCHITIS,

EMPHYSEMA, *see also* PULMONARY EMBOLISM) and the result is that the pressure increases in the right ventricle, enlarging it, producing pain, with the possibility of heart failure.

pulmonary oedema gathering of fluid in the lungs caused by, for example, MITRAL STENOSIS.

pulmonary stenosis a narrowing of the outlet from the heart to the pulmonary artery via the right ventricle, which may be congenital or due, more rarely, to rheumatic fever. Severe cases can produce ANGINA, fainting and enlargement of the heart, with eventual heart failure. Surgery is necessary to clear the obstruction.

pulse the regular expansion and contraction of an artery as a fluid wave of blood passes along, originating with the contraction of the heart and blood leaving the left ventricle. It is detected on arteries near the surface e.g. the radial artery on the wrist, and decreases with a reduction in the size of artery, so that the capillaries are under a steady pressure (hence the reason why venous flow is also steady).

pupil the circular opening in the IRIS which permits light into the lens in the EYE.

purgative drugs or other treatments taken to evacuate the bowels. These may be grouped by their mode of action, LAXATIVES providing a gentle effect. Purgatives work by increasing the muscular contractions of the intestine or by increasing the fluid in the intestine.

pus the liquid found at an infected site (abscess, ulcer, etc.). It is coloured white, yellow or greenish and consists of dead white blood cells, living and dead bacteria and dead tissue.

putrid fever a former name for TYPHUS FEVER.

pyelitis inflammation of part of the kidney, the pelvis. (This is the area from which urine drains into the ureter). The cause is usually a bacterial infection (commonly *E. coli*) and sometimes occurs as a complication of pregnancy. The symptoms include pain in the loins, high temperature and loss of weight, but it does respond to antibiotics. It is usually the case that the infection is not limited to the pelvis but affects all the kidney, hence a more accurate term is *pyelonephritis*.

pyloric stenosis a narrowing of the PYLORUS which limits the movement of food from the stomach to the duodenum, resulting in vomiting. It may be accompanied by distension and peristalsis of the stomach, visible through the abdominal wall. A continuation of the condition causes weight loss, dehydration and ALKALOSIS. It is often due to an ulcer or cancer near the pylorus which requires surgery.

pylorus the lower end of the stomach where food passes into the duodenum and at which there is a ring of muscle, the *pyloric sphincter*.

pyrexia another term for FEVER.

Q

Q fever an infectious disease which produces symptoms resembling pneumonia, including a severe headache, high fever and breathing problems. It is caused by the organism *Coxiella burnetti* and is a disease of sheep, goats and cattle which can be passed to man mainly through unpasteurized milk. The disease is treated with the drug tetracycline, and also chloramphenicol, and is of about two weeks duration.

quadriceps the large thigh muscle, which is divided into four distinct parts, and is responsible for movements of the knee joint.

quadriplegia paralysis of all four limbs of the body.

quarantine a period of time in which a person (or animal) who has, or is suspected of having, an infectious disease is isolated from others to prevent the spread of the infection.

quartan fever the recurrent fever, which usually occurs every fourth day, generally associated with *Malaria*.

quickening the first movements of a baby in the womb which are perceived by the mother usually around the fourth month of pregnancy.

quinine a colourless alkaloid derived from the bark of certain (cinchona) trees which is a strong antiseptic especially effective against the malarial parasite. It was formerly widely used in the treatment of malaria but has now largely been replaced because it is toxic in larger doses. In small amounts it has a stimulating effect and is used in tonic water.

quinsy the medical name for this condition is *pentonsillar abscess* and it is a complication of TONSILLITIS. A pus-filled abscess occurs near the tonsil, causing great difficulty in swallowing, and this may require surgical lancing.

R

rabies (*or* **hydrophobia**)a very severe and fatal disease affecting the central nervous system which occurs in dogs, wolves, cats and other carnivorous animals. Human beings are infected through the bite of a *rabid* animal, usually a dog. The onset of symptoms varies from ten days to up to a year from the time of being bitten. Characteristically, the person becomes irritable and depressed, swallowing and breathing difficulties develop, there are periods of great mental excitement, increased salivation and muscular spasms of the throat. Eventually, even the sight of water causes severe muscular spasms, convulsions and paralysis, and death follows within about four days. Treatment consists of thorough cleansing of the bite and injections of rabies vaccine, antiserum and immunoglobulin. As the UK is currently free of rabies, vigilant quarantine and other regulations involving the movement of animals are in force.

radiation sickness any illness which is caused by harmful radiation from radioactive substances. This may be a complication of radiotherapy for cancer, and produces symptoms of nausea, vomiting and sometimes itchiness of the skin. Antihistamine drugs and tranquillizers such as chlorpromazine are used to alleviate the condition.

radical treatment treatment aimed at the complete cure of a condition (i.e. 'to the root'), rather than the alleviation of symptoms. In contrast, *conservative treatment* is directed towards the minimum interference necessary to keep a condition under control.

radiograph an image produced by X-rays on a film. *Radiography* is the diagnostic technique used to examine the body using X-rays.

radiologist a doctor specialized in the interpretation of X-rays and other diagnostic records.

radiology the branch of medicine concerned with the use of X-rays.

radiotherapy the therapeutic use of penetrating radiation including X-rays, beta rays and gamma rays. These may be derived from X-ray machines or radioactive isotopes and are especially employed in the treatment of cancer. The main disadvantages of radiotherapy is that there may be damage to normal, healthy surrounding tissues.

radium a radioactive metallic element which occurs naturally and emits alpha, beta and gamma rays as it decays. The gamma rays derived from radium are used in the treatment of cancer.

radius the shorter outer bone of the forearm, the other being the *ulna*.

radon a radioactive gas produced when RADIUM decays. *Radon seeds* are small, sealed capsules, which are used in radiotherapy for cancer.

rash an eruption of the skin which is usually short-lived and consists of a reddened, perhaps itchy area or raised red spots.

rat bite fever two types of infectious disease which are contracted following the bite of a rat. The first type is caused by either of two kinds of bacteria and produces symptoms of fever, skin rash and joint and muscle pains. The second type is caused by a fungus and produces similar symptoms and vomiting. Both diseases are treated with penicillin.

Raynaud's disease a circulatory disorder characterized by a numbing and whitening of the body's extremities. The symptoms are caused by spasm of small arteries which cause a temporary interruption of the blood supply to (commonly) the fingers, toes, nose and ears.

recessive gene a gene whose character will only be expressed if paired with a similar gene (allele).

recombinant DNA DNA (deoxyribonucleic acid) containing genes which have been artificially combined by the techniques of GENETIC ENGINEERING. Recombinant DNA technology has become synonymous with genetic engineering.

rectum the final portion of the large intestine between the colon and anal canal in which faeces are stored prior to elimination.

red blood cell *see* **erythrocyte**.

referred pain (*or* synalgia) pain felt in another part of the body at a distance from the site at which it might be expected. An example is certain heart conditions which cause pain in the left arm and fingers. The condition arises because some sensory nerves share common routes in the central nervous system, hence stimulation of one causes an effect in another.

reflex action an unconscious movement which is brought about by relatively simple nervous circuits in the central nervous system. In its simplest form it involves a single *reflex arc* of one receptor and sensory nerve which forms a *synapse* in the BRAIN or SPINAL cord with a motor nerve, which then transmits the impulse to a muscle or gland to bring about a response. However some reflex actions are more complicated than this, involving several neurones. Examples are the *plantar reflex* of the toes, when the sole of the foot is stroked, the *knee-jerk reflex* and the reflex pupil of the eye, which contracts suddenly when a light is directed upon its surface. The presence or absence of reflexes give an indication of the condition of the nervous system and are pointers to the presence or absence of disease or damage.

refractory a condition which does not respond to treatment.

refractory period the time taken for a nerve or muscle cell to recover after an electrical impulse has passed along, or following contraction. During this time, the nerve or muscle cell is unable to respond to a further stimulus.

regimen a course of treatment which usually involves several elements including drugs, diet and lifestyle (such as the taking of exercise), aimed at curing a disease or promoting good health.

registrar a relatively senior hospital doctor responsible for the care of patients and working with consultants.

regression in psychiatry, this refers to a reversion to a more immature form of behaviour. In medicine, the term refers to the stage in the course of a disease when symptoms cease and the patient recovers.

regurgitation the bringing up of swallowed undigested food from the stomach to the mouth (*see also* POSSETING.)

The term is also used to describe the backward flow of blood in the heart if one or more valves is diseased and defective.

rehabilitation the process of restoring (as far as possible) back to normal life a person who has been disabled by injury or physical and/or mental illness. Rehabilitation usually involves various different kinds of therapy and retraining.

Reiter's syndrome (*or* **RS**) a disease of unknown cause, affecting men, which produces symptoms of URETHRITIS, CONJUNCTIVITIS and ARTHRITIS. It may also produce other symptoms, including fever and diarrhoea and it is suspected that the cause may be a virus.

rejection this is a term used in transplant medicine describing the situation in which the immune system of the recipient individual rejects and destroys an organ or tissue grafted from a donor. Various drugs e.g. *cyclosporin A* are given to the recipient to dampen down the immune system and reduce the risk of rejection.

relapse the return of the symptoms of a disease from which a person had apparently recovered or was in the process of recovery.

relapsing fever a disease caused by spirochaete bacteria of the genus *Borrelia*, which is transmitted to man by lice and ticks. The disease is characterized by recurrent bouts of fever, accompanied by headache, joint and muscle pains and nosebleeds. The first attack lasts for about two to eight days and further milder bouts occur after three to ten days. Treatment is by means of bed rest, and with erythromycin and tetracycline drugs.

remission a period during the course of a disease when symptoms have lessened or disappeared.

REM sleep this stands for *Rapid Eye Movement* SLEEP and describes a phase when the eyeballs move rapidly behind closed eyelids. This appears to be the phase during which dreaming occurs.

renal describing or relating to the kidneys.

repetitive strain injury *see* **tendinitis**.

reproductive system the name given to all the organs involved in reproduction. In males these comprise the testes, vasa deferentia, prostate gland, seminal vesicles, urethra and penis. In females, the reproductive system consists of the ovaries, Fallopian tubes, womb (uterus), vagina and vulva (*see individual entries*).

resection a surgical operation in which part of an organ, or any body part, is removed.

resistance the degree of natural immunity which an individual possesses against a certain disease or diseases. The term is also applied to the degree with which a disease or disease-causing organism can withstand treatment with drugs such as a course of antibiotics.

resonance the quality and increase of sound produced by striking the body over an air-filled structure. If resonance is decreased compared to normal this is termed *dullness* and if increased *hyper-resonance*. Tapping the body, often the chest, to determine the degree of resonance is called *percussion*. An opinion may be formed about the condition of underlying organs, i.e. the amount of air present or fluid e.g. in the lungs or if there is any enlargement.

respiration the whole process by which air is drawn into and out of the lungs during which oxygen is absorbed into the bloodstream and carbon dioxide and water are given off. *External respiration* is the actual process of breathing and the exchange of gases which takes place in the lungs. *Internal respiration* is the process by which oxygen is given up from the blood circulation to the tissues, in all parts of the body, and carbon dioxide is taken up to be transported back to the lungs and eliminated.

The process of drawing air into the lungs is known as *inhalation* or *inspiration* and expelling it out as *exhalation* or *expiration*. The rate at which this occurs is known as the *respiratory rate* and it is about 18 times a minute in a static healthy adult.

respirator one of a number of different devices used to assist or take over RESPIRATION, especially when the muscles which should normally be involved are paralysed, as in some forms of POLIOMYELITIS.

respiratory distress syndrome this usually refers to a condition arising in newborn babies, especially those which are premature, being particularly common in infants born between 32 and 37 weeks' gestation. It is also known as *hyaline membrane disease* and is characterized by rapid, shallow, laboured breathing. It arises because the lungs are not properly expanded and lack a substance (known as surfactant) necessary to bring their expansion about.

Adults may suffer from *adult respiratory distress syndrome* in which there is PULMONARY OEDEMA and a high mortality rate.

respiratory syncitial virus (*or* **RS Virus**) this is the main cause of bronchiolitis and PNEUMONIA in babies under the age of 6 months

respiratory system all the organs and tissues involved in RESPIRATION, including the nose, pharynx, larynx, trachea, bronchi, bronchioles, lungs and diaphragm, along with the muscles which bring about respiratory movements (*see individual entries*).

resuscitation reviving a person in whom heartbeat and breathing has ceased. *See* ARTIFICIAL RESPIRATION and CARDIAC MASSAGE.

retardation the slowing down of an activity or a process, often referring to mental subnormality or 'backwardness'.

retina the layer which lines the interior of the eye. The retina itself consists of two layers, the inner one next to the cavity of the eyeball containing the light-sensitive cells, the RODS and CONES, and also nerve fibres. This layer receives light directed onto its surface by the lens. The outer layer of the retina next to the *choroid* contains pigmented cells which prevent the passage of light. *See also* EYE.

retinol *see* **vitamin A**.

retractor one of a number of different surgical instruments designed to pull apart the cut edges of an incision to allow greater operating access.

retroflexion the bending backwards of a part of an organ, particularly the upper portion of the uterus. *Compare* RETROVERSION.

retroversion an abnormal position of the uterus in which the whole organ is tilted backwards instead of forward, as is normally the case. A *retroverted uterus* occurs in about 20% of women. *See* RETROFLEXION.

retrovirus a type of virus containing RNA (ribonucleic acid) which is able to introduce its genetic material into the DNA of body cells. These viruses are suspected causal agents in the development of certain cancers.

Reye's syndrome a rare disorder, of unknown cause, which affects children and seems to follow on from a viral infection such as chicken-pox, often manifesting itself during the recovery phase. The symptoms include vomiting, high fever, delirium, convulsions leading to coma and death, the mortality rate being about 25%. Among those who survive, about half suffer some brain damage. It has been suggested that aspirin may be implicated in the development of this condition and this drug is not now recommended for children under the age of 12.

Rhesus factor *see* **blood groups**.

rheumatic fever a severe disease affecting children and young adults, which is a complication of upper respiratory tract infection with bacteria known as *Haemolytic streptococci*. The symptoms include fever, joint pain and ARTHRITIS, which progresses from joint to joint, a characteristic red rash known as *Erythema marginatum*, and also painless nodules which develop beneath the skin over bony protuberances such as the elbow, knee and back of the wrist. In addition, there is CHOREA and inflammation of the heart, including the muscle, valves and membranes. The condition may lead to rheumatic heart disease, in which there is scarring and inflammation of heart structures. There is sometimes a need for heart valves to be replaced in later life.

The initial treatment consists of destroying the streptococci which cause the disease with antibiotic drugs such as penicillin. Other drugs are also used such as non-steroidal anti-inflammatory drugs (NSAID) and corticosteroids. Surgery may be required later in life to replace damaged heart valves.

rheumatism a general term used to describe aches and pains in joints and muscles.

rheumatoid arthritis the second most common form of joint disease, after OSTEOARTHRITIS, which usually affects the feet, ankles, fingers and wrists. The condition is diagnosed by means of X-rays, which show a typical pattern of changes around the inflamed joints, known as *rheumatoid erosions*. At first there is swelling of the joint and inflammation of the SYNOVIAL MEMBRANE (the membranous sac which surrounds the joint), followed by erosion and loss of cartilage and bone. In addition, a blood test reveals the presence of *serum rheumatoid factor antibody*, which is characteristic of this condition. The condition varies greatly in its degree of severity but at its worst can be progressive and seriously disabling. In other people, after an initial active phase, there may be a long period of remission.

A number of different drugs are used to treat the disease, including analgesics, disease-modifying preparations and anti-inflammatory agents.

rheumatology the branch of medicine concerned with diseases of the joints and associated tissues and structures. The medical specialist in this field is known as a *rheumatologist*.

rhinitis inflammation of the mucous membrane of the nose such as occurs with colds and allergic reactions.

rhinovirus any one of a large number of RNA-containing viruses which cause upper respiratory tract infections, including the common cold.

ribs 12 pairs of thin, slightly twisted and curved bones which form the thoracic rib cage, which protects the lungs and heart. The *true ribs* are the first seven pairs, which are each connected to the STERNUM at the front by a costal CARTILAGE. The *false ribs* are the next three pairs which are indirectly connected to the sternum as each is attached by its cartilage to the rib above. The *floating ribs* are the last two pairs, which are unattached and end freely in the muscle of the thoracic wall. At the backbone, the head of each rib articulates with one of the 12 thoracic vertebrae.

rickets this is a disease affecting children which involves a deficiency of VITAMIN D. Vitamin D can be manufactured in the skin in the presence of sunlight but dietary sources are important especially where sunlight is lacking. The disease is characterized by soft bones, which bend out of shape and cause deformities.

Bones are hardened by the deposition of calcium salts and this cannot happen in the absence of vitamin D. Treatment consists of giving vitamin D, usually in the form of calciferol, and ensuring that there is an adequate amount in the child's future diet. Vitamin D deficiency in adults causes the condition called OSTEOMALACIA.

rickettsiae a group of microorganisms, which share characteristics in common with both bacteria and viruses and are parasites which occur in lice, fleas, ticks and other arthropods. They can be passed to man by the bites of these animals and are the cause of several serious diseases, including TYPHUS, *Rocky Mountain spotted fever* and Q FEVER.

Rift Valley fever a disease caused by a virus which formerly mainly affected domestic animals and rarely human beings in sub-Saharan Africa. However, a widespread outbreak arose in Egypt in 1977, which caused many fatalities and it poses a threat to people throughout the Middle East. A new strain of virus of a more virulent type is thought to be responsible and the infection is characterized by fever, muscle and joint pains, haemorrhages, headache, photophobia and loss of appetite. The virus is transmitted to man by mosquitoes or by direct contact with the carcasses of heavily infected animals. An effective vaccine is available.

rigidity especially used to describe stiffness in a limb which is being moved passively, which is a symptom of PARKINSON'S DISEASE.

rigor a sudden bout of shivering and feeling of coldness, which often accompanies the start of a fever.

rigor mortis the stiffening of the body that occurs within eight hours of death due to chemical changes in the muscles.

Ringer's solution a physiological solution containing sodium chloride (salt), potassium chloride and calcium chloride and some other minerals, in the same proportions as in blood serum. It is injected intravenously in people suffering from dehydration and is used to bathe and maintain organs which have been removed for transplant operations.

ringworm this is an infection caused by various species of fungi and is known medically as Tinea. It is classified according to the area affected e.g. *Tinea capitis* which is ringworm of the scalp. Other areas affected are the beard, groin (dhobi itch) and nails and feet (athlete's foot).

The infection is typically slightly raised, itchy and with a ring-like appearance. It is highly contagious and the commonest form is athlete's foot, which usually begins between the toes. The antibiotic drug, griseofulvin, taken by mouth, is the normal treatment for ringworm, and also antifungal creams applied to the affected areas.

Rinne's test a type of hearing test that uses a vibrating tuning fork which helps to determine whether deafness is *perceptive* (nervous) or *conductive* (indicating an obstruction within the ear).

RNA ribonucleic acid, which is a complex nucleic acid present mainly in the CYTOPLASM of cells but also in the NUCLEUS. It is involved in the production of proteins and exists in three forms, ribosomal (r), transfer (t) and messenger (m) RNA. In some viruses it forms the genetic material. *See also* DNA.

rod one of the two types of light-sensitive cell present in the RETINA of the EYE. The rods enable vision in dim light, due to a pigment called *rhodopsin* (*visual purple*). This pigment degenerates or bleaches when light is present and regenerates during darkness. In bright light all the pigment bleaches and the rods cannot function. Bleaching of the pigment gives rise to nerve impulses, which are sent to the brain and interpreted.

rodent ulcer a slow-growing malignant ulcer, which occurs on the face in elderly people, usually near the lips, nostrils or eyelids. Skin and underlying tissues and bone are destroyed if the ulcer is untreated. Normally, treatment is by means of surgery and possibly radiotherapy.

rosacea a disease of the skin of the face, characterized by a red, flushed appearance and enlargement of the SEBACEOUS GLANDS in the skin. The nose may also enlarge and look red and lumpy (rhinophyma). The cause is unknown but may be aggravated by certain foods or drinks such as an excess of alcohol. Treatment is by means of *tetracycline drugs*.

roseola any rose-coloured rash such as accompanies various infectious diseases e.g. measles.

Rose-waaler test a diagnostic blood test, which is used to detect RHEUMATOID ARTHRITIS.

rotavirus one of a number of viruses which commonly cause gastroenteritis and diarrhoea in young children under the age of six years. They infect the lining cells of the SMALL INTESTINE.

Rotor syndrome a rare inherited liver condition similar to the DUBLIN-JOHNSON SYNDROME.

roughage dietary fibre, which is necessary to maintain the healthy functioning of the bowels and helps to prevent constipation and DIVERTICULOSIS. The eating of sufficient dietary fibre is thought to be important in the prevention of cancer of the colon.

rubella *see* GERMAN MEASLES.

rupture the bursting open of an organ, tissue or structure e.g. ruptured APPENDIX. Also, a popular name for a HERNIA.

S

Sabin vaccine an oral vaccine for POLIOMYELITIS. The appropriate virus is cultured but rendered non-violent while retaining its ability to stimulate production of antibodies.

sac a structure resembling a bag, e.g. the lungs.

sacral nerves nerves that serve the legs, anal and genital region, which originate from the sacral area of the spinal column. There are five pairs of sacral nerves.

sacral vertebrae the five vertebrae that are fused together to form the SACRUM.

sacrum the lower part of the spinal column comprising five fused vertebrae (SACRAL VERTEBRAE) in a triangular shape. The sacrum forms the back wall of the pelvis and articulates with the coccyx below, the lumbar vertebrae above and the hips to the sides.

safe period the days in a woman's menstrual cycle when conception is least likely. OVULATION usually occurs midway through the cycle, about 15 days before onset of menstruation, and the fertile period is about five days before and five after ovulation. Providing periods are regular, it can be calculated when intercourse is unlikely to result in pregnancy.

saliva an alkaline liquid present in the mouth to keep the mouth moist to aid swallowing of food and through the presence of amylase enzymes (ptyalin) to digest starch. It is secreted by the SALIVARY GLANDS and in addition to ptyalin, contains water, mucus and buffers (to minimize changes in acidity).

salivary glands three pairs of glands: parotid, submandibular and sublingual, that produce saliva. The stimulus to produce saliva can be the taste, smell, sight or even thought of food.

Salk vaccine a vaccine against POLIOMYELITIS, administered by injection. The virus is treated with formalin, which renders it unable to cause the disease but it still prompts the production of antibodies.

Salmonella infections FOOD POISONING due to *Salmonella*, a genus of Gram-negative (*see* GRAM'S STAIN) rod-like bacteria.

salpingectomy the surgical excision of a FALLOPIAN TUBE. The removal of both produces sterilization.

salpingitis inflammation of a tube, usually the Fallopian tube, by bacterial infection. It may originate in the vagina or uterus, or be carried in the blood. Peritonitis can ensue. Severe cases may cause a blockage of the Fallopian tubes, resulting in sterility.

salpingostomy the clearing of a blocked FALLOPIAN TUBE, in which the blocked part is removed surgically.

sanatorium a hospital or similar institution for convalescence or rehabilitation.

sandfly fever a viral infection passed to man through the bite of a sandfly. It occurs in much of the tropics and sub-tropics during the warmer months. It is a short-lived infection that resembles influenza in its symptoms.

sanguineous containing blood, covered with or stained with blood.

sarcoma *see* **cancer**.

scab a crust that forms over an injury (scratch, sore, etc.) during the body's healing processes. The scab consists of FIBRIN, dried blood, SERUM or pus, and epithelial cells. Healing occurs beneath the protective scab, which falls off when the process is complete. Scabs due to infections occur e.g. on the face, with no previous sign.

scabies a skin infection causing severe itching. It is due to the mite *Sarcoptes scabiei*, which burrows into the skin and lays eggs, and the resulting larvae cause the itching. The areas of the body affected are the skin between fingers, wrists, buttocks and genitals. An application of special cream is necessary to kill the mites.

scalds *see* **burns**.

scalp the covering of the skull around the top of the head which comprises several layers, from the skin with hair on the outside through fat and fibrous tissue to another fibrous layer (the pericranium) that is attached closely to the skull.

scalpel a small surgical knife with renewable blades, used for cutting tissues.

scan examination of the body using one of a number

of techniques, such as COMPUTERIZED TOMOGRAPHY and ultrasonography. *See* ULTRASOUND.

Also the image produced by a scanning technique

scaphoid bone a bone of the wrist, the outside one on the thumb side of the hand.

scapula (*plural* **scapulae**) the shoulder blade. A triangular bone and one of a pair forming the shoulder girdle.

scar the mark left after a wound heals. It is due to the damaged tissues not repairing completely, and being replaced by a fibrous connective tissue.

scarlet fever (*or* **scarlatina**) an infectious disease, mainly of childhood, caused by the bacterium *streptococcus*. Symptoms show after a few days and include sickness, sore throat, fever and a scarlet rash that may be widespread. Antibiotics are effective and also prevent any complications e.g. inflammation of the kidneys.

schistosomiasis (*or* **bilharziasis**) a parasitic infection caused by blood flukes (*Schistosoma*). Man is infected with the larvae of the fluke that enter through the skin from infected water. The adults then settle in blood vessels of the intestine or bladder. Subsequent release of eggs causes anaemia, diarrhoea, dysentery, enlargement of the spleen and liver and cirrhosis of the liver.

The disease can be treated with drugs but preventative measures are preferable. Schistosomiasis affects millions worldwide, particularly in the Far and Middle East, South America and Africa.

schizophrenia any one of a large group of severe mental disorders typified by gross distortion of reality, disturbance in language and breakdown of thought processes, perceptions and emotions. Delusions and hallucinations are usual, as are apathy, confusion, incontinence and strange behaviour. No single cause is known but genetic factors are probably important. Drug therapy has improved the outlook markedly over recent years.

sciatica pain in the sciatic nerve, and therefore felt in the back of the thigh, leg and foot. The commonest cause is a PROLAPSED INTERVERTEBRAL DISC pressing on a nerve root, but it may also be due to ankylosing SPONDYLITIS and other conditions.

sclera the outer layer of the eyeballs which is white and fibrous save at the front of the eye, when it becomes the transparent CORNEA.

scleritis inflammation of the white of the eye (SCLERA).

scleroderma a condition in which connective tissue hardens and contracts. The tissue may be the skin,

heart, kidney, lung, etc., and the condition may be localized or it may spread throughout the body, eventually being fatal. If the skin is affected, it becomes tough and patchily pigmented and may lead to stiff joints and wasting muscles.

sclerosis hardening of tissue, usually after inflammation leading to parts of organs being hard and of no use. It is applied commonly to such changes in the nervous system (MULTIPLE SCLEROSIS); in other organs it is termed FIBROSIS or CIRRHOSIS.

sclerotherapy a treatment for VARICOSE VEINS. An irritant solution is injected, causing FIBROSIS of the vein lining and its eventual removal by THROMBOSIS and scarring.

screening test a programme of tests carried out on a large number of apparently healthy people to find those who may have a particular disease e.g. cervical smears to detect the precancerous stage of cervical cancer.

scrofula TUBERCULOSIS of the LYMPH NODES in the neck, which form sores and scars after healing. It is now an uncommon condition, but drug treatment is effective.

scrotum the sac that contains the testicles and holds them outside the body, to permit production and storage of sperm at a temperature lower than that of the abdomen.

scrub typhus a disease prevalent in southeast Asia, caused by a parasitic microorganism, *Rickettsia*, transmitted from rodents to man by the bite of mites. It causes chills, headaches, high temperatures, rashes and possibly delirium. An ulcer develops at the initial bite. The condition can be treated with antibiotics.

scrum-pox a bacterial (IMPETIGO) or viral (*herpes simplex*) infection of the face, common to rugby players, occurring probably through facial contact in the scrum or communal changing facilities.

scurvy a deficiency disease caused by a lack of VITAMIN C (ascorbic acid), due to a dietary lack of fruit and vegetables. Symptoms begin with swollen, bleeding gums and then subcutaneous bleeding, bleeding into joints, ulcers, anaemia and then fainting, diarrhoea and trouble with major organs. Untreated, it is fatal, but nowadays it is easily prevented, or cured should it arise, through correct diet or administration of the vitamin.

sebaceous cyst a cyst formed in the duct of a SEBACEOUS GLAND of the skin.

sebaceous gland any of the minute glands in the skin that secrete an oily substance called SEBUM. The glands open into hair follicles. Activity of the glands varies with age, puberty being the most active period.

seborrhoea excessive production of SEBUM by the SEBACEOUS GLANDS producing either a build-up of dry scurf or oily deposits on the skin. The condition often leads to the development of ACNE.

sebum the secretion formed by the SEBACEOUS GLANDS, which forms a thin, oily film on the skin, preventing excessive dryness. It also has an antibacterial action.

secondary sexual characteristics the physical features that develop at puberty. In girls, the breasts and genitals increase in size and pubic hair grows. Boys grow pubic hair and facial hair, the voice breaks and the genitals become adult size.

secretin a polypeptide hormone produced by the lining of the DUODENUM and JEJUNUM in response to acid from the stomach. It stimulates production of alkaline pancreatic juice, and BILE secretion by the liver.

secretion the material produced by a gland.

section cutting in surgery e.g. an abdominal section. Also, a thin slice of a specimen, as used in microscopy.

sedative a drug that lessens tension and anxiety. Sedatives are hypnotic drugs e.g. barbiturates, given in doses lower than would bring on sleep. They may be used to combat pain, sleeplessness, spasms, etc.

semen the fluid that contains the sperm which is ejaculated from the penis during copulation.

senile dementia an organic mental disorder of the elderly involving generalized atrophy of the brain. The result is a gradual deterioration with loss of memory, impaired judgement, confusion, emotional outbursts and irritability. The degree of the condition may vary considerably.

sensation a feeling. The result of stimulation of a sensory receptor producing a nerve impulse which travels on an afferent fibre to the brain.

sensitivity with reference to a SCREENING TEST, the proportion of people with the disease who are identified by the test.

sensitization a change in the body's response to foreign substances. With the development of an allergy, a person becomes sensitized to a certain ALLERGEN and then becomes hypersensitive. Similarly, it may be an acquired reaction when ANTIBODIES develop in response to an ANTIGEN.

sepsis the destruction of tissues through putrefaction by bacteria-causing disease, or toxins produced by bacteria.

septal defect a hole in the SEPTUM or partition between the left and right sides of the heart, whether in the atria (*see* ATRIUM) or VENTRICLES. This condition is a CONGENITAL disorder caused by an abnormal development of the foetal heart. Whether the defect is atrial or ventricular, it allows incorrect circulation of the blood from left to right, from higher pressure to lower. This is called a *shunt*, and results in too much blood flowing through the lungs. PULMONARY HYPERTENSION results and a large shunt may cause heart failure. Surgery can correct the defect, although a small one may not require any treatment.

septic affected with SEPSIS.

septicaemia a term used loosely for any type of blood poisoning. Also, a systemic infection with PATHOGENS from an infected part of the body circulating in the bloodstream.

septic shock a form of shock that occurs due to SEPTICAEMIA. The toxins cause a drastic fall in blood pressure due to tissue damage and blood clotting. Kidneys, heart and lungs are affected and related symptoms include fever, TACHYCARDIA or even coma. The condition occurs most in those who already have a serious disease such as cancer, DIABETES, or CIRRHOSIS. Urgent treatment is vital, with antibiotics, oxygen and fluids given intravenously.

septum a planar dividing feature within a structure of the body; a partition.

serology a laboratory medical subdiscipline involving the study of blood serum and its constituents, including ANTIGEN-ANTIBODY reactions.

serositis inflammation of a SEROUS MEMBRANE.

serous membrane a membrane lining a large cavity in the body. The membranes are smooth and transparent and the surfaces are moistened by fluid derived from blood or lymph serum (hence the name). Examples are the PERITONEUM and the PERICARDIUM. Each consists of two layers: the *visceral,* which surrounds the organs and the *parietal,* which lines the cavity. The two portions are continuous and the surfaces are close together, separated by fluid, which permits free movement of the organs.

serum a serous fluid. More specifically the clear, sticky fluid that separates from blood and lymph when clotting occurs. In addition to water, serum contains albumin and GLOBULIN with salts, fat, sugar, UREA and other compounds important in disease prevention.

Also, a VACCINE prepared from the serum of a hyperimmune donor for use in protection against a particular infection.

serum sickness a hypersensitive reaction that occasionally occurs several days after injection of foreign SERUM, producing rashes, joint pains, fever and swelling of the lymph nodes. It is due to circulating antigen material to which the body responds. It is not a serious condition.

sessile in description of a tumour or growth, one having no stalk.

sex chromosomes CHROMOSOMES that play a major role in determining the sex of the bearer. Sex chromosomes contain GENES that control the characteristics of the individual e.g. testes in males and ovaries in females. Women have two X chromosomes while men have one X and one Y chromosome (*see individual entries*).

sex hormones steroid hormones responsible for the control of sexual development (primary and SECONDARY SEXUAL CHARACTERISTICS) and reproductive function. The ovaries and testes are the organs primarily involved in hormone production, of which there are three main types: ANDROGENS, the male sex hormones; OESTROGENS and PROGESTERONE, the female sex hormones.

sex-linked disorders conditions produced because the genes controlling certain characteristics are carried on the SEX CHROMOSOMES, usually the X chromosome. Some result from an abnormal number of chromosomes, e.g. KLINEFELTER'S SYNDROME affecting only men, and TURNER'S SYNDROME affecting only women.

Other disorders, such as HAEMOPHILIA, are carried on the X chromosome and these manifest themselves in men because although the genes are recessive, there is no other X chromosome to mask the recessive type, as is the case with women.

sexually transmitted disease *see* **venereal disease.**

shingles the common name for Herpes zoster. *See* HERPES.

shock acute circulatory failure, when the arterial blood pressure is too low to provide the normal blood supply to the body. The signs are a cold, clammy skin, pallor, CYANOSIS, weak rapid pulse, irregular breathing and dilated pupils. There may also be a reduced flow of urine and confusion or lethargy. There are numerous causes of shock from a reduction in blood volume as after burns, external bleeding, dehydration, etc., to reduced heart activity, as in CORONARY THROMBOSIS, PULMONARY EMBOLISM, etc.

Certain other circumstances may produce shock, including severe allergic reactions (anaphylactic shock, *see* ANAPHYLAXIS), drugs overdose, emotional shock and so on.

short sight *see* **myopia.**

shoulder the joint formed by the shoulder blade

(SCAPULA) and the upper end of the humerus. It is a ball-and-socket joint, surrounded by a fibrous capsule, strengthened with bands of ligament. The strength of the joint is derived from the associated muscles.

shoulder blade *see* **scapula.**

shoulder girdle *see* **pectoral girdle.**

Siamese twins (*or* **conjoined twins**) when twins are joined together physically at birth. The condition varies from superficial joining, e.g. by the umbilical vessels, to major fusion of head, torso and internal organs. The latter cases are inevitably very much more difficult to separate. The condition is caused by foetuses developing from the same OVUM.

sickle-cell anaemia a type of inherited, haemolytic ANAEMIA (*see* HAEMOLYSIS) that is genetically determined and which affects people of African ancestry. It is caused by a recessive gene and is manifested when this gene is inherited from both parents. One AMINO ACID in the HAEMOGLOBIN molecule is substituted, causing the disease, which results in an abnormal type of haemoglobin being precipitated in the red blood cells during deprivation of oxygen. This produces the distortion of the cells, which are removed from the circulation, causing anaemia and jaundice.

Many people are carriers, due to inheritance of just one defective GENE and because this confers increased resistance to malaria, this gene remains at a high level.

side effect the additional and unwanted effect(s) of a drug, above the intended action. Sometimes side-effects are harmful, and may be stronger than anticipated results of the drug, or something quite different.

sigmoid colon the end part of the COLON, which is S-shaped.

sigmoidectomy surgical excision of the SIGMOID COLON, performed usually for tumours, a long and twisted sigmoid colon or diverticular disease. *See* DIVERTICULITIS, DIVERTICULOSIS.

sigmoidoscopy the examination of the SIGMOID COLON and rectum with a special viewing device. The instrument is tubular, with illumination, although modern forms use fibreoptics, which are flexible.

silicosis a type of PNEUMOCONIOSIS caused by the inhalation of silica as particles of dust. The silica promotes FIBROSIS of the lung tissue, resulting in breathlessness and a greater likelihood to contract tuberculosis. Workers in quarrying, mineral mining, sand-blasting, etc., are most susceptible.

sinew the TENDON of a muscle.

sinoatrial node the natural heart PACEMAKER, which consists of specialized muscle cells in the right atrium. These cells generate electrical impulses, contract and initiate contractions in the muscles of the heart. The AUTONOMIC NERVOUS SYSTEM supplies the node and certain hormones also have an effect.

sinus in general terms, a cavity or channel. Specifically, air cavities in bone, as in the bones of the face and skull. Also a channel, as in the DURA MATER, which drains venous blood from the brain.

sinusitis inflammation of a SINUS. It usually refers to the sinuses in the face which link with the nose and may therefore be due to a spread of infection from the nose. Headaches and a tenderness over the affected sinus are typical symptoms, with a pus-containing discharge from the nose. Persistent infection may necessitate surgery to drain the sinus.

Sjögren's syndrome dryness of the mouth and eyes, associated with rheumatoid arthritis. The syndrome is due to the destruction of the salivary glands (and lacrimal glands).

skeleton the rigid, supporting framework of the body that protects organs and tissues, provides muscle attachments, facilitates movement, and produces red blood cells. There are 206 bones, divided into the axial skeleton (head and trunk) and the appendicular skeleton (limbs). The types of bone are: long (e.g. humerus), short (e.g. carpals), flat (parts of the cranium) and irregular (e.g. the vertebrae).

skin the outer layer of the body comprising an external EPIDERMIS, itself made up of a *stratum corneum* (horny layer) formed of flat cells that rub off, being replaced from below; beneath this are two more layers (*stratum lucidum* and *stratum granulosum*) which act as intermediate stages between the stratum corneum, and a still lower layer, the Malpighian layer.

The Malpighian layer is where the epidermis is produced. The dermis lies beneath the epidermis and then follows subcutaneous tissue composed mainly of fat. The subcutaneous tissue contains glands (sweat, SEBACEOUS, etc.), sensory receptors for pain, pressure and temperature, nerves, muscles and blood capillaries.

The skin is a protective layer against injury and parasites and it moderates water loss. It is a medium of temperature control by means of the sweat glands and blood capillaries and also the hairs (which provide insulation).

skin graft (*see also* GRAFT) a piece of skin taken from another site on the body to cover an injured area, commonly due to burns. The graft is normally taken from elsewhere on the patient's body (*autograft*) but occasionally from someone else (*homograft*). A variety of thicknesses and graft types are used, depending upon the wound.

skull the part of the SKELETON that forms the head and encloses the brain. It is made up of 22 bones, forming the cranium (eight bones) and 14 in the face, and all except the mandible are fused along sutures creating immovable joints. The mandible (lower jaw) articulates close to the ears. A large opening at the base of the skull (FORAMEN magnum) allows the spinal cord to pass from the brain to the trunk of the body.

sleep a state of lower awareness, accompanied by reduced metabolic activity and physical relaxation. When falling asleep, there is a change in the brain's electrical activity. This activity can be recorded by an ELECTROENCEPHALOGRAM (EEG). There are high-amplitude, low-frequency waves (slow-wave sleep) interrupted by short periods of low-amplitude, high-frequency waves. The periods of high-frequency waves are typified by restless sleep with dreams and rapid eye movements, hence the name rem SLEEP, and the EEG is similar to that of a waking person. REM sleep comprises about 25% of the time asleep.

sleeping sickness (*or* **African trypanosomiasis**) a parasitic disease found in tropical Africa, which is spread through the bite of tsetse flies. The organism responsible is a minute protozoan, *Trypanosoma*, and initially the symptoms consist of a recurring fever, a slight rash, headache and chills. Then follows ANAEMIA, enlarged LYMPH NODES and pain in joints and limbs. Then after some time (possibly years), sleeping sickness itself develops. This is due to the parasites occupying minute blood vessels in the brain, resulting in damage, and symptoms of drowsiness and lethargy. Death may follow from weakness or an associated disease. The early stages are curable with drugs. When the brain is affected, arsenic-containing drugs are used and although they are highly active against the parasites, care is necessary due to the toxicity of the compounds.

sling a bandage so arranged as to support an injured limb, usually an arm.

slipped disc *see* **prolapsed intervertebral disc**.

slough dead tissue, usually of limited extent, that after infection separates from the healthy tissue of the rest of the body. In cases of GANGRENE, it is possible for limbs to be lost.

slow virus one of several viruses that show their effects some time after infection, by which time considerable damage of nerve tissue has occurred, resulting ultimately in death. Some years ago such a virus was found to cause scrapie in sheep and recently bovine spongiform encephalopathy in cows. In man a slow virus is thought to be the cause of CREUTZFELDT-JAKOB DISEASE and a type of MENINGITIS.

small intestine *see* **intestine**.

smallpox a highly infectious viral disease that has nonetheless been eradicated. Infection results, after about two weeks, in a high fever, head, and body aches and vomiting. Eventually red spots appear, which change to water, and then pus-filled vesicles, which on drying out leave scars. The person stays infectious until all scabs are shed. Fever often returns, with DELIRIUM, and although recovery is usual, complications often ensue e.g. PNEUMONIA. The last naturally occurring case was in 1977.

smooth muscle *see* **involuntary muscle**.

sneezing the involuntary reflex expulsion of air via the nose and mouth due to irritating particles in the nose e.g. pollen. It is also symptomatic of colds, measles, hay fever, etc. One sneeze can project many thousands of droplets over several metres at great speed (up to 60km/hr) and is therefore instrumental in the spread of infections.

Snellen chart the chart commonly used for testing distant vision. It comprises rows of capital letters that become progressively smaller.

snoring a vibration of the soft palate that produces a hoarse sound. Although breathing through the mouth is essential for snoring, not all those who breathe through their mouth snore. The main cause is a blockage of the nose.

snow blindness an eye disorder due to excessive exposure to ultraviolet light e.g. as reflected from a snowfield. Covering the eyes for 24 hours is usually an effective treatment.

solar plexus a network of sympathetic nerves and ganglia (*see* GANGLION) behind the stomach, surrounding the coeliac artery. It is a major autonomic PLEXUS of the body, where nerves of the sympathetic and parasympathetic nervous system combine (*see individual terms*).

somatic descriptive term meaning relating to the body, as opposed to the mind. More specifically, concerning the *non-reproductive* parts of the body.

somnambulism (*or* **sleep-walking**) walking and performing other functions during sleep with no recollection upon waking.

soporific sleep-inducing. *See also* HYPNOTICS.

sore a common term for an ulcer or open skin wound.

sound an instrument resembling a rod, with a curved end, that is used to explore a body cavity e.g. the bladder, or to dilate STRICTURES.

Southey's tubes very fine tubes for drawing off fluid, e.g. from subcutaneous tissue. They are rarely used today.

spasm a muscular contraction that is involuntary. Spasms may be part of a more major disorder e.g. spastic paralysis or convulsions, or they may be specific, such as cramp or colic, etc. A heart spasm is known as ANGINA.

spasmolytic a drug that reduces spasms (in SMOOTH MUSCLE) in a number of ways. It may generally depress the CENTRAL NERVOUS SYSTEM, act directly on the muscles in question, or modify the nerve impulses causing the spasm. Spasmolytics are used in the treatment of ANGINA and colic and as BRONCHODILATORS.

spastic colon *see* **irritable bowel syndrome**.

spasticity muscular hypertonicity (i.e. an increase in the state of readiness of muscle fibres to contract; an increase in the normal partial contraction) with an increased resistance to stretch. Moderate cases show movement requiring great effort and a lack of normal coordination while slight cases show exaggerated movements that are coordinated.

spastic paralysis weakness of a limb, characterized by involuntary muscular contraction and loss of muscular function. As with SPASTICITY it is due to disease of the nerve fibres that usually control movement and reflexes.

spatula a knife-like instrument with a flat, blunt blade used for spreading or mixing ointments and materials. It is also used to hold down the tongue when the throat is being examined.

speculum an instrument for use in examination of an opening in the body. The speculum holds open the cavity and may also provide illumination.

speech therapy treatment of patients who for whatever reason are unable to speak coherently. Such patients may have congenital conditions or may have suffered an accident or illness producing a condition requiring therapy.

spermatic the term given to any vessel or structure associated with the testicle.

spermatozoon (*plural* **spermatozoa**) the mature male reproductive cell, or gamete. It has a head with the HAPLOID nucleus containing half the CHROMOSOME number, and an acrosome (a structure that aids penetration of the egg). Behind the head comes a midpiece with energy-producing MITOCHONDRIA, and then a long tail which propels it forward. A few millilitres of SEMEN is ejaculated during intercourse, containing many millions of spermatozoa.

spermicide a cream, foam, jelly, etc., that kills spermatozoa, which is used in conjunction with a condom or DIAPHRAGM as a contraceptive.

sphenoid bone a bone in the skull that lies behind the eyes.

sphincter a circular muscle around an opening. The opening is closed totally or partially by contraction of the muscle e.g. the anal sphincter around the anus.

sphygmomanometer the instrument used to measure arterial blood pressure. An inflatable rubber tube is put around the arm and inflated until the blood flow in a large artery stops. This pressure is taken as the SYSTOLIC PRESSURE (i.e. the pressure at each heartbeat). The pressure is then released slowly and the point at which the sound heard in the artery changes suddenly is taken as the diastolic pressure (*see* DIASTOLE).

spina bifida a CONGENITAL malformation in newborn babies in which part of the spinal cord is exposed by a gap in the backbone. Many cases are also affected with HYDROCEPHALUS. The symptoms usually include paralysis, incontinence, a high risk of MENINGITIS and mental retardation. There is usually an abnormally high level of ALPHA FETOPROTEIN in the amniotic fluid and since this can be diagnosed and then confirmed by AMNIOCENTESIS, it is possible to terminate these pregnancies.

spinal anaesthesia generating anaesthesia by injecting the cerebrospinal fluid around the spinal cord. Of the two types, the epidural (*see* EPIDURAL ANAESTHESIA) involves injecting into the outer lining of the spinal cord, while *subarachnoid anaesthesia* is produced by injecting between vertebrae in the LUMBAR region of the vertebral column. Spinal anaesthesia is useful for patients who have a condition that precludes a general anaesthetic e.g. a chest infection or heart disease.

The term is also used for a loss of sensation in a part of the body due to spinal injury.

spinal column (**spine** *or* **backbone** *or* **vertebral column**) the bony and slightly flexible column that forms a vital part of the SKELETON. It encloses the SPINAL CORD, articulates with other bones e.g. the skull and ribs, and provides attachments for muscles.

It consists of bones, the vertebrae, between which are discs of fibrocartilage (the intervertebral discs). From the top, the column comprises 7 cervical, 12 thoracic, 5 lumbar, 5 sacral and 4 coccygeal vertebrae. In adults the last

two groups are fused to from the sacrum and coccyx, respectively.

spinal cord the part of the CENTRAL NERVOUS SYSTEM that runs from the brain, through the SPINAL COLUMN. Both GREY and WHITE MATTER are present, the former as an H-shaped core within the latter. A hollow core in the grey matter forms the central canal which contains the cerebrospinal fluid. The cord is covered by MENINGES and it contains both sensory and motor NEURONS. Thirty-one pairs of spinal nerves arise from the cord, passing out between the arches of the vertebrae.

spirometer an instrument used to test how the lungs are working, by recording the volume of air inhaled and exhaled.

spleen a roughly ovoid organ, coloured a deep purple, which is situated on the left of the body, behind and below the stomach. It is surrounded by a peritoneal membrane and contains a mass of lymphoid tissue. MACROPHAGES in the spleen destroy microorganisms by PHAGOCYTOSIS.

The spleen produces lymphocytes, leucocytes, plasma cells and blood platelets (*see individual entries*). It also stores red blood cells for use in emergencies. Release of red blood cells is facilitated by SMOOTH MUSCLE under the control of the SYMPATHETIC NERVOUS SYSTEM, and when this occurs, the familiar pain called *stitch* may be experienced. The spleen removes worn-out red blood cells, conserving the iron for further production in the bone marrow. Although the spleen performs many functions, it can be removed without detriment and as a result there is an increase in size of the lymphatic glands.

splenectomy removal of the SPLEEN, possibly because of rupture and bleeding.

splenomegaly an abnormal enlargement of the SPLEEN which occurs commonly with blood disorders and parasitic infections.

splint a support that holds a broken bone in the correct and stable position until healing is complete.

spondylitis inflammation of the spinal vertebrae — arthritis of the spine. *Ankylosing spondylitis* is a rheumatic disease of the spine and sacroiliac joints (i.e. those of the sacrum and ilium), causing pain and stiffness in the hip and shoulder. It may result in the spine become rigid (*see* KYPHOSIS).

spondylosis degeneration of joints and the intervertebral discs of the spine, producing pain in the neck and LUMBAR region where the joints may actually restrict movement. OSTEOPHYTES are commonly formed and the space occupied by the discs reduced. Physiotherapy may help sufferers, and collars or surgical belts can prevent movement and give support. Surgery may be required occasionally to relieve pressure on nerves, or to fuse joints.

spongiform encephalopathy a neurological disease caused by a SLOW VIRUS and resulting in a spongy degeneration of the brain with progressive dementia. Examples are CREUTZFELDT-JAKOB DISEASE and kuru (a progressive and fatal viral infection seen in New Guinea highland natives which has decreased with the decline in cannibalism).

sprain an injury to ligaments (or muscles, or tendons) around a joint, caused by a sudden overstretching. Pain and swelling may occur and treatment comprises, in the main, avoiding use of the affected joint.

sprue (*or* **psilosis**) essentially a composite deficiency disease due to lack of food being absorbed because of a disease of the intestine, or a metabolic disorder which means fats cannot be absorbed. The symptoms include diarrhoea, inflamed tongue, ANAEMIA and weight loss.

The condition was considered a disease of tropical climates but other versions have been seen. Treatment involves antibiotics, folic acid (to combat the anaemia), vitamins and a high-protein diet. There may be an immediate improvement on returning to a temperate climate.

sputum saliva and mucus from the respiratory tract.

squint (*or* **strabismus**) an abnormal condition in which the eyes are crossed. There are two types, paralytic and non-paralytic. The paralytic type is due to a muscular or neurological malfunction, while a non-paralytic squint is caused by a defect in the actual relative position of the eyes. Some squints can be corrected by surgery.

stagnant loop syndrome when a segment of the SMALL INTESTINE is discontinuous with the rest or when there is an obstruction, either of which causes slow movement through the intestines. The result is bacterial growth with malabsorption and steatorrhoea (passage of fatty stools).

stammering (*or* **stuttering**) when normal speech falters, with a repetition of the initial consonant of words. Usually it appears first in childhood but often responds to therapy.

starvation *see* **malnutrition**.

stenosis the abnormal narrowing of a blood vessel, heart valve or similar structure.

stent a device used in surgery to help the healing of two structures that have been joined, by draining away the contents.

sterilization the process of destroying all microorganisms on instruments and other objects by means of heat, radiation, etc.

Also, a surgical operation to render someone incapable of producing children. Men usually undergo a VASECTOMY, while in women it can be achieved by cutting and tying the FALLOPIAN TUBES, or removing them. The latter operation is performed via an incision in the abdominal wall or through the vagina.

sternum the breastbone.

steroid one of a group of compounds resembling cholesterol, that are made up of four carbon rings fused together. The group includes the sterols e.g. cholesterol, BILE acids, some HORMONES, and VITAMIN D. Synthetic versions act like steroid hormones and include derivatives of the glucocorticoids used as anti-inflammatory agents for RHEUMATOID ARTHRITIS; oral contraceptives, usually OESTROGEN and PROGESTERONE derivatives; anabolic steroids, such as testosterone, used to treat OSTEOPOROSIS and wasting.

stertor noisy breathing, similar to snoring, often heard in patients who are deeply unconscious.

stethoscope an instrument used to listen to sounds within the body, particularly the lungs and heart. The simplest type consists of earpieces for the examiner, leading via a tube to a diaphragm placed on the body.

Stevens-Johnson syndrome a common hypersensitivity reaction to SULPHONAMIDE antibiotics, and a form of ERYTHEMA. It produces skin lesions and the eyes and mucosa may ulcerate.

stiffness a condition with numerous causes, that results in a reduced movement in joints and muscles. The cause may be quite straightforward e.g. physical injury or it may be due to disease such as RHEUMATISM, MENINGITIS or central nervous system diseases.

stigma a mark or impression upon the skin, possibly one that is typical of a particular disease.

stilboestrol a synthetic OESTROGEN (female sex hormone) with several uses. It relieves menstrual disorders and menopause symptoms. It also proves helpful in treating breast and prostate cancers.

stillbirth the birth of any child that provides no evidence of life.

Still's disease a chronic ARTHRITIS affecting children and causing arthritis in several joints, with fever and a red rash. Some cases develop into ankylosing SPONDYLITIS and there is often muscle wasting. Illness may affect the whole body, complicated by other conditions, e.g. enlargement of the SPLEEN and PERICARDITIS.

stimulant any drug or other agent that increases the rate of activity of an organ or system within the body. This assumes that the target organ is capable of increased activity which merely requires the necessary stimulus.

stitch a sharp pain in the side, often due to cramp after hard exertion. *See also* SPLEE).

Stokes Adams syndrome loss of consciousness as a result of the temporary cessation of the action of the heart, due to asystole or fibrillation.

stoma (*plural* **stomata**) an opening made in the abdominal surface to accommodate a tube from the colon or ileum. This operation is undertaken because of malignancy or inflammatory bowel diseases, e.g. CROHN'S DISEASE.

stomach an expansion of the alimentary canal that lies between the OESOPHAGUS and the DUODENUM. It has thick walls of SMOOTH MUSCLE that contract to manipulate the food, and its exits are controlled by SPHINCTERS, the cardiac anteriorly and the pyloric at the junction with the duodenum (*see* PYLORUS). Mucosal cells in the lining secrete GASTRIC JUICE. The food is reduced to an acidic semi-liquid which is moved on to the duodenum.

The stomach varies in size but its greatest length is roughly twelve inches and the breadth four or five inches. Its capacity is approximately 1 to 1½ litres.

stools *see* **faeces**.

strangulation the constriction or closure of a passage or vessel. This may be due to the intestine twisting (VOLVULUS), or herniation of the intestine. Strangulation of a blood vessel and/or airway affects the organs being supplied and if vital organs are affected, can prove fatal.

strangury the desire to pass water, which can only be done in a few drops and with accompanying pain. It is symptomatic of an irritation of the base of the bladder by a stone, cancer at this site, or CYSTITIS or PROSTATITIS.

strapping the application of layers of adhesive plaster to cover part of the body and maintain moderate pressure, so as to prevent too much movement and provide rest, as with fractured ribs.

streptococcus a genus of Gram-positive (*see* GRAM'S STAIN) spherical bacteria that form chains. Many species are responsible for a variety of infections including scarlet fever, ENDOCARDITIS and pneumonia.

stress fracture a fracture created by making excessive demands on the body, as commonly happens in sport. Treatment involves rest and analgesics for the pain.

stricture a narrowing of a passage in the body e.g. the URETHRA, OESOPHAGUS or URETER. It may result from inflammation, a spasm, growth of a tumour or pressure from surrounding organs. In many cases it is due to ulceration and contraction of the subsequent scar tissue. With a urethral stricture, it becomes increasingly difficult to pass urine.

stridor the noise created on breathing in when there is a narrowing of the upper airway, especially the LARYNX.

stroke (*or* **cerebrovascular accident**) the physical effects, involving some form of paralysis, that result from an interruption to the brain's blood supply. The effect in the brain is secondary and the cause lies in the heart or blood vessels and may be a THROMBOSIS, EMBOLUS or HAEMORRHAGE. The severity of a stroke varies greatly from a temporary weakness in a limb, or tingling, to paralysis, coma and death.

St Vitus' dance the former name for SYDENHAM'S CHOREA.

stye a bacterial infection and inflammation of a gland at the base of an eyelash, resulting in a pus-filled cyst.

subarachnoid haemorrhage bleeding into the SUBARACHNOID SPACE, due often to a ruptured cerebral ANEURYSM. Initial symptoms are a severe headache, stiff neck, followed by vomiting and drowsiness and there may be a brief period of unconsciousness after the event. Brain damage is possible but severe haemorrhages may result in death.

subarachnoid space the space between the arachnoid and pia mater MENINGES covering the brain and spinal cord. It contains cerebrospinal fluid and blood vessels.

subcutaneous general term meaning beneath the skin.

subdural term meaning below the dura mater, and referring to the space between this and the arachnoid MENINGES around the brain.

subphrenic abscess an abscess occurring beneath the diaphragm and commonly on the right side. It may be due to infection after an operation or perforation of an organ, e.g. a peptic ulcer. Surgery is usually necessary, although antibiotics may be effective.

sudden infant death syndrome (*or* **cot death**) the sudden death of a baby, often occurring overnight, from unknown causes. A significant proportion (c. 20% in UK) of infant deaths occur this way. Although the cause is unknown, numerous suggestions have been put forward, from viral infection and allergic reaction to poor breathing control that could be particularly susceptible to mild infections. Research continues.

sulphonamide one of a group of drugs containing the chemical group -SO_2NH_2. These drugs do not kill bacteria, but prevent bacterial growth and are thus very useful in controlling infections. Some side effects may occur but in general these are outweighed by the benefits.

sunburn skin damage caused by exposure to the ultraviolet rays in sunlight. This may vary from a reddening of the skin and itching to formation of blisters which can cause shock if a large area is affected. Fair-skinned people are more susceptible than others and it is advisable to take sun in gradual stages.

sunstroke *see* **heatstroke**.

supine the position in which someone is lying on his or her back, face upwards.

suppository medication prepared in a form which enables it to be inserted into the rectum (or vagina). It may be a lubricant, drugs for treatment in the area of the rectum or anus, or for absorption. The suppository has to be inserted beyond the sphincter muscle to ensure effective retention.

suppuration pus formation, whether on the surface (ulceration) or more deep-seated (as with an ABSCESS).

surgeon a qualified practitioner specializing in surgery.

surgery the branch of medicine that through operation treats disease and injuries or deformities.

susceptibility when there is a lack of resistance to disease, due either to poor general health, or a deficiency in defence mechanism because of another condition e.g. AIDS. Susceptibility can be decreased by vaccination, etc.

suture the means whereby a wound or incision is closed in surgery, using threads of silk or catgut. There are several types of suture to deal with diverse situations.

Also, a type of joint across which there is no movement e.g. in the skull, where there are several sutures.

swab a general term applied to a pad of material used in various ways. It can be used to clean wounds, apply medication, remove blood during operations, and obtain samples from infected areas e.g. throat, for further examination.

sweat *see* **perspiration**.

sweat glands the glands in the EPIDERMIS of SKIN that project into the dermis and are under the control of the sympathetic nervous system (*see also*

PERSPIRATION). The glands occur over most of the body but are especially abundant on the forehead, palms of the hands and soles of the feet and under the arms.

Sydenham's chorea a disorder of the nervous system affecting children over the age of five. The condition is characterized by involuntary jerking movements of the limbs and is associated with RHEUMATISM. Although the condition resolves over a period of time, a percentage of sufferers will develop rheumatism elsewhere in the body or ENDOCARDITIS.

sympathetic the term for a symptom or disease that occurs as a result of disease elsewhere in the body, e.g. injury of one eye and a related inflammation in the other due to them being connected by the lymphatics.

sympathetic nervous system with the parasympathetic nervous system (and acting in opposition to it), this makes up the AUTONOMIC NERVOUS SYSTEM. NORADRENALINE and ADRENALINE are the main NEUROTRANSMITTERS released by its nerve endings. Its functions include raising the heartbeat rate, constricting blood vessels and inhibiting secretion of saliva.

symptom any evidence of a disease or disorder.

synapse the junction between two nerve cells, at which there is a minute gap. A nerve impulse bridges the gap via a NEUROTRANSMITTER (*see also* ACETYLCHOLINE). The chemical diffuses across the gap that connects the axon of one nerve cell to the dendrites of the next. Some brain cells have many thousand synapses.

syncope (*or* **fainting**) a temporary loss of consciousness due to a fall in blood pressure and reduced supply of blood to the brain. It may occur after standing for a long time (particularly in hot weather), or after shock or injury. Typical signs before an attack are sweating and light-headedness.

syndactyly a fusion of fingers or toes which is a CONGENITAL effect. It may affect two or more fingers through webbing, or result in complete fusion of all digits.

syndrome a number of symptoms and signs that together constitute a particular condition.

synovial fluid *see* **synovial membrane**.

synovial membrane (*or* **synovium**) the inner membrane of a capsule that encloses a joint that moves freely. It secretes into the joint a thick lubricating fluid (synovial fluid) which may build up after injury to cause pain.

synovitis inflammation of the SYNOVIAL MEMBRANE that lines a joint capsule. The result is swelling, with pain. It is associated with rheumatic disease, injury or infection e.g. chronic tuberculosis. The treatment depends upon the cause of the condition and often a sample of the synovial fluid is taken for examination.

syphilis an infectious, VENEREAL DISEASE, caused by the bacterium *Treponema pallidum* which shows symptoms in three stages. Bacteria enter the body through mucous membranes during sexual intercourse and an ulcer appears in the first instance. Within a short time the LYMPH NODES locally and then all over the body enlarge and harden and this lasts several weeks.

Secondary symptoms appear about two months after infection and include fever, pains, enlarged lymph nodes and a faint rash, which is usually noticed on the chest. The bacterium is found in enormous numbers in the primary sores and any skin lesions of the secondary stage. The final stage may not appear until many months or years after infection and comprises the formation of numerous tumour-like masses throughout the body (in skin, muscle, bone, brain, spinal cord and other organs such as the liver, stomach etc.). This stage can cause serious damage to the heart, brain or spinal cord resulting in blindness, TABES DORSALIS and mental disability.

CONGENITAL syphilis is much rarer than the former, *acquired*, type. It is contracted by a developing foetus from the mother, across the placenta and symptoms show a few weeks after birth. Treatment of syphilis is with penicillin, but it should be administered early in the development of the disease.

syringe an instrument used for injecting fluids into the body or the removal of body fluids for examination. In such cases, it comprises a hollow needle connected to a piston within a tube. Larger metal syringes are used to wash the outer ear and remove wax.

syrup a mixture of sugar, water and drug, used for the easy administration of medications which may taste unpleasant. It also provides a means of delivering drugs which would otherwise deteriorate when exposed to air.

systemic general term referring to the body as a whole.

systemic lupus erythematosus (*or* **SLE**) an inflammatory disorder which affects the connective tissues of the body. There are a wide range of secondary conditions that are treated symptomatically, such as the enlargement of organs, pulmonary hypertension and haemolytic ANAEMIA. There is as yet no cure for SLE and the specific cause is unknown, although it is believed to be an autoimmune disorder.

systole the contraction of the heart that alternates with the resting phase (diastole). It usually refers to ventricular systole which at 0.3 seconds is three times longer than atrial systole.

systolic pressure *see* **blood pressure**.

T

tabes dorsalis medically known as LOCOMOTOR ATAXIA, this is a complication of syphilis occurring 5 to 20 years after the initial infection. It affects the sensory nerves, especially of the trunk and legs causing stabbing pains and unsteadiness in walking. There is often loss of bladder control and disturbance of vision if the optic nerves are involved. Treatment is by means of penicillin and the condition may be associated with *taboparesis,* which is also called *general paralysis of the insane.*

tachycardia increased rate of heartbeat, which may be caused naturally, as with exercise, or be symptomatic of disease.

talus the ankle bone, which articulates with the lower leg bones (TIBIA and FIBULA) above and also with the heel bone (*calcaneus*) below (*see* TARSUS).

tamoxifen a drug used in the treatment of certain breast cancers.

tampon a plug of compressed gauze or cotton wool inserted into a wound or cavity to absorb fluid or blood.

target cell an abnormal form of ERYTHROCYTE (red blood cell) which is large and has a ringed appearance when stained and viewed microscopically, resembling a target. These cells are present in several kinds of ANAEMIA, including those due to iron deficiency. They are also found when there is liver disease, a small SPLEEN, THALASSAEMIA and haemoglobin abnormalities (haemoglobinopathies).

tarsus a part of the foot in the region of the instep, consisting of seven bones, chiefly the TALUS and the *calcaneus* (heel bone) and also the cuboid, navicular and three cuneiform bones.

taste the perception of flavour which is brought about by chemoreceptors (the TASTE BUDS) situated on the TONGUE. There are four main categories of taste: salt, sour, sweet and bitter.

taste buds the sensory receptors responsible for the perception of taste, located in the grooves around the papillae of the TONGUE, in the epiglottis, parts of the PHARYNX and soft palate. The taste buds are stimulated by the presence of dissolved food in the saliva and messages are sent via nerves to the brain where the information is interpreted and perceived.

taxis the returning to their normal position of displaced organs, parts of organs or bones by manipulation. *See* HERNIA.

teeth *see* **tooth**.

temperature (of the body) the normal body temperature is around 37°C (98.4°F) but it varies considerably both between individuals and in one person throughout the day. In addition, temperature differences occur between various areas of the body being lower in the skin than internally.

temple the side of the head above the level of the eye and the ear.

temporal relating or referring to the temple e.g. *temporal artery.*

temporal lobe one of the main areas of the CEREBRAL CORTEX in each of the CEREBRAL HEMISPHERES of the brain, occurring in the TEMPORAL region of the skull. A cleft known as the *lateral sulcus* separates it from the frontal lobe.

temporal lobe epilepsy EPILEPSY which is centred within the temporal lobe caused by disease within the cortex. It is characterized by hallucinations involving the senses of taste, smell, hearing and sight, and memory disturbances. During an attack, the person usually remains conscious but not fully and normally aware, and afterwards may not have any memory of what has occurred.

tendinitis inflammation of a tendon which often results from excessive or unaccustomed exercise but may also result from infection. Treatment involves rest, possibly splinting of an affected joint and corticosteroid injections, and the taking of ANALGESIC drugs.

tendon a tough and inelastic white cord composed of bundles of COLLAGEN fibres which attaches a muscle to a bone. A tendon concentrates the pull of the muscle onto one point on the bone and the length and thickness varies considerably. The fibres of a tendon pass into, and become continuous with, those of the bone it serves. Many tendons are enclosed in tendon sheaths lined with SYNOVIAL MEMBRANE containing synovial fluid which reduces friction and enables easy movement to occur.

tennis elbow a form of TENDINITIS affecting the tendon at the outer part of the elbow, which becomes inflamed and painful. It is caused by hard and excessive use of the arm and the treatment involves rest and corticosteroid injections.

teratogen a substance or disease or any other factor which causes the production of abnormalities in a foetus. The drugs in this category include thalidomide and alcohol. German measles and cytomegalovirus are among the infections.

teratogenesis the processes which result in the development of physical abnormalities in a foetus.

teratoma a tumour that is composed of unusual tissues not normally found at that site and derived from partially developed embryological cells. Teratomas are most common in the ovary and testicle (particularly if the latter is undescended).

testicle (*or* **testis**) one of the pair of male sex organs which are situated within the SCROTUM and which produce spermatozoa and secrete the hormone TESTOSTERONE. The testicles develop within the abdomen of the foetus but descend around the time of birth into the scrotum.

Each testicle has an outer double membrane layer known as the *tunica vaginalis*. The tunica vaginalis contains an inner fibrous layer called the *tunica albuginea,* which protects the testicle. The bulk of the testicle consists of numerous fine, convoluted tubules, called seminiferous tubules, which are lined with cells that produce the spermatozoa. In addition, other cells known as *sertoli cells* occur, which provide support and possibly nourishment for the developing spermatozoa. The tubules are supported by connective tissue containing nerves and blood vessels and also the *cells of Leydig,* which are responsible for hormone production. The tubules connect with another highly folded tube called the *epididymis,* which is about 7m long and connects with the VAS DEFERENS, which leads to the URETHRA. The spermatozoa are passed by passive movement along the epididymis, completing their development as they go, and are stored in the lower part until EJACULATION.

testis *see* **testicle**.

testosterone the male sex hormone secreted by the TESTES. *See also* ANDROGEN.

tetanus a very serious and sometimes fatal infectious disease, the non-medical name for which is *lockjaw*. It is caused by the bacterium *Clostridium tetani,* spores of which enter through a wound. Rapid multiplication of the bacteria produces a toxin which affects the nerves resulting in rigidity and spasm of muscles. Often there is high fever and the spasms cause extreme agony.

If respiratory muscles are involved death may occur by asphyxia. Effective antitoxin is available, although its effects are not permanent and it needs to be regularly maintained. Antibiotics such as penicillin are also effective against the bacteria.

tetany an abnormal condition due to calcium metabolism disorder, which may occur with a deficiency of vitamin D, hypoparathyroidism or ALKALOSIS. It results in convulsions, cramps and muscle twitching, particularly in the face, feet and hands.

thalamus one of a pair of masses of grey matter located within each side of the forebrain. Each is a centre for coordinating and relaying sensory information concerned with all the senses apart from that of smell.

thalassaemia (*or* **Cooley's anaemia**) this is an inherited form of ANAEMIA in which there is an abnormality in the HAEMOGLOBIN.

There is a continuation in the production of foetal haemoglobin and two forms of the disorder are recognized: T. major, in which the disorder is inherited from both parents (HOMOZYGOUS) and T. minor. The *minor* form is usually asymptomatic but the *major* type causes, in addition to the severe anaemia, bone-marrow abnormalities and enlargement of the spleen. Treatment is by means of repeated blood transfusions. The disease is widespread throughout the Mediterranean, Asia and Africa.

thalidomide a TERATOGENIC drug which was formerly prescribed for treatment of MORNING SICKNESS in pregnancy. It was withdrawn when it was discovered that it caused developmental damage to the foetus, particularly malformation of limbs.

therapeutics the area of medicine concerned with the various methods of healing and treatment.

therapy the treatment of disease.

thermography a method of recording the heat produced by different areas of the body using photographic film sensitive to infrared radiation. Areas with good blood circulation produce more heat and this can occur abnormally if a tumour is present. The record thus obtained is a *thermogram* and this is one of the techniques used to detect breast tumours (*mammothermography*).

thiamine *see* **vitamin B**.

Thiersch's graft a type of skin graft in which thin strips of skin, involving the epidermis and the upper layer of the dermis, are taken from one part of the body and placed on the wound which requires to be healed.

thigh the part of the leg above the knee.

thoracocentesis (*or* **pleuracentesis**) the withdrawal, by means of a hollow needle inserted through the chest wall, of fluid from the pleural cavity.

thorax the chest.

thrombin an enzyme derived from prothrombin, its inactive precursor, which is formed and is active during the final stages of blood clotting (*see* COAGULATION).

thrombocytopenia a reduction in the number of PLATELETS in the blood associated most commonly with tumours (whether benign or malignant) or the reaction of the immune system to drugs. It is a common cause of bleeding disorders.

thromboembolism the situation in which a blood clot (THROMBUS) forms in one part of the circulation, usually a vein in the leg (phlebothrombosis), and a portion breaks off and becomes lodged elsewhere causing a total blockage (EMBOLISM). The embolism often involves the pulmonary artery or one of its branches and this is known as PULMONARY EMBOLISM.

thrombolysis the dissolving of blood clots by enzyme activity. Natural enzymes produced within the body have this effect but drug treatment, especially involving streptokinase, may be used to break up clots following PULMONARY EMBOLISM, CORONARY THROMBOSIS and PHLEBOTHROMBOSIS.

thrombophlebitis inflammation of the wall of a vein along with clot formation in the affected section of the vessel.

This is a complication of pregnancy and may be dangerous, involving a deep vein thrombosis, which can result in PULMONARY EMBOLISM. The condition, known as WHITE LEG (plegmasia alba dolens), is thrombophlebitis, especially of the femoral vein, which can occur after childbirth.

thrombosis the process of clotting within a blood vessel, producing a THROMBUS. It may occur within an artery or vein, often one which is diseased or damaged, and can be very serious or even fatal, e.g. STROKE, CORONARY THROMBOSIS.

thrombus a blood clot within a vessel which partially or totally obstructs the circulation.

thrush an infection caused by the fungus *Candida albicans* which affects the mucous membranes of the mouth and vagina, producing white patches. It is a popular name given to a group of infections known as *candidiasis*.

thymus a gland, divided into two lobes, which is present in the neck and which forms a vital part of the immune system. It is especially large in children and important in the development of the immune response and the production of lymphoid tissue. After puberty, the thymus gradually begins to shrink. Bone-marrow cells, known as *stem cells*, undergo maturation within the thymus and one group, the *T-lymphocytes*, are dependent upon the gland. These are very important cells in the body, which produce ANTIBODIES.

thyroidectomy surgical removal of the thyroid gland.

thyroid gland a bilobed endocrine gland situated at the base and front of the neck. It is enclosed by fibrous tissue and well supplied with blood, and internally consists of numerous vesicles containing a jelly-like colloidal substance. These vesicles produce thyroid hormone, which is rich in iodine, under the control of *thyroid stimulating hormone* (THYROTROPHIN STIMULATING HORMONE) released from the PITUITARY GLAND. Two hormones are produced by the gland, thyroxine and triiodothyronine, which are essential for the regulation of metabolism and growth. *See also* CRETINISM, MYXOEDEMA and HYPERTHYROIDISM.

thyrotoxic adenoma a form of THYROTOXICOSIS or GRAVES' DISEASE.

thyrotoxicosis *see* **Graves' disease**.

thyrotrophin releasing hormone a hormone produced and released from the HYPOTHALAMUS which acts on the anterior lobe of the PITUITARY GLAND, which then releases THYROTROPHIN STIMULATING HORMONE. *See* THYROID.

thyrotrophin stimulating hormone a hormone produced and released by the anterior pituitary gland which stimulates the THYROID GLAND to produce its hormones (*see* THYROID).

thyroxine an important hormone produced by the thyroid gland and used medically to treat conditions resulting from underactivity of this gland e.g. CRETINISM and MYXOEDEMA.

tibia the larger of the two bones in the lower leg, known as the shin bone, articulating above with the FEMUR and with the TALUS of the ankle below.

tinnitus any ringing or buzzing sound in the ear which does not have a real external cause. Many disorders of the ear can cause this e.g hardened wax, Ménière's disease, drugs, including aspirin and quinine, and damage to the auditory nerve. In many cases no underlying cause is found. Tinnitus cannot usually be suppressed altogether, although certain drugs can help to dampen its effects.

tolerance the adaptation of the body to a particular drug or substance so that over a period of time, there is a reduction in the response to a particular dose. Usually a larger dose must now be given to produce the same effect as before.

tomography a particular technique using X-rays or ultrasound so that structures at a given depth are brought into sharp focus while those at other levels are deliberately blurred. In this way, pictures of *slices* of the body are obtained at different levels to build up a three-dimensional image. The image obtained is called a *tomogram*.

tongue the muscular and highly mobile organ attached to the floor of the mouth, the three main functions of which are manipulation of food during chewing prior to swallowing, taste and production of speech. The three areas of the tongue are the tip, body and root and it is covered with a mucous membrane which unites with that of the mouth and pharynx.

The tongue is anchored at the root by various muscles which attach it to the back of the mouth. In addition, the undersurface of the tongue is attached in the midline to the floor of the mouth by a fold of mucous membrane called the *frenulum linguae*. If this is attached too far forward to restrict the movement at the tip it causes the condition known as *tongue tie*.

The tongue has a furred appearance because its surface is covered with minute projections called papillae, of which there are three different kinds, filiform, fungiform and circumvallate. There are grooves surrounding the papillae in which the TASTE BUDS occur. The tongue is well supplied with blood and receives branches from five different nerves on each side.

tonsillectomy surgical removal of the TONSILS.

tonsillitis inflammation of the tonsils, caused by bacterial or viral infection. The symptoms include a severe sore throat causing painful swallowing, accompanied by fever and earache, especially in children. The tonsils are swollen and white in appearance due to infected material exuded from them and glands in the neck are enlarged. Treatment is by means of antibiotics, especially penicillin and erythromycin, along with analgesics for pain relief.

tonsils usually refers to the two small masses of lymphoid tissue situated on either side at the back of the mouth (the *palatine tonsils*). However, another pair occur below the tongue which are the *lingual tonsils,* while the ADENOIDS are the PHARYNGEAL TONSILS. All are part of the body's protective mechanism against infection.

tooth a hard structure used for biting and chewing. Each tooth consists of a *root* embedded in a socket within the jawbone to which it is attached by the fibrous *periodontal membrane*. The projecting part of the tooth is called the *crown,* which is covered with a hard resistant layer of *enamel*, (composed primarily of calcium phosphate and calcium carbonate). The root is covered with a thin hard layer of cementum.

Most of the interior of the tooth consists of *dentine*, a hard ivory-like substance which surrounds the inner core or pulp. The pulp contains blood vessels and nerve fibres and is connected with the dentine by means of fine cellular processes. There are four different types of teeth: canine, incisor, premolar and molar.

torpor a state of physical and mental sluggishness which accompanies various mental disorders and some kinds of poisoning and may be present in elderly people with arterial disease.

torsion twisting, often referring to an abnormal state of the whole or part of an organ which impairs the nerve and blood supply. Examples are a torsion of a loop of bowel or of the spermatic cord of the testicle. Surgery is usually required to correct a torsion.

touch the sense which is conferred by specialized sensory receptors present in the skin (and also in muscles and other areas of the body), which enable sensations of pain, temperature, pressure and touch to be perceived. The sense organs involved are specially adapted to respond to particular sensations conveying their messages to the brain along different nerve pathways.

tourniquet a device used to arrest bleeding, usually from an artery in a limb, which may be a length of bandage, rubber tube or cord tied tightly round, generally as an emergency measure. Direct pressure on a wound is now considered to be preferable as a first aid measure, because a tourniquet can deprive all the tissues of oxygen by arresting the circulation, and there is a risk of damage and gangrene.

toxaemia blood poisoning resulting from the toxins produced by rapidly multiplying bacteria at a localized site of infection such as an abscess. Symptoms are varied, including fever, vomiting and diarrhoea, and a general feeling of being unwell. The source of the infection has to be treated with antibiotic drugs. Toxaemia of pregnancy involves two relatively rare conditions known as ECLAMPSIA and PRE-ECLAMPSIA.

toxicology the scientific study of poisons and their effects.

toxic shock syndrome a state of acute shock due to SEPTICAEMIA and caused by toxins produced by *staphylococcal* bacteria. The symptoms include high fever and skin rash, and diarrhoea can develop very rapidly and prove fatal if not adequately treated with antibiotics, especially PENICILLIN and *cephalosporin*, along with fluid and salt replacement.

The syndrome is associated with the use of tampons by women during menstruation. It is thought that young women or girls whose immune system is not fully developed may be at greater risk, particularly if a tampon is left in place too long. However, the syndrome can also occur in other people and is in all cases rare.

toxin a poison produced by bacteria and by many species of plant and also present in snake venom. In the body, a toxin acts as an ANTIGEN and provokes the production of special antibodies called antitoxins. The antitoxins produced may be used in IMMUNIZATION to protect against the disease, as with tetanus and diphtheria. An *endotoxin* is contained within the bacterial cell and only released when the organism dies and decays. Endotoxins do not provoke antitoxin production. *See* TOXOID.

toxocariasis a disease caused by the larvae of roundworms which normally infect the domestic dog (*Toxicara canis*) and cat (*Toxicara cati*), but can be passed to man by swallowing material contaminated with eggs in infected faeces.

Those most at risk are children, especially at a young age, when hands may become infected while playing. Once swallowed, the larvae which hatch from the eggs travel around the body in the circulation and can cause considerable damage to e.g. the lungs and liver. Also, the larvae may lodge in the retina of the eye causing inflammation and the production of abnormal granulated tissue called granuloma.

Symptoms of the infection include muscular pain, fever, skin rash, respiratory problems, vomiting and convulsions. Treatment is with drugs, such as diethylcarbamazine and thiabendazole.

toxoid a preparation of TOXIN which has been treated with chemicals so that it cannot cause disease but is able to provoke the production of antitoxin.

This is the basis of VACCINES against diphtheria and tetanus.

toxoplasmosis an infectious disease caused by a protozoan organism known as *Toxoplasma*. The infection is either transmitted by eating undercooked meat or through direct contact with contaminated soil or especially with infected cats. This form of the infection is mild and causes few ill-effects. However, a much more serious form of the disease can be passed from a mother infected during pregnancy to her unborn baby. The newborn infant may suffer from HYDROCEPHALUS, mental retardation or blindness, or may even be stillborn. Treatment is by means of sulphonamide drugs and pyrimethamine.

tracer a substance which is marked so that when it is introduced into the body its progress can be followed e.g. radioactive tracers used in the detection of brain tumours and thyroid disease.

trachea the windpipe which is the part of the air passage that is situated between the LARYNX and the bronchi.

tracheitis inflammation of the trachea, often accompanying a viral infection of the upper respiratory tract. The symptoms include a persistent painful cough and sore chest and it often accompanies BRONCHITIS and also DIPHTHERIA.

tracheostomy (*or* **tracheotomy**) a surgical procedure in which a hole is made in the trachea to allow direct access of air to the lower respiratory passages. This may be performed in an emergency if there is an obstruction in breathing. However, usually this operation is carried out in hospital, especially on patients in intensive therapy who require long-term artificial ventilation. This is to avoid the damage to the trachea which is caused by the long-term use of an endotracheal breathing tube (inserted through the nose or mouth) which would normally be used first.

Tracheostomy is also used in cases of diphtheria, where the obstruction is a large tumour or where there is nerve damage. Once the opening has been made a double tube is inserted and held in place by tapes around the neck. The inner tube can be freely withdrawn and replaced and needs to be kept scrupulously clean and free from any obstruction.

traction the use of weights and pulleys to apply a pulling force on a broken bone, to ensure that it is kept correctly aligned while healing takes place.

trance a sleep-like state in which a person ceases to react normally to the environment and loses the power of voluntary movement, but remains aware. It can be induced by HYPNOSIS, meditation, HYSTERIA, CATATONIA and drug abuse.

tranquillizer a drug that has a soothing and calming effect, relieving stress and anxiety. Minor tranquillizers such as diazepam and chlordiazepoxide are widely used to relieve these symptoms which may arise from a variety of causes. There is a danger of dependence with long-term use. Major tranquillizers e.g. chlorpromazine and haloperidol are used to treat severe mental illnesses such as SCHIZOPHRENIA.

transfusion *see* **blood transfusion.**

transient ischaemic attack (*or* **TIA**) a temporary interruption of the supply of blood to the brain, resulting in symptoms including weakness and tingling in the muscles, visual disturbances, giddiness and the slurring of speech. A transient ischaemic attack can be caused by a small EMBOLISM or THROMBUS and is often associated with ATHEROSCLEROSIS.

transplantation the transfer of an organ or tissue from one person to another (called an *allotransplant*) or within the body of an individual (*autotransplant*). It overwhelmingly refers to skin and bone grafting. The person from whom the organ is obtained is known as the *donor* and the one who receives it is known as the *recipient.*

Organ transplants involving the kidney, heart, bone marrow, cornea, lungs and liver have all become more common. Success varies but is improving in all areas especially with the advent of *immunosuppressive* drugs, to prevent organ rejection by the recipient's immune system. *See also* IMMUNOSUPPRESSION and GRAFT.

trauma an event which causes physical damage such as a fracture or an emotional shock brought about by a harmful and upsetting circumstance.

travel sickness *see* **motion sickness.**

tremor involuntary movements which may involve the whole of a muscle or only part of it and produce fine trembling or more pronounced shaking. Tremors are classified according to the type of movement produced and are a symptom of many diseases, including CHOREA, MULTIPLE SCLEROSIS and PARKINSON'S DISEASE.

trench fever an infectious disease, caused by *Rickettsia quintana,* which was epidemic among troops in the First World War and still occurs in Mexico. It is transmitted to man by the body louse and causes fever, rash, leg aches and general weakness.

triceps a three-headed muscle present in the upper arm which extends the forearm.

trichinosis a condition caused by an infestation of the intestine by the *Trichinella spiralis*, the larvae of nematode worms. In humans the condition can be acquired through eating poorly cooked pork (pigs are one of the mammals infested by the larvae). The condition is generally mild but if severe and untreated it can lead to the development of serious complications involving other organs.

trichomoniasis two types of infection caused by a protozoan organism which either attacks the digestive system causing DYSENTERY (*Trichomonas hominis*) or causes vaginal inflammation and discharge (*Trichomonas vaginalis*). In the latter case the infection can be transmitted to a male sexual partner. The drug metronidazole is highly effective.

trichorrhoea the medical name for the falling out of hair which may be due to disease, such as typhoid fever or scarlet fever, or have no apparent cause.

tricuspid valve a valve with three flaps or cusps that controls the passage of blood from the right ATRIUM to the right VENTRICLE of the heart and normally prevents backflow. *See* HEART.

trigeminal nerve the fifth and largest of the cranial nerves, which has three divisions: the *mandibular, maxillary* and *ophthalmic* nerves. The ophthalmic and maxillary are sensory nerves and the mandibular has both sensory and motor functions. Hence the trigeminal nerve is involved in the relaying and perception of sensations (temperature, touch, pain, etc.) from the whole of the face and mouth and also in controlling the muscles involved in chewing.

trigeminal neuralgia (*or* **Tic Douloureux**) a severe form of NEURALGIA, which can affect all the divisions of the trigeminal nerve. It affects women more commonly than men, especially those over the age of 50. It causes severe pain of a burning or cutting nature which can be constant or spasmodic and may be provoked by simple actions such as eating or by heat or cold. The skin of the face may be inflamed and the eye red and watery and the neuralgia is usually confined to one side. The condition is debilitating in that the pain is so intense and interferes with sleeping and eating but the drug carbamazepine is proving to be highly beneficial.

triglycerides fats consisting of three fatty acid molecules combined with glycerol which are the form in which the body stores fat. Triglycerides are derived from the digestion of fats in food.

trophic a term referring to nutrition e.g. trophic fracture which occurs when the bone is weakened due to poor nourishment in the person concerned.

trophoblastic relating to the tissue forming the wall of the BLASTOCYST, the outer of which forms the outer layer of the placenta. Also used, therefore, to categorize related diseases e.g. cancer of the uterus or trophoblastic cancer.

truss a device consisting of a pad attached to a belt with spring straps to maintain its position, which is worn under clothing to support a HERNIA.

trypanosomiasis *see* **sleeping sickness**.

trypsin an important enzyme involved in the digestion of proteins. Its inactive precursor, trypsinogen, is secreted by the PANCREAS and converted to trypsin in the DUODENUM by the action of another enzyme called enteropeptidase.

tubercle either a small rounded knob on a bone e.g. on the ribs or a minute nodular tissue mass (lesion) which is characteristic of TUBERCULOSIS.

tuberculosis (*or* **TB**) a group of infections caused by the bacillus (bacterium) *Mycobacterium tuberculosis* of which pulmonary tuberculosis of the lungs (consumption or phthisis) is the best-known form. The pulmonary disease is acquired through inhalation of air containing the organism from an infected person, or dust laden with bacteria. People infected in this way can show no symptoms but still be carriers. In the lungs, the infection causes formation of a *primary tubercle,* which spreads to lymph nodes to form the *primary complex.*

The disease may wax and wane for years as the body's natural immune system acts against the infection. If the infection is severe, symptoms include fever, wasting, night sweats and the coughing up of blood. The bacteria may enter the bloodstream and spread throughout the body setting up numerous tubercles in other tissues (*miliary tuberculosis*). The organism may also be acquired by eating contaminated food, especially milk, in which case the production of a primary complex in abdominal lymph nodes can lead to PERITONITIS. Rarely, the infection is acquired via a cut from contact with an infected person or animal. Tuberculosis affects people throughout the world (about 6000 new cases each year in England and Wales). Many people acquire the infection and recover without suspecting its presence and the disease is curable with antibiotics e.g. streptomycin. In addition, BCG VACCINATION as a preventive measure is given to children in the UK, in addition to X-ray screening to detect carriers.

tumour any abnormal swelling occurring in any part of the body consisting of an unusual growth of tissue, which may be malignant or benign. Tumours tend to be classified according to the tissue of which they are composed e.g. FIBROMA (mainly fibrous tissue) and MYOMA (largely muscle fibres).

turgor a state of being distended, engorged or swollen.

Turner's syndrome a genetic disorder affecting females in which there is only one X chromosome instead of the usual two. Hence those affected have 45 instead of 46 chromosomes, are infertile (as the ovaries are absent), menstruation is absent and breasts and body hair do not develop. Those affected are short and may have webbing of the neck and other developmental defects. The heart may be affected and there can be deafness and intellectual impairment. In a less severe form of the disorder, the second X chromosome is present but abnormal, lacking in normal genetic material.

tympanic membrane the eardrum which separates the middle and outer ears and which vibrates in response to sound waves transmitting the vibrations to one of the ear ossicles (the *malleus*). *See* EAR.

typhoid fever a severe infectious disease of the digestive system which is caused by the bacterium *Salmonella typhi* and causes symptoms including a rise in temperature, a rash on the abdomen and chest, headache and nosebleeds. The temperature rise occurs in a characteristic fashion known as a *step-ladder temperature*. In severe cases there may be ulceration of the intestinal wall leading to PERITONITIS if an ulcer bursts, or haemorrhage from the bowels and inflammation of the lungs, SPLEEN and bones. In these cases the disease can prove to be fatal. The infection is acquired through ingesting contaminated food or water, hence preventative measures involving high standards of hygiene and sanitation are important. Drug treatment is by means of antibiotics such as chloramphenicol and ampicillin. Inoculation with TAB vaccine confers temporary immunity.

typhus fever *see* **rickettsiae**.

U

ulcer a break on the skin surface or on the MUCOUS MEMBRANE lining within the body cavities that may be inflamed and fails to heal. Ulcers of the skin include BED SORES and varicose ulcers (which are caused by defective circulation). For ulcers of the alimentary tract, *see* DUODENAL ULCER, GASTRIC ULCER and PEPTIC ULCER.

ulna one of the two bones making up the forearm. It is the inner and longer of the two bones (the other being the radius). It articulates with the radius at both ends and additionally with the humerus above, and indirectly with the wrist below.

ultrasound (*or* **ultrasonic waves**) high frequency sound waves (above 20 kHz), beyond the range of the human ear. Ultrasound is used to examine the body's organs, ducts, etc., in addition to assessing the progress of a developing foetus. The patient is not submitted to harmful radiation as with other techniques and no contrast medium is required. It can be used to examine the liver, kidney, bladder, pancreas and ovaries, and is used in diagnosing brain tumours. The vibrations of the sound waves can be used in other ways e.g. breaking up kidney stones.

umbilical cord the cord connecting the foetus to the placenta, containing two arteries and one vein. It is approximately 60cm long. After birth it is severed and the stump shrivels to leave a scar, the navel or UMBILICUS.

umbilicus the navel. *See* UMBILICAL CORD.

unconsciousness the state of being partially or totally unaware of the surroundings and lacking in response to stimuli. Sleep is a natural form of unconsciousness. Unnatural states of unconsciousness can be due to numerous causes, including injuries to the brain resulting in compression or concussion, fainting due to insufficient blood supply to the brain, EPILEPSY, poisoning and various diseases e.g. DIABETES MELLITUS.

undulant fever *see* **brucellosis.**

ungual a term meaning relating to the fingernails or toenails.

unguentum the term in pharmacy for an ointment.

unguis a fingernail or toenail.

uraemia the condition where there is excess UREA in the blood due to kidney disease or failure. Waste products are usually excreted by the kidneys but accumulation in the blood leads to headaches, drowsiness and lethargy, nausea, vomiting and diarrhoea. Eventually, without treatment, death follows. Haemodialysis on a kidney machine may be necessary, or even a renal transplant.

urataemia the presence in the blood of urate compounds (*see* URIC ACID), associated with GOUT, when urates are deposited in the body.

urea a metabolic by-product of the chemical breakdown of protein and the form in which excess nitrogen is removed from the body, in urine. It is formed in the LIVER and taken in the blood to the KIDNEYS. The amount excreted daily is 30-35gm. Although urea is not poisonous in itself, an excess in the blood (URAEMIA) implies a defective kidney, which will cause an excess of other waste products that may be poisonous.

ureaplasma microorganisms responsible for diseases such as PROSTATITIS, non-specific URETHRITIS, infertility and NEONATAL death. The latter can be associated with infection of the placenta by *Ureaplasma urealyticum.*

ureter the tubes joining the KIDNEYS to the bladder and through which urine passes. The muscular ureter walls contract to force urine into the bladder.

ureterectomy surgical excision of a URETER, usually with the removal of the associated kidney.

ureteritis inflammation of the URETER, which usually occurs with bladder inflammations.

ureteroenterostomy the creation by surgery of a link between the URETER and the bowel, thus bypassing the bladder. The join is made at the SIGMOID COLON and is made to bypass a diseased bladder. The urine is then passed with the faeces, thus avoiding an external opening for collection of urine.

ureteroplasty reconstruction of a damaged or diseased ureter by surgery, using bowel or bladder tissue.

ureteroscope an instrument introduced into a dilated URETER, often to locate a stone or remove stone fragments created by ultrasonic destruction of a larger stone.

ureterostomy the creation of an external opening to the URETER whereby the ureter is brought to the surface to permit drainage.

ureterotomy an incision into the URETER, commonly to remove a stone.

urethra the duct carrying urine from the bladder out of the body. It is about 3.5cm long in women and 20cm in men. The male urethra runs through the penis and also forms the ejaculatory duct.

urethritis inflammation of the mucous lining of the URETHRA, which may be associated with CYSTITIS, often being the cause of the latter. The commonest cause of urethritis is GONORRHOEA (*specific* urethritis). Alternatively, it may be due to infection with microorganisms (causing *non-specific* urethritis). The symptoms include a discharge, pain on passing urine, and inflammations in other organs such as the bladder and testicle are possible. Sulphonamide and antibiotic drugs are effective, once the infecting organism is identified.

uric acid an organic acid that contains nitrogen and is the end product of the metabolism of protein. It occurs in the urine but in small amounts (less than 1gm). It is formed in the liver and excreted by the kidneys but in excess, salts (urates) form and occur as stone in the urinary tract. Deposits of urates in joints is a feature of GOUT.

urinary organs the system responsible for the extraction of components from the blood to form urine, its storage and periodic discharge from the body. The organs are the kidneys, ureters, bladder and urethra (*see individual entries*).

urinary tract the system of ducts that permit movement of urine out of the body from the kidneys, i.e. the URETERS, BLADDER and URETHRA.

urination (*or* **micturition**) the discharge of urine from the body via the URETHRA. It is begun by a voluntary relaxation of the sphincter muscle below the bladder.

urine the body's fluid waste excreted by the KIDNEYS. The waste products include UREA, URIC ACID and creatinine (produced by muscles) with salt, phosphates and sulphates and ammonia also present. In a solution with about 95-96% water, there may be 100 or more compounds but the vast majority occur only in trace amounts. Many diseases alter the quantity and composition of urine and its analysis is standard procedure to assist diagnosis of diseases.

urine retention the condition when urine is produced by the kidneys but it is retained in the bladder. This may be due to an obstruction, or a weakness in the bladder. Enlargement of the PROSTATE GLAND is a common cause of blockage. It may also be caused by a STRICTURE, due to injury scar or ulceration.

urinogenital a collective descriptive term relating to all organs and tissues involved in excretion and reproduction, because they are closely linked anatomically and functionally.

urology the subdiscipline of medicine dealing with diseases of the urinary tract, from the kidney to the urethra.

urticaria (*or* **nettle rash**) an allergic reaction by an individual to some substance to which he or she is hypersensitive, in which the allergic response is manifested on the skin. Raised red patches develop which may last for hours or days. There is intense itching.

The sensitivity may be to certain foods e.g. shellfish, and the effect may occur anywhere on the body, but commonly erupts on the face and trunk. If it also affects the tongue or throat, there is danger of a blockage of the airway which would need urgent attention.

uterine relating to the UTERUS.

uterus (*or* **womb**) a vaguely pear-shaped organ within the cavity of the pelvis that is specialized for the growth and nourishment of a foetus. FALLOPIAN TUBES connect to the upper part and the lower part joins the VAGINA at the CERVIX. It has a plentiful blood supply with lymphatic vessels and nerves. During pregnancy it enlarges considerably and the SMOOTH MUSCLE walls thicken. Contractions of the muscular wall push the foetus out via the vagina at childbirth. If there is no pregnancy the lining undergoes periodic changes (MENSTRUATION).

uvea the middle pigmented layer of the EYE, consisting of the IRIS, choroid and ciliary body.

uveitis inflammation of any part of the uvea. The iris and ciliary body are often both inflamed (*anterior uveitis*) producing a painful condition, unlike *posterior uveitis* (when the choroid is affected). The cause of both types is usually different and may follow from affected areas elsewhere in the eye. All types lead to visual impairment and symptoms may include blurred vision with discomfort or pain and diseases or conditions with which it is known to be linked are arthritis, tuberculosis, syphilis and viral and parasitic infections.

V

vaccination the production of immunity to a disease by inoculation with a VACCINE or a specially prepared material that stimulates the production of antibodies. It was used initially to refer only to cowpox virus (which also protected against SMALLPOX) but now is synonymous with inoculation, in immunizing against disease.

vaccine a modified preparation of a BACTERIUM or VIRUS that is no longer dangerous but will stimulate development of antibodies and therefore confer immunity against actual infection with the disease. Other vaccines consist of specific toxins (e.g. tetanus), or dead bacteria (e.g. cholera and typhoid). Live but weakened organisms are used against smallpox and tuberculosis.

vagina the lower part of the female reproductive tract that leads from the uterus to the exterior. It receives the erect penis during sexual intercourse. The semen is ejaculated into the upper part from where the sperms pass through the CERVIX and UTERUS to the FALLOPIAN TUBES. The vagina is a muscular tube lined with mucous membrane.

vaginismus a sudden and painful contraction of muscles surrounding the VAGINA in response to contact of the vagina or VULVA e.g. an attempted intercourse. It may be due to a fear of intercourse or an inflammation.

vaginitis inflammation of the vagina due to infection or deficiency in diet or hygiene. There may be itching, a discharge and pain on urination.

vagotomy the cutting of fibres of the VAGUS nerve to the stomach. The operation can be performed to reduce the stomach's acid and pepsin secretion, in treatment of a PEPTIC ULCER.

vagus the tenth cranial nerve, which comprises motor, sensory, vasodilator and secretory fibres. It supplies the muscles for swallowing and fibres go to the heart, throat, lungs and stomach and other organs in the abdomen. It also carries the taste sensation from the mouth.

valve a structure within an organ or vessel that restricts flow to one direction, whether the fluid be blood or lymph. The valves comprise cusps on the vessel wall. The cusp is like a membranous pocket that fills with blood should it flow back and the cusps distend and close the valve.

valvotomy an operation undertaken to open a stenosed heart valve and render it functional. Several techniques are available including surgery, an inflating balloon or a dilating instrument.

valvular heart disease affects mainly the AORTIC and MITRAL VALVES, which may narrow (STENOSIS) or weaken. Aortic valve disease is associated more with old age while mitral valve disease is rheumatic in origin.

valvulitis inflammation of a valve, particularly in the heart. It is commonly due to rheumatic fever.

vaporizer a device that produces a mist of liquid medication for inhalation. It is commonly used in the treatment of asthma.

varicose veins veins that have become stretched, distended and twisted. The superficial veins in the legs are often affected, although it may occur elsewhere. Causes include congenitally defective valves, obesity, pregnancy and thrombophlebitis (inflammation of the wall of a vein with secondary THROMBOSIS in the affected part of the vein). Elastic support is a common treatment although alternatives are SCLEROTHERAPY and PHLEBECTOMY.

variola a name for SMALLPOX.

vas a vessel or duct, especially those carrying blood, lymph or spermatozoa.

vascular relating to blood vessels; supplied with blood vessels.

vasculitis inflammation of the blood vessels that may cause damage to the linings and cause narrowing. It may result from several conditions, including acute NEPHRITIS and SERUM SICKNESS.

vas deferens (*plural* **vas deferentia**) one of the two tubes that join the testes to the ejaculatory duct via the PROSTATE GLAND. It carries spermatozoa to the URETHRA on ejaculation, aided by contraction of its muscular wall.

vasectomy the cutting of the VAS DEFERENS, which is performed on both ducts causing sterility, although the effect is not immediate.

vasoconstriction the narrowing of blood vessels with a consequent reduction in blood supply to that part of the body supplied. A variety of circumstances can cause vasoconstriction including cold and shock.

vasodilation (*or* **vasodilatation**) the increase in diameter of blood vessels producing a lowering of blood pressure.

vasopressin (*or* **antidiuretic hormone**) a PITUITARY GLAND hormone that constricts blood vessels and reduces urine secretion by increasing the quantity of water reabsorbed by the KIDNEY.

vasovagal attack fainting, precipitated by a slowing of the heart and a fall in blood pressure. This may be due to shock, severe pain, fear, etc., and is caused by excessive stimulation of the VAGUS nerve which participates in the control of breathing and the circulation.

vasovasostomy the reversal of VASECTOMY.

vector commonly, an insect that carries parasitic microorganisms between people, or from animals to people e.g. mosquitoes carrying malaria.

vein one of the numerous blood vessels carrying deoxygenated blood to the right atrium of the heart (the one exception is the PULMONARY vein). Each vein has three tissue layers, similar to the layers of the heart. Veins are less elastic than arteries and collapse when cut. They also contain VALVES to prevent backflow.

vena cava either of two major veins carrying blood from other veins to the right ATRIUM of the heart. The *inferior* vena cava takes blood from the body below the DIAPHRAGM and the *superior* vena cava takes blood from the head, neck, arms and thorax.

venereal disease (*or* **sexually transmitted disease**) a disease transmitted by sexual intercourse. This includes AIDS, SYPHILIS, GONORRHOEA, non-specific URETHRITIS, etc.

venography examination of veins using X-rays after injection of a radio-opaque substance. This enables leaks, blockages or other abnormalities to be identified.

venom the poisonous substance produced by snakes, scorpions, etc., which in humans may produce only localized pain and swelling, or in serious cases cause more general effects and even death.

ventilation the means whereby air passes into and out of the lungs, aided by movement of the diaphragm.

Artificial ventilation is the use of a machine (VENTILATOR) to regulate and perform a person's breathing. This may occur during an operation. Also, damage to the relevant part of the brain, chest injury, lung disease or nerve and muscle disorders may all require the use of artificial ventilation.

ventilator the machine used to provide an air supply to the lungs of patients who cannot breathe normally for themselves. Blood gases and other body functions can be monitored at the same time.

ventouse (*or* **vacuum extractor**) a machine used in childbirth. It comprises a suction cup which is attached to the head of the foetus enabling it to be gently pulled out of the uterus. It is an alternative to the use of forceps.

ventricle one of the two major chambers within the heart. They are thick-walled and muscular and form the main pumping chamber. The right ventricle receives blood from the right ATRIUM and venae cavae and its outflow is the PULMONARY artery. The left ventricle takes blood from the pulmonary vein via the left atrium, and its outflow is the AORTA.

Also, cavities within the brain, filled with cerebrospinal fluid.

ventricular fibrillation a rapid ARRHYTHMIA of the ventricle which is dangerous.

verruca a term for WART.

verrucose covered with warts.

version (*or* **turning**) the procedure to move a foetus in the uterus to a more normal position, to make delivery easier.

vertebra (*plural* **vertebrae**) any of the bones making up the vertebral column. Each has a cavity (the vertebral canal or foramen) and various processes for attachment of muscles or articulation of adjacent vertebrae. The spinal cord passes through the vertebral canal (*see* SPINAL COLUMN).

vertebral column *see* **spinal column**.

vertigo a condition in which a person has a false sensation of imbalance and of the surroundings moving. It is commonly a sensation of spinning but may be as if the ground is tilting. The semicircular canals of the ear are fundamental in the maintenance of balance and vertigo is generally due to some problem with this mechanism or with the appropriate centres in the brain.

vesicular breathing soft, normal sounds of breathing heard in the lung by means of a stethoscope. The sounds change when the lungs are diseased and the different sounds help a doctor diagnose the disease.

vessel any tube that carries fluid, particularly blood or lymph.

vestigial the term applied to an organ that has progressively, over a long time, lost its function and structure to become rudimentary.

viable able to live separately.

villus (*plural* **villi**) *see* JEJUNUM.

Vincent's angina a former name for ulcerative gingivitis and ulcerative inflammation of the throat, caused by bacteria.

viral haemorrhagic fever a viral disease with a high mortality rate. After the incubation period there is headache, fever, severe internal bleeding, diarrhoea and vomiting. Death may follow, usually eight or nine days later. Serum taken from someone recovering from the disease is a useful source of antibodies.

viral pneumonia an acute lung infection caused by one of many viruses. The symptoms include fever, headache, muscle pains and a thick sputum associated with the cough. It often occurs after a viral infection and treatment, in the main, deals with the symptoms only.

virology the study of viruses.

virulence the ability of a bacterium or virus to cause disease, measured by numbers of people infected, the speed with which it spreads through the body, etc.

virus the smallest microbe that is completely parasitic, because it is only capable of replication within the cells of its host. Viruses infect animals, plants and microorganisms. Viruses are classified according to their NUCLEIC ACIDS and can contain double- or single-stranded DNA or RNA. In an infection the virus binds to the host cells and then penetrates the cell membrane to release the viral DNA or RNA which controls the cell's metabolism to replicate itself and form new viruses. Viruses cause many diseases including influenza (single-stranded RNA), herpes (double-stranded DNA), AIDS (a RETROVIRUS, single-stranded RNA) and also mumps, chicken-pox and polio.

viscera the term for organs within the body cavity, usually the abdominal cavity.

vision the capacity for sight. Light enters the EYE through the cornea and the aqueous humour. Next, it passes through the pupil, the lens and the vitreous humour to impinge upon the retina. There the ROD and CONE cells detect light and send impulses to the nerve fibres, impulses which are relayed to the visual cortex in the brain. *Visual acuity* is the sharpness of vision, dependent upon a healthy retina and accurate lens (*see* SNELLEN CHART).

vital capacity the largest volume of air that can be exhaled after breathing in deeply.

vitamin any of a group of organic compounds required in very small amounts in the diet to maintain good health. Deficiencies lead to specific diseases. Vitamins are divided into two groups: vitamins A, D, E and K are fat-soluble while C and B are water-soluble.

vitamin A (*or* **retinol**) a fat-soluble vitamin that must be in the diet as it cannot be synthesized in the body. It occurs in dairy products, egg yolk and liver and is available as a precursor in green vegetables. It is essential for vision in dim light, growth and the maintenance of mucous tissue.

vitamin B any of a group of vitamins that although they are not related chemically, are often found in the same types of food (*see following entries* and BIOTIN).

vitamin B$_1$ (*or* **thiamine**) a vitamin active in the form thiamine pyrophosphate, a deficiency of which leads to BERIBERI. Thiamine can be found in cereals, meat, beans, nuts and potatoes.

vitamin B$_2$ (*or* **riboflavin**) a vitamin important in tissue respiration (enzyme reactions in cells), although a deficiency is not serious. Sources are milk, liver and eggs.

vitamin B$_3$ (*or* **pantothenic acid**) a vitamin that occurs widely in foods and which is therefore unlikely to be lacking in the diet.

vitamin B$_6$ (*or* **pyridoxine**) a vitamin found in many foods (liver, fish, yeast and cereals). It is important in the metabolism of several amino acids.

vitamin B$_{12}$ (*or* **cyanocobalamin**) an important vitamin, in the synthesis of nucleic acids, maintenace of MYELIN surrounding nerve fibres and in the production of red blood cells. It is found in fish, liver, eggs and dairy products. A deficiency produces anaemia and degeneration of the nervous system.

vitamin C (*or* **ascorbic acid**) a vitamin found in citrus fruits and vegetables. Vitamin C is essential in maintaining cell walls and connective tissue and a deficiency leads to fragility of tendons, blood vessels and skin — all characteristic of the disease called scurvy. The presence of ascorbic acid is believed to assist the uptake of iron during digestion.

vitamin D this vitamin occurs as two steroid derivations: D$_2$ or calciferol in yeast and D$_3$ or cholecalciferol which is produced by the action of sunlight on the skin. The dietary source of vitamin D is fish liver oils, eggs and dairy products and it is vital in control of blood calcium levels. It prompts an increase in calcium take-up in the gut, increasing the supply for the production of bone. It also affects phosphorus uptake. A deficiency leads to RICKETS and OSTEOMALACIA.

vitamin E a group of compounds (tocopherols)

thought to prevent damage to cell membranes. Vitamin E is found in cereal grains, green vegetables and eggs. A deficiency is unusual due to its widespread occurrence in foods.

vitamin H *see* **biotin**.

vitamin K a vitamin that is essential for the clotting of blood as it is involved in the formation of prothrombin (the inactive precursor of THROMBIN) in the liver. The main food sources are spinach, leafy vegetables and liver but a deficiency rarely occurs because the vitamin is synthesized by bacteria in the large intestine.

vitreous humour the jelly-like substance occurring between the lens and the retina in the EYE.

vocal cords two membranes in the LARYNX that vibrate to produce sound when air is expelled over them. Tension in the cords is controlled by muscles and tendons, thus changing the sound generated.

Volkmann's contracture a condition often caused by pressure from a cast or tight bandage on the arm. The result is persistent contraction (flexion) of forearm muscles and decreased blood supply to hand and arm. The muscles then swell and become fibrosed.

voluntary muscle (*or* **striated muscle**) muscle that is under conscious control, such as those muscles operating the skeleton. It consists of bundles of elongated fibres surrounded by connective tissue. A tendon at the end of the muscle attaches it to the bone. Each muscle fibre comprises smaller fibres (*myofibrils*) with alternating dark and light bands (*sarcomeres*), which produce the striated appearance and provide the contractile function.

A flexor (*or agonist*) muscle contracts, becoming shorter, thus moving bones closer to each other. An extensor or *antagonist* muscle works in the opposite sense.

volvulus a twisting of part of the bowels which usually results in some obstruction which may reduce the blood supply, ending in gangrene. It may right itself spontaneously or may be righted by manipulation. However, surgery is often necessary.

vomiting (*or* **emesis**) the reflex action whereby the stomach contents are expelled through the mouth, due to the contraction of the diaphragm and abdominal wall muscles. Vomiting is due to stimulus of the appropriate centre in the brain but the primary agent is usually a sensation from the stomach itself e.g. a gastric disease, or some irritant. Other causes may be the action of drugs, some effect on the inner ear (e.g. motion sickness), migraines, etc.

von Recklinghausen's disease a congenital disorder, neurofibromatosis, in which soft tissue tumours form along nerves and beneath the skin. There are often other anomalies such as decalcification of bones, FIBROSIS of the lungs and formation of kidney stones.

vulva the external female genitals comprising two pairs of fleshy folds surrounding the vaginal opening.

vulvectomy surgical removal of the VULVA. The extent of the operation depends upon whether there is a malignant or non-malignant growth.

vulvitis inflammation of the VULVA.

vulvovaginitis inflammation of both the VULVA and the VAGINA.

W

warfarin an anticoagulant given to reduce the risk of EMBOLISM. It may be administered orally or by injection and the significant side effect is bleeding, usually from the gums and other mucous membranes.

wart (*or* **verruca**) a solid, benign growth in the skin, caused by a virus. They are infectious and spread rapidly in schools, etc. There are several types: *plantar*, on the foot; *juvenile*, in children and *venereal*, on the genitals. Warts often disappear spontaneously, but can be dealt with in several ways e.g. cryosurgery (freezing), laser treatment and electrocautery (burning away with an electrically heated wire or needle).

water bed a bed with a water-containing mattress which readily accommodates a patient's posture. This is useful to avoid bed sores.

water on the brain *see* **hydrocephalus**.

weal (*or* **wheal**) an area of the skin that is temporarily raised and coloured red, or pale with red margins. It may be due to an allergy (*see also* URTICARIA), nettle rash or a sharp blow, and in the former cases may be accompanied by itching.

webbed fingers *see* **syndactyly**.

Weber's test assessing a person's deafness using a tuning fork. The stem of a vibrating fork is placed on the forehead or maxillary incisors and if the hearing is normal, the sound is equal in both ears. It helps to diagnose whether hearing loss is due to a middle-ear disorder or a neurosensory loss.

Weil's disease *see* **leptospirosis**.

wen *see* **sebaceous cyst**.

Werthheim's hysterectomy a major form of hysterectomy undertaken to deal with uterine or ovarian cancer. It involves the removal of the uterus, ovaries, Fallopian tubes, upper part of the vagina and the surrounding lymph nodes.

wheeze the sound produced by the long-drawn-out breathing associated with ASTHMA. It also occurs when bronchial tubes are narrowed, as in BRONCHITIS.

whiplash injury damage caused by the sudden jerking backwards of the head and neck, as in a road accident. A severe whiplash can cause death, but injury is the usual outcome. The vertebrae, spinal cord, ligaments and nerves in the neck may all be damaged. Treatment usually involves wearing a special collar to immobilize the affected area.

Whipple's disease a rare disease of the intestines resulting in malabsorption of food. Symptoms include anaemia, weight loss, arthritis, skin pigmentation, chest pain and a non-productive cough. It seems to be caused by microorganisms in the mucosa. It responds to extensive antibiotic treatment.

white leg *see* **thrombophlebitis**.

white matter nerve tissue in the CENTRAL NERVOUS SYSTEM, composed primarily of nerve fibres in light-coloured MYELIN sheaths. In the brain it occupies the central part of the cerebral cortex.

whitlow inflammation of tissues in the finger tip, and usually an abscess affecting the fat and fibrous tissues that comprise the pulp of the finger.

whoop the noisy and characteristic drawing in of breath following a coughing attack in WHOOPING COUGH.

whooping cough (*or* **pertussis**) an infectious disease caused by the bacterium *Bordetella pertussis*. The mucous membranes lining the air passages are affected and after a one-to-two week incubation period, fever, catarrh and a cough develop. The cough then becomes paroxysmal with a number of short coughs punctuated with the 'whooping' drawing in of breath. Nosebleeds and vomiting may follow a paroxysm. After about two weeks the symptoms abate but a cough may continue for some weeks. Whooping cough is not usually serious and immunization reduces the severity of an attack. However, a child may be susceptible to pneumonia and tuberculosis during the disease.

Wilm's tumour a tumour of the kidney (nephroblastoma) in infancy. Early removal of the kidney with radiotherapy and chemotherapy confers a high survival rate.

windpipe *see* **trachea**.

wisdom tooth the last (third) molar tooth on each

side of either jaw. These teeth normally erupt last, around the age of 20 to 25, although some remain impacted in the jaw bone.

withdrawal symptoms a characteristic feature when someone stops using a drug upon which he or she has become dependent. The hard drugs such as heroin and cocaine induce dependence as does alcohol, nicotine and amphetamines. Symptoms include shivering, tremors, vomiting and sweating.

womb *see* **uterus**.

wool sorter's disease *see* **anthrax**.

wound a sudden break in the body tissues and/or organs caused by an external agent. There are four types based upon the result of the injury: incisions, punctures, lacerations and contusions.

wrist the joint between the hand and forearm. The wrist region comprises eight carpal bones and five metacarpal bones joined by strong ligaments. The wrist joint then articulates with the RADIUS and ULNA. The joint can move in all directions with little risk of dislocation.

writer's cramp an involuntary contraction of the hand muscles when writing, but not when using those muscles to undertake other functions. A similar condition may arise with musicians (guitarists and pianists), typists and computer operators.

wryneck (*or* **torticollis**) when the head is twisted to one side due to a scar contracting or, more commonly, to excessive muscle contraction.

X

xanthelasma yellow fatty deposits in the eyelids and skin around the eyes. It often occurs in elderly people, when it is insignificant, but a severe case may be due to a fat metabolism disorder.

xanthochromia a yellow colouring e.g. the skin in jaundice or the cerebrospinal fluid when it contains haemoglobin breakdown products.

X chromosome the sex chromosome present in male and female although women have a pair, and men just one (with one Y CHROMOSOME). Certain disorders such as HAEMOPHILIA are carried as genes on the X chromosome.

xenophobia an abnormal condition in which there is dislike and fear of foreigners.

xeroderma a condition of the skin which manifests itself as a dryness and roughness with the formation of scales. It is a mild form of ICHTHYOSIS.

xiphoid process (*or* **xiphoid cartilage**) the lowest part of the STERNUM. It is a flat cartilage that is progressively replaced by bone, a process completed some time after middle age.

X-rays the part of the electromagnetic spectrum with waves of wavelength 10^{-12} to 10^{-9}m and frequencies of 10^{17} to 10^{21}Hz. They are produced when high-velocity electrons strike a target. The rays penetrate solids to a depth that depends upon the density of the solid. X-rays of certain wavelengths will penetrate flesh but not bone. They are therefore useful in therapy and diagnosis within medicine.

Y

yawning a reflex action when the mouth is opened wide and air drawn into the lungs and slowly released. It is usually, though not exclusively, associated with tiredness or boredom.

yaws an infectious disease of the tropics caused by a spirochaete (a type of bacterium) *Treponema pertenue*, usually in unhygienic conditions. The bacteria enter through abrasions and after about two weeks, during which time there is fever, pain and itching, small tumours appear each with a yellow crust of dried serum. These may eventually form deep ulcers. The final stages may not appear until after several years and include LESIONS of skin and bone. Fortunately, penicillin works dramatically and effectively in this disease.

Y chromosome the small chromosome that carries a dominant gene conferring maleness. Normal males have 22 matched chromosome pairs and one unmatched pair comprising one X and one Y chromosome.

During sexual reproduction the mother contributes an X chromosome, but the father contributes an X or Y chromosome, XX produces a female offspring, XY male.

yellow fever an infectious viral disease in tropical Africa and South America. Transmitted by mosquitoes, it causes tissue degeneration in the liver and kidneys.

Symptoms include headache, back pains, fever, vomiting, jaundice, etc., and an attack can prove fatal. Vaccination will prove effective and anyone recovering from an attack has immunity conferred.

Z

zidovudine an antiviral drug (trade name Retrovir) that is used to treat AIDS. Although it slows the growth of the HIV virus, it does not effect a cure.

Zollinger-Ellison syndrome an uncommon disorder resulting in diarrhoea and multiple PEPTIC ULCERS. The cause is a pancreatic tumour or enlarged pancreas, which in turn leads to high levels of the hormone gastrin, which stimulates excess production of acidic gastric juice, causing the ulceration. Surgery is usually effective.

zoonosis (*plural* **zoonoses**) an infectious animal disease that can be transmitted to man. Some of the 150 or so diseases are: anthrax, brucellosis, bovine tuberculosis, Rift Valley fever, rabies, leptospirosis and typhus (*see individual entries*).

zoophobia an unnatural and strong fear of animals.

zygomatic arch the arch of bone of either side of the face, below the eyes.

zygomatic bone a facial bone and one of a pair of bones that form the prominence of the cheeks.

zygote the cell produced by the fusion of male and female germ cells (GAMETES) during the early stage of fertilization, i.e. an ovum fertilized by a sperm. After passing down the FALLOPIAN TUBE, it implants in the uterus, forming the embryo.

Guide to Symptoms

Symptoms and self-diagnosis—a word of warning

From even a brief study of the contents of this section of the book, it will be apparent that most illnesses and disorders produce a range of symptoms. For any given illness or condition, certain symptoms may be more pronounced in one individual than in another. Diagnosis is a skilled undertaking, which must always be carried out by a doctor and not from the pages of a book. Also, it is overwhelmingly the case that early diagnosis and treatment produce the best results and outlook for the patient. If you are experiencing any symptoms, however slight, that are causing you concern, you should *always* consult your doctor and not attempt to diagnose or treat yourself.

Given the variable nature of the symptoms of many illnesses and disorders, the latter may be listed under more than one heading in the Quick Reference to Symptoms on page 301.

A

abruptio placentae

Description: bleeding from the placenta after the 28th week of pregnancy, which may result in the placenta becoming completely or partially separated from the wall of the uterus (womb).

Persons most commonly affected: females during pregnancy.

Organ or part of body involved: uterus.

Symptoms and indications: these depend upon the degree of separation of the placenta and so range from slight to severe but include bleeding from the vagina, pain in the abdomen and abdominal hardness. In very serious untreated cases: maternal shock and foetal distress with possible fatal outcome for both mother and baby.

Always tell your doctor if you experience bleeding at any time during pregnancy.

Treatment: Admittance to hospital for rest and observation. An ultrasound examination is usually carried out to establish the diagnosis of abruptio placentae as the symptoms are very similar to those of PLACENTA PRAEVIA. If the bleeding is slight, the foetus is in good health and the pregnancy is not near to term, continued bed rest is required until the bleeding stops. If the bleeding worsens, delivery of the foetus by Caesarian section is usually required. (Delivery may sometimes be vaginal if labour has already started.)

Causes and risk factors: the cause is unknown, but abruptio placentae is more likely to occur in women who already have children, who are aged over 35 and who smoke. Also it may result from an accidental blow in the abdominal region.

acne or **acne vulgaris**

Description: a disorder of the skin, especially common in adolescents, characterized by the presence of pustules and blackheads on the face, upper back, chest and shoulders. It is associated with the sebaceous (oil-secreting) glands in the skin.

Persons most commonly affected: adolescents, especially boys.

Organ or part of body involved: skin.

Symptoms and indications: presence on the skin of blackheads, pustules and whiteheads. The surrounding skin may be inflamed, red and sore, especially with scratching.

Treatment: the skin should be carefully and thoroughly washed and dried, and the spots should not be scratched or squeezed to avoid scarring of the skin. Sunlight is helpful, and acne is often worse in the winter months than during the summer. The use of a topical preparation containing benzoyl peroxide, tretinoin (retinoic acid), salicylic acid, vitamin A and/or clindamycin may be recommended by your doctor. Some cosmetics aggravate acne and should be avoided. Also, it is possible that certain foods make the condition worse in some people. Acne in adolescence usually clears up with time.

Causes and risk factors: increased production of androgen hormones at puberty, blockage of sebaceous glands and the breakdown of sebum (the secretion of the glands by bacteria (propionibacterium acnes) seem to be responsible for the inflammation that causes acne.

Addison's disease

Description: a disease caused by the destruction or failure of the cortex of the adrenal glands, so that there is insufficient secretion of the adrenocortical hormones (cortisol, aldosterol and androgens).

Persons most commonly affected: all age groups and both sexes.

Organ or part of body involved: adrenal glands situated above the kidneys.

Symptoms and indications: weakness, fatigue, wasting, anorexia and weight loss, which may be accompanied by gastrointestinal upset including diarrhoea and sickness; low blood pressure with symptoms of dizziness, fainting and feeling cold; dark pigmentation of the skin and loss of underarm hair in women; mood changes, depression.

Treatment: hormone replacement therapy to restore adrenocortical hormones, which effects a complete cure.

Causes and risk factors: in the past, Addison's disease often occurred in patients with tuberculosis, which caused damage to or destruction of the adrenal gland cortex. Today this damage is more commonly caused by disturbances in the immune system (autoimmune damage) and, more rarely, secondary cancerous growths. Damage to the adrenal glands through accidental injury, diabetes mellitus and stress are conditions that may increase the risk of developing Addison's disease.

adult respiratory distress syndrome (ARDS)

Description: severe respiratory failure, which is often fatal, brought about by a number of different disorders. In newborn babies, a similar condition is known as hyaline membrane disease.

Persons most commonly affected: adults and children (except newborn) of both sexes and all ages.

Symptoms and indications: a lack of oxygen in the blood, which is indicated by a blueness (cyanosis) of the skin, an abnormally rapid rate of breathing (tachypnoea) and a raised heartbeat rate (tachycardia). There is pulmonary oedema (a collection of fluid in the lungs) and the substance known as surfactant, which prevents the lungs' sacs (alveoli) from collapsing and allows oxygen to pass in and carbon dioxide to pass out, is lost. These conditions lead to the lungs becoming stiff and ineffective; death follows without emergency medical intervention. A person with signs of this disorder requires urgent medical treatment.

Treatment: intensive care treatment, including mechanical ventilation of the lungs and management of the patient's fluid balance to reduce pulmonary oedema. Also, the underlying cause of the respiratory failure is treated if this is possible. Surfactant may be given by means of a nebulizer or aerosol.

Causes and risk factors: there are a variety of different causes of this disorder, which may be broadly divided into four categories:

1. Physical causes, including injury to the lungs, inhalation of water as in drowning, vomit or other foreign substance.

2. Bacterial, viral or fungal infection of the lungs or other part of the body, as in various diseases including PNEUMONIA, sepsis, poliomyelitis.

3. As a response by the patient's immune system following blood transfusion or cardiopulmonary bypass surgery.

4. Accidental inhalation of poisonous fumes and smoke, ingestion of certain chemicals and drugs.

5. As a complication of various other diseases and disorders, including ASTHMA, EMPHYSEMA, MUSCULAR DYSTROPHY, PANCREATITIS, GUILLAIN-BARRÉ SYNDROME, uraemia, MYASTHENIA GRAVIS.

Patients who receive mechanical ventilation for a long period may develop complications in the form of secondary infections and PNEUMOTHORAX, which require additional treatment. The survival rate for patients with this condition is about 50%, and those who respond well suffer little lung damage. There is a greater likelihood of lung damage in those patients needing prolonged mechanical ventilation.

agranulocytosis

Description: an abnormality of the blood involving white blood cells, called granulocytes or neutrophils, which are a vital part of the body's defence or immune system.

Persons most commonly affected: all age groups and both sexes.

Organ or part of body involved: blood and bone marrow.

Symptoms and indications: fever, aches and pains, sore throat, with ulcers in mouth and throat. Ulcers may also occur in the rectum and vagina. A person with this condition requires prompt medical treatment.

Treatment: admittance to hospital for intensive treatment with antibiotics and, possibly, transfusion of white blood cells. Patient requires to be isolated to avoid or lessen the possibility of acquiring infections. Once the condition is improving, strict attention should be paid to cleanliness and hygiene (particularly oral hygiene) until cured. The condition is usually curable but can be rapidly fatal if a severe and dangerous infection develops.

Causes and risk factors: agranulocytosis is caused by an abnormal fall in or even absence of granulocytes because of destruction of these cells or failure of the bone marrow to produce them. This itself usually results from an adverse reaction to certain drugs, including immunosuppressants and anticancer drugs, sulphonamides, chloramphenicol and others. Certain chemicals may also produce the disease. A person who has recovered from agranulocytosis should avoid drugs or chemicals that were suspected of causing the condition.

Aids

Description: acquired immune deficiency syndrome, first recognized in Los Angeles, USA, in 1981, which affects the body's natural defence or immune system. The person slowly and progressively succumbs to various infections and tumours that eventually prove to be fatal.

Persons most commonly affected: all age groups and both sexes but affected infants acquire the condition at birth from mothers who have Aids.

Organ or part or body involved: the immune system, especially cells known as T-lymphocytes and lymph glands, bone marrow, liver and spleen.

Symptoms and indications: early symptoms include enlargement of lymph glands and spleen, fever, fatigue, bruising and bleeding easily, THRUSH-type infections, diarrhoea and weight loss, dermatitis and respiratory illnesses. Later, a person develops further serious infections or cancers. These include herpes infections, pneumonia, meningitis, serious gastrointestinal disorders (e.g. salmonella infections), Kaposi's sarcoma and non-Hodgkin's lymphoma. A number of illnesses may occur, some of which are particularly associated with Aids and are known as 'Aids indicator conditions'.

Treatment: the symptoms of Aids-related infections can be alleviated with appropriate drug treatments, if not entirely cured. Other drugs, such as dideoxyinosine and zidovudine, may be useful, and many other preparations are helpful depending on the nature of the symptoms.

Causes and risk factors: Aids is caused by a virus called human immunodeficiency virus (HIV), a ribonucleic (RNA) retrovirus. The presence of the virus can be established by a blood test, and it is generally accepted that a person infected with HIV will eventually develop Aids, although there may be a period of many years without signs of illness. HIV is transmitted in blood and body fluids. Those generally accepted to be at risk are sexually active persons who have sexual intercourse with partners infected with HIV. (The use of barrier methods of contraception lessens the risk of infection.) Also, intravenous drug users who share needles that may be contaminated and babies born to mothers who have the HIV virus or Aids. Hospital, dental and medical staff need to follow strict procedures to guard against the possibility of infection. Ordinary social or family contact with a person who has HIV or Aids is generally accepted to pose no risk of the infection being passed on.

alcoholism

Description: a physical and psychological need, and dependence on alcohol to such an extent that

deprivation may result in withdrawal symptoms. The continued and long-term overconsumption (abuse) of alcoholic drink leads to both physical and mental illness. The person's behaviour may become so disordered and disruptive that he or she loses employment, family, friends and home unless counselling and medical help are sought and accepted.

Persons most commonly affected: both sexes and all age groups after adolescence, although more common in males.

Organ or part of body involved: brain, liver, heart.

Symptoms and indications: early indications include the need for an alcoholic drink first thing in the morning before the person does anything else, and it being noticed by others that the person is drinking too much. Also, disturbance of sleep, irritability, attempts to conceal amount being drunk and irritation when overconsumption is suggested. In addition, the person may need to take time off work because of the effects of drinking and may become sexually impotent. Later on, an alcoholic person may become unconscious because of drink, or die from respiratory failure. He or she may suffer from withdrawal symptoms (including hallucinations, fear and imagined persecution, delirium tremens) if drink is withdrawn and experience loss of memory. The person may develop CIRRHOSIS OF THE LIVER, inflammation and ulceration of the gastrointestinal tract and PANCREATITIS. There may be inflammation of peripheral nerves, causing numbness and tingling sensations in hands and feet, and congestive heart failure. A form of DEMENTIA may eventually develop. The physical diseases that result from alcoholism are liable to cause premature death. The unborn child of an alcoholic mother is likely to suffer lasting damage.

Treatment: the success or otherwise of treatment depends on a recognition by the alcoholic person that a problem exists, and a willingness to overcome it. Treatment includes detoxification ('drying out'), counselling and joining a support group such as Alcoholics Anonymous. Physical diseases associated with alcoholism may require appropriate medical and drug therapy and are likely to improve once drinking stops.

Causes and risk factors: the causes are not entirely clear, but some researchers believe that a genetic element exists and some people are more inclined to alcoholism than others. Personality and the environment in which a person lives (e.g. a young person in a family or social group in which alcohol is important) and stress related to work and family and personal relationships are all significant contributory factors. Many people are successfully cured.

allergy

Description: a state of hypersensitivity (or heightened or oversensitivity) in an affected individual to a particular substance, called the 'allergen'. This produces a characteristic response whenever the person is exposed to the allergen.

Persons most commonly affected: both sexes and all age groups.

Organ or part of body involved: various parts of the body depending on the nature of the allergy but including skin, respiratory system, joints and gastrointestinal system.

Symptoms and indications: symptoms usually develop rapidly, within a few minutes, and depend on the nature of the allergy (*see also* ANAPHYLACTIC SHOCK, ASTHMA, DERMATITIS, ECZEMA, HAY FEVER). Common symptoms include nettle rash and skin reactions, swellings and puffiness, e.g. around eyes, wheezing and breathing difficulties, headaches, stomach pains, sickness and diarrhoea. Medical advice should be sought.

Treatment: this depends upon the nature of the reaction but commonly involves the taking of antihistamine drugs. If the allergic response is more serious, as in an asthma attack, hospital treatment may be required, with the administration of bronchodilator and corticosteroid drugs by inhalation. If the allergic response is in the rare form of anaphylactic shock, prompt emergency treatment is necessary with the administration of adrenaline by means of an injection. This condition is fatal unless emergency treatment is promptly received.

Causes and risk factors: in a nonallergic, unaffected person, antibodies present in the bloodstream destroy their particular allergens (antigens). However, in an allergic, affected person this reaction causes some cell damage and there is a release of substances such as histamine and bradykinin, which cause the reaction. Many substances, usually of a protein nature, can be allergens. The list includes many common foods, such as eggs, strawberries and shellfish, colourings and additives used in foods, plants and pollen, mites or dust from animals such as cats, dogs, horses and the feathers of birds. If the allergen is known then it may be possible for the individual to avoid exposure to it. Sometimes it is possible to decrease sensitivity to a particular allergen by gradually increasing exposure under careful medical supervision. However, a person may be allergic to a range of substances. In many people there may be a genetic element, with a family history of allergy.

altitude sickness

Description: also known as mountain sickness, this condition affects individuals (usually mountaineers) who are exposed to high altitudes to which they are unaccustomed.

Persons most commonly affected: both sexes and all age groups (normally adults).

Organ or part of body involved: lungs, respiratory system, blood, brain.

Symptoms and indications: rapid, deep breathing (hyperventilation), nausea, headache, exhaustion, anxiety. In severe cases, there may be breathing difficulties due to PULMONARY OEDEMA, caused by fluid collecting in the lungs, and this is a dangerous condition that may prove fatal.

Treatment: the person must be brought down to a lower altitude for rest and further acclimatization. An individual with pulmonary oedema requires urgent medical treatment in hospital.

Causes and risk factors: the cause is climbing to a high altitude (above 3000 metres) too quickly without giving the body time to adjust to lower oxygen levels and reduced atmospheric pressure. This causes the person to breathe more deeply and rapidly (hyperventilate) with a consequent lowering of CO_2 levels in the blood. It is essential to allow the body to adjust by spending time at a particular altitude and attaining height gradually. Usually, the symptoms are relatively mild, but if they prove to be disabling the climber must return to a lower altitude.

Alzheimer's disease

Description: the commonest cause of DEMENTIA, being a degenerative disease of the cerebral cortex, characterized by gradual and progressive loss of mental faculties.

Persons most commonly affected: both sexes affecting people in middle and old age (over 40).

Organ or part of body involved: brain.

Symptoms and indications: the early indications are forgetfulness and increased difficulty in performing simple, normal tasks to which the person is well accustomed. There may be changes in personality out of character with the person's normal behaviour. There is a progressive deterioration in the person's mental and physical abilities and memory. In the very late stages of the disease, the person is incapable of any task, may be doubly incontinent, may have lost the power of speech, suffer from some paralysis and have total loss of memory. If symptoms are noticed, medical help should be sought.

Treatment: there is no cure or medication to halt the progress of the disease. In the early stages, as much mental activity as possible should be encouraged and carried out. Support and help is needed for the family of a person with Alzheimer's disease. It is usually desirable for the person to be placed in a nursing home in the later stages of the disease when home care becomes too difficult.

Causes and risk factors: the cause is not known but is the subject of ongoing, intensive research. Some researchers believe that there is a connection with the deposition of aluminium in brain cells. It is advisable to avoid cooking acidic fruits in aluminium pans to avoid contamination with aluminium.

anaemia

Description: a decrease in the ability of the blood to carry oxygen because of a reduction in the number of red blood cells and/or the amount of haemoglobin that they contain. Haemoglobin is the pigment within the red blood cells that binds to oxygen. There are a number of different kinds of anaemia, which may be usefully grouped into four main types:

1. microcytic hypochromic anaemia;
2. megaloblastic hyperchromic anaemia (*see* PERNICIOUS ANAEMIA);
3. aplastic anaemia;
4. haemolytic anaemia.

In Britain, the great majority of cases of anaemia (90%) belong to the first group, about 7% to the second group, with the remaining 3% being of the aplastic or haemolytic type.

Persons most commonly affected: all age groups and both sexes but more common in females than in males.

Organ or part of body involved: blood, bone marrow.

Symptoms and indications: the symptoms of anaemia depend to a certain extent on the cause but more especially whether the onset is sudden or gradual. If it is sudden, as in the case of serious haemorrhage, the patient becomes weak and dizzy, may be unable to stand and may lose consciousness. Blood pressure drops, the breathing is fast and laboured, and there is a rapid pulse. In all cases of anaemia, the skin is pale and there is an absence of (or poor) colour inside the inner lower eyelid, if this is gently pulled down. The nails may be concave and brittle, the voice may be husky, and the tongue may be inflamed (glossitis) with accompanying difficulty in swallowing. The person often feels tired and generally weak, and not as well as usual. However, because the changes are sometimes gradual, the person may adapt and not be aware of them until the anaemia has become quite severe. If a person shows signs of anaemia, medical advice should be sought.

Treatment: this depends on the type of anaemia and the cause, but the aim of all treatment is to restore and maintain haemoglobin at normal levels in the blood. A person with serious haemorrhaging will require emergency medical treatment in hospital to stop the bleeding. Hospital treatment may also be required for patients with other forms of anaemia. In severe cases blood transfusions may be needed, but usually iron preparations (in the form of ferrous sulphate) are required until haemoglobin levels and red blood cell counts are normal.

Causes and risk factors: anaemia is caused by a fall in the number of red blood cells and haemoglobin in the blood, so that the oxygen-carrying capacity is reduced. As outlined above, the reasons for this are varied and depend on the type of anaemia. Causes include bleeding caused by injury or illness, menstruation, childbirth, haemophilia, gastrointestinal bleeding, haemorrhoids or piles, iron deficiency in the diet, or malabsorption of iron in the intestine because of disease. Also, some infections, toxins (especially those produced in certain kidney diseases), drugs (anticancer and immunosuppressives, non-steroidal anti-inflammatory drugs, aspirin and chloramphenicol), and chemicals of the benzene type, are causes of anaemia.

anal fissure

Description: an abnormal break or tear in the skin and lining tissue surrounding the anus.

Persons most commonly affected: all age groups and both sexes, but it most often occurs in young children and infants and elderly people aged over 60 years. Also, more common in females than in males.

Organ or part of body involved: anus.

Symptoms and indications: sharp, stabbing pain and bleeding on passing stool with the pain possibly persisting for some time and then subsiding. A person with symptoms of anal fissure should seek medical advice.

Treatment: treatment involves the taking of certain preparations that soften the stool or act as laxatives, and the use of lubricating suppositories to ease stretching and protect the anal tissues. Healing usually occurs naturally after a certain period of time, but occasionally hospital treatment and surgery may be needed. Warm sitz baths (containing salt solution or plain water) are helpful in easing pain.

Causes and risk factors: the cause is thought to be overstretching of the anus from the passage of a hard, large stool, usually caused by constipation. To prevent constipation, plenty of fluids should be drunk and the diet should be high in fibre. An active lifestyle also helps to prevent constipation.

anaphylactic shock

Description: anaphylaxis is a response exhibited by a hypersensitive (highly sensitive) person when confronted with a particular substance or antigen. It results from the release of histamine in body tissues following the antigen-antibody reaction within cells. An allergic reaction is an example of mild anaphylaxis (*see* ALLERGY). Anaphylactic shock is a much rarer and more serious condition that can follow the injection of drugs or vaccines, or a bee sting, to which the person is hypersensitive. Its onset is immediate and results from a widespread release of histamine in the body.

Persons most commonly affected: all age groups and both sexes.

Organ or part of body involved: respiratory and circulatory system, skin and heart.

Symptoms and indications: the symptoms appear rapidly in the form of severe breathing difficulties, swelling (oedema), acute itching and rash (urticaria), a fall in blood pressure leading to fainting, and loss of consciousness. Heart failure leading to shock, cardiac arrest and death. Anaphylactic shock is a medical emergency and requires immediate prompt treatment.

Treatment: the only effective treatment is an intramuscular injection of adrenaline (epinephrine) that should be given as soon as possible. A person receiving prompt treatment usually makes a full recovery.

Causes and risk factors: there are a variety of causes for this condition, including vaccines, drugs and medications, especially if injected, wasp or bee stings and insect bites, and some foods such as peanuts, beans, shellfish, eggs and certain types of fruit. A person with a history of allergy in the form of ECZEMA, ASTHMA or HAY FEVER, or who has had a previous mild reaction to a particular substance, is likely to be at greater risk.

ancyclostomiasis or hookworm disease

Description: a disease caused by infestation with a parasitic nematode worm of which there are two kinds. *Ancyclostoma duodenale*, also called the tunnel worm, occurs mainly in the Mediterranean and the Middle and Far East, while *Necator americanus* is found in the Far East, many parts of Africa and South and Central America. However, because of increasing international travel, cases of hookworm may occur elsewhere.

Persons most commonly affected: all age groups and both sexes.

Organ or part of body involved: intestine via bloodstream and lungs.

Symptoms and indications: gastrointestinal upset, pain in abdomen, diarrhoea, intestinal bleeding causing anaemia, fatigue and general malaise. A person with symptoms of hookworm infestation should seek medical advice.

Treatment: various drugs are effective against hookworm, including mebendazole, kephenium hydroxynaphthoate, and pyrantel embonate. The accompanying anaemia also requires appropriate treatment, and the person may need to rest until fully recovered.

Causes and risk factors: hookworm larvae inhabit the soil and infect people by burrowing through the skin of the feet. Alternatively, they may gain direct access to the gastrointestinal system through the drinking of contaminated water. They enter the bloodstream and travel to the lungs and thence to the intestine via the windpipe and oesophagus. Once in the intestine, the worms mature and burrow into the wall, causing damage and bleeding with the symptoms outlined above. They are a cause of death among poor people suffering from malnutrition, who live in overcrowded and insanitary conditions. Care should be exercised in a country where hookworm is prevalent, with regard to eating, drinking and personal hygiene.

aneurysm

Description: a balloon-like swelling of the wall of an artery that occurs when it becomes weakened or damaged in some way.

Persons most commonly affected: adult persons of both sexes, especially in older age.

Organ or part of body involved: arteries in any part but especially in the brain (circle of Willis), aorta or leg arteries.

Symptoms and indications: these vary a great deal depending on the site and size of the aneurysm. Pain may be present if the aneurysm compresses nerves, and also bulging, which may throb and contract and expand. A thoracic aneurysm may press on the windpipe and cause a hoarseness of the voice and a cough. A brain aneurysm may cause a throbbing headache and changes in the eyes (pupils of different sizes) or disturbances of vision. If the aneurysm affects the heart there may be disturbances of heartbeat rhythm and other symptoms of cardiac failure. Oedema also occurs, causing swelling of the skin because of interference with the circulation. An aneurysm is a medical emergency, and the doctor should be called immediately.

Treatment: hospital treatment and surgery to remove or isolate the aneurysm and restore the circulation by means of a graft or anastomosis (artificial joining of sections of the arteries involved). Anticoagulant drugs may be needed after surgery and penicillin if the aneurysm was caused by SYPHILIS.

Causes and risk factors: aneurysms occur because of a weakness in the walls of the arteries, which is usually caused by atheroma or ATHEROSCLEROSIS (a degenerative disease of the arterial walls with scarring and a build-up of fatty deposits). Syphilis is another cause, especially affecting the aorta in the thorax. More rarely, there may be a congenital weakness affecting the arteries, especially in the case of aneurysms in the circle of Willis (a circle of arteries supplying, and sited beneath, the brain). The danger with aneurysm is that of rupture causing haemorrhage and death, and also the risk of stroke. Some changes in the arteries tend to occur naturally in older people. Atheroma or atherosclerosis is more likely to be a problem in people eating a diet rich in saturated fat. Smoking, obesity, high blood pressure and a sedentary lifestyle are additional contributory factors.

angina pectoris

Description: a pain and feeling of choking felt in the chest, brought on by exercise or exertion and relieved by rest. It occurs when the blood supply to the heart muscle is inadequate.

Persons most commonly affected: more common in men in middle and older age; postmenopausal women.

Organ or part of body involved: coronary arteries.

Symptoms and indications: the main symptom is pain behind the breastbone, brought on by exertion and relieved by rest. The pain may be more or less severe and often passes to the left arm and face. There may be a numbness or feeling of heaviness and tingling in the whole or part of the left arm. Also, there may be a feeling of choking and breathlessness and tightness across the chest. A person with symptoms of angina should always seek medical advice.

Treatment: diagnosis is usually confirmed in hospital by means of an electrocardiogram. Treatment involves rest and avoidance of the exertion that caused the angina attack. The patient needs to keep warm, especially in severe winter weather, and may need to adjust the diet and lose weight. Changes in lifestyle may be necessary to avoid tiredness and stress. Medication in the form of glyceryl trinitrate tablets (or amyl nitrite for inhalation) are used to bring immediate relief during an angina attack. It may be necessary for the patient to undergo coronary-artery bypass surgery or angioplasty.

Causes and risk factors: angina pectoris is caused by an inadequate blood supply to the heart muscle. During exercise, the demand for blood supplied by the coronary arteries is increased and if the supply is insufficient because the arteries are damaged, chest pain results. The most common reason for this damage is atherosclerosis or atheroma, along with spasm of the coronary arteries. Less commonly, aortic valve disease or disease in the aorta itself may be a cause of angina pectoris. Factors thought to contribute to the development of this condition include inadequate exercise, a diet rich in saturated fats and salt, high blood pressure, stress, obesity, smoking and diabetes mellitus. Also, genetic factors, i.e. a family history of coronary-artery disease.

ankylosing spondylitis

Description: a progressive, inflammatory rheumatic disease affecting the spine and hip joints, characterized by stiffening and pain.

Persons most commonly affected: young males, the condition usually beginning between the ages of 10 and 40. It is rare in females.

Organ or part of body involved: sacroiliac region, hips and spine, sometimes affecting joints in the hand, arm and shoulder.

Symptoms and indications: in the early stages there is lower back pain in the lumbar region and stiffness, especially on rising in the morning. Later the disease progresses to involve the whole spine, and fibrous tissue replaces and fuses spinal discs and ligaments. Eventually, the whole spine may become rigid, and the patient's body may be bent forward. This is called a 'bamboo' or 'poker' spine. A person with back pain should seek medical advice.

Treatment: this involves taking non-steroidal anti-inflammatory drugs and physiotherapy, with special exercises designed to maintain the flexibility of the spine. At the present time there is no known cure, and the disease progresses slowly over a number of years. However, symptoms can be alleviated, and it is desirable for an affected person to stay as active as possible. Activities that may stress the back should be avoided, but exercise, especially swimming, is helpful. There is a possibility of other conditions developing in a patient with ankylosing spondylitis.

Causes and risk factors: the cause is unknown, but there is a genetic link and a tendency for the condition to run in families.

aortic valve disease

Description: disease of the aortic valve of the heart, which occurs in two forms—either a narrowing (stenosis) or a widening and scarring causing leaking (incompetence) of the valve. As a result, the left ventricle has to work harder in order to maintain the blood flow into the aorta and become thicker (hypertrophy). In the case of a leaking aortic valve, there is a backflow of blood into the ventricle, causing dilation.

Persons most commonly affected: both sexes and all age groups but more common in older people.

Organ or part of body involved: heart.

Symptoms and indications: these vary in severity according to the extent of damage to the valve. They commonly include breathlessness, ANGINA PECTORIS, dizziness and fainting, and heart murmur. A person with symptoms of heart disease should always seek medical attention.

Treatment: the usual form of treatment in severe cases is surgical, in the form of an operation to replace the defective valve. Also, drugs of various kinds are likely to be required, depending on the nature of the disease. These may include anti-arrhythmic drugs, antibiotics and other heart drugs. A change to a low-salt and low-fat diet may be advised.

Causes and risk factors: in the case of aortic stenosis, the usual cause is a degeneration and calcification that occurs with advancing age. However, the other causes include RHEUMATIC FEVER and a congenital, inherited defect in which the valve has two cusps instead of the normal three. Both of these cause scarring, calcification

and narrowing. The causes of a leaking aortic valve include those listed above but, in addition, syphilis, inflammation (endocarditis) of the heart and aortic ANEURYSM. Also, HYPERTENSION (high blood pressure) and an inherited disease of connective tissue called Marfan's syndrome. A person who has had rheumatic fever in childhood is more likely to be at risk of heart valve disease in later life.

appendicitis (acute)

Description: the vermiform appendix is a blind-ended tube, about 9 or 1 cm long, projecting from the caecum (a pouch), which is the first part of the large intestine. Appendicitis is inflammation of the vermiform appendix, which, in its acute form, is the most common abdominal emergency in the western world.

Persons most commonly affected: all age groups and both sexes, but it is rare in young children under the age of two. It is most common in young people up to the age of 25.

Organ or part of body involved: vermiform appendix.

Symptoms and indications: the symptoms include abdominal pain that often begins over the umbilicus and then moves to the right ileac fossa. The pain is severe and worse with movement e.g. coughing or deep breathing, etc. Also, there may be nausea and vomiting, diarrhoea, loss of appetite and fever. Eventually, there is abdominal swelling and tenderness. A person with symptoms of appendicitis should seek immediate medical attention, as it is an emergency condition.

Treatment: usually appendicitis occurs in the acute form, requiring hospital treatment or appendicectomy—the surgical removal of the appendix. The condition is normally completely cured with prompt surgery but is dangerous if left untreated.

Causes and risk factors: blockage and subsequent infection of the appendix are the causes of appendicitis, which can occur at any time. Danger arises if the condition is left untreated or misdiagnosed. In this instance, the appendix may become the site of an abscess or may become gangrenous and rupture, causing PERITONITIS. This arises because infected material from the burst appendix spreads into the peritoneal cavity, and it is often fatal. Rupture of the appendix is more likely to occur in older patients.

asbestosis

Description: a disease of the lungs that is a form of

PNEUMOCONIOSIS, caused by the inhalation of asbestos dust.

Persons most commonly affected: men in middle or older age who have been exposed to asbestos dust over a number of years.

Organ or part of body involved: lungs.

Symptoms and indications: the early stages of the disease produce symptoms that include breathlessness, tiredness and persistent cough. Later, the person may suffer from severe breathing difficulties, cough up blood, experience disturbance of sleep and pain in the chest, and develop congestive heart failure. There is a serious risk of the development of MESOTHELIOMA or LUNG CANCER, which also produce these symptoms. A person with these symptoms should seek medical advice. The condition is not curable, but various drug treatments can help to alleviate the symptoms. These include bronchodilators, analgesics and antibiotics for infections. Also, bronchial drainage may be needed to remove excess fluid and the use of a humidifier to ease breathing.

Causes and risk factors: asbestos has been used in many industries in the past, although less widely today since the risks have been known. Anyone working with asbestos should keep to strict health and safety procedures, including the wearing of protective clothing and measures to suppress the dust. The particles of asbestos dust cause scarring of the lungs and risks of disease or cancer are greatly increased by smoking.

asphyxia

Description: this translates literally as an absence of pulse but is used in a wider sense to describe the state of suffocation. During the course of this, breathing and heartbeat cease and oxygen fails to reach the tissues and organs. Brain cells are irreparably damaged if deprived of oxygen for more than about four minutes.

Persons most commonly affected: all age groups and both sexes.

Organ or part of body involved: lungs, heart, respiratory and circulatory systems.

Symptoms and indications: in most cases, the person fights and gasps for breath, has a rapid pulse rate, throbbing in the head as blood pressure rises and blueness of the skin. Eventually, there may be convulsions, followed by a state of paralysis, unconsciousness and death. However, in some instances, where the inhalation of toxic fumes such as carbon monoxide is responsible for the asphyxia, death may occur peacefully, without the struggles described above and during sleep. A person suffering from asphyxia requires urgent, prompt treatment if death is to be avoided.

Treatment: this depends on the cause of the asphyxia in the first instance. If the cause is choking because of a piece of food, or other foreign body, becoming lodged in the windpipe, this must be removed. A young child can be held upside down by the legs and struck firmly on the back, as this results in the object being dislodged more easily. In adults, blows on the back over the shoulder blades in time with coughing may help the object to be expelled. However, it may be necessary to perform the Heimlich's manoeuvre. The person carrying out the procedure encircles the patient from behind with his or her arms. A fist is made with one hand slightly above the patient's navel and below the ribs. With the free hand, the fist is thrust firmly into the abdomen with a rapid, upward push, which may need to be repeated several times. As a result of this, the foreign body is expelled through or into the patient's mouth. In the situation outlined above, the patient usually recovers rapidly and resumes normal breathing. If toxic fumes are the cause of asphyxia, the person must be removed into clean air (*see* CARBON MONOXIDE POISONING). In all cases of asphyxia, the essential aim of treatment is to increase the amount of oxygen in the blood. If respiration and heartbeat have stopped, emergency resuscitation methods (mouth-to-mouth breathing and external cardiac massage) must be used. Once respiration and heartbeat have started (or if still present), the person requires further intensive care treatment in hospital.

Causes and risk factors: as indicated above, there are a number of different causes of asphyxia, including drowning, strangulation, choking and inhalation of toxic fumes. Also, swelling leading to obstruction of breathing and asphyxia may occur in certain diseases and conditions, including DIPHTHERIA, ASTHMA, CROUP and infection of a wound.

asthma

Description: a chronic, hypersensitive condition characterized by recurrent bouts of illness or asthma attacks. The affected person has breathing difficulties caused by a narrowing of the airways (the bronchi and bronchioles) leading to the lungs.

Persons most commonly affected: all age groups except newborn babies, often beginning in early childhood. In childhood, more boys than girls suffer from asthma but in adult life both sexes are affected equally.

Organ or part of body involved: airways (bronchi and bronchioles) and lungs.

Symptoms and indications: the main symptoms are breathlessness and a wheezing cough that may be worse at night. The extent to which the bronchi are narrowed varies considerably and governs the severity of the attack. In a severe attack, the breathing rate increases considerably and is rapid and shallow. The pulse rate also increases. In a very severe attack, the person may be so breathless as to make speech impossible and may show signs of cyanosis, i.e. a bluish colour of the skin because of a lack of oxygen in the blood. A severe asthma attack or one that does not respond to the usual controlling medication taken by the patient is an emergency condition and medical help should be sought immediately. Prolonged and repeated attacks of asthma, with no break in between, are called *status asthmaticus*. This also is a serious emergency that can cause death due to exhaustion and respiratory failure.

Treatment: the day-to-day treatment of asthma is one of management to avoid the occurrence of an attack. This includes avoidance of the particular substance or allergen that triggers the asthma, if this is known and if it is possible to do so. Drugs used in the treatment of asthma are of two kinds. Bronchodilators are used to dilate the airways, and these include beta-adrenergic agonists such as salbutamol and anticholinergics such as theophyllines. The second group are anti-inflammatory drugs, which are inhaled corticosteroids and sodium cromoglycate. Most of the drugs used in the management of asthma are inhaled. Patients with severe asthma attacks or status asthmaticus require immediate admittance to hospital and treatment in intensive care.

Causes and risk factors: the cause of asthma is swelling and inflammation of the walls of the airways, and contraction of the muscles, so that the openings are narrowed. This is triggered by a hypersensitive response to a number of different allergens. Common allergens include pollen, dust from mites, domestic pets, birds and farm animals and airborne pollutants from, e.g. car exhaust emissions. An asthma sufferer may have other hypersensitive conditions such as ECZEMA or HAY FEVER, and there may be a genetic element with prevalence within a family. Exercise and stress may also trigger an asthma attack, and the condition is exacerbated by exposure to tobacco smoke.

atherosclerosis and atheroma

Description: a degenerative disease of the arteries in which the inner and middle coats of the arterial walls become scarred and fatty deposits (cholesterol) are built up at these sites. The channel or lumen of the artery becomes progressively narrowed so that the blood circulation is impaired and may become completely blocked.

Persons most commonly affected: adults in middle and older age groups. Less common in women before the menopause than in men in the same age range. However, older (postmenopausal) women experience the same rates of disease as men.

Organ or part of body involved: arteries in any part of the body.

Symptoms and indications: the condition is often well advanced before any symptoms are noticed, and these depend on the arteries involved. If leg arteries are affected, there may be pains and cramps in the legs. If it is the coronary arteries the symptoms could be of ANGINA PECTORIS or CORONARY THROMBOSIS. If the disease involves the arteries in the brain, the person may suffer a STROKE. A person with symptoms of atherosclerosis or atheroma should seek immediate medical help.

Treatment: treatment is aimed at prevention as there is at present no cure for this condition. These measures include eating a low-fat diet that does not contain too much cholesterol or salt, not smoking, taking regular exercise, losing weight if obese and trying to avoid stress. Also, persons suffering from HYPERTENSION or DIABETES MELLITUS should keep strictly to their prescribed treatment. The serious complications that can arise as a result of atherosclerosis obviously require immediate treatment and are described elsewhere.

Causes and factors: the cause of atherosclerosis or atheroma is a build-up of fatty deposits on the inner walls of the arteries leading to reduced blood flow or blockage. The reasons why this occurs are not entirely clear, but there is an association with the western lifestyle, i.e. lack of exercise, smoking, obesity and too high an intake of animal fats. Older persons and those with high blood pressure or diabetes mellitus are also more at risk.

athlete's foot

Description: a fungal infection of the skin of the foot, particularly occurring between the toes and often due to ringworm.

Persons most commonly affected: older children and adults of both sexes and all age groups.

Organ or part of body involved: foot.

Symptoms and indications: the appearance of damp,

white or greyish-coloured skin, red patches and dead skin on the soles of the feet and between the toes.

Treatment: involves paying special attention to hygiene, especially washing and drying the feet thoroughly at least once a day or more frequently if they become sweaty. An antifungal cream, ointment or dusting powder, which may be prescribed by a doctor but can also be bought over the counter, should be applied to affected skin. Socks should be of cotton or other natural fibres, and shoes worn that allow air to circulate as much as possible (ideally, sandals). The condition usually clears up in two or three weeks but may recur.

Causes and risk factors: the cause is a species of fungus (*see also* RINGWORM).

atrial fibrillation

Description: a serious form of arrhythmia affecting the atria (upper chambers) of the heart.

Persons most commonly affected: adults of both sexes in middle and older age, usually with some form of heart disease or damage.

Organ or part of body involved: heart.

Symptoms and indications: irregular, rapid heartbeat and pulse, which are felt as unpleasant palpitations and may cause chest pain, breathlessness, faintness and weakness. There may be symptoms of STROKE because of the formation of blood clots in the heart. In severe cases, this may lead to heart failure and death. Immediate medical help should be sought if a person has these symptoms.

Treatment: emergency medical treatment and intensive care in hospital will be required. This involves attempting to restore a normal heartbeat by means of electric shock and drug treatment. The drugs that may be used include digoxin, betablockers and calcium antagonists. Surgery and the fitting of a pacemaker is sometimes (but rarely) required. Underlying heart disease, responsible for the atrial fibrillation, is also treated, although this is rarely sufficient to restore the normal heartbeat on its own. An exception is if the cause is hyperthyroidism. Later, the patient may be prescribed blood-thinning drugs such as warfarin.

Causes and risk factors: in atrial fibrillation, the output of the heart is maintained by the contraction of the ventricles (the lower, larger chambers) alone. It can arise spontaneously in persons with no apparent heart disease, but often an underlying disorder is present. These diseases include CORONARY ARTERY DISEASE, rheumatic heart disease, ATHEROSCLEROSIS, high blood pressure (HYPERTENSION) and overactive thyroid gland (hyperthyroidism). There is a risk of CORONARY THROMBOSIS because of the formation of blood clots in the heart.

B

Bell's palsy

Description: a sudden paralysis of the facial muscles, usually on one side of the face but sometimes on both.

Persons most commonly affected: usually adults of both sexes and all age groups.

Organ or part of body involved: seventh cranial nerve—the facial nerve.

Symptoms and indications: paralysis on one or both sides of the face, resulting in an inability to move the eyelids and close or open the eyes, smile or close the mouth. The features on the affected side are flat and lacking expression. There may be pain, especially behind the ear, prior to the development of the paralysis. Some people experience loss of the sense of taste, and sounds may seem too loud if hearing is affected. A person affected by symptoms of Bell's palsy should seek medical advice so that the cause of the nerve disorder can be determined.

Treatment: recovery depends on the nature of the damage to the facial nerve, may or may not be complete and may take some time. Treatment includes the use of heat (lamps or compresses) if there is pain and facial massage and exercises for the affected muscles once recovery is under way. While the person is unable to blink, the eyes require additional protection to avoid trauma and injury. This usually involves the wearing of an eye patch or goggles and the use of drops containing methylcellulose. Oral corticosteroid drugs may be prescribed, and in severe cases, which do not recover after six to twelve months, surgery may be performed to improve the function of the facial muscles.

Causes and risk factors: the cause is thought to be inflammation of the facial nerve because of injury or infection or possibly a disorder of the immune system (an autoimmune disease).

bladder stones or calculi (*singular* calculus)

Description: stones occurring in the urinary bladder, which may be of three different types: phosphatic, the most common type, associated with recurrent inflammation and decomposition of the urine contained in the bladder; uratic (particularly in persons suffering from gout); and oxalic. The stones are usually quite small but are too large to be passed with the urine. However, they may occasionally be of considerable size and weight.

Persons most commonly affected: adults of all age groups and both sexes.

Organ or part of body involved: urinary bladder.

Symptoms and indications: the symptoms are those of inflammation of the bladder, including pain on passing urine, feeling the need to urinate frequently although little or nothing is passed, and blood in the urine, or the urine may be cloudy and the person may experience abdominal pain or discomfort and feverishness. A person with symptoms of bladder inflammation should seek medical advice.

Treatment: prompt treatment of any bladder infection that arises, drinking plenty of fluids and adjustment in diet are measures that help to prevent the formation of stones in susceptible people. However, once the stones are formed, and if they are too large to be passed with the urine, the only treatment available is surgical removal. This may be performed in two ways. Lithoplaxy involves passing an instrument (lithotrite) into the bladder via the urethra, which breaks up the stones into small pieces that can pass to the outside. Lithotomy is the name given to direct removal of stones through an incision made in the bladder and is the method needed for larger stones. If infection has been present, antibiotics may be prescribed and possibly drugs to alter the acidity of the urine.

Causes and risk factors: stones grow for a variety of reasons but mainly because of the presence in the urine of an excess of salts or minerals from which they are formed. This may occur because of a number of causes and disorders, including bladder infections, gout and thyroid disorders. Also, excess consumption of certain foods containing the minerals from which stones are formed in susceptible people and some hereditary conditions. Other risk factors include illness or injury to the bladder, and dehydration and inadequate drinking of fluids.

bladder tumour (cancer)

Description: an abnormal growth of cells and tissue in the bladder that is often malignant or cancerous.

Persons most commonly affected: adults of all age groups and both sexes but more common in males and people in middle or older age.

Organ or part of body involved: bladder.

Symptoms and indications: the early signs are those of bladder infection, including pain or burning sensation on passing urine, feeling the urge to urinate frequently but passing little or no urine, blood in the urine. Also, pain in the region of the bladder and eventual weight loss. A person with signs of bladder disorder or infection should seek immediate medical advice.

Treatment: the course of treatment depends upon the nature of the cancer, i.e. whether it is superficial or has invaded deeply into the muscular wall of the bladder. Treatments include radiation therapy and the use of radioactive isotopes, chemotherapy, including the placing of certain drugs into the bladder, and surgery. Also, photoradiation using a light-sensitive dye that releases chemicals that kill the cancer cells is used in some patients with a particular form of superficial malignancy. Preventative measures are directed towards certain industries whose workers are known to be more at risk. This involves following strict health and safety procedures and regular screening of the workforce.

Causes and risk factors: the precise cause remains unclear, but this is regarded as an occupational cancer, with workers in some industries being particularly at risk. These are the chemical and rubber industries, laboratory workers, pest control operators and engineering industries using lubricant oils. The chemicals involved include benzidine, and alpha and beta naphthylamine, and persons exposed to these must follow strict guidelines. Also, people who smoke are more at risk, and there may be a greater risk for those with a family history of the disease.

blepharitis

Description: inflammation of the outer edges of the eyelids.

Persons most commonly affected: adults of all age groups and both sexes.

Organ or part of body involved: eyelids and sometimes the cornea and conjunctiva of the eye.

Symptoms and indications: symptoms include reddening of the eyelids with the appearance of scales caught in the eyelashes. Ulcers may form on the edges of the eyelid and yellowish crusts form on top of these. The lashes become matted and project in various directions, or they may fall out. The conjunctiva and cornea may become reddened and inflamed. A person with symptoms of eye inflammation should seek medical attention.

Treatment: blepharitis is a stubborn condition that is somewhat resistant to treatment but usually clears in time, although it may recur. Treatment involves cleaning the eyes, bathing them with warm water containing sodium bicarbonate and removing the scales. Also, antibiotic eyedrops and solutions of artificial tears may be prescribed by the doctor.

Causes and risk factors: the cause is dry eyes because of lessened tear secretion, along with seborrhoeic dermatitis and infection by staphylococcal bacteria. The risk of developing blepharitis is greater in poor or overcrowded living conditions and possibly in older persons subject to dry eyes.

blood poisoning or septicaemia

Description: a serious and potentially life-threatening condition characterized by the presence of pathogenic microorganisms (especially bacteria) in the blood.

Persons most commonly affected: all age groups and both sexes.

Organ or part of body involved: blood circulation and all body systems.

Symptoms and indications: a temperature that rises rapidly to a high level along with shivering chills, flushing, copious sweating, pains and aches, and a fall in blood pressure. The person feels generally unwell and requires prompt medical attention as there is a risk of shock and death. This is especially the case in a vulnerable person who has an existing illness.

Treatment: involves admittance to hospital and antibiotic therapy. Antibiotics may be required in large amounts until the condition is brought under control. If blood poisoning has arisen as a result of infection in some other organ or part of the body (e.g. the gall bladder), surgery may be necessary to treat this.

Causes and risk factors: blood poisoning may result from infection in a wound or operation site or a tooth abscess. Also as a result of an infection in the gall bladder, appendix, burns or abscesses.

Elderly persons and babies are more at risk, and people with lessened immunity, e.g. those suffering from cancer. Preventative measures include seeking prompt medical attention for infections, wounds and injuries, and having regular dental check-ups and treatment.

boil or furuncle

Description: a skin infection in a hair follicle or gland that produces inflammation and pus. A group of boils that are deeper and more spread are called a carbuncle.

Persons most commonly affected: all age groups and both sexes.

Organ or part of body involved: the skin and its hair follicles and glands.

Symptoms and indications: a painful red swelling or lump, which usually comes up quite quickly and may be fairly large. Also, there is swelling of lymph glands close to the site of the boil and the person may be feverish. The boil usually 'comes to a head' itself and bursts within several days but should be treated by a doctor before this occurs.

Treatment: usually the boil needs to be surgically lanced and the pus drained out. As this is performed by a doctor under clean, aseptic conditions, there is much less likelihood of the pus (which is infective) causing another boil to occur in an adjacent area of skin. Also the boil heals more quickly than if left untreated. Antibiotics may be prescribed to fight the infection that caused the boil.

Causes and risk factors: a boil is caused by a bacterial infection at the base of a hair and the organism involved is usually staphylococcus aureus, or the organism may enter through a small cut or nick in the skin. Occasionally, a boil may cause a more widespread infection, especially in people who are somewhat 'run-down' or with lowered immunity because of illness. Frequent recurrence of boils usually requires further medical investigation to ensure that the patient is not suffering from DIABETES MELLITUS.

bone fracture

Description: any break in a bone, which may be complete or incomplete. There are many different forms of fracture, and these are listed below:

Simple fracture (or closed fracture). In this type, the skin remains more or less intact.

Compound fracture (or open fracture). An open wound connects the bone with the surface. This type of fracture is more serious as it provides a greater risk of infection and more blood loss.

Pathological fracture. A fracture in a diseased bone, which often occurs in people, especially women, with OSTEOPOROSIS.

Stress fracture. Occurs in a bone that suffers recurrent, persistent stress e.g. the march fracture sometimes seen in the second toe of soldiers after long marches.

Greenstick fracture. This occurs only in young children, whose bones are still soft and tend to bend. The fracture occurs on the opposite side to the causal force.

Complicated fracture. This involves damage to surrounding soft tissue including nerves and blood vessels.

Depressed fracture. This refers only to the skull when a piece of bone is forced inwards and may damage the brain.

Comminuted fracture. A serious injury to a bone in which more than one break occurs, accompanied by splintering and damage to the surrounding tissues. It usually results from a crushing force with damage to nerves, muscles and blood vessels, and the bone is difficult to set.

Persons most commonly affected: all age groups and both sexes.

Organ or part of body involved: bones.

Symptoms and indications: symptoms include pain, bruising, swelling and bleeding. Also, if nerves are damaged there may be numbness or even paralysis below the level of the injury. If a limb is fractured there is severe pain on movement and an inability to perform normal activities, and the affected limb may appear deformed or rotated. Occasionally there may be a loss of pulse below the fracture site, particularly in the region of the hands and wrists or feet and ankles. Immediate and often emergency medical attention is needed if a person has a fracture or suspected fracture.

Treatment: involves admittance to hospital where X-rays (radiography) are taken to determine the nature and extent of the injury. Surgery is often necessary to repair or set a fracture and the bone or body part is usually immobilized, generally by means of a plaster cast and splints. Sometimes traction is needed, which involves the use of weights and pulleys to apply a pulling force. This ensures that the bone is kept in correct alignment while healing takes place. Once recovery is well under way, physiotherapy is often needed to restore movement.

Causes and risk factors: with more serious and complex fractures particularly, healing may take a long time or be only partial. Also, there may be shock and death because of haemorrhage if the injury is severe. There may be damage or obstruction of arteries causing problems in blood circulation or EMBOLISM. Fractures are caused by trauma to the bone through accident or injury or repeated stress.

botulism

Description: the most dangerous type of food poisoning, caused by the anaerobic (living without oxygen) bacterium *Clostridium botulinum.*

Persons most commonly affected: all age groups and both sexes but less common in children.

Organ or part of body involved: central nervous system and muscles.

Symptoms and indications: symptoms may appear within a few hours of eating food contaminated by the bacteria and/or their toxin. These include a dry mouth, blurred vision, constipation, retention of urine and dilation of the pupils of the eye. This leads on to muscle weakness and paralysis and may be fatal. Death results from paralysis of the muscles involved in respiration. If botulism is suspected, emergency medical help should be summoned immediately.

Treatment: requires admittance to hospital for intensive care nursing, which may involve the need for a ventilator. Also, drugs that counter the effects of the bacterial toxin are given.

Causes and risk factors: the bacteria that cause botulism grow in tinned foods that have not been properly preserved, especially canned raw meats, fish, vegetables or fruit. Very rarely, infection may occur via an open wound or cut. During its growth the bacteria produce a toxin, one component of which attacks the nervous system and produces the symptoms. The toxin is destroyed by heat so it is a problem only in foods that have not been thoroughly cooked. The toxin has a very small lethal dose, hence it is a wise precaution never to taste suspect food but to discard it immediately.

brain abscess or epidural abscess

Description: a bacterial infection in the brain resulting in an accumulation of pus.

Persons most commonly affected: all age groups and both sexes.

Organ or part of body involved: brain and meninges (membranes) that cover the brain and spinal cord.

Symptoms and indications: early indications may be vague, but eventually the person develops a severe headache, nausea and vomiting, feverishness and often a disturbance of vision.

This is a very serious condition, and a person with these symptoms requires emergency medical treatment.

Treatment: involves admittance to hospital and, usually, surgery to drain the abscess. Antibiotics may be needed to combat infection.

Causes and risk factors: common causes of a brain abscess include injury or wounds on the scalp, an infection that spreads to the brain e.g. from a discharging ear or sinus infection. Also, infection may spread via the blood circulation to the brain, from another infected organ elsewhere in the body. It is wise where possible to prevent the occurrence of a brain abscess. This means that scalp injuries, ear infections, etc., should always be taken seriously and treated properly by a doctor.

brain compression

Description: pressure or squeezing of the brain within the limited space of the skull, due to some form of trauma or injury.

Persons most commonly affected: all age groups and both sexes.

Organ or part of body involved: brain.

Symptoms and indications: symptoms include drowsiness, breathing difficulties, weak pulse, paralysis in one side of the body and unconsciousness. Emergency medical treatment is needed if a person shows signs of brain compression.

Treatment: involves admittance to hospital and a surgical operation (trepanning or trephining of the skull—removal of an area of bone) so that the cause of the compression can be dealt with.

Causes and risk factors: there are various reasons why compression of the brain occurs. These include injury and rupture of a blood vessel producing a clot, tumour and a collection of pus or blood from an infection. As with brain abscess, preventative measures include seeking prompt medical attention for any injury, wound or trauma involving the head and skull.

brain tumour

Description: a growth of abnormal cells in the brain, which may be malignant or nonmalignant and may be fatal. Because of its location, a nonmalignant brain tumour can cause very serious symptoms.

Persons most commonly affected: all age groups and both sexes but more common in adults.

Organ or part of body involved: brain.

Symptoms and indications: symptoms are variable,

depending on the precise location of the tumour in the brain, and may be slow in onset. They include headache, vomiting, nausea, dizziness, poor coordination, disturbance of vision, weakness affecting one side of the body, mental changes and fits. Sometimes a tumour in a particular site may cause a more definite set of symptoms, leading to its presence being suspected. A person with any symptoms of brain disorder should seek medical advice.

Treatment: depends upon the nature and precise site of the tumour. There are a range of treatments, including surgery, radiotherapy and the use of radioisotopes and chemotherapy. Continuing advances in medicine and surgery mean that more brain tumours can now be treated than was possible in the past.

Causes and risk factors: a brain tumour may arise as a secondary growth, resulting from a malignancy elsewhere in the body, or be a primary tumour. A brain tumour can be a result of TUBERCULOSIS or SYPHILIS and these diseases must obviously be treated if present. Preventative measures are primarily avoidance of the known risk factors associated with cancer. The most significant of these is avoidance of smoking.

breast abscess

Description: acute inflammation and infection with a collection of pus within the breast tissue.

Persons most commonly affected: women in the child bearing age group who have recently given birth.

Organ or part of body involved: breast.

Symptoms and indications: redness, heat, inflammation, hardness, tenderness and pain in infected part. Also, enlargement of lymph glands in the armpit and sharp pain when the infant sucks. If left untreated, the skin darkens and the abscess eventually bursts. The person may be feverish and feel unwell. A woman with symptoms of a breast abscess should seek medical treatment.

Treatment: involves supporting and bandaging the affected breast, expressing the milk and not feeding the baby on that side. Also, an antibiotic such as penicillin may be prescribed to fight the infection. Surgery to open and drain the abscess may be necessary and if the infection is very severe, breast-feeding may have to be abandoned.

Causes and risk factors: the cause of a breast abscess is a bacterial infection; usually a staphylococcus or streptococcus is the causal organism. The organisms enter through cracks in

the nipple, particularly at the beginning of breast-feeding before the skin has 'toughened up'. Preventative measures to try to avoid cracking of the nipples include careful cleansing, use of cream or ointment, and not allowing the baby to suck for too long, or to 'comfort suck', especially during the early days of breast-feeding.

breast cancer

Description: a carcinoma (a cancer of the epithelium, the tissue that lines the body's internal organs and skin) or sarcoma (a cancer of the connective tissue), which is the commonest form of cancer in women. The incidence is lowest in countries such as Japan, where breast-feeding is prolonged, as babies are not weaned early, and where the intake of animal fats in the diet is low.

Persons most commonly affected: women, especially after the age of 30 years and more common in postmenopausal women.

Organ or part of body involved: breast and lymph nodes in armpit.

Symptoms and indications: the first sign of breast cancer that is usually noticed is a lump in the breast and/or node in the armpit. In addition, there may be a change in the usual appearance of the breast or a puckering of the skin in the region of the nipple. The breast may feel uncomfortable, and rarely there may be a discharge from the nipple. Most breast lumps are not serious, but a woman who detects a lump should always seek immediate medical attention.

Treatment: involves surgery, radiotherapy and chemotherapy, and usually a combination of these. Sometimes it is possible to remove the lump alone (popularly called 'lumpectomy'), but in other cases, surgery is more radical and the whole breast has to be removed, and lymph nodes under the arm. The degree of surgery depends on the size of the cancer and the extent to which it has spread. In addition to anticancer drugs, other drugs and hormone treatment may be necessary.

Causes and risk factors: as with most cancers, the exact cause is unknown, but some women are more at risk of developing the disease than others. There is a greater risk if a family member (especially mother, aunt or sister) has had breast cancer or if the woman has previously had benign breast tumours. Women who have not had children, and those aged 30 or over at the birth of a first baby, are at greater risk. Women who do not breast-feed are more likely to develop breast cancer. Smokers run a greater risk of developing all forms of cancer than people who do not smoke.

Preventative measures include self-examination of the breasts to check for lumps, which should preferably be carried out just before the monthly period. In this way a woman becomes acquainted with the normal feel and appearance of her breasts and is more likely to detect a change. Also, women over 50 should regularly attend breast-screening clinics. Breast cancer can be completely cured if detected early enough but, as with many cancers, it can spread and set up secondary growths elsewhere. The survival time and treatment for those suffering from breast cancer has improved, and this cancer is a focus for intensive research.

bronchiectasis

Description: a disease of the bronchi (tubes) of the lungs in which, as a result of infection, the passages become blocked with thick secretions causing the walls to dilate and become weakened.

Persons most commonly affected: all age groups and both sexes but more common in adults, although it may originate in childhood.

Organ or part of body involved: lungs and bronchi.

Symptoms and indications: the common, defining symptom is the frequent coughing up of foul, smelly secretions that are thick and green or yellow in colour and may be blood-flecked. The person suffers from frequent respiratory infections and is often breathless and unwell. In addition, the person may be abnormally tired and anaemic. A person with symptoms of bronchiectasis should seek medical treatment.

Treatment: the main treatment is the practice of postural drainage to eliminate the accumulated secretions. The person lies over the edge of the bed with the head hanging down so that the secretions pass into the trachea (windpipe) and can be coughed up. Also, surgery to remove a part of the lung (lobectomy) may be needed, and antibiotics to fight infections. Inhalations of aromatic substances, such as creosote, may be used to eliminate the smell. The person needs yearly immunization against influenza.

Causes and risk factors: the initial damage to the bronchi may result from a number of different causes, including infections of the lungs e.g. pneumonia and chronic bronchitis, allergy (hay fever), inhalation of a foreign body e.g. a tooth, and tuberculosis. The secretions that accumulate lead to blockage and weakening of the bronchial walls, and accumulation of more material and secondary infections, which is bronchiectasis. Preventative measures for a person with bronchiectasis include a good diet, drinking plenty of fluids, avoidance of airborne pollutants (ideally living in an environment where there is clean, fresh air) and trying to avoid respiratory infections.

bronchiolitis or capillary bronchitis

Description: bronchitis (inflammation) affecting the bronchioles, the fine air passages that connect with the minute air sacs of the lungs where oxygen is given up to the blood circulation. This is a serious and potentially fatal condition, especially in young children and elderly persons.

Persons most commonly affected: all age groups and both sexes, especially infants and young children in whom it sometimes occurs in epidemics.

Organ or part of body involved: bronchioles.

Symptoms and indications: bronchiolitis usually develops as a result of a cold or upper respiratory tract infection. The symptoms are respiratory distress characterized by laboured, rapid, shallow breathing, constant hacking cough, flaring of the nostrils, wheezing and seesaw movements (called retractions) of the chest and abdomen. On listening to the chest, there are wheezing, crackling and bubbling sounds. The person may be feverish and restless or a child may be lethargic. Eventually the bronchioles and air sacs become blocked with secretions interfering with the passage of oxygen into the blood. The person shows signs of cyanosis with a bluish tinge to the skin, and death may follow from ASPHYXIA. In the young and old this can occur within 48 hours. A person with symptoms of bronchiolitis requires medical attention. Most patients can be treated at home under the doctor's supervision, but those showing signs of fatigue because of laboured breathing, cyanosis or dehydration need to be admitted to hospital for intensive nursing.

Treatment: at home, involves resting in bed, increasing the humidity in the air by means of steam or a humidifier to ease breathing, and drinking plenty of clear liquids. In hospital, oxygen is likely to be given by means of a tent or a face mask and fluids by intravenous drip. There may be a need for endotracheal intubation (a tube through the mouth or nose directly into the trachea) to deliver oxygen if the person is very ill. The secretions may have to be removed by postural drainage or suction through the trachea. The doctor may prescribe antibiotics if a secondary infection is present.

Causes and risk factors: the cause of the initial infection leading to bronchiolitis is normally a virus, especially respiratory syncytial virus or parainfluenza type 3 virus. Small children who have more than one attack of bronchiolitis may be more likely to develop ASTHMA and allergies.

bronchitis (acute)

Description: inflammation of the bronchi, the tubes that carry air to the lungs.

Persons most commonly affected: all age groups and both sexes.

Organ or part of body involved: bronchi and lungs.

Symptoms and indications: typically, the symptoms begin with those of the common cold but develop with painful coughing, wheezing, throat and chest pains and the production of purulent (pus-containing) mucus. The person is likely to be feverish and feels generally unwell, and crackling, bubbling and wheezing sounds can be heard when listening to the chest. A person with symptoms of bronchitis should seek medical advice.

Treatment: consists of rest and the taking of analgesics or a cough preparation that can be purchased over the counter. Also, inhalation of steam and a heating pad or hot-water bottle on the chest are very effective. Antibiotics may be needed to combat infection.

Causes and risk factors: the cause of bronchitis is a viral and/or bacterial infection, and there is a tendency for the condition to recur. There is a risk of the development of CHRONIC BRONCHITIS or pneumonia. Preventative measures include not smoking, avoiding as far as possible cold, damp conditions and polluted air, drinking plenty of fluids and eating a good diet. Bronchitis is more likely to develop in a person who is 'run-down', with a lower resistance to infections.

bronchitis (chronic)

Description: a chronic inflammation and degeneration of the bronchi in the form of thickening and ulceration, and sometimes dilation of the tubes. It is the commonest cause of death in the UK.

Persons most commonly affected: all age groups and both sexes but more common in elderly persons.

Organ or part of body involved: bronchi and lungs.

Symptoms and indications: a persistent cough that, in the early stages of the disease, tends to occur in the winter months and disappear during the summer. However, as the bronchitis develops, the cough is present most of the time and is at its worst in the morning. There is an excessive, copious production of mucus, and the person is

breathless. The sounds produced on listening to the chest are the same as those in BRONCHITIS (ACUTE). Usually there is less chest pain and feverishness than in the acute form. However, there may be periodic attacks of the acute form of bronchitis, which poses the greatest risk, especially to elderly people.

Treatment: preventative measures and attention to a susceptible person's general state of health are the most important factors. A susceptible person, especially if elderly, will need to be particularly careful with regard to keeping warm, eating a good diet and generally avoiding the risk factors that might worsen the condition.

Causes and risk factors: chronic bronchitis may arise as a result of repeated attacks of the acute form or through some other cause, often as a complication of heart disease. Several parameters are of direct consequence to its cause, including smoking, exposure to air pollutants, cold, wet climate, poor and damp housing, frequent respiratory infections and obesity. Hence, preventative measures involve trying to improve the consequences of these, where possible, particularly in the avoidance of cigarette smoking.

brucellosis or undulant fever or Malta fever or Mediterranean fever

Description: a disease of farm animals (pigs, cattle, goats) that can be passed on to human beings but is rare in Britain.

Persons most commonly affected: all age groups and both sexes.

Organ or part of body involved: liver, spleen, lymph glands, bone marrow.

Symptoms and indications: in humans it is characterized by fever, copious sweats, joint-backache and headache, although the symptoms are not always clear cut. There may be enlargement of the spleen and liver. A person with symptoms of brucellosis should seek medical attention.

Treatment: the treatment consists of relief of the symptoms by means of analgesics and taking antibiotics, particularly tetracyclines, co-trimoxazole or gentamicin, to kill the infection. Sometimes a tetracycline and streptomycin are prescribed if the disease is present in chronic form.

Causes and risk factors: the cause is a species of bacteria belonging to the genus *Brucella*, and humans are usually infected by drinking nonpasteurized milk from cattle or goats with the disease. Hence, preventative measures are of prime importance, particularly the pasteurizing of all milk for human consumption and keeping farm animals free from the disease. Brucellosis itself is rarely fatal, but there may be serious complications in the form of MENINGITIS or PNEUMONIA.

Buerger's disease or thromboangitis obliterans

Description: inflammation of the smaller and medium-sized blood vessels of the legs, especially of the lower limbs. This leads to clot formation and blockage, especially of the smaller arteries.

Persons most commonly affected: younger, adult men aged between about 20 and 45; rare in women.

Organ or part of body involved: arteries (and veins), particularly in lower limbs.

Symptoms and indications: pains in the legs, which come and go because of interruption of the blood circulation, are the main early symptoms. There may be a sensation of numbness, tingling or burning in the legs. GANGRENE may develop, and sometimes ulcers occur on the fingers and toes. A person with symptoms of Buerger's disease should consult a doctor.

Treatment: this is aimed at prevention as there is at present no cure for this condition. The measures recommended are similar to those for ATHEROSCLEROSIS (atheroma) and include not smoking, eating a diet low in cholesterol and salt, taking regular exercise and losing weight if obese. As this is a disease of smokers and is extremely rare in nonsmokers, the most important measure is to give up smoking. The symptoms of the disease can be alleviated in the early stages, and painkillers and drugs to dilate the blood vessels may be prescribed. An affected person should protect himself or herself against cold weather, being especially careful to keep hands and feet warm. Eventually, there may be a need for amputation if gangrene develops.

Causes and risk factors: the cause is unknown, but there is a definite association with smoking. The formation of blood clots in the veins (venous thrombosis) commonly occurs, and there is a risk of CORONARY THROMBOSIS.

burns and scalds

Description: burns are damage to the skin and underlying tissues caused by dry heat, and scalds are similar injuries caused by wet heat. Formerly, burns were categorized by degrees (first, second and third) but are now usually described either as superficial, where sufficient tissue remains to ensure that the skin regrows, or deep, where grafting will be necessary.

Persons most commonly affected: all age groups and both sexes.

Organ or part of body involved: skin and underlying tissues.

Symptoms and indications: symptoms depend on the severity of the burn or scald. If it is relatively minor, there is pain and reddening of the skin, which may later blister or become white and peel off. In more severe burns there are raw wounds from which the skin peels off with a loss of fluid from the injury. Severe wounds of this nature can lead to shock and death, due to fluid loss at the burn site, and infection. All but the most minor burns should be seen by a doctor. In the case of extensive or severe burns and scalds, emergency medical help should be called.

Treatment: depends on the nature and severity of the burn or scald. Minor injuries can be effectively treated by running the affected part under cold water and then covering it with a dressing if needed. Slightly more severe burns should be treated by a doctor and require careful dressing and the use of antiseptics and antibiotics to combat likely infection. Serious and extensive burns are life-threatening and require emergency treatment, the most important part of which is transfusions to counter the fluid loss and maintain the circulation. The person is usually given strong pain relief, such as morphine, and antiseptics and antibiotics are needed to combat infection. Recovery is usually slow, and once the critical period is past, the person is likely to require skin grafting. The greater the extent of the burns and their depth, the poorer the chances of survival, and children and elderly persons are especially vulnerable. Chemical burns require special treatment to counteract the effects of the chemical involved.

Causes and risk factors: burns are caused by dry heat such as fire, sunburn, hot oil or fat in cooking, and also electrical currents and chemicals. Scalds are caused by very hot or boiling water and steam. Small children and the elderly are especially vulnerable to the risk of accidental burns in the home. Hence, the aim should be one of prevention and vigilance to eliminate areas of risk e.g. use of fireguards, cooker guards, safety kettles kept out of reach, fire-retardant clothing (especially pyjamas and nightdresses), installing smoke alarms and general awareness of fire danger.

bursitis

Description: inflammation of a bursa (a fluid-filled hollow surrounding and protecting a joint) e.g. housemaid's knee.

Persons most commonly affected: adults of all age groups and both sexes.

Organ or part of body involved: bursae of joints, especially the knees, elbows, shoulders, wrists, ankles.

Symptoms and indications: pain, especially on moving the affected part, resulting in restriction of normal activity. Also, there may be some swelling and heat. A person with symptoms of bursitis should seek medical advice.

Treatment: the most important aspect of treatment is to rest the affected part and avoid the activity that caused the condition, if this is known. Also, an injection of a corticosteroid preparation into the bursa may be needed to reduce inflammation.

Causes and risk factors: the cause may be obvious, as in the case of housemaid's knee, which is caused by excessive kneeling. Or there may be other repetitive activities that have put the joint under too much strain. However, sometimes the cause of the condition is less easy to discern. Occasionally, there may be infection in the bursa, which is then treated in the same way as an ABSCESS.

C

Caisson disease or **compressed air illness** or **'the bends'**

Description: a condition suffered by persons operating in high pressure in diving bells or divers at depth underwater if they surface too rapidly. Also, those who fly fast, high-performance aircraft.

Persons most commonly affected: adults who are divers or who work in the conditions outlined above e.g. in the oil industry, military aircraft.

Organ or part of body involved: blood and tissues throughout the body.

Symptoms and indications: pains in the joints (the bends), headache and dizziness (decompression sickness), chest pain, breathing difficulties, unconsciousness. Paralysis and death may occur if the person does not receive emergency medical attention.

Treatment: involves admittance to hospital, or a facility with a decompression chamber, until the person has recovered and been slowly readjusted to normal surface pressures.

Causes and risk factors: the cause of this condition is the formation of nitrogen bubbles in the blood, which then accumulate in different parts of the body. The nitrogen bubbles hinder the normal circulation of the blood in supplying the tissues with nutrients and oxygen. Treatment in a decompression chamber forces the nitrogen bubbles to redissolve into the blood. There is a risk of damage to the bones, lungs, brain and heart because of the interruption of the blood circulation, particularly if the person is severely or repeatedly affected. Those working in the occupations listed above, or who take up scuba diving, should receive adequate training and have access to proper medical facilities. The condition can be avoided by returning slowly from high to lower pressure, spending adequate time at each level.

candidiasis or **thrush** or **moniliasis**

Description: an infection of moist areas of the skin, i.e. skin folds or mucous membranes, caused by a fungus. When it occurs in the mouth or vagina it is called thrush.

Persons most commonly affected: young persons and adults of all age groups and both sexes.

Organ or part of body involved: mucous membranes of mouth and vagina; skin folds such as under the arms, breasts, genital area, etc.

Symptoms and indications: itchy, inflamed areas of skin with small pus-filled blisters that may 'weep' and crust over. In the mouth it forms white patches inside the cheeks and on the tongue and throat. Candidiasis is the most commonly occurring fungal infection and affected persons should consult a doctor.

Treatment: is by means of antibiotics, usually nystatin, which, depending upon the site of the infection may be in the form of oral preparations, cream or ointment, pessaries or inhalations.

Causes and risk factors: the causal organism is the fungus *candida albicans* and is generally easy to treat although it may recur. It may occur in people who are 'run-down' or who have recently had to take courses of antibiotics for other illnesses. It also tends to occur in persons with a depressed immune system, who have been taking immunosuppressive drugs, e.g. transplant patients. It may occur in patients suffering from AIDS.

carbon monoxide poisoning

Description: carbon monoxide is an odourless and colourless gas that is highly dangerous when inhaled, leading to carbon monoxide poisoning.

Persons most commonly affected: all age groups and both sexes.

Organ or part of body involved: blood, all tissues and brain.

Symptoms and indications: the symptoms of poisoning include giddiness, flushing of the skin (due to carboxyhaemoglobin in the blood, which is bright red), nausea, headache, raised respiratory and pulse rate and eventual collapse, coma, respiratory failure and death. Carbon monoxide poisoning is an emergency and the person requires immediate medical help.

Treatment: the most important treatment is to immediately remove the person into fresh air and start artificial respiration if needed. Other emergency medical treatment may be needed in the form of giving of oxygen and assisted ventilation.

Causes and risk factors: in the blood, carbon monoxide has a much greater affinity for oxygen (300 times higher) than haemoglobin and converts haemoglobin into carboxyhaemoglobin. (Haemoglobin is the red pigment present in the blood that picks up oxygen in the lungs and carries it in the circulation to all the tissues and organs of the body.) The tissues and organs of the body are quickly deprived of oxygen because there is no free haemoglobin left to pick it up in the lungs. Permanent damage is eventually caused to the ganglia at the base of the brain. Carbon monoxide is present in coal gas fumes and vehicle exhaust emissions. Domestic cases of accidental poisoning usually occur due to inadequate ventilation and ineffective maintenance of boilers and heating systems.

cardiac arrest

Description: the failure and stopping of the pumping action of the heart.

Persons most commonly affected: adults of all age groups and both sexes but particularly middle-aged and elderly persons. Less common in premenopausal women than in men but same incidence in women after menopause as in men.

Organ or part of body involved: heart.

Symptoms and indications: loss of consciousness, breathing and pulse stops, skin is pale and tinged with blue, pupils become dilated. Cardiac arrest or heart attack is a medical emergency and a person requires immediate aid.

Treatment: involves attempting to restart the heart by external cardiac massage (direct depressions of the breastbone) along with artificial respiration (mouth-to-mouth resuscitation). In hospital, defibrillation (electric shock) and direct cardiac massage (the chest wall is opened to allow massage of the heart) may be attempted as a last resort.

Causes and risk factors: causes include various forms of heart disease e.g. CORONARY THROMBOSIS, heartbeat irregularities, serious electrolyte (salts)/fluid imbalance and shock due to severe injury and haemorrhage. Also, electrocution, ANAPHYLACTIC SHOCK, lack of oxygen and respiratory arrest. Stress is believed to be a contributory factor, especially in people with existing heart disease or who are otherwise susceptible.

cardiomyopathy

Description: any disease or disorder of the heart muscle, which may arise from a number of different causes, leading to weak and ineffective pumping of the blood.

Persons most commonly affected: all age groups and both sexes but most common in older adults and in men.

Organ or part of body involved: heart muscle.

Symptoms and indications: the condition may lead to congestive heart failure, the symptoms of which include breathlessness, collection of fluid (oedema) especially in the legs, feet and ankles, palpitations and tiredness. Also, there may be chest pain and a cough. A person with these symptoms should seek medical advice.

Treatment: depends upon whether the cause of the cardiomyopathy can be corrected. Symptoms can, however, be alleviated and drugs that may be prescribed include diuretics, digitalis, vitamin and mineral supplements, especially potassium. Some patients may require a heart transplant.

Causes and risk factors: causes include congenital abnormalities of the heart, dietary deficiencies (especially of potassium and thiamine [vitamin B₄]), viral infections and chronic alcoholism. However, the cause is not always known. Risks increase with severe obesity, smoking and alcoholism, which are reversible factors, and also with increasing age.

carpal tunnel syndrome

Description: a nerve disorder affecting the fingers, thumb and hand.

Persons most commonly affected: adults of both sexes but more common in women aged 30 to 60.

Organ or part of body involved: median nerve supplying hand.

Symptoms and indications: a tingling or burning sensation in the first three or four fingers of one or both hands, pains that may shoot up the arm, numbness and weakness in the hand. The symptoms are usually most severe at night. A person with these symptoms should seek medical advice.

Treatment: includes resting the hand and wrist, sometimes requiring a splint, which often resolves the condition. However, if it does not respond, surgery may be needed to divide the ligament in the wrist that is compressing the median nerve.

Causes and risk factors: the condition is caused by

pressure on the median nerve by an overlying ligament in the wrist. This is brought about by trauma such as a lot of work with the hand and wrist, injury to the wrist or inflammatory conditions, especially arthritis. The condition can often be cured or improved.

catalepsy

Description: a mental disorder in which a person enters a trance-like state.

Persons most commonly affected: adults of both sexes and all age groups.

Organ or part of body involved: brain and central nervous system, whole body.

Symptoms and indications: the body becomes rigid like a statue and the limbs, if moved, stay in the position in which they are placed. There is no sense of recognition or sensation and a loss of voluntary control. The vital body functions are shut down to a minimum level necessary for life and, in fact, may be so low as to resemble death. The condition may last for minutes, hours or, rarely, several days. A person with catalepsy requires medical help.

Treatment: usually occurs in the context of the underlying disease or disorder with which the catalepsy is associated. (*See causes and risk factors*.)

Causes and risk factors: catalepsy may accompany severe mental illnesses such as schizophrenia. Also, it is brought on by severe mental trauma, either as a result of a sudden SHOCK or by a more prolonged depression. Occasionally it may accompany EPILEPSY.

cataract

Description: a condition in which the lens of the eye becomes hard and opaque, resulting in blurring of vision. (The lens is a flexible, clear structure enclosed in a thin capsule within the eye. It is responsible for focusing the incoming light rays onto the retina at the back of the eye where the image is formed.)

Persons most commonly affected: elderly persons of both sexes. Cataracts may affect younger people in certain circumstances and a congenital form can occur in newborn babies. (*See causes and risk factors*).

Organ or part of body involved: lens of one or both eyes.

Symptoms and indications: the main symptom is blurring of vision, which may become progressively worse. A person with symptoms of cataract should consult a doctor.

Treatment: involves surgical removal of the whole or part of the affected lens.

Causes and risk factors: there are various causes of cataract. These include injury to the eye, metabolic disorders especially DIABETES, hypoparathyroidism and some others, congenital disorders, particularly Down's syndrome and GERMAN MEASLES (rubella), which if it affects a mother may cause cataracts in the baby. However, the commonest cause of cataracts is changes that occur in the eye as a result of advancing age. There are natural changes in the protein components of the lens leading to increased opacity and cataract formation. Preventative measures for other than age-related cataracts include seeking prompt attention for any infections or condition involving the eyes, and having regular check-ups and sight tests.

catatonia

Description: a state or syndrome in which a person becomes statue-like, remaining rigid, which is a feature of certain mental illnesses.

Persons most commonly affected: adults of all age groups and both sexes.

Organ or part of body involved: brain, nervous system, with whole body involvement.

Symptoms and indications: symptoms vary to a certain extent but include stereotyped behaviour (an action repeated over and over again in the same way), statue-like rigidity of the limbs, negativism (the person fails to cooperate and does the opposite of what is suggested) and CATALEPSY. A person showing signs of catatonia requires medical help.

Treatment: requires admittance to hospital for drug therapy and psychiatric help and counselling. The drugs that may be used include tranquillizers and, possibly, barbiturates given intravenously along with reassurance and counselling. Electroconvulsive therapy may sometimes be helpful. Patients normally require long-term support and help.

Causes and risk factors: the causes of profound mental disturbance are imperfectly understood. There are likely to be a number of causes at work including genetic factors, upbringing and family background, stressful events in life, physical illnesses and psychological trauma.

cat scratch fever

Description: a mild fever of viral origin resulting in swelling of the lymph glands.

Persons most commonly affected: all age groups and both sexes.

Organ or part of body involved: skin and lymph glands.

Symptoms and indications: swelling and slight infection at the site of a skin puncture. Slight swelling of lymph glands that usually subsides within a few days. Mild feverishness, discomfort and headache. It is advisable to consult a doctor if these symptoms are present.

Treatment: involves rest until the symptoms subside and the person feels better and drinking plenty of fluids. Medication is usually not necessary as the infection is caused by a virus. Occasionally, an ABSCESS may develop at the site of the wound, requiring further treatment. Complete recovery usually takes about one or two weeks.

Causes and risk factors: the cause of the infection is a virus that enters the body following a scratch from a cat, thorn or splinter or other minor injury. In fact, a scratch from a cat is responsible for only about half the cases of cat scratch fever.

cauliflower ear

Description: a thickening of the external part of the ear that can lead to permanent deformity, caused by repeated injury suffered in sport.

Persons most commonly affected: men, especially those who are, or have been, boxers.

Organ or part of body involved: ear.

Symptoms and indications: a collection of blood (haematoma) following a blow or blows on the ear while playing sport. A person with the injury requires medical treatment as soon as possible to prevent permanent deformity.

Treatment: usually requires admittance to hospital where the blood is released to reduce the swelling. A firm bandage, which applies pressure to keep the swelling down, is then used. It is advisable to protect the ears and head during sports activities.

Causes and risk factors: thickening and deformity of the ears is a common injury among boxers.

cerebral palsy

Description: an abnormality of the brain that usually occurs before or during birth and results in severe physical, and often mental, disabilities.

Persons most commonly affected: detected after birth or in infancy and the person is affected for life. Both sexes are affected by congenital cerebral palsy, but it is commoner in boys, and the incidence is in the order of 2 to 2½ per 1000 births. Less commonly, the illness may arise after birth due to a severe infection or trauma, and this type affects equal numbers of girls and boys.

Organ or part of body involved: brain, muscles.

Symptoms and indications: the severity of the symptoms varies greatly. The newborn baby may be floppy and have difficulty sucking but characteristically the child shows spastic paralysis of the limbs. Also, there may be involuntary writhing movements called athetosis, and balance and posture are also affected. There is often mental subnormality and speech impairment and sometimes EPILEPSY. Since a baby is closely monitored from birth, cerebral palsy is usually suspected or detected early on. A parent concerned in any way about the health of a baby should always call a doctor.

Treatment: the treatment required depends upon the severity of the symptoms and the degree to which the child is affected. The outlook is generally favourable and many children are able to enjoy a reasonable or good quality of life. Treatment may involve some surgery but mainly physiotherapy, speech and occupational therapy and special education. It is now considered best to encourage the child to lead as normal and active a life as possible. Also, to expect and help the child to achieve as many aims and goals in life as possible, in spite of disability.

Causes and risk factors: it may arise as a developmental defect in the foetus due to genetic factors, or due to a viral infection during pregnancy. A lack of oxygen during a difficult labour or other trauma to the infant can result in cerebral palsy. After birth, the condition can result from HAEMOLYTIC DISEASE OF THE NEWBORN or infection of the brain e.g. MENINGITIS.

cervical cancer

Description: cancer of the neck or cervix of the womb, which is one of the most common cancers affecting women.

Persons most commonly affected: women who are sexually active.

Organ or part of body involved: cervix—the neck of the womb.

Symptoms and indications: the precancerous and early stages of the disease may produce few or no symptoms. Later symptoms include abnormal vaginal discharge, which usually smells unpleasant and contains blood, and abnormal bleeding. If the cancer has spread to surrounding tissues and organs, further symptoms are likely to occur. Any abnormality in the cervix is normally detected by the cervical smear test offered to all women every three years in the UK. The woman is notified if any such signs occur and is given further investigation and treatment as required.

Treatment: is mainly aimed at prevention by means of the cervical smear test, which detects definite precancerous changes in the cells lining the surface of the cervix before cancer develops. At these early stages, the cancer is readily cured and treatment methods include cryosurgery, diathermy, laser treatment and electrocoagulation. One or a combination of more radical surgery, radiotherapy and chemotherapy are likely to be needed if the cancer has become established or has spread.

Causes and risk factors: the cause of this cancer is unknown but the sexual behaviour of a woman influences her risk of contracting the disease. The cancer does not occur in women who never have sexual intercourse. The earlier a woman or girl starts having sexual intercourse, and the greater the number of partners, are factors now recognized to increase her risk of contracting cervical cancer. However, the cure rate is high (about 95%) if detected and treated at an early stage.

chicken pox (or varicella)

Description: a highly infectious viral disease that is normally mild and of fairly short duration.

Persons most commonly affected: children of both sexes; it can affect adults but this is uncommon.

Organ or part of body involved: skin and mucous membranes.

Symptoms and indications: there is an incubation period of two or three weeks and then usually the child becomes slightly feverish and unwell. Within 24 hours an itchy rash appears on the skin, which consists of fluid-filled blisters that vary in size. These may occur anywhere on the body including the scalp, inside the mouth and on the throat and in the genital area. Eventually these form scabs that fall off after about one week. The blisters are very itchy and tend to leave slight pock marks on the skin after healing, but these are not disfiguring. The symptoms are much more severe in adults accompanied by 'flu-like fever and aches and pains.

Treatment: involves keeping the child at home away from other children and relieving the itching by means of warm baths and soothing preparations. 'After-sun' preparations and calamine lotion are helpful in relieving itching. Children should be encouraged not to scratch, although this is difficult. Once scabs have formed and are drying and falling off, the child can start to resume normal activities but remains infectious until all the spots have gone.

Causes and risk factors: the cause of chicken pox is the varicella zoster virus and a childhood attack confers lifelong immunity as most children are exposed at some stage. Hence, the disease is uncommon in adults. Babies in the first few months of life usually have some immunity from the mother. After recovery from chicken pox the virus may remain within the system and become active later in adult life as SHINGLES.

chilblain or erythema pernio

Description: a round, itchy inflammation of the skin, usually occurring on the toes or fingers in cold weather.

Persons most commonly affected: all age groups and both sexes.

Organ or part of body involved: skin of the toes and fingers and sometimes the ears.

Symptoms and indications: round, red and itchy inflammation of the skin, which is especially troublesome when the feet or hands are warmed after having been chilled outside on a cold day.

Treatment: preventative treatment is best involving wearing good warm gloves and footwear in winter weather. Keeping the feet and hands warm, eating a good diet and taking exercise to improve the circulation are helpful in the prevention of chilblains.

Causes and risk factors: chilblains tend to occur in people with defective circulation and may be an indication of poor health or inadequate nutrition. However, some people are more susceptible than others and in these persons, care and prevention are the best remedy.

cholecystitis or cholangitis

Description: inflammation and infection of the gall bladder and its ducts (bile ducts). Inflammation of the bile ducts is called cholangitis.

Persons most commonly affected: adults of both sexes and all age groups but less common in men. Rare in young people and children.

Organ or part of body involved: gall bladder and bile ducts.

Symptoms and indications: sharp, cramp-like pain in the upper part of the abdomen on the right-hand side. Pain may also be felt elsewhere. Abdominal discomfort, feverishness, nausea and vomiting, flatulence. Sometimes there may be jaundice and itching of the skin, and stools may be pale in colour. A person with symptoms of cholecystitis should seek medical advice.

Treatment: mild attacks may only require rest in bed and a course of antibiotics until the symptoms subside. However, often admittance to hospital and a surgical operation to remove the gall bladder (cholecystectomy) is necessary.

Causes and risk factors: the cause of cholecystitis is usually gallstones causing blockage, inflammation and infection of the bile ducts. Hence, preventative measures to avoid the formation of gallstones are helpful e.g. eating a low-fat diet.

cholera

Description: a severe bacterial infection of the small intestine. Cholera remains a serious killer disease in many countries, especially in conditions of overcrowding and poor sanitation e.g. refugee camps. During epidemics, the death rate exceeds 50% with children and elderly persons being at particular risk. The disease is rare in the UK and such cases that occur are contracted abroad. Strict standards of hygiene, sanitation and nursing ensure that the infection does not spread, and prevent an epidemic. Early and prompt detection and treatment enable most patients to make a full recovery. This vigilance remains necessary because cholera caused thousands of deaths in the last century during widespread epidemics in many countries.

Persons most commonly affected: all age groups and both sexes.

Organ or part of body involved: digestive system — whole body.

Symptoms and indications: there is considerable variation in the severity of symptoms and in the manner in which they present themselves. In mild cases, the patient may hardly feel ill, whereas in those severely affected during epidemics, death may occur very rapidly within a few hours. In most cases, three stages of cholera are recognized. During the first stage, there is copious diarrhoea and vomiting, with the production of characteristic 'rice water stools' containing flakes of fibrin (a protein substance formed in the blood during blood clotting). There are severe pains and cramps, extreme thirst and increasing signs of dehydration. In the second stage, death occurs due to dehydration and collapse. The person's skin is cold and wrinkled, the eyes are sunken, the pulse becomes imperceptible and the voice is a hoarse whisper ('vox cholerica'). During the third stage, the person starts to recover and gradually improve and the symptoms subside. Relapse is still possible at this stage, particularly in the form of a fever. A person who has travelled abroad and has any signs of illness should seek medical advice.

Treatment: requires isolation of the patient and scrupulous attention to hygiene during nursing. This includes treatment and very careful disposal of the body waste of the infected person, to prevent the spread of the disease. Treatment of the patient involves bed rest and the taking of tetracycline or other sulphonamide drugs to kill the cholera bacteria. The patient requires salt solutions to counteract the dehydration that occurs, and these are taken by mouth and/or given intravenously. Prevention of cholera is by means of vaccination but this is only effective for about six months.

Causes and risk factors: the disease is caused by the bacterium vibrio cholerae. It is spread by contamination of drinking water by faeces of those affected by the disease, and also by flies landing on infected material and then crawling on food. In countries where cholera is present, drinking water must be treated or boiled and strict standards of hygiene used in food preparation. Efforts should be made to eliminate flies from houses and to ensure that they do not come into contact with food. Risks remain wherever there are conditions of overcrowding, poverty and poor sanitation.

cirrhosis of the liver

Description: a disease of the liver in which fibrous matter resembling scar tissue is produced as a result of damage and death to the cells. The liver becomes yellow-coloured and nodular in appearance, and there is a loss of its normal function that may eventually lead to complete failure.

Persons most commonly affected: adults of both sexes and all age groups but more common in men.

Organ or part of body involved: liver.

Symptoms and indications: there are various symptoms, which include loss of appetite and weight, digestive upset, weariness, enlargement of liver, ANAEMIA, dark urine, JAUNDICE, haemorrhage and blood in the stools. Also, bruising, fine, red spidery veins in skin, fluid retention, bloating (oedema) and red hands. Also, the spleen enlarges and there may be baldness and breast enlargement in men. Eventually, there may be collapse, coma and death from liver failure. A person with any symptoms of liver disease should seek medical advice.

Treatment: the progress of the disease can be halted if the cause is known, although nothing can be done to repair the damage to the liver that has already taken place. Excess consumption of alcohol is the most common cause of cirrhosis of the liver. Hence, if this is the cause, no more alcohol should be consumed. The affected person should eat a diet that is high in protein and carbohydrates but low in fat and salt. Iron, vitamins, (B and K) and mineral supplements may also be necessary. Provided that the liver damage is not too great, it should be possible for the person to lead a normal life as long as the progress of the disease is halted.

Causes and risk factors: as stated above, the most common cause of cirrhosis of the liver is excess consumption of alcohol over a long period of time. Other causes are viral HEPATITIS (post necrotic cirrhosis) and cirrhosis of unknown cause (cryptogenic cirrhosis). Exposure to toxic chemicals at the workplace is a further potential risk.

coeliac disease or gluten enteropathy

Description: a wasting disease occurring in childhood, an allergic condition in which the intestines are unable to absorb fat.

Persons most commonly affected: begins in infancy when the child is weaned, affecting infants and children of both sexes and remaining throughout life.

Organ or part of body involved: digestive system.

Symptoms and indications: loss of appetite, failure to thrive or weight loss, pains in abdomen, foul-smelling, pale stools, flatulence, dietary deficiencies and possibly anaemia. The symptoms appear after the child is introduced to foods containing gluten, which is found in wheat and rye flour. A baby or child who has symptoms of coeliac disease should be seen by a doctor.

Treatment: consists of eating a gluten-free diet throughout life. The child should start to thrive again once gluten is excluded, but may need vitamin, mineral and iron supplements to regain lost ground.

Causes and risk factors: the cause of coeliac disease is a congenital sensitivity or intolerance to gluten, causing damage to the lining of the intestines. The intestines are then unable to absorb fat, leading to excretion of an excess of fat and then other symptoms described above. There may be a family history of coeliac disease or a link with other allergic conditions. *See also* SPRUE.

cold sores

Description: an infectious inflammation of the skin and mucous membranes, characterized by the development of small blisters.

Persons most commonly affected: both sexes and all age groups, usually first appearing before the age of five. Once present, the virus persists for life.

Organ or part of body involved: skin, lips and mouth area. The lesions sometimes occur on the genitals and, rarely, occur on the cornea or conjunctiva of the eyes.

Symptoms and indications: there is a characteristic development of small, painful, fluid-filled blisters surrounded by a reddish area. In a few days, the eruptions dry up and heal completely, normally without scarring. If the eyes are affected, there may be some scarring and damage to the eye. A person with symptoms of an eye infection should always seek medical advice.

Treatment: various ointments and topical preparations are available without prescription for the treatment of cold sores. Occasionally, a secondary bacterial infection occurs, which requires treatment with an antibiotic preparation. If the eyes are involved, the person requires treatment by an eye specialist and may be prescribed an antiviral agent such as acyclovir.

Causes and risk factors: the cause of the infection is a herpes simplex virus that is contracted from a person already having the virus. The virus is passed on through close physical contact e.g. kissing, and so may affect several members of a family. It often lies dormant for a long period of time before flaring up to produce cold sores. These then tend to occur from time to time throughout life. A person may be more susceptible to infection if 'run-down' or under stress in any way.

colic

Description: spasmodic, severe abdominal pain, which occurs in waves with brief interludes in between. Infantile colic is common in young babies in the first few months of life.

Persons most commonly affected: adults and children of all ages and both sexes. Infantile colic affects babies between the ages of about two weeks and four months.

Organ or part of body involved: digestive tract.

Symptoms and indications: cramping, spasmodic waves of pain; usually the symptoms last for a fairly brief period. Infantile colic characteristically causes the baby to cry loudly for several hours, especially in the evening, and the legs may be drawn up in pain. Colic is painful but usually short-lived. A doctor should be consulted if the symptoms continue for a long time. Infantile colic can be alarming and parents often need reassurance that there is nothing seriously wrong with their baby. However, this condition does not require medical intervention.

Treatment: involves finding the most comfortable position to relieve the pain and resting until the symptoms subside. A hot-water bottle is also helpful. An attack of colic is generally not serious but can result in a twisting of the bowel that must receive immediate medical attention in hospital. Colic-type pain may also be caused by a tumour in the bowel, which again requires urgent medical treatment. Infantile colic is best coped with by general measures to try to comfort the baby. To try to prevent colic, the baby should be 'winded' during feeding and prevented from overfeeding or taking milk too quickly. Infantile colic generally stops after three or four months of age.

Causes and risk factors: the cause of colic is usually the presence of some indigestible food that causes the contraction of the intestinal muscles. Infantile colic is due to wind associated with feeding. In adults, provided that there is no more serious underlying cause, attacks are usually brief and infrequent.

colitis (ulcerative)

Description: inflammation of the colon, that may lead to ulceration and that is a severe chronic condition with a tendency to recur.

Persons most commonly affected: younger adults in the age range 16 to 45, especially women.

Organ or part of body involved: colon, bowel.

Symptoms and indications: abdominal discomfort and pain, watery diarrhoea containing blood, anaemia and fever. Also, there is a lack of appetite and loss of weight and sweating. A person with symptoms of colitis should consult a doctor. Occasionally, there may be serious complications as a result of this condition, which can prove fatal.

Treatment: is by means of bed rest, drug treatment with corticosteroids and sulphasalazine, iron supplements to correct the anaemia and a bland, low-roughage diet. Another drug that may be prescribed is azathioprine and after recovery, it may be necessary to continue with sulphasalazine to prevent the recurrence of the condition. Rarely, surgery may be needed to remove part of the colon. Preventative treatment includes a low-roughage diet and avoidance of cold, damp weather conditions whenever possible.

Causes and risk factors: the cause of colitis is not known but there may be a genetic or family susceptibility, and the risk increases with an overconsumption of alcohol. There is a risk to the

patient's life if the blood loss or wasting is excessive, or if infection such as PERITONITIS sets in as a result of serious ulceration. Also, there is a greater risk of contracting CANCER OF THE COLON.

concussion

Description: a loss of consciousness due to a blow to the head, causing bruising of the brain.

Persons most commonly affected: all age groups and both sexes.

Organ or part of body involved: brain.

Symptoms and indications: the symptoms vary in severity and reflect, to some extent, the force of the blow. There may be confusion, headache and dizziness in a case of mild concussion, or the person may fall into unconsciousness and remain in that state for seconds, hours or even weeks. It may be possible to rouse the person to some extent, but he or she is extremely irritable and does not answer questions correctly and soon becomes unconscious again. When the person comes round from the state of unconsciousness he or she usually suffers from a severe headache and irritability and these symptoms can last for some time. A person suffering from concussion usually needs to be admitted to hospital and a doctor should be called.

Treatment: depending upon the severity of the concussion, the patient requires admittance to hospital for rest and observation. There is a danger of bleeding caused by the blow on the head, which could result in serious, life-threatening damage to the brain. When the unconsciousness persists for some time the person requires careful monitoring, nursing and observation. Once the person has regained consciousness, and even in mild cases of concussion, rest is needed until the headache subsides.

Causes and risk factors: the cause of concussion is a sudden knock to the head causing a compression wave that momentarily interrupts the blood supply to the brain. As indicated above, there is a risk of bleeding and further brain damage. The person normally makes a good and complete recovery but there may be memory loss, irritability and a tendency to headaches, lasting for several months. Also, there may be a risk or tendency in some people to EPILEPSY.

conjunctivitis

Description: inflammation and infection of the mucous membrane (conjunctiva) that lines the inside of the eyelid and covers the front of the eye.

Persons most commonly affected: all age groups and both sexes.

Organ or part of body involved: conjunctiva of the eyes.

Symptoms and indications: reddening, watering and itching of one or both eyes. Discharge from the eye, which may be clear or yellowish, and forms crusts that glue the eyelids together after sleeping. There may be eye pain and discomfort. Symptoms vary according to the cause of the conjunctivitis and some forms are more serious than others. A person with symptoms of conjunctivitis should seek medical advice.

Treatment: depends upon the cause and nature of the condition but usually involves the application of eyedrops or ointment to relieve the symptoms and to kill infection. Drugs used include sodium cromoglycate, chloramphenicol and tetracycline antibiotics, penicillin and acycloguasine. Recovery from the milder forms of conjunctivitis is normally complete.

Causes and risk factors: there are various causes of conjunctivitis, including allergy, bacteria, viruses e.g. Herpes simplex and the microorganism, chlamydia. Chlamydia conjunctivitis (chlamydia trachomatis) is a common cause of blindness in some Third World countries. A baby may be infected by chlamydia or gonococcal infection (GONORRHOEA) as it passes through the birth canal, leading to the development of conjunctivitis in the first weeks of life.

constipation or costiveness

Description: the condition in which the bowels are opened too infrequently and the faeces become dry, hard and difficult and painful to pass.

Persons most commonly affected: all age groups and both sexes.

Organ or part of body involved: colon and rectum.

Symptoms and indications: infrequent opening of the bowels and the faeces passed are hard, dry, very dark and small. There may be bleeding, straining and pain, swelling of the abdomen due to retained faeces and a feeling of bloatedness. A person with persistent constipation should seek medical advice, as the condition itself may be a symptom of an underlying condition.

Treatment: involves making changes to lifestyle, including eating more roughage such as fruit, raw vegetables, wholemeal bread and bran, drinking at least eight glasses of water a day and taking more exercise. In addition, laxatives and enemas may be needed to relieve the condition. It is helpful to respond promptly to the urge to open the bowels and to encourage one daily bowel movement. These measures also help to prevent a recurrence of the condition.

Causes and risk factors: the cause is usually an inappropriate diet, inadequate fluid intake and inattention to the need to open the bowels. Sometimes the cause lies in the colon itself. Too much water may be absorbed quickly (a 'greedy colon'), leading to the production of dry, hard faeces. Or, in the case of a 'spastic colon', the muscles are in spasm (*see* IRRITABLE BOWEL SYNDROME). Sometimes the muscles of the colon do not work properly because of a lack of vitamin B in the food intake. Prolonged bouts of constipation may result in the development of piles or in a HERNIA or prolapse of the rectum or uterus.

convulsions or fits

Description: involuntary and rapidly alternating muscular contractions and relaxations throwing the body and limbs into contortions. Convulsions are themselves a symptom triggered by some underlying cause.

Persons most commonly affected: babies from about the age of six months and young children up to four years. Both sexes may be affected. Convulsions can also affect adults of both sexes.

Organ or part of body involved: brain and central nervous system; muscles.

Symptoms and indications: in young children, convulsions usually accompany a fever. Hence, the child is often already unwell and feverish. During the convulsion itself, there is uncontrolled twitching and jerking of the limbs, body, head and face, and unconsciousness. The person may lose control of bladder and bowel function and be irritable on regaining consciousness. Following the convulsion, the person usually sleeps for several hours. The convulsion normally only lasts for a few minutes. A person who has had a convulsion should be seen by a doctor.

Treatment: depends upon the underlying cause of the convulsion. If triggered by fever, as is often the case in young children, measures to reduce the temperature and treat any infection are usually required. If the underlying cause is EPILEPSY, as is commonly the case in adults, then this requires appropriate treatment. If the convulsions continue, an injection of barbiturates or other sedative drug may be required.

Causes and risk factors: as indicated above, the commonest cause of convulsions in young children is fever. However, breath-holding, which is quite common in infants and very young children, is another cause. Also, breathing difficulties, which may occur, for example, during a bout of WHOOPING COUGH, may trigger a convulsion. More serious causes include inflammation and diseases of the brain such as MENINGITIS and encephalitis, and head injury. In adults, the commonest cause is epilepsy. Convulsions are alarming to observe but unless caused by a serious disease or infection, in themselves they are rarely life-threatening.

corneal foreign bodies

Description: a foreign body lodging on the cornea or outer surface of the eye.

Persons most commonly affected: all ages and both sexes.

Organ or part of body involved: cornea.

Symptoms and indications: intense irritation and watering of the eye and photophobia (profound sensitivity to light).

Treatment: removal of foreign body and application of antibiotic drops or ointment. An eye patch may be worn until any damage has healed (usually about 24 hours).

Causes and risk factors: usually dust or material thrown up by mechanical tools. Can be avoided by wearing suitable eye protection when at risk e.g. when riding a motor cycle or when using power tools. If foreign bodies are not removed quickly from the eye, serious damage may be caused to the sight.

corns (and bunions, hammer toe)

Description: a corn is a small, localized portion of hardened, thickened skin occurring on or between the toes, which is cone-shaped. The point of the cone, known as the 'eye' points inwards and causes pain. A bunion occurs over the joint at the base of the largest toe. The joint between the toe and the first metatarsal bone becomes swollen and forms a lump beneath thickened skin (a callus). A hammer toe is similar but involves the second toe, which becomes bent at the joint to resemble a hammer.

Persons most commonly affected: adults of all groups and both sexes.

Organ or part of body involved: foot

Symptoms and indications: thickened skin and painful lumps or bumps on or between the toes.

Treatment: preventative measures are to ensure that shoes are always of a good fit with plenty of room for the toes. Corns and bunions can be treated at home by soaking in warm water to soften the area of thickened skin and, after drying, rubbing down with a pumice stone. Corn plasters can be used on the corn to reduce pain and pressure on the toe. It is often advisable to have corns and bunions treated professionally by a qualified chiropodist.

Causes and risk factors: the causes of corns and bunions are ill-fitting, tight footwear. There is an overgrowth of cells, due to pressure, leading to a thickening of the skin and the development of a lump.

coronary artery disease or coronary heart disease or ischaemic heart disease

Description: any abnormal condition that affects the coronary arteries that supply blood to the heart and arise from the aorta. The commonest disease is coronary ATHEROSCLEROSIS, resulting in narrowing or blockage that causes serious or fatal damage to the heart.

Persons most commonly affected: adults of both sexes but much less common in premenopausal women. There is equal incidence in adults during later years of life.

Organ or part of body involved: coronary arteries.

Symptoms and indications: often there are no or few symptoms until the arteries are severely narrowed. The disease advances until it causes angina pectoris or coronary thrombosis (which leads to heart attack). These conditions both require immediate medical attention.

Treatment: requires admittance to hospital and balloon angioplasty (a procedure for dilating the arteries), or coronary bypass surgery may be needed. Various drugs may be prescribed, including painkillers, beta-adrenergic blockers, vasodilators, anticoagulants, and nitroglycerin. The diet should be low in fat and salt and the person should undertake a programme of moderate exercise under doctor's advice. Preventative measures include no smoking, eating a low-fat, low-salt diet, taking regular exercise, and measures to avoid stress.

Causes and risk factors: the cause of the disease is not certain but the risk increases with the lifestyle factors mentioned above, i.e. smoking, poor diet, lack of exercise, stress and obesity. Also, persons with DIABETES, high blood pressure (HYPERTENSION) or previous heart problems run a greater risk of developing the disease. The condition is a serious one, which may ultimately shorten life, although many people make a good recovery once the initial crisis has passed.

coronary thrombosis or heart attack or myocardial infarction

Description: a sudden blockage of one of the

coronary arteries by a blood clot or thrombus that interrupts the blood supply to the heart. This causes death of myocardial (heart muscle or myocardium) cells due to interruption of the blood supply.

Persons most commonly affected: men, especially aged over 40, but also occurs in women.

Organ or part of body involved: arteries and heart.

Symptoms and indications: severe and agonizing chest pain that may spread to involve the left arm, upper back, neck and jaw. Breathlessness and a crushing feeling on the chest, vomiting and nausea. A rise in temperature and pale and clammy skin, rapid pulse and collapse. A person suffering a coronary thrombosis requires urgent medical help and the emergency services should be called. If the person stops breathing and the heart stops, mouth-to-mouth resuscitation and external cardiac massage must be given until help arrives. Provided that a person receives prompt medical help, and survives the critical hours following a first heart attack, a good recovery is possible and normal activities can be gradually resumed. However, a severe heart attack may be fatal and the outlook is less favourable if the onset of treatment is delayed.

Treatment: following admittance to hospital, consists of giving strong pain relief, such as injections of morphine, oxygen and thrombolytic drugs to break up blood clots. The person requires intensive nursing in a coronary care unit. Various other drugs designed to restore the function of the heart are likely to be required, including anti-arrhythmics, beta-adrenergic or calcium channel blockers, digitalis, nitroglycerin and other antianginal preparations.

Causes and risk factors: the cause is a final sudden blockage or occlusion of one of the coronary arteries that has previously become narrowed (*see* CORONARY ARTERY DISEASE). This causes an interruption of the blood supply to part of the heart muscle, which dies, and this is known as myocardial infarction. The heart ceases to pump blood effectively, with the symptoms described above. The risk of heart attack increases with smoking, a poor diet high in fat and salt, obesity, high blood pressure, stress, lack of exercise and raised levels of cholesterol in the blood.

Crohn's disease or ileitis

Description: inflammation of a part of the ileum, which is the lower part of the small intestine, leading to ulceration and thickening.

Persons most commonly affected: young adults of both sexes between the ages of 20 and 40.

Organ or part of body involved: ileum, lymph tissue and glands.

Symptoms and indications: spasmodic abdominal pains of a colicky type that may be mistaken for APPENDICITIS. Slight fever, nausea, loss of weight and appetite. There may be diarrhoea and distension of the abdomen with tenderness and pain. There is a thickening of the ileum, which can sometimes be felt externally. A person with symptoms of Crohn's disease should seek medical advice. Attacks of symptoms tend to recur at intervals over a long period of time, although the disease may disappear.

Treatment: consists of rest and eating a low-fibre diet that is high in vitamins. Pain-relieving drugs and vitamin supplements may be prescribed, and also antibiotics and corticosteroid drugs. Occasionally, if there is a complete blockage or a failure to respond to medical treatment, admittance to hospital for surgical removal of the affected part may be necessary.

Causes and risk factors: the cause is unknown, although there may be a tendency for Crohn's disease to occur in families and hence a genetic link. People with food allergies are more likely to develop the disease. There is a possibility of infection or ABSCESS, perforation of the severely inflamed part, FISTULA and increased risk of the development of cancer of the ileum.

croup

Description: a group of diseases characterized by infection, swelling and partial obstruction and inflammation of the entrance to the larynx, occurring in young children.

Persons most commonly affected: young children of both sexes up to the age of about six years.

Organ or part of body involved: larynx, windpipe (trachea) and bronchial tubes (leading to the lungs).

Symptoms and indications: harsh, strained breathing producing a characteristic crowing sound, accompanying a cough and fever. There may be pains in the chest or throat and the child is generally restless and unwell. Attacks usually occur at night. If the child is experiencing severe difficulties in breathing, emergency medical attention is required. Milder cases can be treated at home but a doctor should be consulted.

Treatment: mild cases can be relieved by taking the child into the bathroom and turning on the hot water taps to produce a steamy atmosphere. The condition can be relieved by inhalation of steam from a bowl or basin of hot water to which a soothing preparation, such as tincture of benzoin, can be added. Mild sedatives and/or painkillers may be prescribed by a doctor. The child should be encouraged to drink plenty of fluids. Rarely, the obstruction becomes dangerous and completely blocks the larynx. The outcome is rapidly fatal, unless the child has been admitted to hospital, where nasotracheal intubation or emergency tracheostomy to restore the airway can be carried out.

Causes and risk factors: DIPHTHERIA used to be the most common cause of croup but it now usually results from a viral infection of the respiratory tract (laryngotracheobronchitis), or less commonly, a bacterial infection. A child normally makes a good recovery from croup but attacks are likely to recur. The child should be discouraged from playing outside in cold, damp weather, as this may cause an attack in some cases.

Cushing's syndrome

Description: a metabolic disorder that results from the presence in the body of excessive amounts of corticosteroids, which are hormones produced by the cortex of the adrenal glands. The production and regulation of these hormones is controlled by the pituitary gland at the base of the brain. There may be an inability to regulate adrenocorticotrophic hormone or cortisol, produced by the pituitary gland, which itself controls the production of corticosteroids by the adrenal glands. Or, the problem may lie in the adrenal glands themselves.

Persons most commonly affected: all age groups and both sexes but more common in adults and in women.

Organ or part of body involved: pituitary gland and adrenal glands.

Symptoms and indications: reddening of face and neck with puffiness, growth of body and facial hair, obesity, OSTEOPOROSIS and, possibly, mental disturbances. Also, there may be menstrual irregularities in women, high blood pressure, DIABETES MELLITUS and the development of peptic ulcers. There may be an increased susceptibility to infections and stretch marks on the abdomen. A person with Cushing's syndrome requires careful monitoring and often needs long-term medical treatment.

Treatment: depends upon the source of the problem but may involve surgery to remove a tumour and hormone replacement therapy if glands have to be taken out. Also, drugs to correct high blood pressure and calcium supplements to counteract osteoporosis may be required. Occasionally, treatment may include irradiation of the pituitary gland. Depending upon the cause, Cushing's syndrome can be cured but the person usually needs continuing medication throughout life.

Causes and risk factors: the commonest cause of Cushing's syndrome is a tumour of the pituitary gland or adrenal gland. Also, a malignancy elsewhere e.g. in the lung, which has required extensive and prolonged treatment with corticosteroid drugs can produce Cushing's syndrome. If these are gradually and carefully withdrawn, the symptoms may improve. There is a risk of fractures due to the osteoporosis that accompanies Cushing's syndrome and affected persons should take care to avoid accidental injury.

cystic fibrosis (CF)

Description: an inherited (genetic) disease, the defective gene responsible for it being located on human chromosome no. 7.

Persons most commonly affected: children of both sexes.

Organ or part of body involved: the disease affects all the mucus-secreting glands of the lungs, pancreas, mouth and gastrointestinal tract and also the sweat glands of the skin.

Symptoms and indications: a thick mucus is produced that affects the production of pancreatic enzymes and causes the bronchi to widen (bronchiectasis) and become clogged. The child has a constant, severe cough but the mucus is thick and difficult to cough up. Respiratory infections are common. The stools contain a lot of mucus and are slimy, with a foul smell. The child loses weight and the sweat contains abnormally high levels of sodium and chloride. The liver and spleen become enlarged. The diagnosis of cystic fibrosis is usually made early in the child's life by analysis of the stools, but there is no antenatal test that can detect the condition.

Treatment: the disease is incurable but the outlook for affected children has greatly improved with increasing numbers of patients surviving into adult life. Treatment involves physiotherapy to relieve the bronchial congestion, particularly daily postural drainage that can be carried out at home. Humidifiers may be needed in the home to keep the air moist, which helps to thin the mucus. Any respiratory infection should be treated promptly by a doctor and may require antibiotics. The child may need a special diet that is high in protein and low in fat. Vitamin supplements and pancreatic enzyme tablets are normally required. The child may need frequent admittance to hospital for intensive nursing during infections. The child should be encouraged to lead as normal a life as possible.

Causes and risk factors: the cause is a genetic abnormality that affects about one child in every 2000. Many people carry the gene for cystic fibrosis and if there is a family history of the disease, a couple may need to seek advice before having children.

cystitis

Description: inflammation and infection of the bladder, normally caused by a bacterium.

Persons most commonly affected: females of all age groups. The condition is much less common in males.

Organ or part of body involved: bladder.

Symptoms and indications: characteristically, there is a need to pass urine frequently accompanied by a burning, painful sensation. There may be cramp-like pains in the lower abdomen with dark, strong urine that contains blood. A person with symptoms of cystitis should seek medical advice.

Treatment: involves taking a course of antibiotics and also drinking a lot of fluids, possibly with the addition of bicarbonate of soda which counteracts the acidity of the urine, thereby easing the pain. The increase in fluid makes the urine more dilute, thus helping to flush out the bacteria, making it less likely that they will grow again and cause a further attack. Recovery is usually rapid although cystitis may recur from time to time.

Causes and risk factors: the cause of the infection is usually the common bacterium that normally inhabits the bowel, *E. coli*. The prevalence of cystitis in females is due to the fact that the urethra is much shorter in women than in men, and the bacteria (which are harmless in the bowel) are more likely to gain access both to the urinary tract and vagina. In the bladder, the bacteria cause inflammation and infection with the symptoms of cystitis, as described above. There is a slight risk of the infection spreading up to the kidneys, which is a more serious condition, hence cystitis should always be treated promptly.

D

deafness

Description: partial or total loss of hearing in one or both ears. Deafness may be congenital (present from birth), conductive (an abnormality of the outer or middle ear, preventing the passage of sound waves to the inner ear) or nerve deafness (an abnormality of the inner ear, the auditory nerve or the brain).

Persons most commonly affected: congenital deafness: from birth and both sexes. Conductive deafness: any age and both sexes. Nerve deafness: any age, but increasingly common in people over 50. Both sexes.

Organ or part of body involved: ears.

Symptoms and indications: gradual or sudden loss of hearing. In congenital deafness, this may be noticed as lack of response to sounds, or when the child is older, poor or absent speech.

Treatment: for congenital deafness, early testing of the hearing is important. A hearing aid may be fitted, and special training for parent and child for hearing and speech may be used. Conductive deafness may be treated by an operation, or fitting a hearing aid. Nerve deafness may be helped by use of a hearing aid.

Causes and risk factors: Congenital deafness: in most cases, the cause is unknown, but may be inherited, caused by the mother catching rubella (German measles) in the first 16 weeks of pregnancy, some drugs during pregnancy, brain damage at birth or SYPHILIS in the mother. Vaccination against rubella for girls between the ages of 11 and 14 should give immunity for life, and is an important means of prevention. Conductive deafness: is most commonly caused by OTITIS MEDIA. Nerve deafness: in most cases there is no definite cause, but some are due to exposure to excessive noise, for example, gunfire explosions or working in a very noisy place.

delirium

Description: an acute mental disorder, in which there is disorientation, confusion and hallucination, with several causes.

Persons most commonly affected: all age groups and both sexes.

Organ or part of body involved: brain.

Symptoms and indications: incoherence, confusion, restlessness, fear, anxiety, often hallucinations or illusions and sometimes delusions. If the delirium is caused by ALCOHOLISM, it is called *delirium tremens*.

Treatment: usually by treating the cause. If this is fever, then sponging the patient with tepid water to reduce the temperature will help. Fluid intake and nutrition must be maintained, and if the cause is withdrawal from alcohol dependence, sedation may be required.

Causes and risk factors: a wide range of metabolic disorders, postpartum (after childbirth) or postoperative stress, ingestion of toxic substances (including alcohol), physical or mental stress or exhaustion may all cause delirium.

dementia

Description: mental impairment, caused by a variety of diseases, leading to a permanent deterioration of the brain.

Persons most commonly affected: adults over 60 of both sexes.

Organ or part of body involved: brain.

Symptoms and indications: increasing forgetfulness, especially of recent events, confusion, unpredictable behaviour, loss of interest in events and personal appearance and poor judgement.

Treatment: neurological examination to determine the cause of the dementia. The only help that can be given is in providing care and attention for the sufferer.

Causes and risk factors: the cause is unknown. If the person affected is young or middle-aged, the cause may be ALZHEIMER'S DISEASE.

dengue

Description: also known as break-bone fever or dandy-fever, this is a tropical fever.

Persons most commonly affected: all ages and both sexes.

Organ or part of body involved: skin and joints.

Symptoms and indications: these occur in two stages. In the first, there are normally joint pains, fever, extreme weakness and headache. This is then followed by a day or two of remission and then the fever returns, usually accompanied by a rash.

Treatment: the joint pains can usually be relieved with aspirin, sometimes used together with codeine, although in severe cases, pethidine may be used. Calamine lotion eases the rash. Bed rest is needed and fluid intake should be kept up. In some cases, the fever may return more than once, and the weakness and joint pains may take months to disappear.

Causes and risk factors: the virus causing the fever is transmitted to man by the mosquito *Anopheles*. In areas where there is a risk of being bitten by these mosquitoes, use of an insect repellent and mosquito nets should help to reduce the risk.

dermatitis

Description: an inflammation of the skin that can have many different causes. If the cause is an allergic reaction to something, this form of dermatitis is usually called ECZEMA.

Persons most commonly affected: all ages and both sexes.

Organ or part of body involved: skin.

Symptoms and indications: the skin turns red and in some cases may be itchy. The skin may develop small blisters.

Treatment: the first line of treatment must be to remove the cause of the dermatitis. This may be contact with a substance that irritates the skin (contact dermatitis) or sunlight (light dermatitis). In mild cases, an application of calamine lotion may be sufficient to bring relief, but in more severe cases a topical (applied to the area being treated) corticosteroid may be used. This is an artificial hormone preparation that reduces the body's production of antibodies, which lessens inflammation.

Causes and risk factors: contact dermatitis: is caused by contact between the skin and an irritant substance. There are many substances that may irritate the skin, including soaps and detergents; industrial chemicals; some metals, cosmetics and plants, and for babies, urine, causing nappy rash. People who know that their skin is sensitive to a particular substance must try to avoid further contact with it. Light dermatitis: particularly in children, this may have no specific cause, other than a particular sensitivity to sunlight. However,

in many sufferers, the condition is caused either by use of some drugs, or sometimes, a particular chemical in lipstick or a perfume in cosmetics.

diabetes insipidus

Description: a rare disorder of the pituitary gland (a hormone-producing gland in the brain).

Persons most commonly affected: all ages and both sexes.

Organ or part of body involved: pituitary gland and endocrine (hormone) system.

Symptoms and indications: great thirst and passing of large quantities of pale urine. Dry hands and constipation.

Treatment: if caused by tumour, then surgery is needed, otherwise treatment with antidiuretic hormone, or ADH, (a drug that constricts blood vessels and reduces the passing of urine).

Causes and risk factors: lack of ADH, caused by injury, tumour, intracranial (within the head) bleeding, ANEURYSM or KIDNEY DISEASE.

Diabetes mellitus

Description: a condition in which the body cannot use sugar and carbohydrates (starches) from foods, because the pancreas (an organ in the abdomen, producing digestive juices) does not produce enough of the hormone insulin. This means that sugar accumulates in the blood and body tissues, causing defects in various parts of the body.

Persons most commonly affected: usually people under 30, but it may begin at any age. It can also frequently affect the middle-aged and elderly, particularly if they are obese. Both sexes.

Organ or part of body involved: pancreas.

Symptoms and indications: thirst, fatigue, weight loss, and increased appetite and thirst. Frequent urination, itching genitals, boils, and, if advanced, deterioration of vision.

Treatment: aims to restore the blood sugar level to as near normal as possible. In younger people, the condition is usually more severe and the only treatment is with insulin injections to lower blood sugar levels and by control of the diet to regulate the carbohydrate/insulin balance. In older people diet alone may be sufficient.

Causes and risk factors: the causes are mostly unknown, although there seems to be an inherited tendency to developing diabetes. However, it may be triggered by stress or viral infection. Some women develop diabetes during pregnancy, but it normally disappears after the baby's birth. Missing meals may lead to hypoglycaemia (too low a level of glucose in the blood). The sufferer will be hungry and may sweat and become confused. An immediate intake of glucose will usually return them to normal. Too low a level of insulin may lead to coma and death if not corrected. Sufferers of diabetes are at risk of eye and kidney problems, and they have to be very careful to look after their feet, as any foot infection, if not dealt with immediately, may lead to GANGRENE.

diphtheria
Description: a very contagious, but in western countries, very rare, throat infection.
Persons most commonly affected: people over five. Both sexes.
Organ or part of body involved: throat, skin, heart, central nervous system.
Symptoms and indications: early symptoms are a sore throat, fever and swollen neck glands. If untreated, this may lead to airway obstruction, caused by a film forming in the throat, and shock.
Treatment: the first immediate treatment is an injection of antitoxin, and a course of antibiotics. The patient should be quarantined, and bed rest is required. If the disease is in an advanced stage, a tracheotomy (an incision in the trachea or airway) may be required to help breathing.
Causes and risk factors: a bacterial germ causes the disease, but immunization offers protection against infection.

dislocation
Description: a bone wrenched out of place at a joint is said to be dislocated. If the dislocation is minor, it may be called subluxation.
Persons most commonly affected: all ages, both sexes.
Organ or part of body involved: any joint, but most commonly the jaw, shoulder, knee and spine. Some children are born with hip dislocation.
Symptoms and indications: the joint is very painful and swollen and may show bruising. There is usually difficulty in moving the joint.
Treatment: relocation of the joint by a doctor and then immobilization of the joint for a few weeks. Occasionally, surgery may be required, but this is normally only if dislocations happen repeatedly.
Causes and risk factors: dislocation is usually accidental. It may sometimes be caused by a shallow or poorly formed joint surface (usually congenital) or arthritis.

diverticular disease
Description: diverticulosis is a condition where there are diverticulae (small pouch-like swellings through weak points in the wall of the colon). Diverticulitis is the inflammation or infection of diverticulae.
Persons most commonly affected: adults of both sexes, becoming more common with increasing age.
Organ or part of body involved: colon.
Symptoms and indications: there are usually no symptoms of diverticulosis. However, there may be pain in the left side of the lower abdomen and disturbed bowel habit, caused by muscle spasms in the colon. The symptoms of diverticulitis are intermittent cramping in the abdomen, often becoming severe pain. There is often fever and nausea and there may be tenderness of the affected area.
Treatment: a high-fibre diet. X-rays of the colon are usually taken to ensure that the symptoms are not caused by cancer of the colon. If the diverticulae are infected, treatment with an antibiotic is required. If a diverticula has ruptured, surgery to mend the colon is required.
Causes and risk factors: this disease cannot be prevented, but the risk of getting it can be reduced by making sure that the diet is well balanced, with low salt and fat intake and a high fibre intake.

drowning
Description: the immediate after-effects of prolonged submersion in water.
Persons most commonly affected: all ages and both sexes.
Organ or part of body involved: lungs, blood and heart.
Symptoms and indications: there is a lack of spontaneous breathing. The patient has a blue colour and has no pulse.
Treatment: the patient must be removed from the water. If there are any foreign bodies in the mouth, such as weed, mud or false teeth, they must be removed. A check must be made to determine whether the patient is breathing, and whether he or she a pulse or not. Artificial respiration and external cardiac massage (cardiopulmonary resuscitation or CPR) must be started at once if required, and help sent for. The CPR should be kept up until either the patient recovers enough to breathe unaided, in which case they should be put in the recovery position, or until the emergency services arrive to take over.
Causes and risk factors: water entering the lungs. In 15% of cases, submersion in water causes a spasm of the larynx. To avoid drowning accidents, learn

to swim. Do not swim after drinking alcohol, or too soon after eating. Do not swim in deep water to cool down on a hot summer day, as the water may be very cold, resulting in a sudden and disabling cramp. Do not dive or jump into unknown water; there may be underwater obstructions like weed or rocks, or in a swimming pool, underwater hazards. Do not leave small children alone in the bath, or in gardens with ornamental pools, as a child can drown in just a few inches of water. When taking part in water sports-like boating or water-skiing, wear a life jacket.

drug abuse

Description: the misuse of a mood-changing substance for pleasure, often leading to addiction. Some of the most common substances used are nicotine, alcohol (*see* ALCOHOLISM), amphetamines, barbiturates, cocaine, opium alkaloids, glues and solvents, cannabis and psychedelic drugs. Drugs may also be abused by athletes keen to improve their performance. In this case, it is usually stimulants or anabolic steroids.

Persons most commonly affected: all ages (except early childhood) and both sexes.

Organ or part of body involved: central nervous system, blood, liver and kidneys.

Symptoms and indications: these depend on the substance being abused, but most of them give altered behaviour. There may be increased sensitivity to sights and sounds and unpleasant symptoms when the substance is withdrawn. The use of heroin and cocaine makes the pupils of the eyes contract to pinpoints.

Treatment: the first step in treatment has to be the desire of the abuser to stop. Professional help will probably be needed and counselling. In the case of narcotic abuse, a doctor may prescribe methadone, a less potent drug, to decrease the severity of withdrawal symptoms.

Causes and risk factors: drug abusers risk accidental injury while under the influence of the substance. They risk serious infections if using non-sterile needles for injected drugs, such as HEPATITIS, BLOOD POISONING and HIV. There is a high risk of death caused by overdose, and body organs may suffer irreversible damage. There is also a high risk of losing their job, friends, home and family.

duodenal ulcer

Description: an ulcer (a breach of the membrane,

which does not heal easily) in the duodenum (the tube between the outlet of the stomach and the small intestine).

Persons most commonly affected: adults and both sexes, but especially those of blood group O, or those with a family history of duodenal ulcers.

Organ or part of body involved: duodenum.

Symptoms and indications: a burning, gnawing pain below the ribs. It may wake the sufferer in the early hours. There is usually pain one to two hours after meals, which continues until the next meal and is only relieved by milk, antacids (medicines that reduce the acidity of the stomach) and food.

Treatment: stopping smoking, antacids, barium meal, possibly surgery.

Causes and risk factors: stress. Excess acid. Smoking.

dysentery (amoebic and bacillary)

Description: an inflammation of the intestine, especially the colon, caused by bacteria (bacillary dysentery) or protozoa (amoebic dysentery).

Persons most commonly affected: all ages and both sexes.

Organ or part of body involved: digestive tract, but especially the colon.

Symptoms and indications: bacillary dysentery: severe diarrhoea, with the passage of blood and mucus. There may be nausea, cramp and fever, and the symptoms may last for about a week. Amoebic dysentery: symptoms may appear within a week of infection, or may take years to appear. The onset is very gradual, with weight loss, ANAEMIA and indigestion, and eventually, passing of bloody stools.

Treatment: bacillary dysentery; bed rest, rehydration with plenty of water, and great care to ensure that any soiled clothing or bedding is either destroyed or thoroughly cleaned and disinfected. Amoebic dysentery; treatment with nitroimidazole drugs, followed by diloxamide furoate.

Causes and risk factors: bacterial dysentery is caused by infection from bacteria, amoebic by infection by protozoa. Both can be avoided by protecting food from flies, avoiding contaminated water and taking care to see that sanitation is good. Known carriers of either disease should not be allowed to handle food. Complications in bacillary dysentery only occur in severe cases, when the intestine may perforate and bleed. This may also happen with amoebic dysentery, where there is also a risk of abscesses forming in the liver, brain, bone or testes.

E

eclampsia of pregnancy

Description: convulsions (fits) arising in pregnancy.

Persons most commonly affected: females during pregnancy.

Organ or part of body affected: cardiovascular system (blood system).

Symptoms and indications: an early sign is raised blood pressure, with headaches and marked swelling of the ankles. (Slight swelling of the ankles is quite common in the advanced stages of pregnancy.) There may be an unexplained weight gain. The condition can be confirmed by the presence of protein in the urine. If untreated, convulsions will follow. The condition is usually discovered when the mother is in the early stages of the disease, when it is called PRE-ECLAMPSIA.

Treatment: bed rest is necessary, with careful monitoring of the foetus. If the condition is severe, an emergency Caesarian section may be required.

Causes and risk factors: these are unknown. It is more likely to happen in a first pregnancy, or where the mother is older. The mother may also be obese, have had previous HYPERTENSION or have DIABETES MELLITUS. She may also be carrying twins, or a Rhesus-incompatible baby. No hereditary link has been established but it is recommended that a pregnant woman inform her midwife or doctor of any history of the condition in her family.

ectopic pregnancy

Description: a pregnancy where the fertilized egg grows outside the uterus, usually in one of the Fallopian tubes joining the ovary to the uterus. As the egg grows, it stretches the tube and eventually ruptures it.

Persons most commonly affected: females during pregnancy.

Organ or part of body involved: usually Fallopian tubes.

Symptoms and indications: if a period is two to three weeks overdue, sudden severe pain in the abdomen. Sometimes, there is less severe pain and bleeding from the vagina. If no action is taken at this stage, there may finally be collapse from bleeding into the abdomen.

Treatment: immediate admission to hospital for surgery to remove the affected tube. If the blood loss has been large, a blood transfusion will be necessary.

Causes and risk factors: an ectopic pregnancy is more likely to happen if the Fallopian tube has suffered previous damage from infection. It is also more likely if there is a contraceptive coil in the uterus. As only one tube is affected by an ectopic pregnancy, it is still possible to conceive again.

eczema

Description: an inflammation of the skin, usually caused by allergy. Eczema is a form of DERMATITIS. The most common forms of eczema are atopic or infantile eczema and discoid eczema.

Persons most commonly affected: all ages and both sexes.

Organ or part of body involved: skin.

Symptoms and indications: atopic eczema: this usually starts at the age of three to four months. Reddening of the skin starts on the scalp, spreading to the face and in some cases to other parts of the body. The skin erupts with small spots, which weep and are very itchy. Approximately 70% of children affected by this form of eczema have a family history of ASTHMA, HAY FEVER or eczema. Discoid eczema: in this form of eczema, small coin-shaped patches of skin develop itchy blistered skin. This is more common in young adults or middle life.

Treatment: atopic eczema: the application of 1% hydrocortisone ointment may be prescribed, and if the itching is very severe, a sedative to prevent the sufferer scratching. Discoid eczema: a prescription for coal tar ointment may help the itching.

Causes and risk factors: atopic eczema is usually inherited and the cause of discoid eczema is unknown.

embolism

Description: blocking of a small blood vessel, usually by a THROMBOEMBOLISM, but occasionally by fat after a bone fracture, or by air after an injection or a diving accident. It is usually in the lung (a PULMONARY EMBOLISM), but may be elsewhere.

Persons most commonly affected: all age groups and both sexes.

Organ or part of the body involved: circulatory system.

Symptoms and indications: for a pulmonary embolism, these are shortness of breath, a sudden cough and chest pain that may be slight to very severe. Sometimes the lips turn blue (cyanosis), or there may be blood in the sputum. In severe cases, there may be symptoms of SHOCK or unconsciousness.

Treatment: X-rays are taken to check the position of the embolism, and anticoagulants are given to prevent further clots. In severe cases, a patient may be admitted to hospital for oxygen and anticoagulant therapy, and sometimes surgery may be needed to remove the clot.

Causes and risk factors: it occurs most often after surgery and other treatment involving long stays in bed. It can be partially prevented by moving about as soon as possible after surgery, childbirth or injury. For some operations that carry a higher risk, anticoagulants may be prescribed before treatment. People who have had previous emboli may take regular anticoagulants. Large embolisms can cause sudden death, medium embolisms usually heal, leaving no permanent disability and small embolisms are usually harmless and often heal without their presence being recognized.

emphysema

Description: overinflation of the tiny air sacs in the lungs, which can rupture to form larger sacs. Over time the total surface area available for gaseous exchange is diminished and so less oxygen is available for the body.

Persons most commonly affected: older people of both sexes.

Organ or part of body involved: lungs.

Symptoms and indications: wheezy breathing and shortness of breath, which is even worse after exercise. In severe cases, the patient may become blue, bloated and 'barrel-chested'.

Treatment: oxygen may help and antispasmodics may be of use during attacks of breathlessness.

Causes and risk factors: almost all cases of emphysema are caused by smoking, giving rise to BRONCHITIS. Nothing can be done to reduce existing damage to the lungs. Since a reduced level of oxygen reaches the blood from the damaged lungs, strain may be put on the heart.

encephalitis

Description: inflammation of the brain.

Persons most commonly affected: all age groups and both sexes.

Symptoms and indications: initial symptoms include fever, headache and neck stiffness, generalized aches and pains, fatigue, weakness and irritability. As the condition worsens, the affected person may become confused and disorientated and there may be convulsions, paralysis and eventually coma. Anyone with the symptoms of encephalitis requires emergency medical attention as it is a serious, life-threatening condition.

Treatment: Although there is no specific treatment for encephalitis the condition can be improved by relieving the pressure around the brain (it is increased pressure caused by the inflammation that causes the symptoms). Admittance to hospital is necessary for intensive medical and nursing care.

Causes and risk factors: encephalitis is most commonly caused by a viral infection of the brain which can also lead to the inflammation of the meninges and the development of MENINGITIS. It can also be a complication of a number of infectious diseases such as measles and chicken pox. Japanese encephalitis is caused by the bite of an infectious mosquito. There is a risk of permanent brain damage resulting from the condition.

endocarditis

Description: inflammation of the endocardium (the inner lining of the heart).

Persons most commonly affected: all age groups and both sexes, but bacterial endocarditis is very rare before the age of five.

Organ or part of body involved: heart.

Symptoms and indications: sometimes shows as an unexplained fever, and there are symptoms of HEART BLOCK and/or EMBOLISM.

Treatment: antibiotic therapy.

Causes and risk factors: caused by bacterial or viral infection, usually in a previously damaged heart. This damage may be congenital ('hole in the heart') or caused by RHEUMATIC FEVER. The infection enters the bloodstream and is carried to the damaged heart. This can occur most easily during dental treatment involving extractions or scaling. The condition can be prevented if the dentist is informed and a course of antibiotics taken before treatment. Recovery from endocarditis is not certain.

endometriosis

Description: a condition where cells from the endometrium (the lining of the uterus) are found elsewhere in the body, usually in the Fallopian tubes, ovaries or uterine muscle.

Persons most commonly affected: menstruating females between puberty and menopause.

Organ or part of body involved: reproductive organs, and sometimes bowel.

Symptoms and indications: pelvic pain, often of long duration, usually worse during menstruation. Lower back pain, heavy periods and pain during sexual intercourse.

Treatment: surgery or hormone treatment.

Causes and risk factors: causes are unknown, but the condition may lead to infertility or pelvic cysts.

entropion

Description: inward turning of the eyelid, causing the eyelashes to rub and irritate the cornea.

Persons most commonly affected: both sexes, usually older people.

Organ or part of body involved: eyelid.

Symptoms and indications: sore, watering, red eyes.

Treatment: involves admittance to hospital for surgery to correct the condition.

Causes and risk factors: may be caused by inflammation or scarring following injury, but is usually caused by spasms or slackening of the eyelid muscle, which can occur as the muscles age.

epiglottitis

Description: a relatively rare inflammation and swelling of the epiglottis (the cartilage separating the back of the tongue and the entrance to the airway, which closes off the airway when swallowing).

Persons most commonly affected: both sexes, usually children aged one to six, but may occur in other age groups.

Organ or part of body involved: epiglottis.

Symptoms and indications: fever, noisy difficult breathing, cough, excessive saliva and rapid pulse developing quickly over a few hours.

Treatment: admission to hospital and antibiotic therapy. If obstruction to breathing is severe, the patient may be need to be intubated (have a tube inserted into the airway) or in very severe cases a tracheotomy (an incision into the trachea) may be necessary. Oxygen is usually given.

Causes and risk factors: it is caused by a bacterial infection, but it is rarely transferred between children.

epilepsy (or **falling sickness**)

Description: a neurological disorder characterized by the occurrence of CONVULSIONS or seizures and a loss of consciousness or momentary loss of awareness.

Persons most commonly affected: all age groups and both sexes. Usually, it starts in children between the ages of 2 and 14 and quite frequently below the age of 5.

Organ or part of body involved: brain.

Symptoms and indications: there are several forms of epilepsy and usually the symptoms arise suddenly. Occasionally, the person has a warning that an attack is about to occur. This is called *aura epileptica* and takes the form of odd or unpleasant sensations of sound, sight or smell, a change of mood, or pain or trembling in the muscles.

Grand mal seizure: this affects all age groups and involves a sudden loss of consciousness. The person falls to the ground, the muscles are stiff and he or she has a rapid pulse, poor pallor and dilated pupils. The body is then thrown into spasm by violent jerking of the muscles. The person may gnash the teeth, bite the tongue and froth at the mouth, and the eyes roll in the head. Breathing is noisy and the person may lose control of the bladder and bowel function. The attack usually lasts up to a few minutes and the body then relaxes. The person may regain consciousness to a certain extent but is usually very confused and soon falls into a deep sleep that may last for a few hours. On waking, the person may be restored to normal or feel tired, subdued and depressed.

Petit mal seizure: this often occurs in children and is characterized by a loss of awareness. The person suddenly stops the activity in which he or she is engaged and looks blank and is not aware of his or her surroundings. There may be some odd muscular movements or changes of expression. The attack lasts for a very short time and the person usually comes round and resumes previous activity, often being unaware of the episode.

Temporal lobe epilepsy: the affected person suddenly changes and behaves in an abnormal and inappropriate way, becoming angry or aggressive or agitated. Such behaviour is unusual and abnormal for that person.

Focal epilepsy: one part of the body is thrown into muscular spasm, although this may spread to involve the whole body, but there is no loss of consciousness.

A person who has an epileptic seizure requires immediate medical attention.

Treatment: is tailored to each individual's requirements and the person will require monitoring and periodic check-ups. Various anticonvulsive drugs are used to control epilepsy, including phenytoin, primidone, methoin, clonazepam, sodium valproate and carbamazepine. The type and dose that is most effective varies between individuals. A person who suffers from epilepsy should not drink alcohol and may not be allowed to drive until two years have passed without an attack. Usually, seizures can be prevented and controlled and a person suffering from epilepsy can expect to lead a normal life. However, the condition generally cannot be cured except in those cases where surgery or other treatment can correct a brain disorder.

Causes and risk factors: there are a number of different causes, including brain injury, tumour or inflammation, and infection, disorders of metabolism such as hypoglycaemia, brain haemorrhage and birth trauma. Many people suffer a fit or convulsions at some stage in life, but most do not develop epilepsy.

erythema

Description: any one of a number of skin conditions, characterized by the engorgement of superficial blood vessels and the appearance of red inflamed patches. Types include *erythema ab igne, erythema pernio* (*see* CHILBLAIN), *erythema nodosum, erythema multiformae* and *erythema infectiosum* ('slapped-cheek' disease).

Persons most commonly affected: all age groups and both sexes depending upon type.

Organ or part of body involved: skin, especially legs, arms, hands, face.

Symptoms and indications: erythema ab igne—red inflammation of the legs in a network pattern caused by sitting too close to a fire. Erythema nodosum—more common in females, and characterized by the appearance of painful, red nodules and swellings, which are quite large and usually occur on the lower legs. There may be fever, malaise and swollen, painful ankles and knees. Erythema multiformae—more common in children and young people, especially girls. Red blotches, lumps and blisters appear on the hands, arms and body but the characteristics vary.

Erythema infectiosum—affects children, especially during the months of spring. A bright red rash appears on the cheeks and spreads to other parts of the body. It usually subsides after about three weeks. A person with symptoms of erythema should seek medical advice.

Treatment: depends to a certain extent on the cause and type of erythema and the severity of symptoms. Corticosteroid or non-steroidal anti-inflammatory drugs may be prescribed, along with analgesics. Preparations for bathing affected skin may be recommended along with rest and avoiding extremes of heat and cold.

Causes and risk factors: erythema nodosum—allergic reaction to certain drugs (sulphonamides) and bacterial infections e.g. streptococcus, mycobacterium tuberculosis and sarcoidosis. Erythema multiformae—allergic reaction to the use of some drugs e.g. barbiturates and sulphonamides or caused by a virus. Erythema infectiosum—highly contagious and thought to be caused by a virus.

erythroderma

Description: also known as exfoliative DERMATITIS. It is an abnormal thickening and flaking of the skin.

Persons most commonly affected: both sexes, but three times more common in men than women. It is rare before the age of 50.

Organ or part of body involved: skin.

Symptoms and indications: red patches of skin, which gradually thicken and then peel.

Treatment: corticosteroids.

Causes and risk factors: it occurs half the time in people with existing skin conditions, usually chronic ECZEMA or PSORIASIS. In a third of cases, there is no cause. For the rest, the condition may be as a result of HODGKIN'S DISEASE or LEUKAEMIA.

erythromelalgia

Description: also called red NEURALGIA. It is a condition of red or purple blotches on fingers or toes, which are warm and painful.

Persons most commonly affected: both sexes, mainly middle-aged.

Organ or part of body involved: skin.

Symptoms and indications: a burning sensation and red blotches on hands and feet, occasionally spreading to limbs. It can last for a few minutes to several hours.

Treatment: reduction in temperature by the use of fans and removal of clothes or bedclothes that have triggered the attack. Aspirin usually gives relief.

Causes and risk factors: it may be without cause, but is often associated with HYPERTENSION (high blood pressure). Prevention includes keeping hands and feet cool in summer and by staying out of the sun, and not wearing thick socks or gloves in winter.

Ewing's sarcoma

Description: a rare, very malignant cancer of bone.

Persons most commonly affected: both sexes, children and young adults.

Organ or part of body involved: bone, usually starting in limbs or pelvis.

Symptoms and indications: pain, swelling and tenderness. There may be a high temperature, and the white blood cell count may be raised.

Treatment: irradiation and chemotherapy. Surgical amputation of a limb may be necessary in some cases.

Causes and risk factors: males are more often affected than females and it occurs at a younger age than any other bone tumour, peaking between the ages of 10 and 20 years. Combined therapy results in the cure of over 60% of cases, with localized Ewing's sarcoma.

exophthalmos

Description: forward displacement of one or both eyeballs. Also called 'pop eyes'.

Persons most commonly affected: both sexes, but ten times more common in women than in men. All ages, but most common in the third decade.

Organ or part of body involved: eyeball.

Symptoms and indications: protruding eyes.

Treatment: surgery may be necessary to remove a blood clot, tumour or ANEURYSM. Drugs may be prescribed if the cause is an infection or HYPERTHYROIDISM.

Causes and risk factors: causes include thyrotoxicosis (GRAVES' DISEASE) or a tumour pushing onto the eyeball (in this case, it is only ever one eye).

F

fascioliasis

Description: a disease caused by the liver fluke, *Fasciola hepatica*, which affects the liver and bile ducts.

Persons most commonly affected: all ages and both sexes.

Organ or part of body involved: liver and bile ducts.

Symptoms and indications: the disease is diagnosed by finding eggs of *Fasciola* in the stools. The symptoms include fever, loss of appetite, indigestion and abdominal pain, nausea and vomiting, diarrhoea and coughing. It is possible that the liver may be damaged in more serious or prolonged cases, and there may also be jaundice.

Treatment: most cases are mild and treatment with the drugs chloroquine and bithionol leads to recovery. Emetine may also be used although this can itself irritate the stomach. The most important treatment is preventative, e.g. wild watercress should never be eaten.

Causes and risk factors: the liver fluke is found in cattle and other herbivores and the disease is passed to man via snails. Eggs from the parasite pass out in the faeces of the animal. The eggs are taken up by snails and a larval stage is deposited on vegetation, especially wild watercress, which if eaten causes infection and a renewal of the parasite's life cycle.

favism

Description: a type of haemolytic ANAEMIA, i.e. anaemia caused by the breakdown of red blood cells by the body's own system, but sooner than would normally occur (which is usually at the end of the 'life span' of a red blood cell).

Persons most commonly affected: there is a particular geographic pattern to the disease, those affected most being in Iran, parts of the Mediterranean, a high proportion of Yemenite Jews in Israel and some AfricanAmericans.

Organ or part of body involved: blood.

Symptoms and indications: anaemia with the symptoms fever, headache, dizziness, vomiting, JAUNDICE, diarrhoea.

Treatment: blood transfusion in the case of severe anaemia.

Causes and risk factors: favism is brought on by eating a particular broad bean (*Vicia fava*) because a chemical in the bean causes the haemolysis (breakdown of the red blood cells). However, it only occurs when the affected person has an inherited genetic defect resulting in the absence of an enzyme, glucose-6-phosphate dehydrogenase, which would otherwise protect the red blood cells. The defect is sex-linked and, because it also carries increased resistance against MALARIA, it tends to be perpetuated.

A similar reaction can also occur with the antimalarial drugs primaquine and pamaquine, and other compounds such as sulphonamides and some vitamin K analogues.

fever

Description: a rise in body temperature above normal (37.4°C orally, 37.6°C rectally). Also called pyrexia.

Persons most commonly affected: may affect all ages and both sexes.

Organ or part of the body involved: any part of body may be involved.

Symptoms and indications: at the outset a fever is frequently marked by shivering that can become quite violent. In addition, in the early stages there is accompanying headache, sickness, thirst, diarrhoea or constipation, and possibly back pains. This is usually followed by an increase in pulse and breathing, hot dry skin, a marked thirst and loss of appetite and reduced urination. In severe cases where the body temperature continues to rise, there will be DELIRIUM. Loss of strength and some wasting of muscles may occur in prolonged cases.

Treatment: because a fever is a symptom of another condition or illness, it is vital that the underlying condition is treated. At the same time, some steps may be taken in an attempt to reduce the body temperature directly. The affected person may be sponged with tepid water or placed in a bath in which the water temperature is gradually lowered.

Certain antipyretic drugs, such as paracetamol and quinine, act on the controlling centres of the brain causing greater heat loss through the skin.

Causes and risk factors: fevers are caused primarily by viral or bacterial infections and may occur with any infection, however minor. Fever is the primary outcome of many diseases caused by a toxin in the system e.g. scarlet fever or typhoid, and the toxins are produced by bacteria in the body. Fever may also be associated with tumours, autoimmune diseases or SHOCK.

The risk increases in cases of poor nutrition, in areas with poor sanitation, or where there is polluted water. Delirium occurs above a body temperature of 40.5°C. Excessive fever or hyperpyrexia occurs at 41.1°C and is regarded as dangerous while death usually results if the temperature remains above 41.7–42.2°C.

fibroid

Description: a benign (noncancerous) growth of cells in the wall of the uterus.

Persons most commonly affected: menstruating women over 30. Fibroids do not form after the menopause.

Organ or part of body involved: uterus.

Symptoms and indications: quite often there are no symptoms. However, there may be pain and excessive menstrual bleeding; also more frequent menstruation, bleeding between periods and an increase in vaginal discharge. There may be anaemia.

Treatment: small fibroids may be enlarged by contraceptive pills that have a high oestrogen content, so it may be necessary to change this contraceptive method. If fibroids are troublesome, causing bleeding, discomfort, etc., then they are usually removed surgically. This can be done without removing all of the uterus, but sometimes this is necessary. In addition, if blood loss associated with the fibroids is high, an iron supplement may be necessary.

Causes and risk factors: the cause of fibroids is unknown, but they may be hereditary, and their growth may be enhanced by contraceptive pills containing oestrogen.

In a very small number of cases there may be a malignant change that is indicated by rapid growth. However, this is very rare, occurring in under 0.5% of cases.

fibrositis

Description: also called muscular rheumatism. An inflammation of muscles, particularly in the back, that may also affect the chest, shoulders, arms, hips or thighs. The term fibrositis is to some extent being superseded by fibromyalgia.

Persons most commonly affected: adults, usually over 30 years. It tends to be more common in females.

Organ or part of body involved: muscles.

Symptoms and indications: a gradual onset of stiffness and pain with sudden muscle spasms that can be quite painful. There are tender points, or nodules, which are sensitive to touch. Associated symptoms include fatigue, loss of sleep, IRRITABLE BOWEL SYNDROME symptoms and anxiety.

Treatment: the application of heat to specific areas can help relieve pain whether by means of hot baths, showers, heat lamps or other methods. In addition, gentle massage, exercises and more sleep (encouraged by medication) will all help. In some cases, aspirin may ease discomfort and injection of a local anaesthetic (such as lignocaine) with hydrocortisone can be applied to tender points.

Causes and risk factors: the cause is unknown but there are certain conditions or circumstances that may stimulate the condition. These include stress or trauma, exposure to cold or dampness, muscle injury or a viral infection. Also it may be associated with another disease that causes joint inflammation, such as RHEUMATOID ARTHRITIS. Cases of localized fibrositis develop in men who suffer a strain due to their occupation or participation in sport.

fistula

Description: a channel or connection between an organ or similar natural cavity and the surface, or between two organs or cavities, where no such connection should exist.

Persons most commonly affected: no one group is more susceptible than another.

Organ or part of body involved: depends on the site, commonly the anus.

Symptoms and indications: there are several types of fistula but the commonest is the anorectal, where the connection is from the anal canal to the skin. It may follow a history of abscesses with some discharge. A urinary fistula causes urinary infections and may connect with the skin or elsewhere e.g. uterus, vagina, small intestine or abdominal wall. A salivary fistula causes saliva to run out onto the cheek instead of into the mouth, and an arteriovenous fistula (i.e. a connection between an artery and a vein) will cause arterial or venous insufficiency and a warm mass can be felt if near the surface.

Treatment: in all cases, surgery is the first choice for treatment. In some cases, such as the anorectal fistula, this can be quite difficult if the condition has been present for some time. The operation restores the natural connection and when this is achieved, the fistula heals quite quickly. However, in the case of an anorectal fistula, healing is slowed and complicated by the entrance of material into it from the bowel.

Causes and risk factors: there are numerous causes. It may be congenital but usually is due to injury or illness. An anorectal fistula generally forms due to an abscess and a urinary fistula may occur in women following an injury during a prolonged delivery. Blockage of the salivary duct may lead to a salivary fistula.

food poisoning

Description: poisoning resulting from eating contaminated foods or ingesting poisonous chemicals, fungi or berries. *See also* BOTULISM.

Persons most commonly affected: both sexes and all ages.

Organ or part of body involved: primarily the digestive system.

Symptoms and indications: in general, food poisoning results in nausea and vomiting, diarrhoea, abdominal pain and possibly headache and fever. The symptoms and the time of onset vary with the type of food poisoning, but will usually commence between one and twenty-four hours of intake.

Staphylococcal food poisoning from meat, milk or egg products generates symptoms abruptly within two to eight hours and the attack is usually short-lived (three to six hours) with complete recovery. Only susceptible individuals (young, chronically ill or the elderly) are likely to be at risk. *Clostridium perfringens* is associated with food poisoning from meat and meals that are reheated, and symptoms are produced within eight to twenty-four hours.

Numerous species of *Salmonella* cause food poisoning with symptoms following eight hours to three days after ingestion. Such infections are found in the meat and/or milk of domesticated cows, pigs and poultry and also in uncooked or lightly cooked hen's eggs.

Treatment: in the main, treatment is more preventative than curative, i.e. affected foods should be avoided and preparation and storage of foods should comply with good practice and appropriate regulations. Depending upon the severity of the attack, treatment may just involve bed rest, or, if there is severe vomiting, intravenous infusions of electrolytes may be required. Thereafter, the diet should be bland until recovery is assured.

Causes and risk factors: *Salmonella* (and also *Listeria*) are bacteria causing the symptoms. Although the animals mentioned above may be infected, they do not necessarily display symptoms, but products made from them create the poisoning. *Salmonella* are generally killed by heating to 60°C for about 15 minutes. Staphylococcal and clostridial food poisoning are caused by toxins released by the bacteria and in these cases, heating does not destroy either the toxin (staphylococcal) or the bacteria (clostridial). It is therefore essential that hygienic conditions prevail at all stages of food production.

Although the number of outbreaks of food poisoning has increased over recent years, it is not usually a fatal condition, but certain groups of people will be at greater risk, i.e. babies and the very young, pregnant women, the elderly and the chronically ill.

Friedreich's ataxia

Description: a hereditary disease producing gradual degeneration of the nerve cells of the spinal cord and brain.

Persons most commonly affected: usually children, between the ages of five and fifteen.

Organ or part of body involved: spinal cord and brain.

Symptoms and indications: intitial symptoms include an unsteady walk and loss of the knee-jerk reflex, followed by slurring and other speech difficulties. Progressively, the disease causes some tremor, severe arching of the feet and spinal deformity (curved spine). There may also be progressive heart disease. The sufferer may live for 20 to 30 years, the symptoms becoming gradually worse, leaving the individual quite helpless.

Treatment: there is no treatment.

Causes and risk factors: the disease is caused by a recessive gene on chromosome nine.

frostbite

Description: damage to tissue caused by exposure to freezing conditions.

Persons most commonly affected: no one particular group.

Organ or part of body involved: the extremities: toes, fingers, etc.

Symptoms and indications: the first symptoms of frostbite are when the affected area, be it toes, fingers or face, goes white and numb and all feelings of cold or pain disappear. As the severity of the condition worsens, there can be blisters on the frozen area, with a hardening and blackening of the skin. Swelling of the tissue produces tingling and sometimes severe pain. In very serious cases, the affected part becomes swollen and discoloured (blue/grey) and infection may set in.

Associated symptoms include shivering, slurred speech and possible loss of memory.

Treatment: shelter should be found immediately. The affected area should *not* be massaged, but warmed by putting in warm water, clothing or similar, but not by placing near an open fire or by applying direct heat. A general warming of the body may be required, by means of hot drinks and insulation e.g. a sleeping bag. Any blisters should not be opened and the affected area should be cleaned carefully. It may be appropriate to give antibiotics to combat infection and analgesics to relieve pain. Anyone with a badly affected foot should not walk.

Causes and risk factors: frostbite results from the formation of ice crystals in the tissues causing tissue injury or tissue death in an extreme case. It is therefore essential that anyone who may be at risk is well clothed and equipped for the conditions and if frostbite does occur, can seek shelter and assistance quickly. A possible risk is that dead or infected tissue, be it finger, toe, nose or ear, may have to be amputated, but in mild cases (usually called frosting) full recovery is possible.

frozen shoulder

Description: a painful condition in which the shoulder joint becomes stiff.

Persons most commonly affected: usually between the ages of 50 and 70 in both sexes.

Organ or part of body involved: shoulder.

Symptoms and indications: pain and stiffness that limit considerably the normal movement of the joint.

Treatment: there is no particular treatment but gentle exercise may help. An injection of corticosteroid into the joint may also help in some cases.

Causes and risk factors: the cause is not known and the condition usually occurs gradually for no reason. However, it may also develop after a stroke or myocardial infarction (heart attack).

G

gallstones

Description: stones of varying composition that form in the gall bladder. There are three types of stone: cholesterol, pigment and mixed, the latter being the most common. Calcium salts are usually found in varying proportions.

Persons most commonly affected: adults of both sexes but twice as common in women as in men. They are more common with increasing age, hence more prevalent in middle-aged and older people.

Organ or part of body involved: gall bladder and bile ducts.

Symptoms and indications: in many cases, gallstones may be present for years without causing any symptoms. However, when symptoms do occur they include severe pain of a colic type, particularly on the upper right-hand side of the abdomen. The pain may also be felt in the upper part of the back. There may be nausea, vomiting and indigestion. If the stones pass into the common bile duct, the resulting obstruction can cause JAUNDICE. A person having symptoms of gallstones should seek medical advice.

Treatment: gallstones, particularly small ones, may be treated with ultrasound waves to break them up, or drugs may be prescribed (which are derived from bile salts) to dissolve them. The drugs may need to be taken for about two years before the stones disappear and they can produce some side effects. Surgical treatment to remove the gall bladder may be required and this is carried out either by conventional methods or by making small incisions and using fibreoptic instruments (fibreoptic endoscopy). Prior to surgery, during an attack of pain from gallstones, treatment consists of bed rest and taking painkillers until the symptoms subside. Most patients make a good recovery following cholecystectomy (removal of the gall bladder).

Causes and risk factors: the exact cause is unknown but their formation seems to be due to a change in bile composition, rendering cholesterol less soluble. Stones may also form around a foreign body and calcium salts are usually found in varying proportions. Stones are more likely to form if the gall bladder fails to empty effectively or if any infection of the bile ducts has occurred.

gangrene or mortification

Description: death of tissue due to loss of blood supply or bacterial infection. There are two types of gangrene, dry and moist, and gas gangrene, which is caused by a particular type of bacterial infection.

Persons most commonly affected: all age groups and both sexes.

Organ or part of body involved: gangrene can affect any part of the body and is very serious if it involves the main organs within the abdomen. Often, the fingers, hands, arms, toes, feet and legs are the sites most likely to be affected.

Symptoms and indications: dry gangrene—the affected part becomes cold and turns dark red then brown and black, and there is an obvious line between living and dead tissue. This line of demarcation shows as an area of reddening and slight inflammation. There may be a slight smell but no pain or fever, and eventually, the gangrenous part drops off.

Moist gangrene—there is putrefaction (bacterial decomposition of tissue) and an issuing of fluids from the affected tissues, accompanied by an obnoxious smell but not much pain. The affected area becomes swollen and eventually blackened in places. Its extent is not always clear and is likely to spread. The patient is likely to suffer from a serious fever and there is a risk of death from blood poisoning.

Gas gangrene—this occurs when a wound is present that is infected by a particular form of bacterium that produces gas. The bacteria produce toxins that cause decay and putrefaction with the generation of gas. The gas spreads into muscles and connective tissue, causing swelling, pain, fever and, possibly, toxic DELIRIUM. If untreated, the condition quickly leads to death.

A patient with gangrene requires prompt medical treatment, usually in hospital.

Treatment: usually involves amputation and also the taking of antibiotics if infection is involved. The bacteria causing gas gangrene are anaerobic (exist without air or oxygen). Hence, surgical incisions that allow the penetration of air, along with oxidizing agents, antitoxin and penicillin are all used in treatment to prevent the spread of the gangrene. A person can usually be cured if gangrene is treated early, but is left with disfigurement due to amputation.

Causes and risk factors: dry gangrene is caused purely by loss of blood supply and is a late-stage complication of DIABETES MELLITUS, in which ATHEROSCLEROSIS is present. Moist gangrene is caused by bacterial infection, and gas gangrene by infection with soil bacteria of the genus *Clostridium*. Gangrene may occur following injury, particularly crushing of a limb cutting off the circulation. Also, as a result of atherosclerosis and FROSTBITE.

gastric erosion

Description: degeneration and minor ulceration of the lining of the stomach.

Persons most commonly affected: adults of both sexes and all age groups but more common in men.

Organ or part of body involved: stomach.

Symptoms and indications: black stools owing to the presence of blood. Vomiting blood, which may appear red or as black grains (coffee grounds), anaemia. A person with these symptoms should seek prompt medical advice.

Treatment: involves identifying the cause of the problem, often a drug being taken for some other condition, which may then need to be withdrawn and the prescription changed. Iron supplements and preparations to inhibit the production of acid in the stomach may be required. Foods that may irritate the stomach, and alcohol, should be avoided until the lining heals. Recovery is usually good, and healing may take one or two weeks. However, it may return.

Causes and risk factors: the most common cause is a type of drug that is being taken for some other condition, which may erode the stomach lining in susceptible people. Drugs likely to cause this include those prescribed for arthritic conditions or ASTHMA, aspirin, alcohol and non-steroidal anti-inflammatory drugs. Rarely, serious bleeding or even perforation of the wall of the stomach can occur, which require corrective surgery, and are potentially life-threatening, especially in elderly patients.

gastritis

Description: inflammation and/or infection of the stomach lining (mucosa).

Persons most commonly affected: all age groups and both sexes.

Organ or part of body involved: stomach.

Symptoms and indications: symptoms include vomiting, nausea, diarrhoea, abdominal pains, discomfort and tenderness, wind and loss of appetite. There may be feverishness and the person may feel unwell and generally lethargic. Rarely, there may be vomiting of blood or blood in the stools, which are then black in colour. There may be dehydration due to diarrhoea, which can be serious, especially in children. A person with symptoms of gastritis should seek medical advice.

Treatment: depends upon the cause and if it is drugs, alcohol or other irritant substance, then these need to be withdrawn and avoided. Plenty of fluids should be drunk and food avoided on the first day that gastritis begins. The person should carefully and gradually resume a normal diet, avoiding foods that may irritate, and alcohol. Recovery is normally complete within about one week.

Causes and risk factors: causes include excess consumption of alcohol or indigestible foods, drugs that are being taken for some other condition, and viral infection. There is a slight risk of serious bleeding or perforation of the stomach wall, requiring corrective surgery, which are potentially life-threatening, especially in elderly patients.

gastroenteritis

Description: inflammation and infection of the stomach and intestines.

Persons most commonly affected: all age groups and both sexes.

Organ or part of body involved: stomach and intestines.

Symptoms and indications: diarrhoea and sometimes vomiting, nausea, abdominal pains and tenderness, loss of appetite and fever. There may be dehydration if diarrhoea is severe and prolonged. Young children and elderly persons with gastroenteritis should be seen by a doctor, as should any person showing signs of dehydration.

Treatment: an attack of gastroenteritis is normally short-lived, symptoms subsiding after two to five days. The person should rest in bed and avoid all food but take frequent small quantities of water, gradually increasing the amount as diarrhoea and vomiting subside. Children may need sachets of salts, as prescribed by a doctor, added to drinking water. As symptoms subside, very small quantities of easily digestible solid food can be tried and if this is tolerated, a normal diet can be gradually resumed as the appetite returns. If a person, especially a young child or elderly patient, becomes dehydrated, admittance to hospital may be needed so that fluids can be given by intravenous drip. Scrupulous attention should be paid to hygiene (especially washing hands frequently), as the condition is often very contagious. Recovery is usually good, occurring within a short space of time, although it may be two or three weeks before the person regains a normal appetite.

Causes and risk factors: the most common cause is a bacterial or viral infection but also parasites and food poisoning may be responsible. It is common in persons experiencing a total change of environment, as occurs when visiting a different country. Very young children and babies and the elderly are at greatest risk and this condition is a common cause of death where people are crowded together in poor, inadequate housing with inadequate sanitation.

German measles (rubella)

Description: a highly infectious viral disease, occurring mainly in childhood, which is mild in effect.

Persons most commonly affected: children, but can occur in adults.

Organ or part of body involved: skin, respiratory system, glands in neck.

Symptoms and indications: there is an incubation period of two or three weeks before symptoms appear. These include headache, shivering and a sore throat, with a slight fever. There is some swelling of the glands in the neck and soon after a rash of tiny pink spots appears, initially on the face and/or neck and subsequently spreading over the body. The rash disappears in roughly one week but the condition remains infectious for three or four more days. The symptoms are normally mild and it may be difficult to identify the disease in the early stages. Its most marked feature, although short-lived, is the swelling of the neck. A pregnant woman should consult a doctor if concerned about German measles.

Treatment: no specific treatment is necessary other than keeping the child at home until three or four days after the spots have disappeared and the disease is not infectious. The child can be given mild painkillers, if needed, and bed rest if feeling unwell. Plenty of fluids should be drunk and a

normal diet offered. Recovery is usually complete after a week or ten days.

Causes and risk factors: the cause of the disease is a virus and an attack normally confers lifelong immunity. However, German measles poses a risk of foetal abnormalities in the early stages of pregnancy, if the mother catches the infection. The risk is considered to be greatest during the first 16 weeks of pregnancy. Any woman who has not had the disease in childhood and who is considering pregnancy, should be vaccinated, after a lack of immunity has been established by a simple blood test. Young girls are now routinely immunized around the age of 12 or 13. It is a wise precaution for any pregnant woman to avoid German measles.

giardiasis

Description: inflammation of the duodenum (the first portion of the small intestine) and the upper part of the small intestine.

Persons most commonly affected: all age groups and both sexes, most of which occur in people who have recently travelled in Russia or the Middle East.

Organ or part of body involved: small intestine.

Symptoms and indications: sudden copious diarrhoea, nausea and pain in the abdomen, pale, foul-smelling stools that are fatty, and fever. In some cases there may be little diarrhoea and mild abdominal discomfort. A person with these symptoms should seek medical advice.

Treatment: consists of rest and a course of the drug metronidazole or mepacrine, which kills the causal parasite. Alcohol should be avoided and plenty of fluids should be drunk. Strict attention should be paid to hygiene, especially washing the hands. Recovery is normally good and occurs naturally within about one month, but is much quicker with drug treatment.

Causes and risk factors: the cause is the parasite *Giardia lamblia*, which inhabits the small intestine, often without causing harm. It is contracted from drinking untreated water or water that has not been treated to a high standard, or from streams. To prevent infection, any suspect water should be boiled or treated with purifying tablets. Foods such as fruit or salad vegetables should be washed in treated water. Particular care should be taken when travelling abroad, especially if camping.

glandular fever or infectious mononucleosis

Description: an infectious viral disease, the

symptoms and effects of which can be quite long-lasting.

Persons most commonly affected: adolescents of both sexes in mid-teenage years and young adults under 40 years.

Organ or part of body involved: lymph nodes, liver, spleen, throat.

Symptoms and indications: include a sore throat, swelling of lymph nodes in the neck and also in the armpits and groin, and fever. Also, headache, loss of appetite, and fatigue. The liver and spleen may become enlarged, and occasionally jaundice develops. The person feels generally unwell and tired. A person with symptoms of glandular fever should be seen by a doctor. The disease is diagnosed by the large numbers of monocytes (white blood cells) in the blood.

Treatment: consists of rest in bed and the taking of painkillers to relieve symptoms, as advised by the doctor. Plenty of fluids should be drunk and the patient should try to eat a good balanced diet. Complications are normally rare but total recovery may take many weeks, the person often continuing to feel unusually tired.

Causes and risk factors: the disease is caused by the EPSTEIN BARR VIRUS, which is contracted from close physical contact (such as kissing) with an infected person. It is thought to be prevalent in adolescents because their immune system is not fully mature and also due to the nature of transmission. It is more likely to arise when young people are crowded together and sharing living conditions, as in colleges, student flats, military establishments, etc. A rare complication is a ruptured spleen, requiring surgery and recovery in hospital.

glaucoma (open-angle and narrow-angle)

Description: a serious group of conditions affecting the eyes. They are all characterized by high pressure within the eye (intra-ocular pressure) and may result in blindness.

Persons most commonly affected: adults of both sexes aged over 40 years, with those aged more than 60 being at particular risk.

Organ or part of body involved: eye.

Symptoms and indications: open-angle glaucoma or chronic glaucoma—there are no or few symptoms until the condition is well advanced and then the person normally experiences some form of vision disturbance. This may take the form of partial loss, particularly of peripheral vision or blurring of vision, which tends to get worse. The person may perceive halos around lights and have poor vision in the dark. The intra-ocular pressure within the eye is raised but the angle between the iris and cornea stays open. A person with these symptoms should consult a doctor and will need continuing treatment.

Narrow-angle glaucoma or acute glaucoma—symptoms include seeing a halo of coloured light around lamps, blurring of vision, severe pain around eye and throbbing headache. There is increasing interference with vision, the eyeball is hard and tender and the angle between the iris and cornea is closed. The eye may be red and swollen. The symptoms are caused by increasing pressure in the eye because fluid cannot drain away. This condition requires emergency medical treatment in hospital.

Treatment: open-angle glaucoma or chronic glaucoma—treatment consists of the application of eye drops several times a day, and taking tablets, which cause the intra-ocular pressure to fall. Some patients may require a surgical operation, called trabulectomy, which helps fluid to drain from the eye more easily.

Narrow-angle glaucoma or acute glaucoma—treatment consists of admittance to hospital and intensive use of drops and tablets to lower the intra-ocular pressure. Surgery is then required to prevent the condition occurring again.

Glaucoma can be successfully treated and the symptoms controlled if caught early but failure to do this can result in total blindness.

Causes and risk factors: the cause of all types of glaucoma is a restriction in the outflow of fluid (aqueous humour) within the eye, leading to a build-up of pressure, which causes damage to the retina and optic nerve, resulting in visual loss or blindness. The reason why this occurs is not known but genetic (hereditary) factors, stress, smoking and increasing age are likely to increase the risk of a person developing glaucoma. An eye test carried out at regular intervals can detect glaucoma.

glomerulonephritis (acute, postinfectious and chronic)

Description: inflammation of the glomeruli of the kidneys. A glomerulus is a small round knot of blood capillaries that brings water, salts, urea and other waste products to the kidney tubules, so that the material can be filtered and excreted. Each kidney contains about 1,000,000 glomeruli.

Persons most commonly affected: all age groups and both sexes, but most common in children from one to eleven years.

Organ or part of body involved: kidneys.

Symptoms and indications: acute—symptoms include oedema (fluid retention), with swelling and puffiness of the eyelids, face and ankles, raised blood pressure, reduction in the amount of urine passed that contains protein, blood and albumin. The child is likely to feel generally restless and unwell, may be feverish and have pains and headaches, and suffer from vomiting and nausea, with a lack of appetite. Recovery is normally complete but may take several weeks.

Chronic—this is a very serious condition and the symptoms are those of renal failure. There is nausea and vomiting, pains in muscles and bones, fatigue and the production of large amounts of urine. The person requires kidney dialysis and, eventually, a kidney transplant. A person with symptoms of glomerulonephritis requires medical treatment and may need admittance to hospital, depending upon the nature and severity of the illness.

Treatment: for the acute condition, treatment is aimed at maintenance of the salt/water balance of the body. While the kidneys are producing small amounts of urine, fluid and salt intake need to be restricted. The amount of fluids drunk can be gradually increased as the kidneys recover and the output of urine becomes greater. It is necessary for the person to rest in bed while symptoms persist, as this maintains a good blood supply to the kidneys. Often penicillin or other antibiotic is needed to kill off the initial throat infection. (*See causes and risk factors*).

The chronic disease usually results from different causes and treatment is by means of dialysis and kidney transplant, necessary because of failure of the kidneys.

Causes and risk factors: the cause of acute glomerulonephritis is the deposition of soluble immune complexes in the walls of the fine capillary blood vessels of the glomeruli. These are formed as a result of the activation of the body's immune system by antigens (substances foreign to the body). The antigens responsible are usually streptococcal bacteria, which have already caused a sore throat. The child usually develops glomerulonephritis two or three weeks after an initial streptococcal throat infection. Hence, there is a potential risk of this condition in respiratory infections known to involve streptococcus bacteria.

goitre

Description: a swelling of the neck due to thyroid gland enlargement. There are four main types: simple or endemic, nodular, lymphadenoid and toxic.

Persons most commonly affected: all age groups and both sexes.

Organ or part of body involved: thyroid gland.

Symptoms and indications: a swelling in the front of the neck that may be soft or firmer, depending upon the type of goitre. A person with symptoms of goitre should seek medical advice.

Treatment: depends upon the type and cause of the goitre. It may be due to a deficiency of iodine in the diet and this is remedied by increasing the intake of iodine. Iodine is necessary for the production of thyroid hormones, which are manufactured by the thyroid gland. Thyroid production is itself regulated by the pituitary gland at the base of the brain. This manufactures and releases thyrotrophin stimulating hormone, which stimulates the thyroid gland to produce its hormones. Simple goitres are treated by thyroid hormone replacement therapy with thyroxine, one of the hormones produced by the thyroid. Treatment for nodular goitre consists of surgery to remove the thyroid gland (thyroidectomy) and that for toxic goitre, as in GRAVES' DISEASE. The treatment for lymphadenoid goitre is with thyroid hormone replacement therapy, with thyroxine.

Causes and risk factors: the cause of simple goitres is overproduction of thyrotrophin stimulating hormone by the pituitary gland, which has the effect of producing thyroid gland enlargement. Lymphadenoid and toxic goitres are examples of autoimmune conditions. For reasons that are not understood, the immune system loses its ability to distinguish between 'self' and 'non-self' and produces antibodies against its own tissues. Lymphadenoid goitres are more likely to occur for the first time in people in their 30s and 40s. Simple goitres often arise at times when there is a greater demand by the body for thyroid hormones, such as at puberty and during pregnancy.

gonorrhoea

Description: the most common venereal disease, which is primarily spread by sexual intercourse, i.e. a sexually transmitted infection.

Persons most commonly affected: young adults of both sexes but can affect any age group.

Organ or part of body involved: men—urethra and possibly spreading to affect bladder, prostate gland and testicles. Women—urethra and reproductive organs. The joints, especially wrists and elbows, ankles and knees, are commonly affected. Occasionally, the blood circulation (blood poisoning), heart valves (ENDOCARDITIS) and eyes (CONJUNCTIVITIS) may be affected. The eyes are affected if infected discharge is accidentally passed to them via the hands or a contaminated towel. (*See causes and risk factors*).

Symptoms and indications: men—burning pain on passing urine, which is cloudy and may contain pus, thick yellowish-green discharge from the penis (gleet), enlargement of glands in the groin. If untreated, fibrous tissue may form causing narrowing of the urethra and difficulty in passing urine. There may be pains in the joints and other organs, the bladder, testicles and prostate gland may become inflamed and tender. Women—may have fewer symptoms than men and these include yellowish-green vaginal discharge (gleet), burning pain on passing urine, which may contain pus. Also the Bartholin's glands (which are sited near the opening of the vagina) often become ulcerated and inflamed. If untreated, the infection and inflammation spreads to the main reproductive organs, the womb, Fallopian tubes and ovaries. The damage is likely to cause infertility and other long-term problems, and occasionally, life-threatening peritonitis from an infected Fallopian tube. A person showing any symptoms of gonorrhoea or who has cause for concern should consult a doctor immediately.

Treatment: the patient is usually referred to a hospital clinic specializing in venereal diseases, and diagnosis is confirmed by examination of a sample of the discharge. Treatment is usually very effective through the taking of penicillin, sulphonamides or tetracycline, and can be cured within one or two weeks. The person may need checks for a few more weeks to make sure that the infection has totally cleared. During the course of treatment, the person should refrain from sexual activity, be scrupulous in personal hygiene and not share towels, etc. The person should wash the hands frequently and especially avoid rubbing or touching the eyes. Sexual partners should be informed.

Causes and risk factors: the cause of the infection is the bacterium *Neiseria gonorrhoea*, which is spread mainly by sexual intercourse but occasionally through contact with infected discharge or underwear, towels, etc. The risk of contracting the infection increases if a person has sexual intercourse with many partners, without the use of condoms, but this is a common disease that can affect anyone. There is a danger of sterility and other complications through spread of the infection within the body, especially if it is not caught and treated in the early stages. A

newborn baby may acquire a serious form of conjunctivitis during its passage through the birth canal if the mother has gonorrhoea. This is called ophthalmia neonatorum and was, until recently, a major cause of blindness.

Preventative measures are obviously important, including the use of condoms and non-promiscuity.

gout

Description: a disorder caused by an imbalance of uric acid (an organic acid containing nitrogen, which is the end product of the metabolism of protein) in the body. It leads to deposition of this substance as salts (urates) of the acid, in the joints, causing inflammation.

Persons most commonly affected: adults of both sexes and all age groups, but particularly men aged over 60. Uncommon below 40 years of age unless there is high incidence within a family.

Organ or part of body involved: joints.

Symptoms and indications: inflammation, swelling, reddening, tenderness and severe pain of infected joints (gouty arthritis). The kidneys may also be damaged, with formation of stones. Deposits of the salts (called 'tophi') may reach the stage where they prohibit further use of the joints, causing hands and feet to be 'set' in a particular position. A person with symptoms of gout should seek medical advice.

Treatment: during an attack treatment is usually by taking colchicine, which relieves the inflammation and pain and has been in use (as colchium) for 3000 years. Prevention of future attacks is by means of drugs that increase the excretion of the waste salts or slow their formation, such as probenecid and allopurinol respectively. Also, analgesic and non-steroidal anti-inflammatory drugs may be prescribed for this condition. The person should rest, keeping weight off the affected joint, until the symptoms of the attack subside. Gout cannot be prevented but symptoms and future attacks can be controlled with medication and treatment.

Causes and risk factors: as stated above, the cause is high-circulating blood levels of uric acid leading to the formation and deposition of urates in the joints. There is often a genetic, family predisposition towards the development of the condition, and this is usually the case in a young person with gout. Some blood diseases such as leukaemia and the use of certain drugs and antibiotics may increase the likelihood of a person developing gout.

Granuloma annulare

Description: a chronic skin disease characterized by the appearance of ring-shaped lesions on the lower limbs, hands and feet.

Persons most commonly affected: children of both sexes aged less than 12 years.

Organ or part of body involved: skin on back of hands, arms, elbows, soles of feet, back of lower legs and knees.

Symptoms and indications: formation of raised papules (bumps) that are reddish in colour, do not itch and are arranged in a ring formation. The shape of the rings may change and alter in size as the condition progresses. A person with symptoms of this condition should seek medical advice.

Treatment: the doctor may prescribe topical steroids in order to hasten the healing of the skin. This condition is self-limiting and heals spontaneously in less than two years but treatment speeds up recovery.

Causes and risk factors: the cause is not known but the risk increases with trauma and injury to the skin such as sunburn.

Graves' disease

Description: a disorder characterized by thyroid gland overactivity (HYPERTHYROIDISM), enlargement of the gland (*see* GOITRE) and protruding eyes.

Persons most commonly affected: all age groups and both sexes but particularly people aged over 30 and more common in women than in men.

Organ or part of body involved: thyroid gland.

Symptoms and indications: the symptoms are goitre, protruding eyes and signs of excess metabolism due to hyperthyroidism (because thyroid hormones control the body's metabolism). These symptoms include nervousness, tremor, hyperactivity, rapid heart rate and palpitations, muscular weakness, breathlessness, intolerance of heat and sweating, irritability and blurring of vision. A person with symptoms of Graves' disease requires medical treatment.

Treatment: this may follow one of three courses. Usually, antithyroid drugs are tried first, which inhibit the production of excess thyroid hormones. These include methimazole, carbimazole and propylthiouricil. These can be effective for about two years but often there is a relapse of the condition. Hence, surgery to remove part or three quarters of the thyroid gland (partial thyroidectomy) may be required and this is usually undertaken if the person has a large goitre. The third type of treatment is by means of radioactive iodine therapy, which is taken as a tasteless clear drink. This tends eventually to make the thyroid gland underactive (hypothyroidism), but this can be easily remedied by taking thyroxine tablets (thyroxine is a hormone produced by the thyroid gland). Hence, after treatment with radioactive iodine, the person will need periodic check-ups for the development of hypothyroidism. In general, treatment of Graves' disease is very successful.

Causes and risk factors: Graves' disease is thought to be an example of an autoimmune disorder. For reasons that are not understood, the immune system loses the ability to distinguish between 'self' and 'non-self' and produces antibodies that attack its own tissues. These mechanisms are responsible for the hyperthyroidism and bulging eyes of Graves' disease. There is a family connection and prevalence of autoimmune thyroid disorders among relatives of people with Graves' disease. If the disease is not properly treated or controlled, life-threatening complications can result, due to the effects on the body's metabolism.

Guillain-Barré syndrome or GBS or infectious or acute idiopathic polyneuropathy or polyneuritis

Description: a severe and often rapidly progressive form of polyneuritis (or polyneuropathy) characterized by the development of a symmetric pattern of muscle weakness and paralysis.

Persons most commonly affected: all age groups and both sexes, especially adults between the ages of 30 and 50.

Organ or part of body involved: nerves and muscles.

Symptoms and indications: muscle weakness, which begins in the lower limbs and moves to the arms and other parts of the body within 72 hours. There may be life-threatening involvement of respiratory muscles leading to paralysis and respiratory failure. There may be blood-pressure changes, heartbeat irregularities and complete paralysis. A person with symptoms of Guillain-Barré syndrome requires immediate emergency medical attention.

Treatment: involves admittance to hospital for intensive nursing and, possibly, artificial respiration. Fluid and salt levels require careful monitoring and adjustment. Patients who are seriously ill are given plasmapheresis (blood is drawn off, plasma is removed and blood cells are then returned to the circulation). Heat is used for the relief of pain and, as soon as possible, massage, physiotherapy and exercise of muscles and joints are started. Various mechanical devices are likely to be needed while paralysis persists.

Causes and risk factors: the cause is unknown but it is thought to be an autoimmune disorder. (A condition in which the immune system loses the ability to distinguish between 'self' and 'non-self' and produces antibodies that attack its own tissues). Guillain-Barré syndrome often develops shortly after a mild infection, routine immunization or surgery. Recovery is prolonged, with many patients still having some weakness even after two or three years.

H

haemolytic disease of the newborn

Description: a serious disease affecting foetuses and newborn babies, which is characterized by haemolysis (destruction of red blood cells).

Persons most commonly affected: newborn babies of both sexes.

Organ or part of body involved: blood.

Symptoms and indications: ANAEMIA, JAUNDICE and oedema (fluid retention), which is called hydrops foetalis. The amount of a pigment called bilirubin, derived from haemoglobin in red blood cells, builds up in the baby's blood and can cause brain damage if left untreated.

Treatment: high levels of bilirubin in the blood are treated with ultraviolet light (phototherapy). In severe cases of the disease, it may be necessary to give the baby an exchange blood transfusion. The whole of the baby's blood is replaced with Rhesus negative blood of the right blood group.

Causes and risk factors: the usual cause is incompatibility between the blood of the mother and that of the baby. Generally, the baby has Rh-positive red blood cells (i.e. they contain the Rhesus factor) while that of the mother is Rh-negative. The mother produces antibodies to the Rh factor present in the foetal blood and these are passed to the foetus in the blood circulation via the placenta. This then causes the destruction or haemolysis of the baby's red blood cells.

The incidence of the disease has been greatly reduced by giving a Rh-negative mother an injection of anti-D immunoglobulin following the birth of a Rh-positive baby. This prevents the formation of the antibodies that would harm a subsequent baby and is also given to Rh-negative women following miscarriages or abortions.

haemophilia

Description: a hereditary disorder of blood coagulation in which the blood clots very slowly. There are two types of haemophilia, due to a deficiency of either one of two coagulation factors in the blood. Haemophilia A is caused by deficiency of factor VIII and haemophilia B by deficiency of factor IX, called Christmas factor. The severity of the disease depends upon how much less of the coagulation factor than normal is present in the blood.

Persons most commonly affected: males; the disease is a sex-linked recessive disorder carried on the X chromosome.

Organ or part of body involved: blood.

Symptoms and indications: the severity of the symptoms depends upon the extent of the deficiency of the coagulation factor. Symptoms are prolonged, severe bleeding following wounds or injury and bleeding into joints, muscles and other tissues. In severe cases, there may be spontaneous internal bleeding and serious bleeding after only a minor wound.

Those less severely affected only bleed seriously after a greater wound or injury. Haemophilia is likely to be diagnosed at an early stage and the child will require ongoing treatment throughout life.

Treatment: is by means of injections of transfusions of plasma containing the missing coagulation factor. Freeze-dried preparations can be kept at home in a refrigerator for reconstitution and injection intravenously, when required. Special pre-operative treatment is required for haemophiliacs needing planned surgery to raise the levels of coagulation factor in the blood. In the past, haemophiliacs suffered great pain due to internal bleeding, which caused deformity of joints and muscles. Many did not survive into adult life. Now, the outlook is good, although the person obviously has to be aware of, and take greater precautions against, the dangers of accidental injury. However, with care, a sufferer can hope to lead a much more normal life.

Causes and risk factors: as stated above, haemophilia is a sex-linked recessive condition carried on the X chromosome; hence, it affects males, with females being the carriers. Half the daughters of a mother carrying the haemophilia gene will also be carriers and half of her sons will be haemophiliacs. The sons of a haemophiliac father and non-carrier mother will not have haemophilia but half of the daughters will be carriers.

haemorrhage

Description: haemorrhage means bleeding—a flow of blood from a ruptured blood vessel, which may occur externally or internally. A haemorrhage is classified according to the type of vessels involved: arterial H—bright red blood spurts in pulses from an artery. Venous H—a darker coloured steady flow from a vein. Capillary H—blood oozes from torn capillaries at the surface of a wound. In addition, a haemorrhage may be primary, i.e. it occurs at the moment of injury. Or, it is classed as reactionary when it occurs within 24 hours of an injury and results from a rise in blood pressure. Thirdly, a secondary haemorrhage occurs after a week or ten days as a result of infection (sepsis). Haemorrhage at specific sites within the body are designated by special names, e.g. haematuria (from the kidney or urinary tract), haemoptysis (from the lungs) and haematemesis (from the stomach).

Persons most commonly affected: all age groups and both sexes.

Organ or part of body involved: any blood vessel.

Symptoms and indications: the symptoms are, obviously, bleeding from the blood vessels involved but this may only be apparent if the haemorrhage is external. Internal haemorrhage may produce a range of symptoms depending upon the part of the body involved and the person is likely to be seriously ill. Haemorrhage from a major artery is the most serious kind, as large quantities of blood are quickly lost and death can occur within minutes from organ failure and SHOCK. A person with a haemorrhage needs emergency medical treatment and admittance to hospital.

Treatment: is aimed at arresting the bleeding. For an external haemorrhage there are four approaches to stopping the bleeding.

1. Direct pressure on the point of the bleeding.
2. Direct pressure on the artery or blood vessel.
3. Raising the wounded part (if a limb).
4. Application of substances (called styptics) to help the blood to clot or to constrict the blood vessels.

Hot water at a temperature between 46° and 49°C and, also, water that is ice cold, can be helpful in this respect.

For internal haemorrhage, it is important to keep the person lying down, as the heart then pumps the blood with less force and the blood pressure is lowered. Also, the patient should be kept calm and warm until emergency medical help arrives. Morphine is often given by injection.

A person with haemorrhage will require further treatment in hospital, which may include surgery and blood transfusions, depending upon the nature of the injury or other cause of the condition.

Causes and risk factors: the most obvious cause of haemorrhage is a wound or other injury. However, there are many others, including ulcers or drugs that may cause inflammation or bleeding in the digestive tract, haemorrhage after childbirth and certain diseases or conditions, such as haemophilia.

haemorrhoids or piles

Description: varicose and inflamed veins around the lower end of the bowel, situated in the wall of the anus. They are classified as internal, external and mixed, depending upon whether they appear beyond the anus.

Persons most commonly affected: adults in middle and older age of both sexes.

Organ or part of body involved: veins at the lower end of the bowel (called the haemorrhoidal veins) in the wall of the anus.

Symptoms and indications: symptoms include bleeding, pain and itching, and the distended vein, may be felt as a lump. Bleeding is generally slight but can occasionally be more persistent and cause anaemia. A person with haemorrhoids should seek medical advice.

Treatment: is by means of creams, injections and suppositories. Attention should be paid to lifestyle, especially the diet and taking regular exercise. It is important to eat a healthy diet containing plenty of fibre and to drink water to avoid constipation. Also, taking regular exercise to improve the blood circulation, and avoiding sitting down for long periods are helpful in preventing and improving piles. In severe cases that do not respond to these measures, admittance to hospital for surgical removal of haemorrhoids may be needed. Symptoms of piles can normally be successfully relieved, although there is a tendency for the condition to recur.

Causes and risk factors: piles are commonly caused by constipation and straining when passing stools, especially in middle-aged and elderly persons. Hence it is important to avoid constipation and a sedentary life style. They are also common in pregnancy, disappearing again after the baby is born. However, piles may be a symptom of other disorders affecting the bowel or blood circulation. They often occur in persons with liver disease, such as CIRRHOSIS, heart and congestive disorders.

hand, foot and mouth disease

Description: a highly contagious viral infection affecting the mucous membranes within the mouth, the feet and hands.

Persons most commonly affected: infants and young children of both sexes.

Organ or part of body involved: mucous membranes of the mouth, throat, feet, especially the toes, and palms of the hands.

Symptoms and indications: painful blisters and ulcers that appear in the areas described. The child often has a sore throat and fever and loss of appetite. A child with hand, foot and mouth disease should be seen by a doctor.

Treatment: consists of bed rest, encouraging the child to drink plenty of fluids and use of pain-relieving drugs such as paracetamol. Sucking ice cubes and eating ice cream or sipping iced drinks will help to relieve the pain from mouth and throat ulcers and help fluid intake. Complete recovery usually takes about four or five days. Special care should be taken with hygiene and washing of utensils used by the child.

Causes and risk factors: the cause of the infection is a virus, the Coxsackie A16 virus, which is highly infectious. Hence, there is usually an outbreak among a number of children and the incubation period, before symptoms appear, is three to five days.

hay fever

Description: an allergic reaction to pollen e.g. that of grasses, trees and many other plants, which affects numerous individuals.

Persons most commonly affected: all age groups and both sexes.

Organ or part of body involved: nose, throat, eyes, respiratory system.

Symptoms and indications: symptoms include a blocked and runny nose, sneezing, watering eyes that are itchy and red and may swell. The person may sometimes wheeze and have slight breathing difficulties. A person with severe symptoms of hay fever should seek medical advice.

Treatment: is by means of antihistamine drugs and if the allergen (the substance causing the symptoms) can be identified, desensitization may be successful. This involves injecting or exposing the individual to controlled and gradually increasing doses of the allergen until antibodies are built up.

Causes and risk factors: the cause of the symptoms is the release of a naturally occurring chemical substance in the body, called histamine. This is widely found throughout all the body tissues and is responsible for the dilation of blood vessels (small arterioles and capillaries) and the contraction of smooth muscle, including that of the bronchi of the lungs.

headache

Description: a pain felt within the head. Most people experience headaches at one time or another and the causes and significance of these vary tremendously. *See* MIGRAINE.

Persons most commonly affected: all age groups and both sexes.

Organ or part of body involved: head.

Symptoms and indications: pain or ache in the head, the site of which varies according to the cause of the headache. A headache is often a symptom of illness or disorder. In this case, it may well be accompanied by other symptoms, such as nausea and vomiting. A person with a severe headache should seek medical advice if the pain persists or if worried in any way.

Treatment: depends upon the underlying cause. If the headache is a symptom of an underlying disease or disorder, then this must be identified and treated. Other forms of headache can be relieved using painkillers such as paracetamol.

Causes and risk factors: there are many causes of headache and some are more serious than others. Common causes are stress, tiredness, feverishness accompanying an infection such as a cold, an excess of close work involving the eyes, dyspepsia (indigestion and digestive disorders), overexposure to hot sun (sunstroke or heatstroke) and hunger. Other more serious causes include uraemia and kidney failure, high blood pressure, rheumatic diseases, GLAUCOMA, brain disorders and infections such as MENINGITIS, encephalitis, small inflammation of the brain, TUMOUR and ANEURYSM. Also, a headache is a common symptom following brain injury or CONCUSSION. The arteries that supply it with blood, meninges (membranes) that cover it and the fibrous partitions within the brain are capable of transmitting the sensation of pain. It is thought that stretching and dilation, or other pressure on the arteries (called the intracranial arteries) may be the cause of headaches due to the disorders or diseases listed above.

head injury

Description: any injury to the head that may or may not be accompanied by a wound or fracture of the skull.

Persons most commonly affected: all age groups and both sexes.

Organ or part of body involved: head.

Symptoms and indications: the danger of a head injury lies with possible damage to the brain itself. Hence, there may be bleeding and swelling if there is a wound, but also other symptoms that indicate that the brain has suffered trauma. These include drowsiness, nausea and vomiting, confusion and memory loss, blurring of vision, lapses into unconsciousness, headaches, effects on the pupils of the eyes and irritability (*see also* CONCUSSION). A person who has suffered a head injury should always be seen by a doctor and may require emergency treatment and admittance to hospital.

Treatment: the person requires admittance to hospital for observation, and may need further treatment, including surgery, depending upon the nature of the injury and development of symptoms.

Causes and risk factors: normally caused by an accident of some sort. It is important to wear proper protective headgear and helmets when taking part in various sporting activities, such as cycling, horse riding, etc.

heart attack *see* coronary thrombosis.

heart block

Description: a condition in which there is a failure in the conduction of electrical impulses from the natural pacemaker (the sinoatrial node) through the heart, which can lead to a slowing of the pumping action. There are three types: in first, degree (partial or incomplete) heart block, there is a delay in conduction between the atria (the two thin-walled, upper chambers of the heart) but this does not cause slowing. In second-degree heart block, there is intermittent slowing because not all the electrical impulses are conducted between the atria and ventricles (the lower thick-walled, muscular main pumping chambers of the heart). In third-degree (or complete) heart block, there is no electrical conduction, the heartbeats are slow and the ventricles beat at their own inbuilt low rhythm.

Persons most commonly affected: men in middle and older age and postmenopausal women. However, can occur in people in younger age groups.

Organ or part of body involved: the electrical conduction system of the heart, which regulates the contraction of heart muscle.

Symptoms and indications: slow, irregular heartbeats, blackouts (Stokes Adams syndrome) and possible heart failure. A person with symptoms of heart block requires medical treatment.

Treatment: for second- and third-degree heart block, treatment involves admittance to hospital and the fitting of an artificial pacemaker that overrides and replaces the natural pacemaker of the heart. Although there can occasionally be a problem with electrical interference to the artificial pacemakers, the treatment is, on the whole, highly successful and abolishes all symptoms.

Causes and risk factors: heart block is more common in elderly people where degenerative changes have occurred (*see* ATHEROSCLEROSIS). However, it is sometimes an inborn (congenital) disorder or may accompany other forms of heart disease, such as myocarditis (inflammation of the heart muscle), CORONARY THROMBOSIS, CARDIOMYOPATHY and heart valve disease. As with many forms of heart disease, risks increase with smoking, a poor diet which is high in salt and cholesterol, stress and lack of fitness and exercise. Also, persons with high blood pressure (HYPERTENSION), DIABETES MELLITUS, an imbalance of salts (electrolytes) within the body and previous heart disease are at a greater risk of developing heart block. The use of certain drugs such as quinidine, digitalis and beta-adrenergic blockers increase the risk of heart block.

heartburn

Description: a burning pain or discomfort felt in the region of the heart and often rising upwards to the throat.

Persons most commonly affected: adults of all ages and both sexes. Pregnant women.

Organ or part of body involved: stomach and oesophagus (gullet).

Symptoms and indications: unpleasant burning sensation in stomach, gullet and throat.

Treatment: the treatment is relieved by taking antacid tablets or alkaline substances such as sodium bicarbonate.

Causes and risk factors: the cause is usually regurgitation of the stomach contents, the burning being due to the acid in the gastric juice. Also, it may be caused by inflammation of the oesophagus (oesophagitis) or ulcers in the oesophagus. In order to prevent heartburn, it is advisable to avoid overeating or food and drink that might lead to an increased production of stomach acid. These foods include spicy curries, acid fruits, alcohol and coffee. The risk of developing heartburn increases with age, obesity, excess consumption of alcohol, poor diet and some drugs, such as aspirin and preparations taken for ARTHRITIS.

heat exhaustion

Description: exhaustion and collapse due to overheating of the body and loss of fluid following unaccustomed or prolonged exposure to excessive heat.

Persons most commonly affected: all age groups and both sexes but more common in elderly persons.

Organ or part of body involved: all body systems.

Symptoms and indications: in the mildest form, which is heat collapse, blood pressure and pulse-rate fall and this is accompanied by fatigue, light-headedness and, possibly, muscular cramps. The person urinates less frequently and is usually pale, but the skin may be moist and the temperature near to normal. A person showing these symptoms should receive treatment immediately and be seen by a doctor.

Treatment: involves rest in the shade away from the sun and taking extra fluids. Drinks of salt solution may be required, or this may need to be given intravenously. Recovery is normally good, occurring in about one or two days.

Causes and risk factors: the cause of heat exhaustion is unaccustomed or prolonged exposure to excessive heat. It is more common in hot climates and results from excessive sweating, leading to loss of fluids and salts and disturbance of the electrolyte balance in body fluids. It can be prevented by gradual acclimatization to the heat, especially if hard physical work is to be carried out, and drinking lots of fluids. The risk increases with gastrointestinal disorders where there has been vomiting and diarrhoea, and if conditions are humid as well as hot. Any illness such as diabetes may make this condition more likely to occur and elderly people should be especially careful (*see also* HEATSTROKE).

heatstroke or heat hyperpyrexia

Description: a severe condition that follows overexposure of the body to excessive heat.

Persons most commonly affected: all age groups and both sexes with elderly persons most at risk.

Organ or part of body involved: all body systems.

Symptoms and indications: failure of sweating and all temperature regulation, headache, muscular cramps, hot, dry skin and high body temperature. The heartbeat rate is rapid, and there is a loss of consciousness, followed by coma and death, which can occur quite quickly. The person requires immediate emergency attention to save his or her life and admittance to hospital.

Treatment: the body is overheated and must be cooled immediately by sponging or immersion in cool water, and fanning. The body may be wrapped in wet sheets. Once the temperature has returned to just above normal (38.9°C), the person should be dried and wrapped in a dry blanket. When consciousness returns, drinks and salt solutions are needed or may have to be given intravenously. Convalescence may take some time and it may not be possible for the person to continue former activities in the prevailing climate.

Causes and risk factors: the cause of the symptoms is loss of fluid and salt through excessive sweating, leading to disruption of the salt/water balance, lowered blood volume, metabolic disturbance and shock. Preventative measures include taking enough time for acclimatization to the heat and increasing the amount of fluids drunk. People who are required to carry out hard, physical work need to drink salt solutions to compensate for the loss that occurs in profuse sweating.

hepatitis

Description: inflammation of the liver due to the presence of toxic substances or infection caused by viruses. Hepatitis may be 'acute', causing a flare-up of symptoms, or chronic, with similar symptoms that persist for years. Other forms of hepatitis are designated A, B, C, D and E, according to the type of virus that causes them. Fulminant hepatitis is a rare and very severe form that is often fatal.

Persons most commonly affected: all age groups and both sexes.

Organ or part of body involved: liver.

Symptoms and indications: acute and chronic hepatitis—symptoms include abdominal pain, JAUNDICE, nausea, itching, malaise and fever. The chronic condition may persist for years and eventually lead to CIRRHOSIS. Hepatitis A (infectious hepatitis) and Hepatitis E—these produce symptoms of fever, sickness, malaise and jaundice. Serum hepatitis (viruses B, C and D)—the symptoms include chills, fatigue, headaches and jaundice.

All these viruses may persist in the blood for a long time and if B is involved, the condition is known as chronic type B hepatitis.

Fulminant hepatitis—the symptoms are very severe with great destruction of liver cells, retention of fluid, unconsciousness, serious jaundice and liver and kidney failure. Coma and death may follow unless a liver transplant can be carried out. A person with any symptoms of hepatitis should always seek immediate medical advice.

Treatment: treatment for many forms of hepatitis includes bed rest and drinking plenty of fluids. Various drugs are used to combat viral hepatitis, including interferon. Surgery in the form of a liver transplant operation may be the only option in severe forms of the disease. Recovery from many types of hepatitis is good and complete although may take some time. Infection with and recovery from viral hepatitis normally confers immunity from a future attack.

Causes and risk factors: causes are various and include those viruses listed above. Also, other viral infections, such as glandular fever and HIV can produce symptoms of hepatitis. Some drugs cause liver inflammation and hepatitis, especially alcohol and paracetamol in excess. Alcohol abuse is the most common cause of hepatitis in the UK. Infectious hepatitis is transmitted by eating food contaminated by a person who has the virus and is common in conditions of poor hygiene and sanitation. With serum hepatitis, the route of infection is blood or blood products and is most common where infected needles have been shared among drug addicts. The infection may also be passed on by tattooing needles and also through sexual intercourse with an infected individual.

hepatoma or heptocellular carcinoma

Description: a malignant tumour of the liver that is rare in western countries except among persons with CIRRHOSIS. It is prevalent in parts of the Far East and Africa.

Persons most commonly affected: adults of both sexes but more prevalent in men.

Organ or part of body involved: liver.

Symptoms and indications: malaise, loss of appetite and weight, abdominal discomfort, jaundice, retention of fluid in the abdomen, feverishness. There may be an enlargement of the spleen and it may be possible to detect a hard mass in the abdomen. There may be unexplained bleeding from the gastrointestinal tract. A person with symptoms of hepatoma should seek medical treatment as soon as possible.

Treatment: may involve admittance to hospital and surgery to remove the tumour, if possible. Also,

various drugs including painkillers may be prescribed to relieve the symptoms. The disease is incurable but ongoing research is being carried out to further understanding and to improve treatment methods.

Causes and risk factors: the risk of this form of cancer increases with excessive consumption of alcohol and cirrhosis of the liver. Also, there is a greater risk with previous HEPATITIS, particularly infection with the hepatitis B virus. Hepatoma is common in parts of the Far East and Africa and a suspected cause is the aflatoxin (produced in the spores of the fungus *Aspergillus flavus*) which contaminates stored peanuts and cereals. Hepatoma often produces alpha fetoprotein (a type of protein normally produced in the liver and gut of a foetus), which is detectable in the blood and can be tested for as an indicator of the presence of the malignancy. Preventative measures include not drinking alcohol, especially for those who have had previous liver diseases.

hernia

Description: the protrusion of a part or whole of an organ from out of its normal position within the body cavity. Most commonly, a hernia involves part of the bowel. There are various types of hernia described according to their nature and origin.

Congenital hernia—present at birth, a common one being an 'umbilical hernia', in which abdominal organs protrude into the umbilical cord.

Acquired hernia—occurs after birth, a common example being an 'inguinal hernia' in which part of the bowel bulges through a weak part of the abdominal wall (known as the inguinal canal).

HIATUS HERNIA—the stomach passes through the hiatus (a hole allowing passage of the oesophagus) from the abdomen into the chest cavity.

Reducible hernia—one that is freely movable and can be returned by manipulation into its proper place.

Irreducible hernia—one that cannot be returned by manipulation into its proper place.

Incarcerated hernia—one that has become swollen and fixed in its position.

Obstructed hernia—one involving the bowel. The contents of the hernia are unable to pass further down and are held up and obstructed.

Strangulated hernia—the most dangerous type, in which the blood supply has been cut off due to the protrusion itself.

Persons most commonly affected: all age groups and both sexes.

Organ or part of body involved: any organ may be involved except the liver and pancreas. Usually, however, a hernia involves the bowel and digestive tract.

Symptoms and indications: a protruding lump that often can be returned to its normal position by manipulation. (However, not all hernias produce a lump that can be felt on the body's surface.) There may be slight discomfort or pain and a feeling of weakness. A strangulated hernia is a life-threatening condition causing severe pain, feverishness and vomiting, and eventually turning gangrenous. This requires immediate emergency surgery as there is a risk of PERITONITIS and death. A person with symptoms of a hernia should always seek medical advice.

Treatment: a reducible hernia may be treated by pushing back into place and support. Curative treatment is by means of surgery to return and retain the protrusion in its proper place (hernioplasty). It may be necessary for a person to go on a diet or have other treatment to reduce the size of a large hernia before surgery is performed. Treatment and recovery from all but a strangulated hernia is usually good and complete.

Causes and risk factors: the cause of a hernia is a weakness or injury in retaining muscles or connective tissue. There may be a congenital weakness, or stretching and tearing may occur along a line of weakness, such as a previous operation scar (incisional hernia). The risk of development of a hernia increases with age, pregnancy and obesity, and also inappropriate lifting and straining. In the latter case, the hernia may appear suddenly but usually its development is gradual.

herpes simplex infection or genital Herpes

Description: an infection of the genital region caused by a herpes virus.

Persons most commonly affected: sexually active adults of both sexes and all age groups.

Organ or part of body involved: genitals.

Symptoms and indications: itching of genital area, followed by the development of small, painful blisters or ulcers. The person feels generally unwell, the lymph glands are enlarged and there may be slight fever. Urination is painful due to the presence of the ulcers. A person with genital herpes should consult a doctor.

Treatment: involves rest until symptoms subside and possibly the antiviral drug acyclovir. Scrupulous attention should be paid to personal hygiene and warm baths may help to relieve symptoms. The virus remains in the body throughout life and tends to flare up from time to time, although some people are more susceptible to recurrent attacks than others. These are more likely to occur when the person is suffering from, or recovering from, some other debilitating condition when the body has been under stress. During an attack, the person should refrain from sexual intercourse until one month after all symptoms have disappeared. Also, it is advisable to use condoms.

Causes and risk factors: the cause of the infection is herpes simplex viruses types I and II. Herpes type I virus causes COLD SORES. The virus is transmitted by sexual relations with a person who has an active herpes infection (either cold sores or genital herpes). The infection is especially damaging in those taking anticancer drugs or other drugs that suppress the immune system. A newborn baby who acquires the virus from an infected mother during birth may become seriously ill with a general infection. Hence, a pregnant woman who has previously had an active infection should inform the doctor.

hiatus hernia

Description: a hernia in which part of the stomach passes through the hiatus (a hole allowing the passage of the oesophagus through the diaphragm) from the abdomen into the chest cavity.

Persons most commonly affected: adults of both sexes over the age of 50 but can affect younger people.

Organ or part of body involved: oesophagus, diaphragm, stomach.

Symptoms and indications: the symptoms are usually felt after eating a meal and include heartburn, wind and discomfort. A person with symptoms of hiatus hernia should seek medical advice.

Treatment: includes the taking of antacid preparations to alleviate the symptoms of heartburn, eating small meals, avoidance of hot, spicy foods and, as with all hernias, avoidance of straining. Corrective surgery may be required to repair the hernia.

Causes and risk factors: there may be a congenital or inborn weakness in the diaphragm or this may be due to pressure or injury. The symptoms of heartburn are caused by backflow of gastric juice from the stomach into the oesophagus. The risk of the development of a hiatus hernia increases with age, obesity and inappropriate lifting or straining of the abdominal muscles.

hip fracture

Description: the hip joint is a 'ball-and-socket' joint made up of the head of the femur (thigh bone), which rests inside a deep, cup-shaped cavity (the acetabulum) in the hip bone. The hip bone (or innominate bone) is itself made up of three fused bones, the pubis, ischium and ilium, which form part of the pelvis. A hip fracture involves a break of some sort in the femur.

Persons most commonly affected: all age groups and both sexes but especially older persons, particularly women with OSTEOPOROSIS.

Organ or part of body involved: femur and other elements of the hip joint.

Symptoms and indications: severe pain, swelling and inability to walk following a fall or injury. A person suffering this injury requires immediate emergency medical treatment in hospital.

Treatment: is by means of surgery to repair the joint, securing the damaged portions by means of steel pins. Elderly patients may need a hip-replacement operation. Convalescence and recovery may take some time especially in older people.

Causes and risk factors: the cause is an accidental injury or, in the elderly, a fall. Care should be taken to avoid the possibility of falls and the diet should include adequate amounts of calcium. Women should consider hormone replacement therapy after the menopause to minimize the risk of osteoporosis. As with all injuries of this nature, there is a risk of poor healing, infection, and damage to nerves and blood vessels, especially if the fracture is severe or complicated. These are particularly dangerous in elderly people.

Hodgkin's disease

Description: a malignant disease affecting the lymphatic system in which there is a gradual and increasing enlargement of lymph glands and nodes throughout the body.

Persons most commonly affected: both sexes and all age groups but more common in men and rare in young children under ten years.

Organ or part of body involved: lymphatic system including nodes, glands and spleen.

Symptoms and indications: loss of weight, sweating, anaemia and a characteristic type of fever (known as Pel-Ebstein fever). This is an intermittent type of fever, coming on for a short period then subsiding for a few days before returning again. The person becomes gradually weaker and the glands enlarge and may attain a very great size. A person with symptoms of Hodgkin's disease requires immediate medical treatment.

Treatment: is by means of surgery, radiotherapy and chemotherapy (a combination of drugs being used). The outlook is generally good, especially if the disease is detected early. Some treatment methods may cause side effects, usually relatively short-lived.

Causes and risk factors: the cause of the disease is unknown but there is a possibility that a virus may be involved in some cases. There are no particular preventative measures but it is wise not to smoke.

Huntington's chorea

Description: an inherited condition characterized by DEMENTIA and involuntary jerking movements.

Persons most commonly affected: the usual age for symptoms to develop is between 35 and 45 and it affects people of both sexes. A few people develop symptoms at a much younger age.

Organ or part of body involved: nervous system, brain, muscles.

Symptoms and indications: early symptoms include behavioural changes such as apathy, increased irritability and, in some cases, more profound psychiatric disturbances. Early physical signs include flicking movements of fingers and toes, unsteadiness in walking, contortion of facial muscles and muscle spasms. The disease progresses inexorably over a number of years, leaving the person completely mentally and physically disabled. A person with symptoms of Huntington's chorea should seek medical advice.

Treatment: there is no treatment to cure or halt the progress of the disease but drugs can be used to diminish the muscle spasms (chorea).

Causes and risk factors: the cause is unknown and the disorder cannot be prevented. Each child of an affected parent has a 50% chance of developing the disease and should receive genetic counselling before having children.

hydrocephalus

Description: an abnormal collection of cerebrospinal fluid within the skull.

Persons most commonly affected: children of both sexes but can occur in adults.

Organ or part of body involved: brain.

Symptoms and indications: in children, the chief indication is a gradual abnormal increase in the size of the head, the growth being disproportionate to that of the rest of the body. Other symptoms are drowsiness, irritability and eventual mental subnormality. In severe cases there may be loss of vision and hearing, paralysis and death. The condition is often congenital and is usually detected during medical and developmental checks on the child.

Treatment: involves surgery to redirect the fluid but this is not always successful. About 50% of children survive if the progress of the condition is halted and one third of these go on to enjoy a normal life with little or no physical or mental impairment.

Causes and risk factors: hydrocephalus results either from an excessive production of fluid or from a defect in the mechanism for its reabsorption, or from a blockage in its circulation. The cause is frequently congenital and it often accompanies spina bifida in babies, or infection (MENINGITIS), or the presence of a tumour. The collection of fluid in hydrocephalus causes pressure on the brain, with the resultant damage and loss of mental and physical abilities.

hyperemesis gravidarum

Description: a rare condition of pregnancy characterized by severe vomiting, which is greatly in excess of that of 'morning sickness'.

Persons most commonly affected: pregnant women.

Organ or part of body involved: gastrointestinal tract.

Symptoms and indications: severe vomiting leading to dehydration, disturbance of the electrolyte/fluid balance in the body and damage to the liver. If untreated, it can result in coma and death. The person suffers severe vomiting, may have a headache and pale dry skin, show signs of confusion and have a rapid heartbeat rate. A pregnant woman with any of these symptoms requires immediate medical treatment.

Treatment: involves replacement of fluids and electrolytes. This may need to be carried out in hospital by means of an intravenous drip. Recovery is normally good if the person is treated early.

Causes and risk factors: the cause is not known but is more likely with a multiple pregnancy and may be linked to the production of high levels of the hormone human chorionic gonadotrophin. There is a possibility that it may recur in any subsequent pregnancy.

hypernephroma or renal cell carcinoma or Grawitz tumour

Description: a malignant growth affecting kidney cells, which resembles tissue of the adrenal glands (suprarenal glands) and was thought at one time to originate from them.

Persons most commonly affected: adults of both sexes, especially men in middle and older age groups.

Organ or part of body involved: kidney.

Symptoms and indications: the malignancy may be present for some time without causing symptoms. Eventually symptoms are produced, including feverishness, lower abdominal pain, blood in the urine, possibly vomiting and enlargement of the abdomen. The tumour may go on to cause KIDNEY FAILURE if not detected and treated early, and is liable to spread and produce secondary growths elsewhere. A person with any symptoms of kidney disease should seek medical advice.

Treatment: involves surgery to remove the tumour and, possibly, radiotherapy, chemotherapy and use of hormones (testosterone and progestogens) to inhibit growth. The outcome is generally favourable if the tumour is dealt with early and has not spread.

Causes and risk factors: the cause is not known. There is a likelihood of spread of the tumour via the blood system and small growths can occur along the renal vein. Other organs affected include the liver, lungs (where a characteristic growth is produced), bones and brain. These secondary growths may already be present before the hypernephroma is diagnosed.

hypertension or high blood pressure

Description: an increase above normal in the pressure exerted by blood circulating through the arteries. It may be a condition in itself or a symptom of underlying disease. There are two types: essential hypertension and malignant hypertension (which may be an end stage of essential hypertension).

Persons most commonly affected: essential hypertension—adults aged over 40 years, especially males, most commonly occurring or between 50 and 60 years. Malignant hypertension—younger adults of both sexes. Hypertension affects people in western countries far more commonly than those in the east.

Organ or part of body involved: heart, blood vessels (arteries), kidneys.

Symptoms and indications: both forms of hypertension may present no symptoms in the early stages. Symptoms arise because complications have developed (see below).

Essential hypertension—later stages or when symptoms are present, headache, especially on waking but wearing off through the day and returning in the evening. The headache is often felt at the back of the head. There may be noise or ringing in the ears (tinnitus) and dizziness. If not treated, death may follow, due to kidney failure, heart attack, stroke or cerebral haemorrhage.

Malignant hypertension—as well as the above symptoms, characteristically there is a high diastolic blood pressure. (Diastole is the point at which the heart relaxes between contractions, when the ventricles fill with blood. It usually lasts about half a second, at the end of which the ventricles are about three quarters full. Diastolic blood pressure is that exerted during this period and it should normally be at the lowest point). Also, there is swelling of the first part of the optic nerve in the eye (called the optic disc, or papilla) because of high intracranial pressure within the head. This is called papilloedema. Malignant hypertension is fatal in a short period of time if it is not treated, often due to kidney failure. A person with symptoms of hypertension should seek immediate medical advice.

Treatment: involves lifestyle changes particularly as regards diet (a low-salt, low-saturated-fat diet is usually recommended), exercise and avoidance of stress. Smoking should be avoided and those who are obese usually need to lose weight. Many antihypertensive drugs are available including beta adrenoreceptor blockers, thiazide diuretics, angiotensin inhibitors such as captopril, guanethedine, methyldopa and others. Some drugs produce side effects. With early detection and treatment of hypertension the outcome is usually good and the development of fatal complications can be averted.

Causes and risk factors: the cause is generally unknown but the risk of the development of hypertension increases with stress, smoking, obesity, a high salt, high saturated fat diet, and the lack of exercise and fitness. Also, there are hereditary factors in many cases. Preventative measures include avoidance of the risk factors outlined above.

hyperthyroidism

Description: excessive activity of the thyroid gland—an overactive thyroid. *See also* GRAVES' DISEASE.

Persons most commonly affected: adults of both sexes in younger age groups below 50. More common in women than in men.

Organ or part of body involved: thyroid gland—an important endocrine (hormone-producing) gland essential for the regulation of metabolism and affecting many body functions.

Symptoms and indications: symptoms include flushing, sweating and feeling warm, itchy skin, anxiety and overactivity, insomnia, rapid heartbeat, breathlessness, weight loss or gain, gastrointestinal upset, protrusion of eyes, goitre and weariness. A person with symptoms of thyroid gland disorder should seek medical advice.

Treatment: includes the taking of antithyroid drugs to depress thyroid gland activity. Also, radioactive iodine therapy and surgery to remove part of the thyroid gland may prove to be necessary.

Causes and risk factors: causes include a tumour of the thyroid gland, pituitary gland disease or other disorder, and there may be a family history of hyperthyroidism.

hyperventilation

Description: breathing at an abnormally rapid rate when at rest, resulting in a fall in the concentration of carbon dioxide in the blood.

Persons most commonly affected: all age groups and both sexes.

Organ or part of body involved: respiratory system, central nervous system and whole body.

Symptoms and indications: hyperventilation is characterized by rapid, shallow breathing and the person may be agitated and then feel faint with tingling or numbing sensation in the hands, feet and face. If not checked, the person falls into unconsciousness. A person suffering from these symptoms should seek medical advice.

Treatment: hyperventilation often accompanies extreme anxiety. The affected person must be reassured and helped to calm down and breathe normally. Breathing into and out of a paper bag is helpful (the expired air contains more carbon dioxide). Hyperventilation may also occur if the carbon dioxide level in the blood is abnormally high due to impaired gas exchange in the lungs, as in PULMONARY OEDEMA and PNEUMONIA, and subsides when these conditions are treated and controlled.

Causes and risk factors: hyperventilation may occur as a result of extreme stress or anxiety or a sudden shock, as a symptom of a panic attack. The person may need counselling to deal with stress if the condition is a recurring problem.

hypothermia

Description: hypothermia describes the bodily state when the core temperature falls below 35°C due to prolonged exposure to cold.

Persons most commonly affected: all age groups and both sexes but especially likely in elderly persons.

Organ or part of body involved: whole body—all metabolism.

Symptoms and indications: early signs of hypothermia include shivering and the heart works harder to increase the flow of blood around the body. The person feels cold, the body temperature drops and there is mental confusion and tiredness. Eventually, shivering ceases and, with increasing chilling, the function of the body organs becomes disturbed and cardiac output falls. The tissues require less oxygen as their functions start to fail, but eventually the heart is unable to supply even this reduced demand. The symptoms are a further drop in body temperature and unconsciousness, leading to death. A person suffering from even mild hypothermia requires emergency medical treatment.

Treatment: consists of warming the person to restore body temperature to normal. If the core temperature has fallen very low (below 28°C) great care has to be exercised in moving the patient, who is susceptible to ventricular FIBRILLATION. Warming is done by means of insulating blankets, warm water baths, heating pads, etc. The person may be given warm moist air or oxygen to breathe. However, peritoneal, gastric or bladder dialysis with warm saline solutions may be needed to save the life of an unconscious patient who is very severely chilled. The salt and water balance of the body is disrupted and requires careful monitoring and appropriate treatment along with ECG monitoring of the output of the heart. The person requires intensive care treatment and nursing until consciousness returns and the body temperature approaches a normal level.

Causes and risk factors: the cause of hypothermia is prolonged exposure to severe cold. This is an obvious problem outdoors in winter especially if there is a cold wind. However, people may suffer from hypothermia when wet, even if the weather is not severely cold, or in accidents involving falling into the sea or other very cold water. Elderly persons can suffer hypothermia in their own homes when heating is inadequate. Preventative measures include the obvious ones of preparing for outdoor winter activities by wearing adequate protective clothing. Elderly people must keep their homes warm or live and sleep in one room that can be kept adequately heated. In some surgical operations (heart and brain surgery) a state of deliberate hypothermia may be induced while a particular procedure is carried out.

I

ichthyosis

Description: a generally hereditary skin condition, in which the skin is very dry and looks cracked, producing a resemblance to fish scales.

Persons most commonly affected: both sexes, present for life.

Organ or part of body involved: skin.

Symptoms and indications: there are various types of ichthyosis and the appearance of the skin varies according to the severity of the condition and the parts affected. The skin lacks oil and looks rough and dry, and dirt collects easily in the cracks. The scales may be quite thin, or thicker, depending upon the type and severity of the icthyosis. The skin may improve in summer and be especially hard in winter. A person with this condition often requires prolonged treatment to improve the condition and appearance of the skin.

Treatment: the most important treatment is the ongoing use of emollient preparations, particularly petroleum-based or mineral oils, to replace the natural oils the skin lacks. Special bath preparations and creams and ointments containing vitamin A acid and retinoic acid may be prescribed. Synthetic tretinoin preparations (vitamin A) taken by mouth, such as etretinate and isotretinoin may be prescribed under specialist supervision.

Causes and risk factors: the cause of ichthyosis is generally genetic, although it may occur in some other disease, such as leprosy, LYMPHOMA, AIDS and hypothyroidism. Inherited forms are due to a defect in keratinization (a natural process in which the nails, hair and outer layers of the skin become filled with keratin, a fibrous protein).

ileitis

Description: inflammation of the ileum (the lower part of the small intestine).

Persons most commonly affected: younger adults of both sexes but can occur in other age groups.

Organ or part of body involved: ileum and gastrointestinal tract.

Symptoms and indications: generally similar to those of CROHN'S DISEASE, including abdominal pains and tenderness, bowel irregularity and loss of weight. The intestine may become thickened and this can sometimes be felt externally. If the thickening is to a great extent, a blockage may occur, necessitating an immediate emergency operation. A person with symptoms of ileitis should seek medical advice.

Treatment: involves bed rest, eating a low-fibre diet that is high in vitamins, and taking various medications, which may include corticosteroids, antibiotics, analgesics and vitamin supplements. An operation to remove the thickened part of the ileum (ileostomy) may be needed. Treatment is relatively successful in relieving symptoms but the condition may recur.

Causes and risk factors: the specific cause is not known but ileitis may occur in association with TUBERCULOSIS, bacterial infection (by *Yersinia enterocolitica*), Crohn's disease, ulcerative colitis and TYPHOID FEVER. Complications arising from this condition are similar to those of Crohn's disease, including blockage of the ileum, abscess formation, bleeding and ANAEMIA.

impetigo

Description: a common, infectious bacterial skin disease.

Persons most commonly affected: babies and children of both sexes but can occur in older persons e.g. scrum-pox in players of rugby football. A severe form in infants is called pemphigus neonatorum.

Organ or part of body involved: skin on face and limbs.

Symptoms and indications: the infection starts as a red patch that forms pustules that join to create crusted yellowish sores. The contents of the sores are highly infectious and easily spread by direct contact or via towels, etc. The scabs usually dry up, fall off and do not cause scarring. However, in pemphigus neonatorum serious blistering of the skin occurs, and treatment should begin as soon as possible. A person or child with this condition requires prompt medical treatment.

Treatment: is by means of scrupulous attention to hygiene and taking a course of antibiotics such as penicillin. Treatment should begin as soon as possible as the infection may spread and continue for months if not treated. Special solutions and lotions may be prescribed for treating the affected areas of skin. The condition usually responds well to antibiotic treatment. Affected children should be kept away from others until the infection has completely cleared.

Causes and risk factors: the cause is usually a staphylococcus bacterium, although, occasionally, a streptococcus may be involved.

influenza

Description: a highly infectious disease caused by a virus that affects the respiratory tract.

Persons most commonly affected: all age groups and both sexes.

Organ or part of body involved: respiratory tract.

Symptoms and indications: symptoms include headache, weakness, fever, sneezing and coughing, sore throat, aches and pains in limbs and joints, and loss of appetite. It may be necessary to seek medical advice if the symptoms are very severe or if the patient is elderly.

Treatment: the symptoms subside more quickly with complete rest. Painkillers such as paracetamol can be taken to relieve the symptoms and plenty of fluids should be drunk. The person should endeavour to eat some light meals until the appetite returns. In the absence of complications, symptoms usually subside in one or two weeks.

Causes and risk factors: the cause of the infection is usually one of three main strains of influenza virus, designated A, B and C, which are each sometimes responsible for epidemics of the disease occurring in cycles. Characteristically, infection with one strain does not confer immunity against another. Also, the virus quickly produces new variants or characteristics so that an attack of one is unlikely to provide protection against a later bout of the disease. Sometimes, complications can arise as a result of influenza in the form of secondary lung infections. These can be dangerous in elderly people and may require treatment with antibiotics and, possibly, admittance to hospital. In Britain, virus A is responsible for the majority of outbreaks.

intestinal obstruction and intussusception

Description: an obstruction of some part of the intestine or bowel, preventing the passage of food material. Intussusception is an obstruction caused by one part of the bowel slipping inside another part beneath it, much as a telescope closes up.

Persons most commonly affected: all age groups and both sexes. Intussusception is more common in young children.

Organ or part of body involved: the small and large intestine or bowel.

Symptoms and indications: abdominal swelling and constipation, severe cramping pain that comes and goes, and characteristic vomiting. At first the vomit is normal but later it contains bile and is green, and later still resembles faeces (faecal vomiting). Symptoms of intussusception are similar, but a child passes a jelly-like blood-stained mucus. A person with these symptoms requires immediate, prompt medical treatment as a delay may be dangerous or even fatal. Nothing should be taken by mouth.

Treatment: involves admittance to hospital and, usually, surgery to remove the cause of the obstruction or barium enema (intussusception). Recovery is usually good and complete in the case of intussusception, provided that the child receives prompt and early attention. Surgery to correct intestinal obstruction is also normally successful, especially when diagnosis and treatment begins early. However, a cure depends upon the underlying cause of the condition.

Causes and risk factors: intestinal obstruction has a number of causes, including the presence of a tumour pressing upon the area either within the bowel or in a near organ, scar tissue from previous lesions, infections or operations (adhesions), a swallowed object, e.g. a fruit stone or internal body such as a hard mass of faeces and a twisted bowel. There is a risk of abscess, perforation and PERITONITIS, which can prove fatal, particularly if treatment is delayed.

iritis

Description: inflammation of the iris, the coloured part of the eye, which is a muscular disc controlling the entry of light.

Persons most commonly affected: adults of both sexes, especially those aged under 60.

Organ or part of body involved: the iris.

Symptoms and indications: symptoms include eye pain, which may be severe, reddening and watering of the eye, sensitivity to light and blurring of vision. A person with symptoms of eye disorder should seek prompt medical advice.

Treatment: consists of mydriatic eyedrops that dilate the pupil, and anti-inflammatory cortisone (steroid) eyedrops. Occasionally, steroid tablets may be prescribed. The eye should be rested as much as possible and the condition usually improves in one or two weeks.

Causes and risk factors: the cause may not be known but this condition is associated with SYPHILIS, viruses, TUBERCULOSIS, some disorders of the bowel, various forms of arthritis and some parasitic and fungal infestations and infections. There is a risk of permanent eye damage or the development of CATARACTS or GLAUCOMA.

irritable bowel syndrome or IBS

Description: (also known as spastic colon, irritable colitis or mucous colitis) a condition caused by abnormal muscular contractions (or increased motility), producing effects in the large and small intestine.

Persons most commonly affected: all age groups and both sexes.

Organ or part of body involved: bowel.

Symptoms and indications: symptoms include pain and discomfort in the abdomen, which changes location, disturbed bowel movements with

diarrhoea, then normal movements or constipation, heartburn and a bloated feeling due to wind. These symptoms are produced without any signs of structural disorder or obvious cause. A person with these symptoms should seek medical advice. A series of tests are usually made to rule out other disorders (such as cancer) before the diagnosis is made.

Treatment: involves some drug therapy, including anticholinergic preparations to inhibit movement in the bowel. Also, drugs that reduce diarrhoea, such as codeine phosphate and Lomotil, may be prescribed. In addition, measures to reduce stress and anxiety and adjustments to the diet and lifestyle may prove helpful.

Causes and risk factors: the cause is usually not known but the condition sometimes develops after a gastrointestinal tract infection. Stress and anxiety are believed to be contributory factors and certain foods or drinks may make the symptoms worse in some people. If this is known to be the case, then these should obviously be avoided.

J

jaundice

Description: a condition characterized by the unusual presence of bile pigment (bilirubin) in the blood. The bile (produced in the liver and stored in the gall bladder) passes into the blood instead of the intestines and because of this there is a yellowing of the skin and the whites of the eyes. Jaundice is a symptom of an underlying cause, disease or disorder, rather than a disease in itself.

There are several types of jaundice: obstructive jaundice is due to bile not reaching the intestine because of an obstruction such as a GALLSTONE. Haemolytic jaundice is where red blood cells are destroyed by haemolysis, with the production of a yellow pigment in the blood. Hepatocellular jaundice occurs in liver diseases, such as HEPATITIS, which renders the liver incapable of using the bilirubin. Neonatal jaundice is quite common in newborn infants and is due to physiological immaturity of the liver. It usually only lasts for a few days.

Persons most commonly affected: all age groups and both sexes.

Organ or part of body involved: liver, gall bladder, bile ducts, blood circulation.

Symptoms and indications: the characteristic sign of jaundice is yellowing, first of the whites of the eyes and then the skin. The colour varies from a pale yellow to a bronze colour like a suntan. The urine may be dark and there may be a loss of appetite and a bitter taste in the mouth. The tongue may be furred and faeces may be pale and foul-smelling. The person may experience nausea and the skin may itch. There may be lethargy, a slow pulse rate and confusion. Jaundice should always be investigated so that the underlying cause or disorder can be treated. An affected person should seek medical advice.

Treatment: depends upon the nature of the causal illness or disorder. In general, the person requires admittance to hospital, bed rest and a diet high in protein and carbohydrates but very low in fat. Vitamin supplements may be needed. In severe cases of neonatal jaundice, the infant is exposed to blue light, which converts bilirubin to biliverdin, another (harmless) bile pigment.

Causes and risk factors: as indicated above, jaundice may be due to liver diseases such as HEPATITIS or obstruction of the bile ducts by GALLSTONES. Also, CIRRHOSIS OF THE LIVER, cancer of the pancreas or enlargement of glands close to the liver are causes of jaundice. Some infectious diseases, including MALARIA, TYPHOID FEVER and LEPTOSPIROSIS, cause jaundice. Many drugs and toxins that have adverse effects on the liver may cause jaundice, including snake venom and mercury. The risk of liver damage and jaundice increases with excess alcohol consumption.

K

Kaposi's sarcoma

Description: a condition in which there are malignant skin tumours that form from the blood vessels. The disease is common in Africa, but less so in western countries. It does, however, occur in persons suffering from AIDS.

Persons most commonly affected: adults of both sexes and all age groups, especially children and young men. Persons with Aids.

Organ or part of body involved: skin, especially of feet, ankles, hands and arms. It affects the gastrointestinal and respiratory tracts in Aids patients, and also the lymph nodes.

Symptoms and indications: purple-coloured lumps due to tumours form on the feet and ankles and spread to arms and hands. In Aids patients the tumours form in the respiratory and gastrointestinal tracts and cause bleeding and anaemia. A person with symptoms of this disease requires medical treatment, which should start as early as possible.

Treatment: is in the form of radiotherapy, which is usually effective in mild cases of the disease. However, chemotherapy (anticancer drugs) is also required for those more severely affected in order to retard the growth and spread of the tumours.

Causes and risk factors: the cause is not known but this disease is a significant cause of death in some African countries. The form of the disease associated with Aids is especially aggressive and the outlook for these patients is poor. Kaposi's sarcoma may occasionally accompany malignant LYMPHOMA, DIABETES and some other diseases.

Kawasaki disease (or mucocutaneous lymph node syndrome)

Description: a disease affecting young children, first reported in Japan but now widespread in other countries.

Persons most commonly affected: children of both sexes under five years but can occur in young adults.

Organ or part of body involved: lymph nodes, skin, coronary arteries of the heart.

Symptoms and indications: the disease usually passes through a number of stages, beginning with fever, tiredness, fretfulness and, sometimes, pains in the abdomen. A rash develops about one day later and after several days there may be conjunctivitis and changes to mucous membranes such as a red (strawberry) tongue and dry, cracked lips. Lymph glands in the neck are enlarged. During the first week of the illness the nails may become pale and there is reddening and hardening of the soles of the feet and palms of the hands. The skin may peel off revealing new skin underneath. Provided that the disease does not affect the coronary arteries (*see causes and risk factors*), recovery is normally good and complete within a few weeks. A child with this disease must receive medical treatment and monitoring because of the risk of coronary artery involvement, which occurs in 5–20% of all cases.

Treatment: there is no specific treatment but aspirin is usually prescribed for this disorder to reduce the risk of coronary artery disease. The child will require checks on the heart and coronary arteries for several months, including ECG and echocardiography.

Causes and risk factors: the cause of this disorder is not known and, as indicated above, the main danger arises from the risk of coronary artery and heart disease. There are fatalities in about 1–2% of cases, and these can occur some time after the original infection. The complications that can arise include inflammation of the coronary arteries, ANEURYSM, myocarditis (inflammation of the heart muscle), heart failure, THROMBOSIS, PERICARDITIS (inflammation of the membrane called the pericardium, which is a sac surrounding the heart), and heart rhythm disorders (arrhythmias). If these develop, then the appropriate treatment is necessary.

keratitis

Description: inflammation and/or infection of the cornea of the eye, which may arise from a number of different causes. (The cornea is the outermost,

218

transparent exposed layer of the eye that lies over the iris and lens.)

Persons most commonly affected: all age groups and both sexes.

Organ or part of body involved: cornea of the eye.

Symptoms and indications: reddening, inflammation, watering and severe pain and blurring of vision. There may be a yellow discharge. A person with symptoms of keratitis should seek immediate medical treatment as the bacterial form can rapidly lead to a loss of sight.

Treatment: depends on the cause of the keratitis. If it is bacterial, the person requires admittance to hospital for intensive antibiotic therapy in the form of eyedrops and tablets. If the cause is a virus, antiviral eyedrops will be required. Other treatments include the use of artificial tears and wearing a patch to rest the eye until the condition clears. Some conditions may require corrective surgery. With prompt treatment at an early stage most forms of keratitis can be cured. However, there is a danger of permanent damage and loss of vision in some cases, especially if treatment is delayed.

Causes and risk factors: as indicated above, the cause may be a bacterial infection (usually staphylococcus, streptococcus, enterobacteria or pseudomonas) or a virus (often *herpes simplex*). Other causes include dry eyes (exposure keratitis, due to a failure of tear production and spread by blinking), paralysis of the facial nerve so that the eyelids are unable to blink, previous injury, and scarring of eyelids and protrusion of the eye so that the eyelids do not completely close. All these are likely to increase the risk of the development of exposure keratitis.

keratosis

Description: a condition or disease of the skin in which there is a thickening and overgrowth of the horny layer (called the stratum corneum) of the skin. There are two types: actinic keratosis, which is usually induced by prolonged exposure to sunlight and seborrhoeic keratosis, which develops to a certain extent in most people with increasing age.

Persons most commonly affected: adults of both sexes and all age groups. If sun-related, the age at which it develops depends upon the climate and degree of exposure to the sun.

Organ or part of body involved: skin.

Symptoms and indications: actinic keratosis—scaly patches of dry, reddish-brown skin, which are not painful and do not itch. Seborrhoeic keratosis—

small, raised, yellow-brown warts or papules that vary in colour.

A person with symptoms of keratosis should seek medical advice. Actinic keratosis may be a precancerous condition and an affected person may require periodic skin check-ups.

Treatment: actinic keratosis—preventative and ongoing treatment is avoidance of overexposure to the sun. If only small areas of skin are affected, freezing with liquid nitrogen provides rapid and successful treatment (cryotherapy). For larger areas, treatment with topical preparations (creams, ointments or solutions) containing 5-fluorouracil is very effective but there are unpleasant side effects, in the form of burning, inflammation and scaling of the skin. These are uncomfortable and disfiguring while treatment lasts.

Seborrhoeic keratosis—the warts or papules are not harmful and can be left unless they are itchy, troublesome or unsightly. Methods of removal include cryosurgery (freezing with liquid nitrogen or carbon dioxide, 'dry ice') or chemocautery (surgical removal after an injection into the area of 1% lidocaine).

Causes and risk factors: as indicated above, actinic keratosis is caused by overexposure to sunlight and is more likely to occur in those who regularly sunbathe or who work outdoors. Seborrhoeic keratosis tends to affect most adults to a slight extent by the time they reach middle or older age, but the cause is not known.

kidney failure

Description: either a sudden failure of the kidneys to perform their usual function of eliminating waste products from the body (acute kidney failure) or a more slow and gradual development of this state (chronic kidney failure). Kidney failure is, in itself, caused by a wide range of diseases and disorders.

Persons most commonly affected: all age groups and both sexes.

Organ or part of body involved: kidney.

Symptoms and indications: acute kidney failure—symptoms include a reduction in the amount of urine produced and the urine contains blood and albumin (a protein made in the liver). There may be nausea, vomiting, diarrhoea and headaches and the person becomes lethargic and later collapses into unconsciousness. The skin may be intensely itchy, with bruising and bleeding. There may be convulsions. Symptoms develop due to electrolyte imbalances and acidosis caused by the failure of the regulatory function of the kidneys to filter the blood and eliminate waste products. The general state is called 'uraemia', which means an excess of urea in the blood. Other symptoms are likely to be present depending upon the cause of the acute kidney failure. (*See causes and risk factors*).

Chronic kidney failure—this may be well advanced before symptoms become apparent. These include itchy skin, fluid retention, tiredness and lethargy, pains, bleeding, ANAEMIA and HYPERTENSION. A person with symptoms of kidney failure requires immediate medical attention.

Treatment: depends upon the cause and degree of the kidney failure. It may include medication and/or surgery to correct the underlying disease or disorder. Kidney dialysis and/or a transplant operation will be needed if the disorder cannot be treated.

Causes and risk factors: there are a variety of causes of kidney failure, including heart and artery diseases, severe urinary tract infections, congenital kidney disorders, accidental kidney damage, GLOMERULONEPHRITIS, abuse of certain drugs and chemicals, and others. Persons suffering from some diseases or disorders, such as GOUT and DIABETES, are more at risk of developing kidney failure, as are those who have only one kidney due to previous surgery.

kidney stones or calculi (*singular* calculus)

Description: deposits of hard material, varying in size, that may form and collect within the kidneys and pass into the ureters (the tubes that carry urine to the bladder). The deposits are composed of calcium phosphate, calcium oxalate, ammonium phosphate, calcium carbonate, uric acid or urates.

Persons most commonly affected: adults of both sexes aged over 30 years but more common in men than women. They affect about 2% of adults in Britain, especially those in sedentary occupations.

Organ or part of body involved: kidneys and ureters.

Symptoms and indications: severe stabbing pain in the back that comes and goes, nausea, and there may be slight amounts of blood in the urine (haematuria). A person with symptoms of kidney stones should seek medical advice.

Treatment: depends upon whether the stones are small enough to be passed spontaneously with the urine. Large stones require surgical removal or ultrasound treatment to break them up so that they can be passed naturally. A person with kidney stones should drink plenty of fluids to help them to be passed naturally. Stones may form due to a change in the acidity or alkalinity of the urine hence, preparations to alter this may be prescribed. If they are mainly of calcium, bendrofluazide may be prescribed. Dietary changes to avoid foods high in calcium or phosphorus may be advised.

Causes and risk factors: there are various causes or factors that favour the formation of kidney stones. These include a high level of calcium (hypercalcuria) in the urine, a change in the acidity or alkalinity of the urine, concentration of the urine, which may occur if too little fluid is drunk or if sweating is excessive as in a hot climate. Also, GOUT (uric acid stones), a family tendency, kidney infections, a diet deficient in vitamin A and an overactive parathyroid gland are all factors that may lead to the formation of stones. Persons with an inactive lifestyle are more at risk.

L

labyrinthitis

Description: inflammation and infection of the inner ear affecting the membranous labyrinth of the semicircular canals and associated structures and the central cavity of the cochlea. These are organs of hearing and balance.

Persons most commonly affected: adults of all age groups and both sexes.

Organ or part of body involved: inner ear.

Symptoms and indications: severe dizziness and nystagmus (involuntary, quick movements of the eyes from side to side, up and down or circular). Also, loss of hearing, nausea, vomiting, falling and complete loss of balance. This is a serious condition and the person requires immediate medical attention.

Treatment: depends on cause, but may involve surgery for drainage of fluid from the labyrinth or removal of infected bone cells from the mastoid process (a part of the temporal bone), which is called mastoidectomy. Intensive therapy with antibiotics or antiviral drugs may be required, possibly given intravenously. With prompt treatment, recovery of hearing and from symptoms is usually good but complications can arise (*see causes and rish factors*). The person should rest in bed until all symptoms have disappeared.

Causes and risk factors: the cause is usually a viral or bacterial infection of the inner ear or one from the middle ear that has spread. Labyrinthitis may follow a viral infection such as CHICKEN POX, MUMPS or MEASLES. If the infection is caused by bacteria (purulent labyrinthitis) there is a risk of MENINGITIS and intravenous antibiotics are then necessary.

laryngeal cancer

Description: malignant growth in the larynx (vocal cords and surrounding tissues).

Persons most commonly affected: adults of both sexes in middle age or older, especially men.

Organ or part of body involved: larynx.

Symptoms and indications: persistent hoarseness and sore throat, with pain or difficulty in swallowing and a feeling that there is something caught or an obstruction in the throat. The lymph glands in the neck may also be enlarged and tender. Any person with hoarseness or sore throat that persists should seek medical advice.

Treatment: involves admittance to hospital for radiotherapy and possible removal of the larynx (laryngectomy). In the latter case, the person requires therapy and counselling to learn to communicate without the vocal cords. As with many cancers, the outlook is best if the cancer is caught early before it has spread.

Causes and risk factors: the cause is linked with smoking; hence, the best preventative measure is not to smoke. Risks also increase with overconsumption of alcohol. There is a danger that the cancer will spread to other parts of the body, eventually causing death.

laryngitis

Description: inflammation and/or infection of the mucous membrane that lines the larynx and vocal cords. There are two forms: acute laryngitis accompanies infections of the upper respiratory tract; chronic laryngitis may be due to recurrence of the acute form or to other factors (*see causes and risk factors*). The symptoms are as for acute laryngitis, but with more permanent changes in the vocal cords.

Persons most commonly affected: all age groups and both sexes.

Organ or part of body involved: larynx (the part of the air passage connecting the pharynx with the trachea [or windpipe], and also the organ producing vocal sounds). It is situated high up in the front of the neck.

Symptoms and indications: hoarseness and loss of the voice. There may be a sore throat and difficulty in swallowing or a feeling of a lump in the throat. The person may be feverish. Sometimes the loss of the voice is the only symptom and the person otherwise feels quite well. A person with persistent symptoms of laryngitis should seek medical advice (*see* LARYNGEAL CANCER).

Treatment: the best treatment is to completely rest

the voice and inhalations of moisture-laden air (steam inhalation) are also helpful. Painkillers such as paracetamol may be used to relieve other symptoms. Recovery is usually good, within ten days to two weeks, although it may take some time for the complete range of the voice sounds (i.e. high singing notes) to return. Antibiotics are only effective if a bacterial infection is known to be present. Preventative measures include not smoking and not straining the voice, especially when the person has a cold or upper respiratory tract infection.

Causes and risk factors: the usual cause is a viral infection, although sometimes laryngitis is bacterial in origin. Allergies that produce respiratory symptoms, excessive straining or use of the voice as in shouting or singing and (rarely) cancer of the larynx may cause the condition. Chronic laryngitis is often attributable to excessive smoking with the effects exacerbated by overconsumption of alcohol. Wise preventative measures are not to smoke and to drink alcohol in moderation.

Lassa fever

Description: a serious and highly contagious viral infection first reported from Lassa in Nigeria. Outbreaks tend to occur in some African countries, but imported cases have been reported in the UK and the USA.

Persons most commonly affected: all age groups and both sexes.

Organ or part of body involved: whole body and all body systems except the central nervous system.

Symptoms and indications: the incubation period for this disease is usually about ten days but may be shorter or longer. Early symptoms are less severe and include fever, headache, sore throat, chills, muscle pains and lethargy. Later, vomiting, loss of appetite and weight and severe pains in the chest tend to develop. The sore throat worsens and may show a yellow-white discharge from the tonsils and vomiting worsens, with severe abdominal pains. There may be swelling of neck, face and conjunctiva of the eyes, due to fluid collection, ringing in the ears, rash, bleeding, blood pressure and heart rate changes. Fluid and electrolyte balances are disturbed. Death may follow rapidly, mortality being especially high among pregnant women or those who have just given birth (50%). A person who has returned from an African country where this disease is present should seek immediate medical advice.

Treatment: there is little that can be done to combat the virus itself, so treatment is aimed at alleviation of the symptoms. The correction of fluid and electrolyte imbalance is particularly important. One antiviral agent that appears to be promising and has been used in trials is ribavirin. The person must be kept in isolation and barrier methods of nursing have to be used.

Causes and risk factors: the cause of Lassa fever is an arena virus that is harboured and spread by rats. In Africa, most people are probably infected by contamination of food with rat urine, but person to person infection can occur via body waste, blood or saliva.

Legg-Calvé Perthes' disease

Description: a condition belonging to a group of disorders known as the osteochondroses. These affect the epiphyses, or heads of the long bones, which are separated from the main shaft of these bones in children and fuse and disappear when growth is complete. Legg-Calvé Perthes' disease is the most common form of the osteochondroses and affects the epiphysis at the head of the femur (thigh bone) at the hip joint. There is localized death and degeneration of epiphyseal cells leading to a gradual weakening of the hip joint.

Persons most commonly affected: children between the ages of five and ten years, especially boys.

Organ or part of body involved: epiphysis at head of femur and hip joint, usually on one side.

Symptoms and indications: stiffness and pain in the region of the hip joint and leg, development of a peculiar lopsided gait or limp. Wasting of the thigh muscles. The symptoms develop gradually and slowly. A child with these symptoms requires medical treatment.

Treatment: involves prolonged orthopaedic care. The child may need to be confined to bed for a long period of time, with the use of traction, splints and plaster casts. Surgery may sometimes be needed. Once the child is allowed to use the leg, braces or crutches are likely to be needed for a period of time. The child requires additional help and support in coming to terms with a long period of immobilization. Treatment may be needed for three or four years.

Causes and risk factors: the cause is unknown and may involve a number of different factors. There is a risk of further problems, particularly degenerative OSTEOARTHRITIS, in the affected joint in adult life.

Legionnaire's disease (*Legionella pneumophilia bronchopneumonia*)

Description: an influenza-like illness that is a

bacterial infection and a form of pneumonia. It was named after an outbreak in America in 1976 at the American Legion Convention.

Persons most commonly affected: all age groups and both sexes, especially men.

Organ or part of body involved: lungs, respiratory system.

Symptoms and indications: symptoms appear after a two-to-ten day incubation period and include fever, chills, headaches, muscular aches, cough and breathing problems that may progress to chest pains and PLEURISY. A person with these symptoms should seek medical advice as treatment should begin as soon as possible.

Treatment: is by means of antibiotic drugs, usually erythromycin and rifampicin. Bed rest and the taking of painkillers is helpful to relieve pain and chills. The illness can usually be cured if caught early but may prove fatal in some cases.

Causes and risk factors: the bacterium responsible is called *Legionella pneumophila* and is commonly found in water and soil. Static water provides ideal conditions for multiplication and inhalation of water in aerosol form is the usual means of infection. Air-conditioning cooling towers are a particular source of infected water and the organism may be able to grow at the outlets of taps or showers. If the organism is found to be present, it is vital that infected water tanks, air-conditioning systems, etc., are cleaned and chlorinated.

Leishmaniasis or Kala-azar

Description: a common tropical and sub-tropical disease (in Africa, Asia, South America), caused by minute parasitic organisms, protozoa belonging to the genus *Leishmania*. These organisms are transmitted to human beings by the bites of sandflies. There are two types of the disease, visceral and cutaneous leishmaniasis, which are caused by different varieties of *Leishmania*.

Persons most commonly affected: all age groups and both sexes. Depending upon the country or region, one age group may be more affected than another.

Organ or part of body involved: visceral leishmaniasis—internal organs, liver, spleen, glands, bone marrow. Cutaneous Leishmaniasis—skin, and in some cases, nose, throat and nasal passages.

Symptoms and indications: visceral Leishmaniasis—the person may show symptoms quite rapidly or become gradually unwell. The symptoms are fever and general enlargement of glands and liver and spleen. If not treated, three quarters of those affected will eventually die.

Cutaneous leishmaniasis—skin ulcers, spreading to involve the nose and throat in some cases and countries (South America). There may be erosion of the nasal passages and cartilage in the nose.

A person who has recently travelled to an area where leishmaniasis is prevalent and who shows signs of illness should seek medical advice.

Treatment: the person requires bed rest and good nutrition and intake of fluids. Drugs used include sodium stibogluconate and other pentavalent antimony compounds and pentamidine. These are usually given intravenously but may produce side effects of vomiting and nausea. Recovery is normally good with treatment but fatalities occur in untreated cases.

Causes and risk factors: the cause of leishmaniasis is a number of species of *Leishmania*, which have sandflies as their secondary host and are transmitted to humans via the bite of these insects.

leptospirosis

Description: an acute infection caused by bacteria in the genus *Leptospira*. It is relatively uncommon but some cases occur each year in the UK.

Persons most commonly affected: all age groups and both sexes, especially males. However, adults in certain occupations (*see causes and risk factors*) are most at risk.

Organ or part of body involved: respiratory system and, in the more severe form, the liver, kidneys and central nervous system may be involved.

Symptoms and indications: symptoms in the early stages resemble those of influenza, including fever, headache, chills, aches and pains. The disease may involve the liver causing severe damage and serious jaundice, the central nervous system (meningitis) or the kidneys. A person with symptoms of leptospirosis, especially in an occupation where contact with the organism is a possibility, should seek immediate medical treatment.

Treatment: involves the taking of antibiotics, particularly penicillin, ampicillin or tetracyclines and these must be given as soon as possible. Intravenous doses will be needed in those patients who are seriously ill. As serious metabolic disturbance takes place in the severe form of the disease, the person requires intensive nursing and treatment to correct fluid and electrolyte imbalances. Preventative measures include informing workers about the disease, wearing of protective clothing and, particularly, covering up cuts and abrasions through which the organisms can enter. Bathing or swimming in static water that may be contaminated should be avoided. Also, recent trials suggest that doxycycline might prevent the infection from developing.

Causes and risk factors: the causal organisms are found in the urine of many animals, including dogs and rats. Farmers, sewage workers and veterinary workers are all at greater risk, due to the nature of their occupation. The organisms can enter through cuts in the skin but also via the mucous membranes of the mouth, nose and eyes. Hence some people are infected by swimming in contaminated water. Pregnant women are at risk of aborting the foetus if they become infected, even during recovery from the illness. One particular species of the organism, *L. icterohaemorrhagiae,* is transmitted by rats and is responsible for WEIL'S DISEASE.

As early and less severe symptoms of the infection resemble a respiratory illness like mild influenza, there may be many more cases of the disease than are currently reported. Often medical help is only sought when the disease has advanced and the person has become more seriously ill.

leukaemia

Description: any one of a number of malignant diseases in which there is an uncontrolled proliferation of leucocytes (white blood cells) in the bone marrow. The cells fail to mature to adult cells and thus cannot function as part of the defence mechanism or immune system of the body in fighting infections. Leukaemia is described as acute or chronic forms. In addition, it is further classified by the predominant type of white blood cell involved e.g. acute lymphoblastic leukaemia (lymphoblasts), acute myeloblastic leukaemia (myeloblasts), etc.

Persons most commonly affected: depends upon the type of leukaemia. Acute lymphoblastic leukaemia mainly affects children, especially boys between the ages of two and five. Another form, chronic lymphocytic leukaemia, mainly affects people in middle or older age.

Organ or part of body involved: white blood cells, bone marrow, spleen, lymph glands, liver, eventually affecting the whole body if the disease is not checked.

Symptoms and indications: anaemia, pallor, fatigue, bruising easily and, occasionally, nosebleeds or bleeding from the gums or gastrointestinal tract.

Also, enlargement of the spleen, lymph nodes and liver. A person with symptoms of leukaemia requires immediate medical treatment that should begin as soon as possible.

Treatment: involves chemotherapy with such drugs as methotrexate, vincristine, mercatopurine, cyclophosphamide and cortisone, in some cases, for other acute forms of leukaemia. Other types of leukaemia may be treated with busulphan, mercatopurine, cyclophosphamide or chlorambucil. Also, surgery in the form of a bone-marrow transplant or radiotherapy may be needed. The outlook for patients with leukaemia has improved dramatically over recent years. Although there is still no cure, both short- and long-term survival rates have continued to improve and the outlook is now much more optimistic, especially for children.

Causes and risk factors: the cause of leukaemia is unknown, although there is a suspected link, for some forms of the disease, with ionizing radiation, viruses, toxic chemicals, such as benzene, and genetic factors.

lipoma

Description: a common type of benign tumour made up of fat cells.

Persons most commonly affected: adults of both sexes and all age groups, especially women.

Organ or part of body involved: subcutaneous layers beneath the skin surface or in other fibrous tissues.

Symptoms and indications: a lump develops, usually beneath the skin of the arms or upper body but can occur anywhere. It can be moved about and is relatively soft and painless. A person should seek medical advice if concerned about a lipoma or if its characteristics undergo a change.

Treatment: lipomas are harmless and do not require any treatment unless disfiguring or troublesome in any way. In the latter case, they can be removed by surgery or liposuction.

Causes and risk factors: the cause is not known and there is little evidence of lipomas being in any way connected with malignancy.

listeriosis

Description: an infectious and contagious disease of animals that can be transmitted to man.

Persons most commonly affected: all age groups and both sexes. Newborn babies may acquire the infection from the placenta if the mother has the infection.

Organ or part of body involved: respiratory system

and possibly affecting the central nervous system.

Symptoms and indications: early symptoms are similar to those of influenza, including fever, headache, aches and pains, chills, tiredness. However, it often causes inflammation of the central nervous system (especially MENINGITIS) and encephalitis (or inflammation of the brain). The eyes may be inflamed and lymph glands and nodes are enlarged. A person with symptoms of listeriosis requires admittance to hospital for intensive antibiotic treatment.

Treatment: is by means of antibiotics, especially penicillin, given intravenously. This treatment is usually effective but elderly persons, the very young and pregnant women are most at risk and the disease can be fatal.

Causes and risk factors: the cause is the bacterium *Listeria monocytogenes*, which infects farm animals. People acquire the organism either through eating infected foods or directly through contact with infected animals (particularly abattoir workers, butchers, vets and farmers). The bacteria are able to grow and survive on food stored in a refrigerator. If the infection is contracted during pregnancy, it may result in abortion or damage to the foetus.

liver abscess

Description: a collection of pus in the liver, which may develop as a complication of some other disease or condition.

Persons most commonly affected: all age groups and both sexes.

Organ or part of body involved: liver.

Symptoms and indications: symptoms include fever, general malaise, nausea, severe pain in the abdomen and tenderness, especially in the area of the liver. Pain may also be felt in the right shoulder and there may be pronounced shivering (rigor). The liver is greatly enlarged. There is loss of weight and appetite. A person with symptoms of liver inflammation or abscess requires immediate medical treatment.

Treatment: is by means of antibiotic drugs, including the nitroimidazole group, usually metronidazole, if the cause of the abscess is amoebic DYSENTERY. The person requires bed rest and adequate intake of fluids. With treatment, recovery is normally good but may take some time.

Causes and risk factors: the cause is usually amoebic dysentery and the abscess may develop some time after disease symptoms have disappeared. Further causes include inflammation in the river due to other diseases or conditions or

as a result of blood poisoning. It may be necessary for the abscess to be drained by aspiration of its contents through a needle under local anaesthetic. However, this is less likely to be performed than formerly and antibiotics are the usual first choice of treatment.

liver cancer or hepatocellular carcinoma or hepatoma

Description: uncontrolled proliferation of malignant cells in the liver, which may either be primary (hepatoma) or a secondary growth resulting from a cancer elsewhere in the body. Primary liver cancer is rare in western countries but more common in Africa and Asia. (*See also* HEPATOCELLULAR CARCINOMA, HEPATOMA.)

Persons most commonly affected: adults of both sexes but more likely to occur in men aged 60 and over.

Organ or part of body involved: liver.

Symptoms and indications: enlargement of the liver with lumps that may be able to be felt externally. Malaise, severe loss of weight and appetite, fluid retention (oedema), JAUNDICE and abdominal pain. A person with symptoms of liver disease should seek immediate medical treatment.

Treatment: the condition is not considered to be curable but treatment with anticancer drugs or surgery may be needed. Other drugs to control symptoms, especially pain, will also be needed.

Causes and risk factors: secondary liver cancer may occur as a result of spread of a primary cancer elsewhere in the body (metastasis). Tumours involved include those of the breast, colon, lung, stomach and pancreas. Sometimes, the secondary growth is discovered before the primary tumour is located.

lung abscess

Description: a relatively uncommon condition in which there is inflammation and a collection of pus in one or more areas of a lung.

Persons most commonly affected: all age groups and both sexes.

Organ or part of body involved: lung.

Symptoms and indications: symptoms include fever, malaise and chills with sweating. The person may have a cough, producing sputum that may contain pus or blood and be foul-smelling. The person may have pain in the chest. If pus is coughed up, it indicates that the abscess has burst and is discharging into the lung or bronchial tube. A person with symptoms of a lung abscess requires prompt medical treatment.

Treatment: consists of taking antibiotic drugs to kill the bacteria causing the abscess. The organism may first need to be isolated (from the sputum) and grown in order to prescribe the most effective antibiotic. Several courses of antibiotics for quite a long period may be needed to clear up the abscess and prevent a recurrence of the infection. The person may be required to practise postural drainage to rid the lungs of the secretions. Occasionally surgery may be needed to drain the abscess of pus and enable healing to take place.

Causes and risk factors: the cause may be mechanical, i.e. a foreign body such as a small piece of food that finds its way down into the lung setting up inflammation and infection. Or, it may result from PNEUMONIA, blood poisoning or TUBERCULOSIS or a wound in the lung allowing bacteria to penetrate.

lung cancer

Description: uncontrolled growth of malignant cells in the lung.

Persons most commonly affected: adults of both sexes aged over 40 but especially men.

Organ or part of body involved: lung.

Symptoms and indications: severe, permanent cough producing sputum that may be flecked with blood. Wheezing, pain in chest and abnormal tiredness. Unexplained weight loss. Any person with a persistent cough or other symptoms of lung cancer should seek medical treatment as soon as possible.

Treatment: may involve chemotherapy, radiotherapy, or occasionally, surgery. Pain-relieving drugs may also be prescribed. Lung cancer is incurable although symptoms can be relieved.

Causes and risk factors: in almost all cases, the cause is smoking—usually direct smoking of cigarettes but also 'passive smoking'. It may be caused by breathing airborne pollutants, especially asbestos dust, but smoking is widely recognized to be the main preventable reason for this disease. Hence the most obvious preventative measure is not to take up, or to stop, smoking. A smoker who gives up the habit immediately lessens his or her chance of developing the disease. Lung cancer causes thousands of premature deaths each year, more than any other form of the disease.

lupus erythematosus and lupus vulgaris or discoid lupus erythematosus or DLE

Description: lupus describes a number of skin disorders of which there are two main kinds, lupus erythematosus and lupus vulgaris (rare). The two types are not related.

Persons most commonly affected: lupus erythematosus—women, particularly those in their 30s but can also affect men. Lupus vulgaris—young people of both sexes below the age of 20, but lasts throughout life.

Organ or part of body involved: lupus erythematosus (discoid)—skin, especially of face, but also neck, scalp, ears and arms. If it affects the scalp, it may cause bald patches to appear. There may be some mild inflammation and pain in the joints. Lupus vulgaris—skin, especially of face and neck but also mucous membranes within the mouth and nose.

Symptoms and indications: lupus erythematosus—round, raised patches of reddened skin that may merge at the fringes, when they are described as 'butterfly' lesions. They are unsightly and may cause scarring.

Lupus vulgaris—appearance of a small, yellow, transparent nodules that gradually proliferate and are called 'apple jelly' nodules. The skin becomes ulcerated and thickened and, if not treated, over a number of years can even be eaten away in places. The lesions leave considerable scarring. A person with symptoms of lupus should seek medical advice. Tests are needed to confirm the diagnosis.

Treatment: lupus erythematosus (discoid)—the condition is made worse by exposure to sunlight, hence this should be avoided as far as possible and sunscreen products may need to be used. The patches are treated with ointments and creams containing corticosteroids. Sometimes, local injection of the lesions with triamcinolone acetonide may be required. A daily oral dose of hydroxy-chloroquine (an antimalarial drug) may be prescribed, which helps to control the symptoms.

Lupus vulgaris—this is treated with antituberculous drugs and nodules may occasionally be surgically removed.

Causes and risk factors: lupus erythematosus (discoid)—the cause is unknown but it is thought to be an autoimmune disease. About 10% of patients with this disorder go on to develop SYSTEMIC LUPUS ERYTHEMATOSUS (SLE).

Lupus vulgaris—this is caused by the bacterium responsible for tuberculosis, *Mycobacterium tuberculosis*. It is a rare manifestation of tuberculosis and can be effectively prevented and treated.

Lyme disease

Description: an inflammatory disorder that

produces a wide range of symptoms over a period of time.

Persons most commonly affected: all age groups and both sexes.

Organ or part of body involved: skin, joints, heart, central nervous system.

Symptoms and indications: the first symptoms in most affected persons is the development of a small, raised red bump or papule, usually on the buttock, thigh or under the arm, which spreads and may become quite large. Other skin lesions may then appear. Accompanying symptoms include fever and chills, fatigue, headache, muscle and neck aches and general malaise. Nausea, vomiting, sore throat, backache and enlargement of spleen and lymph glands may occur. Within weeks or months about half of those affected develop symptoms of ARTHRITIS, especially in the knee joint. This may persist and cause problems for years. Less commonly, within weeks or months of acquiring the disease, inflammation of the central nervous system, particularly aseptic MENINGITIS and BELL'S PALSY may occur. Also, inflammation and enlargement of the heart resulting in conduction disorders may rarely occur.

Lyme disease occurs in many countries, especially in the autumn. A person with symptoms of this disease or who has received a tick bite should seek medical advice.

Treatment: is by means of antibiotics, especially penicillins and erythromycin. If complications arise, these are treated with other appropriate drugs, including aspirin and other NSAIDs (non-steroidal anti-inflammatory drugs). Skin symptoms may respond and clear within two weeks with early antibiotic treatment. Other symptoms may persist and only slowly subside and may have a tendency to recur.

Causes and risk factors: the cause of Lyme disease is a spirochaete bacterium *Borrelia burgdorfen*, transmitted by ticks that are parasites of a variety of mammals including deer. The risk increases for those living in wooded or other areas where ticks may be present.

lymphoma or lymphosarcoma, non-Hodgkin's lymphoma

Description: a tumour, usually malignant, of the lymph glands and nodes.

Persons most commonly affected: all age groups and both sexes, especially elderly persons aged 60 to 70.

Organ or part of body involved: lymph system— glands, nodes, vessels and spleen.

Symptoms and indications: enlargement of lymph glands anywhere in the body; this may be most obvious in the armpit, groin and neck. The swellings are usually not painful. The person is tired, with general malaise and loss of appetite and weight. The spleen and liver become enlarged, with symptoms of JAUNDICE and ANAEMIA. A person with symptoms of lymphoma should seek immediate medical advice.

Treatment: is by means of radiotherapy and chemotherapy. The outlook depends upon the type of lymphoma, with some responding better than others.

Causes and risk factors: the cause is unknown but there may be a link with viruses in some cases. There are no known preventative measures but it is wise not to smoke.

M

malaria

Description: an infection caused by minute parasites in the blood and characterized by recurring bouts of fever. It cannot be contracted in the UK but infection can be acquired by those travelling abroad.

Persons most commonly affected: all age groups and both sexes.

Organ or part of body involved: blood (red blood corpuscles or cells), liver and central nervous system.

Symptoms and indications: depending upon the type of malarial parasite, symptoms develop from about one to four weeks after a bite by an infected mosquito. The person may feel somewhat unwell for one or two days before the onset of an attack, which typically passes through three stages, although these are not always apparent. The first stage (cold stage) is marked by extreme shivering and feeling very cold although the person has a high temperature. After about one hour, this is followed by the hot stage. The person is burning with fever, has a very high temperature, a headache, nausea, giddiness and pain, and may become delirious. The final, sweating stage is marked by profuse perspiration and a fall in temperature. The aches and pains subside and the person, although weak, feels better. Depending upon the type of parasite, there is a lapse of a certain period of time (two or three days or a few hours) before the next attack.

There may be widespread destruction of red blood cells, especially with recurrent attacks, and if the disease becomes chronic the person may become severely anaemic. The person becomes jaundiced and the liver and spleen are enlarged. Usually over a few weeks, even without treatment, the number of parasites in the blood drops to a low level and no more attacks occur. However, they can become active again and multiply to produce further bouts of fever.

Any person returning from a country where malaria occurs, who develops these symptoms should seek immediate medical treatment.

Treatment: complete bed rest and adequate intake of fluids is important. There are various drugs used for the prevention of malaria, and it is necessary to consult a doctor to obtain a course of these before travelling to a country where the disease occurs. The drugs afford some degree of protection but are not totally effective and infection may still occur. Treatment involves the taking of various antimalarial drugs, especially chloroquinine, but may vary according to the area in which the infection was acquired. (The parasites have developed resistance to some of the drugs used in certain areas.) Treatment is normally effective for most forms of malaria. However, life-threatening complications can arise and some people may require intensive treatment in hospital.

Causes and risk factors: the cause of malaria is infection by any one of four types of protozoan organisms. These belong to the genus *Plasmodium* and are *P. falciparium, P. malariae, P. vivax* and *P. ovale*. These organisms complete some stage of their lifecycle within female *Anopheles* mosquitoes. The mosquito acquires the organisms by biting an infected person. It passes them on in its saliva when it bites an uninfected person. The parasite passes in the blood circulation to the liver and multiplies there. Eventually they return to the blood and occupy red blood cells, further enlarging and multiplying in the process. Finally, they rupture and destroy the red blood cells. The bouts of fever correspond with the rupturing of the red blood cells and the parasites that are released go on to invade new cells. In some type of malaria (*P. vivax* and *P. ovale*) the parasite persists within the liver. A person may die due to the high fever that can occur during a malarial attack. Also, the parasites may be so numerous as to block small blood vessels in the brain, which again can be fatal (cerebral malaria). A very dangerous complication is blackwater fever, characterized by high fever, severe ANAEMIA, great destruction of red blood cells and the presence of haemoglobin (the red blood pigment) in the urine. Malaria is likely to be more dangerous if treatment is inadequate and does not eradicate the organisms. Also in people who are poorly nourished or otherwise ill or run-down from some other cause.

mastitis

Description: acute inflammation and infection of the breast. Cystic mastitis is another form that does not involve inflammation but the presence of cysts (thought to be caused by hormonal factors) that make the breasts lumpy.

Persons most commonly affected: breast-feeding mothers of any age, especially during the first two months of nursing.

Symptoms and indications: some discomfort and hardness in the breast is usually noticed first. If not treated, the whole breast may become swollen, hard, red and painful, especially when suckling the baby, and the mother may be feverish. A woman with symptoms of mastitis should seek immediate medical advice.

Treatment: is by means of antibiotics, especially penicillin as soon as possible to prevent the formation of an abscess. Pain relief can be used as directed by a doctor. The breasts should be kept well supported and clean but it is usually not necessary to stop breast-feeding. If an abscess forms, breast-feeding must be stopped on the affected side and, in severe cases, finished completely by giving hormones to halt the production of milk. The abscess needs to be surgically opened and drained and antibiotic treatment given. Milk production often stops naturally in women who develop a breast abscess. Preventative measures include keeping the breasts scrupulously clean with careful washing and drying and use of creams. This is especially important at the start of breast-feeding when cracked nipples are more likely to occur, as the skin is not accustomed to suckling. If cracked nipples occur a cream should be used, as recommended by a doctor.

Causes and risk factors: the usual cause is bacteria that gain access through cracks in the nipples; often staphylococcus or streptococcus organisms are involved.

measles or **rubeola** or **morbilli**)

Description: an extremely infectious disease, characterized by the presence of a rash, and usually occurring in children in epidemics every two or three years.

Persons most commonly affected: children of both sexes but can occur at any age in people not immunized or previously exposed to the infection.

Organ or part of body involved: skin and upper respiratory tract, eyes.

Symptoms and indications: after an incubation period of 10–15 days, the initial symptoms are those of a cold, with coughing, sneezing, red, watery eyes and high fever. It is at this stage that the disease is most infectious and spreads from one child to another in airborne droplets before measles has been diagnosed. This is the main factor responsible for the epidemic nature of the disease. Small red spots with a white centre (known as Koplik spots) in the mouth, on the inside of the cheeks. Then a characteristic rash develops on the skin, spreading from behind the ears and across the face and also affecting other areas. The small red spots may be grouped together in patches and the child's fever is usually at its height while these are developing. The spots and fever gradually decline and no marks are left upon the skin, most children making a good recovery. The infection is not, however, without risk and complications can arise (*see causes and risk factors*). A child with symptoms of measles should be seen by a doctor and the diagnosis confirmed.

Treatment: involves keeping the child at home and in bed while he or she is feverish and unwell. Plenty of fluids should be drunk and pain relief in a form designed for children may be given, as advised by the doctor. If the symptoms worsen, particularly if there is a very high temperature, earache or severe headache or any signs of breathing difficulties, the doctor should be called immediately. Preventative treatment in the form of a vaccine is available and protects children from the severe symptoms and complications of measles. It is normally advisable for all children to be immunized.

Causes and risk factors: the cause of measles is a virus and it is an unpleasant infection that makes the child feel quite ill. Complications can occur, especially PNEUMONIA and middle-ear infections that can result in DEAFNESS. Also, inflammation of the brain (encephalitis) or MENINGITIS can occur as a result of measles, and the infection may prove fatal in some children.

melanoma

Description: any one of several extremely malignant tumours of the melanocytes, the cells in the skin that produce melanin. Melanomas are also found, although less commonly, in the mucous membranes and in the eye. A highly malignant form can also arise from the pigmented cells of moles on the skin.

Persons most commonly affected: adults of all age groups, particularly white-skinned people and both sexes. It is rare in dark-skinned people. The incidence of malignant melanoma is increasing in the UK.

Organ or part of body involved: skin but may spread to other body organs, especially the liver and lymph nodes.

Symptoms and indications: appearance of a raised or flat, painless skin lesion that may be of a variety of colours and may bleed slightly. A person with a skin lesion or mole, especially one that is active and undergoing change, should seek immediate medical advice.

Treatment: if malignant melanoma is diagnosed early, treatment in the form of surgical removal of the lesion is highly successful and the condition can be cured. However, if the melanoma has spread, the outlook is less favourable. Treatment with radiotherapy and chemotherapy may be recommended in these cases. Preventative measures include, most importantly, protecting the skin from exposure to the sun. This involves wearing clothing and a hat to cover or shade the skin, avoiding the sun during the hottest part of the day and using sunscreen products. These measures are particularly important in young children and fair-skinned people. Sunbathing should be avoided as should exposure to ultraviolet light (i.e. the use of sun lamps, sun beds, etc).

Causes and risk factors: there is a link between the development of malignant melanoma and exposure to the sun, especially harmful ultraviolet radiation. The fact that the incidence of the condition is rising has been linked by some with the formation of holes in the ozone layer that screens the earth from UV radiation. Any person whose work or leisure activities involves excessive exposure to the sun runs an increased risk of developing this form of cancer. Hence it is wise to be aware of and practise the preventative measures outlined above.

Ménière's disease

Description: a disease first described by the Frenchman, Prosper Ménière in 1861, which affects the inner ear causing a range of symptoms.

Persons most commonly affected: both sexes in middle age but slightly more common in men.

Organ or part of body involved: the membranous labyrinth of the inner ear, usually affecting one side only.

Symptoms and indications: this usually begins with some hearing loss in one ear, followed after a period of months by a severe attack of giddiness or vertigo. This occurs suddenly, often waking the person up from sleep at night, and is accompanied by ringing in the ear (tinnitus). This is usually followed by vomiting and sweating. The symptoms usually subside in a few hours but the person is unsteady with loss of balance for some days afterwards. Another attack may follow in about one week or after some months. With each attack, the loss of hearing becomes worse until the person is completely deaf in the affected ear. A person with symptoms of Ménière's disease should seek medical advice.

Treatment: involves a variety of different drugs to control symptoms and also, possibly, surgery. An affected person should rest in bed until symptoms have subsided. Diuretic drugs to prevent fluid accumulation may be prescribed. No method of treatment is completely successful but some symptoms can be relieved.

Causes and risk factors: the cause is unknown but the symptoms are due to an overaccumulation of fluid in the labyrinth of the inner ear. It has been suggested that this may be an allergic reaction or due to spasm of tiny blood vessels supplying the inner ear.

meningitis

Description: inflammation of the meninges (membranes) of the brain (cerebral meningitis) or spinal cord (spinal meningitis) or the disease may affect both regions. Meningitis may affect the dura mater membrane, the outermost layer or meninx, in which case it is known as pachymeningitis. Or, it often results as a secondary infection due to the presence of disease elsewhere, as in the case of tuberculous and syphilitic meningitis. Meningitis that affects the other two membranes (the piaarachnoid membranes) is known as leptomeningitis, which is more common and may be either a primary or a secondary infection. Meningitis is also classified according to its causal organism (viral or bacterial).

Persons most commonly affected: all age groups and both sexes.

Organ or part of body involved: central nervous system.

Symptoms and indications: the symptoms include a severe headache, sensitivity to light and sound, muscle rigidity, especially affecting the neck, Kernig's sign (an inability to straighten the legs at the knees when the thighs are at right angles to the body), vomiting, confusion and coma, leading to death. These are caused by inflammation of the meninges and by a rise in intracranial pressure. One of the features of meningitis is that there is a change in the constituents and appearance of the cerebrospinal fluid and the infective organism can usually be isolated from it and identified. One of the most feared aspects of (bacterial) meningitis is that the onset of symptoms can be very rapid and death can also follow swiftly. A person with symptoms of meningitis requires admittance to hospital for urgent medical treatment.

Treatment: depends upon the cause of the meningitis, which is established by analysis of the cerebrospinal fluid. If the cause is a virus, the disease is usually less severe but may still prove fatal in some cases. Mild cases may recover spontaneously with bed rest in a darkened room. Some cases require treatment by means of antiviral drugs, such as acyclovir, given intravenously. If the cause is a fungal or yeast infection, the drug amphotericin B is normally given intravenously. Various bacteria may cause meningitis, especially those responsible for TUBERCULOSIS, PNEUMONIA and SYPHILIS. Treatment is by means of intensive doses of appropriate antibiotics and sulphonamide drugs given intravenously. The person requires additional treatment to correct dehydration and electrolyte disturbances and to lower fever.

Causes and risk factors: three types of bacteria are responsible for most cases of bacterial meningitis. These are *Haemophilus influenzae* type b, *Neisseria meningitidis* (meningococcus) and *Streptococcus pneumoniae* (pneumococcus). Meningococcus occurs in the nose and throat of about 5% of the population, who are carriers of the organism but rarely become ill themselves. Meningococcal meningitis is the most common form of the disease in children aged one year or under. Pneumococcal meningitis is the most common type in adults. In general, the very young and the very old are most at risk from meningitis but modern treatments and drug therapy have improved the outlook for recovery considerably.

mesothelioma

Description: a usually malignant tumour of the pleura of the chest cavity (a membrane that covers the lungs and inside of the chest wall). It may also affect the pericardium (the membrane surrounding the heart) or the peritoneum (the membrane lining the abdominal cavity).

Persons most commonly affected: men in middle age who have previously worked with asbestos but can affect adults of either sex.

Organ or part of body involved: lungs and lining membranes.

Symptoms and indications: early indications include breathlessness on exercise, and there may be chest pain and a cough and symptoms of bronchitis. The breathlessness continues to get worse, ultimately leading to respiratory failure and death as the cancer spreads. A person with symptoms of breathlessness, persistent cough, etc., should seek early medical advice.

Treatment: most mesotheliomas are in sites that are inoperable, although occasionally surgery may be possible. Chemotherapy and radiotherapy may be used, although success is limited. Treatment is mainly aimed at relieving symptoms and easing breathing difficulties.

Causes and risk factors: the cause of malignant mesothelioma is usually previous exposure to asbestos dust, especially the form called crocidolite. Even a brief period of exposure of as little as six months to two years may be sufficient to cause problems in later life. Less common, benign mesothelioma of the pleura is not related to asbestos dust. The risk of developing all forms of lung cancer is greatly increased in persons who smoke cigarettes. Preventative measures for those who have to work with asbestos include dust suppression and the wearing of protective clothing. *See also* ASBESTOSIS.

methahaemoglobinaemia

Description: the presence in the blood of an excess of methahaemoglobin. Methahaemoglobin is derived from the blood pigment haemoglobin, and is formed when the iron this contains is oxidized from ferrous to ferric form. Methahaemoglobin cannot combine with oxygen in the lungs and so is unable to carry this in the blood circulation to the body tissues. There are two types of methahaemoglobinaemia, hereditary and toxic. A third form, infantile methahaemoglobinaemia, may rarely occur in bottle-fed babies due to high level of nitrates in the water used to make the baby's feed.

Persons most commonly affected: all age groups and both sexes.

Organ or part of body involved: blood circulation—affecting all body systems.

Symptoms and indications: a blue tinge to the lips,

tips of the ears, cheeks and nails and then the whole of the skin (cyanosis), tiredness, headache, sickness and nausea, giddiness and breathlessness. A person with these symptoms should seek immediate medical treatment.

Treatment: for the toxic form, the drug that is suspected to have caused the condition should be immediately stopped, if the symptoms are severe. The person may require ascorbic acid (vitamin C) or methylene blue and these are used to treat the inherited form of the condition.

Causes and risk factors: the cause of the inherited form is an abnormality of the haemoglobin molecule in the blood. The toxic form is caused by certain drugs that cause the iron atoms in the haemoglobin molecules to become oxidized. These include sulphonamides, phenacetin, acetanilide, benzocaine and prilocaine (local anaesthetics), polyphenols and dinitrophenol. An excess of nitrates in some foods, e.g. spinach and carrots, and bakery products containing excess nitrobenzene may also cause the formation of methahaemoglobin in the blood. Serious cases of the infantile form of the condition have mainly affected people with a private water supply. Guidelines exist to ensure that if public water supplies are likely to exceed the recommended safety levels for nitrate, alternative arrangements can be made.

migraine

Description: a very severe, throbbing headache, usually on one side of the head, and often accompanied by other symptoms.

Persons most commonly affected: adolescents and adults of both sexes but especially premenopausal women.

Organ or part of body involved: head, eyes, gastrointestinal tract.

Symptoms and indications: early symptoms of a migraine attack may be nausea and disturbance of vision in the form of seeing flickering bright lights (the aura of migraine). A severe, throbbing pain develops, often sited over one eye, nausea continues and there may be vomiting. The person is sensitive to light and sound, which make the condition worse.

Treatment: consists of rest in bed in a darkened, quiet room until the symptoms subside (up to 24 hours), and taking pain-relieving drugs. Other drugs that may be prescribed are ergotamine tartrate and metoclopramide. An affected person may have to experiment to find which pain-relieving drugs are the most helpful. Usually, they

are most effective if taken during the period when an attack is felt to be coming on.

Causes and risk factors: the cause is unknown but is thought to involve constriction followed by dilation of blood vessels in the brain and an outpouring of fluid into surrounding tissues. Migraine is a common condition and seems to be triggered by any one or several of a number of factors. These include anxiety, fatigue, watching television or video screens, loud noises, flickering lights (e.g. strobe lights) and some foods such as cheese and chocolate, and alcoholic drinks. There may be an inherited tendency for migraine and the most common time of onset is puberty. In women, attacks may no longer occur after the menopause.

mitral incompetence or mitral regurgitation

Description: a condition in which the mitral valve of the heart is defective and allows blood to leak back from the left ventricle (larger, lower chamber) into the left atrium (smaller, upper chamber). It may be a congenital condition or result from disease of the valve. The mitral valve, formerly known as the bicuspid valve, is located between the atrium and ventricle of the left side of the heart, attached to the walls at the opening between the two. It has two cusps or flaps that normally allow blood to pass into the ventricle from the atrium but prevent any backflow.

Persons most commonly affected: adults of both sexes in middle or older age groups, or newborn babies if a congenital condition.

Organ or part of body involved: mitral valve of heart.

Symptoms and indications: if mild, there may be few or no symptoms. In more severe cases, there is breathlessness, especially at night, wheezing, changes in heartbeat rhythm (atrial fibrillation) and a tendency for clots to form (EMBOLISM). The left ventricle is forced to work harder and enlarges but eventually may be unable to cope and this can result in left-sided heart failure. A person with symptoms of mitral valve disease should seek medical advice.

Treatment: a person with mild or moderate mitral incompetence should not undertake hard physical exercise. Treatment with antibiotics may be required to prevent endocarditis (inflammation of the endocardium, a membrane lining the heart, and heart valves and muscle). Intensive antibiotic treatment may be needed before dental work is carried out. If the cause of the condition is RHEUMATIC FEVER, then daily doses of penicillin may be needed to prevent a flare-up of the condition, risking further damage to the mitral valve. In more severe cases, surgery to replace the defective valve may be required (mitral prosthesis).

Causes and risk factors: as indicated above, the cause may be a congenital abnormality or due to scarring and damage to the valve caused by rheumatic fever. Also, heart disease, a previous heart attack, infection or inflammation may be responsible for mitral valve incompetence. *See also* MITRAL STENOSIS.

mitral stenosis

Description: a condition in which the opening between the left atrium (smaller, upper chamber of the heart) and left ventricle (lower, larger chamber of the heart) is narrowed, due to scarring and adhesion of the mitral valve. The mitral valve, formerly known as the bicuspid valve, is located between the atrium and ventricle of the left side of the heart, attached to the walls at the opening between the two. It has two cusps or flaps that normally allow blood to pass into the ventricle from the atrium, but prevent any backflow.

Persons most commonly affected: adults of both sexes between the ages of 30 and 40 who have previously (in childhood) had RHEUMATIC FEVER.

Organ or part of body involved: mitral valve of heart.

Symptoms and indications: the condition may be symptomless, even in patients with quite considerable mitral valve stenosis. Symptoms, when present, are similar to those found in MITRAL INCOMPETENCE but there is also a diastolic murmur. (Diastole is the point in the cycle of heart contraction when the heart relaxes between contractions and the ventricles fill with blood.) A person with symptoms of mitral stenosis should seek medical advice.

Treatment: various drugs may be prescribed for those patients with a mild or moderate degree of mitral stenosis, in order to manage the condition. These include calcium antagonists or betablockers, digitalis, anticoagulants, warfarin and aspirin. In more severe forms of the disease, the condition may be treated surgically by widening the stenosis (mitral valvotomy) or by valve replacement (mitral prosthesis).

Causes and risk factors: the cause of this condition is almost always previous rheumatic fever and it may be many years before the damage to the mitral valve becomes apparent (10–20 years), and symptoms are noticed. The cause may occasionally be congenital but an affected infant does not usually survive.

multiple sclerosis (MS)

Description: a disease of the brain and spinal cord, which affects the myelin sheaths (protein and phospholipid coverings) of nerves and disrupts their function.

Persons most commonly affected: adults of both sexes in younger age group between the ages of 20 and 40.

Organ or part of body involved: the brain and spinal cord (the central nervous system).

Symptoms and indications: the disease is characterized by the presence of patches of hardened (sclerotic) connective tissue irregularly scattered through the brain and spinal cord. At first the fatty part of the nerve sheaths breaks down and is absorbed, leaving bare nerve fibres, and then connective tissue is laid down. Symptoms depend upon the site of the patches in the central nervous system and the disease is characterized by periods of progression and remission. However, they include unsteady gait and apparent clumsiness, tremor of the limbs, involuntary eye movements, speech disorders, loss of bladder and bowel control, paralysis and male impotence. A particular reflex sign, known as Babinski sign, is shown when the sole of the foot is firmly stroked. This is an abnormal reaction of the toes (the large toe curls upwards and the other toes spread outwards, whereas normally all the toes curve downwards) that is exhibited by people with multiple sclerosis. A person with symptoms of multiple sclerosis should seek medical advice.

Treatment: there is no specific treatment and since the progress of the disease is marked by periods of remission (which may last for months or even years), followed by relapse, the effectiveness of drugs is difficult to determine. Prednesone, dexamethasone and corticosteroids may be prescribed during periods when the symptoms are active. The affected person should lead as normal and active a life as possible but avoid stress and becoming overtired. Massage and physiotherapy are helpful, as are all physical and mental activities that help the person to maintain an optimistic outlook on life.

Causes and risk factors: the cause is unknown but is the subject of ongoing research. It is not clear whether there is a hereditary factor involved or, possibly, infection by a slow virus may be implicated. There may be some abnormality in the immune system that makes certain people susceptible or multiple sclerosis may be an autoimmune disorder.

mumps

Description: an inflammatory and infectious disease of childhood caused by a virus.

Persons most commonly affected: children of both sexes between the ages of 5 and 15 but can occur in older age groups.

Organ or part of body involved: parotid salivary glands, other salivary glands and, possibly, the pancreas, breasts, testes, ovaries, meninges of the brain and spinal cord.

Symptoms and indications: the incubation period, following infection, is two to three weeks before symptoms start to appear. These include feverishness, headache, sore throat and vomiting before, or along with, a swelling of the parotid gland on one side of the face. (The parotid glands are a pair of salivary glands, one situated in front of each ear and opening inside on the cheek near the second last molar of the upper jaw.) The swelling may be confined to one side or spread to the other side of the face, and may also go on to include the submaxillary and sublingual salivary glands beneath the jaw. Generally after a few days, the swelling subsides and the child recovers but remains infectious until the glands have returned to normal. If a child has symptoms of mumps it is advisable to consult a doctor.

Treatment: there is no specific treatment, other than keeping the child isolated from others until no longer infectious, and in bed while the symptoms are at their height. Pain relief suitable for children may be given, as advised by a doctor, and the child should be encouraged to drink plenty of fluids. However, acidic foods and drinks (fruit juices, etc.) should be avoided. Food should be soft, to reduce the pain of chewing and swallowing. Complications may arise, especially in adults and young people past puberty. About 20% of males develop inflammation of the testes (orchitis) which, in rare cases, can cause sterility. The testes may need to be supported and ice packs applied to relieve pain and, occasionally, corticosteroid drugs may be prescribed by the doctor. A smaller proportion of females develop inflammation of the ovaries (oophoritis), which is generally treated with appropriate pain relief. PANCREATITIS (inflammation of the pancreas) may occur, causing vomiting and nausea. If this is severe, the patient may become dehydrated and require salt and dextrose solutions by intravenous drip to restore fluid and electrolyte balance. Also, inflammation of the brain and meninges (membranes) or meningoencephalitis, may arise as a complication of mumps, requiring appropriate treatment in hospital.

Preventative treatment for mumps is in the form of the MMR (measles, mumps, rubella) vaccine which, in the UK, is routinely offered to children usually in their second year.

Causes and risk factors: the cause is a virus affecting the salivary glands.

muscular dystrophy or myopathy

Description: any one of a group of diseases that involve wasting of muscles and in which a hereditary factor is involved. The disease is classified according to the groups of muscles that it affects and the age at which it first appears. The commonest form is Duchenne muscular dystrophy, which is a sex-linked, recessive disorder. (It is carried on the X chromosome and affects males because they have the sex chromosomes XY, females being XX.) The genes responsible are recessive, but in males there is no other X chromosome to mask them and so they are able to be expressed and cause the disorder.) The mother is the carrier but has no symptoms of the disease herself; however, half of her sons are likely to be affected.

Persons most commonly affected: (Duchenne muscular dystrophy) boys between the ages of three and seven years.

Organ or part of body involved: muscles, usually attacking the pelvic girdle first (hips) and the shoulder girdle.

Symptoms and indications: the disease causes muscle fibres to degenerate and be replaced by fatty and fibrous tissue. Early symptoms are a peculiar waddling gait, numerous falls, difficulty in standing up and going up and down stairs. The spine curves inwards, a condition known as lordosis, and the child walks on his toes rather than placing the heel down first. The muscles appear large and firm but this is due to the internal changes that are taking place. Muscles become progressively weaker and usually the child is confined to a wheelchair by about the age of 12. Some other forms of muscular dystrophy are, however, less severe. A child with muscular dystrophy requires ongoing support and therapy.

Treatment: there is no specific drug treatment at present although trials on the corticosteroid drug prednisone are being carried out. Therapy is aimed at keeping the child as physically and mentally active as possible. Methods used include physiotherapy, massage and orthopaedic measures. There is no cure for this disorder, and the outlook depends upon the type of disease, discovered by tests (muscle biopsy and electromyography).

Causes and risk factors: the cause is a genetic mutation resulting in a lack of a protein called dystrophin, which is essential for the normal functioning of muscle cells. In the severest form, Duchenne muscular dystrophy, serious life-threatening complications can arise, especially chest and other infections, such as pneumonia. Most children also develop heart abnormalities. In other types of muscular dystrophy, degrees of disability and complications may be less severe. Persons with a family history of the more severe forms of muscular dystrophy should seek genetic counselling.

myalgic encephalomyelitis (ME)

Description: a disorder that has been the subject of much controversy, and is characterized by extreme tiredness and certain other symptoms. It appears to follow on from viral infections such as influenza and those affecting the gut; hence, it is also called postviral fatigue syndrome.

Persons most commonly affected: all age groups and both sexes.

Organ or part of body involved: whole body— physical and psychological effects.

Symptoms and indications: symptoms include muscular pain, extreme weariness and fatigue, depression, loss of memory and concentration and panic attacks. There are no physical signs of disease.

Treatment: there is no specific cure or treatment but rest is usually essential as the affected person has very little energy. Recovery may be prolonged and the person may only slowly return to normal after months or even longer.

Causes and risk factors: the cause is not understood but there appears to be a link with infection by certain viruses, the enteroviruses. An enterovirus is one that enters via the gut, where it multiplies and goes on to attack the central nervous system.

myasthenia gravis

Description: a serious and chronic disorder characterized by great muscular weakness and fatigue.

Persons most commonly affected: young people and young adults, especially women. Males usually develop the disease after the age of 40.

Organ or part of body involved: muscles—skeletal muscles and those for breathing and swallowing, etc.

Symptoms and indications: muscle weakness that may be noticed in the face leading to 'flatness' of expression and drooping of eyelids, swallowing and breathing difficulties and speech disorder. There may be flare-ups of symptoms, followed by periods of improvement. There is no wasting of the muscles, only weakness. A person with symptoms of myasthenia gravis should seek medical advice and requires referral to a skilled specialist in this disorder.

Treatment: is by means of various kinds of drugs. These include anticholinesterase drugs, which inhibit the action of the enzyme, cholinesterase. This is the enzyme that removes excess acetylcholine (a chemical substance that is a neurotransmitter and transmits nerve impulses to the muscles). Anticholinesterase drugs, e.g. pyridostigmine, increase the amount of acetylcholine available to transmit nerve impulses, so that muscles can continue to contract. Other drugs used are immunosuppressives, which suppress the production of antibodies. Two types that are used are azathioprine and corticosteroids but these may need to be taken for some time before an improvement can be discerned. Rest and avoidance of any unnecessary exertion is very important in myasthenia gravis in order to conserve muscle strength. Treatment may also involve removal of a whole or part of the thymus gland (thymectomy) (*see causes and risk factors*) which is helpful for many persons with this disease.

Causes and risk factors: myasthenia gravis is believed to be an autoimmune disorder, i.e. a failure of the immune system, in which the body develops antibodies that attack its own tissues. For reasons that are not understood, the immune system loses the ability to distinguish between 'self' and 'non-self'. In this case, the antibodies produced interfere with acetylcholine receptors in the nerve endings of the muscles, causing a reduction in their number or rendering them ineffective. The thymus gland is thought to be the site of production of the acetylcholine receptors. Some patients with myasthenia gravis are found to have a tumour of the thymus gland and the condition goes into remission if this is removed. There is a risk of myasthenic crisis, when symptoms of muscular weakness (especially involving the respiratory muscles) become particularly acute. This can occur during the course of drug treatment and may be life-threatening, causing serious respiratory distress. If this occurs, the person requires assisted ventilation in an intensive care unit.

Myasthenia gravis cannot be cured but symptoms can be managed and controlled.

myeloma or **multiple myeloma** or **myelomatosis**

Description: a malignant disease of the bone marrow in which tumours are present in more than one bone at the same time. Characteristically, when the bones are X-rayed, they appear to have holes in them due to the presence of typical deposits. The bone marrow contains an abnormal quantity of malignant plasma cells. The blood often contains abnormal protein (an immunoglobulin), which is usually produced to combat infection. An unusual amount of protein may also be present in the urine.

Persons most commonly affected: both sexes but more common in persons over 40 years of age.

Organ or part of body involved: bone marrow especially of ribs, pelvis, skull and spine.

Symptoms and indications: the patient may suffer from bone pain that can be severe and abnormal tiredness due to ANAEMIA. He or she may be subject to recurrent bacterial infections, especially of the respiratory tract, e.g. pneumococcal pneumonia. There may be kidney failure and the weakened bones are susceptible to fractures, or vertebrae may collapse, causing spinal cord damage and paralysis. A person with symptoms of myeloma requires immediate medical treatment.

Treatment: involves radiotherapy, chemotherapy and the use of painkilling drugs and antibiotics to fight infections. The person should remain as active as possible and should drink plenty of fluids. The use of bone-marrow transplants for this disease is under investigation in some hospitals.

Causes and risk factors: the cause is not known and the disease is not considered curable. However, symptoms can be relieved and a majority of patients show improvements with treatment.

Myelomatosis is the process of production of myeloma in the bone marrow.

myxoedema

Description: a common disease caused by underactivity of the thyroid gland, known as hypothyroidism, which may arise from a variety of different causes.

Persons most commonly affected: adults of both sexes between the ages of 30 and 60 years but more common in women.

Organ or part of body involved: thyroid gland—affecting the metabolism of the whole body.

Symptoms and indications: myxoedema affects both physical and intellectual abilities. There is intellectual impairment, with slow speech, mental dullness and lethargy. Physical symptoms include a characteristic development of a dry, yellow, coarse skin and swelling of subcutaneous tissue (beneath the skin). Also, weight gain and constipation, thinning of hair, which becomes brittle, with bald patches appearing, and pains in the muscles. Some deafness in the middle ear and CARPAL TUNNEL SYNDROME may occur. A person with symptoms of myxoedema should seek medical advice.

Treatment: the symptoms are caused by a lack of the thyroid hormones thyroxine and triodothyronine, which control metabolic processes in the body. Treatment is in the form of hormone replacement therapy with thyroxine. A small dose is given each day at first, and is gradually increased as necessary.

Causes and risk factors: there are various causes for underactivity of the thyroid gland, including goitre, and congenital factors such as rare enzyme deficiencies and cretinism. The most usual cause is an autoimmune disorder, chronic thyroiditis, in which the thyroid gland becomes fibrous and shrinks and has very little or no functional ability. Also, the condition may arise due to previous drug treatment or surgery for the opposite condition, an overactive thyroid gland (HYPERTHYROIDISM). Some of these causes are primary and others are secondary, i.e. the condition results from another disorder or disturbance.

A rare, life-threatening complication may arise, which is myxoedema coma, requiring immediate emergency medical treatment. It tends to occur in patients with a long medical history of hypothyroidism and is precipitated by a variety of factors including chilling or physical trauma, infections and treatment with drugs that act on the central nervous system.

N

narcolepsy

Description: a rare condition in which a person has a tendency to fall asleep a few times each day for several minutes or hours.

Persons most commonly affected: all age groups and both sexes but continues throughout life.

Organ or part of body involved: central nervous system.

Symptoms and indications: falling asleep for several minutes or longer (usually about a quarter of an hour). These may occur at times likely to induce sleep e.g. in a warm, quiet room after a meal, but also on other occasions, such as during a conversation. The person is easily woken and feels refreshed and the 'attacks' of sleep may occur several times in a day. They may occur during laughter or when the person is carrying out routine, monotonous activity. Eventually, after a period of time that may be years later, the condition becomes associated with attacks of cataplexy (a condition in which there are transient bouts of muscle weakness or momentary paralysis). A person with symptoms of narcolepsy should seek medical advice.

Treatment: drugs of the amphetamine type (dexamphetamine) may be prescribed to be taken on special occasions when an attack would be particularly inappropriate or embarrassing. For cataplexy, the drugs clomipramine or imipramine are usually prescribed. A person with narcolepsy may have to avoid risky activities, such as driving, or hazardous sports. If an attack is triggered by laughter or monotonous activity, then these should be avoided as much as possible.

Causes and risk factors: the disorder is present for life and the cause is unknown, although there is a tendency for narcolepsy to run in families. Recent research suggests that narcolepsy is a disorder related to the immune system.

nephrotic syndrome

Description: a disorder of the kidneys in which there is an excess of protein in the urine, low levels of albumin in the blood and swelling of the tissues due to considerable fluid retention or oedema. There are high levels of cholesterol in the blood. Nephrotic syndrome has a number of different causes and may be a primary or secondary disorder.

Persons most commonly affected: all age groups and both sexes. In children it is most common between the ages of one and five and in boys rather than girls.

Organ or part of body involved: kidneys.

Symptoms and indications: an early symptom is production of frothy urine. Oedema or fluid retention occurs, which may be localized e.g. in the knees, eyes, ankles, chest (where it can cause breathing difficulties) or abdomen (where it may cause pain). Frequently, the site may change, involving the eyelids first thing in the morning and then the ankles once the person has got up and walked about. There is a loss of appetite and weight, muscle wastage and general malaise and weakness. There is a reduction in the amount of urine produced and some patients develop kidney failure. A person with symptoms of nephrotic syndrome should seek medical advice.

Treatment: depends upon the underlying cause of the nephrotic syndrome and whether it is primary or secondary (i.e. arising out of another disorder). If the underlying disorder is treatable, then the outlook is generally favourable and the condition can be controlled. These varieties of nephrotic syndrome usually respond well to treatment with corticosteroid drugs e.g. prednisone but there may be a tendency for relapses to occur. Other types of nephrotic syndrome, which respond less well to corticosteroids alone, may be treated with prednisone and a cytotoxic drug on alternate days in order to control the condition. Some patients with types of nephrotic syndrome that do not respond to drug treatment go on to develop KIDNEY FAILURE, which requires dialysis or organ transplant. Patients with nephrotic syndrome often require a special diet low in salt and saturated fats.

Causes and risk factors: there are a number of

different causes and diseases with which the syndrome is associated. These include GLOMERULONEPHRITIS, DIABETES MELLITUS, cancers such as LYMPHOMAS and LEUKAEMIAS, SYSTEMIC LUPUS ERYTHEMATOSUS, autoimmune disorders, infections including HIV and syphilis and certain drugs and naturally occurring toxins e.g. snake venom. Some types have a hereditary factor involved. A number of complications can arise accompanying this disorder, including kidney failure, heart and central nervous system disorders, THROMBOSIS, HYPERTENSION, susceptibility to recurrent infections including PERITONITIS and a tendency for relapses to occur.

neuralgia

Description: this strictly describes pain in some part, or the whole, of a nerve without there being any physical change in that nerve. However, neuralgia is used more widely to describe any pain in a nerve or its branches, whatever the cause. It occurs in several forms and is named accordingly; trigeminal neuralgia affects the face and intercostal neuralgia the ribs. *See also* SCIATICA.

Persons most commonly affected: intercostal neuralgia: adults of both sexes, but more common in women over 50 years, especially in persons who are already in poor health. Trigeminal neuralgia: adults of both sexes.

Organ or part of body involved: any nerve or its branches, usually the trigeminal (facial) nerve, nerves that arise from the spinal cord and run between the ribs (intercostal) and the sciatic nerve.

Symptoms and indications: intercostal neuralgia: pain, usually on the left side, especially where the nerve leaves the spine in the back and in the front where it branches into the skin. The pain may come in intense bursts and may occur more often at a particular time of the day or night. There may be other symptoms, such as tingling, numbness or paralysis, and loss of appetite and muscle wastage.

Trigeminal neuralgia (tic douloureux) usually on one side of the face; severe pain of a burning or cutting nature, which may be constant or spasmodic and may be provoked by simple actions such as eating or by heat or cold. The skin of the face may become inflamed and the eye on the affected side red and watery. The condition is very debilitating in that the pain can be so intense as to interfere with sleeping and eating. Hence, the person may suffer from loss of appetite and weight.

A person with symptoms of neuralgia should seek medical advice.

Treatment: various treatments may be tried according to the type of neuralgia. Externally, heat in the form of a hot bath or rubbing in liniment (ABC liniment containing aconite, belladonna and chloroform) may be helpful and also, diathermy and the application of blisters (button cautery). Drugs used include pain-relieving analgesics, with carbamazepine being especially effective in the treatment of trigeminal neuralgia. If other treatments prove ineffective, injections to freeze the nerve or surgery to destroy a whole or a part of it may become necessary.

Causes and risk factors: sometimes the cause of neuralgia may be inflammation or pressure on the nerve but often the cause cannot be discovered. Neuralgia attacks tend to recur from time to time in an affected person, especially if the overall state of health is low.

neuritis

Description: inflammation of and degeneration of one or more nerves, which may be localized (localized neuritis) or widespread, when it is known as polyneuritis, multiple neuritis or peripheral neuritis.

Persons most commonly affected: adults of both sexes and all age groups. Polyneuritis, if caused by alcohol, is more common in women than in men.

Organ or part of body involved: nerves.

Symptoms and indications: localized neuritis: symptoms depend upon whether the nerve involved is sensory (i.e. carrying sensations to the central nervous system) or motor (carrying electrical impulses from the central nervous system to a muscle to make it contract). If a sensory nerve is involved the main symptom is pain, as in NEURALGIA. If a motor nerve is involved, the main symptom is a degree of paralysis of the muscle that is supplied by that nerve. The overlying skin may become shiny or ulcerated, the nails ridged or pitted, and OSTEOPOROSIS may develop.

Polyneuritis: symptoms are often slow to develop and generally vague but include tingling, numbness and pains in the limbs, hands and feet, a peculiar stepping gait and drooping wrists, and there may be breathing difficulties and effects on the heart.

A person with symptoms of neuritis should seek medical advice.

Treatment: for localized neuritis, depends upon the cause but is, in general, the same as that for neuralgia. Treatment of polyneuritis primarily involves identifying the cause and/or removing the toxin that is affecting the nerves. Rest in bed, massage and physiotherapy, and electrical treatments are all used to preserve and then strengthen weakened nerves and muscles.

Causes and risk factors: the cause of localized neuritis may be an infection e.g. DIPHTHERIA, injury or other disease, such as DIABETES MELLITUS. Polyneuritis may be caused by a nutritional deficiency e.g. beriberi, which results from a lack of thiamine (vitamin B12), metabolic disease or disorder e.g. diabetes mellitus, hypothyroidism and PORPHYRIA, infectious disease, autoimmune disorder, cancer or long-term ingestion or exposure to a toxin such as lead, mercury, many solvents and alcohol. *See also* GUILLAIN-BARRÉ SYNDROME.

non-specific urethritis (NSU)

Description: sexually transmitted inflammation and infection of the urethra, caused by various types of microorganism.

Persons most commonly affected: sexually active adults of both sexes.

Organ or part of body involved: urethra, pelvic organs, cervix, possibly pharynx and anus.

Symptoms and indications: men: discomfort and pain in the urethra, mild pain on urination, increased frequency of urination and slight or more profuse discharge. The urethra is red and inflamed. Symptoms vary from mild to more severe. Women: there may be few or no symptoms but, if they do occur, include pain on urination, frequency of urination and pain in the pelvic region. Also vaginal discharge, which may be yellowish and thick, and pain during sexual intercourse.

A person with symptoms of non-specific urethritis should seek medical advice. The affected person and his or her sexual partner require treatment.

Treatment: diagnosis requires bacteriological examination of urethral sample or urine to exclude other causes of infection, such as GONORRHOEA. Treatment is by means of antibiotics including tetracycline, doxycycline or erythromycin, usually for one week, but longer if infection persists or if complications arise (*see causes and risk factors*). Patients should refrain from sexual intercourse and are usually given a follow-up examination to ensure that the infection has cleared.

Causes and risk factors: the microorganisms commonly responsible for the infection are chlamydia trachomatis and ureaplasma urealyticum but the causal organism is not always known. In both men and women, if there has been anal or oral sexual activity, inflammation of the anus (proctitis) and pharynx (throat—PHARYNGITIS) can occur. In men there may be inflammation of the sperm ducts in the testes (epidydimitis), producing symptoms of pain, feverishness and swelling, and also narrowing or stricture of the urethra. In women, there may be inflammation or the development of cysts on the Bartholin's glands (secretory vaginal glands), inflammation of the Fallopian tubes (salpingitis) and perihepatitis. These complications can cause sterility or increased risk of ectopic pregnancy and even death in some cases. A serious complication that can arise, especially in men, is REITER'S SYNDROME (an arthritic disorder with CONJUNCTIVITIS, inflammation of the uveal tract of the eye and urethritis). A newborn baby may acquire an infection of the eye (called ophthalmia neonatorum) during passage through the birth canal if the mother has non-specific urethritis. This is treated with antibiotic (chlortetracycline) eye ointment.

O

oesophageal cancer or cancer of the oesophagus

Description: a malignant growth of abnormal cells in the oesophagus (gullet—the tube that takes food from the mouth to the stomach). It most frequently occurs at the lower end of the tube near the opening into the stomach.

Persons most commonly affected: adults of both sexes, especially men, in middle or older age.

Organ or part of body involved: oesophagus.

Symptoms and indications: symptoms include difficulty in passing food from the oesophagus into the stomach, which gradually becomes worse. Loss of weight, weakness and tiredness, swelling of lymph glands in the neck. A person with symptoms of oesophageal cancer should seek medical advice.

Treatment: involves admittance to hospital for radiotherapy, surgery and chemotherapy. The person may require food in liquid form or in extreme cases an operation to introduce food directly into the stomach (gastrostomy).

Causes and risk factors: the cause is not known but it is wise not to smoke.

oesophageal stricture

Description: a narrowing of the oesophagus (or gullet) which may arise for a number of different reasons and causes difficulty in the passage of food.

Persons most commonly affected: adults of all age groups and both sexes.

Organ or part of body involved: oesophagus.

Symptoms and indications: discomfort and pain in swallowing and regurgitation of (undigested) food back into the mouth, weight loss and weakness. A person with symptoms of oesophageal stricture should seek medical advice.

Treatment: depends upon the cause and extent of the stricture. The aim of treatment is to enlarge the opening so that food can pass down into the stomach. Treatment may involve dilation by means of special instruments, surgery or radiotherapy, if the cause of the stricture is cancer.

Causes and risk factors: causes of oesophageal stricture include scarring from a previous injury (due to infection or swallowing of a drink that is too hot or corrosive substance), cancer and some serious nerve diseases. Also, a condition known as cardiospasm in which the cardiac sphincter (a ring of muscle located at the lower end of the oesophagus) fails to relax when food is swallowed to allow its passage into the stomach. Treatment consists of passing special instruments called bougies down the oesophagus to widen the opening, before a meal is eaten. The treatment is tedious as it may be needed for several months, but it is usually ultimately successful.

Osgood-Schlatter's disease

Description: a condition belonging to a group of disorders known as the osteochondroses. These affect the epiphyses, or heads of the long bones, which are separated from the main shaft of these bones in children, and fuse and disappear when growth is complete. Osgood-Schlatter's disease affects the tibial tubercle (a bony nodule) of the knee.

Persons most commonly affected: children, especially boys, between the ages of 10 and 15.

Organ or part of body involved: knee.

Symptoms and indications: swelling, warmth, tenderness and pain in the knee, especially when the leg is straightened. A child with these symptoms should see a doctor.

Treatment: resting the affected leg, and avoidance of activities that are liable to stress the knee, especially sports, are necessary until recovery takes place. Rarely, some surgical procedures, injections of hydrocortisone into the knee or encasing the leg in plaster, may be required. Painkillers suitable for children may be recommended by the doctor.

Causes and risk factors: the cause is believed to be excessive stress on the tibial tubercle, which may be pulled out of line, caused by overuse of the quadriceps muscle. This is often due to excessive participation in vigorous sporting activities. Sports can be cautiously resumed once the knee has recovered completely.

osteoarthritis

Description: an imprecise term generally describing a form of arthritis involving joint cartilage with accompanying changes in the associated bone. It usually involves the loss of cartilage and the development of osteophytes (bony spurs or projecting knobs) at the bone margins. Osteoarthritis is a painful condition affecting the function of the affected joint.

Persons most commonly affected: adults of both sexes aged over 45. All persons are affected by changes in the joints with advancing years but not all have serious or disabling symptoms.

Organ or part of body involved: joints, especially toes, fingers, ankles, knees, hips and spine.

Symptoms and indications: stiffness and pain in affected joints. The aching may be weather-affected and worse when it is cold and damp. There is a loss of dexterity and movement in the affected joint. There may be a cracking or grating sound with movement and the joint may show signs of swelling. Persons with symptoms of osteoarthritis should seek medical advice.

Treatment: is aimed at maintaining movement and relieving pain. Analgesics may be prescribed and, possibly, non-steroidal anti-inflammatory drugs for acute phases of osteoarthritis. Surgery to replace the affected joint may ultimately be required.

Causes and risk factors: there are a variety of causes including overuse and stress of the joints, injury and natural processes of ageing. Some occupations are likely to pose a greater risk, e.g. certain sports, ballet and dance or other activities that put joints under stress.

osteogenesis imperfecta or brittle bone disease

Description: an uncommon hereditary disease that results in the bones being unusually fragile and brittle. There are several forms but that which affects newborn babies (osteogenesis imperfecta congenita) is the most severe. The form that is usually diagnosed slightly later (osteogenesis imperfecta tarda) is usually somewhat less severe.

Persons most commonly affected: children of both sexes. Babies born with this condition may not survive.

Organ or part of body involved: skeleton.

Symptoms and indications: symptoms include fractures that occur with the slightest degree of trauma, joints that are unusually mobile, transparent teeth and bluish sclera (eyeballs that normally appear white). In addition there may be DEAFNESS and dwarfism, as the bones are so severely affected. Symptoms range from very severe to relatively mild and in the latter form, often become apparent when the child starts to walk. A parent who is concerned about the development of a child should always seek medical advice.

Treatment: there is no effective medical treatment or cure for this condition. The child requires orthopaedic support to limit the adverse effects of brittle bone disease and other measures to encourage life to be as normal as possible.

Causes and risk factors: the cause is an inherited abnormality of collagen (a protein substance that is widely found in large amounts in the body in connective tissue, tendons, skin, cartilage, bone and ligaments).

osteomyelitis

Description: inflammation and infection of bone marrow and bone, which may be an acute or chronic condition.

Persons most commonly affected: both sexes and all age groups. In children, it more commonly occurs in those aged between 5 and 14.

Organ or part of body involved: bones. The infection may be localized or more general. In children, it usually occurs in the long bones of the arms and legs, and in adults, in the spine or pelvis.

Symptoms and indications: symptoms include worsening pain in the affected bone, swelling, fever and muscle spasm, redness and warmth. The pain is usually increased when a nearby joint is moved. A person with symptoms of osteomyelitis requires immediate medical attention.

Treatment: may require admittance to hospital for high doses of antibiotics, which may need to be delivered intravenously. Bed rest is needed until the infection has cleared and symptoms have subsided. Antibiotics are likely to be needed for several weeks. Appropriate pain relief is normally prescribed by the doctor.

Causes and risk factors: the infection is usually caused by staphylococcal bacteria, which enter the bone via the bloodstream following injury or surgery or an infection elsewhere, such as a BOIL. Sometimes after an acute attack, chronic myelitis may develop with a periodic flare-up of symptoms. This may be due to bits of dead bone or sequestra that have been left behind, perhaps after injury, which are sites of irritation and infection.

osteoporosis

Description: a loss of bone tissue, due to it being

resorbed, resulting in bones that become brittle and likely to fracture.

Persons most commonly affected: loss of bone density is a feature of ageing and affects older people of both sexes. However, problems mainly occur in postmenopausal women, especially those with a small frame.

Organ or part of body involved: bones.

Symptoms and indications: there may be few symptoms but those that may occur include backache, loss of height and deformation of the spine. Also, bones that fracture easily with minor falls. Persons with symptoms of osteoporosis should seek medical advice.

Treatment: is mainly preventative and for women, hormone replacement therapy in the form of oestrogen after the menopause, is effective, especially in the first few years. A good diet that is high in calcium is also essential. Calcium and vitamin D supplements may be prescribed. Remaining active and taking regular exercise, particularly walking, is helpful in maintaining the condition and strength of the bones.

Causes and risk factors: the cause in women appears to be related to the decline in oestrogen levels after the menopause, or if the ovaries have been removed due to disease. Patients with CUSHING'S SYNDROME or who have had prolonged treatment with corticosteroid drugs are also at risk of osteoporosis, as are women who have undergone radiotherapy for ovarian cancer. Those with poor nutrition and especially a low calcium intake are more at risk of developing osteoporosis. The main complications that arise, and can be life-threatening in the elderly, are bone fractures, which occur easily. Eliminating the risks to minimize the the possibility of accidents in the home are important for elderly persons with osteoporosis.

osteosarcoma

Description: the commonest and most malignant form of bone tumour.

Persons most commonly affected: older children of both sexes and young adults (ages 10 to 20).

Organ or part of body involved: bones. About half affect the femur near the knee and others may occur in the long bones of the arm. Secondary tumours (metastases) commonly occur, especially in the lungs.

Symptoms and indications: symptoms include pain and swelling around the site of the tumour. A person with symptoms of osteosarcoma should seek immediate medical advice.

Treatment: involves admittance to hospital for chemotherapy and surgery. Formerly, amputation of the limb was standard treatment but newer surgical techniques often enable the tumour to be removed and the limb reconstructed. Radiotherapy may also be needed.

Causes and risk factors: the cause is not known and this is a serious and life-threatening disease. Much research is being carried out into treatment regimes and control of symptoms to improve the outlook and quality of life of patients.

otitis media

Description: an infection of the middle ear.

Persons most commonly affected: both sexes and all ages, but mostly children.

Organ or part of body involved: ear.

Symptoms and indications: the patient complains of earache. In small babies, this may be shown by frequent rubbing of the affected ear. They are often feverish, and there may be partial deafness, or sometimes tinnitus (a ringing or buzzing sound in the ear, with no real source).

Treatment: antibiotics are prescribed, and sometimes external heat (for example, a hot-water bottle) may help to reduce the pain. In exceptional cases, if the antibiotics do not give fast relief, it may be necessary to make an incision in the eardrum, in order to allow pus to escape. This relieves the pressure in the ear, and therefore reduces the pain.

Causes and risk factors: otitis media often develops as a result of a cold or SINUSITIS, when infection spreads from the nasal passages via the Eustachian tubes that connect them with the middle ear. It can also follow jumping or diving into water without holding the nose, when infection can be forced into the ear by the same route. It is very important for the doctor to follow up the course of the infection, as repeated infections or incomplete clearance of the infection may lead to secretory otitis media, which is the main cause of glue ear in children, which is itself a cause of DEAFNESS.

otitis externa

Description: an infection of the outer ear.

Persons most commonly affected: all ages and both sexes.

Organ or part of body involved: ear.

Symptoms and indications: pain, discharge from the outside of the ear and itching.

Treatment: usually, syringing with warm saline (salt solution) and packing with a soothing lotion are all that is required. The application of mild heat may help relieve the pain.

Causes and risk factors: this infection is most common in hot countries, but it may happen anywhere. It can be caused by scratching the ear with dirty fingers, or by the use of a badly cleaned, ill-fitting hearing-aid earpiece. It sometimes occurs after swimming in chlorinated water.

otosclerosis

Description: a hereditary disorder in which abnormal bone is deposited in the middle ear, which fixes the stapes (one of the three small bones in the ear). The stapes can no longer vibrate and transmit sound waves, resulting in loss of hearing.

Persons most commonly affected: usually becomes apparent in young people between the ages of 15 and 30 and is more common in women.

Organ or part of body involved: bones of the middle ear.

Symptoms and indications: progressive loss of hearing and tinnitus (ringing in the ears). A person experiencing these symptoms should seek medical advice.

Treatment: involves admittance to hospital for microsurgery to remove the stapes and to fit an artificial replacement. The loss of hearing can usually be, at least partially, restored by this procedure. Some patients may require a hearing aid.

Causes and risk factors: the cause is a dominant genetic factor that affects about 10% of White people although not all develop a loss of hearing. In pregnancy, the course of the disease may accelerate rapidly and become apparent for the first time.

ovarian cyst

Description: a growth in the form of a sac, filled with fluid or other more solid material, that develops in the ovary and is nearly always nonmalignant.

Persons most commonly affected: women of all age groups.

Organ or part of body involved: ovary.

Symptoms and indications: often there are no symptoms until the cyst has grown to a large size and exerts pressure on nearby organs. Symptoms that can occur include abdominal pain, interference with bladder function or pain on urination, painful sexual intercourse and vaginal discharge. A person with these symptoms should seek immediate medical advice.

Treatment: usually involves admittance to hospital for surgical removal of the affected ovary, and this is most successful if carried out at an early stage, before the cyst has grown too large. In other cases, the cyst itself may be removed or drained.

Causes and risk factors: the cause is hormonal and ovarian cysts may be triggered by hormonal changes during pregnancy. If an ovarian cyst grows too large it may form adhesions (bands of tissue) that attach to other pelvic organs causing a range of symptoms. Surgery tends to be less successful if this occurs. Ovarian cysts vary in their nature. There is a danger of rupture in thinner-walled types, or twisting, which causes severe pain, fever and vomiting, requiring emergency surgery. This is a life-threatening situation that can cause death due to PERITONITIS or haemorrhage within the abdomen.

ovarian tumours

Description: a solid tumour in the ovary, which may be either benign or malignant.

Persons most commonly affected: women of all ages but more common in those between 45 and 65.

Organ or part of body involved: ovary, often one but possibly both.

Symptoms and indications: the tumour usually produces few symptoms until it has grown to a relatively large size. The symptoms of malignancy include abdominal discomfort and pain, digestive upset and, later, more severe pain and ANAEMIA, a hard mass that can be felt, deepening of the voice and hair growth. A woman with any symptoms, however vague, of ovarian tumour should seek immediate medical advice.

Treatment: involves admittance to hospital and surgery to remove the tumour or, usually, the ovary and Fallopian tube. In some cases of malignancy, hysterectomy may be required. Chemotherapy and/or radiotherapy are likely to be needed if the tumour is cancerous. There may be a need for more than one type of anticancer (cytotoxic) drug to be taken.

Causes and risk factors: the cause is not known. The outcome may be fatal if the cancer spreads to other parts of the body and secondary growths occur.

P

Paget's disease of bone or osteitis deformans

Description: a chronic disease, particularly affecting the long bones, skull and spine, which results in the bones becoming thickened, disorganized, soft and weak.

Persons most commonly affected: adults of both sexes over the age of 40 but more common in men.

Organ or part of body involved: bones, especially of the limbs, skull and spine.

Symptoms and indications: symptoms include bone pain, which is of an aching nature and can be very severe, especially at night. Also, the bones become enlarged and deformed and movement is impaired. The skull may become enlarged, nerves compressed and damaged (especially if the spine is involved), causing some degree of paralysis. There may be bowing of the spine or legs and the bones are liable to fracture. The person may experience headaches and loss of hearing. The symptoms may be vague or absent in the early stages of the disease, which tends to progress in active phases with quiescent periods in between. A person with symptoms of Paget's disease should seek medical advice.

Treatment: there is no cure for the disease and treatment is aimed at the relief of pain. Various drugs may be used, including salicylates, non-steroidal anti-inflammatory drugs, calcitonin and diphosphonates. Some patients may require orthopaedic surgery and devices to increase mobility. Heat in the form of hot baths, heating pads, etc., are helpful in the relief of pain and bed rest is necessary during the acute phases of the disease.

Causes and risk factors: the cause is not known but is more likely in those with a family history of the disease. Various complications can arise, including compression of the brain by the enlargement of the skull, HYPERTENSION and heart disease. Paget's disease may be misdiagnosed as secondary bone cancer (especially from primary breast or prostate gland cancer) or an overactive parathyroid gland (hyperparathyroidism).

pancreatic cancer or cancer of the pancreas

Description: an abnormal malignant proliferation of cells in the pancreas, which is an increasingly common type of cancer in Britain.

Persons most commonly affected: adults of both sexes in middle or older age but more common in men.

Organ or part of body involved: pancreas (a gland located behind the stomach between the duodenum and spleen, which produces digestive enzymes and the hormone insulin).

Symptoms and indications: in the early stages there may be few or no symptoms and by the time they appear, the cancer may have spread to the lymph nodes, lungs or liver. Symptoms include abdominal pain that radiates to the back and lessens if the person bends forward, JAUNDICE, loss of weight, and haemorrhage (bleeding) in the gastrointestinal tract. The jaundice often causes severe itching of the skin. A person with symptoms of cancer of the pancreas should seek immediate medical treatment.

Treatment: involves admittance to hospital for chemotherapy, radiotherapy and, possibly, surgery. In addition, pain-relieving drugs, pancreatic enzymes and preparations to relieve itching may be needed. Insulin may also be needed.

Causes and risk factors: the cause is not known but the risk increases in those who have chronic PANCREATITIS, DIABETES MELLITUS, excessive consumption of alcohol and smoking. The condition is incurable but symptoms can be relieved.

pancreatitis

Description: inflammation of the pancreas, which can arise from a variety of causes and may be either acute or chronic.

Persons most commonly affected: adults of all age groups and both sexes.

Organ or part of body involved: pancreas.

Symptoms and indications: acute pancreatitis; very severe abdominal pain, fever, sweating, vomiting, which may lead to SHOCK and collapse. This is a life-threatening disorder and the patient requires immediate emergency medical treatment in hospital. Chronic pancreatitis: symptoms include pain that varies in intensity and may last for one day or several days with repeated attacks over a period of time. The function of the pancreas in secreting important digestive enzymes may be impaired and abnormal fatty stools are produced. Also, the cells that secrete the hormone insulin become ineffective and the person is likely to develop DIABETES MELLITUS. A person with symptoms of chronic pancreatitis should seek immediate medical attention.

Treatment: for acute pancreatitis, admittance to an intensive care unit is necessary. The person has to be maintained in a fasting state and requires various solutions given intravenously. Usually, the person has a nasogastric tube (a tube through the nose into the stomach) through which antacids can be given to neutralize stomach acid and prevent the possible development of ulcers. The patient may need to be starved for two to four weeks and other body systems and functions (e.g. heart) require careful monitoring. For less severe cases, fasting is still likely to be needed and fluids may be required intravenously. Various painkillers may be prescribed along with other drugs, such as pancreatic enzymes. Depending upon the cause of the pancreatitis, some surgery may be needed. In all cases of pancreatitis, alcohol must be avoided.

Causes and risk factors: causes include excess consumption of alcohol, GALLSTONES and disease of the gall bladder and bile duct. Also, injury and disease of the pancreas, such as cancer, and as a complication of surgery (especially of the stomach, gall bladder and bile ducts) or other metabolic diseases and disorders. Hereditary factors may be involved in some people or it may arise as a complication of an infection e.g. MUMPS. The risk of developing pancreatitis increases with abuse of alcohol and with the taking of certain drugs, especially chlorothiazide, sulphasalazine, azathioprine, valproic acid and furosemide. Abuse of alcohol over a prolonged period is responsible for many cases of the disease.

Parkinson's disease or Parkinsonism

Description: a progressive condition occurring in mid to later life, due to a degenerative change in a part of the brain. It results in a rigidity of muscles and tremor when resting and unsteadiness in walking.

Persons most commonly affected: elderly adults of both sexes but more common in men.

Organ or part of body involved: part of the brain (ganglia located at the base of the cerebrum) that controls certain muscle movements.

Symptoms and indications: early symptoms include a fixed expression of the face and lack of blinking, resulting in a mask-like look, tremor of the hand when sitting still, which reduces with movement and does not occur when the person is sleeping. This may also affect the arms and legs. Movements eventually become slow, and there is a loss of the postural reflexes that help to maintain the person in an upright position. The person develops a typical shuffling gait and the body stoops. There is a tendency to fall forward or backwards or to break into a run to prevent falling. Voice and speech may be affected and there may be difficulty in swallowing. A person with symptoms of Parkinson's disease should seek medical advice.

Treatment: the condition cannot be cured but symptoms can be managed and relieved by means of various drugs, the most important of which is levodopa (a precursor of 'dopamine'—*see causes and risk factors*). The drugs used in the treatment of Parkinson's disease must be individually tailored to the needs of each patient and are administered under specialist medical care. Side effects from drug treatment may occur and should be immediately reported to the doctor. Also, the patient's response to the drugs may vary over a period of time and treatment requires monitoring and possible alteration with time.

Causes and risk factors: the cause is believed to be a degenerative change in the basal ganglia of the brain, resulting in a deficiency of the naturally occurring substance, dopamine, which transmits nerve impulses. However, in some cases, it may result from a lack of other 'neurotransmitters' (chemical substances that are naturally present in the body). Parkinson's disease also arises as a result of the taking of certain (neuroleptic) drugs, e.g. phenothiazine tranquillizers and reserpine. Parkinson's disease may arise after inflammation of the brain (encephalitis), brain tumours, injuries or degenerative diseases, ingestion of manganese or carbon monoxide and HYDROCEPHALUS. Drug abusers may develop Parkinson's disease from injecting a form of heroin.

pelvic inflammatory disease (PID)

Description: any acute or chronic inflammation and infection of the female reproductive organs.

Persons most commonly affected: women of all age groups; the most common form affects those who are sexually active under the age of 35.

Organ or part of body involved: ovaries, Fallopian tubes, cervix.

Symptoms and indications: symptoms may be slight or severe. These include pain, which often increases in severity and usually starts during menstruation, malaise and fever, foul-smelling vaginal discharge, abnormal bleeding, pain during intercourse and vomiting. If an abscess develops, this can be felt as a soft, movable mass. Rupture of such an abscess produces severe symptoms of pain, shock and collapse and is a life-threatening condition requiring emergency medical treatment. A person with any symptoms of pelvic inflammatory disease should immediately seek medical treatment.

Treatment: often involves admittance to hospital for antibiotics given at first intravenously and then by mouth for two to four weeks. Surgery may be necessary in some cases. Recovery is normally good if caught and treated early but may take several weeks, according to severity of symptoms.

Causes and risk factors: the cause is a bacterial infection, especially chlamydia trachomatis or Neisseria gonorrhoeae, contracted through sexual intercourse. However, infection elsewhere e.g. in the appendix, which spreads either directly or via the blood circulation, caused by other organisms, is sometimes responsible. Women are more at risk after childbirth, abortion or surgery involving reproductive organs. Also, women who have an intrauterine contraceptive device (IUD) are more likely to develop the infection. There is a risk of permanent sterility if the disease is not diagnosed and treated at an early stage.

pemphigus

Description: a group of disorders, known as bullous diseases, including a serious but rare disease of the skin and mucous membranes, pemphigus vulgaris. It is locally common in some countries, particularly Brazil and parts of South America.

Persons most commonly affected: adults of both sexes in middle and older age.

Organ or part of body involved: skin and mucous membranes with possible systemic (whole body) involvement.

Symptoms and indications: there is the development of bullae, which are thin-walled blisters containing clear fluid, and usually these occur first in the mouth and later on the skin. These rupture and leave raw and painful areas that render the person susceptible to serious infection. There is a loss of weight, malaise and weakness. A person with symptoms of pemphigus requires immediate medical treatment.

Treatment: is aimed at prevention of the development of new blisters. In all but mild cases, admittance to hospital is necessary for large doses of corticosteroid drugs such as prednisone. Long-term maintenance doses of these drugs, and others such as cyclophosphamide, methotrexate and azathioprine are often needed to prevent a relapse, but there is a risk of side effects. If complications arise in the form of other infections these require appropriate antibiotic treatment.

Causes and risk factors: pemphigus is an autoimmune disorder (i.e. one in which the body's immune system fails to recognize 'self' and 'non-self' and produces antibodies that attack its own tissues). Characteristically, the blood serum and skin contains IgG antibodies or 'ABs' and the amount of these may be related to the severity of the symptoms produced.

pericarditis

Description: inflammation of the pericardium, the smooth membranous sac surrounding the heart.

Persons most commonly affected: all age groups and both sexes.

Organ or part of body involved: pericardium.

Symptoms and indications: pain in the chest, which varies in severity and worsens with movement. The inflammation causes roughening of the sac and the pain results from the heart rubbing against it as it contracts. The rubbing can be heard as a scratching noise through a stethoscope and is called pericardial or friction rub. The person is feverish and breathing is rapid and shallow. Fluid may collect within the pericardial sac and this is called pericardial effusion. The resultant pressure that this exerts on the heart may cause blood pressure to fall and failure of the circulation. Chronic constrictive pericarditis—an uncommon condition in which there is a thickening of the pericardium—produces symptoms similar to those of heart failure. There is oedema and collections of fluid in the peritoneal cavity (ascites), which may cause the abdomen to swell. A person with symptoms of pericarditis should seek medical treatment.

Treatment: depends upon the underlying cause, but will normally require admittance to hospital. Pericardial fluid needs to be drawn off or aspirated by means of a needle inserted through the chest wall. Surgery may be required in some cases, e.g. in chronic constrictive pericarditis to remove the pericardium. Pain-relieving drugs are likely to be prescribed but other medication depends upon the cause of the condition.

Causes and risk factors: a common cause is infection by a virus but also pericarditis may result from RHEUMATIC FEVER, TUBERCULOSIS, cancer, LUPUS ERYTHEMATOSUS and kidney failure. Other causes can be a complication resulting from chest or heart injury or surgery or heart attack.

peritonitis

Description: inflammation and, usually, infection of the peritoneum, a serous membrane (one lining a large cavity in the body) that lines the abdominal cavity. It may be acute or chronic (rare), localized or general. Acute, general peritonitis is the most dangerous form.

Persons most commonly affected: all age groups and both sexes.

Organ or part of body involved: peritoneum.

Symptoms and indications: pain in the abdomen, which usually rapidly becomes severe. There is shivering, chills and high fever, and the skin is hot. The abdomen swells and the muscles become rigid. Breathing is shallow and rapid, blood pressure falls and heartbeat rate rises. The symptoms may lead to shock and collapse and can prove rapidly fatal. A person with symptoms of peritonitis needs immediate emergency medical treatment in hospital.

Treatment: the underlying cause of the peritonitis must be identified and treated and this may involve surgery. Antibiotics are required to fight infection and fluids and nourishment are given intravenously. Recovery is likely, providing treatment begins at an early stage.

Causes and risk factors: the cause is usually bacterial infection, the organisms responsible gaining access either from an external wound (especially a deep stab wound) or from perforation of any of the digestive organs within the abdomen. Hence, inflammation of the stomach, gall bladder and bile duct (GALLSTONES), bowels (obstruction or twisting), HERNIA (which may become strangulated), ulcers in the digestive tract that may rupture, APPENDICITIS, ECTOPIC PREGNANCY, PELVIC INFLAMMATORY DISEASE, PANCREATITIS, abscesses or cysts e.g. in the ovaries or Fallopian tubes, and infection following abdominal surgery all carry a potential risk of peritonitis. A form known as puerperal fever may occur in the first two days after childbirth, but is rarely serious, provided that the mother has access to hygienic conditions and good medical care. The chronic form of peritonitis is normally the result of TUBERCULOSIS. A variety of bacteria can cause peritonitis, particularly *E. coli*, which is normally present in the gut, staphylococci and streptococci.

Adhesions or scar tissue may form as a result of peritonitis, causing symptoms and problems later on.

pernicious anaemia

Description: a type of anaemia due to a deficiency in vitamin B_{12}.

Persons most commonly affected: all age groups and both sexes, depending upon underlying cause. More common in elderly persons.

Organ or part of body involved: blood, bone marrow, peripheral nerves, spinal cord.

Symptoms and indications: symptoms include weight loss, a burning feeling in the tongue, ANAEMIA that becomes progressively worse, leading to pallor, diarrhoea and constipation, numbness or tingling in the fingers and toes, fever and malaise. If the spinal cord is affected (rare), there may be unsteadiness, disorders of movement and spasticity. Persons with symptoms of pernicious anaemia should seek medical advice.

Treatment: consists of regular injections (once a month) of vitamin B_{12}.

Causes and risk factors: in pernicious anaemia, there is a failure to produce the substance (intrinsic factor) that enables vitamin B_{12} to be absorbed from the bowel. Or, the symptoms may arise from a dietary lack of this vitamin, vegans being at particular risk. The failure to produce sufficient intrinsic factor may be an autoimmune disorder (one in which the body fails to recognize 'self' and 'non-self' and produces antibodies that destroy its own tissues). In this case, the parietal cells in the stomach, which secrete the intrinsic factor (the carrier protein for vitamin B_{12} that enables it to be absorbed in the small intestine), are attacked and rendered ineffective. GASTRITIS, removal of part of the stomach (gastrectomy) or small intestine, ILEITIS (inflammation and infection of the ileum, where absorption of vitamin B_{12} takes place), enteritis, PANCREATITIS, malabsorption syndrome, COELIAC DISEASE, SPRUE, parasitic infestation, some other disorders and congenital factors may all be responsible for vitamin B_{12} deficiency. The deficiency of vitamin B_{12} in the body causes a lack of red blood cell production and the presence of abnormal large cells (megaloblasts) in the bone marrow. Before the discovery of vitamin B12 and its role in the body, pernicious anaemia invariably resulted in the death of the sufferer but the condition can now be successfully treated.

phaeochromocytoma

Description: a tumour of the adrenal gland (one of a pair of 'endocrine' or hormone-secreting glands each situated above a kidney). The tumour is normally benign and usually located in the inner part of the gland, the medulla. The tumour is usually a few centimetres in diameter but, occasionally, can be of a much greater size and weight.

Persons most commonly affected: all age groups and both sexes but especially in adults aged 30 to 50.

Organ or part of body involved: one or both adrenal glands.

Symptoms and indications: symptoms include hypertension, headaches, vomiting and nausea, weight loss, palpitations, clammy skin, anxiety and nervousness, rapid heartbeat (tachycardia) rate, disturbance of vision, hypotension on rising, fainting and sweating. Some or all of these symptoms may be present more or less frequently, i.e. each day or every few weeks. A person with symptoms of phaeochromocytoma should seek immediate medical advice.

Treatment: analysis of urine samples for the presence of catecholamines (the breakdown products of adrenal gland hormones) confirms the diagnosis. Treatment involves admittance to hospital and, usually, monitoring of the patient's condition, along with drugs to block hormone secretions for a few days before surgery to remove the tumour. Surgery is usually effective.

Causes and risk factors: the presence of the tumour causes excess production of the hormones noradrenaline and adrenaline, producing the symptoms described above. The cause is unknown, although there may be a connection with some other types of disorder. The high blood pressure that is the main feature of phaeochromocytoma carries a risk of death through stroke or heart disease.

pharyngitis

Description: inflammation and infection of the pharynx or throat.

Persons most commonly affected: all age groups and both sexes except young babies.

Organ or part of body involved: throat and tonsils.

Symptoms and indications: symptoms include a sore throat, difficult, painful swallowing, a feeling of a lump in the throat and possibly fever and swollen glands. The throat may look red and inflamed or be covered by a grey-coloured membrane with pus discharge. A person with symptoms of pharyngitis should seek medical advice.

Treatment: involves bed rest, and plenty of fluids should be drunk. Liquid foods may be needed if swallowing is painful. Appropriate pain relief may be prescribed by the doctor and antibiotics, if the pharyngitis is caused by bacteria. Penicillin is given for streptococcal pharyngitis to prevent the possible complication of RHEUMATIC FEVER. Pharyngitis caused by a virus usually clears up with bed rest and supportive measures.

Causes and risk factors: the cause may be a virus or various bacteria, especially species of the streptococcus genus, *Chlamydia pneumoniae* or *Mycoplasma pneumoniae*.

pituitary gland tumour

Description: a benign or malignant abnormal growth of cells in the pituitary gland. The pituitary is a small, but very important endocrine (hormone-secreting) gland situated at the base of the brain. The hormones it produces control the activity of other endocrine glands. A malignant tumour of the pituitary gland does not usually spread.

Persons most commonly affected: all age groups and both sexes but more common in adults aged 30 to 50.

Organ or part of body involved: pituitary gland.

Symptoms and indications: in children, there are likely to be effects on growth, which is either accelerated (gigantism) or retarded (dwarfism). (The tumour may cause either an overproduction or an underproduction of growth hormone). The tumour may affect the production of gonadotrophic hormones, which stimulate the testes and ovaries to produce their hormones. In this case, puberty does not take place or, at a later stage, there is an absence of menstruation in females and depression of libido in both sexes.

In adults, if the tumour causes an excessive production of growth hormone, a condition known as acromegaly occurs in which there is abnormal enlargement of hands, feet, ears and face. There may be hypothyroidism, CUSHING'S SYNDROME and a form of diabetes (diabetes insipidus). The person may experience fits, gastrointestinal upset, headaches and vision disturbance, if the tumour exerts pressure on the nerves supplying the eye. A person with symptoms of a pituitary gland tumour should seek medical advice.

Treatment: involves admittance to hospital for radiation therapy and/or surgical removal of the tumour. After treatment, hormone imbalance is likely to persist and preparations of hormones are needed.

Causes and risk factors: the cause is not known but hereditary factors may be involved.

placenta praevia

Description: attachment of the placenta in the bottom part of the uterus (womb) so that it may partly or completely cover the cervix. It occurs in about 1 in every 200 pregnancies.

Persons most commonly affected: pregnant women.

Organ or part of body involved: placenta (the temporary organ that develops during pregnancy and attaches the embryo to the uterus. It consists of both maternal and embryonic tissues and allows oxygen and nutrients to pass from the mother's blood to that of the developing baby. It secretes hormones that regulate the pregnancy and is expelled after the birth of the baby as the afterbirth.)

Symptoms and indications: there is a sudden onset of bleeding late in the pregnancy, which, although painless, may become severe. Bright red blood is passed. A pregnant woman with bleeding of this nature requires emergency admittance to hospital.

Treatment: placenta praevia resembles ABRUPTIO PLACENTA and normally, an abdominal ultrasound scan is necessary to confirm the diagnosis. If the bleeding is not severe but only minor, and the pregnancy is not near to term, the patient is usually kept in bed for observation. If the bleeding is severe, the mother will require blood transfusions and the baby is delivered, usually by Caesarian section. Occasionally, vaginal delivery may be possible.

Causes and risk factors: the cause is not known but the risk increases in women who have had several pregnancies, have FIBROIDS in the uterus or other abnormalities e.g. scarring that prevents normal attachment, and are in an older age group. The bleeding occurs because the placenta partially or completely detaches from the uterus, and may be triggered by changes as the pregnancy nears full term, such as dilation of the cervix, which occurs just before labour begins. There is a risk to the life of the mother due to the blood loss if admittance to hospital is delayed. The baby may not survive if very premature at the time of delivery.

pleurisy or pleuritis

Description: inflammation of the pleura, the serous membrane (one that lines a body cavity) that covers the lungs (visceral) and the inside of the chest wall (parietal). The membranes normally have a smooth surface that is moistened to allow them to slide over each other.

Persons most commonly affected: all age groups and both sexes.

Organ or part of body involved: pleura.

Symptoms and indications: generally, a chest pain that starts suddenly and varies in severity from relatively mild to intense. The pain is of a stabbing nature and is worse with movement, breathing, and coughing. Hence, breathing is shallow and rapid and, eventually, a characteristic sound called pleural frictional rub may develop, which can be heard with a stethoscope. The sound may be of a crackling, rasping or grating nature. Fluid may collect between the two layers, called pleural effusion, and this tends to deaden the pain but may decrease lung volume through pressure so that breathing is even more laboured. Sticky fibrous material may be discharged onto the surface of the pleura, which can cause adhesions, although this does not occur in all forms of pleurisy. A person with symptoms of pleurisy should seek medical advice.

Treatment: depends upon the underlying cause of the pleurisy, and is likely to require admittance to hospital. It involves the use of various drugs, including analgesics, antibiotics and bronchodilators. Strapping of the whole chest with elastic bandages and the use of heat may be needed to ease pain. Measures to ease the coughing up of bronchial secretions (such as the use of humidifiers) may be advised. In some cases, drawing off or aspiration of pleural effusion is required via a small incision in the chest wall. This relieves distressed breathing by enabling the lung(s) to expand properly once more.

Causes and risk factors: there are a variety of causes of pleurisy including injury, especially fracture of a rib, respiratory tract infections e.g. PNEUMONIA, BRONCHITIS and TUBERCULOSIS, other diseases including SYSTEMIC LUPUS ERYTHEMATOSUS (SLE), RHEUMATOID ARTHRITIS, cancer and asbestos-related disorders. There is a risk of pneumonia, collapse of the lungs and scarring as a result of pleurisy.

pneumoconiosis

Description: a general term for a chronic form of lung disease caused by inhaling dust while working. Most of the cases are coal miner's pneumoconiosis or anthracosis, ASBESTOSIS and SILICOSIS.

Persons most commonly affected: men in middle age or older who have been exposed to dust at work. Can affect adults of both sexes.

Organ or part of body involved: lungs.

Symptoms and indications: in the early stages there may be few or no symptoms; e.g. coal dust can be deposited in the lungs without causing much disruption of lung tissue. However, this situation may change and the patient may develop progressive massive fibrosis in which there is damage to the lungs and disruption of respiratory function. The person may be breathless, have a cough, pains in the chest, and shadows on the lungs revealed by X-rays. A person with symptoms of pneumoconiosis should seek medical advice.

Treatment: preventative measures are mainly aimed at suppression of dust in the workplace and monitoring of workers. If X-rays reveal changes in the lungs that are a cause for concern, the person should no longer work in this environment. Treatment includes the use of various drugs such as bronchodilators and analgesics. Any infections should be promptly treated with antibiotics and the person should rest in bed during attacks, until symptoms subside.

Causes and risk factors: the cause of this disorder is various types of industrial dusts, especially coal dust, but also beryllium (berylliosis), tin, barium and iron oxide. Berylliosis is a rare, severe form that appears to develop in those hypersensitive to the dust. The risk of more serious lung disease and complications is greater in those who smoke. There is a risk of LUNG CANCER, PLEURISY and congestive heart failure.

pneumonia

Description: a severe inflammation and infection of the lungs caused by many different kinds of bacteria, viruses and fungi. Most cases are caused by bacteria. It results in the filling of the air sacs (alveoli) of the lungs with fluid and pus so that they become solid and air can no longer enter.

Persons most commonly affected: all age groups and both sexes.

Organ or part of body involved: lungs, bronchi, bronchioles (the major and minor air passages supplying the lungs).

Symptoms and indications: symptoms vary in intensity depending upon how much of the lung is affected. They include chills and shivering, high fever, sweating, breathlessness, chest pain, coughing and there may be cyanosis. (In cyanosis, there is a blue appearance of the skin due to

insufficient oxygen within the blood and tissues.) A sputum is produced that is often rust-coloured or may be thicker and contain pus. Breathing is laboured, shallow and painful. The patient may become drowsy and confused if cyanosis occurs and convulsions can occur in children. A person with symptoms of pneumonia requires immediate medical attention.

Treatment: may require admittance to hospital for antibiotics, which may need to be given intravenously in the first instance. The patient may require oxygen and analgesics to relieve pain, and measures such as tepid sponging to reduce fever. Fluids may need to be given intravenously. Amantadine and acyclovir may be given for viral pneumonia. Recovery from pneumonia depends upon the severity of the illness, and whether it occurs in a person who was previously well, or as a complication of existing illness. The elderly and very young and those with previous illness are most at risk, and it remains a major cause of death.

Causes and risk factors: pneumonia is usually caused by a bacterial infection and numerous different kinds may be responsible. Commonly, *Streptococcus pneumoniae*, *Staphylococcus aureus*, *Chlamydia pneumoniae* or *Mycoplasma pneumoniae* are the causal organisms. The elderly and very young, persons with a depressed immune system e.g. transplant patients and those who have been treated for cancer, AIDS patients, those with ALCOHOLISM and people with respiratory disorders, such as obstructive airways disease (asthma), are most at risk from pneumonia. The infection is usually caught by inhalation of airborne deposits containing the bacteria.

pneumothorax

Description: air in the pleural cavity between the two layers of the pleura (the double serous membrane that covers the lungs and the inside of the chest wall), which exerts pressure and causes the lung to collapse.

Persons most commonly affected: all age groups and both sexes (depending upon the cause).

Organ or part of body involved: lungs and pleura.

Symptoms and indications: symptoms vary greatly depending upon the nature and extent of the pneumothorax and whether underlying lung disease is present. They include a sharp pain in the chest that comes on suddenly and may travel to the shoulder and abdomen, breathlessness and a dry, barking cough. If severe lung disease is present there may be collapse and shock with respiratory and circulatory failure. A person with symptoms of pneumothorax should seek medical advice.

Treatment: depends upon the nature and degree of severity of the pneumothorax. A patient with a simple, small pneumothorax and who has no existing lung disease requires no special treatment other than to rest until symptoms subside. The air is reabsorbed naturally and the affected part of the lung re-expands. If a larger area of lung is involved, this may take some time and the person requires monitoring to ensure that there is no leak of fluid (pleural effusion) or development of fibrous deposits. For a more severe or complicated pneumothorax, where there has been an injury or the person has existing lung disease, or is elderly and generally at greater risk, admittance to hospital is needed. The person may require a chest tube and various drugs including pain relief. In some emergency cases, the air may need to be drawn off rapidly by means of a needle or catheter into the chest wall, in order to save life. A person who has more than one pneumothorax on the same side may eventually require surgery.

Causes and risk factors: causes include a penetrating external wound or internal injury e.g. a lung punctured by a fractured rib. Also, rupture of one or more small air sacs inside the lung due to diseases such as EMPHYSEMA, ASTHMA, TUBERCULOSIS, CYSTIC FIBROSIS, inflammation and infection e.g. abscess or FISTULA in the lung. A simple pneumothorax may occur for no apparent reason or be associated, in some people, with taking part in high-altitude flight or deep diving.

Polyarteritis nodosa or periarteritis nodosa

Description: a disease in which there is inflammation and death of sections of medium-sized arteries, with the development of small ANEURYSMS and nodules in their muscular walls. The tissues supplied by these arteries suffer from a decreased blood supply (ischaemia). This is a disorder of collagen (a collagen vascular disease), an important protein substance that is the major constituent of all connective tissue.

Persons most commonly affected: all age groups and both sexes, especially adults aged between 40 and 50 years but more common in men.

Organ or part of body involved: any part of the body may be involved.

Symptoms and indications: the symptoms are variable and imprecise, and can mimic those of other disorders, because any part of the body or

organ can be affected. Commonly, the gastrointestinal tract, heart, kidneys and liver are affected. The most common symptoms include fever, pain in the abdomen, numbness and tingling in the feet and hands due to peripheral nerves being affected, loss of weight, general weakness and malaise, retention of fluid (oedema), high blood pressure, a reduction in the quantity of urine passed and presence of urea in the urine. Also, gastrointestinal upset, bleeding in the gastrointestinal tract and nausea and vomiting, headaches, muscle and joint pains. A person with symptoms of polyarteritis should seek immediate medical advice.

Treatment: depends to some extent upon the area of the body that is affected. However, it may require admittance to hospital and, usually, high doses of corticosteroids (e.g. prednisone) and/or immunosuppressive drugs are needed. Complications and conditions caused by the effects of the disease on particular organs require appropriate treatment. The drugs used in treatment may themselves be responsible for certain side effects, especially when used for an extended period of time.

Causes and risk factors: the cause is not known but it is believed to be a hypersensitivity disorder in susceptible individuals. Bacterial infections such as those caused by staphylococcus or streptococcus, viral infections e.g. HIV, influenza and serum HEPATITIS and the use of some drugs and vaccines may trigger off the disease in some people. There is a risk of death from failure of major organs (especially of the kidneys), if these are affected, or from rupture of an ANEURYSM. Immunosuppressive drugs used in treatment make potentially dangerous infections more likely to occur.

polycystic disease of the kidney or polycystic kidney disease or PKD

Description: one of a group of abnormal disorders of the kidney characterized by the development of cysts in the kidneys. These disorders are inherited and may be either dominant or recessive.

Persons most commonly affected: all age groups and both sexes. Different types of disease may be present at or even before birth, in childhood or in adult life.

Organ or part of body involved: kidneys.

Symptoms and indications: the kidneys enlarge but have a reduced ability to perform their normal functions. Normal tissue is replaced by diseased cysts that are expanded portions of kidney tubules. The cysts may cause low back pain or sharp pain of a colicky nature in the kidneys. Also, there may be blood in the urine, high blood pressure and, in some patients, ANEURYSMS or subarachnoid haemorrhage, which is a dangerous and life-threatening condition. Patients are likely to suffer from frequent urinary tract infections and cysts may also occur in the liver. Persons with symptoms of polycystic kidney disease should seek medical advice.

Treatment: depends upon the severity of the symptoms and is aimed at maintaining kidney function, treating infections and managing high blood pressure. Dialysis or a kidney-transplant operation may eventually be necessary.

Causes and risk factors: the cause of the disorder is usually a mutant gene located on chromosome 16. The disease tends to reduce life expectancy and some affected persons die from ruptured ANEURYSMS, causing brain haemorrhage, or eventually from KIDNEY FAILURE. People with a family history of this disease should seek genetic counselling before having children.

polycythaemia (rubra vera and secondary polycythaemia)

Description: an excessive production of red blood cells in the blood. Primary polycythaemia or polycythaemia rubra vera is a rare disorder in which red blood cells, white blood cells and platelets are all produced in excessive amounts. Secondary polycythaemia arises as a result of some other disorder.

Persons most commonly affected: adults of both sexes but more common in men aged 60 years or over.

Organ or part of body involved: bone marrow and blood.

Symptoms and indications: symptoms include headache, weariness, breathlessness, disturbance of vision, itching, flushed skin, bleeding and enlargement of the spleen. Complications may arise, including symptoms of peptic ulcer, pain in the bones, THROMBOSIS, GOUT and KIDNEY STONES and liver disorder (Budd-Chiari syndrome). Some patients have no symptoms. A person with symptoms of polycythaemia should seek medical advice.

Treatment: may involve admittance to hospital for phlebotomy (the incision of a vein to allow blood to be collected, now usually known as 'venesection'). Also, chemotherapy with cytotoxic drugs and radiotherapy with radioactive phosphate may be required. Treatment is tailored to the individual needs of the patient and one or more methods may be needed, depending upon response. Also, other drugs such as aspirin and preparations to relieve itching may be needed. Primary polycythaemia is not curable, although the symptoms can be relieved. Secondary polycythaemia can be cured if the underlying disorder can be treated.

Causes and risk factors: the cause of primary polycythaemia rubra vera is not known. Secondary polycythaemia may arise as a result of smoking, living at a high altitude for a long period of time, chronic lung disease or tumours in the kidneys, liver, brain or uterus. There is a risk of death from thrombosis, bone marrow abnormality, haemorrhage and development of LEUKAEMIA.

Polymyalgia rheumatica and temporal arteritis

Description: pain and stiffness in certain groups of muscles, which may, in some patients, be associated with temporal arteritis (or giant-cell or cranial arteritis), which is an inflammatory disease of large arteries.

Persons most commonly affected: adults of both sexes aged over 50 but is twice as common in women.

Organ or part of body involved: muscles of shoulder and hip girdles and the neck. Temporal arteritis usually involves the carotid and cranial arteries (temporal arteries) and sometimes peripheral and heart arteries.

Symptoms and indications: symptoms of polymyalgia rheumatica include stiffness and pain in the neck, shoulders, back or hips, which is usually worse on rising in the morning or after sitting still and wears off through the day. There is no degeneration or disease of the muscles. There may also be feverishness, weight loss, loss of appetite, fatigue and malaise. In temporal arteritis, there is, additionally, a severe and pounding headache, disturbance of vision, tenderness of the head and weakness of the muscles of the tongue and jaw. Patients with any symptoms of these conditions should seek immediate medical advice.

Treatment: is by means of steroid drugs in the form of prednisone, which may be needed in high doses at the start of treatment. Treatment should begin immediately if temporal arteritis is suspected, to prevent the risk of blindness.

Causes and risk factors: the cause is not known but treatment is usually successful within two years. Long-term use of steroid drugs may produce side effects. Without treatment or if this is delayed, temporal arteritis poses a risk of blindness, STROKE or heart disease.

polymyositis or dermatomyositis

Description: a disease of connective tissue, with inflammation and degeneration of many muscles (polymyositis) and also the skin (dermatomyositis). It leads to weakness and atrophy of muscles, especially those of the limbs, shoulders and hips.

Persons most commonly affected: both sexes and all age groups but twice as common in females as in males. In children, it usually first appears between the ages of 5 to 15 and in adults, between 40 to 60 years.

Organ or part of body involved: muscles, skin, connective tissue.

Symptoms and indications: the symptoms may be slight or more acute and may be preceded by an infection. In children, the symptoms are more likely to appear in an acute form. Symptoms include muscle weakness, especially noticed in the shoulder and hip girdles and also in those of the throat, leading to swallowing difficulty, regurgitation of food and voice changes. The weakness may be severe so that the person is unable to undertake normal activities. There may be a raised, dusky skin rash that is itchy and can occur on the face, neck, trunk and limbs. There may be muscle tenderness and pain and eventually the limbs may become contracted. A person with these symptoms should seek immediate medical advice.

Treatment: is likely to involve admittance to hospital for treatment with corticosteroid drugs, especially prednisone, during the acute stages of the disease. Some patients may require treatment with immunosuppressive drugs if corticosteroid therapy is not effective. Other medication may be needed, including potassium supplements and antacids. Appropriate exercises are likely to be needed to combat muscle contracture.

Causes and risk factors: the cause is not known, but it may be an autoimmune disease (one in which the body fails to recognize the difference between 'self' and 'non-self' and produces antibodies that attack its own tissue). Sometimes, a preceding infection seems to precipitate the disorder. The outlook is extremely variable and difficult to predict but tends to be more favourable in children, in whom there may be a remission or cure. Most patients become confined to a wheelchair and death may occur due to heart and lung disease, inflammation of blood vessels of the bowel, malnutrition and malignancy.

porphyria

Description: a group of rare inherited metabolic disorders in which there is an increased production of porphyrins within the body. (Porphyrins are naturally-occurring chemical compounds found throughout the plant and animal kingdom in many different types of living tissue.)

Persons most commonly affected: all age groups and both sexes, some types being more common in women.

Organ or part of body involved: whole body.

Symptoms and indications: symptoms include abdominal pain, which may be severe, and there may be gastrointestinal upset such as vomiting and nausea, diarrhoea or constipation. There may be high blood pressure, a raised heartbeat rate and feverishness. There is muscle weakness, due to neuropathy of motor nerves and this especially affects the hands, feet, arms and legs. There is a sensitivity to sunlight, blistering and itching of the skin, production of a dark urine due to the presence of excreted porphyrins and mental disturbances, including depression. There may be liver damage in some forms of the disease. A person with symptoms of porphyria should seek medical advice.

Treatment: is usually aimed at preventing attacks. This involves avoidance (as far as possible) of precipitating factors, including certain drugs, alcohol, sunlight and prompt treatment of infections. Also, the person should have a good diet and plenty of fluids, use sun screen products, and wear a hat and protective clothing when going outside. In some patients, transfusions of packed red blood cells, the taking of beta-carotene (to increase tolerance to the sun) and removal of the spleen may be helpful in reducing the severity of symptoms. Supportive care in hospital may be needed during a severe attack.

Causes and risk factors: the cause is an inherited disorder and is not curable, although symptoms can be relieved and managed. Various drugs including hormones used in oral contraceptives and hormone replacement therapy, alcohol, barbiturates and sunlight may precipitate an attack in a person with porphyria.

pre-eclampsia of pregnancy

Description: a complication of pregnancy arising after the 20th week and characterized by high blood pressure, fluid retention (oedema) and the presence of a protein (albumin) in the urine.

Persons most commonly affected: pregnant women.

Organ or part of body involved: whole body.

Symptoms and indications: the symptoms of pre-eclampsia are a blood pressure of 140 over 90mm of mercury (or greater), or a rise in systolic blood pressure of 30mm or diastolic blood pressure of 15mm of mercury. Also, fluid retention causing swelling, especially of the hands and/or face and the presence of albumin in the urine. The symptom that is most likely to be noticed by the patient is the fluid retention and this, and any other symptoms, should immediately be reported to the doctor. Other symptoms may be detected during routine antenatal check-ups.

Treatment: in very mild cases of pre-eclampsia, the woman may be treated at home, requiring complete bed rest and careful monitoring until blood pressure falls and symptoms improve. If the woman's condition does not respond or in any other than very mild cases, admittance to hospital is necessary. The patient is usually given a salt solution intravenously and also magnesium sulphate. The aim is to stabilize the woman's condition, to lessen the risk of convulsions and bring about a fall in blood pressure, and then to deliver the child. Other drugs may additionally be needed. Once the patient's condition has improved, labour may be induced and the baby delivered normally, or a Caesarian section may be required.

Causes and risk factors: the cause is unknown but is more likely to occur in a first pregnancy and in women with a history of high blood pressure or blood vessel disorders. There is a danger of the development of ECLAMPSIA OF PREGNANCY and also, ABRUPTIO PLACENTAE, both of which are potentially fatal conditions. With prompt treatment, the outlook for mother and child is usually good.

prolapsed intervertebral disc or slipped disc

Description: intervertebral discs are thick, fibrous cartilaginous discs that connect and lie between adjacent vertebrae of the backbone. They permit rotational and bending movements of the back and make up approximately 25% of the length of the backbone, acting as shock absorbers and providing cushioning for the brain and spinal cord. Each disc has an outer fibrous layer over a pulpy centre. A slipped or prolapsed disc is caused by the inner layer being pushed through the fibrous layer to impinge upon a neighbouring spinal nerve-causing pain.

Persons most commonly affected: adults of both sexes in middle or older age.

Organ or part of body involved: intervertebral disc, usually either between the last two lumbar vertebrae (lumbago) or the lowest lumbar vertebrae and the five fused sacral vertebrae that form the sacrum (sciatica).

Symptoms and indications: pain in the lower part of the back, which may come on and worsen gradually or, more usually, is sudden and occurs during an activity that involves bending or sudden twisting of the backbone. A person with symptoms of a slipped disc should seek medical advice.

Treatment: depends upon the severity of the condition but involves bed rest on a flat, firm surface, possibly with manipulation and physiotherapy at a later stage. Epidural anaesthesia (an injection of local anaesthetic into the spine) may be required to relieve pain. Occasionally, surgical removal of the disc may be carried out.

Causes and risk factors: a slipped disc is more likely to occur in middle or later adult life and may be related to degenerative changes that take place. However, the condition is not unknown in younger adults. It is sensible to take extra care when carrying out movements or activities that might stress the back.

prostate gland cancer

Description: a malignant growth of cells in the prostate gland, which is a fairly common form of cancer in men. The prostate is a gland in the male reproductive system that is located below the bladder, opening into the urethra. Upon ejaculation, it secretes an alkaline fluid into the semen, which aids the movement of sperm.

Persons most commonly affected: men aged 50 years or over.

Organ or part of body involved: prostate gland.

Symptoms and indications: the cancer normally grows very slowly and causes no symptoms in the early stages. Later there may be urinary obstruction due to pressure of the growth on the bladder outlet or ureter (one of a pair of tubes each leading from a kidney to the bladder). If the tumour has spread and there are secondary growths, there may be pain in the bones. Other symptoms include the presence of blood and white blood cells in the urine. A person with any symptoms of prostate cancer should seek immediate medical advice.

Treatment: involves admittance to hospital for possible surgery to remove the prostate gland (prostatectomy) and sometimes, the testes (orchidectomy), and/or radiation therapy. Also, treatment with hormones (oestrogens, especially diethylstilboestrol) is effective in controlling the cancer and relieving the symptoms. The condition can be cured if caught and treated in the early stages. Even at a later stage, symptoms can be relieved and life prolonged with treatment. A regular rectal examination after the age of 40 may detect the cancer at an early stage and is a possible preventative measure.

Causes and risk factors: the cause is not known but does not appear to be connected with ENLARGEMENT of the prostate gland, which commonly occurs in elderly men.

prostate gland enlargement or prostatic hypertrophy or benign prostatic hypertrophy

Description: benign enlargement of the prostate gland. (The prostate is a gland in the male reproductive system that is located below the bladder, opening into the urethra. Upon ejaculation, it secretes an alkaline fluid into the semen, which aids the movement of the sperm.)

Persons most commonly affected: men aged over 50 years.

Organ or part of body involved: prostate gland.

Symptoms and indications: increased frequency of urination, especially during the night, causing sleep disturbance. There may be a poor flow of urine and inability to empty the bladder completely and accompanying pain. There may be dribbling and some degree of urinary incontinence and a greater likelihood of urinary tract infection. A man with these symptoms should seek immediate medical advice.

Treatment: usually involves admittance to hospital for surgical removal of the prostate gland, normally by the method of transurethral resection. (This is carried out via the urethra, using a cytoscope, an electric current being used to cauterize and remove the gland. No surgical incision is necessary with this method, and recovery is normally good with less likelihood of postoperative complications. Before surgery is carried out, it may be necessary for any infection to be treated and for the bladder to be completely drained using a catheter. Also, catheter drainage is usually needed for the first few days after surgery.

Causes and risk factors: the cause of prostate gland enlargement is not known but may be associated with hormonal changes accompanying ageing.

psittacosis

Description: a bacterial infection of psittacine birds, e.g. parrots, budgerigars, lovebirds, canaries, pigeons and some seabirds, which is contagious and can be transmitted to human beings.

Persons most commonly affected: both sexes and all age groups.

Organ or part of body involved: lungs, respiratory system.

Symptoms and indications: the symptoms include headache, shivering, feverishness, chills, malaise, loss of appetite and weight, cough and breathlessness. The cough may be dry at first but eventually produces a pus-containing sputum. A person with these symptoms who has recently been in contact with birds, should seek immediate medical advice.

Treatment: consists of complete bed rest and taking tetracycline antibiotics for ten days or longer. Other drugs such as codeine for treatment of the cough may be indicated. The patient should be kept in isolation, as inhalation of airborne droplets may cause a spread of the infection. Preventative measures include keeping imported birds in quarantine and treating them (via their feed) with chlortetracycline. People who routinely handle birds should exercise care and be well informed about this disease. The infection can progress to life-threatening PNEUMONIA if not treated, but usually responds well with recovery in two to three weeks.

Causes and risk factors: the cause is a microorganism called *Chlamydia psittaci* that is transmitted to man by inhalation of dust from feathers or droppings or directly via the bite of an infected bird. There is a particular danger from some virulent forms of the disease and the mortality in human beings can be quite considerable, especially if the disease is not caught and treated early enough.

psoriasis

Description: a chronic skin disorder that tends to remain throughout life and is characterized by alternating active and quiescent periods.

Persons most commonly affected: usually beginning in adolescence or early adulthood and continues throughout life affecting people of both sexes.

Organ or part of body involved: skin.

Symptoms and indications: the appearance of raised, red, roughened patches covered by silvery, shiny scales. These usually first appear on the elbows and knees but may affect other areas of the trunk, arms, legs, scalp and back. The nails may also be affected, with thickening, pitting and splitting, which may be confused with a fungal infection. A person with symptoms of psoriasis should seek medical advice.

Treatment: is by means of various creams and ointments containing coal tar, corticosteroids, salicylic acid and anthralin. Sunlight (but not sunburn) is helpful and also synthetic vitamin A may be prescribed. Ultraviolet light (known as PuVA therapy) may be used to treat more extensive or severe psoriasis, under strict medical supervision. In very severe cases, or where there is additional psoriatic arthritis or exfoliative psoriatic dermatitis (*see causes and risk factors*), methotrexate (a potent antimetabolite drug) may be prescribed.

Treatment is usually effective in controlling the symptoms, although the condition itself cannot be cured. Stress or anxiety seems to exacerbate psoriasis and bring on an attack of the symptoms in some people. Hence, this should be avoided if possible and the person may require counselling and advice to learn to adjust his or her life to the condition.

Causes and risk factors: the cause is not known, but there is often a family history of psoriasis. It is much more common among White races of people. The symptoms of thickening and scaling of the skin are caused by changes in the epidermis with the production of a greater number of cells. Usually, psoriasis does not affect the person's overall health. However, in some people it is associated with a severe and disabling form of arthritis. In others, the skin may be much more severely and extensively affected, leading to a profound deterioration in general health, and this condition is known as exfoliative psoriatic dermatitis. Patients with the most severe forms of the disease may require periods of treatment in hospital.

ptosis

Description: drooping of the eyelid.

Persons most commonly affected: both sexes and all age groups.

Organ or part of the body involved: eyelid; one or both eyes may be involved.

Symptoms and indications: eyelid drooping over the eye and poor blinking reflex.

Treatment: depends on cause. Surgery may be required, or treatment of underlying disorder.

Causes and risk factors: may result from damage or weakness of the muscles or nerve supply of the eyelid, or may be because of restriction of the eyelid by scarring, cysts or a tumour. Other conditions that cause ptosis are MYASTHENIA GRAVIS, birth trauma, MUSCULAR DYSTROPHY, brain tumour, DIABETES.

pulmonary embolism

Description: a condition in which the pulmonary artery (leading from the heart to the lung) or a branch of it, becomes blocked by a clot or embolus, which is usually of blood, and rarely a clump of fat cells. The clot usually originates as a phlebothrombosis of a deep vein in the leg or pelvis. The seriousness of the condition is related to the size of the clot. The clot moves through the circulation, ultimately lodging in a part of a pulmonary artery. Large pulmonary emboli can be fatal, while smaller ones may cause tissue death of parts of the lung, breathing difficulties and symptoms of PLEURISY.

Persons most commonly affected: adults of both sexes but can affect people of all ages.

Organ or part of body involved: a pulmonary artery or one of its branches.

Symptoms and indications: there is a sudden and often severe pain in the chest, breathlessness and a cough that may result in the bringing up of blood. There is a rapid heartbeat rate and the person feels anxious and restless. The person may be feverish or faint and there may be shock and death if the clot is large. Often there are symptoms of PULMONARY HYPERTENSION. A person with symptoms of pulmonary embolism requires immediate emergency medical attention.

Treatment: involves admittance to hospital. Anticoagulant drugs such as heparin may be prescribed in less severe cases, or streptokinase to dissolve the clot. In other cases, emergency surgery may be needed to remove the clot. Pulmonary embolism occasionally arises as a complication of surgery, injury, especially bone fractures, pregnancy and childbirth, due to the formation of a clot in a deep vein of the leg or pelvis. Preventative measures for hospital patients include the wearing of elastic stockings and encouraging leg exercises and walking as soon as possible after surgery, and also the use of drugs to thin the blood.

Causes and risk factors: The risk of phlebothrombosis and pulmonary embolism is greater in those who smoke or are overweight and in older women taking oral contraceptives. Also, it is more likely in those with existing heart and circulatory disorders, in elderly persons aged over 60 years, and in those with SICKLE CELL ANAEMIA and some other diseases (POLYCYTHAEMIA).

pulmonary hypertension

Description: a considerable rise in blood pressure in the pulmonary artery due to increased resistance to the flow of blood, usually caused by diseases of the lung or PULMONARY EMBOLISM. The result is that the right ventricle (one of the larger lower chambers of the heart) has to work much harder to maintain the flow of blood and enlarges.

Persons most commonly affected: all age groups and both sexes.

Organ or part of body involved: heart, a pulmonary artery or its branches.

Symptoms and indications: there is chest pain or discomfort, fainting and light-headedness and, possibly, convulsive episodes and heart failure. A person with these symptoms requires immediate emergency medical attention.

Treatment: depends upon the underlying cause of the pulmonary hypertension. Admittance to hospital for diagnostic tests is followed by an appropriate course of treatment. (*See* PULMONARY EMBOLISM, BRONCHITIS, EMPHYSEMA.)

Causes and risk factors: the cause is usually underlying lung disease, as described above. There is a risk of death from heart failure, depending upon the severity of the condition.

pulmonary oedema

Description: a gathering of fluid in the lungs arising for a variety of reasons, especially as a result of congestive heart failure or MITRAL STENOSIS. It produces severe and life-threatening symptoms.

Persons most commonly affected: adults of both sexes, especially those in middle or older age groups.

Organ or part of body involved: lungs and heart.

Symptoms and indications: great breathing difficulties with shallow, rapid breaths, cyanosis (a lack of oxygen in the blood), anxiety, restlessness, and a feeling of suffocation. Also, there may be sweating, a cough, dry at first but then producing a pink-stained frothy sputum, a weak or pounding pulse and characteristic crackling sounds from the lungs (called rales) that can be heard through a stethoscope. There may be a collection of fluid in the hands and feet, low blood pressure (hypotension), and veins may become engorged and prominent. A person with these symptoms requires emergency medical treatment.

Treatment: admittance to hospital is required for immediate treatment aimed at saving life. This involves the giving of oxygen, and various drugs may be required including narcotics (morphine sulphate), nitroglycerin, diuretics, e.g. frusemide or ethacrynic acid, digitalis and dopamine. The underlying condition responsible for the pulmonary oedema will require appropriate treatment. The outlook is more favourable if treatment begins promptly.

Causes and risk factors: the usual cause is failure of the left ventricle of the heart (one of the lower larger chambers) or MITRAL STENOSIS. Other causes include poisoning with some drugs, such as barbiturates or opiates, fluids and blood given intravenously, KIDNEY FAILURE, STROKE, head injury, inhalation of toxic fumes and near-drowning.

pulmonary valve stenosis

Description: narrowing of the pulmonary valve, which controls the outlet from the right ventricle (one of the large upper chambers of the heart) to the pulmonary artery leading to the lungs. This leads to obstruction and a reduction of normal heart function.

Persons most commonly affected: both sexes and all age groups. The congenital form is likely to become apparent at or shortly after birth.

Organ or part of body involved: heart.

Symptoms and indications: symptoms are those of ANGINA, along with fainting and signs of congestive heart failure. These include breathlessness, fatigue, fluid retention and a cough which may produce a pink and frothy sputum. Part of the heart may become enlarged. A person with symptoms of pulmonary valve stenosis should seek medical advice.

Treatment: unless the symptoms are very mild, treatment usually involves admittance to hospital for surgery to clear the obstruction and widen the valve.

Causes and risk factors: the cause is usually congenital but rarely it arises as a result of RHEUMATIC FEVER.

pyelitis

Description: inflammation and infection of a part of the kidney, the pelvis. (This is the area from which urine drains into the ureter). It is usually the case that the infection is not limited to the pelvis but involves all the kidney, hence a more accurate term is pyelonephritis.

Persons most commonly affected: females of all age groups but can affect males, especially the elderly and those with underlying disorders such as kidney stones.

Organ or part of body involved: kidney.

Symptoms and indications: the symptoms include pain in the loins, high temperature, chills and shivering, loss of appetite and weight and malaise.

There may be frequency of urination and the urine is acidic and may contain pus. A person with these symptoms should seek medical advice.

Treatment: is by means of antibiotics, which may need to be given intravenously in hospital in the first instance. The person requires bed rest, and a high intake of fluids. Pain relief may be prescribed and oral antibiotics may be needed for some time to prevent a recurrence of infection. Investigative procedures are likely to be needed to detect any underlying disease or abnormality that may have caused the inflammation. If this is present, it will require further appropriate treatment.

Causes and risk factors: the usual organism responsible (in three quarters of the cases) is the common gut bacterium *E. coli*. There is an increased risk of this condition occurring during pregnancy and in patients who have had investigations of the bladder, using instruments, or urinary catheters. Also, patients being treated with immunosuppressive drugs or corticosteroids are at greater risk of developing this type of infection.

pyloric stenosis

Description: a narrowing of the pylorus (the lower end of the stomach, the opening from which food passes into the duodenum and which is controlled by a ring of muscle, the pyloric sphincter).

Persons most commonly affected: both sexes and all age groups. A congenital form is present at birth and particularly affects baby boys. This usually becomes apparent in the first two to five weeks after birth.

Organ or part of body involved: pylorus (stomach).

Symptoms and indications: there is vomiting and distension of the stomach, the muscular movements (peristalsis) of which may be visible through the abdomen. Without intervention, the person loses weight, becomes dehydrated and blood and body fluids become alkaline (alkalosis), due to acid loss following prolonged vomiting. In the congenital type, the thickened pyloric muscle can be felt externally. A person with these symptoms requires immediate medical attention.

Treatment: requires admittance to hospital for surgery to correct the condition. In babies, the surgical procedure is called pyloromyotomy or Ramstedt's procedure, and involves dividing the thickened muscle. The baby normally makes a good and complete recovery, with no recurrence of symptoms. In adults, surgery relieves the symptoms but the long-term outlook depends upon the underlying cause of the condition. Further treatment may be needed.

Causes and risk factors: the congenital form of pyloric stenosis is caused by a thickening of the muscle of the pylorus, which eventually closes the outlet to the duodenum. In adults, the cause is usually a peptic (pyloric) ulcer or cancerous growth that is responsible for the narrowing of the channel.

Q

Q fever

Description: an infectious disease of sheep, goats and cattle and some other mammals and birds (which do not exhibit symptoms), that can be passed to man producing a pneumonia-like disease.

Persons most commonly affected: all age groups and both sexes; persons in close contact with animals.

Organ or part of body involved: lungs, respiratory system.

Symptoms and indications: the symptoms usually begin suddenly and include a severe headache, high fever, breathing difficulties, chills, muscle and chest pains, cough and general malaise. A person with these symptoms should seek immediate medical advice. The illness lasts for about two weeks.

Treatment: is by means of antibiotics, especially tetracycline and chloramphenicol, and the person should be kept in isolation, rest in bed and drink plenty of fluids. An effective vaccine is available for those who may be at risk.

Causes and risk factors: the cause of the infection is a microorganism named *Coxiella burnetti*, which is present in the droppings, urine, milk and tisssues (especially the placenta) of infected animals. Transmission to humans is usually by means of inhalation of airborne droplets, but also through drinking unpasteurized milk. In slaughterhouses and other industries connected with animals, strict standards of hygiene, and health and safety measures including dust suppression, should be employed.

R

rabies

Description: a very severe and fatal disease affecting the central nervous system, which occurs in dogs, wolves, cats and many other mammals. Human beings are infected through the bite of a rabid animal, usually a dog. The UK is currently free of rabies but it occurs in many countries throughout the world.

Persons most commonly affected: all age groups and both sexes.

Organ or part of body involved: brain and central nervous system.

Symptoms and indications: symptoms may begin from ten days up to a year, following a bite from a rabid animal. Usually, however, they begin after four to eight weeks, starting with depression and irritability. Swallowing and breathing difficulties develop, and feverishness, and there are periods of great mental excitement, increased salivation and muscular spasms of the throat that are very painful. Eventually, even the sight of water causes severe muscular spasms, convulsions and paralysis, with death following in about four days. A person who is bitten by an animal that may be rabid should immediately thoroughly cleanse the wound with soap or detergent and antiseptic to remove all traces of saliva, being especially careful about deep punctures. The wound should be covered with a clean dressing and then medical advice should be sought. The appropriate authorities should also be notified so that the animal can be caught and dealt with.

Treatment: is by means of injections of rabies vaccine, antiserum and immunoglobulin. A person who has previously received rabies vaccine as a preventative measure, and who receives a bite, requires further injections. The incubation period for rabies enables effective treatment to be given. However, if symptoms start, the outcome is normally fatal (in 80% of cases), although some people survive with vigorous supportive treatment.

Causes and risk factors: the cause of rabies is a virus that is present in populations of wild and feral animals in many countries of the world. Rabid animals exhibit one of two forms of behaviour, known as 'mad' or 'furious' rabies and dumb rabies. In the former, the animal may exhibit wild, uncontrolled behaviour, running around and snapping and biting if it is a dog, or losing its normal fear of humans and behaving unusually, in the case of a wild creature. In the other form, which is a more advanced stage of the furious type, the animal is more or less paralysed and drags itself around but may bite if cornered. Preventative treatment with rabies vaccine is advisable for all those living, working or visiting countries where rabies is endemic and who are likely to be in contact with animals. If prompt medical care is available, rabies is uncommon in human beings but remains one of the most feared diseases.

radiation sickness

Description: any illness that is caused by harmful radiation from radioactive substances. It often occurs as a complication of radiotherapy for cancer.

Persons most commonly affected: all age groups and both sexes; cancer patients.

Organ or part of body involved: any part of the body may be involved, depending upon site and degree of exposure to radiation.

Symptoms and indications: the symptoms vary a great deal, depending upon the site and nature of the exposure to radiation. Symptoms due to radiotherapy for cancer are usually relatively short-lived. These include nausea and vomiting, loss of appetite and weight, diarrhoea, a reddened and itchy skin. Also, there may be hair loss, increased likelihood of other infections, bleeding and ANAEMIA. These symptoms should be reported to a doctor.

Treatment: antihistamine drugs and tranquillizers, such as chlorpromazine, are used to alleviate the condition, and also soothing preparations to relieve itching. The person should have plenty of rest and endeavour to eat a nutritious diet and drink plenty of fluids. A liquid diet may be needed for a time, or fluids given intravenously.

Causes and risk factors: the cause is radiation from radioactive substances and high doses (related to accidents in the nuclear power industry or nuclear weapons industries) may prove fatal. There is a risk of the development of cancer, sterility, genetic abnormalities and birth defects in those accidentally exposed to high doses of radiation.

rat bite fever

Description: two types of infection, with similar symptoms, that may be transmitted to man following a bite from a rat, mouse or possibly some other animal e.g. a weasel. Occasionally, drinking unpasteurized milk that is contaminated with the causative microorganisms is responsible for this infection.

Persons most commonly affected: all age groups and both sexes.

Organ or part of body involved: skin, respiratory system, gastrointestinal tract, joints.

Symptoms and indications: the symptoms usually develop about ten days after a rat or mouse bite. They include fever, headache, chills, malaise, vomiting, joint pains and skin rash. A person with these symptoms should seek medical advice and you should always consult a doctor following a bite from a wild animal.

Treatment: is by means of penicillin or erythromycin and the person should rest in bed until the symptoms subside.

Causes and risk factors: the causal organisms are *Streptobacillus moniliformis* or *Spirillum minus*. Persons most at risk are those likely to come into contact with rats, such as workers in sewage-treatment plants, laboratories or those in poor or overcrowded living conditions.

Raynaud's disease and Raynaud's phenomenon

Description: a disorder of the circulation, in which there is a periodic interruption in the blood supply to outlying parts of the body, due to spasm of the small arteries involved.

Persons most commonly affected: women below the age of 40.

Organ or part of body involved: small arteries in the fingers, toes, ears and nose.

Symptoms and indications: pale, numb and deadened fingers or toes, ears or nose. If the disease is prolonged, the skin becomes taut and ulcers appear. There is often cyanosis in the affected parts, i.e. a lack of oxygen causing a bluish colouration of the skin. When the spasm

passes, and on warming, normal colour returns to the affected part. Raynaud's disease is defined as being present for two or more years without becoming worse, and in the absence of any evidence of underlying disorder. It is a primary disease. Raynaud's phenomenon produces similar symptoms but is secondary to another disease such as ATHEROSCLEROSIS or SCLERODERMA. It usually develops within two years and there may be thickening of the skin and ulcers.

Treatment: in mild cases of Raynaud's disease, protecting the hands, feet, head and face from the cold and avoiding stress (which both precipitate the onset of symptoms) may be all that is required. The person must stop smoking as this is another precipitating factor, causing blood vessels to contract. Various drugs may be prescribed that are vasodilators or calcium antagonists. Some patients may benefit from surgery to cut sympathetic nerves to the affected parts. This usually relieves symptoms for one or two years and is more effective in those with primary Raynaud's disease. Treatment for the underlying cause of Raynaud's phenomenon is also likely to be needed.

Causes and risk factors: the cause is spasms of the small arteries supplying the affected area, due to sensitivity to cold, or precipitated by stress or smoking. Raynaud's phenomenon is associated with diseases of connective tissue and arteries, myxoedema, Buerger's disease and pulmonary hypertension. Also, the taking of certain drugs such as clonidine, beta blockers and those containing ergot alkaloids, all of which cause constriction of blood vessels and may exacerbate the condition.

rectal abscess or abscess of the rectum or anorectal abscess

Description: an inflamed and infected part of the rectum, the final portion of the large intestine in which faeces are stored prior to elimination via the anus.

Persons most commonly affected: all age groups and both sexes.

Organ or part of body involved: rectum.

Symptoms and indications: a superficial abscess in the lower part of the rectum usually causes swelling, heat, tenderness and pain that may be severe, and can sometimes be felt on examination. A person with symptoms of a rectal abscess should seek medical advice.

Treatment: normally involves admittance to hospital for surgery to drain the abscess. Antibiotics may be prescribed and recovery is normally good.

Causes and risk factors: the cause is usually a number of bacteria producing a mixed infection, and these include streptococcus and staphylococcus, *E. coli* and *Proteus vulgaris*. One complication of the surgical procedure is that a FISTULA may develop in some patients.

rectal prolapse or prolapse of the rectum

Description: a protrusion of a greater or lesser portion of the rectum to the outside through the anus.

Persons most commonly affected: children of both sexes and women aged over 60 years.

Organ or part of body involved: rectum.

Symptoms and indications: these include a discharge of mucus that may be tinged with blood and protrusion of a firm mass, especially following a bowel movement. A person with symptoms of this disorder should seek medical advice.

Treatment: the disorder is sometimes associated with straining; hence, measures to correct constipation, including attention to diet and possible use of laxatives may be needed. In children, strapping the buttocks together after a bowel movement for a period of time and correcting diarrhoea or constipation, are usually all that is needed to correct the prolapse. In adults or children with a more extensive prolapse, some surgery may be needed.

Causes and risk factors: the risk increases with age and loss of muscle tone and previous surgery in the region of the rectum. Exercises to strengthen the pelvic floor muscles may be helpful in preventing the occurrence of this condition.

rectal tumour or benign growth and cancer of the rectum

Description: a benign growth of cells or a polyp within the rectum, or a proliferation of malignant cells. Cancer of the rectum is a fairly common form of malignancy.

Persons most commonly affected: adults of both sexes in late middle and older age. It is rare in younger people.

Organ or part of body involved: rectum, abdominal lymph glands, liver.

Symptoms and indications: symptoms vary but include bleeding and pain or discomfort.

Cancer—in the early stages there may be few or no symptoms but later there is diarrhoea alternating with constipation, bleeding and watery, blood-stained discharge, fatigue and weakness, loss of weight and lower back pain. The tumour may be felt as a projecting mass. A person with any of these symptoms should seek medical advice.

Treatment: for both benign and malignant tumours, usually involves admittance to hospital for surgery. Patients with cancer may require removal of a considerable portion of the whole of the rectum and part of the colon with the production of a colostomy. This is an operation to produce an artificial opening of the colon through the abdominal wall, which then acts as an anus. Patients who have a colostomy require help and counselling to learn to cope with the situation. Recovery is usually good and the person can expect to lead a near-normal life. In addition to surgery, a cancer patient may require chemotherapy and radiotherapy.

Causes and risk factors: the cause is not known, although it is generally accepted that there is a connection with a diet containing too much refined food and little fibre. This disease is more common in people in western countries, where refined foods are more readily available.

Reiter's syndrome (RS)

Description: a disease that produces symptoms of urethritis, CONJUNCTIVITIS and ARTHRITIS (reactive arthritis, i.e. inflammation of the joints resulting from infection elsewhere).

Persons most commonly affected: males aged 12 to 40 years. It is rare in females and younger children.

Organ or part of body involved: urethra, eyes, joints and, sometimes, the skin.

Symptoms and indications: early symptoms include feverishness, frequent need to pass water, discharge that may contain pus, reddened, watering eyes, pains in the joints, and there may be raised, reddened areas on the skin (keratitis). Small painful ulcers may develop on the mucous membranes of the mouth and at the tip of the penis. A person with these symptoms should seek medical advice.

Treatment: is by means of antibiotics such as tetracycline or erythromycin for urethritis, and non-steroidal anti-inflammatory drugs for arthritis. Symptoms of arthritis may continue for some time and physiotherapy and exercises for the affected joints may be needed. With the sexually transmitted form of Reiter's syndrome, the patient's partner should also be given antibiotics. *See causes and risk factors*.

Causes and risk factors: there are two forms of Reiter's syndrome, one of which is thought to be sexually transmitted and the other as a result of infections in the gastrointestinal tract (dysenteric RS). Women, children and elderly persons are usually affected by the dysenteric form, which is less common. There is evidence of a genetic tendency for this disease, as many of those affected have a particular tissue antigen designated HLA-B27. This is human leucocyte antigen, a genetic marker located at a particular point on chromosome 6. There are known associations between some HLA types and certain diseases.

relapsing fever

Description: a disease caused by spirochaete bacteria of the genus *Borrelia*, which exists in two forms. One type of infection is transmitted to human beings by lice and the other by ticks. The former type is endemic in some sub-tropical and tropical countries, while the latter is more widely spread and occurs in Europe and the USA. It tends to occur in populations affected by war and hunger, where there is malnutrition, overcrowding and a lack of hygiene. Characteristically, there are bouts of fever followed by periods without symptoms related to the development and release of the parasitic microorganisms in the body.

Persons most commonly affected: all age groups and both sexes.

Organ or part of body involved: brain, joints, gastrointestinal tract, skin.

Symptoms and indications: symptoms usually appear about six days after a bite from a tick or louse but may occur at any time between three and ten days following infection. They include severe headache, chills, high fever, pains in muscles and joints, vomiting and nosebleeds. Heartbeat rate rises and a raised, reddish rash may appear. Eventually as the disease progresses there may be enlargement of the liver and spleen and jaundice, especially in the louse-transmitted type. The fever and other symptoms usually subside after three to five days and there is a period of several days before they return again. There may be anything from two to ten periods of relapse but eventually the illness subsides as the patient develops immunity. However, there is a risk of death from complications and in people who are already suffering from debility. A person with these symptoms, especially having visited a country where relapsing fever occurs, should seek medical advice.

Treatment: is by means of bed rest and antibiotics, especially tetracycline or erythromycin, which may need to be given intravenously, along with fluids in severe cases. Doxycycline is also effective and treatment needs to be given at the start of the fever or after this has subsided, but not when it is at its height. This is due to the risk of the development of the Jarisch-Herxheimer reaction, a sudden rise in temperature with possible shock and collapse. This is a feature particularly of tick-transmitted relapsing fever (and also LEPTOSPIROSIS and SYPHILIS), which may follow once antibiotic treatment has begun. Its effects can be lessened by giving another drug, acetaminophen, before and after the first doses of antibiotics.

Causes and risk factors: the cause of relapsing fever is species of *Borrelia spirochaete* bacteria. Insecticide chemicals to eliminate lice are highly effective but it is more difficult to control ticks. Ideally, good-fitting, protective clothing should be worn to lessen the likelihood of a tick bite.

renal carbuncle

Description: an abscess that develops in a kidney.

Persons most commonly affected: elderly persons, especially men, but can affect people of other age groups and both sexes. Especially likely in those with a debilitating illness, DIABETES MELLITUS and existing bladder infection.

Organ or part of body involved: kidney.

Symptoms and indications: symptoms include pain, feverishness, malaise, chills and possibly symptoms of septicaemia (blood poisoning). Symptoms may appear suddenly or more gradually. A person with symptoms of a renal carbuncle should seek immediate medical advice.

Treatment: is likely to involve admittance to hospital for surgery to drain the carbuncle of pus, and antibiotics to combat the infection. The person may require further treatment for underlying illness or infection. The condition can be cured, although the outcome may depend upon the overall health of the patient.

Causes and risk factors: usually the cause is a bladder infection that spreads upwards to the kidney or it may be caused by a staphylococcal infection elsewhere in the body.

renal tuberculosis

Description: tuberculosis affecting the kidney.

Persons most commonly affected: adults of both sexes, especially men.

Organ or part of body involved: kidney.

Symptoms and indications: there may be few or no symptoms for a considerable period of time. Eventually, there may be symptoms of kidney inflammation and infection (PYELITIS or PYELONEPHRITIS), including fever, chills, pain, shivering, loss of appetite and weight, and malaise. A person with these symptoms should seek medical advice.

Treatment: the diagnosis is likely to be made after other causes of the symptoms have been ruled out. In men, it can usually be confirmed following analysis of urine samples in which the organism, *Mycobacterium tuberculosis* is likely to be present. In women, other tests may be needed. Treatment is by means of antituberculosis drugs e.g. rifampicin.

Causes and risk factors: the cause of renal tuberculosis is the bacterium Mycobacterium tuberculosis. In both men and women there is a risk of the infection spreading to involve reproductive organs.

retinal detachment or detachment of the retina of the eye

Description: a hole or tear in the retina, the layer that lines the interior of the eye and contains light-sensitive cells and nerve fibres. The retina consists of two layers and when the tear is produced, the inner one becomes separated from the outer one and retinal detachment occurs. This is caused by fluid (vitreous humour) leaking through the hole, forcing the inner layer to become detached from the outer layer.

Persons most commonly affected: all age groups and both sexes, especially males.

Organ or part of body involved: retina, usually of one eye only.

Symptoms and indications: symptoms include the appearance of floating spots (floaters) before the eye, blurring of vision, flashes of light and loss of sharpness in the centre of the image. The person may appear to see a veil or curtain in the affected eye. Any person with these symptoms requires immediate emergency medical treatment in order to preserve sight in the affected eye.

Treatment: consists of admittance to hospital for surgery to seal the hole or repair the separation of the retina by means of electric current, which produces heat (diathermy) or cold (cryotherapy) using liquid nitrogen or solid carbon dioxide. At an early stage, laser treatment may be the preferred method. Occasionally it may be necessary to alter the shape of the eye to bring about healing. The condition can usually be cured if treated at an early stage but a delay in treatment may result in permanent partial or complete loss of vision.

Causes and risk factors: the causes are eye injury or a complication of eye surgery (especially the removal of cataracts) and the risk increases in those with short-sightedness (myopia) and DIABETES MELLITUS. Also, older persons are at greater risk, as are those with a history of this condition. Malignant tumours of the eye may also be a cause of retinal detachment.

Reye's syndrome

Description: a rare and serious disease of childhood that seems to follow on from a viral infection such as CHICKEN-POX or INFLUENZA, often becoming apparent during the recovery phase of the illness.

Persons most commonly affected: children of both sexes, rare in adults.

Organ or part of body involved: brain, liver.

Symptoms and indications: the symptoms usually appear during recovery from an upper respiratory tract infection. They include nausea and vomiting, and mental disturbances that may manifest themselves in a number of ways. The child may be confused, forgetful and lethargic or excited and agitated. Eventually, this leads to unresponsiveness, progressing to coma, with fits and, possibly, fixed, dilated pupils, respiratory collapse and death. In many cases, enlargement and damage to the liver occurs and other organs, such as the pancreas, kidneys, spleen, heart and lymph nodes may be affected. A child with these serious symptoms requires immediate emergency medical attention.

Treatment: since the cause is unknown, there is no specific regime of drug treatment. The child requires admittance to hospital for intensive supportive nursing and may need intravenous fluids, assisted ventilation and monitoring and control of all body functions. Various drugs may be needed to maintain the child in a stable condition. The outlook varies according to the severity of the symptoms but is more favourable in those who receive early treatment.

Causes and risk factors: the cause of the disorder is unknown but aspirin may be implicated in the development of Reye's syndrome. This drug is no longer recommended for children under the age of 12 years. The overall mortality rate is about 21% and children who lapse into the deeper stages of coma are most at risk. The outlook for those less severely affected is generally good. About 30% of survivors have residual brain damage, especially those who suffered fits or were in a deeper stage of coma. Others make a full recovery and the condition is not likely to recur.

rheumatic fever

Description: a severe disease, mainly occurring in childhood or adolescence, which is a complication of infections with the Group A streptococcus bacteria. It generally occurs in those who have had a streptococcal infection of the upper respiratory tract and produces a wide range of symptoms.

Persons most commonly affected: children of both sexes between the ages of 4 and 18.

Organ or part of body involved: joints, heart, skin, central nervous system.

Symptoms and indications: the child may develop a fever, pains, loss of appetite and malaise. Usually there are symptoms of ARTHRITIS with joint pain that progresses from joint to joint. Affected joints are swollen, tender, hot and painful and normally, the wrists, elbows, ankles and knees are involved. Other joints may also be affected. Painless nodules may develop beneath the skin over bony protuberances such as the elbows, knees and wrists. In addition, there may be chorea (involuntary, jerking movements of the muscles) and the development of a transient characteristic rash called Erythema marginatum. A serious set of symptoms that often accompanies rheumatic fever is inflammation of the heart (carditis), which can include the muscles, valves and membranes. The condition may cause rheumatic heart disease, in which there is scarring and inflammation of heart structures. In later adult life, there may be a need for surgery to replace damaged heart valves. A child with symptoms of rheumatic fever requires immediate medical attention.

Treatment: depends upon symptoms but rest in bed is needed until the attack subsides. Initially, treatment consists of destroying the streptococci that cause the disease, with antibiotics such as penicillin. For arthritis symptoms, analgesics, non-steroidal anti-inflammatory drugs or corticosteroids may be prescribed. Those with heart symptoms are likely to require admittance to hospital for special care and treatment with aspirin or salicylate drugs, corticosteroids and other drugs. Following recovery, low doses of antibiotics may need to be continued to prevent any further streptococcal infections. Patients with known damage to heart valves require intensive courses of antibiotics before dental treatment or other surgical procedures.

Causes and risk factors: the cause of rheumatic fever is previous streptococcal infection but there are likely to be factors making some individuals more susceptible than others. In general, children living in poor, overcrowded living conditions with inadequate nutrition are more likely to develop this disorder but this is by no means always the case. The incidence of rheumatic fever is declining in most developed countries.

rheumatoid arthritis

Description: the second most common form of joint disease (after OSTEOARTHRITIS), which usually affects the feet, ankles, fingers and wrists. The condition is diagnosed by means of X-rays, which show a typical pattern of changes around the inflamed joints, known as rheumatoid erosions. At first there is swelling of the joint and inflammation of the synovial membrane (the membranous sac that surrounds the joint), followed by erosion and loss of cartilage and bone. In addition, a blood test reveals the presence of serum rheumatoid factor antibody, which is characteristic of this condition.

Persons most commonly affected: all age groups and both sexes but especially women and more common in those aged 30 to 50.

Organ or part of body involved: joints.

Symptoms and indications: symptoms usually arise slowly and insidiously, but may occasionally be rapid in onset. There is inflammation, tenderness or pain in the affected joints, and stiffness, especially on first getting up in the morning. By the afternoon, the person may feel unusually tired or unwell. Deformities of affected joints are likely to develop. In other people, after an initial active phase, there may be a long period of remission. A person with symptoms of rheumatoid arthritis should seek medical advice.

Treatment: rest in bed during active phases of the disease is essential, and adequate rest and good nutrition are important at all times. Drugs used in treatment include aspirin and salicylates, non-steroidal anti-inflammatory preparations and slow-acting agents including penicillamine, sulphasalazine, gold and hydroxychloroquine. Many patients improve with treatment and the condition varies greatly in its degree of severity. At its worst, it is progressively and severely disabling, whereas others, less seriously affected, are able to enjoy a relatively normal life.

Causes and risk factors: the cause is not known but there appear to be genetic factors involved. Most affected people have a particular antibody— HLA-DR4, but there are likely to be other factors involved, including a family tendency for the disease.

ringworm

Description: an infection caused by various species of fungi, known medically as tinea. It is contagious from person to person, either through direct contact or from an infected surface such as a floor, face flannel, towel, etc.

Persons most commonly affected: adolescents and adults of both sexes but more common in males.

Organ or part of body involved: feet—tinea pedis or athlete's foot; groin—tinea cruris or dhobi itch; scalp—tinea capitis, tinea favosa favus or honeycomb ringworm; body—tinea corporis; chest and trunk—tinea versicolor; nails—tinea unguium; beard—tinea barbae.

Symptoms and indications: typically, slightly raised, itchy patches on the skin with a ring-like appearance. Blisters and scabs often occur. Ringworm affecting the nails causes a greenish or grey discolouration, with thickening, the nails becoming brittle and somewhat deformed. A person with symptoms of ringworm should seek medical advice.

Treatment: the usual treatment for ringworm, which is, in general, highly effective, is the antibiotic drug griseofulvin, taken by mouth. In addition, various other antifungal creams or ointments may be prescribed. Careful attention to hygiene, wearing clothing and footwear made of natural rather than synthetic materials and keeping the skin dry are important measures. Warm, moist, sweaty conditions favour the growth of ringworm fungus. Ringworm can usually be successfully treated in a few weeks but may recur. Ringworm of the nails is more difficult to treat and it may take longer to cure.

Causes and risk factors: the cause is various types of fungus, which are fairly prevalent. Athlete's foot is a very common type of infection.

Rocky Mountain spotted fever

Description: a serious acute infection transmitted to man by the bite of a tick and prevalent in many states of the USA. It is absent from the UK.

Persons most commonly affected: all age groups and both sexes.

Organ or part of body involved: central nervous system, skin, gastrointestinal tract, muscles—whole body symptoms.

Symptoms and indications: the symptoms appear between 3 and 12 days after the bite of an infected tick. They include fever, severe headache, vomiting and nausea, muscular stiffness and pain, chills and the appearance of a characteristic red rash that eventually spreads over much of the body. This may eventually darken and ulcerate. The person shows symptoms of mental confusion, agitation, DELIRIUM leading to coma and possibly death. A person with symptoms of this disease requires immediate, urgent medical treatment.

Treatment: is by means of antibiotics such as chloramphenicol or tetracycline, which should begin as soon as possible once symptoms appear. The disease is usually curable if caught and treated early but may be fatal if treatment is delayed. Preventative measures include the wearing of protective clothing in areas where the disease is endemic and the use of tick-repellent chemicals such as deet (diethyltoluamide).

Causes and risk factors: the cause of the infection is a microorganism called *Rickettsia rickettsii*, transmitted by the bite of ticks that are parasitic on many wild animals as well as man. There are similar feverish infections transmitted by ticks in European countries (*see* TYPHOID FEVER).

rodent ulcer

Description: a slow-growing malignant ulcer generally occurring on the face.

Persons most commonly affected: middle-aged and elderly persons of both sexes.

Organ or part of body involved: the face, especially the edges of the nostrils, eyes and lips.

Symptoms and indications: the symptoms and appearance of rodent ulcers vary greatly and they can be confused with other skin conditions such as dermatitis or PSORIASIS. Usually, it appears as a shiny papule that gradually enlarges and often alternately bleeds and forms a scab. A person with symptoms of a rodent ulcer should seek medical advice.

Treatment: involves admittance to a specialist unit for biopsy and tests. Usually, some form of surgical procedure is required and occasionally, radiotherapy. Recovery is normally good, although occasionally there may be a recurrence.

Causes and risk factors: the cause is not known but fair-skinned European people living in a hot climate may be more at risk. Rodent ulcers do not normally cause secondary growths elsewhere but can destroy underlying healthy tissue, which, in rare cases, may be sufficiently serious to cause death.

rosacea or acne rosacea

Description: a disease of the skin of the face characterized by a red, flushed appearance and engorgement.

Persons most commonly affected: adults of both sexes aged over 30 years but more common in women.

Organ or part of body involved: face.

Symptoms and indications: in the early stages there is a red, raised rash (erythema) that comes and goes, usually appearing upon exposure to the sun or after eating a meal. This causes a hot, burning or tingling sensation. Eventually, this becomes permanent and there may be pimples and pustules. In some cases, the sebaceous glands become involved and greatly enlarge, especially in the region of the nose. The skin becomes thickened and uneven and the nose is very red, large and prominent. This condition is called rhinophyma. A person with symptoms of rosacea should seek medical advice at an early stage, in order to prevent the development of rhinophyma.

Treatment: is by means of antibiotic drugs, especially tetracycline, taken by mouth, or isotretinoin, in less responsive cases. Also, topical ointments or creams containing the antibiotic metronidazole may be prescribed. Occasionally, surgery may be needed to correct rhinophyma. Antibiotic treatment is usually very effective in controlling the condition.

Causes and risk factors: the cause is not known but it tends to affect fair-skinned people. Exposure to the sun, excess alcohol consumption and certain foods may exacerbate the condition, although this is not certain.

roseola infantum or **pseudorubella** or **exanthem subitum**

Description: an acute fever and skin rash that is highly contagious and affects babies and young children.

Persons most commonly affected: babies and young children aged six months to three years.

Organ or part of body involved: central nervous system, skin.

Symptoms and indications: the child suddenly develops a high fever of 103° to 105°F or 39.5° to 40.5°C, for which there is no obvious cause. The fever usually lasts about three to five days and convulsions may occur. The child is irritable and unwell. The fever normally reaches a peak and then subsides and this coincides in some, but not all cases, with the development of a red rash, mainly on the chest and abdomen. This normally subsides quite soon and by this time the child is evidently feeling much better. A child who develops a high fever should always be seen by a doctor. The doctor should be summoned urgently if the child has a convulsion or shows signs of dehydration.

Treatment: consists of measures to reduce fever,
including the use of medicines containing paracetamol that are designed for young children, tepid sponging and cooling fans. The child should be encouraged to drink plenty of fluids. In rare cases, admittance to hospital may be required. The child normally recovers well after a few days.

Causes and risk factors: the cause is now thought to be, in many cases, human herpes virus type 6 (HHV-6), although there may be others.

roundworms or **ascariasis**

Description: an illness caused by infestation with a parasitic type of worm (which resembles an earthworm) called *Ascaris lumbricoides*. It is prevalent in warm climates in overcrowded conditions with poor hygiene and sanitation. The larvae of the worm pass through the lungs and may cause respiratory symptoms. They ascend to the throat and are swallowed, maturing into adult worms in the gastrointestinal tract where they may cause further abdominal symptoms.

Persons most commonly affected: children of both sexes.

Organ or part of body involved: lungs and gastrointestinal tract.

Symptoms and indications: during the passage of the larvae through the lungs, there may be coughing, wheezing and fever. Coughed-up sputum may contain the larvae. In the intestine, particularly if there is a heavy infestation, the adult worms may cause pains in the abdomen, loss of appetite and weight, tiredness and, possibly, diarrhoea and vomiting. Sometimes an adult worm is vomited up or passed in faeces. A person with symptoms of roundworm infestation should seek immediate medical treatment.

Treatment: consists of drugs to kill the worms, either pyrantel pamoate or mebendazole. The latter should not be taken by pregnant women and the doctor should be informed if pregnancy is a possibility. The drugs used in treatment are highly effective.

Causes and risk factors: people, especially children, become infected by playing in dirt contaminated by the eggs of the parasite and putting their hands in their mouths. Hence, roundworms are a problem in conditions of poor sanitation and hygiene. Also, eating vegetables (especially raw) that have been washed in contaminated water, and directly drinking contaminated water are other sources of infection. Anyone visiting an area where such conditions exist should be scrupulous about hygiene, food and drinking water. Domestic animals (dogs and cats) may be infested with roundworms and should be wormed regularly. Children should be taught to wash their hands after touching animals, and pets should not be allowed near food for human consumption. There is a risk (rare) of obstruction of the gut by adult worms, if the infestation is heavy, requiring urgent medical treatment.

ruptured eardrum

Description: a hole that may develop in the eardrum because of infection or injury. It may also be called perforated eardrum.

Persons most commonly affected: all ages and both sexes.

Organ or part of body involved: ear.

Symptoms and indications: there may be sudden deafness following acute OTITIS MEDIA or injury.

Sometimes, there may be sudden relief of the pain of otitis media. There may be a discharge from the ear, and sometimes sufferers complain of tinnitus.

Treatment: a doctor will usually clean the middle ear and prescribe a course of antibiotics. The ear should be protected while showering. In children, a ruptured eardrum usually heals within two weeks; in adults, this may take a little longer.

Causes and risk factors: it can be caused by severe or untreated otitis media. It may also be caused by sudden high pressure applied to the eardrum, either while diving, from a slap on the ear, or by a sudden very loud noise. It may be avoided by wearing ear protectors in a very noisy environment. Otitis media should always be treated and cleared up, and no-one should scuba-dive without training.

S

salivary gland enlargement

Description: enlargement of one or more salivary glands due to an infection, salivary duct stone or tumour.

Persons most commonly affected: adults of both sexes.

Organ or part of body involved: salivary glands, ducts, nearby lymph glands.

Symptoms and indications: salivary gland infection: swelling and pain in the affected gland, either sublingual (beneath the tongue), submandibular (beneath the jaw) or parotid (behind the ear). Lymph glands in the neck may also be swollen and tender and there may be malaise and feverishness. Salivary duct stone: this usually affects the submandibular glands, causing swelling and pain, especially when eating. Lymph glands may be swollen and tender in the neck and there may be malaise and feverishness. Salivary gland tumour: swelling due to mass of tumour growth, which is tender and painful.

A person with enlargement and pain in a salivary gland should seek medical advice.

Treatment: salivary gland infection—treatment is by means of antibiotics and pain-relieving drugs. Salivary duct stone—treatment may involve admittance to hospital for surgical removal of the stone. Antibiotics and pain-relieving drugs may be prescribed. Salivary gland tumour—treatment involves admittance to hospital for surgical removal of the tumour. If the growth is malignant, tumours may require radiotherapy and chemotherapy. The outlook is usually quite good if the tumour is caught at an early stage.

Causes and risk factors: infections are caused by one or other of many different types of bacteria e.g. staphylococcus. Salivary duct tumours may arise as a result of a change in the composition of the saliva. The cause of a salivary gland tumour is unknown. The risk of developing a salivary gland disorder increases with poor nutrition, a lack of vitamins in the diet, inadequate fluid intake leading to dehydration and inattention to oral hygiene. It is important to clean the teeth thoroughly at least twice each day and to visit the dentist regularly.

sandfly fever or phlebotomus fever

Description: a viral infection characterized by fever of short duration, which is transmitted to humans through the bite of a sandfly. It occurs in many warm countries including parts of the Mediterranean.

Persons most commonly affected: all age groups and both sexes.

Organ or part of body involved: central nervous system, whole body symptoms.

Symptoms and indications: the symptoms resemble those of influenza and appear about three to seven days after a bite. They include headache, chills, fever, pains in muscles and joints, flushing and bloodshot eyes. The fever subsides in about three days but the person may be left feeling weak and take some time to fully recover.

Treatment: consists of rest in bed, painkilling drugs and adequate fluid intake until symptoms subside. Preventative measures include the use of insect repellent preparations, protective clothing and sandfly netting.

Causes and risk factors: the cause of the infection is a virus transmitted by the sandfly *Phlebotomus paparasi*.

scabies

Description: a contagious skin infection caused by a mite and characterized by severe itching.

Persons most commonly affected: all age groups and both sexes.

Organ or part of body involved: skin between the fingers, wrists, buttocks, genitals and under the arms, breasts, elbows.

Symptoms and indications: the burrows of the mites are visible on the skin as thin, dark lines, each with a small pimple at one end. These may soon be obscured by scarring due to scratching. There is severe itching, which is particularly marked when the person is in bed. A person with symptoms of scabies should seek immediate medical advice.

Treatment: consists of cream or ointment to kill the mites, which is applied to the whole surface of the body and is left in place for at least 12 hours and preferably longer. It is usually a preparation of 5% permethrin or Lindane gamma-benzene hydrochloride, although for babies or pregnant women other ointments (containing sulphur) may be prescribed. Clothing and bed linen should be carefully washed although, as the mites do not survive for long off the human body, spread is more likely to be due to direct skin contact between people.

Causes and risk factors: the cause is a mite called *Sarcopetes scabei*. The female burrows into the skin, lays eggs and the larvae, which hatch in a few days, cause the itching and are mature mites in about three weeks. Secondary bacterial skin infections may occur due to scratching, which may require further antibiotic treatment. The risk of contracting scabies is greater among those living in poor, overcrowded conditions, where cleanliness and hygiene are more difficult to maintain.

scarlet fever or scarlatina

Description: an infectious disease, mainly of childhood, characterized by a bright red skin rash that generally follows and is caused by a preceding throat infection due to streptococcus bacteria. Scarlet fever used to be the major cause of death in young children in Britain but is now rare and less severe, due to the availability of antibiotics.

Persons most commonly affected: children of both sexes aged two to ten.

Organ or part of body involved: throat and surrounding tissues, skin, central nervous system, whole body symptoms.

Symptoms and indications: symptoms appear after an incubation period of about three days. There is a high fever (up to 104°F [40°C]), chills, headache, vomiting, rapid pulse and a very sore throat. The tonsils and lymph glands in the neck are usually swollen and tender. Within 24 hours, a bright red rash appears on the face and spreads to include other parts of the body. The rash fades and disappears after about one week, with peeling of the skin. When it is at its height, the tongue is usually a bright strawberry red, as is the face apart from a pale white area around the mouth. Also characteristic are dark red lines in skin folds and creases. Usually, a child with a streptococcal throat infection receives early antibiotic treatment and scarlet fever does not develop. If symptoms of this illness do appear, the child should be seen by a doctor.

Treatment: consists of bed rest and a course of antibiotics, usually penicillin or erythromycin. The child should be encouraged to drink plenty of fluids. Prompt treatment with antibiotics generally ensures that complications do not arise (*see causes and risk factors*) and recovery is usually complete in about ten days to two weeks.

Causes and risk factors: the cause of scarlet fever is erythrogenic toxin produced by Group A streptococcus bacteria. If left untreated, serious complications can arise, particularly inflammation of the kidneys (GLOMERULONEPHRITIS), heart (ENDOCARDITIS), middle ear and joints (ARTHRITIS or rheumatism).

schistosomiasis or bilharziasis

Description: a very severe disease caused by parasitic blood flukes, which affects many millions of people in tropical countries, especially in the Far and Middle East, South America and Africa.

Persons most commonly affected: all age groups and both sexes.

Organ or part of body involved: urinary tract or gastrointestinal tract, spleen, liver.

Symptoms and indications: depending upon the species, the flukes settle in blood vessels of the rectum or bladder. Intestinal symptoms include diarrhoea, with passing of blood, ANAEMIA, DYSENTERY, enlargement of the spleen and liver and CIRRHOSIS OF THE LIVER. Urinary tract symptoms are those of CYSTITIS, with blood in the urine, bladder stones and an increased likelihood of cancer of the bladder. A person with any of these symptoms should seek immediate medical advice.

Treatment: may involve admittance to hospital and is by means of various drugs, depending upon the type of schistosome parasite. Drugs used include praziquantel, metriphonate and oxamniquine. The parasite is acquired through the skin by contact with infected water. Preventative measures are therefore extremely important, especially not swimming or bathing in water that may be suspected of containing the parasites.

Causes and risk factors: the cause of the disease is schistosome blood flukes (*Trematoda*) of various species, which complete a part of their life cycle within freshwater snails. The larvae of the parasite burrow through the skin of humans and mature to cause symptoms of the illness. People engaged in planting rice crops or bathing in water containing snails and parasites are especially at risk. The disease affects millions of people and control is by means of education, attempts to eradicate the snail hosts and drug treatment for those affected.

sciatica

Description: pain in the sciatic nerve, which is felt in the back of the thigh, leg and foot.

Persons most commonly affected: adults of both sexes aged under 60.

Organ or part of body involved: sciatic nerve, affecting leg and foot.

Symptoms and indications: the symptoms may develop rapidly, due to an awkward, strained or twisting movement, such as lifting a heavy object. Or, they may begin more gradually, due to an underlying condition causing pressure on the sciatic nerve. Symptoms include stiffness and pain in the back, leg and foot, which can be severe. A person with symptoms of sciatica should seek medical advice.

Treatment: may be in the form of bed rest and painkilling drugs until the symptoms improve. Persistent pain and weakness may require admittance to hospital for corrective surgery depending upon the underlying cause of the condition.

Causes and risk factors: the cause may be inadvertent stressing of the back, due to an awkward movement. However, the commonest cause of sciatica is a PROLAPSED INTERVERTEBRAL DISC pressing on the nerve root, but it may also be due to ANKYLOSING SPONDYLITIS or some other conditions e.g. spinal tumour.

scleritis

Description: deep inflammation of the sclera, the outer white fibrous layer of the eyeball.

Persons most commonly affected: all age groups and both sexes but more common in adults.

Organ or part of body involved: one or both eyes.

Symptoms and indications: pain in the eye, which can be extremely severe, with purple discolouration of parts of the sclera. A person with symptoms of scleritis should seek immediate medical advice.

Treatment: is usually in the form of a corticosteroid drug, such as prednisone, taken by mouth. However, if scleritis occurs in conjunction with rheumatic disorders or does not respond to corticosteroid treatment, immunosuppressive drugs such as azathioprine or cyclophosphamide may be prescribed by a specialist. In this case, the patient requires careful monitoring, due to the potent effects of these drugs.

Causes and risk factors: the cause is not known but scleritis is sometimes associated with rheumatic conditions such as rheumatoid arthritis. It may also occur in connection with CROHN's DISEASE. There is a risk of perforation of the eyeball and loss of the eye. If perforation occurs, admittance to hospital for surgery to preserve the eye is necessary. Even if the eye is saved, there is likely to be some loss of vision.

scleroderma or progressive systemic sclerosis or PSS

Description: a condition in which connective tissue gradually and progressively hardens and contracts. The tissue affected may be the skin, heart, kidney, lung, etc., and the condition may be localized or it may spread throughout the body, eventually becoming fatal. If the skin is affected it becomes thickened and rough with patchy pigmentation. There may be stiffening of joints and wasting of muscles.

Persons most commonly affected: adults of both sexes but four times more common in women.

Organ or part of body involved: skin (e.g. of fingers and face), oesophagus, joints, gastrointestinal tract, body organs, particularly heart, lungs and kidneys, blood vessels.

Symptoms and indications: there are a wide range of symptoms depending upon the nature and extent of the disease. There may be RAYNAUD's PHENOMENON, which is often an early indication of the disease. Other symptoms include thickening, stiffening, pigmentation and shiny skin, ulcers on the fingers, swallowing difficulty due to effects on the oesophagus, with symptoms of heartburn and indigestion. There may be stiffening and contraction of joints, especially the fingers, wrists, elbows and knees. There may be malaise and loss of weight. If fibrosis of organs occurs, particularly of the lungs, heart or kidneys, a range of serious symptoms may occur, including pulmonary and renal HYPERTENSION, heart and kidney failure. Eventually, most patients have some degree of organ involvement but many years may elapse before symptoms occur as the disease tends to progress in a slow and unpredictable fashion. A person with any symptoms of scleroderma should seek immediate medical advice.

Treatment: the disease is not considered to be curable but a wide range of drugs are available to control and limit symptoms. These include corticosteroids, penicillamine and nifedipine, preparations to relieve digestive symptoms, analgesics, skin lubricants and drugs to improve heart, lung and kidney function. The person should keep warm and other helpful measures include eating frequent small meals and raising the end of the bed (to prevent reflux of stomach acid).

Causes and risk factors: the cause is not known but it may be an autoimmune disease. (This is one in which the immune system, for some reason, fails to recognize the difference between 'self' and 'non-self' and produces antibodies that attack its own tissues.) Serious, life-threatening symptoms can occur but other patients are less severely affected, hence the outcome is difficult to predict.

senile macular degeneration

Description: age-related loss of vision due to changes in the retina of the eyes.

Persons most commonly affected: elderly persons aged 65 years and over of both sexes. It is more common in White races of people.

Organ or part of body involved: one or both eyes.

Symptoms and indications: there is a rapid or more slowly worsening loss of sharpness and accuracy of vision in the centre of the visual field. Peripheral and colour vision remain and large objects can be seen but detailed central vision is lost. A person who experiences these symptoms should seek medical advice.

Treatment: there is little effective treatment for this condition. The aim is to preserve and enhance the vision that remains with the use of glasses, etc. Laser treatment may help some patients.

Causes and risk factors: the cause is not known but hereditary factors may be involved. There is, at present, no way of preventing the development of this condition.

shingles or herpes zoster

Description: an infection produced by the virus that causes CHICKEN POX in children. The infection affects the central nervous system (dorsal root ganglia), running along the course of a nerve, producing severe pain and small yellowish blisters on the skin.

Persons most commonly affected: adults of all age groups and both sexes, especially those over 50 years.

Organ or part of body involved: sensory nerve of the skin. It affects the course of a nerve on one side only.

Symptoms and indications: early symptoms include chills, headache, slight fever and a general feeling of malaise. Blisters then appear on the skin following the route of a nerve, often in a semicircle around one side of the chest, side and back. There is pain, which may be very severe. The blisters form scabs that drop off and heal in about two weeks but pain may persist for some time (post-herpetic neuralgia). A person with symptoms of shingles should seek medical advice.

Treatment: there is no specific treatment but pain-relieving drugs, along with tranquillizers when the pain is very severe, may be prescribed. Corticosteroids have been used in some cases and antiviral drugs, such as acyclovir, may be prescribed for certain patients, particularly those with a suppressed immune system. Warm compresses and heat may be helpful for pain. Most people make a full recovery and have immunity from future attacks.

Causes and risk factors: the cause of shingles is the *Varicella-zoster* virus, which is also responsible for chicken pox in children. It is thought that the virus may be dormant in the body until some factor causes it to flare up as shingles. Most adults affected by shingles have had chicken pox in their childhood years. Those most at risk of developing shingles are people who are generally somewhat ill or 'run-down', those under stress or who have received treatment with immunosuppressive drugs. People with HODGKIN'S DISEASE are also at greater risk of developing this illness.

shock

Description: acute, circulatory failure due to blood pressure in the arteries falling so low that blood is no longer supplied to all parts of the body. Hence the normal functions of the body can no longer take place and there is a risk of death.

Persons most commonly affected: all age groups and both sexes.

Organ or part of body involved: blood circulatory system and heart.

Symptoms and indications: shock may develop as a result of injury or illness. The signs are a cold, clammy skin, pallor, cyanosis (blue-coloured skin due to a lack of oxygen in the blood), weak, rapid pulse, irregular breathing and dilated pupils. The person may feel anxious or suffer from confusion or lethargy and there is a lack of urination. Blood pressure falls to a low level and may not be detectable by normal methods. A person in shock requires immediate, emergency medical attention.

Treatment: depends upon the underlying cause of

the shock. If due to bleeding or loss of fluid, this must be halted and the person is likely to require blood transfusion and fluids given intravenously. If it is due to severe infection, large doses of antibiotics are likely to be needed. The person may be given drugs to raise blood pressure. General measures include keeping the person warm and calm and lying down with the legs raised. The patient should be accompanied at all times and emergency artificial respiration may be needed if breathing stops.

Causes and risk factors: there are numerous causes of shock, including a reduction in blood volume due to internal or external bleeding, and loss of fluid from burns or illnesses that cause dehydration and fluid/salt imbalance. Also, reduced heart activity as in CORONARY THROMBOSIS, PULMONARY EMBOLISM and heart rhythm disorders, blood poisoning and ANAPHYLACTIC SHOCK. Shock is a serious, life-threatening condition and the outcome depends upon the severity of the cause and response to treatment.

sickle-cell anaemia

Description: a type of inherited haemolytic anaemia that is genetically determined and that affects people of African ancestry. It is caused by a recessive gene, so people can be carriers of the sickle-cell trait without themselves showing any sign of illness. The anaemia occurs in a child who inherits the gene from both parents. The red blood cells have a characteristic distorted sickle shape and there are periods of crisis when the anaemia is especially severe.

Persons most commonly affected: present at birth in babies of both sexes, with symptoms usually becoming apparent by the age of six months. The illness is present for life.

Organ or part of body involved: bone marrow, blood, spleen, liver, thymus gland, lymph glands.

Symptoms and indications: the child fails to thrive, has frequent infections, and is anaemic, with symptoms of pallor, fatigue, breathlessness and JAUNDICE. There are episodes of joint and bone pain and fever. In children, pains in the feet and hands are characteristic. The child fails to grow properly and there may be chest and abdominal pain and vomiting. Skin ulcers may occur particularly on the ankles and there are nerve disorders and impairment of lungs, heart and kidneys. The bones are distorted and the spleen and heart become enlarged. A child with symptoms of sickle-cell disease requires ongoing medical help.

Treatment: is aimed at the relief of symptoms as there is no cure for the condition. Blood transfusions may be necessary for severe bouts of anaemia and drugs used include painkillers and courses of antibiotics to treat infections. Any infection should be treated promptly and antibiotics and immunization given to prevent infection e.g. against PNEUMONIA.

Causes and risk factors: the cause of the disease is a recessive gene, resulting in an abnormal type of haemoglobin (the blood pigment in red blood cells that binds to oxygen and carries it to all parts of the body). The abnormal haemoglobin causes distortion of the red blood cells, resulting in anaemia and the other symptoms described above. Improved supportive and antibiotic treatment has improved the outlook for sufferers of this disease. However, the illness shortens life and victims are at greater risk of a STROKE and other complications. People with a family history of sickle-cell disease are advised to seek genetic counselling before having children. Many people are carriers of the defective gene and because this confers increased resistance to MALARIA, the gene persists at a high level.

silicosis or 'potter's asthma'

Description: a type of PNEUMOCONIOSIS caused by the inhalation of silica (quartz) as particles of dust. The silica causes fibrosis of lung tissue and a greatly increased risk of contracting tuberculosis.

Persons most commonly affected: adults of either sex could be affected. In practice, this is an occupational disease of men aged over 40 years who have been long-term workers in certain industries and exposed to silica dust over a prolonged period (20 to 30 years). These industries include sandstone and granite cutting, sand-blasting, tin and anthracite mining, metal grinding and pottery manufacture.

Organ or part of body involved: lungs.

Symptoms and indications: symptoms include increasing breathlessness and coughing, chest pains, hoarseness, fatigue and malaise. There is likely to be a loss of appetite and disturbance of sleep. A person with these symptoms should seek medical advice.

Treatment: is aimed at the relief of symptoms and includes the use of drugs such as bronchodilators (inhalers), antibiotics and analgesics.

Causes and risk factors: the cause is inhaled particles of silica, which lodge in the alveoli (minute air sacs) of the lungs and cause the formation of fibrous tissue, resulting in loss of lung elasticity and function. People with silicosis are three times more likely to develop TUBERCULOSIS and are at risk of PULMONARY HYPERTENSION, which may prove fatal. Effective measures can now be taken in most industries to suppress dust. Workers can also wear protective hoods with breathing equipment and should be monitored by means of regular health checks and chest X-rays.

sinusitis

Description: inflammation of a sinus (one of a number of air cavities in the bones of the face and skull). It usually refers to the sinuses in the face that link with the nose. Hence, the cause of the inflammation is often due to a spread of infection from the nose.

Persons most commonly affected: all age groups and both sexes.

Organ or part of body involved: sinuses.

Symptoms and indications: there is usually a preceding upper respiratory tract infection. Symptoms include headache, blocked nose with a greenish infected discharge, a feeling of heaviness and pain inside the head and face and, possibly, disturbance of sleep. Depending upon the location of the affected sinus, there may be eye pain and inflammation. A person with symptoms of sinusitis should seek medical advice.

Treatment: is by means of antibiotics and also decongestants, usually in the form of nasal drops. Painkillers may be taken to relieve headache and pain. Rarely, if the problem is persistent and severe, admittance to hospital for surgery to drain the affected sinus may be necessary. The condition usually improves but may recur.

Causes and risk factors: the cause is usually an upper respiratory tract infection such as a cold, which spreads to the sinus.

sinus node disease or sinoatrial node disease

Description: any disorder of the sinus node or sinoatrial node, the natural pacemaker of the heart. This consists of specialized muscle cells in the right atrium (upper smaller chamber) of the heart. These cells generate electrical impulses, contract and initiate contractions in the muscles of the heart and hence are responsible for the heartbeat. Some disorders may be inherited and others may be acquired.

Persons most commonly affected: all age groups and both sexes.

Organ or part of body involved: heart.

Symptoms and indications: depending upon the type of disorder, there may be either a speeding up or a slowing down of heartbeat rhythm. This may not be perceived by the patient or may be felt as palpitations. The person may experience anxiety, fainting or dizziness. Any person who is aware of heartbeat irregularity should seek medical advice.

Treatment: usually, the person is admitted to hospital for monitoring of the heartbeat (Holter 24-hour ECG monitoring). Treatment methods include the use of a number of different drugs and surgery to install an artificial heart pacemaker.

Causes and risk factors: causes may be congenital or due to disease or disorder of the node. The condition can often be corrected but the outlook may depend upon the extent and nature of any underlying disease.

skin cancer or squamous cell carcinoma

Description: a growth of malignant cells in the outer epithelial layer of the skin.

Persons most commonly affected: middle-aged and older adults of both sexes.

Organ or part of body involved: skin, especially a part that has been exposed to the sun.

Symptoms and indications: a small, hardened, red, raised lump develops on the skin, which is neither itchy nor painful but has a crusty, scaling surface. Eventually it ulcerates and spreads to affect the surrounding tissues of the skin. The appearance of the lump can vary considerably, and it may also occur on a part of the skin that has not been exposed to the sun. A person with symptoms of skin cancer should seek immediate medical advice.

Treatment: a biopsy is first performed to confirm the diagnosis. Treatment in hospital is usually by means of surgical removal, curettage or scraping and electrodesiccation or, less commonly, the use of X-ray radiation. This type of skin cancer can normally be successfully, treated especially if caught early.

Causes and risk factors: the cause appears to be an overexposure of the skin to sunlight over many years. There is a possibility that the cancer will spread to other areas if left untreated but the risk is generally considered to be fairly low.

sleeping sickness (African trypanosomiasis) and Chagas' disease (South American trypanosomiasis)

Description: a parasitic disease found in tropical Africa, which is spread through the bite of tsetse flies. Chagas' disease is a South American form, which is spread through the bite of bugs called assassin bugs. The organisms responsible are minute parasitic protozoans called trypanosomes.

Persons most commonly affected: all age groups and both sexes.

Organ or part of body involved: small blood vessels, lymph vessels and glands, brain.

Symptoms and indications: a few days after the bite of an infected tsetse fly, the person develops a fever and reddish skin rash. The fever gradually becomes more severe but there are periods when it subsides and the person is somewhat better. Gradually, the person becomes weakened, and there is ANAEMIA, fluid retention and enlargement of lymph glands, which are swollen and painful. Eventually, the brain is involved, and the person becomes lethargic and apathetic, with an increased tendency to sleep, and suffers headaches and, possibly, convulsions. Eventually, these symptoms can lead to coma and death. In Chagas' disease, inflammation of heart muscle (myocarditis) often occurs and may cause death. The early symptoms may occur for years before the brain becomes affected. Any person who develops symptoms of sleeping sickness should seek medical advice. (*See causes and risk factors.*)

Treatment: is by means of various drugs including eflornithine and suramin. In the later stages of the disease, when the brain is affected, arsenic-containing drugs such as melarsoprol is used but great care is necessary due to the toxicity of the compounds. Preventative measures are the key to the control of sleeping sickness. These include measures to eliminate the habitat of the tsetse flies, insecticides to combat the flies or bugs, avoidance of high-risk areas and wearing protective clothing. Drug treatment for Chagas' disease is not very effective and the outlook is often poor, although some forms of the disease are more severe than others. The African forms of the disease also vary in their severity and drugs are more effective in the early stages.

Causes and risk factors: the cause of the symptoms is the multiplication of the parasites in blood vessels and lymph glands. Eventually, the parasites reach the brain, producing the severe symptoms of sleeping sickness. Anyone travelling to an area where sleeping sickness is known to occur should seek advice on how to avoid the possibility of a bite, and take sensible precautions. Visitors are generally at a low risk of acquiring sleeping sickness.

small intestine tumours

Description: any abnormal growth of cells in a part of the small intestine. The great majority of these growths are benign.

Persons most commonly affected: adults of both sexes.

Organ or part of body involved: small intestine.

Symptoms and indications: there may be few or no symptoms but those that occur include bleeding, with the occurrence of black stools, fatigue, loss of weight and paleness. There may be partial or complete obstruction of the bowel, with symptoms of pains, vomiting and fever. A person with symptoms of a tumour in the small intestine should seek immediate medical advice.

Treatment: depends upon the site and nature of the tumour but usually involves admittance to hospital for destruction of the tumour by heat, electric current, laser beam or surgical removal, or resection of a portion of the small intestine. Treatment of benign tumours is usually successful but malignant ones can spread to other organs.

Causes and risk factors: the cause of these tumours is unknown but the risk of developing them increases with certain diseases e.g. CROHN'S DISEASE.

spinal cord tumour

Description: an abnormal growth of cells that compresses the spinal cord or the nerve roots that arise from it. The tumour may be malignant or nonmalignant. If malignant, it may be either primary (rare) or, quite commonly, be a secondary growth arising from a malignancy elsewhere in the body e.g. cancer of the breast or lung.

Persons most commonly affected: adults of all age groups and both sexes but can occur in children.

Organ or part of body involved: part of the spinal cord and associated nerves.

Symptoms and indications: symptoms include pain in the back, numbness, weakness and wasting of the muscles supplied by nerves affected by the tumour. There may be a loss of sensation in areas of the body below the level of the tumour. The nerve supply to the sphincter muscles that control the bowel and bladder may be affected and there may be incontinence. The symptoms vary considerably in their severity, depending upon the site and nature of the tumour. A person with symptoms of a spinal cord tumour should seek medical advice.

Treatment: depends upon the site and nature of the tumour. It may involve admittance to hospital for surgery to remove the tumour and/or bone to relieve pressure on the spinal cord. Drugs that may be prescribed include pain relief and corticosteroids to reduce swelling.

Causes and risk factors: the cause of primary

tumours is unknown but secondary malignant growths arise as a result of a number of different types of cancer.

spondylosis

Description: degeneration of the intervertebral discs (fibrous discs of cartilage that connect adjacent vertebrae) and joints of the spine. It is characterized by pain in the neck and lumbar region, where the movement may become restricted.

Persons most commonly affected: middle-aged and older adults of both sexes.

Organ or part of body involved: intervertebral discs and joints of the spine.

Symptoms and indications: pain in the neck, lower back, leg and, possibly, the arm. There may be muscle weakness and difficulty in movement if the spinal cord becomes compressed. A person with symptoms of spondylosis should seek medical advice.

Treatment: is by means of physiotherapy, including the wearing of a neck collar, support belt in the lumbar region of the spine and traction. Also, pain-relieving drugs, muscle relaxants and anti-inflammatory preparations may be prescribed. Occasionally, admittance to hospital for surgery to relieve pressure on nerves may be needed.

Causes and risk factors: there is a degeneration of the discs along with the formation of osteophytes (bony projections), so that the space occupied by the discs is reduced. There appears to be a tendency for these changes to occur due to the process of ageing. The symptoms can be relieved, although the degenerative processes cannot be halted.

sporotrichosis

Description: a fungal infection of the skin and lymph nodes, characterized by the presence of abscesses and ulcers.

Persons most commonly affected: adults of both sexes, especially those working with plants and soil.

Organ or part of body involved: skin, superficial lymph channels and nodes. Rarely, it affects the lungs and some deeper tissues, such as the synovial membranes that line the joints.

Symptoms and indications: a small nodule appears under the skin, which can be moved and is not painful. This gradually increases in size and finally becomes pink and ulcerates. After a period of days or weeks, other nodules appear under the skin, following the course of a lymph channel,

and these usually appear on the hand or arm. Rarely, if the fungus is inhaled, symptoms of PNEUMONIA may result. If the fungus spreads to other tissues within the body, particularly the bones, joints and their membranes and rarely, other organs, more serious life-threatening symptoms can occur. A person with symptoms of sporotrichosis should seek medical advice.

Treatment: is by means of saturated potassium iodide solution that is usually taken diluted in drinks. Some persons may experience an allergic reaction (iodism) with skin rashes, respiratory symptoms (e.g. BRONCHITIS and LARYNGITIS) or CONJUNCTIVITIS. For a person with the rare systemic form of the infection, admittance to hospital for treatment with antifungal drugs such as amphotericin B, given intravenously as needed.

Causes and risk factors: the cause is a fungus named *Sporothrix schenckii*, which is found especially associated with sphagnum moss, mulches, barberry bushes and rose bushes. Those most at risk are gardeners and horticultural and farm workers.

sprue or psilosis

Description: this is essentially a composite deficiency disease due to poor absorption of food substances. Primarily, it is a metabolic disorder in which the person is unable to absorb fats, carbohydrates, minerals and vitamins. It was once considered to be a disease of tropical climates (tropical sprue) but versions of it (nontropical sprue and COELIAC DISEASE) have been recognized in temperate countries.

Persons most commonly affected: all age groups and both sexes. Tropical sprue is more common in adults, especially women, and is usually seen in Europeans after a prolonged period of residence in a tropical country.

Organ or part of body involved: gastrointestinal tract, blood, tongue—whole body symptoms.

Symptoms and indications: symptoms include a loss of appetite and weight, diarrhoea and the production of frothy, pale, fatty stools, red, inflamed sore tongue, swallowing difficulty and the development of severe ANAEMIA. A person with symptoms of sprue should seek medical advice.

Treatment: for tropical sprue, consists of bed rest and a high-protein diet, as the person is able to tolerate protein more readily than other food substances. Vitamin supplements, especially vitamin B complex and A and D, are usually required, along with folic acid, to combat anaemia. Nontropical sprue is treated by eating a strict gluten-free diet and also with vitamin, mineral and folic acid supplements, if these are needed.

Causes and risk factors: the cause of these diseases is an inability to absorb certain food substances from the small intestine. In the case of COELIAC DISEASE and nontropical sprue, there is an intolerance to gluten, a wheat protein, which causes the symptoms. In adults, symptoms may be triggered by some other illness or surgery. Tropical sprue is an acquired disease resulting in an inability to absorb many different food substances. It is thought that it may be triggered by gastrointestinal infection, food toxins, vitamin or mineral deficiency or infestation by parasites. There is a risk of death for those severely affected by these diseases, especially if the condition is not recognized early enough. Some patients fail to respond to treatment or develop life-threatening complications.

Still's disease or juvenile rheumatoid arthritis

Description: a chronic ARTHRITIS affecting children, which may involve several joints in a symmetric fashion.

Persons most commonly affected: children of both sexes under the age of 16 years. Usual age is between two and five years.

Organ or part of body involved: joints and sometimes the blood, glands, eyes, membranes.

Symptoms and indications: symptoms may occur gradually or develop rapidly. They include pain and inflammation in both small and large joints. Often this begins in the fingers and then spreads to other joints in a characteristic symmetrical fashion, usually the wrists, elbows, knees and ankles. Sometimes only one joint is involved. Accompanying the arthritis there may be fever, a characteristic skin rash, eye inflammation, blood changes (an increase in the number of white blood cells), and an enlargement of the spleen and other glands. If the spine is involved there may be a stiff neck and there is muscle wastage, retardation of growth and a receded chin. Some children show the symptoms of rash and fever, etc., before any arthritis develops. A child with symptoms of Still's disease should be seen by a doctor.

Treatment: includes bed rest and the use of certain drugs such as aspirin and, possibly, other non-steroidal anti-inflammatory agents. Gold salts may also be prescribed and, in general, treatment methods are the same as for adults. The outlook in children is usually much better than in adults, and three quarters of those affected experience a total remission of symptoms. However, there is a tendency for relapses to occur and the condition may persist for some years.

Causes and risk factors: the cause is not known but some children go on to develop ANKYLOSING SPONDYLITIS.

stomach cancer

Description: a proliferation of malignant cells in the stomach.

Persons most commonly affected: adults of both sexes from age 40 onwards but more common in men. In general, more common in people with blood group A.

Organ or part of body involved: stomach.

Symptoms and indications: early symptoms are those of indigestion, with discomfort or pain, nausea and vomiting, wind and a feeling of fullness. In the later stages there is poor appetite, loss of weight, pain in the upper part of the abdomen, passage of black stools due to the presence of blood, and vomiting of blood. Sometimes a hard mass can be felt in the upper part of the abdomen. A person with symptoms of stomach cancer should seek medical advice.

Treatment: is by means of surgery to remove the tumour whenever this is possible and, possibly, chemotherapy and radiotherapy. The outlook varies considerably but treatment can relieve symptoms.

Causes and risk factors: the cause is not known but there is a greater risk with increasing age, excess consumption of alcohol, a family history of the disease and blood group A. In the later stages of gastric cancer there may be secondary growths in other organs with enlargement of the liver, retention of fluid (ascites), JAUNDICE, nodules in the skin and bone fractures.

stomach ulcer or gastric ulcer or peptic ulcer

Description: a broken inflamed portion of the lining or mucosal membrane of the stomach. The ulcer is usually small (about 15 to 25mm across) and is round or oval in shape. In most cases, the ulcer is situated near the point where the stomach opens into the duodenum (the first part of the small intestine) on the lower posterior wall. One or more ulcers may be present.

Persons most commonly affected: adults of both sexes in middle or older age, especially men.

Organ or part of body involved: stomach.

Symptoms and indications: symptoms may be quite vague or more definite and vary in their severity. They include pain felt either at the front or in the back, which may be more severe before a meal.

Also, there may be nausea and a feeling of bloatedness after meals. Sometimes, instead of pain there is discomfort felt as a feeling of emptiness or hunger or of an aching nature. A person with symptoms of gastric ulcer should seek medical advice.

Treatment: diagnostic techniques include endoscopy, analysis of gastric secretions and X-ray studies using barium. Treatment is by means of a number of different drugs including antacids, carbenoxolone and histamine H₂ receptor antagonists e.g. cimetidine, famotidine, rantidine and nizatidine. Most gastric ulcers respond fairly well to treatment, although there is a tendency for healing and relapse to occur. The person should eat a light diet and irritant foods or drinks should be avoided. These include spicy foods containing pepper, fatty foods, coffee and alcohol. The person should avoid smoking and stress. Complications can arise in the form of blockage of the stomach outlet (pylorus), due to the formation of scar tissue, perforation through to an adjacent space or organ (a medical emergency) and haemorrhage (indicated by the vomiting of blood and passing black, tarry faeces containing blood). In the event of these arising, admittance to hospital for surgery to remove the ulcer and a part of the stomach may prove to be necessary. A person with symptoms of a gastric ulcer should seek medical advice.

Causes and risk factors: the exact cause is not known but is believed to be linked with changes in the mucous-membrane lining of the stomach, mucus secretion, and acid and pepsin (an enzyme) production. Some drugs, particularly aspirin and other non-steroidal anti-inflammatory drugs and corticosteroids, encourage the formation of an ulcer. The risk of developing a stomach ulcer increases with age whereas a duodenal ulcer may occur in younger adults.

stroke or apoplexy

Description: the physical effects, involving some form of paralysis, that result from damage to the brain due to an interruption in its blood supply. The effect in the brain is secondary and the cause lies in the heart or blood vessels and may be a thrombosis, embolus or haemorrhage. The severity of a stroke varies greatly from a temporary weakness in a limb, or tingling, to paralysis, coma and death.

Persons most commonly affected: elderly adults of both sexes although younger people may occasionally be affected.

Organ or part of body involved: brain.

Symptoms and indications: symptoms vary according to the nature and severity of damage to the brain and may be gradual or sudden in their onset. They include loss of control over movement, numbness or tingling on one side of the body, loss of speech, mental confusion and disturbance of vision, headache, loss of consciousness, with noisy breathing. The unconscious person may appear flushed and have a slow pulse rate, and the pupils of the eyes are unequally contracted. A person with symptoms of a stroke requires emergency medical treatment in hospital.

Treatment: is in the form of intensive nursing aimed at maintaining the person in as stable a state as possible. Some drugs might be given depending upon the nature of the stroke and the patient's condition. These include drugs to lower blood pressure, anticoagulants or heparin and nimodipine. Physiotherapy and exercises of paralysed limbs, etc., are usually begun as soon as possible. A severe stroke often proves fatal. Patients who survive are likely to suffer physical and possibly mental disability and require a great deal of continuing help, support and encouragement.

Causes and risk factors: the cause of stroke is usually ATHEROSCLEROSIS, or hardening and narrowing of the arteries, which occurs with increasing age. This can result in a blockage of a small artery by a blood clot interrupting the blood flow to the brain (THROMBOSIS). Or, there may be an EMBOLISM in which a clot or plug is carried from the heart or an artery elsewhere, via the circulation to lodge in a vessel of the brain and cause blockage. Another cause of stroke is haemorrhage of a blood vessel within the brain, causing an escape of blood into the brain tissue. The blood vessels may already have become diseased and the leakage of blood may be due to rupture of an ANEURYSM. In a younger person who suffers a stroke, the cause is usually the rupture of an aneurysm (which has occurred due to some congenital weakness) leading to a SUBARACHNOID HAEMORRHAGE.

stye

Description: a bacterial infection and inflammation of the follicle (small sac) at the base of an eyelash, resulting in a painful, pus-filled abscess.

Persons most commonly affected: all age groups and both sexes.

Organ or part of body involved: eyelid of one eye.

Symptoms and indications: early symptoms are a red, shiny swelling on the edge of an eyelid, which is painful and tender. The 'head' of the stye usually develops around the base of the eyelash and more than one stye may develop. A person with symptoms of a stye should seek prompt medical treatment.

Treatment: is by means of hot compresses to encourage the stye to come to a head, removal of the eyelash so that pus can drain out and application of antibiotic eyedrops or ointment containing chloramphenicol. Care should be taken not to rub or touch the eye so as not to spread the infection. The infection usually clears up within about a week although there is a tendency for recurrence.

Causes and risk factors: the usual cause is a local infection with staphylococcus bacteria. Styes sometimes occur in people who are somewhat 'run-down' or with lowered resistance to infection. The person's general state of health may need attention.

sùbarachnoid haemorrhage

Description: bleeding into the subarachnoid space of the brain. (The subarachnoid space occurs between two of the membranes or meninges that cover the brain, the arachnoid and pia-mater membranes. The space usually contains cerebrospinal fluid.)

Persons most commonly affected: adults of both sexes between the ages of 25 and 50 but can affect people in any age group.

Organ or part of body involved: brain.

Symptoms and indications: symptoms include a sudden, very severe headache, nausea and vomiting, dizziness, fainting and coma. Sometimes the person may suffer fits and heartbeat and breathing rates are erratic. Within 24 hours, the person develops a stiff neck and certain other muscle and reflex responses (called Kernig's sign and Babinski's sign). During the first few days after the haemorrhage, the person continues to suffer from headache and confusion and has an elevated temperature. There may be paralysis on one side of the body (hemiplegia). A person with symptoms of a subarachnoid haemorrhage requires emergency medical treatment in hospital.

Treatment: following admittance to hospital, diagnostic tests and scans are carried out to determine the nature of the haemorrhage. Treatment is usually by means of surgery to stop the bleeding e.g. by clipping an ANEURYSM. The outlook is best in patients who are well enough to undergo surgery within the first 72 hours. A majority of patients survive a first subarachnoid haemorrhage but there is a risk of a second one occurring, especially within the first few weeks. Surgery reduces the risk of subsequent haemorrhage. Patients who recover may be left with residual brain damage. There may be some degree of paralysis or muscular weakness, difficulties with speech or mental confusion. Hence, recovery and rehabilitation are likely to take some time.

Causes and risk factors: the commonest cause of subarachnoid haemorrhage is accidental head injury. Other causes are rupture of an aneurysm, with ATHEROSCLEROSIS and high blood pressure being significant contributory factors. After a subarachnoid haemorrhage there is a risk of raised intracranial pressure and HYDROCEPHALUS.

subconjunctival haemorrhage

Description: bleeding under the conjunctiva (the lining of the eyelid and the white of the eye).

Persons most commonly affected: all ages and both sexes, but it is spontaneous usually only in the middle-aged or elderly.

Organ or part of body involved: conjunctiva.

Symptoms and indications: the white of the eye becomes partially or totally bright red.

Treatment: none. This condition disappears after a few days.

Causes and risk factors: it can result from inflammation or injury, but is usually spontaneous in the elderly, due to the blood vessels becoming fragile.

subdural haemorrhage and haematoma (acute and chronic)

Description: bleeding or haemorrhage that occurs into the space between the outer (dura mater) and middle (arachnoid mater) membranes that surround the brain, causing a collection or clot of blood, a haematoma. An acute subdural haematoma is a common occurrence following a serious head injury and occurs soon after the event. A chronic subdural haematoma may occur some weeks after a seemingly trivial head injury. The following relates to the chronic condition.

Persons most commonly affected: adults of both sexes aged over 50 years but can occur at any age.

Organ or part of body involved: brain.

Symptoms and indications: symptoms may not arise until some weeks after a relatively minor head injury. They include worsening headaches that occur each day, periods of drowsiness and confusion, muscular weakness on one side of the body. In babies, there may be an enlargement of the head if the haematoma is large. A person with symptoms of a subdural haematoma requires immediate emergency medical treatment.

Treatment: involves admittance to hospital where diagnostic tests and scans will first be carried out. Surgery is then needed to remove the clot and relieve the compression of the brain that is responsible for the symptoms. Once pressure is relieved, the brain may slowly recover or there may be some permanent damage. The outlook is best in those patients who receive prompt surgical intervention.

Causes and risk factors: the cause is previous trauma to the head that results in internal bleeding, even though the injury may appear to have been minor. The risk is greatest in older people or in those who abuse alcohol. There is a risk of death or permanent disability but other patients make a good recovery.

Sydenham's chorea (St Vitus' dance)

Description: a childhood disorder of the nervous system, which is characterized by involuntary, jerky, purposeless movements and which is associated with acute rheumatism. The disorder is self-limiting and symptoms disappear over a period of time leaving no residual ill effects. However, about one third of affected children develop rheumatism elsewhere in the body and this usually involves the heart.

Persons most commonly affected: children aged over five years, especially girls.

Organ or part of body involved: brain, central nervous system, muscles.

Symptoms and indications: the symptoms are jerky, involuntary movements that can involve any muscles but especially the face, shoulders and hips. The child contorts the face and intentional movements are poorly coordinated. The symptoms tend to start slightly and gradually increase, and usually last between three and eight months. Sometimes, the flailing movements of the limbs are so excessive that the child needs to be sedated. The movements do not occur when the child is asleep. The symptoms of chorea may not appear until up to six months after a rheumatic infection such as RHEUMATIC FEVER. About one-third of children also develop rheumatism, which commonly affects the heart and may cause problems in later life. If a child shows symptoms of chorea, medical advice should be sought.

Treatment: consists of rest and possibly giving mild sedatives if the uncontrolled movements are particularly violent. Reassurance for the child, family, school, etc, is especially important. The child should continue to lead a normal life as the symptoms subside over a period of time without any physical or intellectual impairment. If the child has rheumatic symptoms or if the heart is affected, the treatment is as for rheumatic fever.

Causes and risk factors: the cause is thought to be the same streptococcal bacteria responsible for rheumatic disorders but causing an autoimmune response involving the central nervous system. In temperate countries it is more common in the summer and early autumn months. This correlates with the peak incidence of rheumatic fever, in the spring and first part of the summer.

syphilis (**acquired** and **congenital**)

Description: acquired syphilis is a venereal disease caused by a bacterium that produces symptoms in three stages. If left untreated, the final stages may not appear for months or even years and the disease causes widespread damage throughout the body. Congenital syphilis is a much rarer form that is contracted by a developing foetus from the mother via the placenta. Symptoms begin to show a few weeks after birth.

Persons most commonly affected: congenital syphilis—newborn babies of both sexes; acquired form—persons of either sex who have had sexual contact with an infected person.

Organ or part of body involved: reproductive organs, central nervous system, skin and other organs.

Symptoms and indications: first, or primary stage,—bacteria enter the body through the mucous membranes of the genital organs, rectum or mouth. After a few days or weeks, a small ulcer develops at the site of infection. This may be inflamed, or painless and relatively insignificant, but is highly infectious, and is called the primary sore or chancre. Within a short time, the lymph nodes (at first those near the sore and then all over the body), enlarge and harden and this stage lasts for several weeks. The ulcer eventually heals and the swelling subsides. Secondary stage—secondary symptoms appear about two months after infection and include fever, pains, loss of appetite and a red rash that is usually noticed on the chest. The bacteria are found in enormous numbers in the spots of this rash and so this stage is also highly contagious. Third, or tertiary, stage (noninfectious)—the final stage may not appear until many months or years after infection, and symptoms are more likely to occur in untreated or inadequately treated people. In this stage numerous tumour-like masses, called gummas, form and may occur in the skin or within the muscles, bones, brain, spinal cord, heart, liver, stomach, etc. The serious damage that can be caused to tissues and organs may result in blindness, paralysis, tabes dorsalis (a disease of the nerves characterized by weakness of muscles, stabbing pains, unsteadiness in walking, incontinence, loss of vision) and mental disability. Also, there may be heart and artery disease and ANEURYSM. In congenital syphilis, the child is highly infectious and a few weeks after birth, develops second-stage symptoms of the disease.

Any person who suspects that he or she may have contracted syphilis should seek immediate medical advice.

Treatment: is preceded by diagnostic tests on blood serum or fluid from the sore. Treatment should begin as soon as possible after the infection has been acquired, and is necessary both for the person and his or her sexual partners. Courses of antibiotics are needed, mainly penicillin, unless the person is known to be allergic to this. The condition can usually be cured in a few weeks. The person should refrain from sexual intercourse until the infection has cleared, and should receive periodic check-ups for some time afterwards. Preventative measures include the use of condoms, and penicillin is the treatment for all stages of the disease.

Causes and risk factors: the cause of syphilis is the bacterium *Treponema pallidum*. Modern antibiotic treatment has greatly improved the outlook for people with syphilis but it remains a serious and life-threatening disease.

systemic lupus erythematosus (SLE)

Description: an inflammatory disease of connective tissues, believed to be an autoimmune disorder. It is generally a chronic disorder, characterized by active and quiescent periods that may last for years.

Persons most commonly affected: younger women aged between 20 and 50 years (90%), although can affect males and other age groups.

Organ or part of body involved: connective tissue—whole body is affected.

Symptoms and indications: symptoms vary considerably with some people being more severely affected than others. They may arise abruptly or more gradually and include malaise, fever, arthritic and joint pains and a rash, especially on the face, neck, chest or arms. The rash is of a particular 'butterfly' pattern and there may be a reddening and mottling of the skin on the fingers, palms and hands. Mouth ulcers can develop and there can be increased sensitivity to light. The spleen and other organs may become enlarged. The kidneys may be affected with protein in the urine and inflammation that can prove fatal. Other serious symptoms of PULMONARY HYPERTENSION, inflammation of the pericardium (the membrane surrounding the heart) and PLEURISY can occur. Also, changes in the blood, haemolytic ANAEMIA and mental disorders can occur. A person with symptoms of this disorder should seek medical advice.

Treatment: it may take some time and a series of tests for diagnosis of systemic lupus erythematosus to be made. Treatment very much depends upon the severity and the nature of the disorder and is aimed at relief of symptoms. Various drugs may be prescribed, including non-steroidal anti-inflammatory agents, aspirin, antimalarial preparations, corticosteroids and immunosuppressives. Infections that arise should be promptly treated with antibiotics. This disorder cannot be cured but effective relief of symptoms can be achieved and the outlook for sufferers is generally improving.

Causes and risk factors: systemic lupus erythematosus is believed to be an autoimmune disorder, i.e. one in which the body fails to recognize the difference between 'self' and 'non-self'. The immune system attacks its own tissues, in this case connective tissue throughout the body.

T

tapeworms

Description: symptoms of illness caused by infestation with parasitic tapeworms. Several species of tapeworm can affect man and some produce few symptoms whereas others may be responsible for serious illness.

Persons most commonly affected: all age groups and both sexes.

Organ or part of body involved: depends upon the type of tapeworm involved—gastrointestinal tract, muscles, brain, eyes, liver, lungs.

Symptoms and indications: (and route of infection) *Taenia saginata*—the beef tapeworm (many countries including Europe). People are infected by eating undercooked beef containing the larval stages of the parasite. The worm develops into an adult inside the intestine of the infected person. Many people experience few or no symptoms. Those that can occur include pains, hunger, weight loss, gastrointestinal upset and passing segments of the worm in the stools.

Taenia solium—the pork tapeworm (many countries including Europe). People are infected by eating undercooked pork containing the larval stages (cysts) of the parasite. The larvae of this tapeworm tend to migrate and form cysts in various body tissues. Cysts may form in organs such as the brain, causing serious symptoms resembling those of a BRAIN TUMOUR.

Echinococcus granulosus—dog tapeworm (sheep-rearing countries where dogs are used; Australia, New Zealand, South Africa, Middle East, Europe, USA). The disease produced is called hydatid disease. Human beings, often children, are infected by swallowing the eggs of the tapeworm, which are present in the faeces of dogs. An infected dog may pass the eggs to a person by licking or a child may pick up the eggs on the fingers while playing on ground that is contaminated. Inside the body, the parasite larvae are carried in the blood circulation and lodge in the liver, kidneys, lungs, brain or other organs. They form cysts, called hydatids, that gradually become larger and cause symptoms due to the pressure they exert. Symptoms vary according to the organ or tissue affected. There may be chest pain, cough and coughing up of blood if the lungs are affected, JAUNDICE and abdominal pain, if it is the liver, blindness and EPILEPSY if the brain. The cysts may rupture causing serious allergic responses including rash, fever or anaphylaxis.

Diphyllobothriasis—fish tapeworm (Europe, USA, Canada, Africa, Japan). People are infected by eating raw or undercooked fish. Symptoms are usually absent or mild but include gastrointestinal upset and, occasionally, severe ANAEMIA. Eggs can be seen in the stools.

Any person who has symptoms of tapeworm infestation should seek medical advice.

Treatment: in most cases is by means of drugs to kill and expel the parasite including niclosamide and praziquantel. For hydatid disease, treatment involves admittance to hospital for surgical removal of the cysts, if this is possible. Drugs, including mebendazole and albendazole, are also used in treatment, and relieve symptoms. Most tapeworm infestations can be successfully dealt with but others may cause lasting tissue and organ damage that can prove fatal. Preventative measures include vigilance when travelling abroad, in eating only meat or fish that has been verified as having been thoroughly cooked. Domestic animals and pets should be wormed regularly and strict standards of hygiene observed, especially to protect young children.

Causes and risk factors: the cause of symptoms are various types of tapeworm, as described above. Tapeworms pose a threat to human health in many countries of the world. (*See also* TOXOCARIASIS).

tendinitis

Description: inflammation of a tendon, which is a tough and inelastic white cord, composed of bundles of collagen fibres, that attaches a muscle to a bone. A tendon concentrates the pull of the muscle onto one point on the bone, and the length and thickness varies considerably. The fibres of a tendon pass into, and become continuous with, those of the bone it serves. Many tendons are enclosed in membrane (synovial membrane)—lined sheaths containing synovial fluid that reduces friction during movement.

Persons most commonly affected: young people and adults of both sexes.

Organ or part of body involved: tendons, joints. Tennis elbow is tendinitis of the tendon on the outer part of the elbow.

Symptoms and indications: pain and restriction of movement around a joint with heat and swelling. A person with symptoms of tendinitis should seek medical advice.

Treatment: consists of rest and, possibly, splinting of an affected joint, steroid injections and the taking of painkillers or non-steroidal anti-inflammatory drugs. The use of heat or ice packs may be helpful to relieve pain and inflammation. Preventative measures include avoiding stressing a tendon or joint, especially building up gradually when taking up a new sporting activity.

Causes and risk factors: the cause is often excessive or unaccustomed exercise, which places the tendon under stress. However, it may also result from an infection or as a complication of a rheumatic or connective tissue disorder. Care should be taken when engaged in sporting or other physical activities to avoid exposing a tendon or joint to unaccustomed or excessive stress.

testicular cancer

Description: a proliferation of malignant cells in a testicle. There are several different types of malignancy and some are more virulent than others.

Persons most commonly affected: adolescent youths and young men under the age of 30 years.

Organ or part of body involved: testicle.

Symptoms and indications: a firm mass or lump in the scrotum that gradually increases in size and is only rarely painful. Any person who finds such a lump should seek immediate medical advice.

Treatment: following diagnostic tests, treatment is by means of surgery to remove the affected testicle and, possibly, chemotherapy and radiotherapy. The outlook depends upon the type of malignancy and how soon it is detected and treated. Many forms of testicular cancer can be successfully treated, especially if detected early but this is the most common form of cancer in young men.

Causes and risk factors: the cause is unknown but young men with an undescended testicle (cryptorchidism) in infancy are at a greater risk of developing this malignancy. This appears to remain true, even when the testicle has been brought down by surgical operation at a young age. Preventative measures (as with breast cancer in women) involves self-examination of the testicles each month. If one testicle has to be removed, the remaining one is sufficient to maintain fertility and normal sexual function.

tetanus or lockjaw

Description: a very serious and sometimes fatal disease caused by bacteria that enter through a wound.

Persons most commonly affected: all age groups and both sexes.

Organ or part of body involved: motor nerves, spinal cord, muscles.

Symptoms and indications: symptoms usually appear about two or three weeks after the person has received a wound, often after this has healed. In the early stages, there is usually stiffening and rigidity of muscles near the site of the wound. Later, there is rigidity and spasm of muscles in other parts of the body, which cause extreme agony. Characteristically, the muscles of the face and jaw are affected. The person is unable to open the mouth and finds it very difficult to swallow. The spasms in the muscles of the face give a characteristic appearance, exposing the teeth, called risus sardonicus. The muscular seizures occur at the slightest stimulus and cause extreme agony. The muscles involved in breathing and respiration may be so severely affected that the person dies from ASPHYXIA and exhaustion. Frequently, there is accompanying high fever and profuse sweating. The person experiences great anxiety, as the symptoms are painful and frightening.

A person with symptoms of tetanus requires immediate emergency medical treatment. Also, a person who receives a wound, especially while outdoors, or who has a wound contaminated with soil or manure, and who is unsure about his or her state of immunity, should seek medical advice. A person who has a wound requiring medical attention is usually given tetanus antitoxin as a precaution unless it is certain that immunization is up to date.

Treatment: involves admittance to hospital and rest in bed in a quiet and darkened room. Tetanus antitoxin is given by means of injection, and muscle relaxants and sedatives may also be needed. Other antibiotics may be prescribed. The outcome depends upon the severity of the symptoms, the patient's age and state of immunity and how soon treatment begins. Tetanus can be successfully cured in most cases and the incidence of the disease and numbers of deaths have been greatly reduced by immunization. Preventative measures, including routine immunization of children, is by means of a course of three antitetanus injections with a booster every ten years.

Causes and risk factors: the cause is a bacterium with a characteristic shape called *Clostridium tetani*. It is found in soil, especially that which has been treated with manure, but also may occur in other circumstances. People engaged in any outdoor sporting activity, farming, gardening, forestry, etc., should take care to keep tetanus immunizations up to date.

thalassaemia or Cooley's anaemia

Description: an inherited form of severe ANAEMIA that affects people in Mediterranean, Middle Eastern and Far Eastern countries. There is an abnormality in the haemoglobin (the red blood pigment that carries oxygen) and it is especially common in Italy and Greece. Two forms of the disease occur, thalassaemia major, in which the defective gene is inherited from both parents, and which produces symptoms, and thalassaemia minor, in which the person has only one defective gene and is a carrier, but usually does not show any symptoms.

Persons most commonly affected: all age groups and both sexes.

Organ or part of body involved: blood.

Symptoms and indications: symptoms include malaise, fatigue, pallor, anaemia, blood in the urine, JAUNDICE, and there may be enlargement of the spleen. Ulcers may develop on the legs. A person with symptoms of thalassaemia should seek medical advice.

Treatment: is aimed at relief of symptoms as there is no known cure. This takes the form of blood transfusions when symptoms are particularly severe and also the giving of analgesic drugs for the relief of pain. The disorders shorten life expectancy.

Causes and risk factors: the cause is an inherited genetic abnormality affecting the haemoglobin. Persons with a family history of thalassaemia or who may be at risk should seek genetic counselling before having children.

threadworms or pinworms or seatworms also called enterobiasis or oxyuriasis

Description: a common intestinal infestation by parasitic nematode worms, which affects people, especially children, throughout the world.

Persons most commonly affected: young children of both sexes but any age group can be affected.

Organ or part of body involved: large intestine, skin around the anus.

Symptoms and indications: there may be no symptoms but when they do occur the commonest indication is itching around the anus, especially at night. The child may scratch extensively and cause the skin to become irritated and inflamed. In girls, the worms may enter the vulva causing irritation and a discharge. Occasionally, the child may experience abdominal pains and a loss of appetite. Rarely, it is possible that the worms are responsible for APPENDICITIS. A parent who is concerned that a child may have threadworms should seek medical advice.

Treatment: is by means of drugs such as mebendazole and pyrantel pamoate. The whole family should be treated at the same time but, since the eggs of the worm can survive for about three weeks in the home environment, re-infestation is common.

Causes and risk factors: the cause is tiny nematode worms, only a few millimetres long. Female worms in an infested person migrate to the rectum and lay their eggs in the skin around the anus. If the child scratches, the eggs are transferred to the fingers and deposited on toys, etc., or find their way onto clothing, bedding, the toilet seat or other objects. The minute eggs are easily transferred to a new host and swallowed, and mature into adult worms in the large intestine. Eggs may float in the air and be inhaled and swallowed, and they remain viable for about three weeks outside the body of a host. It is very rare for these worms to cause harm and it is probable that many people have the infestation without realizing that this is the case.

It is thought that the body somehow rids itself of the worms after a period of time, even without treatment, or they die out for reasons that are not known. It is advisable to maintain a high standard of hygiene, to encourage children to wash their hands and not to allow children to put their fingers in their mouth.

thrombocytopaenia

Description: a condition in which the quantity of platelets (disc-shaped cells involved in blood clotting) in the blood is reduced. Due to this, there is an increased tendency for bruising and bleeding to occur as the blood is less likely to clot.

Thrombocytopaenia may be a symptom of an underlying disease or arise from a different cause.

Persons most commonly affected: all age groups and both sexes.

Organ or part of body involved: blood.

Symptoms and indications: irrespective of the cause, thrombocytopaenia generally produces a pattern of unexplained bleeding. There tends to be the appearance of petechiae, which are minute reddish or purple spots that appear like a rash. These are due to minute haemorrhages within the skin and often appear on the legs below knee level. Also, bleeding in the mouth, nosebleeds, vaginal bleeding and heavy bleeding following surgery may occur. Unexpected areas of bruising occur following very slight trauma, and gastrointestinal and urinary tract bleeding indicated by black stools and blood in the urine. The spleen may become enlarged if the bleeding is prolonged, symptoms of ANAEMIA may occur, such as pallor and fatigue. A person with symptoms of thrombocytopaenia should seek medical advice.

Treatment: depends upon the primary condition or disorder (*see causes and risk factors*), which must first be established. This is likely to require admittance to hospital for various diagnostic tests and the person may need transfusions of blood platelets given intravenously. The outcome depends upon the underlying cause but can be successfully treated in many cases.

Causes and risk factors: thrombocytopaenia may arise as a result of a failure in the production of platelets or from disorders that cause their destruction or increase their utilization or dilution in the blood. Causes include SYSTEMIC LUPUS ERYTHEMATOSUS, CIRRHOSIS OF THE LIVER and enlarged spleen, excess consumption of alcohol, certain drugs, especially heparin but also antidiabetic drugs taken by mouth, quinidine, rifampicin, gold salts and some others. Also, surgery and blood transfusions, BLOOD POISONING, LEUKAEMIA, some forms of ANAEMIA, malignancy, some obstetric conditions and HIV infection.

thromboembolism

Description: the situation in which a blood clot (thrombus) forms in one part of the circulation, usually a vein in the leg (phlebothrombosis), and a portion breaks off and becomes lodged elsewhere, causing a total blockage (EMBOLISM). The embolism often involves the pulmonary artery (to the lung) or one of its branches, and this is known as a PULMONARY EMBOLISM.

Persons most commonly affected: adults of all age groups and both sexes.

Organ or part of body involved: arteries anywhere in the body.

Symptoms and indications: the symptoms depend upon the site of the embolism. In a limb or extremity, symptoms include numbness and tingling, pain and weakness and a weak pulse. In the brain there are symptoms of STROKE that vary in severity. In the kidneys, there are symptoms of KIDNEY FAILURE and high blood pressure. If the gastrointestinal tract is involved, there is severe pain, nausea and vomiting, and SHOCK may occur. (*See also* PULMONARY EMBOLISM.) A person with the symptoms of thromboembolism requires emergency medical treatment.

Treatment: involves admittance to hospital and, possibly, surgery to remove the clot or bypass a damaged artery. Drugs that may be prescribed include anticoagulants, aspirin and vasodilators to widen blood vessels. Many patients are prescribed anticoagulant drugs before and after planned surgery to lessen the risk of thromboembolism. The condition may prove fatal, depending upon the part of the body that is affected but in other cases it can be cured.

Causes and risk factors: the cause is a blood clot or part of a blood clot that forms in a vein and travels in the circulation to lodge in an artery. The risk increases with conditions such as HYPERTENSION (high blood pressure), ATHEROSCLEROSIS, increased age, DIABETES MELLITUS, surgery, injury to blood vessels, pregnancy, smoking, disorders of the circulatory system and a previous history of thromboembolism.

thrombophlebitis (superficial)

Description: inflammation of the wall of a vein, along with clot formation in the affected section of the vessel. It is very rare for these clots to break away and travel in the circulation to cause THROMBOEMBOLISM. *Compare* THROMBOSIS.

Persons most commonly affected: adults of both sexes, especially women.

Organ or part of body involved: superficial veins.

Symptoms and indications: the affected vein becomes hard and cord-like with reddening heat and tenderness or localized pain. The person may become feverish. A person with symptoms of thrombophlebitis should seek medical advice.

Treatment: may involve surgical removal of the clot and the wearing of a firm elastic stocking. The person should move the legs as much as possible, especially when resting, and avoid crossing the legs or ankles. It may be helpful to rest with the legs raised. Non-steroidal anti-inflammatory drugs may be prescribed. Recovery is usually complete in about two weeks.

Causes and risk factors: causes include injury or trauma to the vein in which the lining membrane is damaged, an increased tendency for the blood to clot and a decrease in the rate of blood flow. The risk increases with VARICOSE VEINS, smoking and the use of oral contraceptives. A person who develops superficial thrombophlebitis should refrain from smoking and should not use contraceptive pills.

thrombosis (deep vein)

Description: the process of clotting within a vein so that the vessel becomes partially or completely blocked by the clot or thrombus. There is a risk of the clot breaking away and travelling to the lung to cause a PULMONARY EMBOLISM.

Persons most commonly affected: adults of both sexes.

Organ or part of body involved: veins, especially the deep veins of the calves (lower legs).

Symptoms and indications: symptoms include pain, swelling, tenderness, warmth, redness and the superficial veins may become enlarged and prominent. However, this condition can occur with few or no symptoms, as the lower legs are served by three main veins and thrombosis in one does not affect the functioning of the others. The person usually experiences pain on walking or standing still, which disappears when resting with the leg raised. A person with symptoms of deep vein thrombosis requires immediate medical treatment.

Treatment: the person usually needs to be admitted to hospital for tests, including venography (or phlebography), which produces X-ray images of veins using injected radio-opaque dye. Treatment is by means of anticoagulant drugs, usually heparin, given intravenously, followed by coumarin taken by mouth. The condition can usually be successfully treated, provided that pulmonary embolism does not occur. A person who has had this condition may be advised to wear elasticated stockings, to rest with the feet and lower legs raised, and to avoid sitting with the feet or legs crossed.

Causes and risk factors: the cause of deep vein thrombosis is probably a combination of factors, including damage to the lining of the vein, a pooling of blood due to a decrease in the rate of flow and an increase in the clotting tendency. Risks increase with prolonged bed rest, as occurs after serious illness, injuries or surgery, immediately following childbirth, smoking, taking oral contraceptives and long journeys (especially by air), when a person is sitting for an extended period of time. A person who has to be confined to bed should try to move the legs as much as possible. People who are to undergo planned surgery are frequently given small doses of anticoagulants to lessen the risk of thrombosis.

thyroid gland tumour

Description: a benign or malignant growth of cells in the thyroid gland. The early stages of these tumours tend to produce similar symptoms.

Persons most commonly affected: all age groups and both sexes. There are various types of growth and some are more common in certain age groups than in others. Malignant forms are more common in females.

Organ or part of body involved: thyroid gland.

Symptoms and indications: generally, the person reports to his or her doctor with a painless lump or swelling in the neck. Some forms are painful and there may be difficulty in swallowing and symptoms of either hypo- or hyperthyroidism. A person with symptoms of a thyroid gland tumour should seek medical advice.

Treatment: usually requires admittance to hospital for specialist surgery to remove the lump and/or a part or the whole of the thyroid gland (thyroidectomy). Some malignant forms require removal of nearby lymph nodes and also treatment with radioactive iodine. The person may require antithyroid drugs or thyroid hormone replacements, depending upon the type of tumour and nature of the treatment. Most thyroid tumours, even malignant ones, can be successfully treated if detected early enough—one form (more common in elderly persons) is highly malignant and tends to have a fatal outcome.

Causes and risk factors: the cause is unknown but the risk increases with exposure to radiation of the chest, neck and head during childhood. In the past, radiation therapy was used to treat some fairly minor childhood complaints, such as tonsillitis, as well as more serious illnesses e.g. HODGKIN'S DISEASE. The thyroid gland was irradiated during this treatment. It is now known that this form of treatment, even though very small doses of radiation were involved, increased the risk of later development of a thyroid tumour. In the majority of cases, these tumours are benign.

tonsillitis

Description: inflammation of the tonsils caused by bacterial or viral infection. The term tonsils usually refers to two small masses of lymphoid tissue situated on either side at the back of the mouth (the palatine tonsils). However, another pair, situated below the tongue, are the lingual tonsils, while the adenoids are the pharyngeal tonsils, located at the back of the nose. All are part of the body's protective mechanism against infection and are larger during childhood.

Persons most commonly affected: children of both sexes after infancy and before puberty, but can affect other age groups.

Organ or part of body involved: tonsils, pharynx (throat).

Symptoms and indications: symptoms include a severe sore throat that makes swallowing very painful, accompanied by fever and earache, especially in children. The tonsils are usually swollen and white in appearance, due to infected material exuded from them, and lymph glands in the neck are enlarged. There is malaise and loss of appetite and, rarely, an abscess may develop on a tonsil. A person with symptoms of tonsillitis requires immediate medical treatment.

Treatment: complete bed rest is necessary and the person should drink as much fluid as possible. Tonsillitis is usually a bacterial infection and treatment is by means of antibiotics, especially penicillin or erythromycin, along with analgesics for pain relief. Recovery is usually good and complete within about one week or ten days. In some cases, a child may suffer recurrent bouts of tonsillitis, or the tonsils and adenoids may become permanently enlarged so that breathing is affected. If this occurs, surgery to remove the tonsils and adenoids may become necessary.

Causes and risk factors: tonsillitis is usually caused by streptococcal bacteria, although it can be viral in origin. In the past, tonsillitis often preceded RHEUMATIC FEVER or inflammation of the kidneys. Due to the advent of antibiotic drugs (and improvements in living conditions), this is now much less common in western countries. If an abscess develops on a tonsil, admittance to hospital for surgery is likely to be necessary.

tooth abscess

Description: a bacterial infection causing an abscess around the root of a tooth where it is embedded in the bone of the jaw.

Persons most commonly affected: all age groups and both sexes.

Organ or part of body involved: root of tooth and surrounding tissues of mouth and face.

Symptoms and indications: early symptoms include mild pain or toothache and sensitivity to hot and cold. Later the pain becomes severe, there is swelling at the base of the tooth and the face may become red and puffy on the affected side. There may be fever and malaise and the pain is usually of a throbbing nature. There is a loss of appetite, as chewing is painful. If the abscess bursts into the mouth, there is a foul taste and bad breath but other symptoms are relieved. A person with symptoms of a tooth abscess should seek immediate dental treatment.

Treatment: involves draining the abscess by means of a small incision into the gum or tooth canal. Often, a small wick or tube is inserted to allow the abscess to drain completely. Alternatively, the tooth may need to be extracted to allow the abscess to drain. Antibiotics and pain-relieving drugs may be prescribed and the person should refrain from eating on that side until healing is complete. Recovery is normally good and complete within a few days. Preventative measures include attention to dental hygiene, especially brushing the teeth thoroughly to help prevent decay. Also, regular dental check-ups are necessary so that any problems, especially signs of decay, can be dealt with at an early stage.

Causes and risk factors: the cause is usually a bacterial infection that spreads from the mouth to the base of a tooth. If the abscess occurs in the upper jaw there is a risk that it may rupture into a sinus, or infected material may spread in the bloodstream, causing infection elsewhere in the body.

torsion of a testis or testicle

Description: twisting or rotation of the spermatic cord and testicle, leading to irreversible damage if not treated promptly.

Persons most commonly affected: young adolescent males between the ages of 12 and 20 but can occur at any age.

Organ or part of body involved: testicle—usually only one is affected.

Symptoms and indications: the symptoms may arise for no apparent cause or as a result of strenuous physical activity. Symptoms include severe pain in the testicle, hardening, swelling and reddening of the scrotum, nausea and vomiting, fever and sweating, raised heartbeat rate. A person with these symptoms requires emergency treatment in hospital.

Treatment: is by means of surgery to correct the torsion and to attach the testicle to the wall of the scrotum to prevent a recurrence. Often, the unaffected testicle is similarly fixed at the same time as a precaution. Provided that prompt surgical treatment is carried out, recovery is normally good.

Causes and risk factors: the cause is not known but is sometimes present at birth. If treatment is delayed, the blood supply to the testicle is interrupted, leading to irreversible damage. If this occurs, the testicle and spermatic cord are removed by surgery. The remaining testicle produces sufficient hormones to ensure sexual maturation and fertility.

toxic shock syndrome

Description: a state of acute shock, due to a form of blood poisoning, caused by toxins (poisons) produced by staphylococcal bacteria. The syndrome is generally associated with the use of tampons by women during menstruation, but it may arise for other reasons in males as well as females. It is a rare occurrence, whatever the cause.

Persons most commonly affected: females during menstruation but can affect people of both sexes and all age groups.

Organ or part of body involved: respiratory system, blood, organs.

Symptoms and indications: symptoms include a sudden high fever, diarrhoea, red skin rash, anxiety, headache, fall in blood pressure, mental changes, and confusion and thirst. A person with symptoms of toxic shock syndrome requires emergency medical treatment.

Treatment: involves admittance to hospital for intensive supportive nursing. The person requires high doses of antibiotics (especially penicillin and cephalosporin), fluids and electrolytes all given intravenously until symptoms subside. The condition can be cured if caught and treated early but may prove fatal in some cases.

Causes and risk factors: the cause is toxins released by staphylococcus bacteria into the blood circulation. The syndrome can arise as a result of an infection within the body or from a wound, as well as from the use of tampons. Women should wash their hands before and after the insertion of a tampon and change tampons frequently. It is thought that young women or girls in whom the immune system is not fully developed may be at greater risk, particularly if a tampon is left in place too long.

toxocariasis

Description: a disease caused by a parasitic infestation with the larvae of roundworms that normally infect the domestic dog (*Toxocara canis*) or cat (*Toxocara cati*). The parasites are passed to man by swallowing eggs that are deposited in the faeces of infected pets.

Persons most commonly affected: young children of both sexes but may occur in older persons also.

Organ or part of body involved: various body tissues and organs, including the eyes, liver, lungs, central nervous system, heart.

Symptoms and indications: there are a variety of symptoms, depending upon which tissues are affected and whether allergic reactions take place. They include eye lesions and uveitis (an inflammation of the uveal tract of the eye, the iris, choroid and ciliary body). This usually occurs as the only symptom when the infestation has been with just a few larvae. Also, there may be wheezing, cough, symptoms of PNEUMONIA and lung inflammation, enlargement of the liver and spleen, blood changes, skin rash, muscular pains, vomiting, convulsions and fever. A person with symptoms of toxocariasis should seek medical advice.

Treatment: if the eyes alone are affected, treatment is by means of corticosteroids alone. Drugs that are likely to be prescribed for other manifestations include mebendazole (vermox), prednisone and diethylcarbamazine. The activity of the parasites and course of the disease lasts for about 6 to 18 months, when the larvae die off and do not mature into adults. Hence, the outlook is generally good, although the lesions produced by the larvae may remain. Preventative measures include excluding dogs from children's play areas and regularly de-worming pets. Care should be taken to ensure that small children wash their hands after playing or handling pets, especially before eating.

Causes and risk factors: the cause of the disease, as indicated above, is the larvae of toxocara roundworms. After the eggs have been swallowed, the larvae hatch in the intestine and pass through the wall into the blood circulation. They disperse and lodge in other tissues and organs in the body and may cause considerable damage and allergic reactions. The body responds to the presence of the larvae by producing a form of scar tissue (called granulation tissue). In the eye, this leads to the formation of a small nodule or nodules called granuloma(s). It is thought that about 2% of people in the UK may be affected by this parasite, but many do not exhibit symptoms.

toxoplasmosis

Description: a disease caused by a protozoan organism known as *Toxoplasma*. The disease occurs in two ways, an acquired infection that is generally mild and a much more serious and often fatal congenital form passed from mother to baby during pregnancy.

Persons most commonly affected: all age groups and both sexes. The illness may be severe in AIDS patients or others with a suppressed immune system, and newborn babies.

Organ or part of body involved: lymph nodes and vessels, muscles, central nervous system, eyes, liver, blood.

Symptoms and indications: in the case of acquired toxoplasmosis, often there are no symptoms. When they are present they include malaise, muscular pains, slight fever and enlargement of lymph nodes and glands. Also, liver and blood changes, ANAEMIA and low blood pressure may occur. These symptoms may be present for several weeks or longer and then subside and disappear. A chronic form of toxoplasmosis occurs that produces eye inflammation as its main symptom. Patients with a suppressed immune system (due to some other medical condition or illness) tend to have more severe symptoms, including chills, skin rash, high temperature, lung, heart, kidney or brain inflammation. Similarly, patients with Aids may exhibit severe symptoms, especially encephalitis (inflammation of the brain), with headache, muscle weakness in one half of the body, tremor, visual and hearing disturbance, confusion and coma.

Congenital toxoplasmosis—symptoms vary from mild to extremely severe and may appear shortly after birth or be delayed until later in childhood. They include eye problems, loss of sight and hearing, mental retardation, HYDROCEPHALUS (water on the brain), convulsions, JAUNDICE, enlarged liver and spleen, inflammation of the lungs and heart and skin rashes. Toxoplasmosis may cause abortion or stillbirth and, in general, is more severe in those infected during the early stages of pregnancy.

A person with symptoms of toxoplasmosis should seek medical advice.

Treatment: for those with symptoms is by means of various drugs, especially sulphonamides and pyrimethamine, folinic acid and corticosteroids. The outlook is good for those with slight symptoms of the acquired disease, but is poor in immunosuppressed and Aids patients, and in the severe congenital form. Children identified as having congenital toxoplasmosis require ongoing monitoring and treatment. Preventative measures are in the form of education. Pregnant women and those trying to conceive should avoid soil or cat litter contaminated with cat faeces, wash hands after handling raw meat or garden produce and eat only well-cooked meat.

Causes and risk factors: the cause is the protozoan organism *Toxoplasma gondii*, which is common throughout the world, affecting about 8% of human populations. The infection is transmitted by eating undercooked meat or through direct contact with soil contaminated by infected cat faeces. The organism undergoes sexual reproduction in cats, the eggs passing out in faeces. In other animals and birds, it reproduces asexually within the cells of its host. The host's immune system attacks the organism and renders it ineffective within a period of weeks or months. Hence, the disease is usually mild or produces no symptoms requiring blood tests for diagnosis, except in the more serious cases described above.

transient ischaemic attack (TIA)

Description: a temporary decrease in the normal supply of blood to a part of the brain. Usually the artery involved is partially blocked by a small plaque of material due to ATHEROSCLEROSIS, or a blood clot or embolus.

Persons most commonly affected: middle-aged and elderly adults of both sexes but can affect younger people and children with heart and circulatory disease.

Organ or part of body involved: one of the arteries supplying the brain, especially a branch of the carotid artery (in the neck) or the vertebral-basilar system of arteries.

Symptoms and indications: symptoms come on abruptly and last for two minutes to one or two hours (rarely longer). They include muscular weakness and numbness or tingling in the limbs, disturbance of vision or loss of sight in one eye, slurred speech or loss of the ability to speak, giddiness and confusion. The person remains conscious throughout the episode. Attacks tend to recur and vary in frequency from two or three each day to one or two over several years. A person with symptoms of a transient ischaemic attack should seek medical advice.

Treatment: depends, to a certain extent, upon the patient's condition and whether any underlying disorders are discovered or known to be present. The person is likely to be examined for high blood pressure (HYPERTENSION), DIABETES MELLITUS, and heart disease, and a blood sample may be taken to check for raised levels of fats (lipids) and polycythaemia (an abnormal increase in the number of red blood cells). If the attack is an isolated one or a rare occurrence, the person is usually treated with a small daily dose of aspirin. For more frequent attacks, anticoagulants such as heparin may be prescribed, or antiplatelet drugs. Some patients may require surgery to remove atherosclerotic deposits or plaques from a carotid artery. A person who experiences a transient ischaemic attack should have regular medical check-ups and monitoring.

Causes and risk factors: the cause of the condition is a partial temporary blockage of an artery supplying the brain by a fatty deposit, piece of arterial wall or blood clot. The risk increases in those who smoke, who are obese or who have high blood pressure, DIABETES MELLITUS, high levels of cholesterol or other fats in the blood, ATHEROSCLEROSIS or polycythaemia. There is an increased risk of STROKE in those who have transient ischaemic attacks and treatment is aimed at preventing the occurrence of this serious condition. A stroke is probably more likely to occur in a person who does not receive treatment for a transient ischaemic attack.

trichinosis

Description: a parasitic infestation with larvae of nematode worms that normally live in a number of different mammals including pigs.

Persons most commonly affected: all age groups and both sexes except young babies.

Organ or part of body involved: gastrointestinal tract, blood, lymph vessels and glands, muscles.

Symptoms and indications: symptoms vary greatly in severity, depending upon the overall health of the person and number of parasites that invade the body. Many people experience no, or few, mild symptoms whereas in others they may be severe. The parasites enter the digestive system and, after a few days, the females burrow into the intestinal wall and produce larvae. There may be few gastrointestinal symptoms but if they do occur, they include pains, sickness, diarrhoea and loss of appetite. The larvae of the parasites are then spread throughout the tissues of the body. A characteristic symptom is swelling of the upper eyelids due to fluid retention (oedema), which occurs about 11 days after infection. There may be bleeding into the tissues of the eyes and beneath the tongue, sensitivity to light, muscular pains, high fever and profuse sweating, thirst and

painful, irritated skin. The person is generally weak and experiences pain and difficulty in swallowing, chewing and speaking, these muscles often being greatly affected. There is an increase in the number of a certain type of white blood cells (eosinophils) in the blood (an immune response), which reach a peak and then gradually decline. Most symptoms gradually decline and disappear after about three months. The larvae of the parasites die, except in skeletal muscle where they encyst and may remain alive for several years. The person may be affected by muscular pains and fatigue for many months after the infection.

A person with symptoms of trichinosis should seek medical advice.

Treatment: is by means of drugs to kill the parasites, usually mebendazole or thiabendazole. Complete bed rest is necessary and analgesics, and corticosteroids (for those with allergic symptoms or where the heart or central nervous system is involved) may be necessary. Plenty of fluids should be drunk. The outlook is normally good but is more serious in those who develop severe complications (*see causes and risk factors*). Most affected persons recover completely but some deaths have occurred. People with severe symptoms require admittance to hospital for intensive supportive care. Preventative measures are making sure that all pork meats and products are thoroughly cooked before being eaten.

Causes and risk factors: the cause of the infection is a species of nematode worm, *Trichinella spiralis*, which infests various mammals, including pigs.The larvae of the parasite encyst in muscle tissue and human beings are infected by eating poorly cooked pork, especially sausages. The disease is generally mild but a few people develop serious complications involving the heart, lungs and central nervous system. These include MENINGITIS, encephalitis (inflammation of the brain), myocarditis (inflammation of the heart muscle), pneumonitis (lung inflammation), PLEURISY, disorders of vision and hearing.

tuberculosis (TB)

Description: a group of infections caused by a bacterium (bacillus) of which pulmonary tuberculosis of the lungs (consumption or phthisis) is the best-known form. In the lungs, the infection causes the formation of a primary tubercle that spreads to lymph nodes to form the primary complex. Later, the bacteria may enter the lymph and blood system and spread throughout the body, setting up numerous tubercles in other tissues (miliary tuberculosis). The tubercles of tuberculosis are minute, nodular masses of tissue that gradually change and fuse together and destroy surrounding healthy tissue.

Persons most commonly affected: all age groups and both sexes.

Organ or part of body involved: lungs (usually) but may spread to other tissues and organs.

Symptoms and indications: there may be few or no symptoms in the early stages. X-ray examinations and post-mortem studies have revealed that many people are affected by tuberculosis (showing the presence of old calcified tubercles and scarring in the lungs) but recover without suspecting that they have the disease.

If symptoms develop at an early stage, they resemble those of INFLUENZA or upper respiratory tract infections. Later, more serious symptoms may develop, including fever and copious sweating (especially at night), wasting, with loss of appetite and weight, malaise and tiredness. A severe cough develops with a thick sputum often containing blood, there is chest pain and breathing difficulty and, in some cases, the production of discoloured, red, cloudy urine. A person with symptoms of tuberculosis requires immediate medical treatment.

Treatment: is by means of antituberculous drugs, especially ethambutol, rifampicin, isoniazid (INH) and streptomycin. The person should rest in bed until symptoms subside, and drink plenty of fluids. It is advisable to limit contact with other people as much as possible but it is now thought that the disease is likely to have been spread before diagnosis. An infected person is thought to become noninfectious after about two weeks of drug treatment. Treatment may need to continue for some months with periodic check-ups to make sure that the TB is inactive. Most people make a full and complete recovery but complications can arise, and the disease may prove fatal in those who do not receive treatment. Preventative measures in the UK are the BCG vaccination given to children and X-ray screening to detect carriers.

Causes and risk factors: the cause of the infection is a bacterium, the bacillus *Mycobacterium tuberculosis*. The route of infection, especially in developed countries, is almost always by inhalation of airborne droplets containing the bacteria from an infected person, resulting in the pulmonary form of the disease. The organism may also be acquired by eating contaminated meat or milk, as a form of the disease occurs in cattle. However, bovine tuberculosis is rigorously screened for, and controlled in developed countries, so this route of infection is rare.

A further rare route of infection is via a cut, the bacteria gaining direct access from an infected person or animal. Tuberculosis can affect almost any organ or tissue and serious complications can arise. One of the most severe is tuberculous meningitis, which particularly affects children and the elderly. Other serious complications can occur in the kidneys, peritoneum (PERITONITIS), pericardium (the smooth membrane surrounding the heart) causing inflammation, lymph nodes, bones and joints and Fallopian tubes. Persons most at risk are those with suppressed immunity or who are otherwise ill, and AIDS patients. Also, those living in poor and overcrowded living conditions, suffering from DIABETES MELLITUS, people who are alcoholics and, as with many diseases, young children and the elderly.

In some countries there are worrying signs of the emergence of drug-resistant forms of the disease and, worldwide, the incidence of tuberculosis is increasing. There are about 6000 new cases each year in England and Wales. Hence, there is a continuing need for vigilance and prompt treatment of this disease.

typhoid fever

Description: a severe infectious disease of the gastrointestinal tract that is caused by a bacterium. It is more likely to occur in conditions of poor water sanitation, where there is inadequate disposal of sewage. It is uncommon in developed countries.

Persons most commonly affected: all age groups and both sexes.

Organ or part of body involved: gastrointestinal tract, skin, sometimes the lungs, spleen, tongue, bones, central nervous system.

Symptoms and indications: symptoms vary considerably in their severity depending upon the number of organisms swallowed. Some persons are carriers who do not show signs of the illness and in others, a mild attack may be mistaken for GASTROENTERITIS. Early symptoms include malaise, headache, nosebleeds, joint pains, sore throat, abdominal aches and tenderness. If not treated, there is a rise in temperature, occurring in steps and known as a stepladder temperature. Changes in the appearance of the tongue, thirst, diarrhoea that may contain blood and a characteristic pink rash of 'rose spots' on the abdomen and chest (in some cases). When the fever is at its height, the person is weak and unable to rise and there may be a lowering of heartbeat rate. There may be enlargement of the spleen, disturbance of liver function, ANAEMIA, blood changes and protein in the urine. Usually, the symptoms gradually subside, but in some severe cases, there may be ulceration of the intestinal wall, which can lead to PERITONITIS if an ulcer bursts, or serious haemorrhage from the bowels. Other complications include PNEUMONIA, acute HEPATITIS, CHOLECYSTITIS, MENINGITIS, tissue abscesses, ENDOCARDITIS (inflammation of the endocardium, the fine membrane lining the heart, and heart valves and muscle) and kidney inflammation. These complications may prove fatal in some cases. A person with symptoms of typhoid fever requires medical treatment.

Treatment: may necessitate admittance to hospital if the illness is severe, and is by means of antibiotics and, possibly, fluids, salts and nutrition given intravenously. Antibiotics used include chloramphenicol, ampicillin, ceftriaxone and cefoperazone. Scrupulous attention to hygiene is needed to prevent the spread of infection, including treatment of faeces, and the person may need to be isolated. Clothing and bedding may need to be sterilized. The patient and those involved in nursing care must wash their hands frequently. Recovery is usually good, with prompt treatment, unless complications occur. The person should rest in bed and may take some time to recover completely. Follow-up tests are needed for some time to ensure that the person is clear of the infection and is not a carrier of the organism. A preventative measure against typhoid fever is available in the form of a vaccine that gives temporary immunity. Anyone travelling to an area or country where the disease is known to occur should be vaccinated.

Causes and risk factors: the cause of the illness is the bacterium *Salmonella typhi*. The infection is acquired by swallowing food or water contaminated by the organisms. Water may easily become contaminated where standards of sanitation and sewage disposal are poor. Food may be contaminated directly by an infected person or one who is a carrier. In countries where typhoid fever occurs, raw foods, such as salads, which may have been washed in contaminated water, should be avoided. Food eaten should be thoroughly cooked and eaten immediately, and all drinking water boiled or treated with sterilizing tablets. Persons identified as carriers should not handle food and may also require treatment to eradicate the organism.

U

urethra (stricture of)

Description: a narrowing of the urethra, the narrow tube carrying urine from the bladder to the outside of the body. It is about 3.5cm long in women and 20cm in men. The stricture may be spasmodic, which is a temporary, reversible condition and is not serious or progressive, or chronic, which is more severe.

Persons most commonly affected: both sexes and all age groups.

Organ or part of body involved: urethra.

Symptoms and indications: the symptoms are those of urethritis (*see* NON-SPECIFIC URETHRITIS) including pain or burning feeling on urination, frequent need to urinate even though little is passed, and a discharge. As the urethra becomes progressively more narrow, there may be an occasional complete blockage, causing severe pain due to distension of the bladder from accumulated urine. As this is a progressive condition, there is a tendency for inflammation and infection of the bladder to occur and this may spread to involve the kidneys. A person with these symptoms should seek prompt medical advice.

Treatment: involves admittance to hospital for tests to establish the extent and position of the stricture. An operative procedure is usually required to widen the stricture, which may involve the passage of special instruments called bougies or surgery. Follow-up procedures are usually required to ensure that the passage does not contract again. Antibiotics may be prescribed to fight off infection.

Causes and risk factors: the cause of the stricture is usually a previous injury or recurrent or chronic inflammation and infection. These lead to the formation of scar tissue that contracts and causes the narrowing of the urethra.

uterine cancer or cancer of the uterus

Description: a growth of malignant cells in the uterus or womb, which is a relatively common form of cancer in women.

Persons most commonly affected: older women past the menopause, especially those aged 50 to 60.

Organ or part of body involved: uterus (or womb).

Symptoms and indications: the main symptom is unusual, abnormal bleeding. In postmenopausal women this occurs after menstruation has ceased and may be preceded by a watery or mucus-containing discharge that may be streaked with blood. In premenopausal women, abnormal bleeding occurs that is not connected with menstruation. A woman with symptoms of abnormal vaginal bleeding should seek medical advice.

Treatment: involves admittance to hospital for surgery to remove the womb (hysterectomy) and also, usually, the ovaries and Fallopian tubes. Also, radiotherapy and treatment with progesterone (a hormone) may be necessary. With prompt treatment, the outlook is quite good for the majority of patients.

Causes and risk factors: the cause is unknown but the risk of developing cancer of the uterus increases with DIABETES MELLITUS, a family history of cancer of the breast or ovaries, menstrual cycles in which an egg is not released and there is no input of progesterone, and oestrogen therapy. Also, those who are overweight or who have high blood pressure (HYPERTENSION) or disorders of hormonal imbalance are at greater risk. There is a risk that the cancer will spread to set up secondary growths elsewhere (metastases), which are likely to be fatal.

V

vaginal cancer or **cancer of the vagina**

Description: uncontrolled growth of malignant cells in the vagina.

Persons most commonly affected: adult women aged between 45 and 65 but can occur at any age. One form (embryonal rhabdomyosarcomas) can affect babies and girls in childhood.

Organ or part of body involved: vagina; often spreads to rectum and bladder.

Symptoms and indications: symptoms include abnormal vaginal bleeding especially with sexual intercourse (which may be painful), or internal examination by a doctor. There may be a thin, watery discharge and, if the cancer spreads to the bladder or rectum, a frequent need to empty these organs accompanied by pain. A person with symptoms of cancer of the vagina should seek medical advice.

Treatment: consists of admittance to hospital for surgery to remove the affected part and, possibly, hysterectomy and removal of lymph nodes in the pelvis. Radiotherapy, both external and internal (by means of implants of radium or caesium) is likely to be needed. The outlook varies, depending upon the extent of the cancer but symptoms can be relieved.

Causes and risk factors: in most cases, the cause is unknown but in children, the cancer is linked to exposure to oestrogen (diethylstilboestrol) taken by the mother during pregnancy. It is thought that exposure to human papilloma virus (HPV) may influence the development of other forms of this cancer. Risks increase in women with family members who developed cancer of the reproductive organs.

vaginitis

Description: inflammation and, frequently, infection of the vagina, often involving the vulva. Usually, the condition is accompanied by a vaginal discharge.

Persons most commonly affected: females of all age groups, depending upon cause.

Organ or part of body involved: vagina and vulva.

Symptoms and indications: symptoms include vaginal discharge that may be thick, discoloured (yellow or greenish) or white and can be foul-smelling. Also, itching of the skin or burning in the region of the vulva, reddening, discomfort and pain. The symptoms may vary in severity, depending upon the cause of the condition. A person with symptoms of vaginitis should seek medical advice.

Treatment: depends upon the cause, which is established by means of a physical examination and discussion, and may involve obtaining a swab so that infective organisms can be cultured. Treatment for inflammation without infection may be by means of soothing creams or anti-inflammatory preparations such as hydrocortisone. Bacterial infections are treated with appropriate antibiotics such as doxycycline erythromycin and metronidazole, which is also used for infections caused by the parasite *Trichomonas*. If the cause is *Candida* (*see* CANDIDIASIS), treatment is by means of miconazole or clotrimazole. In older, postmenopausal women, in whom the vaginitis may be atrophic (due to the thinning of tissues, with or without infection) the treatment is usually hormone replacement therapy with oestrogen. The condition can usually be successfully treated.

Causes and risk factors: include bacterial and fungal infections, infestation with a minute protozoan parasite, *Trichomonas vaginalis*, mechanical or chemical irritation, e.g. by tight clothing, use of deodorants, foam baths, body sprays and detergents, etc., or presence of a foreign body, and atrophic changes due to ageing. CANCER OF THE VAGINA may also be the cause. Various factors may make vaginitis more likely to occur, including general poor health, DIABETES MELLITUS, hot, humid conditions that favour infections, taking oral contraceptives and exposure to human papilloma virus.

varicose veins

Description: veins that have become stretched,

distended and twisted. The superficial veins in the legs are often affected, although it may occur elsewhere.

Persons most commonly affected: adults of all age groups and both sexes.

Organ or part of body involved: veins.

Symptoms and indications: early symptoms include discomfort and aching legs after a prolonged period of standing still, and there may be cramp-like pains. Later, the veins become enlarged and visible as bluish cords beneath the skin. The feet and ankles may swell and the person may be unusually tired. Eczema and ulceration of the skin may occur. A person with symptoms of varicose veins should seek medical advice.

Treatment: in mild cases, the wearing of elasticated stockings provides effective treatment. More serious cases may require surgical removal of the affected vein (phlebectomy). Another form of treatment is sclerotherapy. An irritant substance, usually sodium tetradecyl sulphate, is injected into the vein, which causes fibrosis of the vein lining, with clot formation and scarring, leading to the obliteration of the vein. This treatment is usually very successful, with few side effects or complications. Varicose veins can be treated but new veins may become affected. Treatment is aimed at relief of symptoms and to improve appearance. If ulcers are present, they are treated with compresses and dressings. Preventative measures include taking regular exercise to improve the flow of blood through the veins.

Causes and risk factors: the cause is distension and failure of the valves in the vein so that blood does not drain properly. This may occur due to congenital factors, obesity, pregnancy, THROMBOPHLEBITIS (inflammation of the wall of a vein, with secondary thrombosis in the affected part), and also prolonged standing. Varicose veins that develop during pregnancy usually go down after the birth of the child.

vasovagal attack

Description: intense activity in the vagus (the tenth cranial nerve, which supplies various organs and has motor sensory and secretory functions). This causes a slowing of the heartbeat and a fall in blood pressure, resulting in fainting (syncope).

Persons most commonly affected: all age groups and both sexes.

Organ or part of body involved: vagus nerve, heart, blood circulation, brain.

Symptoms and indications: the episode is preceded by a sudden unpleasant event. Symptoms include weakness, disturbance of vision, sweating, nausea followed by fainting, usually from an upright position. As there are many causes of fainting, it is usually advisable for a person who has experienced such an attack to be seen by a doctor.

Treatment: depends upon the cause of the fainting and overall condition of the patient. Usually, gently and slowly raising the person to a sitting position, along with reassurance, brings the episode to an end. Further treatment depends upon the nature of the patient's condition.

Causes and risk factors: there are various causes of a vasovagal attack, usually involving severe emotional shock, or sudden intense pain or fear. The attack normally involves a person who is otherwise apparently healthy. However, fainting may be a symptom of underlying diseases or disorders and it is advisable to seek medical advice.

W

warts or verrucas

Description: small, solid benign growths on the skin, caused by a virus, which are contagious and may spread rapidly from one person to another. There are several types: plantar, on the foot; juvenile, in children, and venereal, on the genitals. Warts often disappear spontaneously but can be dealt with in various ways. In adults, flat parts may persist for years.

Persons most commonly affected: all age groups and both sexes.

Organ or part of body involved: skin.

Symptoms and indications: one or more small raised bumps, or they may be fairly flat, that occur on the skin. Colour varies, in adults flat warts may be dark brown. A person affected by warts or who notices any change in a wart should seek medical advice.

Treatment: depends upon the type and site of a wart; some may not require treatment unless they are troublesome or unsightly. Others disappear spontaneously after a period of time. Treatment that may be given includes painting or coating the wart with chemical cauterant solutions, and removal by cryosurgery (freezing), laser beam or electrocautery (burning away with an electrically heated wire or needle).

Causes and risk factors: the cause is a virus that infects the skin, the human papilloma virus. The infection may be acquired directly from contact with another person or from the floor of changing rooms e.g. public swimming pools.

whooping cough or pertussis

Description: an infectious disease of childhood, caused by a bacterium producing a characteristic cough and other respiratory symptoms. Due to immunization, the incidence and severity of the disease is generally less severe than formerly.

Persons most commonly affected: children of both sexes aged under ten years but can occur in other age groups.

Organ or part of body involved: respiratory tract, bronchial tubes, lungs.

Symptoms and indications: the mucous membranes lining the air passages are affected and after a one, or two-week incubation period, fever, catarrh and a cough develop. The cough then becomes paroxysmal, with continual bouts lasting up to one minute. At the end of each bout the child draws in the breath with a characteristic whooping sound. Nosebleeds and vomiting may follow a bout of coughing, with diarrhoea and fever. After about two weeks the symptoms start to lessen, although the cough may persist for some time. Subsequent respiratory infections may produce a similar paroxysmal type of cough that is not a recurrence of whooping cough itself. A child with symptoms of whooping cough should receive medical attention.

Treatment: the child should be kept in bed, and isolated from others, while symptoms are at their height, and encouraged to drink plenty of fluids. Salt solutions may be needed if the child has been continually sick. In general, medication such as antibiotics are not recommended except for infants who are seriously ill or patients with complications. Treatment in hospital is necessary for those more seriously affected. Recovery normally takes about six weeks. Prevention is by means of vaccination given in infancy.

Causes and risk factors: the cause of whooping cough is a bacterium, *Bordetella pertussis*, and infection is by inhalation of airborne droplets coughed out by an infected person. Patients are not infectious after the paroxysmal stage. Whooping cough is serious in small children aged less than two years, and in elderly persons, but generally not so in other age groups unless complications arise. Infants may suffer from ASPHYXIA, bronchopneumonia and convulsions. Other serious complications include rupture of blood vessels in the brain (cerebral haemorrhage) or eye, and RETINAL DETACHMENT due to the violent coughing, TUBERCULOSIS and encephalitis (inflammation of the brain). Some children may sustain lung damage, leading to EMPHYSEMA or ASTHMA. Severe complications can result in death or permanent brain damage, but vaccination provides protection and should be given to all children (with rare exceptions).

Wilm's tumour or congenital nephroblastoma

Description: a malignant tumour of the kidney, which is present at birth and is usually diagnosed in children aged under five years. Occasionally, symptoms may appear later in childhood or, rarely, in adults.

Persons most commonly affected: children of both sexes aged under five years.

Organ or part of body involved: kidney (normally only one).

Symptoms and indications: the usual symptom that is first noticed is an abdominal mass that can be felt through the skin. There may be fever, pain in the abdomen, blood in the urine, loss of appetite and weight, vomiting and nausea. Blood pressure may be high. A child with these symptoms requires immediate medical attention.

Treatment: involves admittance to hospital for tests and scans to confirm the diagnosis and evaluate the extent of the tumour. Treatment is by means of surgical removal of the diseased kidney, chemotherapy with anticancer drugs and, possibly, radiotherapy. The outlook depends upon the nature and extent of the tumour and whether it has spread, and the age of the child. Younger children usually have a more favourable prognosis and in some cases the condition can be cured.

Causes and risk factors: the cause is not known but there is an association with some other congenital abnormalities. In rarer cases (about 4%) both kidneys may be affected. There is a risk of secondary growths occurring in other organs, which can cause death.

Wolf-Parkinson White syndrome

Description: a tachycardia (increased heartbeat rate) caused by abnormally fast electrical conduction in an accessory pathway. This links the atria and ventricles (the upper and lower chambers) of the heart while bypassing the normal pacemaker system.

Persons most commonly affected: all age groups and both sexes.

Organ or part of body involved: heart.

Symptoms and indications: the condition is a complex one but symptoms include chest pain, dizziness and temporary loss of consciousness. More serious symptoms of ATRIAL FIBRILLATION can occur. A person with any symptoms of heart abnormality requires immediate medical attention.

Treatment: involves admittance to hospital for tests and electrophysiological studies to determine the best course of treatment. Anti-arrhythmic drugs are used with extreme caution and, usually, a surgical procedure to correct the condition is required. This is a skilled procedure but one that produces excellent results.

Causes and risk factors: the cause is an abnormality in the electrical conducting system of the heart, involving accessory pathways.

Y

yaws or pian or framboesia

Description: an infectious bacterial disease of tropical countries, particularly occurring in the West Indies and Africa, and characterized by the appearance of small tumours on the skin. Similar infections occur in South America.

Persons most commonly affected: all age groups and both sexes.

Organ or part of body involved: skin, usually on the legs at first and then hands, feet, face, buttocks. Bones may be affected especially the tibia (leg) and nasal bone.

Symptoms and indications: the bacteria enter through cuts and abrasions on the skin, often the legs. Following an incubation period of two or more weeks, a lesion appears at the site of infection, which usually heals. This is followed by the eruption of more small tumours on the skin, each with a yellow crust of dried serum. During the incubation period the person suffers fever, pain, itching and general malaise. The tumours may form painful deep ulcers if the condition remains untreated e.g. on the face and soles of the feet. Ultimately, possibly after several years, there may be deep lesions of the skin and bone, especially of the face and leg. A person with symptoms of yaws requires immediate medical treatment.

Treatment: is by means of penicillin, which works dramatically and effectively in this disease and also can be used as a preventative measure.

Causes and risk factors: the cause of this and similar diseases are species of spirochaete bacteria belonging to the genus *Treponema*. They are spread by direct bodily contact with an infected person or via contaminated clothing or bedding, usually in poor, unhygienic conditions. Anyone visiting or working in an area where yaws occurs should receive preventative treatment with benzathine penicillin.

yellow fever

Description: a severe viral infection, occurring in Africa and South America, that is transmitted to humans via the bite of mosquitoes.

Persons most commonly affected: all age groups and both sexes.

Organ or part of body involved: gastrointestinal tract, central nervous system, muscles, liver, kidneys.

Symptoms and indications: symptoms appear in stages and vary greatly in severity.

First stage: symptoms appear rapidly and include high fever, an initial rise in pulse rate and then this becomes slow, flushing of the face, bloodshot eyes and furring of the tongue. Also, vomiting, nausea and constipation, irritability, headache and muscle pains. The amount of urine passed decreases and it contains protein, indicating inflammation of the kidneys. In mild cases, these symptoms gradually subside and the person recovers.

Second stage: symptoms subside and the person feels better and this period of remission usually lasts from a few hours to a few days.

Third stage: characteristically there is the development of JAUNDICE (hence yellow fever), the bringing up of black vomit (containing blood), slow pulse (bradycardia) and fever. The person is extremely weak, urine production may cease and the urine contains protein, and there may be haemorrhages from mucous membranes. The person may suffer DELIRIUM, convulsions and coma, leading to death. The kidneys, liver and gastrointestinal tract are inflamed and undergo degenerative changes. A person with symptoms of yellow fever should seek medical advice.

Treatment: in mild cases, rest in bed and drinking plenty of fluids may be all that is necessary, and it is thought that many cases go undiagnosed. In more severe cases, admittance to hospital for supportive nursing treatment is necessary, aimed at reducing the severity of symptoms. Preventative measures are by means of immunization and control of mosquitoes. Vaccination is effective and gives protection for ten years. A person travelling to an area in which yellow fever occurs should be vaccinated. Also, a person who recovers from an attack of yellow fever acquires natural immunity.

Causes and risk factors: the cause is a virus transmitted by the bite of *Aedes aegypti* mosquitoes, which acquire the organism from an infected person or monkey or ape. Wild primates act as a reservoir for the virus in areas where yellow fever occurs.

Quick Reference to Symptoms

sudden or severe abdominal pain
Possible cause:
appendicitis
cholecystitis
colic
colitis
Crohn's disease
diverticular disease—diverticulitis
ectopic pregnancy
gallstones
ileitis
intestinal obstruction and intussusception
liver abscess
ovarian cyst (ruptured)
pancreas cancer
pancreatitis
peritonitis
porphyria

behavioural changes, dementia, psychological disturbance or disorder
Possible cause:
alcoholism
Alzheimer's disease
brain tumour
catalepsy
catatonia
concussion
Cushing's syndrome
delirium
drug abuse
epilepsy—temporal lobe epilepsy
head injury
Huntington's chorea
myxoedema
narcolepsy
porphyria
rabies
Reye's syndrome
(stroke)
syphilis
(transient ischaemic attack)

bleeding from the rectum, blood in faeces, pain
Possible cause:
anal fissure
cirrhosis of the liver
colitis
constipation
dysentery
gastric erosion
haemorrhoids
hepatoma
Polyarteritis nodosa
rectal abscess
rectal prolapse
rectal tumour
small intestine tumour
stomach cancer
stomach ulcer
thrombocytopaenia

abnormal vaginal bleeding
Possible cause:
Abruptio placentae (pregnancy)
ectopic pregnancy
endometriosis
fibroid
pelvic inflammatory disease
Placenta praevia (pregnancy)
uterine cancer
vaginal cancer

unexplained or sudden bleeding. *See also* ANAEMIA, abnormal vaginal bleeding, bleeding from rectum
Possible cause:
AIDS
bone fracture
cirrhosis of the liver
haemophilia
haemorrhage
leukaemia
radiation sickness

subconjunctival haemorrhage (eye)
thrombocytopaenia

breathlessness, wheezing, breathing difficulty
Possible cause:
allergy
asbestosis
asthma
emphysema
hay fever

chest pain
Possible cause:
aneurysm
Angina pectoris
aortic valve disease
atrial fibrillation
coronary artery disease
coronary thrombosis (heart attack)
heartburn
pericarditis
pleurisy
pneumothorax
pulmonary embolism
pulmonary hypertension
pulmonary valve stenosis

chest pain with breathlessness, breathing difficulty, cough
Possible cause:
Angina pectoris
aortic valve disease
asbestosis
atrial fibrillation
bronchiolitis
cardiomyopathy
emphysema
mesothelioma
pericarditis
pneumoconiosis
silicosis
tapeworms

convulsions (fits)
Possible cause:
asphyxia
brain tumour
eclampsia of pregnancy
epilepsy
fever—and any infections that cause fever
head injury
meningitis
Reye's syndrome

pulmonary hypertension
Roseola infantum

abnormal discharge from vagina or penis
Possible cause:
AIDS
fibroid in uterus
gonorrhoea
nonspecific urethritis
ovarian cyst
pelvic inflammatory disease
Reiter's syndrome
uterine cancer
vaginitis

symptoms of ear disorder e.g. discharge, pain, ringing in ears (tinnitus), vertigo, nausea, vomiting, deafness
Possible cause:
deafness
labyrinthitis
Menière's disease
Otitis externa
Otitis media
otosclerosis
ruptured eardrum

fluid retention causing swelling (oedema)
Possible cause:
adult respiratory distress syndrome (pulmonary oedema)
allergy
altitude sickness (pulmonary oedema)
anaphylactic shock
aneurysm
cardiomyopathy
cirrhosis of the liver
eclampsia of pregnancy
glomerulonephritis
haemolytic disease of the newborn
hepatitis
hepatoma
hydrocephalus
kidney failure
liver cancer
nephrotic syndrome
Polyarteritis nodosa
pre-eclampsia of pregnancy
pulmonary oedema
pulmonary valve stenosis
sleeping sickness (tropical disease)
trichinosis

gastrointestinal symptoms—e.g. nausea,

vomiting, diarrhoea, abdominal pains, loss of appetite and weight, abnormal stools, fever

Possible cause:
ancyclostomiasis
Addison's disease
cholera
cirrhosis of the liver
coeliac disease
diverticular disease—diverticulosis
duodenal ulcer
fascioliasis
food poisoning
gastritis
gastroenteritis
giardiasis
irritable bowel syndrome
Lassa fever
ovarian tumour
Polyarteritis nodosa
radiation sickness
roundworms
sprue
stomach ulcer
tapeworms

headache that may be accompanied by other symptoms, e.g. numbness or weakness, nausea and vomiting, confusion, vision disturbance

Possible cause:
aneurysm
brain abscess
brain tumour
Caisson disease (compressed air illness)
carbon monoxide poisoning
concussion encephalitis
glaucoma
head injury
heatstroke
hypertension
meningitis
migraine
temporal arteritis—*see* Polymyalgia rheumatica and temporal arteritis.
sinusitis
subarachnoid haemorrhage
subdural haemorrhage ·

symptoms of hormonal disorders— unexplained weight gain or loss, gastrointestinal upset, menstrual changes in women, unusual growth of body hair or enlargement of breasts, retarded or

accelerated growth, swelling, palpitations, anxiety

Possible cause:
Addison's disease
Cushing's syndrome
Grave's disease
hyperthyroidism
myxoedema
ovarian tumour
phaeochromocytoma
thyroid gland tumour

inflammation of eyes or eyelids e.g. reddening, itching, pain, discharge

Possible cause:
blepharitis
conjunctivitis
corneal foreign body
entropion
iritis
keratitis
ptosis
scleritis
stye
subconjunctival haemorrhage

influenza-like symptoms e.g. headache, chills, shivering, fever, aches and pains, malaise, sore throat, swollen glands. Many diseases have early symptoms resembling those of influenza.

Possible cause:
AIDS
bronchitis
brucellosis
cat scratch fever
croup
dengue
diphtheria
glandular fever
Hodgkin's disease
influenza
Kawasaki disease
Lassa fever
Legionnaire's disease
leptospirosis
lung abscess
malaria
mumps
pneumonia
psittacosis
Q fever
sandfly fever
sinusitis

tonsillitis
toxocariasis
toxoplasmosis
tuberculosis
whooping cough

**kidney symptoms; including pain in the
lower back or abdomen, fever, blood or pus
in urine, nausea, vomiting, chills, malaise,
headache, fatigue, decrease or increase in
amount of urine passed, oedema (fluid
retention) and swelling**
Possible cause:
glomerulonephritis
hypernephroma
kidney failure
kidney stones
myeloma
nephrotic syndrome
Polyarteritis nodosa
polycystic disease of the kidney
pyelitis
Reiter's syndrome
renal carbuncle
renal tuberculosis
scleroderma
systemic Lupus erythematosus
Wilm's tumour

**symptoms of liver disorder; jaundice, loss of
appetite and weight, fluid retention, fatigue,
anaemia, dark coloured urine, digestive
upset, itching skin**
Possible cause:
cirrhosis of the liver
fascioliasis
hepatitis
hepatoma
leptospirosis
liver abscess
liver cancer
lymphoma
schistosomiasis (tropical disease)
tapeworms
thalassaemia

**symptoms of lung infection or inflammation;
including cough with sputum or blood,
chest pain, breathlessness, breathing
difficulty, fever, chills, malaise**
Possible cause:
asbestosis
bronchiectasis
bronchitis

chronic bronchitis
emphysema
Legionnaire's disease
lung abscess
lung cancer
pleurisy
pneumoconiosis
pneumonia
psittacosis
pulmonary oedema
Q fever
silicosis
tuberculosis

**mass or lump, including swollen glands that
can be felt externally**
AIDS (glands)
boil (skin)
breast abscess (breast and armpit)
breast cancer (breast and armpit)
cat scratch fever (glands)
cauliflower ear (ear)
cirrhosis of liver
corns
diphtheria (glands in neck)
Ewing's sarcoma (bones)
glandular fever (glands in neck, armpits, groin)
Grave's disease (neck)
haemorrhoids (piles)
hepatoma (liver—abdomen)
hernia (usually abdomen, groin)
Hodgkin's disease (all glands)
hyperthyroidism (thyroid—neck)
ileitis (abdomen)
intestinal obstruction (abdomen)
Kaposi's sarcoma (feet, ankles, hands, arms, lymph
   glands)
Kawasaki disease (neck glands)
laryngeal cancer (lymph glands in neck)
leishmaniasis (tropical disease)
leukaemia (lymph glands, spleen, liver)
lipoma (skin)
listeriosis (lymph glands)
liver abscess (abdomen)
liver cancer (abdomen)
lymphoma
mastitis (breast)
mumps (salivary glands in face, neck)
oesophageal cancer (glands in neck)
osteosarcoma (bones, especially leg or arm)
ovarian tumour (abdomen)
pharyngitis (throat)
pyloric stenosis (stomach)
rectal abscess (rectum)

rectal prolapse (rectum)
rectal tumour (rectum)
salivary gland enlargement (mouth, neck)
sleeping sickness (tropical disease, lymph glands)
sporotrichosis (skin)
stomach cancer (upper abdomen)
syphilis (lymph glands)
testicular cancer (testis, scrotum)
thyroid gland tumour (neck)
tonsillitis (neck, throat)
tooth abscess (face)
torsion of a testis (scrotum)
toxoplasmosis (lymph glands)

abnormal involuntary muscular twitches or spasms
Possible cause:
cerebral palsy
convulsions
epilepsy
Huntington's chorea
multiple sclerosis
Parkinson's disease

nerve pain; pain along the course of a nerve
Possible cause:
Bell's palsy (face)
carpal tunnel syndrome (hands, arms)
neuralgia
neuritis
sciatica
shingles

numbness or weakness, tingling, unsteadiness, paralysis, speech disorder, confusion
Possible cause:
Bell's palsy (facial muscles)
brain compression
carpal tunnel syndrome (fingers, hands, arms)
cerebral palsy
Friedreich's ataxia
Guillain-Barré syndrome
Huntington's chorea
multiple sclerosis
muscular dystrophy
myasthenia gravis
Paget's disease of bone
Parkinson's disease
Polyarteritis nodosa
polymyositis
ptosis
spondylosis
stroke

syphilis
transient ischaemic attack

pain, stiffness and inflammation around a joint with heat, swelling and, possibly, other symptoms such as fever, malaise etc.
Possible cause:
bursitis
dislocation
Ewing's sarcoma
frozen shoulder
gout
Legg-Calvé Perthes disease
Osgood-Schlatter's disease (knee)
osteoarthritis
psoriasis (psoriatic arthritis)
rheumatic fever
rheumatoid arthritis
scleroderma
Still's disease
systemic Lupus erythematosus
tendinitis

pain in the back with restriction of movement or stiffness
Possible cause:
ankylosing spondylitis
bone fracture
osteoarthritis
osteoporosis
Paget's disease of bone
Polymyalgia rheumatica
prolapsed intervertebral disc
spondylosis
Still's disease

pains in the legs
Possible cause:
atherosclerosis
Buerger's disease
thromboembolism
thrombophlebitis
thrombosis (deep vein)
varicose veins

respiratory distress, e.g. breathing difficulty, breathlessness, cyanosis (blue tinge to skin), rapid, laboured breathing, chest pain, raised heartbeat rate.
Possible cause:
adult respiratory distress syndrome
anaphylactic shock
asphyxia
asthma (severe attack)

bronchiolitis
croup (severe attack)
diphtheria
pneumothorax (severe)
pulmonary oedema
shock

skin lesions or ulcers; there may be accompanying symptoms of illness, e.g. fever, malaise, aches and pains, chills, headache
Possible cause:
agranulocytosis
AIDS
athlete's foot
boil or furuncle
Buerger's disease
burns and scalds
candidiasis (thrush)
chilblain
cold sores
corns and bunions
dermatitis
diabetes mellitus
eczema
erythema
erythroderma
erythromelalgia
frostbite
Granuloma annulare
hand, foot and mouth disease
Herpes simplex infection
icthyosis
impetigo
Kaposi's sarcoma
keratosis
Lupus erythematosus
melanoma
pemphigus
psoriasis
Raynaud's disease
Reiter's syndrome
ringworm
rodent ulcer
scabies
scleroderma
shingles
skin cancer
sporotrichosis
syphilis
thalassaemia
varicose veins
warts
yaws

skin rash; with or without accompanying symptoms of fever, malaise, chills, aches and pains, headache
Possible cause:
allergy
anaphylactic shock
chicken pox
German measles
Lassa fever
Lupus erythematosus
Rocky Mountain spotted fever
rosacea
Roseola infantum
scarlet fever
systemic Lupus erythematosus
thrombocytopaenia

severe or persistent sore throat, hoarseness, voice changes
Possible cause:
diphtheria
glandular fever
laryngeal cancer
laryngitis
pharyngitis
scarlet fever
tonsillitis

thirst
Possible cause:
Diabetes insipidus
Diabetes mellitus

vision disturbance or loss of vision
Possible cause:
brain tumour
cataract
glaucoma
Grave's disease
head injury
hydrocephalus
iritis
migraine
phaeochromocytoma
polycythaemia
retinal detachment
senile macular degeneration
stroke
tapeworms
thromboembolism
toxoplasmosis
transient ischaemic attack
trichinosis

vomiting
Possible cause:
Hyperemus gravidarum (in pregnancy)
pyloric stenosis
vomiting of blood
Possible cause:
gastric erosion
gastritis
stomach cancer
yellow fever (tropical disease)

urinary tract symptoms; urinary frequency, pain on passing urine, blood in urine
Possible cause:
bladder stones
bladder tumour
cystitis
fistula (urinary)
glomerulonephritis
gonorrhoea
hypernephroma
nonspecific urethritis
ovarian cyst
prostate gland cancer
prostate gland enlargement
schistosomiasis (tropical disease)
urethra, stricture of
vaginal cancer

Prescription Drugs

A

Accupro

Description: a proprietary preparation of the antihypertensive drug, quinapril; used in conjunction with a diuretic or cardiac glycoside. Available as brown tablets (oval, round or triangular according to strength).

Used for: hypertension and congestive heart failure, especially after other treatments have been tried.

Dosage: in adults only starts at 2.5mg per day usually increasing to 10–20mg per day. The maximum daily dose is 40mg.

Special care: all elderly patients, impairment of kidney function, haemodialysis, severe congestive heart failure, some types of vascular disease and in patients having anaesthesia.

Avoid use: children, pregnant and nursing mothers, some kidney and heart valve diseases.

Possible interaction: potassium-containing supplements, diuretic drugs, NSAIDs, tetracyclines.

Side effects: numerous including hypotension, abdominal, chest and muscle pains, headache, nausea, dizziness, rhinitis, upper respiratory tract infection and allergic reactions.

Manufacturer: Parke-Davis.

Acepril

Description: an ACE inhibitor and preparation of the antihypertensive drug captopril available as white tablets and marked A (12.5mg strength), or ACE and strength (for 25 and 50mg strengths).

Used for: an addition to diuretic drugs and where appropriate digitalis in congestive heart failure. After heart attacks when there is a disorder of the left ventricle.

Dosage: 6.25 or 12.5mg for heart failure, maintenance 25mg two or three times per day. Maximum 150mg per day. treatment to be commenced under close supervision. Diuretics to be reduced or stopped before treatment. Post heart attack-6.25mg, increasing slowly to 150mg per day in divided doses. Start 3 days after attack. For children, contact manufacturer.

Special care: severe congestive heart failure, haemodialysis, kidney disease, anaesthesia, monitor kidney function, white cell count and urinary protein.

Avoid use: pregnancy, lactation, narrowing of the aorta.

Possible interaction: potassium supplements or potassium-sparing diuretics, vasodilators, NSAIDs, lithium, allopurinol, clonidine, probenecid, immuno-suppressants.

Side effects: anaemia, loss of taste, hypotension, proteinuria, pancreatitis, rash, angioneurotic oedema, neutropenia, thrombocytopenia.

Manufacturer: Squibb.

Acezide

Description: a combined diuretic/ACE inhibitor anti-hypertensive preparation. Contains captopril (50mg) and hydrochlorothiazide (25mg) in a white, scored tablet, code AZE 50/25.

Used for: mild to moderate hypertension.

Dosage: 1 tablet daily (maximum 2) (in patients who have first become accustomed to the two components given in the same amounts separately).

Special care: patients with renal disorders or undergoing haemodialysis.

Avoid use: in children, pregnant and breast feeding mothers, outflow obstruction of the heart, aortic stenosis and renovascular disease.

Possible interaction: NSAIDs, potassium-containing supplements, antihypertensives, vasodilatory and immunosuppressant drugs.

Side effects: protein in urine (proteinuria), rash, loss of sense of taste, fatigue, changes in constitution of the blood and, very unusually, a cough.

Manufacturer: Squibb.

Achromycin

Description: a preparation of the antibiotic tetracycline hydrochloride used to treat a variety of conditions. Available as orange tablets. Also, as intramuscular injection and via intravenous drip. Effective against the bacterium *Haemophilus influenzae*.

Used for: complications of chronic bronchitis.

Dosage: 1 or 2 tablets at 6 hourly intervals.

Special care: patients with any liver or kidney

disease. May require avoidance of use in cases of renal impairment.

Avoid use: in cases of impaired kidney function. It is absorbed into growing bone and stains teeth, hence must not be given to children less than 12 years or to pregnant women or nursing mothers.

Possible interaction: consumption of milk which reduces absorption of tetracycline, contraceptive pill, antacids, iron, magnesium and calcium mineral supplements.

Side effects: digestive upset—diarrhoea and vomiting, nausea, headache, disturbance of vision, possible allergic response.

Also used for: acne vulgaris.

Description: achromycin topical ointment containing 3% tetracycline hydrochloride.

Used for: moderate to severe acne and effective against the bacterium *Propionbacterium acnes*.

Dosage: apply to affected skin once a day or as directed by physician.

Special care: in patients with kidney and liver disorders or perforated ear drum.

Avoid use: as above.

Possible interaction: as above.

Side effects: possible additional infection, especially thrush. Occasionally diarrhoea.

Also used for: mild bacterial skin infections.

Dosage: apply once daily to affected area or as directed.

Side effects: possible super infection (infection caused by different microorganism, or a strain of the bacterium causing the original infection which has become resistant to Achromycin).

Also available as sterile ointment containing 1% tetracycline hydrochloride.

Used for: bacterial infections of the outer ear (otitis extrema) which are sensitive to tetracycline.

Dosage: once or twice daily or as directed.

Special care: patients with perforated ear drum and for short-term use.

Side effects: localized allergic reactions and possible superinfection (see above).

Also used for: infections of eyelids, e.g. styes, surface infections, e.g. conjunctivitis and chlamydial opthalmia (along with antibiotic preparations taken orally). Also following minor abrasions to the surface of the eye to prevent infections.

Dosage: every 4 hours or as directed by physician.

Special care: generally as above.

Side effects: possible superinfection.

Manufacturer: Lederle.

Aclacin

Description: a class II anthracycline, cytotoxic,

antibiotic drug. It contains aclarubicin hydrochloride in the form of a powder (20mg) which is reconstituted as a fluid for rapid infusion.

Used for: non-lymphocytic leukaemia especially in patients who are resistant to other forms of chemotherapy or who have relapsed from these treatments.

Dosage: as infusion, directed by physician.

Special care: elderly, impairment of liver and kidney functions, heart disorders. Monitoring of cardiac function is essential during treatment. High cumulative doses can lead to cardiac dysfunction.

Side effects: possible tissue damage to healthy cells adjacent to cancer cells through interference with cell division. Severe nausea and vomiting, loss of hair, suppression of bone marrow so blood cell formation is impaired.

Manufacturer: Lundbeck.

Actilyse

Description: a fibrinolytic (disperses blood clots) drug available as a powder for reconstitution and injection. It can only be used under close medical supervision.

Used for: thrombosis, embolisms and particularly myocardial infarction.

Dosage: a total of 100mg, given intravenously over a 2 hour period in adults only.

Special care: in patients with liver or kidney disease, diabetes or hypertension.

Avoid use: in children, pregnant and nursing mothers, those with any form of bleeding (e.g. menstruation), recent surgery including dental treatment, or haemorrhage, any condition likely to bleed, e.g. active peptic ulcer or case of pancreatitis. Should not be administered to those having allergic reactions to streptokinase and anistreplase or who have recently been treated with these.

Possible interaction: with other plasma protein-bound drugs, i.e. anticoagulants.

Side effects: mainly nausea, vomiting and bleeding usually confined to puncture site but can occur elseshere including intracerebral haemorrhage. Severe bleeding necessitates halting of treatment and possible administration of drugs to counter the fibrinolytic. Hence close monitoring is essential during treatment.

Manufacturer: Boehringer Ingelheim.

Actinac

Description: an antibacterial steroid (corticosteroid) preparation with skin softening properties, available as a powder with solvent to be made up as a lotion. Contains the broad spectrum antibiotic chloramphenicol (4%), hydrocortisone acetate (4%) and also sulphur precipitate, allantoin and butoxyethyl nicotinate.

Used for: acne.

Dosage: apply to affected skin morning and night for 4 days then at night only for up to 3 weeks, continuing for 3 days after spots have disappeared.

Special care: pregnant women, avoid contact with jewellery.

Side effects: possible erythema, which may be severe.

Manufacturer: Roussel

Acupan

Description: an analgesic non-narcotic drug available in the form of white tablets or as a solution for injection. Contains 30mg nefopam hydrochloride, tablets being marked APN. (Injection contains 20mg nefopam hydrochloride per ml in each ampoule).

Used for: relief of moderate and severe pain, e.g. following surgery, muscle and joint pain, dental cancer.

Dosage: tablets 3 times per day, adults only, total dose in the order of 30–90mg. Injection—one 20mg dose intramuscularly 3 times a day.

Special care: elderly patients (1 tablet, 3 times a day initially), pregnant women, patients with kidney or liver disorders or suffering from urine retention.

Avoid use: children, history of convulsions or heart attack (myocardial infarction) and also glaucoma.

Possible interaction: drugs including sympathomimetics, tricyclics, anticholinergics and MAOIs (antidepressants).

Side effects: nervousness, irritability, dry mouth, dizziness and nausea, headaches. Occasionally insomnia, irregular heartbeat and sweating. Urine may be tinged pink.

Manufacturer: 3M Health Care.

Adalat

Description: a calcium antagonist and vasodilator, available as liquid-filled orange capsules, containing the active ingredient nifedipine (5mg and 10mg). Also as sustained release tablets and as a preparation for injection.

Used for: angina and Raynaud's phenomenon.

Dosage: 10mg 3 times a day (5mg in elderly patients) in first instance, depending upon response, up to 60mg a day thereafter. Capsules taken with or immediately after food.

Special care: patients with significant left ventricle disorders or congestive heart failure, low blood pressure, kidney and liver disease.

Avoid use: if pain worsens during treatment, pregnant and nursing mothers, children, patients with very low blood pressure.

Possible interaction: antihypertensive drugs; quinidine and cimetidine.

Side effects: dizziness, flushing, nausea, palpitations, sweating, headaches, fluid retention, digestive upset, increased frequency of urination, drowsiness and insomnia. Rarely jaundice and swelling of gums.

Manufacturer: Bayer. Nifedipine capsules also produced by Norton, Evans, APS, Ashbourne (Angiopine), CP, Eastern (Calcilat ®), Kerfoot, Cox.

Adcortyl

Description: a potent topical steroid preparation (a corticosteroid), containing the active ingredient triamcinolone acetonide 0.1%, as cream or ointment.

Used for: eczema and psoriasis, which has proved unresponsive to less potent preparations of corticosteroids. Can also be used to treat external ear infections and neurodermatitis.

Dosage: apply sparingly to affected area 2–4 times each day and less frequently as condition improves.

Special care: for children and babies, especially face and neck.

Avoid use: acne (including acne rosacea), any skin conditions caused by ringworm, fungi, viruses, tuberculosis, leg ulcers, pregnant women and long term use. Also fungal or bacterial infections which have not been treated.

Side effects: suppression of adrenal gland function, skin thinning and retention of fluid.

Also available: adcortyl witth graneodin (an antimicrobial agent) which includes the antibiotic neomycin. This contains 0.1% triamcinolone acetonide, 0.25% neomycin (as sulphate) and 0.025% gramicidin as cream. It is used as above but where a bacterial infection may additionally be present.

ADCORTYL IN OROBASE is available as an oral paste used to treat mouth ulcers and other oral inflammations. It is applied 2 to 4 times daily and should not be used long term or by pregnant women. Adcortyl containing 10mg/ml triamcinolone acetonide is available for injection intradermally or into a joint. Used intradermally to treat scaly skin diseases, alopecia areata (patchy hair loss). Used intraarticularly to treat joint pain, stiffness and swelling caused especially by rheumatoid arthritis, bursitis, tenosynovitis and osteoarthrosis (osteoarthritis).

Manufacturer: Squibb

Adifax

Description: a preparation containing dexfenfluramine hydrochloride (fenfluramine is chemically related to amphetamine but is not a central nervous system stimulant and is less likely to cause dependence). It is an appetite suppressant which appears to affect the levels of serotonin (a naturally occurring compound in the body) in the brain. It is available in the form of 15mg white capsules marked S5614.

Used for: severe obesity alongside other treatments, mainly control of diet.

Dosage: 1 tablet in the morning and evening, at mealtimes.

Special care: treatment should be limited to three months with gradual withdrawal over 1 or 2 weeks. Elderly patients.

Avoid use: in children, pregnant and nursing mothers, patients with history of psychiatric illness, drug/alcohol abuse, anorexia, glaucoma, epilepsy, liver and kidney disorders.

Possible interaction: anorectic drugs; MAOIs, antidepressants, sedatives, antihypertensive drugs, antidiabetics.

Side effects: dependence effects possible on withdrawal including depression, breathlessness, headache, nervousness and irritability, sleep disturbance, dry mouth, dizziness, nausea, diarrhoela, constipation, more frequent urination.

Manufacturer: Servier

Adizem

Description: a calcium antagonist and vasodilator containing the active ingredient diltiazem hydrochloride. Available as tablets in 3 forms:
Adizem 60—coded 60/DL, 60mg white capsules.
Adizem-SR—white 90mg; brown 120mg; white/brown 180mg. Also as 120mg white tablets (DL/120). All continuous-release capsules.
Adizem XL—pink/blue 120mg; pink/blue 180mg; red/blue 240mg; maroon/blue 300mg. All continuous-release capsules marked with strength.

Used for: angina and hypertension.

Dosage: 60mg 3 times a day increasing if required to a maximum of 480mg. Elderly, twice a day in first instance.

Special care: patients with heart block, reduced function in left ventricle of heart, bradycardia, diabetes.

Avoid use: in children, pregnant and nursing mothers, severe heart block or bradycardia, impairment of kidney and liver function.

Possible interaction: digoxin, ß-blockers, antihypertensive drugs, cardiac depressants, diazepam, cyclosporin, cimetidine, theophylline, cartamazepine.

Side effects: swelling of ankles, nausea, headache, bradycardia, rash, first degree heart block.

Manufacturer: Napp

Aerolin Autohaler

Description: a preparation of a selective Beta₂-agonist (beta receptor stimulant) salbutamol which causes dilation or expansion of air passages in the lungs. Salbutamol (as sulphate) is present as 100 µg per dose.

Used for: prevention (prophylaxis) and treatment of bronchial asthma and breathing difficulties associated with bronchitis.

Dosage: Aerolin is administered by means of a breath-activated aerosol inhalant which delivers a metered dose. Dose is 1–2 puffs 3–4 times daily for prevention. Half dose for children.

Special care: thyroid gland disorders (hyperthyroidism) hypertension, heart disorders, e.g. myocardial insufficiency, during pregnancy and breast-feeding. May cause thyrotoxicosis with associated symptoms.

Possible interaction: corticosteroids—increased risk of hypokalaemia with high doses.

Side effects: headache, nervousness and irritability, fine tremor (in hands), vasodilation in peripheral areas of body.

Manufacturer: 3M Health Care

Akineton

Description: an anticholinergic preparation containing the active ingredient biperiden hydrochloride, used to counter the effects of Parkinson's disease. It is available as white, scored tablets with Knoll logo, containing 2mg biperiden hydrochloride and as a preparation containing biperiden lactate 5mg/ml, for slow intravenous or intramuscular injection.

Used for: Parkinson's disease and treatment of symptoms of drug-induced Parkinson's disease.

Dosage: *Tablets*: in adults, 1mg twice daily in first instance gradually increasing to 2mg 3 times a day. After initial period, the usual daily dose is in the order of 3–12mg 3 times a day. *Injection*: 2.5–4mg per ml up to 4 times per day.

Special care: in patients with liver, kidney or heart disease. Treatment must be discontinued gradually.

Avoid use: children, pregnant and nursing mothers, some types of glaucoma, patients with untreated urine retention or gastrointestinal obstruction.

Possible interaction: CNS depressant drugs and other anti-Parkinson's disease drugs.

Side effects: dry mouth, drowsiness, blurred vision and gastrointestinal disorders. More rarely, urine retention and tachycardia and possible allergic reactions.

Manufacturer: Knoll.

Aknemin

Description: an antibiotic drug, containing minocycline hydrochloride, available as 50mg red/fawn coloured capsules and 100mg red capsules.

Used for: acne.

Dosage: adults, twice daily dose of 50mg or 100mg. Tablets required for a minimum period of 6 weeks to 3 months with improvement not expected until after first month.

Special care: liver or kidney disorders.

Avoid use: pregnant and nursing mothers, children, kidney failure, SLE.

Possible interaction: alcohol, antacid stomach preparations, mineral supplements, anticoagulant drugs, penicillin.

Side effects: skin rashes, dizziness, blood abnormalities. Possible intracranial hypertension—drug should be discontinued.

Manufacturer: Stiefel.

Aldactide

Description: a proprietary preparation containing a potassium-sparing diuretic (encourages potassium to be retained and not eliminated in kidney) combined with a thiazide (a drug which inhibits the reabsorption of chloride and sodium in the kidney). The preparation is available in two strengths. **Aldactide 25** contains 25mg spironalactone and 25mg hydroflumethiazide in buff-coloured tablets marked Searle 101. **Aldactide 50** (Gold Cross) contains 50mg of each drug.

Used for: congestive heart failure.

Dosage: *Aldactide 25*: adults, 4 tablets daily with food in first instance with a maximum of eight. *Aldatide 50*: two tablets daily with a maximum of four. In children: 1.5–3mg per kg of body weight given at intervals through the day.

Special care: elderly, liver and kidney disorders, pregnant mothers, diabetic patients, gout, long-term use in young people. Blood tests and monitoring of electrolyte levels may be required.

Avoid use: nursing mothers, patients with liver or kidney failure, hypercalcaemia, hyperkalaemia, Addison's disease, sensitivity to sulphonamide drugs.

Possible interaction: potassium supplements, other potassium-sparing diuretic drugs, NSAIDs, anti-diabetic drugs, antihypertensive drugs, ACE inhibitors and cardiac glycosides.

Side effects: metabolic disorders, disturbance of electrolyte balance in blood, rash, drowsiness, sensitivity to light, gastrointestinal upset, menstrual irregularities, deepening of voice.

Manufacturer: Searle.

Aldactone

Description: a diuretic, potassium-sparing preparation containing spironolactone. Tablets available: 25mg buff marked Searle 39, 50mg off-white (Searle 916), 100mg buff (Searle 314).

Used for: congestive heart failure, oedema caused by cirrhosis of the liver, malignancy or nephrotic syndrome, primary aldosteronism (overproduction of the adrenal hormone, aldosterone).

Dosage: in adults with congestive heart failure, 100mg daily in first instance increasing to 400mg taken with food. Thereafter, 75–200mg per day. Children, 3mg per kg of body weight in first instance in several doses.

Special care: pregnant mothers, long-term use in young people patients with liver or kidney disorders. Blood electrolyte levels may need to be monitored.

Avoid use: nursing mothers, patients with kidney failure, Addison's disease, and hyperkalaemia.

Side effects: gastrointestinal upset, rash, headache, disturbance of electrolyte levels, metabolic disturbance, breast enlargement, deepening of voice, menstrual irregularities, confusion, ataxia (unsteadiness).

Manufacturer: Searle.

Aldomet

Description: a centrally acting (on central nervous system), antihypertensive preparation containing the drug methyldopa. It is available as tablets or in ampoules for injection. May be used in combination with a diuretic drug. Aldomet tablets are available in three strengths all marked Aldomet and coloured yellow: Aldomet 125mg code 135; Aldomet 250mg code 401, Aldomet 500mg code 516.

Used for: hypertension, especially useful for hypertension of pregnancy.

Dosage: in adults, 250mg 2 to 3 times a day in first instance with an eventual maximum of 3 grams at 2-day intervals. In children, 10mg per kg of body weight each day in 2 to 4 separate doses.

Special care: history of liver disease, kidney disorders, haemolytic anaemia, undergoing anaesthesia.

Avoid use: liver disease, a disease of the adrenal glands called phaeochromocytoma, patients with depression.

Possible interaction: sympathomimetics, other hypertensives, MAOIs, tricyclic antidepressants, lithium and phenothiazines.

Side effects: depression, sleepiness, headache, dry mouth, nasal congestion, gastrointestinal upsets, bradycardia, jaundice, haemolytic anaemia, positive Coombs test.

Manufacturer: MSD.

Alexan

Description: a preparation of the antimetabolite, cytotoxic drug, cytarabine. It is available as ampoules for intravenous injection in two strengths, 20mg/ml and 100mg/ml (**Alexan 100**).

Used for: acute kind of leukaemia, especially myeloblastic leukaemia, to induce remission.

Dosage: as directed by cancer specialist.

Special care: careful monitoring of the blood is essential as this drug significantly reduces the ability of the bone marrow to manufacture blood cells.

Side effects: hair loss, nausea, vomiting.

Manufacturer: Pfizer.

Alfa D

Description: a manufactured form of vitamin D containing alfacalcidol (1a-hydroxycholcalciferol), a hydroxylated derivative. Since the conversion of vitamin D to its active form (which can be used by the body) requires hydroxylation by the kidneys, alfacalcidol is especially useful for patients suffering from any form of renal disorder. Alfa D is available in two strengths and contains 0.25 μg of alfacalcidol in a pink capsule or 1 μg in an orange capsule, each marked appropriately.

Used for: rickets and osteomalacia (adult rickets, possibly caused by liver disease or malabsorption of vitamin D), overactivity of the parathyroid glands (and bone disease) (hyperparathyroidism), underactivity of the parathyroid glands (hypoparathyroidism), renal osteodystrophy (bone disease associated with chronic kidney failure).

Dosage: adults: 1 μg each day in first instance, adjusted according to response. Elderly patients: 0.5 μg at first followed by adjustment of dose. Children over 20kg weight, 1 μg daily, then adjusted dose.

Special care: pregnant and breast-feeding mothers; vitamin D is passed into breast milk and can cause hypercalcaemia in infants. Patients with kidney failure. Monitoring of blood plasma levels of calcium is essential during treatment.

Avoid use: children under 20kg body weight.

Possible interaction: barbiturate and anticonvulsant drugs, digitalis, danazol, thiazides, mineral supplements, cholestyramine, sucralfate, colestipol.

Side effects: (associated with overdose) diarrhoea, vomiting, nausea, weight loss, vertigo, headache, sweating, lethargy, thirst, elevated levels of calcium and phosphate in urine.

Manufacturer: Du Pont

Algitec

Description: a preparation, containing the H₂-receptor antagonist, cimetidine, which acts to reduce the production of gastric acid in the stomach. It is also a reflux suppressant which is available in chewable tablets called Chewtab and as a liquid suspension. Algitec tablets are off-white in colour and contain 200mg cimetidine and 500mg alginic acid and are marked ALGITEC 120. Also, **Algitec Suspension** containing 100mg cimetidine and 250mg sodium alginate in each 5ml.

Used for: gastric and duodenal ulcers, Zollingen-Ellison syndrome, reflux oesophagitis.

Dosage: adults, one to two tablets chewed four times a day following meals, or 10–20mls of suspension, and at night time, for four to eight weeks.

Special care: the presence of gastric cancer should first be eliminated. Patients suffering from kidney disorders and pregnant and nursing mothers.

Avoid use: not for children.

Possible interaction: oral anticoagulants, warfarin, phenytoin, theophylline or aminophylline.

Side effects: generally few but dizziness, fatigue, rash, diarrhoea may occur, and rarely, headache, confusion, joint and muscle pains, reversible liver damage and gynaecomastia (breast enlargement).

Manufacturer: SK & F.

Alimix

Description: a preparation containing the active ingredient, asapride, which acts to promote stomach and intestine motility and emptying. It is thought to work by promoting the release of acetylcholine in the wall of gastrointestinal tract. It is available as white scored tablets, marked J/Y and C and containing 10mg of cisapride (as monohydrate).

Used for: gastro-oesophageal reflux, delayed gastric emptying accompanying such conditions as diabetes, systemic sclerosis and autonomic neuropathy (nerve supply to gastrointestinal tract is disrupted), non-ulcer dyspepsia (short-term treatment).

Dosage: depending upon condition being treated but usually 1 tablet 3 or 4 times daily, a quarter or half an hour before meals, for 6–12 weeks.

Special care: nursing mothers, elderly patients, kidney and liver disorders.

Avoid use: children and pregnant women, gastrointestinal bleeding, obstruction or perforation. Any condition where stimulation of gastrointestinal tract might prove to be harmful.

Possible interaction: anticholinergic drugs, anticoagulants, sedatives, opiod analgesics, antimuscarines.

Side effects: diarrhoea and abdominal pains, borborygmi (stomach and abdominal rumbling caused by fluid and gas), rarely headaches and convulsions.

Manufacturer: Janssen.

Alkeran

Description: a preparation of the alkylating, cytotoxic drug melphalan, for use by a physician skilled in cancer chemotherapy. It is available in tablets of two strengths, a white tablet coded A2A (2mg), and a white tablet coded B2A (5mg). Also available as a powder for reconstitution, containing 50mg melphalan (as hydrochloride), for injection.

Used for: myeloma (or multiple myeloma, myelomatosis) a malignant bone marrow disease, ovarian and breast cancer.

Dosage: 150–300 µg per kg of body weight each day for four to six days. This may be repeated after four to eight weeks.

Special care: bone marrow suppression occurs but not immediately. Hence blood counts must be checked before each stage of treatment. Dose must be reduced in patients with impaired kidney function.

Possible interaction: antibacterial drugs, nalidixic acid cyclosporin.

Side effects: nausea, vomiting, hair loss, bone marrow suppression.

Manufacturer: Wellcome.

Allegron

Description: a TCAD, nortriptyline, available in tablets of two strengths. It has less of a sedative efect than some other TCAD drugs. It is available as white scored tablets marked DISTA, containing 10mg nortriptyline hydrochloride, and orange scored tablets marked DISTA (25mg).

Used for: depressive illnesses and bed-wetting in children.

Dosage: adults, 20 to 40mg each day in divided doses, increasing to 100mg if required. Maintenance, 30 to 75mg a day. Elderly persons; 10mg three times daily in first instance. Children (for bed-wetting), seven to ten years, 10 to 20mg, 11 to 16 years, 25 to 50mg, given half an hour before bedtime.

Special care: patients with heart disease, elderly people (reduced doses), nursing mothers, those with diabetes, thyroid disease, liver disorders, tumours of the medulla of adrenal glands, epilepsy, glaucoma, urine retention, psychosis, suicidal tendencies. Withdrawal should be gradual. May reduce ability to perform skilled tasks such as driving.

Avoid use: pregnant mothers, heart block, heart attack, serious liver disorders.

Possible interaction: alcohol, MAOIs, barbiturate drugs, anticholinergic drugs, other antidepressant and antihypertensive drugs, adrenaline, noradrenaline, oestrogens, cimetidine.

Side effects: drowsiness, blurred vision, dry mouth, insomnia, urine retention, palpitations and shakiness, low blood pressure, weight changes, skin reactions, jaundice, blood changes, loss of libido.

Manufacturer: Dista.

Almevax

Description: a preparation of vaccine against German measles (Rubella) containing the live, but attenuated, strain Wistar RA 27/3 virus. It is available in one and ten dose vials for injection.

Used for: immunization against Rubella in non-pregnant women and girls aged 10–14 who have not received MMR vaccine.

Dosage: one dose given intramuscularly or subcutaneously.

Special care: contraceptives should be used during the first three months although there is thought to be little risk of harm to the foetus.

Avoid use: pregnancy, cancer, acute fevers, hypogamma globulinaemia (gamma globulin blood deficiency).

Possible interaction: other live vaccines, transfusions, irradiation, cytotoxic drugs, corticosteroids, immunoglobulins.

Side effects: sore throat, rash, malaise, aching joints, possible anaphylaxis.

Manufacturer: Evans.

Alomide

Description: a preparation containing lodoxamide tromethamine with additives benzalkonium chloride and disodium edetate, available as 1% solution.

Used for: allergic conjunctivitis.

Dosage: one to two drops in each eye four times daily.

Special care: pregnant and nursing mothers.

Avoid use: those who wear soft contact lenses, children under four years of age.

Side effects: irritation, stinging, watering of eyes.

Manufacturer: Galen.

Alphaderm

Description: a moderately strong steroid with a hydrating agent (to moisten the skin). Alphaderm combines 1% hydrocortisone, 10% urea in a slightly oily cream.

Used for: dermatitis and eczema.

Dosage: wash and dry affected skin and apply thinly twice a day.

Special care: short-term use only (especially in children or on face).

Avoid use: acne, scabies, tuberculosis, ringworm, untreated bacterial and fungal infections, viral skin diseases, leg ulcers, pregnant mothers.

Side effects: usually few but skin thinning, adrenal gland suppression, fluid retention possible.

Manufacturer: Procter and Gamble.

Alphosyl HC

Description: a preparation of coal tar and hydrocortisone used in the treatment of psoriasis. It contains 5% coal tar extract, 0.5% hydrocortisone and 2% allantoin in a water-based cream.

Used for: psoriasis.

Dosage: adults and children over 5 years, apply to affected skin twice each day.

Special care: use should be limited to 5 days with children or on face. If treatment in adults is prolonged, withdrawal should be gradual.

Avoid use: extensive or prolonged use in pregnant women, acne or untreated fungal and bacterial infections, tuberculosis, viral skin disease, leg ulcers, ringworm. Children under 5 years.

Side effects: thinning of skin, suppression of adrenal glands, fluid retention.

Manufacturer: Stafford-Miller.

Alrheumat

Description: a NSAID preparation available as capsules and suppositories. Alrheumat contains 50mg ketoprofen and propionic acid in off-white cream-coloured capsules or as anal suppositories.

Used for: pain and inflammation caused by musculoskeletal diseases and rheumatoid and osteoarthritis, acute gout, pain following orthopaedic surgery, ankylosing spondylitis.

Dosage: capsules—adults one 2–4 times each day with food. Suppositories—100mg at bedtime. Combined capsules and suppositories no more than 200mg daily.

Special care: pregnancy and lactation, patients with heart, kidney or liver diseases, elderly people.

Avoid use: children, patients with asthma, allergy to aspirin or NSAIDs, active peptic ulcer or history of peptic ulcer, gastrointestinal haemorrhage.

Possible interaction: high doses of methotrexate, sulphonamide antibiotic drugs, quinolones, hydantoins and anticoagulant drugs.

Side effects: gastrointestinal upsets, rash, rectal irritation (suppositories).

Manufacturer: Bayer.

Alupent

Description: a bronchodilator, containing the partially selective drug orciprenaline sulphate. It is available as off-white scored tablets marked A7 containing 20mg orciprenaline sulphate. Also available as alupent sugar-free syrup (10mg/5ml of solution) and alupent aerosol containing 0.75mg per metered dose.

Used for: bronchial spasm due to asthma, chronic bronchitis and emphysema.

Dosage: tablets and syrup: adults, one tablet or 10mls four times a day. Children under 1 year 2.5 to 5mls three times daily; 1–3 years, 2.5 to 5mls four times daily; 3–12 years, 5mls four times daily up to 10mls three times daily depending on age and symptoms. Aerosol: adults, 1–2 puffs which can be repeated after 30 minutes if required. Maximum dose 12 puffs in 24 hours. Children, 6 years and under, one puff, 6–12 years, one or two puffs. Must not be repeated within 30 minutes and maximum dose is four puffs in 24 hours.

Special care: patients with diabetes or hypertension. Patients should follow instructions carefully.

Avoid use: acute heart disease, hyperthyroidism or cardiac asthma.

Possible interaction: sympathomimetic drugs, tricyclic antidepressants, MAOIs.

Side effects: tachycardia, arrythmia, fine tremor, headache and nervous tension, dilation of blood vessels.

Manufacturer: Boehringer Ingelheim.

Ambaxin

Description: a broad-spectrum antibiotic preparation, containing a form of penicillin, available as scored, oblong-shaped tablets marked Upjohn and 130.

Used for: respiratory, ear, nose, throat, soft tissue and skin infections. Also urinary tract infections and venereal diseases such as gonorrhoea. Para-typhoid fever.

Dosage: adults, 1–2 tablets, 2 or 3 times a day. Venereal disease, 4 tablets plus 1g of probenecid as a single dose. Children over 5 years, half a tablet 3 times daily.

Special care: patients suffering from liver and kidney diseases or infectious mononucleosis (glandular fever).

Avoid use: children under five years. Allergy to penicillin.
Side effects: gastrointestinal upsets, possible allergic responses, e.g. rash (discontinue treatment).
Manufacturer: Upjohn.

Amfipen

Description: a broad-spectrum antibiotic penicillin, ampicillin, available as capsules, Amfipen syrup and in vials for injection; Amfipen capsules are grey/red and available in 2 strengths containing 250mg and 500mg, marked with name and strength. **Amfipen Syrup** is also available in 2 strengths and contains 125mg and 250mg ampicillin per 5ml.
Used for: respiratory and ear, nose and throat infections. Also, soft tissue, urinary tract and veneral infections (gonorrhoea).
Dosage: adults, 250mg–1g 4 times each day. Children, half adult dose.
Special care: patients with kidney disease or glandular fever (infectious mononucleosis).
Avoid use: allergy to penicillin.
Side effects: gastrointestinal upsets, allergic responses, e.g. rash (discontinue treatment).
Manufacturer: Brocades

Amikin

Description: a preparation of the aminoglycoside antibiotic drug, amikacin, produced in the form of solutions for intramuscular or slow intravenous injection or infusion. Amikin contains 500mg per 2mls. **Amikin Paediatric** contains 100mg amikacin (as sulphate) per 2ml.
Used for: serious bacterial infections particularly those caused by Gramnegative bacteria which are resistant to the more usual aminoglycosides, gentamicin and tobramycin.
Dosage: adults, 15mg per kg of body weight intramuscularly or intravenously in two divided doses for up to 10 days. Maximum total dose 15g. For urinary tract infections, 7.5mg per kg of body weight each day in two divided doses. Children, 10mg–15mg per kg of body weight daily in two divided doses.
Special care: patient should receive adequate fluid intake, caution with kidney disease. Monitor for toxicity.
Avoid use: pregnant women.
Possible interaction: anaesthetics, neuromuscular blocking drugs, ethacrynic acid, frusemide.
Side effects: temporary kidney impairment and irreversible deafness can occur with prolonged or too high dosage.
Manufacturer: Bristol-Myers.

Amil-Co

Description: a potassium-sparing diuretic available in the form of peach-coloured, diamond-shaped tablets with the name and logo. They contain 5mg amiloride hydrochloride and 50mg hydrochlorothiazide (co-amilozide 5/50).
Used for: cirrhosis of the liver (with fluid retention), congestive heart failure, hypertension.
Dosage: adults, 1–2 tablets each day increasing up to 4, if required, in single or divided dose.
Special care: patients with gout, kidney or liver disease, diabetes, acidosis.
Avoid use: children, pregnant and nursing mothers, hyperkalaemia, severe or progressive kidney failure.
Possible interaction: other potassium-sparing diuretics, potassium supplements, antihypertensive drugs, ACE inhibitors, lithium, digitalis (digoxin).
Side effects: gout, rash, sensitivity to light, blood dyscrasias.
Manufacturer: Baker-Norton.

Amoxil

Description: preparations of the broad-spectrum antibiotic, amoxycillin, which is a derivative of ampicillin and available as maroon/gold capsules (250mg or 500mg amoxycillin trihydrate), marked with name and strength; dispersible, sugar-free tablets containing 500mg; **Amoxil Fiztab** chewable tablets, sugar-free (125mg). Not suitable for children under 3 years of age; **Amoxil Syrup SF** sugar-free, containing either 125mg or 250mg per 5ml for reconstitution with water; **Amoxil Paediatric Suspension**, 125mg amoxycillin (as trihydrate) per 1.25ml; **Amoxil 3g Sachets SF**—3g in sucrose-free sorbitol base as a powder in a sachet. **Amoxil 750mg Sachet SF** containing 750mg in sugar-free, sorbitol base as a powder in a sachet; **Amoxil Injection**—Either 250mg, 500mg or 1g amoxycillin (as sodium salts), in a vial as a powder for reconstitution.
Used for: one or more of the different forms are used for soft tissue infections, urinary tract infections, respiratory, ear, nose, throat, infections, gonorrhoea, dental abscess and to prevent endocarditis during dental treatment. Glandular fever.
Dosage: infants under 6 months, Amoxil Paediatric suspension is appropriate. Adults, 250–500mg three times each day, children half adult dose. Injection, (used for glandular fever), adults, 500mg intramuscularly at 8-hour intervals or 1g intravenously at 6-hourly intervals if infection is severe. Children, 50–100mg per kg of body weight in divided doses.
Special care: patients with allergy to penicillin.

Side effects: gastrointestinal upsets, allergic responses, e.g. rash, especially in patients with glandular fever, HIV virus, lymphatic leukaemia.
Manufacturer: Bencard.

Ampiclox

Description: a broad-spectrum antibiotic ampicillin with cloxacillin available as capsules, black/purple (250mg ampicillin trihydrate) and 250mg cloxacillin (as sodium salt); Also **Ampiclox Syrup** containing 125mg/125mg per 5ml, available as powder for reconstitution; **Ampiclox Neonatal**, a sugar-free suspension containing 60mg/30mg per 0.6ml when reconstituted; **Ampiclox Neonatal Injection** containing 50mg/25mg as powder for reconstitution; **Ampiclox Injection** containing 250mg/250mg as powder for reconstitution.

Used for: emergency treatment of serious bacterial infections of urinary tract, ear, nose, throat, upper respiratory tract while bacteriology is being investigated. Also as a preventative against infection when the patient is to undergo major surgery.

Dosage: adults, capsules, 1–2 every four to six hours; syrup, 10–20ml every four to six hours. Children, babies under one month, neonatal suspension, 0.6ml every four to six hours or neonatal injection intravenously or intramuscularly, 1 vial three times a day. Children 1 month to 2 years 2.5ml–5ml Ampiclox syrup both every 4 to 6 hours. Adults, Ampiclox injection, intravenously or intramuscularly, 1 to 2 vials every 4 to 6 hours. Children 1 month to 2 years, one-quarter adult dose, children 2 to 10 years, half adult dose.

Special care: allergic patients, kidney disease, rashes especially in glandular fever, HIV, chronic lymphatic leukaemia.

Avoid use: patients with known penicillin allergy.

Side effects: gastrointestinal upsets, allergic responses.

Manufacturer: Beecham.

Amsidine

Description: a cytotoxic, antibiotic, anti-cancer preparation containing amsacrine. This is available as a preparation for intravenous infusion for use by a physician skilled in cancer therapy. Amsidine concentrate contains 5mg amsacrine (as lactate) per ml when reconstituted.

Used for: acute myeloid leukaemia.

Dosage: as directed by physician. Usually no more than 450mg/m² of body surface area as a total cumulative dose.

Special care: patients with cardiac disorders, liver or kidney disease (reduced doses), elderly people, pregnant women. Caution in handling as irritant to tissues and skin; glass apparatus should be used for mixing. Cardiac monitoring and monitoring of electrolyte levels is essential during treatment.

Side effects: suppression of bone marrow function (myelosuppression), hair loss, mucositis. Rarely, tachycardia associated with ventricles of heart. Heart disease and potentially fotal heart failure.

Manufacturer: Parke-Davis

Amytal

Description: a barbiturate preparation containing amylobarbitone, available as white tablets containing 50mg amylobarbitone.

Used for: severe intractable insomnia of a persistent nature for use by those patients already taking barbiturates.

Dosage: adults, 100–200mg at bedtime.

Special care: extremely dangerous, addictive drug with narrow margin of safety. Liable to abuse by overdose leading to coma and death or if combined with alcohol. Easily produces dependence and severe withdrawal symptoms. Drowsiness may persist next day affecting driving and performance of skilled tasks.

Avoid use: should be avoided if possible in all patients. Not to be used for children, young adults, pregnant and nursing mothers, elderly pesons, those with drug or alcohol related problems, patients with liver, kidney or heart disease, porphyria, insomnia where the cause is pain.

Possible interaction: alcohol, central nervous system depressant drugs, Griseofulvin, metronidazone, rifampicin, phenytoin, chloramphenicol. Anti-coagulant drugs of the coumarin type, steroid drugs including contraceptive pill.

Side effects: hangover with drowsiness, shakiness, dizziness, headache, anxiety, confusion, excitement, rash and allergic responses, gastrointestinal upsets, urine retention, loss of sexual desire.

Manufacturer: Kite.

Anafranil

Description: a TCAD containing clomipramine hydrochloride, available as capsules, syrup and in ampoules for injection. There are three strengths: yellow/caramel (10mg), orange/caramel (25mg), grey/caramel (50mg) all marked Geigy. Also **Anafranil SR** sustained release pink capsules containing 75mg, marked Geigy on one side and GD on the other. In addition, **Anafranil Syrup** containing 25mg per 5ml. Also, **Anafranil Injection**, containing 25mg per 2ml in ampoules.

Used for: depression, phobic and obsessional states.
Dosage: adults, capsules for depression, 10mg each day gradually increasing to 30–150mg (maximum 250mg) in divided doses or as a single dose at bedtime. Obsession and phobia, 25mg at first increasing to 100–150mg daily. Elderly, 10mg each day at first increasing to a maximum of 75mg. Intramuscular injection, 25mg–50mg each day increasing by 25mg to 100–150mg. Intravenous infusion, 25–50mg then about 100mg for 7–10 days.
Special care: nursing mothers, elderly, psychoses or suicidal tendencies. Persons with heart disease, liver disorders, thyroid disease (hyperthyroidism), epilepsy, diabetes, urine retention, glaucoma, tumour of the adrenal glands. Blood tests are advisable during therapy.
Avoid use: children, pregnant women, patients with heart block, heart attack, serious liver disease.
Possible interaction: MAOIs or within 14 days of their use, other antidepressant drugs, anticholinergic drugs, alcohol, adrenaline, noradrenaline (or anaesthetics containing these), antihypertensive drugs, barbiturates, cimetidine, oestrogens.
Side effects: gastrointestinal disturbances such as constipation, blurred vision, dry mouth, anxiety, drowsiness, insomnia, urine retention, sweating, tremor, disturbance of heartbeat rate, weight gain or loss. Also low blood pressure, allergic skin reactions, jaundice, loss of libido and impotence may occur. Occasionally, symptoms of schizophrenia and mania may be activated particularly in elderly persons.
Manufacturer: Geigy

Anapolon 50
Description: a preparation containing the anabolic steroid drug, oxymethalone. Available as white scored tablets containing 50mg and marked Syntex 50.
Used for: certain types of anaemia (especially aplastic anaemias and hypoplastic anaemias which have not improved after other therapy).
Dosage: children over 2 years, 2–4mg per kg of body weight daily. Adults, 2–5mg per kg of body weight in first instance reducing to half or less as condition improves. All in divided doses.
Special care: patients with diabetes, cardiac failure, enlarged prostate gland in men. Liver tests should be carried out during therapy.
Avoid use: children under 2 years, pregnant and nursing mothers, liver or kidney disease, men with breast or prostate cancer, women with breast cancer and hypercalcaemia.
Possible interaction: anticoagulant and corticosteroid drugs.

Side effects: vomiting, nausea, diarrhoea, sleeplessness, muscle cramps. Toxic effect on liver including jaundice, pruritis (itching), tumours, hepatic coma. Also oedema, congestive heart failure, masculinization in women and pre-pubertal children, loss of menstruation (amenorrhoea) in women, changes in blood, hypercalcaemia (therapy should be halted).
Manufacturer: Syntex.

Androcur
Description: an anti-androgen hormonal preparation containing cyproterone acetate, for use under hospital supervision. Available as white, scored tablets (50mg), marked BV in a hexagon.
Used for: male sexual deviation and severe hypersexuality. (Also, acne and abnormal hair growth in women, prostate cancer in men).
Dose: adult men only, 1 tablet in morning and evening after food.
Special care: patient consent is vital. Drug inhibits sperm production resulting in reversible infertility. Abnormal sperm are produced and liver tumours have been produced in animals. Ability to drive and perform skilled tasks impaired. Ineffective where hypersexuality is caused by chronic alcoholism. Special care in patients with diabetes mellitus and disorders of adrenal glands. Blood (haemoglobin) and sperm tests and monitoring of liver and adrenal gland function is advisable.
Avoid use: males under 18 years of age or those in whom bones and testes are not fully matured. Patients with thrombosis, embolism, severe liver disease, malignant or wasting diseases. Severe chronic depression.
Side effects: depression, tiredness, weight gain, breast enlargement, changes in hair growth, rarely, osteoporosis.
Manufacturer: Schering H.C.

Anectine
Description: a depolarizing muscle relaxant, the effect of which lasts for only 5 minutes and is used during anaesthesia. It is available as ampoules for injection, and contains 50mg suxamethonium chloride per ml.
Used for: muscle relaxation during anaesthesia to facilitate the insertion, e.g. of a ventilator, into the windpipe.
Dosage: according to body weight, usually 0.3–1.1mg/kg depending on degree of muscle relaxation needed.
Special care: premedication with atropine is desirable. More prolonged muscle paralysis may

occur in patients with dual block (after several doses of suxamethonium) and in those with low pseudocholinesterase enzymes in blood plasma, requiring continued artificial ventilation until normal muscle function is resumed.

Avoid use: patients with burns and those with serious liver disease.

Manufacturer: Wellcome.

Anexate

Description: an antagonist to the effects of benzodiazepines used in anaestheseia, diagnostic procedures and intensive care. It contains 100 µg of flumazenil per ml of solution and is administered by means of intravenous injection or infusion.

Used for: reversal of sedative effects of benzodiazepines in anaesthesia, intensive care and diagnostic investigations.

Dosage: by injection, 200µg given over 15 seconds. Repeated doses of 100µg at one minutes intervals if needed. Usual dose in the order of 300–600µg with a maximum of 1mg (possibly 2mg in intensive care procedures). By infusion (if drowsiness persists after initial injection), 100–400µg per hour according to patient response.

Special care: rapid injection should be avoided especially in patients who have had major surgery, head injury or liver disorders.

Avoid use: epileptic patients who have received sustained doses of benzodiazepines.

Side effects: vomiting, nausea, flushing. If wakening is too rapid patient may be anxious, agitated and fearful. Intensive care patients may have short-lived increase in heart rate and blood pressure. Rarely, convulsions may occur especially in epileptic patients.

Manufacturer: Roche.

Anhydrol Forte

Description: an anti-perspirant solution containing 20% aluminium chloride hexahydrate in an alcohol base. It is available as a solution in a bottle with a roll-on applicator.

Used for: excessive sweating (hyperhidrosis) of armpits, hands and feet.

Dosage: apply at night to dry skin and wash off the following morning. Use less as condition improves.

Special care: avoid bathing immediately before use or use of depilatory creams and shaving of armpits within 12 hours of applying. Should only be used on feet in children.

Avoid use: contact with eyes, broken or inflamed skin. Contact with clothing and jewellery.

Manufacturer: Dermal.

Anquil

Description: an antipsychotic drug available as white tablets containing 0.25mg (butyrophenone) benperidol marked Janssen, A and 0.25.

Used for: antisocial, deviant sexual behaviour.

Dosage: adults, 0.25mg to 1.5mg per day in divided doses. Elderly or debilitated patients, half adult dose.

Special care: patients with epilepsy, Parkinson's disease, heart disease, kidney or liver disorders, glaucoma, acute infections, elderly persons, pregnant or nursing mothers. Also, those with history of jaundice, underactive thyroid gland, myasthenia gravis, enlarged prostate gland. Regular blood counts and tests of liver function should be carried out during extensive therapy.

Avoid use: children, symptoms of central nervous system disturbance (pyramidal or extrapyramidal effects).

Possible interaction: alcohol, antihypertensive, antidepressant and anticonvulsive drugs, analgesic drugs, central nervous system depressants, levodopa and antidiabetic drugs.

Side effects: muscle spasms of eyes, neck, back, face, Parkinson-like symptoms (tremor and rigidity), dry mouth, nasal stiffness, irregular heartbeat, palpitations, blurring of vision, blood changes, jaundice, drowsiness, fatigue, low blood pressure, weight gain, impotence, breast enlargement, hypothermia (in elderly), constipation, rarely, fits.

Manufacturer: Janssen.

Antabuse

Description: a preparation containing the drug disulfiram, an enzyme (aldehyde dehydrogenase) inhibitor used in the treatment of alcoholism. It is available as white, scored tablets (200mg) marked ANY 200 and CP.

Used for: adjunct in therapy for alcohol dependence.

Dosage: adults, 800mg as single dose on first day. Afterwards reducing to 200–100mg over period of five days. Should not be used for longer than six months.

Special care: liver or kidney disease, respiratory disease, diabetes mellitus, epilepsy. Careful counselling of patient essential before use as reaction of disulfiram with even a minute quantity of alcohol causes extremely unpleasant and possibly fatal consequences due to accumulation of acetaldehyde in body. With small amounts of alcohol reactions include severe throbbing headache, palpitations, nausea, vomiting, raised heartbeat, flushing of face. The quantity of alcohol in many medicines may be sufficient to precipitate this. Larger quantities of alcohol can cause hypotension, heart arrhythmias and collapse. No alcohol should be consumed until one week after stopping the drug or for 24 hours prior to start of treatment.

Avoid use: patients with heart failure, coronary artery disease or high blood pressure. Children and pregnant women. Patients with severe mental disorders or suicidal tendencies.

Possible interaction: alcohol, some TCADs, paraldehyde, warfarin, barbiturate drugs, antiepileptic drugs, metronidazole (antibacterial drug).

Side effects: fatigue and drowsiness, vomiting and nausea, bad breath (halitosis), reduced libido, allergic skin reactions, liver damage. Rarely, mental disturbances (mania, paranoia, schizophrenia, depression).

Manufacturer: CP Pharmaceuticals.

Antepsin

Description: a cytoprotectant (cell-surface protectant) preparation available in the form of tablets and suspension. The tablets are scored, white, oblong in shape and contain 1g sucralfate, marked Antepsin on one side and WY39 on reverse. **Antepsin Suspension** contains 1g/5ml of solution.

Used for: gastric and duodenal ulcers, chronic gastritis, prevention of haemorrhage from stress, ulceration in patients who are seriously ill.

Dosage: tablets, adults 2g twice a day in the morning and at bedtime or 1g four times a day one hour before meals. Maximum dose 8g per day. Treatment period usually 4–6 weeks, sometimes up to 12 weeks. Prevention (prophylaxis) of stress ulceration, 1g suspension 6 times a day with a maximum of 8g daily.

Special care: patients with kidney failure, pregnancy and lactation.

Avoid use: children and patients with severe kidney failure.

Possible interaction: antibacterial drugs (ciprofloxcin, ofloxacin, norfloxacin and tetracycline), warfarin, antiepileptics (phenytoin).

Side effects: gastrointestinal upsets—constipation, diarrhoea, indigestion, nausea, dry mouth, rash, back pain, dizziness, sleeplessness, drowsiness, vertigo are possible.

Manufacturer: Wyeth.

Anthranol

Description: an ointment available in three strengths, containing 0.4%, 1% and 2% dithranol, and also 0.5% salicylic acid. Dithranol is the most potent of the preparations used in the treatment of psoriasis and must be applied with caution.

Used for: psoriasis.

Dosage: starting with low concentrations initially once a day, ointment is applied to skin lesions and washed off after ten minutes. The concentration and time period may be gradually increased (the ointment may be left on for half an hour), depending upon the response of the patient's condition.

Special care: may cause severe skin irritation in some people (especially those with fair skin) even at low concentrations hence must be used with caution. Stains clothing and skin.

Avoid use: acute psoriasis, pustular psoriasis.

Side effects: skin irritation which may be severe, burning, allergic reactions.

Manufacturer: Stiefel.

Anturan

Description: a preparation containing the active ingredient, sulphinpyrazone, which promotes the excretion of uric acid by preventing its reabsorption in the kidney tubules. Anturan is available in the form of yellow, sugar-coated tablets marked Geigy in 2 strengths, (100mg and 200mg).

Used for: hyperuricaemia (high blood levels of uric acid), chronic gout, recurrent gouty arthritis.

Dosage: adults, 100mg to 200mg with food per day at first increasing over a 2–3 week period to 600mg. After this the amount is reduced (once uric acid level has dropped) to a maintenance dose which may be as low as 200mg daily.

Special care: pregnant and breast-feeding mothers, kidney disease or heart failure. Plenty of fluids should be taken during treatment and blood and kidney function tests may be necessary.

Avoid use: children. Patients with known allergies to anti-inflammatory drugs, severe liver or kidney disease, acute gout, history of peptic ulcers or acute peptic ulcer, blood disorders, porphyria.

Possible interaction: salicylates, aspirin, hypoglycaemic drugs, anticoagulants, sulphonamides, penicillins, phenytoin, theophylline.

Side effects: gastrointestinal upset and bleeding, ulcers, acute gout, kidney stones, renal colic, liver and kidney disorders, rash, blood changes (treatment should stop).

Manufacturer: Geigy.

Anugesic H-C

Description: a preparation containing corticosteroid combined with antiseptic and soothing properties, available in the form of a cream and as suppositories. The cream contains 1.25% benzyl benzoate, 0.875% bismuth oxide, 0.5% hydrocortisone acetate, 1.85% Peru balsam, 1% pramoxine hydrochloride and 12.35% zinc oxide.

Anugesic H-C Suppositories contain 33mg benzyl benzoate, 24mg bismuth oxide, 59mg bismuth subgallate, 5mg hydrocortisone acetate, 49mg Peru balsam, 27mg pramoxine hydrochloride and 296mg zinc oxide.

Used for: haemorrhoids, anal itching and other ano-rectal disorders.

Dosage: adults, 1 suppository or application of cream morning and night and after bowel movement.

Special care: pregnant women. Avoid prolonged use—no more than 7 days.

Avoid use: children. Fungal and viral infections. Tuberculosis.

Side effects: systemic (affecting body as a whole) corticosteroid effects.

Manufacturer: Parke-Davis.

Anusol HC

Description: an astringent antiseptic with soothing properties in the form of an ointment and suppositories. The ointment contains 1.25% benzyl benzoate, 0.875 bismuth oxide, 2.25% bismuth subgallate, 0.25% hydrocortisone acetate, 1.875% Peru balsam, 10.75% zinc oxide. The suppositories contain 33mg benzyl benzoate, 24mg bismuth oxide, 59mg bismuth subgallate, 10mg hydro-cortisone acetate, 49mg Peru balsam and 296mg zinc oxide.

Used for: haemorrhoids, ano-rectal inflammation.

Dosage: adults, one application of ointment or one suppository night and morning and after bowel movement.

Special care: pregnant women. Not to be used for longer than 7 days.

Avoid use: children, patients with fungal or viral infections or suffering from tuberculosis.

Side effects: systemic (affecting whole body) corticosteroid effects.

Manufacturer: Parke-Davis.

Apisate^{CD}

Description: a preparation which combines an appetite suppressant with vitamin B. It contains the central nervous system stimulant, and sympatho-mimetic agent, diethylproprion, which should only be taken for a few days as it can cause dependence and psychiatric effects. Apisate is available in the form of two-layer yellow, sustained-release tablets marked Wyeth containing 75mg diethylproprion hydrochloride, 5mg thiamine hydrochloride, 4mg riboflavine, 2mg pyridoxine hydrochloride, 30mg nicotinamide.

Used for: patients suffering from obesity.

Dosage: adults, 1 daily in early morning or mid-afternoon.

Special care: patients with severe liver or kidney disorders, peptic ulcer, angina, heart arrhythmias, high blood pressure, enlargement of prostate gland, depression, first three months of pregnancy. May affect the performance of skilled tasks such as driving. Prolonged use should be avoided.

Avoid use: children and elderly persons, patients with a history of psychiatric illness, drug or alcohol abuse, arteriosclerosis, glaucoma, severe high blood pressure, hyperthyroidism.

Possble interaction: sympathomimetic drugs, MAOIs, psychotropic drugs, guanethidine, methyldopa, other anoretics.

Side effects: dependence and tolerance, psychiatric disorders, anxiety, insomnia, agitation and nervousness.

Manufacturer: Wyeth.

Apresoline

Description: a vasodilator available in the form of tablets of two strengths and as a powder for reconstitution for injection. It contains hydralazine hydrochloride. Yellow tablets (25mg) are sugar-coated and marked CIBA and GF, while the deep pink tablets are marked in the same way and contain 50mg. **Apresoline Injection** contains 20mg hydralazine hydrochloride as a powder in an ampoule for reconstitution.

Used for: moderate and severe chronic heart failure. Also used for moderate to severe hypertension.

Dosage: for hypertension in adults (along with ß-blocker and thiazide diuretic), 25mg twice a day at first increasing to a maximum of 200mg daily. For cardiac failure in adults (with diuretics and cardiac glycosides), 25mg 3–4 times each day increasing to 50–75mg 4 times a day every second day.

Special care: patients with coronary or cerebro-vascular disease, liver disorders, severe kidney failure, nursing mothers. Withdrawal should be gradual.

Avoid use: children, first half of pregnancy, patients with certain heart disorders (aortic, mitral stenosis, tachycardia, idiopathic SLE, constructive pericarditis, dissecting aortic aneurysm, cor pulmonale).

Possible interaction: anaesthetics, TCADs, MAOIs, antihypertensive drugs, diazoxide, CNS depressants.

Side effects: hypotension, tachycardia, angina, headache, flushes, especially with daily dose exceeding 100mg. Protein in urine, blood in urine, kidney failure, urine retention. Possible though rare, liver damage, nerve disorders and blood changes.

Manufacturer: CIBA

Aprinox

Description: a thiazide preparation which has

diuretic properties and is available as white tablets of two strengths containing 2.5mg or 5mg of bendrofluazide.

Used for: hypertension, oedema such as occurs in mild to moderate heart failure.

Dosage: adults, for oedema, 5–10mg in morning or on alternate days at first and then 5–10mg once or twice per week for maintenance. For hypertension, 2.5–5mg once each day.

Special care: pregnancy and breast-feeding, elderly persons. Patients with liver or kidney disease, liver cirrhosis, gout, diabetes, SLE. Advisable to monitor fluid, electrolytes and glucose levels.

Avoid use: children. Patients with severe liver or kidney failure, hypercalcaemia, Addisons disease, allergy to sulphonamide drugs.

Possible interaction: alcohol, opioids, barbiturates, antidiabetic drugs, NSAIDs, corticosteroids, tubocurarine, carbenoxolone, cardiac glucosides, lithium.

Side effects: metabolic disturbance and upset of electrolyte balance, gastrointestinal disturbance, blood changes, rash, dizziness, impotence, pancreatitis, anorexia.

Manufacturer: Boots.

Aramine

Description: a sympathomimetiuc amine that acts as a vasoconstrictor available as ampoules for injection containing 10mg metraminol tartrate per ml.

Used for: acute hypotension such as may occur in patients in severe shock or during general anaesthesia.

Dosage: 15–100mg according to response.

Special care: possible localized tissue death at injection site.

Avoid use: pregnancy, heart attack.

Side effects: reduced blood flow to kidneys, heart arrhythmias and tachycardia.

Manufacturer: MSD.

Aredia

Description: a preparation of the disophonate drug disodium pamidronate available as a powder for reconstitution and intravenous infusion. Vials contain 15mg or 30mg.

Used for: hypercalcaemia caused by malignancy.

Dosage: adults, depending upon levels of calcium in blood plasma, maximum dose of 90mg each treatment given by slow infusion at a rate not exceeding 30mg in two hours. Dose may be divided over 2–4 days.

Special care: severe kidney disorders, may cause convulsions due to disturbance of electrolyte balance.

Avoid use: pregnancy and breast-feeding.

Possible interaction: other infusions containing calcium disophonates, drugs for hypocalcaemia, plicamycin.

Side effects: diarrhoea, nausea, short-lived rise in body temperature, hypocalcaemia, lowering of magnesium levels, decrease in number of white blood cells (lymphocytes) in blood.

Manufacturer: CIBA

Arelix

Description: a powerful diuretic (a *loop diuretic*) which acts on the parts of the kidney tubules known as the loops of Henle. It is available as orange/green sustained release capsules containing 6mg of piretanide.

Used for: mild to moderate hypertension.

Dosage: 1 or 2 capsules taken in the morning with food.

Special care: hypokalaemia may develop and monitoring of electrolyte levels may be necessary especially in patients with impaired kidney or liver function. Also, in patients with enlarged prostate gland or impaired urination. Pregnancy and nursing mothers, persons with diabetes or gout.

Avoid use: patients with severe imbalance of electrolytes, liver cirrhosis, children.

Possible interaction: antihypertensive drugs, NSAIDs, digoxin, lithium, cephalosporin antibiotic drugs, aminoglycosides.

Side effects: electrolyte imbalance, rarely gastrointestinal upset, muscle pain after high doses.

Manufacturer: Hoechst.

Arfonad

Description: trimetaphan camsylate, a ganglion blocker, available in ampoules for injection or infusion (50mg per ml).

Used for: controlled lowering of blood pressure (hypotension) during surgery.

Dosage: by intravenous infusion at a rate of 3–4mg per minute in first instance and thereafter adjusted according to the patient's response.

Special care: patients with impaired liver or kidney function, coronary disease, cerebral vascular disease, degenerative conditions of the central nervous system, Addison's disease, reduced adrenal gland function. Also in elderly persons and patients with diabetes mellitus.

Avoid use: pregnant women, serious heart disease, severe arteriosclerosis, pyloric stenosis.

Side effects: depression of breathing (especially in combination with muscle relaxant drugs), tachycardia, dilation of pupils, increased intraocular pressure in eyes, constipation.

Manufacturer: Cambridge.

Arpicolin

Description: an anticholinergic preparation of the drug procyclidine hydrochloride available in the form of a syrup in two strengths, containing 2.5mg or 5mg per 5ml.

Used for: Parkinson's disease, including that which is drug-induced.

Dosage: 2.5mg–5mg 3 times each day at first. This is increased at 2 to 3 day intervals to a usual maximum of 30mg daily (exceptionally, 60mg).

Special care: patients with obstruction of gastrointestinal tract, enlarged prostate gland, heart disease, narrow-angle glaucoma. Drug should be withdrawn gradually.

Avoid use: children, patients with a movement disorder called tardive dyskinesia.

Possible interaction: antidepressant and anti-histamine drugs. Phenothiazines.

Side effects: anticholinergic effects, with high doses there may be mental confusion.

Manufacturer: R.P. Drugs.

Artane

Description: an anticholinergic containing benhexol hydrochloride, an antimuscarine drug used in the treatment of Parkinson's disease. White-scored tablets are available in two strengths (2mg and 5mg) coded 4434 and 4436 respectively. Both are marked Lederle.

Used for: Parkinson's disease including drug-induced Parkinson's disease.

Dosage: first day, 1mg, second day, 2mg, then increased by 2mg daily every 3 to 5 days. The maintenance dose is usually 5–15mg per day.

Special care: patients with obstruction of gastrointestinal tract, kidney or liver disease, heart disorders, enlargement of prostate gland, narrow angle glaucoma.

Avoid use: children.

Possible interaction: antihistamine and anti-depressant drugs. Phenothiazine drugs.

Side effects: anticholinergic effects. After high doses, agitation and confusion.

Manufacturer: Lederle.

Arthrotec

Description: an NSAID containing diclofenac sodium, a phenylacetic acid prostaglandin analogue. Arthrotec tablets contain 50mg diclofenac sodium, 200 μg misoprostol and are marked with a symbol and Searle 1411.

Used for: osteoarthritis, rheumatoid arthritis.

Dosage: adults, one tablet twice a day with food increasing to one three times a day if required.

Special care: women of childbearing age should use effective contraception. Patients with gastric or duodenal ulcer, heart disease, coronary, cerebro-vascular, peripheral vascular disease, kidney or liver disorders. Patients taking the drug for a long period should be monitored.

Avoid use: children, pregnant women or those planning pregnancy, breast-feeding. Patients with gastrointestinal bleeding, those with allergy to aspirin or other anti-inflammatory drugs.

Possible interaction: NSAIDs, anticoagulants, quinolone, methotrexate, digoxin, lithium, steroids, diuretic drugs, oral hypoglycaemics.

Side effects: gastrointestinal upset, erosion of gastrointestinal tract, heavy menstrual bleeding and intermenstrual bleeding, dizziness, headache, oedema, nausea, skin reactions.

Manufacturer: Searle.

Arythmol

Description: a class I antiarrhythmic drug used to treat disturbances of heart rhythm. Arythmol contains propafenone hydrochloride and is available in tablets of two strengths (150 and 300mg) which are white, scored and film-coated.

Used for: treatment and prevention of ventricular arrhythmias.

Dosage: adults, 150mg 3 times daily in first instance, gradually increasing at 3-day intervals to 300mg twice a day. Maximum dose is 300mg 3 times a day.

Special care: patients with heart failure or who are fitted with pacemakers, those with liver or kidney disorders, elderly persons.

Avoid use: children, pregnant women, some particular forms of heart rhythm disturbance, patients with uncontrolled congestive cardiac failure, electrolyte balance disturbances, obstructive lung disease, severe hypotension, myasthenia gravis.

Possible interaction: other class I antiarrhythmic drugs, myocardial (heart muscle) depressant drugs, warfarin, digoxin, cimetidine rifampicin, propranolol, metoprolol.

Side effects: gastrointestinal upset including constipation, diarrhoea, vomiting, nausea, unpleasant bitter taste, fatigue, headache, allergic skin rashes, disturbances of heart rhythm.

Manufacturer: Knoll.

Asacol

Description: a preparation of the salicylate drug, mesalazine, available as tablets and suppositories. Tablets (400mg strength) are oblong, red and resin-coated. Suppositories are available in two strengths containing 250mg and 500mg. Also, **Asacol foam enema** is available.

Used for: to induce and maintain remission in ulcerative colitis and to treat acute attacks of this condition.

Dosage: adults, tablets, acute attack, 6 daily in divided doses. For maintenance, 3–6 tablets daily in divided doses. Asacol suppositories, adults 750–1500mg daily in divided doses with last dose at night.

Special care: elderly persons, pregnant and nursing mothers, patients with kidney disease, elevated blood urea levels, proteinuria.

Avoid use: children, patients with severe kidney disease.

Possible interaction: lactulose, substance which increases acidity of motions.

Side effects: gastrointestinal upset, blood changes, headache, kidney failure.

Manufacturer: S.K. & F.

Asendis

Description: a TCAD preparation containing amoxapine, available in tablets of various strength, all seven-sided, scored tablets: 25mg, white, marked LL25; 50mg, orange, marked LL50; 100mg, blue, marked LL100 and 150mg, white, marked LL150.

Used for: depression.

Dosage: 100–150mg per day at first increasing to a maintenance dose in the region of 150–250mg. Maximum daily dose is 300mg. Elderly persons, 25mg twice a day at first increasing, after 5–7 days, to 50mg 3 times daily if required.

Special care: patients with psychoses or suicidal tendencies, elderly persons, pregnant and nursing mothers, people with cardiac disorders, epilepsy, hyperthyroidism, urine retention, closed angle glaucoma, liver disease, tumours of adrenal gland, diabetes.

Avoid use: children, patients with recent heart attack, heart arrhythmias, heart block, porphyria (rare blood disorder).

Possible interaction: alcohol, barbiturate drugs, local anaesthetics (containing adrenaline or nor-adrenaline), antihypertensive and sympathomimetic drugs, anticholineric drugs, cimetidine, oestrogens.

Side effects: anticholinergic effects including urine retention, dry mouth, constipation, blurred vision, rapid heartbeat, palpitations, nervousness, insomnia, sweating, dizziness, fatigue, weight changes, jaundice, blood changes, allergic skin rashes, changes in libido, breast enlargement and impotence.

Manufacturer: Novex.

Aspav

Description: a combined salicylate and opiate analgesic containing aspirin and papaveretum available as dissolvable tablets. Aspav white tablets contain 500mg aspirin, 10mg papaveretum.

Used for: relief of postoperative pain and chronic pain caused by inoperable cancers.

Dosage: adults, 1–2 tablets in water every four to six hours. Maximum daily dose, 8 tablets in 24 hours.

Special care: women in labour, pregnant women and nursing mothers, elderly persons. Patients with head injury, liver or kidney disease, gastrointestinal ulcers, heart failure, hypothyroidism, history of bronchospasm or allergy to anti-inflammatory drugs.

Avoid use: children, patients in comatose states with depressed breathing, or obstructed airways.

Possible interaction: central nervous system depressants, NSAIDs, anticoagulants, MAOIs, sulphonamide antibiotics, hypoglycaemic drugs, uric acid-lowering drugs, methotrexate.

Side effects: allergic responses, asthma, bleeding of gastrointestinal tract, confusion, nausea, constipation.

Manufacturer: Roussel.

Atarax

Description: an antihistamine preparation containing hydroxyzine hydrochloride available as sugar-coated tablets of two strengths (10 and 25mg) coloured orange and green respectively and in the form of a syrup. **Atarax Syrup** contains 10mg hydroxyzine hydrochloride per 5ml.

Used for: anxiety (short-term treatment) and itching caused by an allergy (chronic urticaria and dermatitis).

Dosage: anxiety, adults only, 50–100mg 4 times each day. Itching, adults, 25mg taken at night increasing to 25mg 3–4 times a day if required. Children, 6 months to 6 years, 5–15mg daily increasing to 50mg in divided doses if required; 6 years and over, 15–25mg daily increasing to 50–100mg in divided doses if required.

Special care: patients with kidney disease. Patients must be warned that judgement and dexterity is impaired. Children should be given reduced doses for itching only.

Avoid use: pregnant women.

Possible interaction: central nervous system depressants, alcohol.

Side effects: drowsiness, anticholinergic effects, if high doses are taken there may be involuntary muscle movements.

Manufacturer: Pfizer.

Ativan

Description: an anxiolytic benzodiazepine, lorazepam, which is for short-term use only as it carries a risk of dependency. It is available as tablets of two strengths and also in the form of ampoules for injection. Blue, oblong, scored tablets, marked A1 contain 1mg and yellow, oblong, scored tablets, marked A2.5 contain 2.5mg. **Ativan injection** contains 4mg lorazepam per ml.

Used for: anxiety, status epilepticus (a condition where a person with epilepsy suffers a series of fits in close succession and is deprived of oxygen), a sedative premedication prior to full anaesthesia.

Dosage: tablets, adults, for anxiety, 1–4mg each day in divided doses. Elderly persons, 0.5mg–2mg each day. For status epilepticus, adults, 4mg by intravenous injection, children half the adult dose. For premedication, adults, tablets, 2–4mg 1 or 2 hours prior to operation or 0.05mg per kg of body weight intravenously about 30–45 minutes before operation.

Special care: women in labour, pregnancy, breast-feeding, elderly, liver or kidney disorders, lung disease. Short-term use only, withdraw gradually.

Avoid use: children, acute lung diseases, depression of breathing, those with chronic psyc‌ es, obsessional states and phobias.

Possible interaction: CNS depressant drugs, alcohol, anticonvulsants.

Side effects: light-headedness, drowsiness, vertigo, confusion, unsteadiness in walking, gastrointestinal upset, disturbance of vision, rash, retention of urine, changes in libido, low blood pressure. Rarely, blood changes and jaundice. Risk of dependence especially with high doses.

Manufacturer: Wyeth.

Atromid-S

Description: an isobutyric acid derivative which lowers the concentration of cholesterol and other fats (lipids) found in blood plasma. It is available as red, gelatin-coated capsules, marked ICI, containing 500mg of clofibrate.

Used for: elevated plasma lipid levels (hyperlipidaemias) of types IIb, III, IV and V which have not been lowered by dietary changes or other appropriate treatments.

Dosage: adults, 20–30mg per kg of body weight two to three times daily after meals in divided doses.

Special care: patients with low levels of albumin (protein) in blood serum. Regular blood checks may be carried out.

Avoid use: children, pregnant women, patients with diseases of the gall bladder, liver or kidney disorders.

Possible interaction: hypoglycaemics, phenytoin, anticoagulants.

Side effects: gastrointestinal upset, muscle pains, gallstones.

Manufacturer: Zeneca.

Atrovent

Description: an anticholinergic containing ipratropium bromide available available in various forms: aerosol inhalation, 20 µg per dose delivered by metered dose inhaler; **Atrovent Autohaler**, 20 µg per dose delivered by breath-actuated metered dose aerosol; **Atrovent Forte**, 40 µg per dose delivered by metered dose inhaler; **Atrovent Solution**, 250 µg per ml, in preservative-free isotonic solution in unit dose vials for use with nebulizer.

Used for: severe obstruction of airways, especially that caused by chronic bronchitis.

Dosage: adults, inhaler, 1–2 puffs three or four times a day. Children under 6 years, one puff, 6–12 years, 1–2 puffs, both three times a day. Adults, Atrovent Forte, 1 or 2 puffs three to four times daily; children 6–12 years, 1 puff three times daily. Adults, Atrovent solution, 0.4–2ml nebulised up to four times each day. Children over 3 years, 0.4–2ml nebulised up to three times each day.

Special care: patients with enlarged prostate gland (prostate hypertrophy), glaucoma.

Side effects: urine retention, constipation, dry mouth.

Manufacturer: Boehringer Ingelheim.

Audicort

Description: a combined antibacterial, antifungal and anti-inflammatory (corticosteroid) preparation available in the form of ear drops. Audicort contains 1mg triamcinolone acetate and neomycin undecylenate (antibiotic) (equivalent to 3.5mg neomycin base).

Used for: chronic and acute inflammation and/or bacterial infection of the outer ear.

Dosage: adults, 2–5 drops three of four times each day.

Special care: pregnant and nursing mothers avoid prolonged use.

Avoid use: children, patients with perforated ear drum.

Side effects: localized irritation, additional infection.

Manufacturer: Lederle.

Augmentin

Description: a broad-spectrum, penicillin-like antibiotic, amoxycillin as the trihydrate, with clavulanic acid as the potassium salt. The latter makes the antibiotic effective against a wider range of infections by combating certain enzymes produced by some bacteria. Available as white film coated tablets, Augmentin 375mg (250mg/125mg) and 625mg (500mg/125mg). Also, **Augmentin Dispersible** (250mg/125mg), white tablets marked Augmentin. Also **Augmentin Suspension 125/31 SF** (sugar-free) contains 125mg amoxycillin as trihydrate, 31mg clavulanic acid as potassium salt, per 5 ml when reconstituted with water. Similarly, **Augmentin Suspension 250/62 SF** (250/62mg). **Augmentin Intravenous** is a powder for intravenous injection available in 2 strengths containing amoxycillin as sodium salt and clavulanic acid as potassium salt (500/100mg, and 1g/200mg).

Used for: respiratory tract and ear, nose and throat infections, skin and soft tissue infections, urinary tract infections.

Dosage: adults, tablets, 375mg three times a day (severe infections 625mg) for 14 days. Children, use suspension, under 6 years use lower strength 125/31. Under one year 25mg per kg body weight each day; 1–6 years, 5ml three times a day for 14 days. 6–12 years use 250/62 suspension, 5ml 3 times each day for 14 days.

Intravenous injection: adults, 1.2g or by intermittent infusion 6 to 8-hourly for 14 days. Children, under 3 months, 30mg per kg of body weight every 12 hours in newborns increasing to every 8 hours in older infants. 3 months–12 years, 30mg per kg of body weight every 8 or 6 hours. By intravenous or intermittent infusion for up to 14 days.

Special care: pregnant and breast-feeding mothers, patients with liver and kidney disease, glandular fever. Review after 14 days.

Avoid use: allergy to penicillin.

Side effects: gastrointestinal upset, allergic responses, rarely cholestatic jaundice, hepatitis, phlebitis at site of injection.

Manufacturer: Beecham.

Aureocort

Description: a combined antibacterial and steroid preparation available in the form of cream or ointment, containing 0.1% of the corticosteroid triamcinolone acetonide and 3% of the tetracycline antibiotic, chlortetracycline hydrochloride.

Used for: inflammation and irritation of the skin where infection is present also.

Dosage: apply sparingly to affected skin two or three times daily.

Special care: limit use to a short time period. In children and on face, treatment should not exceed 5 days.

Avoid use: on extensive areas of skin or for long time periods or for prevention. Acne (including rosacea), urticaria, scabies, leg ulcers, viral skin infections, tuberculosis, ringworm.

Side effects: thinning of skin and skin changes, adrenal gland suppression, fluid retention.

Manufacturer: Lederle.

Aureomycin

Description: a broad-spectrum antibiotic preparation, containing chlortetracycline hydrochloride, available as cream and ointment both of which contain 3% chlortetracycline hydrochloride. Aureomycin is also available as an eye ointment containing 1% tetracycline hydrochloride.

Used for: superficial skin infections with bacterial origin. Eye infections sensitive to tetracycline.

Dosage: skin infections, apply on gauze once or twice daily. Eye infections, apply into eye every two hours then reduce frequency as condition improves. Continue to use for 48 hours after symptoms have disappeared.

Avoid use: Possible interaction:

Side effects: additional infections.

Manufacturer: Lederle.

Aventyl

Description: a TCAD, nortripyline hydrochloride, available in capsules of two strengths: white/yellow capsules coded H17 (10mg) and white/yellow capsules coded H19 (25mg). All marked Lilly.

Used for: depression and also bed-wetting in children.

Dosage: depression, adults, 20–40mg each day in divided doses increasing to 100mg daily if necessary. Usual maintenance is in the order of 30–75mg. Elderly persons, 10mg three times daily. Bed-wetting in children over six years, 10–35mg 30 minutes before bedtime.

Special care: patients with heart disease, tumours of adrenal gland, enlarged thyroid gland, liver disease, diabetes, epilepsy, glaucoma, urine retention. Persons with psychoses or suicidal tendencies. Also, in nursing mothers.

Avoid use: children under six years, pregnant women, serious liver disease, heart attack, heart block.

Possible interaction: other antidepressants, MAOIs, alcohol, barbiturates, local anaesthetics containing adrenaline or noradrenaline, anticholinergics, antihypertensives, oestrogens, cimetidine.

Side effects: constipation, urine retention, dry mouth, blurred vision, raised heartbeat, palpitations, insomnia, anxiety, drowsiness, tremor, sweating, dizziness, fatigue, unsteadiness, weight changes, low blood pressure. Allergic skin rashes, blood changes, jaundice, heart arrhythmias, changes in libido, impotence. Mania and schizophrenic symptoms may be activated especially in elderly persons.

Manufacturer: Eli Lilly.

Avloclor

Description: an antimalarial drug containing chloroquine phosphate, available as white, scored tablets containing 250mg chloroquine phosphate.

Used for: prevention and treatment of malaria, rheumatoid arthritis, lupus erythematosus (inflammatory disease of skin and some internal organs), amoebic hepatitis.

Dosage: prevention of malaria; adults, 2 tablets as one dose on the same day each week commmencing 2 weeks before entering affected area and continuing for 4 weeks after leaving. Children should take in the same way at a dose rate of 5mg per kg of body weight. Treatment of hepatitis, adults only, four tablets each day for two days then one tablet twice daily for two to three weeks.

Special care: pregnancy, liver or kidney disease, breast-feeding, patients with epilepsy and some other neurological conditions, psoriasis, porphyria, severe gastrointestinal disorders. Regular eye tests may be needed during treatment.

Side effects: gastrointestinal upset, headache, hair loss, loss of pigment, skin rashes, blurred vision, opacity of cornea, retinal damage.

Manufacturer: Zeneca.

Axid

Description: a preparation containing nizatidine (an H_2 blocker) available in the form of capsules: pale, yellow/dark yellow, coded 3144 (150mg) and yellow/brown coded 3145 (300mg). **Axid Injection** contains 25mg nizatidine per ml.

Used for: duodenal and benign gastric ulcers and their prevention. Gastro-oesophageal reflux disease.

Dosage: adults, for duodenal and gastric ulcers, 300mg taken in the evening or 150mg morning and evening for 4–8 weeks. Prevention, 150mg in evening for up to one year. Adults, for gastro-oesophageal reflux disease, 150mg–300mg twice a day for up to 12 weeks. Axid injection, adults, dilute before use, 100mg by slow intravenous injection three times each day or 10mg per hour by intravenous infusion. Maximum 480mg per day.

Special care: patients with liver or kidney disease, pregnant or breast-feeding mothers.

Avoid use: children.

Possible interaction: salicylates.

Side effects: sweating, **sleepiness, itchiness,** headache, muscle and joint pain, jaundice, raised levels of liver enzymes, hepatitis, anaemia.

Manufacturer: Lilly.

Axsain

Description: a topical counter-irritant analgesic preparation available as a cream containing 0.075% capsaicin.

Used for: post-herpetic neuralgia.

Dosage: adults only, massage in 3 to 4 times daily once lesions have healed.

Avoid use: children, on broken, irritated skin.

Side effects: local skin irritation.

Manufacturer: Euroderma.

Azactam

Description: a powder for injection and infusion, containing 500mg aztreonam available as 1g or 2g powder in vials.

Used for: serious infections caused by Gram-negative bacteria, including those of the lower respiratory tract and lung infections in cystic fibrosis sufferers. Also, soft tissue, skin, joint, bone, gynaecological and abdominal infections. Urinary tract infections and gonorrhoea, meningitis (where *H. influenzae* or *N. Menigitidis* is the causal organism), septicaemia and bacteraemia (bacteria in blood indicating infection).

Dosage: adults, 1g by intramuscular or intravenous injection every eight hours or 2g intravenously every 12 hours. If infection is severe, 2g six to eight hourly intravenously. Maximum daily dose is 8g. For urinary tract infections, 0.5–1g intramuscularly or intravenously every eight to twelve hours. For cystitis, 1g intramuscularly as a single dose. Children, one week to two years, 30mg per kg of body weight every six to eight hours. Severe infections in children over two years, 50mg per kg of body weight every six to eight hours. Maximum dose is 8g each day.

Special care: patients with allergy to penicillin or cephalospoin. Persons with kidney or liver disease.

Avoid use: children under one year, pregnant or breast-feeding mothers.

Side effects: gastrointestinal upset, vomiting and diarrhoea, local skin inflammation at injection site.

Manufacturer: Squibb.

Azamune

Description: an immunosuppressant, cytotoxic preparation containing azathioprine available as yellow, scored tablets marked AZA 50 (50mg).

Used for: to lessen the likelihood of rejection following organ transplants and donor skin grafts. Also, some autoimmune diseases.

Dosage: adults and children, following transplant, 5mg per kg of body weight at first then 1–4mg per kg of body weight each day for 3 months in divided doses. For chronic hepatitis, 1–1.5mg per kg of body weight daily. Autoimmune diseases, 2–2.5mg per kg of body weight daily.

Special care: Azathioprine causes suppression of bone marrow function, hence careful monitoring of blood count for toxic effects is necessary and dosage must be adjusted accordingly. Pregnant women, patients with over-exposure to sun, any infection, kidney disorders.

Avoid use: toxic hepatitis, stoppage of bile flow.

Possible interaction: muscle relaxant drugs, cytostatics, allopurinol.

Side effects: bone marrow suppression, liver toxicity, gastrointestinal upset, rashes.

Manufacturer: Penn Pharmaceuticals.

B

Bactrim

Description: a preparation combining an antibacterial sulphonamide with a folic acid inhibitor. Elongated, orange, film-coated capsules marked Roche contain 80mg trimethoprim and 400mg sulphamethoxazole. Also, **Bactrim Dispersible**: yellow tablets, scored, containing 480mg co-trimoxazole.

Bactrim Double Strength: white scored tablets containing 160mg trimethoprim and 800mg sulphmethoxazole and marked Roche 800 and 160. **Bactrim Adult Suspension** is a yellow syrup containing 480mg co-trimoxazole per 5ml and **Bactrim Paediatric Syrup** contains 40mg trimethoprim and 200mg sulphmethoxazole per 5ml (sugar-free and fruit-flavoured).

Used for: urinary tract infections, infections of joints, bones and skin, gastrointestinal and respiratory tract.

Dosage: adults, ordinary strength tablets, 1–3 tablets twice each day; children 6 to 12 years, 1 twice a day. Children under 6 years use paediatric syrup. Six weeks to 5 months, 2.5ml; 6 months to 5 years, 5ml. Six to 12 years, 10ml, all doses twice each day. Adults, double strength tablets, $^1/_2$ to $1^1/_2$ tablets twice each day.

Special care: breast-feeding, elderly, kidney disease (reduce dose, increase interval between doses). Regular blood tests should be carried out.

Avoid use: children under 6 weeks, pregnant women, patients with severe kidney or liver disease or blood changes.

Possible interaction: antidiabetics, anticoagulants, antiepileptic drugs, antimalarial drugs, cyclosporin, cytotoxics, folate inhibitors.

Side effects: vomiting, nausea, blood changes, skin rashes, inflammation of the tongue (glossitis), folate (folic acid) deficiency. Rarely, Lyell syndrome, erythema multiformae (circular red patches on skin).

Manufacturer: Roche

Bactroban

Description: a broad-spectrum antibiotic preparation containing 2% mupirocin in the form of an ointment. **Bactroban Nasal** is an ointment containing 2% mupirocin in a soft white paraffin base.

Used for: bacterial skin infections. Nasal ointment, infections of the nose and nostrils caused by staphlocci bacteria.

Dosage: ointment, apply to skin 3 times a day for up to 10 days. Nasal ointment, apply to the inner surface of nostrils 2 or 3 times daily.

Special care: patients with kidney disorders, avoid eyes.

Side effects: may sting on application.

Manufacturer: Beecham.

Bambec

Description: a preparation containing bambuterol hydrochloride which is a selective ß$_2$-agonist used in the treatment of asthma. Bambec is available as tablets of 2 strengths containing 10mg (marked A/BA) and 20mg (marked A/BM). Tablets are oval, white and scored.

Used for: asthma (bronchospasm) and reversible airways obstruction.

Dosage: 10mg as one dose taken at night increasing to 20mg once a day if necessary. If the patient has been used to treatment with a ß$_2$–agonist, then 20mg may be taken from the start.

Special care: pregnant women and breast-feeding mothers, diabetics, moderate or severe kidney disorders, heart disorders, thyrotoxicosis. In cases of severe asthma, potassium levels in blood should be monitored.

Avoid use: children.

Possible interaction: Other ß-blockers, suxamethonium.

Side effects: headache, palpitations, cramps, tremor, hypokalaemia.

Manufacturer: Astra.

Baratol

Description: an antihypertensive, alpha-adrenoreceptor blocking drug, indoramin hydrochloride, available in 2 strengths, blue tablets

(25mg, marked MPL020 and 25) and green tablets (50mg, marked MPL 021 and 50). Both are film-coated and scored.

Used for: hypertension (high blood pressure).

Dosage: adults, 25mg twice each day at start increasing by 25mg or 50mg each fortnight. Maximum dose is 200mg per day in 2 or 3 divided doses.

Special care: patients with liver or kidney disorders, Parkinson's disease, epilepsy, history of depression. Patients with incipient heart failure should be treated with digoxin and diuretics. Performance of skilled tasks such as driving may be impaired.

Avoid use: children, cardiac failure.

Possible interaction: alcohol, antihypertensive drugs, MAOIs.

Side effects: drowsiness, dizziness, depression, dry mouth, blocked nose, weight gain, failure to ejaculate.

Manufacturer: Monmouth.

Baxan

Description: a cephalosporin antibiotic preparatiton available as tablets and as powder for reconstitution with water, in 3 strengths. Baxan white capsules contain 500mg cefadroxil (as monohydrate) and are marked 7244. **Baxan Suspension** contains either 125mg, 250mg or 500mg per 5ml when reconstituted with water, available as powder to make 60ml.

Used for: various infections of skin, urinary and respiratory tracts, ear and soft tissues.

Dosage: adults, 500mg–1g twice each day (1 to 2 tablets); children under 1 year, 25mg per kg of body weight in divided doses; 1 to 6 years, 250mg twice each day; 6 years and over, 500mg twice each day.

Special care: patients with penicillin allergy or kidney disease.

Avoid use: cephalosporin allergy, porphyria.

Possible interaction: some diuretics.

Side effects: gastrointestinal upset, allergic responses.

Manufacturer: Bristol-Myers.

Baycaron

Description: a thiazide-like diuretic preparation, mefruside, available as white scored tablets marked Bayer and L/1 (strength 25mg).

Used for: oedema and hypertension.

Dosage: 1-2 tablets as a single dose taken in the morning for 10-14 days, then 1 daily or on alternate days for maintenance. Maximum dose for oedema is 4 tablets daily.

Special care: elderly, pregnancy and breast-feeding, liver or kidney disease, gout, diabetes, liver cirrhosis. Fluid, electrolytes and glucose levels should be monitored.

Avoid use: children, patients with liver or kidney failure, Addison's disease, hypercalcaemia, sensitivity to sulphonamide drugs.

Possible interaction: alcohol, opioids, barbiturates, NSAIDs, antidiabetic drugs, tubocurarine, lithium, corticosteroids, cardiac glycosides, carbenoxolone.

Side effects: gastrointestinal upset, rash, blood changes, disturbance of electrolyte levels and metabolism, dizziness, sensitivity to light, pancreatitis, anorexia, impotence.

Manufacturer: Bayer.

Beclazone

Description: a corticosteroid preparation containing either 50 or 100µg beclomethasone dipropionate per dose, delivered by metered dose aerosol. Also **Beclazone 250**, containing 250µg per metered dose.

Used for: chronic reversible obstructive airways disease (asthma).

Dosage: adults, 100µg 3 to 4 times each day. If very severe, 600–800µg (maximum 1g) in divided doses each day. Children, 50–100µg 2 to 4 times each day. Beclazone 250, adults only, 500µg twice each day or 250µg 4 times each day. This may be increased to 1500–2000µg each day in divided doses if required.

Special care: pulmonary tuberculosis, pregnant women, patients who have been taking systemic steroid drugs.

Side effects: hoarseness, fungal infections of throat and mouth.

Manufacturer: Baker Norton.

Becloforte

Description: a corticosteroid preparation in a variety of forms for inhalation containing 250µg beclomethasone dipropionate per dose delivered by metered dose aerosol. **Becloforte VM** is available as a pack consisting of 2 Becloforte inhalers and Volumatic. Also, **Becloforte Diskhaler** consisting of blisters containing 400µg beclomethasone dipropionate per dose delivered by breath-actuated inhaler.

Used for: patients with chronic and severe asthma, emphysema or chronic bronchitis who require high doses of Beclomethasone.

Dosage: adults only, 500µg twice each day or 250µg 4 times a day. May be increased to 500µg 3 or 4 times each day if necessary. Diskhaler, adults, 2 blisters each day.

Special care: pregnancy, patients with active or quiescent pulmonary tuberculosis, those transferring from systemic steroids.

Avoid use: children.
Side effects: hoarseness, fungal infections of throat and mouth.
Manufacturer: A & H.

Becodisks

Description: a corticosteroid preparation available as a dry powder for inhalation with Diskhaler. Beige disks contain 100µg beclomethasone dipropionate; brown disks contain 200µg; light brown disks contain 400µg.
Used for: bronchial asthma.
Dosage: adults, 400µg twice each day or 200µg 3 to 4 times each day. Children, 100µg 2 to 4 times each day or 200µg twice each day.
Special care: pregnant women, patients with active or quiescent pulmonary tuberculosis, those transferring from systemic steroids.
Side effects: hoarseness, fungal infections of throat and mouth.
Manufacturer: A & H.

Becotide

Description: a corticosteroid preparation, beclomethasone diproprionate, available in the form of an aerosol of different strengths for inhalation. Becotide-50 (50µg per metered inhalation), Becotide-100 (100µg) and Becotide-200 (200µg).
Used for: bronchial asthma.
Dosage: adults, 400µg each day in 2, 3 or 4 divided doses. If asthma is severe, 600–800µg may be required in first instance in daily divided doses. This should be reduced as condition improves. Children, 400µg twice each day using Becotide-50 or 100 only.
Special care: pregnant women, patients with active or quiescent pulmonary tuberculosis, those transferring from systemic steroids.
Side effects: hoarseness, fungal infections of throat and mouth.
Manufacturer: A & H.

Becotide Rotacaps

Description: a corticosteroid preparation, beclomethasone diproprionate, available as a dry powder in capsules for inhalation: buff/clear (100µg), brown (200µg), dark brown/clear (400µg), all marked with name and strength and each is a single dose for use with a Rotahaler.
Used for: bronchial asthma.
Dosage: adults, 400µg twice each day or 200µg 3 or 4 times each day. Children, 100µg 2 or 4 times each day or 200µg twice each day.
Special care: pregnant women, patients with active

or quiescent pulmonary tuberculosis, those transferring from systemic steroids.
Side effects: hoarseness, fungal infections of throat and mouth.
Manufacturer: A & H.

Benemid

Description: a uricosuric preparation (one which enhances the excretion of uric acid from the kidneys), available as white, scored tablets containing 500mg probenecid, and marked MSD 501.
Used for: gout, hyperuricaemia (elevated uric acid levels in blood). Also, with certain antibiotics (e.g. penicillin) to prolong their effects and maintain high blood levels. This occurs because excretion of the antibiotic is inhibited.
Dosage: for gout and hyperuricaemia, half a tablet twice a day for 1 week then 1 twice daily. Adults, with certain antibiotics, 4 tablets daily in divided doses. Children over 2 years, with antibiotics, 25mg per kg of body weight, then 40mg per kg each day in divided doses.
Special care: pregnancy, elderly, history of peptic ulcer or kidney disorders. Plenty of fluids should be taken.
Avoid use: children under 2 years, patients during acute attack of gout (the start of treatment should be delayed), uric acid stones in kidneys, blood changes.
Possible interaction: ß lactam antibiotics, methotextrate, indomethacin, sulphonamides, salicylates, pyrazinamide, sulphonylureas.
Side effects: gastrointestinal upset, headache, sore gums, flushes, frequency of urination, hypersensitivity, kidney colic, kidney stones, acute gout.
Manufacturer: M & D.

Berotec 100

Description: a proprietary bronchodilator and short-acting ß2-agonist that acts rapidly to relax smooth muscle in the walls of the airways and relieves symptoms for about 3 to 6 hours. Berotec is produced in the form of an aerosol of 2 strengths or as a solution for use with a nebulizer, for inhalation. Berotec 100 contains 0.1mg fenoterol hydrobromide per metered dose inhalation. **Berotec 200** contains 0.2mg per metered dose inhalation. **Berotec Nebulizer** solution contains 0.5% fenoterol hydrobromide.
Used for: reversible obstruction of airways as in bronchial asthma, emphysema and bronchitis.
Dosage: adults, aerosol starting with lower strength (100), 1 to 2 puffs up to 3 times each day with a

maximum of 2 puffs every 6 hours. Berotec 200, 1 to 2 puffs up to 3 times each day with a maximum of 2 puffs every 6 hours. Nebulized solution, 0.5–1.25mg us to 4 times a day with strength adjusted as necessary by dilution with sterile sodium chloride solution. Children, lower strength 100 aerosol, over 6 years of age, 1 puff up to 3 times each day with a maximum of 2 puffs every 6 hours. Berotec 200 and nebulizer solution should not be given to children under 16 years of age.

Special care: pregnant women, patients with hypertension, heart arrhythmias, heart disorders, angina, hyperthyroidism.

Avoid use: children under 6 years.

Possible interaction: sympathomimetic drugs.

Side effects: headache, dilation of blood vessels in skin, nervousness.

Manufacturer: Boehringer Ingelheim.

Beta-Adalat

Description: a cardio-selective ß-blocker/Class II calcium antagonist containing atenolol and nifedipine available as red-brown capsules marked with the Bayer cross and name and containing 50mg atenolol and 20mg nifedipine.

Used for: hypertension, angina (where therapy with a calcium-channel blocker or beta-blocker alone proves to be ineffective).

Dosage: for hypertension, 1 capsule each day increasing to 2 if required. Elderly persons, 1 capsule. Angina, 1 capsule twice each day.

Special care: weak heart, liver or kidney disease, diabetes, anaesthesia.

Avoid use: children, pregnancy, breast-feeding, heart block, heart shock or heart failure.

Possible interaction: cardiac depressant drugs, cimetidine, quinidine.

Side effects: headache, dizziness, flushing, dryness of eyes, skin rashes, oedema, swelling of gums, allergic jaundice.

Manufacturer: Bayer.

Beta Cardone

Description: a non-cardioselective ß-blocker, sotalol hydrochloride, available as tablets in 3 strengths: green-scored tablets marked Evans/BC4 (40mg) ; pink-scored tablets marked Evans/BC8 (80mg) and white-scored tablets marked Evans/BC20 (200mg).

Used for: heart arrhythmias, angina, hypertension and as an additional therapy for thyrotoxicosis.

Dosage: heart arrhythmias, 40mg 3 times daily for 7 days increasing to 120–240mg each day either all at once or in divided doses. Angina, 80mg twice each

day in first instance for 1 week to 10 days, increasing to 200–600mg daily either all at once or in divided doses. Hypertension, 80mg twice each day in first instance for 1 week to 10 days, increasing to 200–600 mg daily, either all at once or in divided doses. Thyrotoxicosis, 120–240 mg each day as a single amount or in divided doses.

Special care: patients with diabetes, liver or kidney disorders, those undergoing general anaesthesia (drug may need to be stopped). Pregnant women and nursing mothers. Patients with weak hearts may need to be treated with digitalis and diuretic drugs.

Avoid use: children, patients with asthma or history of bronchospasm, those with heart block, heart attack, heart shock and some other cardiac disorders. Drug should be stopped gradually.

Possible interaction: verapamil, clonidine withdrawal, hyperglycaemics, class I anti-arrhythmic drugs, some anaesthetics, reserpine, sympathomimetics, antidepressants, ergotamine, indomethacin, cimetidine.

Side effects: slow heartbeat, disruption of sleep, cold hands and feet, fatigue in exercise, gastrointestinal upset, wheezing, heart failure, skin rash, dry eyes (withdraw drug gradually).

Manufacturer: Evans.

Betagan

Description: a ß-blocker in the form of eye drops containing 0.5% levobunolol hydrochloride and 1.4% polyvinyl alcohol, and as single dose units.

Used for: chronic simple open-angle glaucoma, reduction of intraocular pressure.

Dose: adults, 1 drop once or twice each day.

Special care: patients with breathing disorders, breast-feeding mothers, diabetics.

Avoid use: children, patients with asthma, pregnant women, those with various heart disorders including heart block, heart failure, heart shock, slow heartbeat, history of obstructive lung disease.

Possible interaction: ß-blockers, reserpine.

Side effects: local allergic irritation or dry eyes, respiratory difficulties, dizziness, headache, ß-blocker effects.

Manufacturer: Allergan.

Beta-Prograne

Description: a non-cardioselective ß-blocker produced in the form of sustained-release capsules which are white and contain 160mg propranolol hydrochloride. Also available, **Half Beta-Prograne** white sustained-release capsules containing 80mg propranolol hydrochloride.

Used for: angina, high blood pressure, as additional

therapy for overactive thyroid gland (thyrotoxicosis), prevention of migraine.

Dosage: angina, 80–160mg each day increasing to a maximum of 240mg if needed. Hypertension, 160mg each day increasing to 320mg by 80mg each day if necessary. Thyrotoxicosis, 80mg to 160mg each day increasing to 240mg if necessary. Prevention of migraine, 80mg–160mg each day increasing to 240mg if necessary.

Special care: pregnancy and lactation, diabetes, liver or kidney disease, metabolic acidosis, those undergoing general anaesthesia, patients with weak hearts should be treated with digitalis and diuretics. The drug should be stopped gradually.

Avoid use: children, patients with various heart disorders including heart shock, heart block, heart failure, asthma.

Possible interaction: some anaesthetics, antidiabetic drugs, antihypertensives, sympathomimetics, sedatives, indomethacin, reserpine, class I antiarrhythmics, verapamil, clonidine withdrawal.

Side effects: disturbance of sleep, cold feet and hands, slow heartbeat rate, fatigue with exercise, wheezing, heart failure, gastrointestinal disorders; dry eyes or skin rash (gradually withdraw drug).

Manufacturer: Tillomed.

Betaloc

Description: a cardioselective ß-blocker, metaprolol tartrate, available as tablets of 2 strengths, as modified-release tablets and in ampoules for injection. Betaloc tablets are white, scored and contain 50mg (marked A/BB) or 100mg (marked A/ME). Also, **Betaloc-SA** modified-release tablets (Durules®), containing 200mg and marked AMD. Also, **Betaloc Injection** containing 1mg per ml in 5ml ampoules.

Used for: heart arrhythmias, angina, maintenance therapy in heart attack, hypertension, additional therapy in thyrotoxicosis, prevention of migraine.

Dosage: heart attack, 200mg each day; heart arrhythmias, 50mg 2 or 3 times each day increasing to maximum daily dose of 300mg. Angina, 50–100mg twice or three times each day. Hypertension, 50mg twice each day at first increasing to 400mg if required. Thyrotoxicosis, 50mg 4 times each day; migraine prevention, 100mg–200mg each day in divided doses.

Special care: pregnancy, breast-feeding, liver or kidney disease, diabetes, metabolic acidosis, those undergoing anaesthesia; patients with weak hearts should be treated with digitalis and diuretics. Drug should be stopped gradually.

Avoid use: children, patients with asthma, various forms of heart disease including heart block, heart shock, slow heartbeat rate, heart failure.

Possible interaction: cardiac depressant, anaesthetics, reserpine, sedatives, antihypertensives, sympathomimetics, cimetidine, indomethacin, ergotamine, class I antiarrhythmic drugs, verapamil, clonidine withdrawal, hypoglycaemics.

Side effects: sleep disturbance, cold feet and hands, slow heartbeat, fatigue on exercise, wheeziness, heart failure, gastrointestinal disorders; dry eyes or skin rash (stop use gradually).

Manufacturer: Astra.

Bethanadine

Description: an antihypertensive drug, bethanidine sulphate, which acts by blocking the release of noradrenaline (a neurotransmitter) from nerve endings. It is available in the form of tablets containing 10mg bethanidine sulphate.

Used for: hypertension, especially that which has failed to respond to other antihypertensive drugs. It is usually used in conjunction with a diuretic (e.g. a thiazide) or beta-blocker.

Dosage: adults, 10mg, 3 times each day after food at first increasing by 5mg once a week to a maximum daily dose of 200mg.

Special care: kidney disease, pregnant women, asthma, peptic ulcer or history of peptic ulcer, cerebral or coronary arteriosclerosis. Low blood pressure when rising from a prone position may cause falls in elderly people.

Avoid use: children, patients with kidney or heart failure, phaeochromocytoma.

Possible interaction: tricyclic antidepressants, sympathomimetics, MAOIs.

Side effects: low blood pressure associated with lying down (postural hypotension), blocked nose, headache, drowsiness, oedema, failure of ejaculation.

Betim

Description: a non-cardioselective beta-blocker available as white, scored tablets containing 10mg timolol maleate and marked with 102 and symbol.

Used for: prevention of second heart attack following initial episode, angina, hypertension, prevention of migraine.

Dosage: adults, prevention of secondary heart attack, 5mg twice each day for first 2 days, thereafter 10mg twice each day. Angina, 10mg twice each day at first, adjusted according to response to a maximum of 60mg. Hypertension, 10mg a day at first in single or divided dose increasing by 10mg every 3 to 4 days to a maximum of 60mg. Usual maintenance dose is in the order of 10–30mg. Prevention of migraine, 10–20mg each day in 1 or 2 divded doses.

Special care: pregnancy, breast-feeding, liver or kidney disease, diabetes, those undergoing general anaesthesia, patients with weak hearts should receive digitalis and diuretics. Drug should be stopped gradually.

Avoid use: children, patients with asthma or history of breathing difficulties, those with various forms of heart disease including heart block, heart shock, slow heartbeat, heart failure.

Possible interaction: class I antiarrhythmics, cardiac depressant anaesthetics, ergotamine, sedatives, sympathomimetics, cimetidine, indomethacin, reserpine, hypoglycaemic drugs, clonidine withdrawal, verapamil.

Side effects: sleep disturbance, cold feet and hands, slow heartbeat, fatigue in exercise, wheeziness, heart failure, gastrointestinal upset, dry eyes or skin rash (stop drug gradually).

Manufacturer: Leo.

Betnelan

Description: a corticosteroid preparation containing the glucocorticoid betmethasone, in the form of white, scored tablets (0.5mg strength) and marked with the name and Evans.

Used for: allergic conditions, severe asthma, rheumatoid arthritis, collagen diseases.

Dosage: adults, 0.5mg–5mg daily then reduce to effective maintenance dose according to response. Children, 1 to 7 years, quarter to half adult dose, 7 to 12 years, half to three-quarters adult dose.

Special care: pregnant women, patients who have recently undergone intestinal surgery, some cancers, inflamed veins, peptic ulcer, active infections and those with viral or fungal origin, tuberculosis. High blood pressure, kidney diseases, osteoporosis, diabetes, glaucoma, epilepsy, underactive thyroid, liver cirrhosis, stress, psychoses. Patients should avoid contact with chicken pox or *Herpes zoster* virus while on steroid treatment and for 3 months afterwards. In the event of exposure to chicken pox, patients should be immunized within 3 days (if chicken pox is contracted specialist care is required). Drug should be stopped gradually.

Avoid use: children under 12 months.

Possible interaction: NSAIDs, anticoagulants taken by mouth, diuretics, hypoglycaemics, cardiac glycosides, anticholinesterases, phenobarbitone, phenytoin, rifampicin, ephedrine.

Side effects: mood swings (euphoria and depression), hyperglycaemia, osteoporosis, peptic ulcers, Cushing's syndrome caused especially by high doses.

Manufacturer: Evans.

Betnesol

Description: a corticosteroid containing the glucocorticoid betmethasone (as sodium phosphate), available as soluble tablets— pink, scored and marked with the name and Evans and containing 0.5mg. Also, **Betnesol Injection** containing 4mg per ml in 1ml ampoules.

Used for: allergic conditions, severe asthma, rheumatoid arthritis, collagen diseases. Injection: adrenal crisis and shock.

Dosage: adults, 0.5mg–5mg in water as daily dose reducing to minimum effective dose for maintenance. Children, 1 to 7 years, one quarter to half adult dose; 7 to 12 years, half to three-quarters adult dose. Injection: adults, 4–20mg intravenously 3 or 4 times a day if needed. Children, 1 year and under, 1mg; 1 to 5 years, 2mg; 6 to 12 years, 4mg by intravenous injection.

Special care: pregnancy, recent intestinal surgery, some cancers, inflamed veins, peptic ulcer, active infections and those with fungal or viral origin, tuberculosis, high blood pressure, kidney diseases, osteoporosis, diabetes, glaucoma, epilepsy, underactive thyroid, liver cirrhosis, stress, psychoses. Patients should avoid contact with chicken pox or *Herpes zoster* while on steroids and for 3 months after treatment has ceased. In the event of exposure to chicken pox, patients should be immunized within 3 days. (If chicken pox is contracted, specialist care is required). Drug should be stopped gradually.

Avoid use: children under 12 months.

Possible interaction: NSAIDs, oral anticoagulants, diuretics, hypoglycaemics, cardiac glycosides, anticholinesterases, phenobarbitone, phenytoin, rifampicin, ephedrine.

Side effects: mood swings (cuphoria and depression), hyperglycaemia (elevated blood sugar levels), osteoporosis, peptic ulcers, Cushings syndrome, especially caused by high doses.

Manufacturer: Evans.

Betnovate

Description: a group of moderate to potent corticosteroid preparations containing betamethasone and available as ointment, cream or lotion. Betnovate cream and ointment both contain 0.1% betmethasone (as valerate); **Betnovate Scalp Application**, (0.1%) **Betnovate C** cream and ointment contains an antimicrobial drug (antifungal and antibacterial), 3% clinoquinol and 0.1% betmethasone (as valerate); **Betnovate N** cream and ointment also contain an antimicrobial (antibacterial) drug, 0.5% neomycin sulphate and 0.1% betmethasone (as valerate). **Betnovate RD** cream and ointment are less potent containing 0.025% betmethasone (as valerate).

Used for: eczema, seborrhoeic and contact dermatitis, psoriasis, other skin disorders (lichen simplex and planus). For infected conditions, Betnovate C or N are used depending upon causal organism.

Dosage: adults, apply sparingly 2 or 3 times each day. More potent preparations may be used first with Betnovate RD then used for maintenance treatment. Children over 1 year same as adult dose.

Special care: should not be used extensively or for a prolonged period. Should be used for only 5 days on children or on face. Stop use gradually.

Avoid use: children under 1 year, continuous use especially by pregnant women, any conditions caused by ringworm, fungi, viruses, tuberculosis, acne, leg ulcers, scabies.

Side effects: thinning of skin, suppression of adrenal glands, hair growth, symptoms associated with Cushings syndrome, e.g. reddening of skin on face and neck.

Manufacturer: Glaxo.

Betnovate Rectal

Description: a steroid, vasoconstrictor and local anaesthetic preparation produced in the form of an ointment with applicator. The ointment contains 2.5% lignocaine hydrochloride, 0.1% phenylephrine hydrochloride and 0.05% betmethasone valerate.

Used for: haemorrhoids and mild proctitis (inflammation of the rectum).

Dosage: adults, apply 2 or 3 times daily at first and then once each day.

Special care: avoid use for a long period, especially pregnant women.

Avoid use: children, patients with tuberculosis, bacterial, viral or fungal infections.

Side effects: systemic corticosteroid effects.

Manufacturer: Glaxo.

Betoptic

Description: a cardio-selective beta-blocker that reduces pressure within the eye. Betoptic contains 0.5% betaxolol hydrochloride in the form of eye drops.

Used for: chronic open angle glaucoma and hypertension of eyes.

Dosage: 1 drop twice each day into eye.

Special care: patients with diabetes, thyrotoxicosis, blocked airways disease, those undergoing general anaesthetic.

Avoid use: children, patients with certain heart diseases including heart shock, cardiac failure, slow heart beat, those using soft contact lenses.

Side effects: passing slight discomfort, rarely staining or reddening of cornea and decreased sensitivity of cornea.

Manufacturer: Alcon.

Bezalip

Description: a preparation used to reduce high levels of fats (lipids) in the bloodstream, and available in the form of white, film-coated tablets marked BM/G6, containing 200mg bezafibrate. **Bezalip-Mono** are white, film-coated, modified-release tablets marked BM/D9 containing 400mg bezafibrate.

Used for: hyperlipidaemias (high blood levels of lipids, classified as type IIa, IIb, III, IV and V) which are resistant to changes in diet.

Dosage: adults, Bezalip-MONO, 1 tablet after food at night or in morning. Bezalip, 1 tablet 3 times each day with food.

Special care: patients with kidney disease.

Avoid use: children, patients with serious kidney or liver disease, nephrotic disease, pregnant and breast-feeding women.

Possible interaction: MAOIs, antidiabetic and anticoagulant drugs.

Side effects: gastrointestinal upset, rash, muscle pain.

Manufacturer: Boehringer Mannheim.

Bicillin

Description: a preparation of 2 types of penicillin used in the treatment of a variety of infections. Bicillin is available as a powder for reconstitution and injection containing 1.8g procaine penicillin and 360mg benzylpenicillin (300mg procaine penicillin, 60mg benzylpenicillin per ml).

Used for: gonococcal, streptococcal, pneumococcal, meningococcal infections, gas-gangrene, anthrax, syphilis, tetanus, diphtheria, yaws, Lyme disease in children. Other penicillin-sensitive infections where prolonged effect of antibiotic in tissues is desirable.

Dosage: adults, 1ml given by intramuscular injection once or twice each day. Early syphilis, 3ml by intramuscular injection (or 4ml for patients over 80kg), each day for 10 days. Gonorrhoea, up to 12ml as a single intramuscular injection. Children, under 25kg body weight dose adjusted in proportion to that given to a light adult. Over 25kg, same as adult dose.

Special care: patients with history of allergy or kidney disease.

Avoid use: patients with penicillin allergy.

Side effects: allergic responses including rash, fever, joint pains (anaphylactic shock in patients with penicillin allergy), gastrointestinal upset.

Manufacturer: Brocades.

Bicnu

Description: an alkylating cytotoxic drug used in the treatment of certain cancers and produced in the form of a powder for reconstitution and injection. Bicnu contains 100mg carmustine as a powder in a vial, with 3ml sterile ethanol for reconstitution.

Used for: leukaemia, lymphomas, myelomas, brain tumours.

Dosage: as directed by skilled cancer specialist.

Special care: patients should receive regular checks for blood count.

Side effects: vomiting and nausea, hair loss, bone marrow suppression (onset of which is delayed) necessitating regular blood checks, adverse effects on fertility. Possible kidney and liver damage may occur.

Manufacturer: Bristol-Myers.

Binovum

Description: a combined oestrogen/progesterone oral contraceptive preparation produced as a course of 21 tablets: 7 white tablets marked C over 535 contain 0.5mg (500µg) norethisterone and 35µg ethenyloestradiol; 14 peach tablets, marked C over 135, contain 1mg nore-thisterone and 35µg ethinyloestradiol.

Used for: oral contraception.

Dosage: 1 tablet each day starting with white tablets on first day of period. There are 7 tablet-free days before the process is repeated.

Special care: hypertension, asthma, diabetes, varicose veins, multiple sclerosis, Raynaud's disease, kidney dialysis, chronic kidney disease, obesity, severe depression. Family history of heart disease, inflammatory bowel disease, Crohn's disease. Risk of arterial thrombosis especially in older women, those who smoke and those who are obese. Regular checks on blood pressure, breasts and pelvic organs should be carried out at intervals.

Avoid use: pregnancy, history of heart disease or thrombosis, hypertension, sickle cell anaemia, liver disease, cholestatic jaundice of pregnancy, abnormalities of liver function, porphyria, undiagnosed vaginal bleeding, some cancers, (hormone-dependent ones), infectious hepatitis, recent trophoblastic disease.

Possible interaction: barbiturates, tetracycline antibiotics, rifampicin, griseofulvin, carbamezapine, chloral hydrate, primidone, phenytoin, ethosuximide, glutethimide, dichloralphenazone.

Side effects: oedema and bloatedness, leg cramps, reduction in sexual desire, headaches, depression, weight gain, vaginal discharge, breakthrough bleeding, cervical erosion, nausea, chloasma (brownish patches on skin).

Manufacturer: Ortho.

Bioplex

Description: a cytoprotectant produced in the form of granules for reconstitution with water to form a mouthwash. Bioplex contains 1% carbenoxolone sodium (20mg per 2g sachet).

Used for: mouth ulcers.

Dosage: use as mouthwash 3 times each day and at night.

Special care: do not swallow.

Manufacturer: Thames

Biorphen

Description: an antimuscarine or anticholinergic preparation used in the treatment of Parkinson's disease. It is thought that antimuscarine drugs act to correct the excess of acetylcholine believed to be the result of dopamine deficiency in Parkinson's disease. Biorphen is produced as a sugar-free liquid containing 25mg orphenadrine hydrochloride per 5ml.

Used for: Parkinson's disease including drug-induced symptoms.

Dosage: adults and children, 150mg each day at first in divided doses, increasing by 25–50mg every 2 or 3 days. Usual maintenance dose is in the order of 150–300mg.

Special care: heart disorders, gastrointestinal blockage, liver or kidney disease, avoid abrupt withdrawal of treatment.

Avoid use: narrow or closed angle glaucoma, enlarged prostate gland, some disorders of movement (tardive dyskinesia).

Possible interaction: antidepressants, antihistamines, phenothiazines.

Side effects: euphoria, agitation, confusion, anticholinergic effects and rash (high doses).

Manufacturer: Bioglan.

Blocadren

Description: a non-cardioselective beta-blocker produced in the form of blue scored tablets, marked MSD 135, containing 10mg timolol maleate.

Used for: prevention of secondary heart attack, angina, prevention of migraine, hypertension.

Dosage: adults, prevention of secondary heart attack, starting 1 to 4 weeks after first heart attack, 5mg twice each day for 2 days, then 10mg. Adults, angina, 5mg 2 or 3 times each day at first, increasing if required to 10–15mg daily every 3 days. Usual maintenance dose is in the order of 35–45mg. Adults, hypertension, 10mg each day at first as single or divided doses, increasing to a maximum of 60mg daily if required. Adults, prevention of migraine, 10–20mg each day, either as a single or as divided doses.

Special care: patients with kidney or liver disease, diabetes, metabolic acidosis, those undergoing general anaesthesia, pregnant women and nursing mothers. Persons with weak hearts should receive diuretics and digitalis. May need to halt drug before planned surgery. Withdraw gradually.

Avoid use: children, patients with asthma, heart block, heart failure, slow heartbeat, heart shock, severe peripheral arterial disease.

Possible interaction: cardiac depressant anaesthetic drugs, antihypertensives, sedatives, class I antiarrhythmic drugs, verapamil, clonidine withdrawal, ergotamine, cimetidine, indomethacine, sympathomimetics.

Side effects: disturbance of sleep, cold hands and feet, fatigue on exercise, slow heartbeat, bronchospasm, heart failure, rash, dry eyes (withdraw gradually).

Manufacturer: MSD

Bolvidon

Description: a tetracyclic antidepressant available in various strengths, containing 10mg mianserin hydrochloride (coded CT4); 20mg marked CT6, 30mg marked CT7. All tablets are white film-coated and marked ORGANON.

Used for: depressive illnesses, particularly those requiring sedation.

Dosage: adults, 30–40mg each day either as divided doses or a single one taken at night. May be gradually increased over a period of days to a maintenance dose in the order of 30–90mg each day according to response. Elderly persons, 30mg each day which may be carefully increased over a period of days if required.

Special care: elderly persons, pregnant women, patients with heart block or heart attack, enlarged prostate gland, epilepsy. Regular blood counts may be required.

Avoid use: children, breast-feeding mothers, patients with serious liver disease, those suffering from mania.

Possible interaction: alcohol, MAOIs, anticoagulant drugs.

Side effects: blood changes, drowsiness, if signs of influenza-like infection, convulsions, jaundice, hypomania occur, the drug should be withdrawn gradually.

Manufacturer: Organon.

Bonefos

Description: a preparation of the drug, sodium clodronate (a diphosphonate) which affects bone metabolism, preventing the increased rate of bone turnover associated with certain malignant conditions. Bonefos is available in the form of capsules and as a solution for intravenous infusion. Yellow capsules contain 400mg and intravenous solution contains 60mg per ml in 5ml ampoules.

Used for: hypercalcaemia of malignancy. Bone pain and lesions associated with secondary bone growths as a result of multiple myeloma (malignant bone marrow disease) or breast cancer.

Dosage: adults, 4 tablets each day as single or divided dose avoiding food for 1 or 2 hours before and after treatment, especially anything containing calcium, mineral supplements or iron. Infusion, adults, 1500mg as single infusion over 4 hours or 300mg given by slow intravenous infusion for up to 7 days. Afterwards, capsules should be taken.

Special care: moderate kidney disorders. Ensure adequate fluid intake, monitor blood calcium levels and kidney function.

Avoid use: children, pregnancy, breast-feeding, severe kidney failure.

Possible interaction: other diphosphonates, NSAIDs, mineral supplements, antacid preparations.

Side effects: skin rashes, gastrointestinal upset, disturbance of kidney function, parathyroid hormone, lactic acid dehydrogenase, creatinine, transaminase, alkaline phosphatase (enzymes) levels may be elevated for a time. Rarely, there may be hypocalcaemia which does not cause symptoms. There may be transient proteinurea.

Manufacturer: Boehringer Ingelheim.

Brelomax

Description: a bronchodilator of a type known as a selective β_2-agonist. It is available as white scored tablets, marked with logo, contain 2mg tulobuterol hydrochloride.

Used for: prevention and control of bronchospasm in reversible airways disease (asthma).

Dosage: adults, 1 tablet twice each day at first increasing to 1 tablet 3 times daily if needed. Children over 10 years, $^1/_2$ to 1 tablet twice daily.

Special care: patients with diabetes, epilepsy, mild

kidney failure, hypertension, heart-circulatory disease (cardio-vascular disease), hyperthyroidism.
Avoid use: children under 10 years, serious liver disease or liver failure, moderate to severe kidney failure.
Possible interaction: Other ß-blockers, corticosteroids, theophylline (increased risk of hypokalaemia with high doses).
Side effects: hypokalaemia, which may be serious, raised heartbeat rate, palpitations, headache, tremor, nervous tension.
Manufacturer: Abbott.

Bretylate

Description: a proprietary class III antiarrhythmic drug used to treat irregularities of heartbeat. Available in the form of a solution for injection containing 50mg bretylium tosylate per ml in 10ml ampoules.
Used for: heartbeat irregularities (ventricular arrhythmias) especially those resistant to other forms of treatment.
Dosage: 5–10mg per kg of body weight at first given intramuscularly or intravenously and repeated after 1–2 hours if necessary. The treatment is continued every 6 to 8 hours for up to 5 days.
Special care: patients with kidney disorders.
Avoid use: children, patients with phaeochromo-cytoma.
Possible interaction: noradrenaline, other sympatho-mimetics.
Side effects: passing worsening of arrhythmia, hypotension, vomiting and nausea.
Manufacturer: Wellcome.

Brevibloc

Description: a cardio-selective beta-blocker available in the form of a solution for injection. Brevibloc contains either 10mg esmolol hydrochloride per ml in a 10ml vial or 250mg per ml (for dilution before use) in 10ml ampoules.
Used for: cardiac arrhythmias of various types, (sinus tachycardia; atrial flutter, atrial fibrillation), raised heartbeat rate and hypertension.
Dosage: 50–200μg per kg body weight per minute by intravenous infusion.
Special care: women in late pregnancy, breast-feeding, liver disease, kidney disease, angina, diabetes.
Avoid use: asthma, history of obstructive airways disease, heart failure, heart block, heart shock.
Possible interaction: other antiarrhythmic drugs.
Manufacturer: Gensia.

Brevinor

Description: a combined oestrogen/progestogen contraceptive preparation available as white tablets, marked B and Syntex contain 35μg ethinyloestradiol and 0.5mg norethisterone.
Used for: contraception.
Dosage: 1 each day for 21 days starting on 5th day of period, then 7 tablet-free days.
Special care: women with asthma, hypertension, Raynaud's disease, diabetes, multiple sclerosis, chronic kidney disease, kidney dialysis, varicose veins, depression, smoking, age and obesity increase the risk of thrombosis.
Avoid use: pregnant women, patients with history of thrombosis or who may be at risk of this, heart disease, sickle cell anaemia, liver diseases, infectious hepatitis, history of cholestatic jaundice (caused by a failure of bile to reach the small intestine), porphyria, chorea, osteosclerosis, haemolytic uraemic syndrome, hormone-dependent cancers, recent trophoblastic disease, undiagnosed vaginal bleeding.
Possible interaction: tetracycline antibiotics, barbiturates, chloral hydrate, griseofulvin, rifampicin, carbamazepine, phenytoin, primidone, dichloralphenazone, ethosuximide glutethimide.
Side effects: oedema and bloatedness, leg cramps, enlargement of breasts, loss of libido, headaches, nausea, depression, weight gain, breakthrough bleeding, cervical erosion, vaginal discharge, brownish patches on skin (chloasma).
Manufacturer: Syntex.

Bricanyl

Description: a bronchodilator and a selective ß$_2$–agonist (a selective beta receptor stimulant) and muscle relaxant containing terbutaline sulphate. Bricanyl is available as tablets, a syrup and as a variety of preparations suitable for use with different kinds of inhaler.
Dosage: Bricanyl white scored tablets, marked 5 contain 5mg. Adult dose: 1 tablet twice each day or at 8-hour intervals. Children: 7 to 15 years, half adult dose. Young children under 7 should use syrup.
Also, **Bricanyl SA** (sustained release) tablets, white, marked A/BD, contain 7.5mg. Adult dose: 1 twice each day. Aerosol inhalation, capsules contain 0.25mg per metered dose aerosol. Adults and children: 1 to 2 puffs as required, maximum dose 8 puffs in 24 hours. **Bricanyl Turbohaler** is a breath-actuated dry powder inhaler containing 0.5mg per metered dose. Adults and children, 1 inhalation as needed with a maximum of 4 in 24 hours. **Bricanyl Spacer Inhaler** (with extended mouthpiece which is collapsible) contains 0.25mg per dose. Adults and

children, 1 to 2 puffs as required with a maximum of 8 in 24 hours. **Bricanyl Respules** (for use with nebulizer) contain 5mg per 2ml solution as single dose units. Adults: 5–10mg 2, 3 or 4 times each day. Children over 25kg body weight: 5mg 2, 3 or 4 times daily. Both with nebulizer.
Bricanyl Respirator Solution (for use with power-operated nebulizer) contains 10mg per ml (diluted before use with sterile physiological saline). Adults and children 2–10mg diluted and used with nebulizer. **Bricanyl Syrup** (sugar-free) contains 1.5mg per 5ml. Adults: 10–15ml; children under 3 years: 2.5ml; 3 to 7 years, 2.5–5ml, 7 to 15 years, 5–10ml. All at 8-hour intervals.
Bricanyl Injection contains 0.5mg per ml in ampoules. Adults; 0.25–0.5mg by subcutaneous, intramuscular or slow intravenous injection. Children; 2 to 15 years, 10µg per kg of body weight, subcutaneously, intramuscularly or by slow intravenous injection.
Special care: pregnancy, angina, heart disorders and arrhythmias, hypertension, hyperthyroidism. Caution in diabetic persons if given intravenously.
Possible interaction: sympathomimetics.
Side effects: headache, nervous tension, trembling, dilation of blood vessels.
Manufacturer: Astra.

Britaject

Description: a dopamine agonist used in the treatment of Parkinson's disease. Britaject contains 10mg apomorphine hydrochloride per ml in ampoules for injection.
Used for: treatment of involuntary muscle movements in Parkinson's disease which have not responded to other methods of treatment.
Dosage: as directed by hospital physician.
Special care: patients require 3 or more days of treatment prior to start of therapy.
Manufacturer: Britannia

Britiazem

Description: a vasodilator which is a class III calcium antagonist, available as white tablets, scored on one side contain 60mg diltiazem hydrochloride.
Used for: angina.
Dosage: 1 tablet 3 times daily increasing if required to a maximum of 6 each day in divided doses. Elderly, 1 tablet twice each day.
Special care: monitoring of heartbeat rate may be required during therapy especially in elderly patients, those with a slow heartbeat and those with kidney or liver disorders.

Avoid use: children, pregnant women, those with marked bradycardia, heart block (2nd- and 3rd-degree atrio-ventricular block) sick sinus syndrome.
Possible interaction: beta-blockers, carbamazepine, digoxin, cardiac depressants, other antihypertensive drugs, cyclosporin, diazepam, lithium, cimetidine, dantrolene infusion.
Side effects: bradycardia, 1st degree heart block (atrio-ventricular block), headache, rash, nausea, swelling of ankles caused by oedema.
Manufacturer: Thames

Britoflex

Description: a preparation acting on the central (sympathetic) nervous system available as peach, film-coated tablets with 0.2mg lofexidine hydrochloride.
Used for: control of withdrawal symptoms in patients undergoing detoxification from opioid drug dependency.
Dosage: adults, 1 tablet twice each day in first instance increasing by 1 or 2 daily if necessary. Maximum daily dose is 12 tablets. Therapy usually should be carried out over a period of 7 to 10 days and then is gradually withdrawn over 2 to 4 days.
Special care: pregnancy, breast-feeding, heart and circulatory diseases, recent heart attack or chronic kidney failure, severe bradycardia, depression.
Avoid use: children.
Possible interaction: alcohol, sedatives.
Side effects: dry mouth throat and nose, drowsiness, hypotension, rebound hypertension on withdrawal.
Manufacturer: Britannia.

Brocadopa

Description: a preparation of the drug, Levodopa, which is a dopamine precursor. Levodopa is converted into dopamine inside the body, and it is a lack of dopamine in the brain which is associated with Parkinson's disease. Brocadopa is produced in capsule strengths 125mg, 250mg and 500mg.
Used for: Parkinson's disease but not drug-induced.
Dosage: 250mg each day in divided doses at first, gradually increasing by 250mg every 3 to 4 days until best response is achieved. Usual dose is in the order of 1–8g in divided doses.
Special care: pregnancy, heart, lung, liver, kidney diseases, disorders of the endocrine (hormones) system, wide angle glaucoma or peptic ulcers. Heart, liver and kidney function should be monitored and blood checks carried out.
Avoid use: children, patients with narrow angle glaucoma, history of malignant melanoma, severe psychoses.

Possible interaction: sympathomimetics, MAOIs, drugs affecting amine levels in central nervous system, pyroxidine, ferrous sulphate antihyptertensive drugs.
Side effects: vomiting and nausea, anorexia, low blood pressure on rising from sitting or lying down (postural hypotension), heart and central nervous system disturbance, involuntary movements, discolouration of urine.
Manufacturer: Yamanouchi.

Broflex
Description: an antimuscarine or anticholinergic preparation, produced in the form of a pink syrup containing 5mg benzhexol hydrochloride per 5ml.
Used for: Parkinson's disease including drug-induced.
Dosage: adults, 1mg each day at first increasing over a period of days by 1 or 2mg to a usual maintenance dose of 5–15mg. Maximum daily dose is 20mg.
Special care: narrow angle glaucoma, enlarged prostate gland, obstruction of gastrointestinal tract, heart, liver or kidney disease. Withdraw drug slowly.
Avoid use: children, tardive dyskinesia (movement disorder), closed angle glaucoma, severe gastrointestinal obstruction, untreated urinary retention.
Possible interaction: antidepressants, antihistamines, phenothiazines.
Side effects: gastrointestinal disturbances, dry mouth, dizziness, blurred vision, sometimes nervousness, hypersensitivity, tachycardia (raised heart beat rate), urinary retention. In susceptible patients and/or with higher doses, psychiatric disturbances, mental confusion, excitability which may require treatment to be discontinued.
Manufacturer: Bioglan.

Bronchodil
Description: a bronchodilator and selective beta$_2$-agonist available in the form of an aerosol containing 0.5mg reproterol hydrochloride per metered dose inhalation.
Used for: reversible airways obstruction in bronchitis, bronchial asthma and emphysema.
Dosage: adults, 1 or 2 puffs every 3 to 6 hours. Prevention of symptoms, 1 puff 3 times each day. Children, 6 to 12 years, 1 puff 3- to 6-hourly; prevention of symptoms, 1 puff 3 times each day.
Special care: pregnant women, patients with weak hearts, heart arrhythmias, hypertension, angina, hyperthyroidism.
Avoid use: children under 6 years.

Possible interaction: sympathomimetics.
Side effects: headache, dilation of blood vessels, fine tremor of hands, nervous tension.
Manufacturer: ASTA Medica.

Brufen
Description: an NSAID used as an analgesic to treat a variety of disorders and available as tablets, granules and syrup containing ibuprofen: magenta-coloured, oval, sugar-coated tablets are available in 3 strengths; coded Brufen (200mg);coded Brufen 400 (400mg) and coded Brufen 600 (600mg). **Brufen Granules** are effervescent, orange-flavoured granules in sachet containing 600mg. **Brufen Syrup** contains 100mg per 5ml and **Brufen Retard**, contain 800mg as white, oval film-coated sustained release tablets.
Used for: pain and inflammation in such conditions as rheumatic disorders, joint pain, juvenile arthritis, periarticular disorders, rheumatoid arthritis, seronegative arthritis, ankylosing spondylitis, osteoarthrosis, postoperative pain, period pain, soft tissue injuries.
Dosage: adults, 1200–1800mg each day in divided doses (after food) with a maximum daily dose of 2400mg. A maintenance dose in the region of 600–1200mg may be sufficient. Children, over 7kg body weight, use syrup. Age 1 to 2 years, 2.5ml; 3 to 7 years, 5ml; 8 to 12 years, 10ml. All 3 to 4 times each day.
Special care: pregnancy, nursing mothers, elderly, asthma, gastrointestinal disorders, heart, liver or kidney disease. Patients on long-term therapy should receive monitoring.
Avoid use: patients with known allergy to aspirin or anti-inflammatory drugs, those with peptic ulcer. Children under 7kg body weight.
Possible interaction: quinolones, anticoagulants, thiazide diuretics.
Side effects: gastrointestinal upset and bleeding, rash, low levels of blood platelets.
Manufacturer: Boots.

Buccastem
Description: an anti-emetic and dopamine antagonist belonging to a group called the phenothiazines, available as pale yellow (buccal) tablets containing 3mg prochlorperazine maleate.
Used for: severe nausea, vomiting, vertigo due to labyrinthine disorders or Ménière's disease.
Dosage: 1 to 2 tablets twice each day, the tablet being placed high up between upper lip and gum and left to dissolve.
Special care: pregnancy, nursing mothers.

Avoid use: children under 14 years of age (may cause dystonia, a movement disorder, and other extra-pyramidal symptoms in children and young people). Patients with Parkinson's disease, blood changes, narrow angle glaucoma, enlarged prostate gland, liver or kidney disease, epilepsy.

Possible interaction: alcohol, alpha-blockers, CNS depressants (sedatives).

Side effects: hypotension (low blood pressure), especially in elderly persons or dehydrated patients, anticholinergic effects, drowsiness, skin reactions, insomnia. Rarely extra-pyramidal symptoms may occur and parkinsonism, especially in elderly patients.

Manufacturer: Reckitt & Colman.

Burinex

Description: a loop diuretic preparation, (acting on the part of the kidney tubules called loops of Henle), available in the form of tablets, liquid and in ampoules for injection containing bumetanide. White, scored tablets marked 133 and with logo contain 1mg, those marked with strength contain 5mg. **Burinex Liquid** contains 1mg per 5ml. **Burinex Injection** contains 0.5mg per ml in ampoules.

Used for: oedema caused by congestive heart failure, liver and kidney disease including nephrotic syndrome.

Dosage: adults, tablets or liquid, 1mg daily according to response of patient's condition. Injection, 1–2mg given intravenously (for pulmonary oedema), repeated after 20 minutes if necessary.

Special care: pregnancy, breast-feeding, diabetes, gout, liver or kidney disease, enlarged prostate gland, impaired micturition (urination). Potassium supplements may be needed.

Avoid use: children, patients in precomatose states as a result of liver cirrhosis.

Possible interaction: digoxin, lithium, antihypertensives, aminoglycosides.

Side effects: gastrointestinal upset, cramps, skin rash, blood changes, enlarged breasts, thrombocytopenia.

Manufacturer: Leo.

Burinex A

Description: a combined loop and potassium-sparing diuretic preparation available as scored, cream, oval-shaped tablets, marked with lion and 149, containing 1mg bumetanide and 5mg amiloride hydrochloride.

Used for: patients requiring immediate diuresis,

especially those in whom hypokalaemia may be a problem.

Dosage: adults, 1 to 2 tablets each day.

Special care: pregnancy, breast-feeding, diabetes, impaired micturition (urination). Blood electrolyte levels should be monitored.

Avoid use: children, patients with severe imbalance of electrolyte levels (salts), kidney or liver disease, disorders of adrenal glands, hepatic pre-coma.

Possible interaction: antihypertensive drugs, digitalis, potassium supplements, potassium-sparing diuretics, lithium, ACE inhibitors, cephalosporins, aminoglycosides.

Side effects: gastrointestinal upset, skin rash, cramps, thrombocytopenia.

Manufacturer: Leo.

Burinex K

Description: a combined loop diuretic, potassium supplement preparation available in the form of white, oval tablets, containing 0.5mg bumetanide, and 573mg potassium in a slow release wax core.

Used for: oedema accompanying congestive heart failure, kidney and liver disease in which a potassium supplement is needed.

Dosage: adults, 1 to 4 tablets each day.

Special care: pregnancy, breast-feeding, gout, diabetes, kidney or liver disorders, enlarged prostate gland, impaired micturition (urination).

Avoid use: children, patients with Addison's disease, hyperkalaemia, precomatose states in liver cirrhosis.

Possible interaction: aminoglycosides, digitalis, lithium, antihypertensives, potassium-sparing diuretics.

Side effects: gastrointestinal upset, cramps, skin rash, enlarged breasts, thrombocytopenia. Drug should be discontinued if obstruction of ulceration of small bowel occurs.

Manufacturer: Leo.

Buspar

Description: an anxiolytic (anxiety-relieving) preparation, and an azapirone. It is thought to be less open to abuse than the benzodiazepine drugs which are also used to relieve severe anxiety, and also to be less sedating in its effect. Buspar is produced in tablets of 2 strengths, containing 5mg or 10mg buspirone hydrochloride. The tablets are white, oval-shaped and marked with strength.

Used for: short-term relief of severe anxiety, i.e. that which is causing extreme distress and inability to function normally. This may or may not be accompanied by depression.

Dosage: adults, 5mg 2 or 3 times each day at first,

increasing every 2 or 3 days to a usual dose in the order of 10mg twice daily. Maximum dose is 45mg daily.

Special care: if patient has been taking a benzodiazepine this should be slowly withdrawn before starting Buspirone therapy. Special care in patients with liver or kidney disorders.

Avoid use: children, patients with severe kidney or liver disease, epilepsy, pregnant women, breast-feeding mothers.

Possible interaction:

Side effects: headache, nervous tension, dizziness. Rarely, confusion, fatigue, dry mouth, chest pain, tachycardia.

Manufacturer: Bristol-Myers.

C

Cafergot

Description: an analgesic preparation containing ergotamine which is available as white, sugar-coated tablets containing 1mg ergotamine tartrate and 100mg caffeine. **Cafergot Suppositories** contain 2mg ergotamine tartrate and 200mg caffeine.

Used for: migraine.

Dosage: 1 or 2 tablets at start of attack with no more than 4 in 24 hours; should not be repeated within 4 days. Suppositories, 1 at start of attack with maximum of 2 in 24 hours. Must not repeat within 4 days.

Avoid use: children, pregnancy, breast-feeding, liver or kidney disease, coronary, occlusive or peripheral vascular disease, sepsis, severe hyptertension.

Possible interaction: ß-blocker, erythromycin.

Side effects: vomiting, nausea, abdominal pains, impairment of circulation, weakness in legs. If pleural or retroperitoneal fibrosis occurs drug should be immediately stopped.

Manufacturer: Sandoz.

Calciparine

Description: an anticoagulant available in the form of pre-filled syringes containing 25,000 units heparin calcium per ml for use as subcutaneous injection only.

Used for: deep vein thrombosis, pulmonary embolism and prevention of these before surgery.

Dosage: 5000 units 2 hours before surgery then every 8 to 12 hours for 7 days.

Special care: pregnancy, kidney or liver disease. Blood platelet counts are required and therapy should be halted in patients who develop thrombocytopenia.

Avoid use: patients with allergy to heparin, those with haemophilia, haemorrhagic disorders, severe hypertension, peptic ulcer, cerebral aneurysm, recent eye surgery or concerning central nervous system, serious liver disease.

Side effects: haemorrhage, thrombocytopenia, allergic reactions. After prolonged use, osteoporosis and rarely, baldness may occur.

Manufacturer: Sanofi Winthrop.

Calcitare

Description: a preparation of thyroid hormone (derived from pig), available as a powder for reconstitution and injection, consisting of 160 units porcine calcitonin in a vial with gelatin diluent.

Used for: Paget's disease of bone, hypercalcaemia.

Dosage: Paget's disease, 80 units 3 times a week to 160 units daily in single or divided doses, but subcutaneous intramuscular injection. Hypercalcaemia, 4 units per kg of body weight daily by subcutaneous or intramuscular injection, adjusted according to response. Children per kg of body weight in similar way but should not receive treatment for periods exceeding a few weeks.

Special care: if history of allergy, scratch skin test should be carried out. Pregnant women, breast-feeding mothers.

Possible interaction: cardiac glycosides.

Side effects: vomiting and nausea, tingling in hands, flushing, unpleasant taste in mouth.

Manufacturer: Theraplix.

Calmurid HC

Description: a topical, moderately potent steroid with keratolytic and hydrating agents which have a softening and moistening effect on the skin. Available as a cream containing 1% hydrocortisone, 10% urea and 5% lactic acid.

Used for: dry eczemas and dermatoses.

Dosage: wash and dry affected skin, apply thinly twice a day at first and reduce frequency as condition improves.

Special care: limit use in children to 5 to 7 days, use extreme care with infants (napkin rash and infantile eczema). Also, use on face should be limited to 5 to 7 days. If stinging occurs, dilute to half-strength with water-based cream for 1 week before reverting to full strength preparation.

Avoid use: long-term use especially in pregnant women, patients with acne or skin conditions caused by tuberculosis, viral, fungal, bacterial infections which are untreated or ringworm, leg ulcers.

Side effects: not usually severe but thinning of skin, lines in skin (striae), blotchy red patches caused by distended blood vessels (capillaries) (telangiectasia), suppression of adrenal glands may occur.

Manufacturer: Novex.

Calsynar

Description: a manufactured form of a hormone, calcitonin, which is concerned with the regulation of calcium levels in the body. It is produced in ampoules for injection and contains 100 units salcatonin per ml in saline, (salcatonin is synthetic salmon calcitonin). Calcitonin lowers levels of calcium in blood plasma by inhibiting resorption of bone.

Used for: osteoporosis in post-menopausal women, Paget's disease, hypercalcaemia, in bone cancer, bone pain resulting from cancer.

Dosage: hypercalcaemia, 5–10 units per kg of body weight each day to 400 units 6- to 8-hourly according to response, by subcutaneous or intramuscular injection. Paget's disease of bone, 50 units 3 times each week to 100 units daily in single or divided doses, by subcutaneous or intramuscular injection. Post-menopausal osteoporosis, 100 units each day by subcutaneous or intramuscular injection along with 600mg calcium and 400 units vitamin D taken by mouth. Bone pain in cancer, 200 units every 6 hours or 400 units every 12 hours, for 48 hours by subcutaneous or intramuscular injection. Children should not receive therapy for more than a few weeks, as directed by physician.

Special care: history of allergy, perform scratch skin test. Pregnant women, breast-feeding mothers.

Possible interaction: cardiac glycosides.

Side effects: vomiting and nausea, tingling sensation in hands, flushing, allergic responses, unpleasant taste in mouth.

Manufacturer: Theraplix.

Camcolit

Description: an antidepressant preparation of lithium salts available as tablets of 2 strengths. Camcolit 250® tablets are white, scored, film-coated and contain 250mg lithium carbonate (equivalent to 6.8mmol Li$^+$). **Camcolit 400®** tablets are white, scored, modified release, film-coated and contain 400mg lithium carbonate (10.8mmol Li$^+$), marked S and CAMCOLIT.

Used for: treatment and prevention of mania, recurrent bouts of depression, manic depression, aggressive and self-mutilating behaviour.

Dosage: adults, prevention 0.5–1.2g each day at first (elderly patients 0.5–1g). Maintain serum levels of lithium in range of 0.5 to 1mmol per litre.

Treatment: 1.5 to 2g each day at first, (elderly patients, 0.5 to 1g). Maintain serum levels of lithium in range of 0.6 to 1.2 mmol per litre. Camcolit 250 should be given in divided doses; Camcolit 400 in single or divided doses.

Special care: treatment should be started in hospital with monitoring of plasma lithium concentrations at regular intervals. (Overdosage usually with plasma concentrations in excess of 1.5mmol Li$^+$ per litre can be fatal). Adequate fluid and salt intake should be maintained. Monitor thyroid function.

Avoid use: children, pregnancy, breast-feeding, heart or kidney disease, hypothyroidism, Addison's disease, imbalance in sodium levels.

Possible interaction: NSAIDs, diuretics, haloperidol, phenytoin, metodopramide, carbamazepine, flupenthixol.

Side effects: oedema, hypo and hyperthyroidism, weight gain, gastrointestinal upset, diarrhoea and nausea, trembling in hands, muscular weakness, heart and central nervous system disturbance, skin reactions, intense thirst, large volumes of dilute urine.

Manufacturer: Norgine.

Canestan-HC

Description: a mildly potent steroid with an antifungal and antibacterial drug in the form of a cream containing 1% hydrocortisone and 1% clotrimazole.

Used for: fungal infections accompanied by inflammation.

Dosage: apply to affected skin twice each day.

Special care: limit use on face or in children to 5 to 7 days, especially on infants. Withdraw gradually, short term use only.

Avoid use: prolonged or extensive use on pregnant women, patients with untreated bacterial or fungal infections, acne, leg ulcers, scabies, viral skin infections, tuberculosis, ringworm, peri-oral dermatitis.

Side effects: slight burning or irritation, allergic reactions.

Manufacturer: Bayer.

Cantil

Description: an anticholinergic preparation which acts as a smooth muscle relaxant, available as tablets which are yellow, scored and contain 25mg mepenzolate bromide.

Used for: spasm and overactivity of smooth muscle of the lower gastrointestinal tract.

Dosage: adults, 1 to 2 tablets 3 or 4 times daily.

Special care: enlarged prostate gland.

Avoid use: children, pregnancy, breast-feeding, glaucoma, myasthenia gravis, unstable angina, tachycardia, liver and kidney disease, ulcerative colitis, reflux obstructive disease, hiatus hernia.

Possible interaction: antihistamines, tricyclic antidepressants, benzodiazepines.

Side effects: gastrointestinal upset, nausea, constipation, vomiting, dry mouth, difficulty in swallowing (dysphagia), tachycardia, flushing, blurred vision, insomnia, weakness, retention of urine.

Manufacturer: Boehringer Mannheim.

Capastat

Description: a peptide antituberculous preparation available as a powder for reconstitution and injection. Capastat consists of 1 mega unit (million units) of capreomycin sulphate (equivalent to approximately 1g capreomycin).

Used for: treatment of tuberculosis which has failed to respond to other drugs.

Dosage: usually 1g each day given by deep intramuscular injection for a period of 60–120 days. Thereafter, 1g 2 or 3 times a week by intramuscular injection.

Special care: pregnancy, breast-feeding, kidney and hearing disorders, history of liver disease or allergy. Liver, kidney and vestibular (concerned with balance and controlled by organs in the inner ear) functions should be monitored and hearing tests carried out.

Avoid use: children.

Possible interaction: other antibacterial drugs, streptomycin, viomycin, vancomycin, colistin, aminoglycosides.

Side effects: allergic reactions, e.g. skin rash and urticaria, changes in blood (thrombocytopenia, leucocytosis—an increased number of white blood cells, leucopenia), nephrotoxicity (toxic effects on the kidney), ototoxicity (damage to the organs of hearing and balance), liver damage, electrolyte level disturbances, loss of hearing accompanied by tinnitus and vertigo.

Manufacturer: Dista.

Capoten

Description: an antihypertensive preparation, captopril, which is an ACE inhibitor, produced in tablets of 3 strengths: white (12.5mg); mottled white square (25mg); mottled white oval (50mg).

Used for: mild to moderate hypertension (with diuretics and digitalis), severe hypertension, where other methods have not been successful, congestive heart failure, heart attack, diabetic nephropathy in insulin-dependent diabetes.

Dosage: adults, mild to moderate hypertension, 12.5mg twice each day at first with usual maintenance dose in the order of 25mg twice daily. Maximum dose is 50mg twice each day. Addition of a thiazide may be needed. Severe hypertension, 12.5mg twice each day at first, increasing to a maximum of 50mg 3 times each day if needed. Diabetic nephropathy, 75–100mg each day in divided doses. Heart failure, 6.25–12.5mg daily at first increasing to usual maintenance in the order of 25mg 2 or 3 times each day. Maximum dose is 150mg each day. N.B. therapy should be initiated in hospital under strict medical supervision with any diuretics being stopped or reduced before treatment begins. Post heart attack, 6.25mg daily at first beginning 3 days after attack increasing to 150mg daily in divided doses.

Special care: severe congestive heart failure, kidney disease, reno-vascular hypertension, undergoing dialysis or anaesthesia. Those with collagen vascular disease. White blood cell counts and checks on protein in urine and kidney function should be carried out before and during therapy. Contact manufacturer before use in children.

Avoid use: pregnancy, breast-feeding, various heart disorders (aortic stenosis, outflow obstruction).

Possible interaction: NSAIDs, potassium supplements, potassium-sparing diuretics, immunosuppressants, vasodilators, allopurinol, probenecid, clonidine, procainamide.

Manufacturer: Squibb.

Capozide

Description: a combined thiazide diuretic with an ACE inhibitor, produced in the form of white, scored tablets marked SQUIBB containing 25mg hydrochlorothiazide and 50mg captopril. **Capozide LS** tablets are white, scored and contain 12.5mg hydrochlorothiazide and 25mg captopril and are marked SQUIBB 536.

Used for: mild to moderate hypertension in patients who are stable when taking the same proportions of captopril and hydrochlorothiazide individually.

Dosage: adults, 1 tablet daily with a possible maximum of 2. Capozide LS, 1 tablet each day.

Special care: patients with kidney disease or receiving dialysis, liver disease, gout, collagen vascular disease, diabetes, undergoing asnaesthesia. Kidney function, urinary protein and white blood cell count shoudl be checked before and during treatment.

Avoid use: pregnant women, breast-feeding mothers, patients with certain heart diseases (aortic stenosis, outflow obstruction), anuria.

Possible interaction: NSAIDs, potassium supplements, potassium-sparing diuretics, immunosuppressants, vasodilators, allopurinol, probenecid, clonidine, procainamide.

Side effects: blood dyscrasias (blood changes), hypotension, rash, proteinuria, loss of sensation of taste, sensitivity to light, pancreatitis, tiredness, rarely, a cough.

Manufacturer: Squibb

Carace

Description: an ACE inhibitor produced in the form of blue, oval tablets marked NSD15 containing 2.5mg lisinopril; white, oval, scored tablets contain 5mg lisinopril; yellow, oval, scored tablets contain 10mg lisinopril; orange, oval, scored tablets contain 20mg lisinopril. All except 2.5mg tablets are marked with name and strength.

Used for: congestive heart failure (in conjunction with diuretics and possibly digitalis), hypertension.

Dosage: adults, congestive heart failure, (reduce dose of any diuretic being taken before start of treatment) 2.5mg once each day at first increasing gradually to maintenance dose in the order of 5–20mg once daily, after 2 to 4 weeks. Hypertension, (discontinue any diuretic being taken 2 to 3 days before treatment starts); 2.5mg once a day increasing to a maintenance dose in the order of 10–20mg once daily. Maximum daily dose, 40mg.

Special care: breast-feeding, patients with kidney disease, receiving dialysis, renovascular hypertension, severe congestive heart failure, undergoing anaesthesia. Kidney function should be monitored before and during treatment. Treatment should begin under hospital supervision for heart failure patients.

Avoid use: pregnancy, children, patients with various heart disorders (aortic stenosis, outflow obstruction), cor pulmone (a lung disorder), angioneurotic odema as a result of previous ACE inhibitor treatment.

Possible interaction: potassium supplements, potassium-sparing diuretics, antihypertensives, indomethacin, lithium.

Side effects: headache, dizziness, diarrhoea, nausea, tiredness, palpitations, hypotension, rash, angioedema, asthenia (weakness), cough.

Manufacturer: DuPont.

Carace Plus

Description: an ACE inhibitor with a thiazide diuretic produced in the form of blue, hexagonal tablets marked 145 containing 10mg lisinopril and 12.5mg hydrochlorothiazide. **Carace 20 Plus** are yellow, hexagonal scored tablets containing 20mg lisinopril and 12.5mg hydrochlorothiazide.

Used for: mild to moderate hypertension in patients who are stable when taking the same proportions of lisinopril and hydrochlorothiazide individually.

Dosage: adults, 1 Carace Plus or Carace 20 Plus each day with a possible maximum of 2 tablets.

Special care: patients with liver or kidney disease receiving dialysis, heart and circulatory diseases, gout, hyperuricaemia (excess uric acid levels in blood), undergoing anaesthesia or surgery, with imbalances in salts (electrolytes) or fluid levels, children.

Avoid use: pregnancy, breast-feeding, anuria, angioneurotic oedema as a result of previous ACE inhibitor treatment.

Possible interaction: potassium supplements, hypoglycaemics, NSAIDs, lithium, tubocurarine.

Side effects: cough, headache, nausea, weariness, hypotension, diarrhoea, angio-neurotic oedema, impotence, dizziness.

Manufacturer: Du Pont

Carbo-Cort

Description: a mildly potent topical steroid combined with a cleansing agent, produced in the form of an antipsoriatic cream. Carbo-Cort contains 0.25% hydrocortisone and 3% coal tar solution.

Used for: eczema, lichen planus (a type of skin disease).

Dosage: apply to affected skin 2 or 3 times each day.

Special care: use in children or on face should be limited to 5 to 7 days. Special care in infants. Extensive or prolonged use should be avoided and the preparation withdrawn gradually.

Avoid use: patients with acne, untreated fungal or bacterial infections, tuberculosis, ringworm, viral skin infections, leg ulcers, scabies, peri-oral dermatitis.

Side effects: adrenal gland suppression, skin thinning, striae (lines on skin), telangiectasia (red blotches on skin).

Manufacturer: Lagap.

Cardene

Description: a Class II calcium antagonist produced in the form of capsules: blue/white capsules contain 20mg nicardipine hydrochloride and pale blue/blue capsules containing 30mg .

Used for: chronic angina which is stable.

Dosage: adults, angina, 20mg 3 times each day in first instance increasing with 3-day intervals to a maintenance dose in the order of 30mg 3 times daily. Maximum daily dose, 120mg.

Special care: congestive heart failure, liver or kidney disease, weak heart.
Avoid use: children, pregnancy, breast-feeding, advanced aortic stenosis (a heart valve disease).
Possible interaction: cimetidine, digoxin.
Side effects: headache, dizziness, nausea, palpitations, flushing and feeling of warmth; chest pain within half an hour of taking dose or on increasing dose, drug should be withdrawn.
Manufacturer: Syntex.

Cardene SR

Description: a Class II calcium antagonist produced in the form of sustained-release capsules: white capsules marked SYNTEX 30 contain 30mg nicardipine hydrochloride; blue capsules marked SYNTEX 45 contain 45mg.
Used for: mild to moderate hypertension.
Dosage: adults, 30mg twice each day at first increasing to 60mg twice daily if required.
Special care: congestive heart failure, liver or kidney disease, weak heart.
Avoid use: children, pregnant women, breast-feeding mothers, patients with advanced aortic stenosis (a heart valve disease).
Possible interaction: cimetidine, digoxin.
Side effects: headache, dizziness, nausea, palpitations, flushing and feeling of warmth; chest pain within half an hour of taking dose or on increasing dose, drug should be withdrawn.
Manufacturer: Syntex

Cardura

Description: an antihypertensive alpha-blocker, doxazosin mesylate, available as white, pentagonal tablets, marked DXP1 (1mg); white, oval tablets, marked DXP2 (2mg); white, square tablets, marked DXP4 (4mg). All tablets are marked Pfizer.
Used for: hypertension.
Dosage: adults, 1mg once a day at first increasing to 2mg after 1 or 2 weeks and then to 4mg once each day if needed. Maximum daily dose is 16mg.
Special care: pregnant women.
Avoid use: children, breast-feeding.
Side effects: headache, weariness, dizziness, vertigo, postural hypotension, asthenia (weakness), oedema.
Manufacturer: Invicta.

Carisoma

Description: a carbamate preparation which acts as a muscle relaxant and available as white tablets containing 125mg carisoprodol and white tablets marked with P in a hexagon contain 350mg carisoprodol.

Used for: muscle spasm resulting from bone and muscle disorders.
Dosage: 350mg, elderly, 125mg, both 3 times each day.
Special care: history of drug abuse or alcoholism, liver or kidney disease. Long term treatment should be avoided and the drug withdrawn gradually.
Avoid use: children, pregnancy, breast-feeding, acute intermittent porphyria.
Possible interaction: oral contraceptives, steroids, CNS depressants, tricyclics, griseofulvin, phenothiazines, rifampicin, phenytoin, anticoagulants.
Side effects: nausea, constipation, flushes, rash, weariness, drowsiness, headache.
Manufacturer: Pharmax.

Catapres

Description: an antihypertensive preparation, clonidine hydrochloride, produced in the form of tablets of 2 strengths, modified release capsules and in ampoules for injection. White scored tablets, marked with symbol and C over C, contain 0.1mg; white scored tablets marked with symbol and C over 03C, contain 0.3mg . Also, **Catapres Perlongets** are yellow/red sustained-release capsules marked with name, 11P and symbol and contain 0.25mg. Additionally, **Catapres Injection** contains 0.15mg per ml in ampoules.
Used for: hypertension.
Dosage: tablets, 0.05–1mg 3 times each day, gradually increasing every second or third day. Perlongets, 1 at night increasing, if required, to 1 tablet night and morning.
Special care: breast-feeding, depression, peripheral vascular disease. Tablets should be stopped gradually especially if beta-blockers are being withdrawn.
Avoid use: children.
Possible interaction: other antihypertensives, tricyclics, CNS depressants, alpha-blockers.
Side effects: dry mouth, oedema, drowsiness, dizziness.
Manufacturer: Boehringer Ingelheim.

CCNU

Description: an alkylating cytotoxic preparation produced in the form of blue/white capsules containing 10mg lomustine, and blue capsules containing 40mg lomustine.
Used for: Hodgkin's disease and some solid tumours.
Dosage: 120–130mg per square metre of body surface every 6 to 8 weeks.

Side effects: nausea, vomiting, bone marrow suppression, the onset of which is delayed.
Manufacturer: Lundbeck.

Cefizox

Description: a cephalosporin antibiotic preparation available as powder in vials for reconstitution and injection. Cefizox contains cefizoxime in the form of sodium salts as 500mg, 1g and 2g powder in vials.
Used for: septicaemia, urinary tract infections and gonorrhoea, skin and soft tissue infections and those of the lower respiratory tract.
Dosage: by intravenous infusion, deep intramuscular injection or slow intravenous injection, 1–2g 8- to 12-hourly increased in severe infections to a maximum of 8g daily, in 3 divided doses. Children over 3 months old, 30–60mg per kg of body weight each day in 2 to 4 divided doses. When infection is severe, 100–150mg per kg of body weight may be required.
Special care: patients with known allergy to penicillins and those with kidney disorders.
Avoid use: patients with allergy to cephalosporins, those with porphyria.
Possible interaction: amino glycosides, loop diuretics.
Side effects: allergic reactions, pain at site of injection, gastrointestinal upset, rise in level of liver enzymes and urea in blood, candidosis eosinophils (increase in blood of number of eosinophils, a variety of white blood cell), thrombocytopenia, neutropenia. Positive Coomb's test.
Manufacturer: Wellcome.

Celance

Description: a dopamine agonist, pergolide mesylate, produced in the form of tablets: ivory, marked 4131 contain 0.05mg , green marked 4133, contain 0.25mg, and pink tablets, marked 4135 contain 1mg. All are rectangular, scored and marked LILLY.
Used for: additional therapy (to levodopa) in treatment of Parkinson's disease.
Dosage: 0.05mg each day at first increasing every third day by 0.1–0.15mg for a period of 12 days. Then the dose is increased by 0.25mg every third day until the best response is achieved. Maximum daily dose is 5mg. Levodopa dose should be carefully reduced.
Special care: pregnancy, breast-feeding, heart disease, heart arrhythmias, history of hallucinations. Drug should be gradually withdrawn.
Avoid use: children.

Possible interaction: anticoagulants, antihypertensives, other dopamine antagonists.
Side effects: disturbances of heartbeat, movement disorder (dyskinesia), drowsiness, hypotension, inflammation of the nose, dyspepsia, nausea, dyspnoea (laboured breathing), diplopia.
Manufacturer: Lilly

Celectol

Description: an antihypertensive preparation which is a cardioselective beta₁-blocker and partial beta₂-agonist. It is produced in heart-shaped tablets of 2 strengths, yellow scored tablets contain 200mg celiprolol hydrochloride and white tablets contain 400mg. The tablets are film-coated and marked with logo and strength.
Used for: mild to moderate hypertension.
Dosage: adults, 200mg once each day half an hour before food, maximum dose 400mg.
Special care: pregnancy, nursing mothers, anaestheseia or planned surgery, diabetes, liver or kidney disease, metabolic acidosis. Patients with weak hearts should receive diuretic and digitalis. Patients with history of bronchospasm. Drug should be gradually withdrawn.
Avoid use: children, patients with various forms of heart disease including heart block, heart failure, slow heart beat rate; sick sinus syndrome, peripheral arterial disease. Patients with obstructive airways disease (unless absolutely no alternative).
Possible interaction: sympathomimetics, central nervous system depressants, indomethacin, antihypertensives, ergotamine, reserpine, cimetidine, cardiac depressant anaesthetics, hypoglycaemics, verapamil, Class I antiarrhythmics, clonidine withdrawal.
Side effects: gastrointestinal disorders, fatigue with exercise, cold feet and hands, disruption of sleep, slow heartbeat rate. If dry eyes or skin rash occur, drug should be gradually withdrawn.
Manufacturer: Rhône-Poulenc Rorer.

Ceporex

Description: a cephalosporin antibiotic produced in the form of tablets, capsules and syrup. Pink, film-coated tablets, containing 250mg, 500mg and 1g cephalexin are marked GLAXO and with name and strength. **Ceporex Capsules** coloured grey/caramel contain 250mg and 500mg and are marked GLAXO and with capsule name and strength. **Ceporex Orange Syrup** (produced as granules for reconstitution), contains 125mg, 250mg and 500mg per 5ml when made up with water. **Ceporex Suspension** coloured yellow, contains 125mg or

250mg per 5ml. **Ceporex Paediatric Drops** coloured orange contain 125mg per 1.25ml solution (produced as granules for reconstitution with 10ml water).

Used for: urinary tract infections, gonorrhoea, middle ear infections, respiratory tract, skin and soft tissue infections.

Dosage: adults, 1–2g daily in 2, 3 or 4 divided doses. Children, under 3 months, 62.5mg–125mg twice each day; 4 months to 2 years, 250–500mg each day; 3 years to 6 years, 1–2g each day, all in 2, 3 or 4 divided doses.

Special care: patients with allergy to penicillins or kidney disease.

Side effects: allergic reactions, gastrointestinal upset.

Manufacturer: Glaxo.

Cesamet

Description: an anti-emetic preparation, which is a cannabinoid drug thought to have an effect in the central nervous system involving opiate receptors. It is produced as blue/white capsules, for hospital use only, containing 1mg babilone.

Used for: nausea and vomiting caused by cytotoxic drugs.

Dosage: 1mg twice each day increasing to 2mg twice daily if required. First dose is taken the night before and the second, 1 to 3 hours before cytotoxic therapy begins. Maximum dose is 6mg in 3 divided doses. If necessary, it may be continued for 48 hours after cytotoxic therapy has ceased.

Special care: elderly persons, patients with heart disease, severe liver disorders, hypertension, history of psychiatric disorders. Performance of skilled tasks, e.g. driving may be affected.

Possible interaction: alcohol, hypnotics and sedatives (enhances the effect of drowsiness).

Side effects: dry mouth, disturbance of vision, headache, drowsiness, vertigo, inability to concentrate, sleep disturbances, unsteady gait, hypotension, nausea. Mental disturbances including confusion, euphoria, disorientation, hallucinations, psychosis, depression, lack of coordination, loss of appetite, increased heartbeat rate, tremor, abdominal pain.

Manufacturer: Lilly.

Chemotrim Paediatric

Description: an antibiotic preparation produced in the form of a suspension specifically intended for children. It combines a sulphonamide with a folic acid inhibitor, containing 200mg sulphamethoxazole and 40mg trimethoprim per 5ml of suspension.

Used for: urinary tract, skin, respiratory and gastrointestinal infections.

Dosage: children 6 weeks to 5 months, 2.5ml; 6 months to 5 years, 5ml; 6 years to 12 years, 10ml. All twice each day.

Special care: elderly, breast-feeding, kidney disease (reduce and/or increase time between doses). During long-term therapy, regular blood counts should be carried out.

Avoid use: neonates (babies from birth to 1 month of age), pregnancy, patients with serious liver or kidney disease or blood changes.

Possible interaction: hypoglycaemics, anticoagulants, anticonvulsants, folate inhibitors.

Side effects: skin rashes, glossitis (inflammation of tongue), nausea, vomiting, blood changes, folate deficiency. Rarely erythema multiforme, Lyell syndrome.

Manufacturer: RP Drugs.

Chendol

Description: a bile acid preparation produced in the form of orange/ivory capsules, marked CHENDOL contain 125mg chenodeoxycholic acid.

Used for: to dissolve cholesterol gallstones which are not calcified.

Dosage: adults 10–15mg per kg of body weight as a single nightly dose or divided doses. Continue for 3 months after gallstones have been dissolved.

Special care: liver function should be carefully monitored.

Avoid use: children, women planning a pregnancy, patients with chronic liver disease or inflammatory intestinal disease.

Possible interaction: oral contraceptives.

Side effects: pruritis (itching), diarrhoea.

Manufacturer: CP Pharmaceuticals.

Chenofalk

Description: a bile acid preparation produced in the form of tablets and available as white capsules containing 250mg chenodeoxycholic acid.

Used for: to dissolve cholesterol gallstones which are not calcified.

Dosage: adults, 15mg per kg of body weight each day in divided doses. Should be continued for 3 to 6 months after stones have been dissolved.

Special care: liver function should be carefully monitored.

Avoid use: women planning pregnancy or who are not using contraception. Patients with non-functioning gall bladder, inflammatory intestinal disease, chronic liver disease.

Possible interaction: oral contraceptives.

Side effects: pruritis (itching), diarrhoea.
Manufacturer: Thames.

Chlorasept
Description: a proprietary disinfectant preparation available as a pink solution and containing 0.05% chlorhexidine acetate.
Used for: cleansing of wounds.
Dosage: apply as required.
Manufacturer: Baxter

Chlordiazepoxide
Description: an anxiolytic and long-acting benzodiazepine produced in the form of tablets of strengths 5mg, 10mg and 25mg chlordiazepoxide. Also, **Chlordiazepoxide Hydrochloride** tablets are available in strengths of 5mg, 10mg and 25mg and **Chlordiazepoxide Capsules**, available in strengths of 5mg and 10mg.
Used for: relief of anxiety.
Dosage: adults, 30mg each day in divided doses increasing to 40–100mg if symptoms are severe. Elderly persons, 10mg each day at first, carefully increased if needed.
Special care: use for short-term relief of severe and disabling anxiety (for a period of 2–4 weeks). Lowest possible dose and withdraw drug gradually. Special care needed for elderly persons, pregnant women, breast-feeding mothers, women in labour. Patients with lung, liver or kidney disease.
Avoid use: patients with severe lung disease or depressed respiration. Those with psychiatric disorders including obsessional and phobic states and psychosis.
Possible interaction: alcohol, CNS depressants, anticonvulsant drugs.
Side effects: gastrointestinal upset, drowsiness, light headedness, unsteadiness, vertigo, confusion, impaired judgment and dexterity. Disturbance of vision, hypotension, skin rashes. Urine retention, changes in libido. Rarely, jaundice and blood changes. Risk of dependency with higher doses or longer period of use.
Manufacturer: non-proprietary.

Chloromycetin
Description: a broad-spectrum antibiotic, chloramphenicol, produced in the form of capsules, as a suspension and as a powder for reconstitution and injection. White/grey capsules marked PARKE-DAVIS contain 250mg, **Chloromycetin Palmitate Suspension** contains 125mg per 5ml. **Chloromycetin Injection** produced as a powder in vials contains cholamphenicol (as sodium succinate).

Used for: severe infections where there are no effective alternatives, typhoid fever, influenzae meningitis.
Dosage: adults, 50mg per kg of body weight each day in divided doses at 6 hourly intervals. Children under 2 weeks of age, half adult dose; over 2 weeks, same as adult.
Special care: regular blood tests are advisable during course of treatment.
Avoid use: for minor infections or for prevention.
Possible interaction: paracetamol, anticonvulsants, anticoagulants.
Side effects: gastrointestinal upset, allergic reactions, blood changes, neuritis, and optic (eye) neuritis with prolonged use. Newborn babies may develop Grey syndrome.
Manufacturer: Parke-Davis.

Chloromycetin Eye Ointment
Description: a broad-spectrum antibiotic eye ointment containing 1% chloramphenicol and also eye drops, **Chloromycetin Redidrops**, containing 0.5% chloramphenicol.
Used for: bacterial conjunctivitis.
Dosage: 2 drops or apply ointment every 3 hours or more often if needed. Continue for 2 days after symptoms have gone.
Side effects: rarely, aplastic anaemia (caused by bone marrow failure) a form of anaemia in which there is a lack of all blood elements.
Manufacturer: Parke-Davis.

Chloromycetin Hydrocortisone
Description: a proprietary antibiotic and corticosteroid ointment containing 1% chloramphenicol and 0.5% hydrocortisone acetate.
Used for: eye infections.
Dosage: apply to eye once an hour if infection is severe, or less frequently if infection is less severe.
Special care: infants or prolonged use.
Avoid use: glaucoma, viral, fungal or purulent infections.
Manufacturer: Parke-Davis

Cicatrin
Description: an aminoglycoside, antibacterial preparation available in the form of a cream, dusting powder and aerosol. The cream and powder contain 3300 units neomycin sulphate, 250 units bacitracin zinc, 2mg l-cysteine, 10mg glycine and 1mg threonine per g. The aerosol contains 16,500 units neomycin sulphate, 1250 units bacitracin zinc, 12mg l-cysteine, 60mg glycine/g in the form of a spray powder.
Used for: minor bacterial skin infections.

Dosage: adults and children, cream, aerosol and dusting powder, apply 3 times each day to affected skin for 3 weeks.

Special care: on large areas of affected skin. Do not repeat for 3 months.

Side effects: allergic responses, ototoxicity (damage to organs of hearing and balance).

Manufacturer: Wellcome.

Cidomycin

Description: an aminoglycoside antibiotic preparation containing gentamicin as sulphate and produced in a variety of different forms for injection. Cidomycin injection contains 40mg gentamicin (as sulphate) per ml produced in ampoules and vials. **Cidomycin Paediatric Injection** contains 10mg/ml in 2ml vials. **Cidomycin Intrathecal Injection** contains 5mg/ml in ampoules.

Used for: serious infections sensitive to gentamicin; urinary tract infections.

Dosage: adults, 5mg per kg of body weight by intramuscular or intravenous injection each day in 3 or 4 divided doses. Children, up to 2 weeks of age, 3mg per kg of body weight at 12 hour intervals; over 2 weeks, 2mg per kg of body weight at 8-hour intervals. Both intramuscularly or intravenously for a period of 7–10 days.

Special care: patients with kidney disease, myasthenia gravis; regular blood tests are necessary as blood concentrations over 10μg per ml can cause damage to the organs of hearing and balance.

Avoid use: pregnant women.

Possible interaction: anaesthetics, neuromuscular blocking drugs, frusemide, ethacrynic acid.

Manufacturer: Roussel.

Cidomycin Topical

Description: an aminoglycoside antibiotic preparation containing 0.3% gentamicin (as sulphate) in the form of a cream or ointment.

Used for: skin infections (including impetigo), of a primary and secondary nature.

Dosage: apply to affected skin 3 or 4 times each day.

Special care: large areas of affected skin.

Side effects: allergic reactions, ototoxicity.

Manufacturer: Roussel.

Cidomycin Eye and Ear Drops

Description: an antibiotic preparation containing 0.3% gentamicin (as sulphate) in the form of ear and eye drops. Also, **Cidomycin Eye Ointment** containing 0.3% gentamicin as sulphate.

Used for: bacterial infections of the external ear and eye.

Dosage: ear drops, adults and children, 2 to 4 drops 3 or 4 times each day and at night. Eye drops and ointment, adults and children, 1 to 3 drops or applications of ointment 3 to 4 times each day.

Avoid use: ear infections where drum is perforated.

Side effects: risk of superinfection (another infection occurring during treatment).

Manufacturer: Roussel.

Cilest

Description: a combined oestrogen/progestogen contraceptive preparation containing 35μg ethinyloestradiol and 0.25mg norgestimate in the form of blue tablets marked C250.

Used for: oral contraception.

Dosage: 1 tablet each day for 21 days starting on first day of period, followed by 7 tablet-free days.

Special care: patients with asthma, diabetes, Raynaud's disease, varicose veins, hypertension, serious kidney disease, kidney dialysis, multiple sclerosis, hyperprolactinaemia (an excess of prolactin, a hormone, in the blood), serious depression. The risk of thrombosis increases with age and if woman smokes or is obese. Pelvic organs, breasts and blood pressure should be checked regularly during the time oral contraceptives are being taken.

Avoid use: pregnancy, history of thrombosis or at risk, those with various forms of heart disease, heart valve disease and angina. Patient with sickle cell anaemia, infectious hepatitis, certain liver and kidney disorders, hormone-dependent cancers, undiagnosed vaginal bleeding.

Possible interaction: tetracyclines, barbiturates, carbamazepine, primidone, griseofulvin, phenytoin, chloral hydrate, glutethimide, ethosuximide, dichloralphenazone.

Side effects: nausea, headaches, bloatedness due to fluid retention, enlargement of breasts, cramps and leg pains, reduction in libido, depression, weight gain, bleeding, vaginal discharge, erosion of cervix.

Manufacturer: Ortho.

Cinobac

Description: a quinolone antibiotic drug produced as green/orange capsules containing 500mg cinoxacin and marked LILLY 3056.

Used for: infections of the urinary tract.

Dosage: 1 tablet twice each day for 7 to 14 days. For prevention of infection, 1 tablet at night.

Special care: patients with kidney disorders or history of liver disease.

Avoid use: children, pregnancy, breast-feeding, severe kidney disorders.

Possible interaction: NSAIDs, anticoagulant drugs taken by mouth, theophylline.
Side effects: gastrointestinal upset, disturbance of CNS, allergic reactions.
Manufacturer: Lilly

Ciproxin

Description: A 4-quinolone antibiotic preparation, ciprofloxacin hydrochloride monohydrate, produced in the form of tablets of 3 different strenths and as a solution for infusion. White, film-coated tablets, marked with BAYER logo and CIP 250 contain 250mg; BAYER logo and CIP 500 (500mg); marked with BAYER logo and CIP 750 (750mg). **Ciproxin Infusion** contains 2mg ciprofloxacin (as lactate) per ml.
Used for: ear, nose, throat, respiratory tract infections. Skin, bone, joint, soft tissue and eye infections. Also, pelvic and gastrointestinal infections, gonorrhoea and pneumonia caused by Gram-negative bacteria. Prevention of infection in endoscopy and surgery on upper gastrointestinal tract.
Dosage: adults, tablets, 250mg to 750 mg twice each day for 5 to 10 days. For gonorrhoea, one 250mg dose. For prevention of infection, 750mg 1 hour to 1½ hours before operation. Infusion, 100–200mg twice each day by intravenous infusion for 5 to 7 days. For gonorrhoea, 100mg by intravenous infusion.
Special care: severe kidney and liver disorders, epilepsy or disorders of central nervous system, history of convulsions. Plenty of fluids should be drunk.
Avoid use: children and adolescents (except in exceptional circumstances), pregnancy, breast-feeding.
Possible interaction: alcohol, NSAIDs, opiates, theophylline, cyclosporin, glibenclamide, iron, magnesium or aluminium salts.
Side effects: headache, tremor, dizziness, confusion, impaired judgment and dexterity (ability to drive and operate machinery may be affected), disturbance of sleep, convulsions. Sensitivity to light, skin rash, pains in joints, disturbance of vision, tachycardia. There may be changes in liver, kidneys and in blood.
Manufacturer: Bayer.

Citanest

Description: a local anaesthetic preparation produced as solutions of various strengths, for injection and containing prilocaine hydrochloride. Citanest is available in strengths of 0.5% (5mg prilocaine hydrochloride per ml), 1% (10mg per ml), 2% (20mg per ml) and 4% (40mg per ml). Also, **Citanest with Octapressin** containing 3% and 0.03 units per ml of felypressin.
Used for: local anaesthesia.
Dosage: adults, (adjusted according to patient response and nature of operation), maximum 400mg if used alone or 600mg with felypressin or adrenaline. Children according to body weight and nature of operation.
Special care: patients with liver, kidney or respiratory disorders, epilepsy or conduction disturbances.
Avoid use: patients with anaemia, methaemoglobinaemia (presence in the blood of methaemoglobin derived from the blood pigment, haemoglobin, which results in a lack of oxygen being carried in the blood and various symptoms arising from this).
Side effects: allergic reactions, rarely, whole body (systemic) effects.
Manufacturer: Astra.

Claforan

Description: a cephalosporin antibiotic preparation produced in the form of a powder for reconstitution and injection. Claforan contains 500mg, 1g or 2g of cefotaxime (as sodium salt), as powder in vials.
Used for: urinary tract and soft tissue infections, septicaemia, meningitis and respiratory tract infections.
Dosage: adults, 1g by intravenous or intramuscular injection at 8-hourly intervals. For serious infections dose may need to be increased to 6g (maximum 12g) daily in 3 or 4 divided doses. The 2g dose should be given intravenously. Children, newborn babies, 50mg per kg of body weight daily in 2, 3 or 4 divided doses; older infants and children, 200mg per kg of body weight daily in 2, 3 or 4 divided doses.
Special care: pregnancy, breast-feeding, penicillin allergy and serious kidney failure.
Possible interaction: aminoglycosides, loop diuretics.
Side effects: gastrointestinal upset, pain at injection site, allergic reactions, candidosis, blood changes, haemolytic anaemia, rise in liver enzymes and blood urea.
Manufacturer: Roussel.

Clarityn

Description: an antihistamine preparation produced in the form of oval, white, scored tablets containing 10mg loratadine, and marked with strength and logo. Also, **Clarityn Syrup** containing 5mg per 5ml.

Used for: relief of symptoms of allergic rhinitis, e.g. hay fever, urticaria.

Dosage: adults, 1 tablet each day, or 10ml syrup. Children, syrup only, 2 to 7 years, 5ml; 7 to 12 years, 10ml, both once each day.

Avoid use: children under 2 years of age, pregnancy, breast-feeding.

Side effects: headache, nausea, fatigue.

Manufacturer: Schering-Plough.

Clexane

Description: an anticoagulant preparation produced in pre-filled syringes for injection containing either 20mg (low molecular weight heparin) enoxaparin per 0.2ml or 40mg enoxaparin per 0.4ml.

Used for: prevention of deep vein thrombosis especially associated with orthopaedic and general surgery. Prevention of blood clot formation during haemodialysis.

Dosage: adults, low to medium risk of thrombosis (in general surgery), 20mg 2 hours before operation by deep subcutaenous injection and then 20mg once each day for 7 to 10 days. High risk of thrombosis (orthopaedic surgery), 40mg 12 hours before operation by deep subcutaenous injection, and 40mg once a day for 7 to 10 days. Haemodialysis, 1mg per kg of body weight with a further dose of 0.5 to 1mg/kg if process lasts for longer than 4 hours.

Special care: pregnancy, breast-feeding, hypertension, history of liver disorders or ulcers.

Avoid use: children, patients with peptic ulcer, serious bleeding disorders (e.g. haemophilia), those at risk of haemorrhage, thrombocytopenia, cerebral aneurysm, severe liver disease. Patients who have had recent CNS or eye surgery.

Possible interaction: aspirin, NSAIDs, dextran, anticoagulants taken by mouth, antiplatelet drugs.

Side effects: effects on liver, thrombocytopenia, less commonly, bruising and haemorrhage.

Manufacturer: Rhône-Poulenc Rorer.

Climagest

Description: a combined oestrogen, progestogen hormonal preparation, produced in the form of tablets. Climagest 1mg consists of 16 blue-grey tablets containing 1mg oestradiol valerate, coded E1, and 12 white tablets, containing 1mg oestradiol valerate and 1mg norethisterone, coded N1. Also, **Climagest 2mg** consists of 16 blue tablets containing 2mg oestradiol valerate, coded E2, and 12 yellow tablets containing 2mg oestradiol valerate

and 1mg norethisterone, coded N2.

Used for: relief of menopausal symptoms.

Dosage: 1 tablet daily starting with oestradiol valerate (coded E) on first day of period (if present), and finishing with the 12 tablets (coded N), containing norethisterone.

Special care: patients considered to be at risk of thrombosis, those with diabetes, epilepsy, hypertension, multiple sclerosis, migraine, fibroids in uterus, ostosclerosis, tetany, liver disease, porphyria, gallstones. Regular examination of breasts and pelvic organs should be carried out and blood pressure checked. Drug should be stopped if there are any signs of jaundice, headaches which are severe, migraine, rise in blood pressure before planned surgery.

Avoid use: pregnancy, breast-feeding, hormone-dependent cancers, breast or uterus cancer, endometriosis, undiagnosed vaginal bleeding, sickle cell anaemia. Serious heart, kidney or liver disease, thrombosis. Patients suffering from Dublin-Johnson syndrome or Rotor syndrome.

Possible interaction: drugs which induce liver enzymes.

Side effects: weight gain, enlargement and tenderness of breasts, fluid retention, cramps, gastrointestinal upset, nausea and vomiting, headaches, breakthrough bleeding, dizziness.

Manufacturer: Sandoz.

Climaval

Description: a hormonal oestrogen preparation produced in tablets of 2 strengths. Climaval 1mg are grey/blue tablets containing 1mg oestradiol valerate marked E1; Climaval 2mg are blue tablets containing 2mg oestradiol valerate and marked E2.

Used for: treatment of menopausal symptoms in women who have had a hysterectomy.

Dosage: 1 tablet each day either 1mg or 2mg according to response. May be taken continuously for up to 2 years.

Special care: only in elderly women for post-menopausal symptoms, otherwise avoid use; patients considered to be at risk of thrombosis, those with diabetes, epilepsy, hypertension, multiple sclerosis, migraine, fibroids in uterus, ostosclerosis, tetany, liver disease, porphyria, gallstones. Regular examination of breasts and pelvic organs should be carried out and blood pressure checked. Drug should be stopped if there are any signs of jaundice, severe headaches and migraine, a rise in blood pressure and before planned surgery.

Avoid use: pregnancy, breast-feeding, hormone-dependent cancers, breast and uterine cancer, endometriosis, undiagnosed vaginal bleeding, sickle cell anaemia, serious heart, kidney or liver disease, thrombosis. Patients suffering from Dublin-Johnson syndrome or Rotor syndrome.

Possible interaction: drugs which induce liver enzymes.

Side effects: weight gain, enlargement and tenderness of breasts, fluid retention, cramps, gastrointestinal upset, nausea and vomiting, headaches, dizziness.

Manufacturer: Sandoz.

Clinoril

Description: a proprietary analgesic NSAID produced in the form of hexagonal yellow scored tablets containing 100mg or 200mg sulindac and marked MSD 943 and MSD 942 respectively.

Used for: inflammation and pain in rheumatic diseases including gout, rheumatoid arthritis and osteoarthritis.

Dosage: adults, 200mg twice each day with food or drink.

Special care: elderly persons with history of lithiasis (gallstones, kidney stones, stones in lower urinary tract), patients with heart failure, liver or kidney disease, history of gastrointestinal haemorrhage or ulcers. Plenty of fluids should be taken and liver function monitored.

Avoid use: children, pregnancy, breast-feeding, allergy to aspirin or anti-inflammatory drugs, those with gastrointestinal bleeding or peptic ulcer.

Possible interaction: aspirin, anticoagulants, diflunisal, hypoglycaemic drugs, methotrexate, dimethyl sulphoxide, cyclosporin.

Side effects: allergic responses including liver failure and fever (stop drug immediately). Disturbance of vision, central nervous system effects, heart arrythmias, changes in blood, kidney stones and disturbance of kidney function, pancreatitis, hyperglycaemia, gastrointestinal bleeding and upset. Also rash, dizziness, glossitis (inflammation of tongue), tinnitus, muscle weakness, effects on urine including discolouration, proteinuria (protein in urine), crystals in urine (crystalluria), oedema.

Manufacturer: MSD.

Clobazam

Description: an anxiolytic long-acting benzodiazepine drug also used as an additional treatment for epilepsy. It is produced in the form of capsules containing 10mg clobazam.

Used for: short-term relief of symptoms of anxiety; additional therapy for epilepsy.

Dosage: anxiety, 20–30mg each day in divided doses or as 1 dose taken at night. In severe cases (under hospital supervision) dose may be increased to 60mg each day in divided doses. Elderly or debilitated persons, reduced daily dose of 10–20mg. Adults, epilepsy, 20–30mg each day (maximum 60mg) in divided doses. Children, for epilepsy only, age 3 to 12 years, half adult dose.

Special care: children under 3 years (epilepsy) and not for children in cases of anxiety, pregnancy, women in labour, breast-feeding, elderly (reduced dose), patients with liver or kidney disease or respiratory disorders. Prolonged use and abrupt withdrawal of drug should be avoided.

Avoid use: severe respiratory or lung disorders.

Possible interaction: CNS depressants, alcohol, anticonvulsant drugs.

Side effects: impaired judgment and dexterity interfering with performance of skilled tasks, lightheadedness, confusion, drowsiness, unsteadiness, vertigo. Also disturbance of vision, gastrointestinal upset, retention of urine, skin rashes, change in libido, hypotension. Rarely, jaundice and blood changes.

Manufacturer: non-proprietary but available from Hoechst as **Frisium**.

Clomid

Description: an anti-oestrogen hormonal preparation produced in the form of pale yellow scored tablets, containing 50mg clomiphene citrate, and marked with a circle containing the letter M.

Used for: treatment of sterility in women due to failure of ovulation.

Dosage: 1 tablet each day for 5 days starting on the fifth day of menstruation.

Special care: ensure patient is not pregnant before and during the course of treatment.

Avoid use: women with large ovarian cyst, cancer of the womb, undiagnosed uterine bleeding, liver disease.

Side effects: hot flushes, enlargement of ovaries, abdominal discomfort, blurring of vision (withdraw drug).

Manufacturer: Merrell Dow.

Clopixol

Description: an antipsychotic drug and thioxanthene produced in the form of tablets and as solutions for injection. Tablets are produced in various strengths and all are film-coated; pink tablets contain 2mg zuclopenthixol hydrochloride; light brown tablets contain 10mg; brown tablets contain 25mg.

Clopixol Injection contains 200mg per ml (as oily

injection) contained in ampoules and vials. **Clopixol Concentrated Injection** contains 500mg per ml (as oily injection) contained in ampoules. **Clopixol Acuphase** contains 50mg per ml (as oily injection) contained in ampoules.

Used for: psychoses, particularly schizophrenia and especially when accompanied by aggression and agitated behaviour.

Dosage: tablets, 20–30mg each day in divided doses in first instance. Usual maintenance dose is in the order of 25–50mg each day with a maximum daily dose of 500mg. Clopixol injection, 200–400mg every 2 to 4 weeks by deep intramuscular injection with a maximum weekly dose of 600mg. Clopixol concentrated injection, 250–500mg every 1 to 4 weeks by deep intramuscular injection with a maximum weekly dose of 600mg. Clopixol acuphase (for immediate treatment of acute psychoses), 50–150mg by deep intramuscular injection repeated after 1, 2 or 3 days if required. Maximum total dose is 400mg and maintenance should be by means of tablets or other Clopixol injections.

Special care: pregnancy, breast-feeding, heart and circulatory disorders, liver or kidney disease, Parkinson's disease, an intolerance to neuroleptic drugs taken by mouth.

Avoid use: children, coma, states of withdrawal and apathy.

Possible interaction: alcohol, antidiabetic drugs, levodopa, anticonvulsant drugs, analgesics, CNS sedatives, antihypertensive drugs.

Side effects: Parkinson's disease-like effects, spasms in muscles and involuntary, repetitive movements, rapid heartbeat rate, vision disturbance, tremor. Also hypotension, changes in weight, difficulty in passing urine, dry mouth and stuffiness in nose, impotence, enlargement of breasts, hypothermia (especially in elderly persons). There may be blood changes, dermatitis, weariness and lethargy, fits and jaundice.

Manufacturer: Lundbeck.

Clostet

Description: a preparation of tetanus toxoid vaccine (40iu per 0.5ml) adsorbed onto aluminium hydroxide and contained in pre-filled (0.5ml) syringes.

Used for: immunization against tetanus and for 'booster' injections to reinforce immunity.

Dosage: adults, a course of 0.5ml by subcutaneous or intramuscular injection given a total of 3 times at 4 week intervals. After 10 years, a 'booster' reinforcing dose of 0.5ml may be given by subcutaneous or intramuscular injection. If an injury

is received which might give rise to tetanus, a booster reinforcing dose should be given to patients previously immunized. Those who have not, should be given a first dose of the primary course and an injection of antitetanus immunoglobin at a different site. Children normally receive a combined triple vaccine consisting of adsorbed tetanus, diphtheria and pertussis (whooping cough) vaccine, and can later receive booster reinforcing doses against tetanus.

Special care: allergic reactions especially in persons receiving vaccine within 1 year of receiving a previous booster dose. Normally, 10 years should have elapsed before a reinforcing dose is given.

Avoid use: patients with serious infections unless there is a wound likely to be prone to tetanus.

Side effects: malaise, fever, slight soreness and local reactions.

Manufacturer: Evans.

Clozapril

Description: an antipsychotic drug and dibenzodiazepine, clozapine, produced as yellow scored tablets (25mg strength) and marked CLOZ 25, and 100mg strength, marked CLOZARIL 100.

Used for: schizophrenia which has failed to respond to, or patient is intolerant of other conventional antipsychotic drugs.

Dosage: first day, 12.5mg once or twice. Second day, 25mg once or twice; dose is gradually increased over a period of 2 to 3 weeks by 25–50mg each day until patient is receiving 300mg daily in divided doses. Depending upon response, a further increase may be required by giving an additional 50–100mg every 4 to 7 days to a maximum of 900mg each day in divided doses. Usual maintenance dose is in the order of 150–300mg in divided doses. Elderly persons, 12.5mg each day in first instance slowly increasing by 25mg daily.

Special care: patient, prescribing doctor and pharmacist must be registered with Sandoz Clorazil Patient Monitoring Service (CPMS). Patients should report signs of infection and must take contraceptive precautions. Special care in pregnant women, patients with enlarged prostate gland, liver disease, glaucoma, paralytic ileus. Persons with epilepsy should be monitored. Regular blood counts of leucocytes should be carried out before and during treatment. Drug should be immediately withdrawn if whole blood count falls below 3000/mm^3 or neutrophil (a type of white blood cell) count below 1500/mm^3.

Avoid use: children; patients with history of drug induced blood disorders—neutropenia, agranulocytosis (a serious fall in the number of white blood cells called eosinophils, basophils and neutrophils), bone marrow disorders. Also, patients with history of drug intoxication, toxic and alcoholic psychoses, CNS depression or those in comatose states. Avoid use in breast-feeding mothers, persons with serious kidney or liver disease or circulatory collapse and cardiac failure.

Possible interaction: benzodiazepines, alcohol, MAOIs, CNS depressants, other drugs which cause agranulocytosis, anticholinergics, antihistamines, hypotensive drugs, lithium, phenytoin, warfarin, cimetidine.

Side effects: neutropenia leading to agranulocytosis (characterized by fever, collapse, bleeding ulcers of vagina, rectum and mouth) which may be fatal, effects on heart muscle and brain activity, tachycardia, fits, fatigue, dizziness, headache, overproduction of saliva in mouth, retention of urine, gastrointestinal upset, disturbance of body temperature regulation.

Manufacturer: Sandoz

Co-Betaloc

Description: an antihyptertensive preparation combined with a cardioselective ß-blocker with a thiazide diuretic produced in the form of white scored tablets, marked A/MH, contain 100mg metoprolol tartrate and 12.5mg hydrochloro-thiazide. Also **Co-Betaloc SA** are yellow, film-coated tablets, marked A/MC, containing 200mg metoprolol tartrate and 25mg hydrochlorothiazide and having a sustained-release core.

Used for: mild to moderate hypertension.

Dosage: adults, 1 to 3 tablets each day in single or divided doses, or 1 Co-Betaloc SA tablet daily.

Special care: pregnancy, breast-feeding, diabetes, kidney or liver disorders, metabolic acidosis, undergoing general anaesthesia, (may need to be withdrawn before planned surgery). Monitor electrolyte levels. Patients with weak hearts may need treatment with digitalis and diuretics. Drug should be gradually withdrawn. Potassium supplements may be required.

Avoid use: children, patients with history of obstructive airways disease, bronchospasm, asthma, heart block, heart shock, heart failure, severe peripheral arterial disease, sick sinus syndrome, severe kidney failure, anuria.

Possible interaction: sympathomimetics, cardiac depressant anaesthetics, clonidine withdrawal, hypoglycaemics, class I antiarrhythmic drugs, other antihypertensives, verapamil, ergotamine, reserpine, indomethacin, cimetidine, CNS depressants, lithium, digitalis.

Manufacturer: Astra.

Co-Danthramer

Description: a preparation which combines a stimulant laxative and faecal softener produced in the form of a liquid. It contains 200mg of Poloxamer '188' and 25mg of danthron per 5ml of liquid. Also, **Strong Co-Danthramer** which contains 1g Poloxamer '188' and 75mg danthron per 5ml of liquid.

Used for: treatment and prevention of constipation in terminally ill persons (which has been caused by analgesic drugs). Also, constipation in elderly persons and patients with coronary thrombosis or cardiac failure.

Dosage: adults, 5–10ml Co-Danthramer or 5ml Strong Co-Danthramer taken at night. Children, 2.5–5ml Co-Danthramer only, taken at night.

Special care: pregnant women, patients suffering from incontinence (avoid prolonged contact with skin as irritation and soreness may occur).

Avoid use: babies in nappies, breast-feeding, severe painful abdominal disorders, any intestinal obstruction.

Side effects: red discolouration of urine and skin with which urine comes into contact.

Manufacturer: non-proprietary, available from Napp as variations of **Codalax**.

Co-Danthrusate

Description: a preparation which combines a stimulant laxative and faecal softener produced in the form of capsules and as a suspension. The capsules contain 50mg danthron and 60mg docusate sodium and **Co-Danthrusate Suspension** contains 50mg danthron and 60mg docusate sodium per 5ml.

Used for: treatment and prevention of constipation in terminally ill patients (which has been caused by analgesic drugs). Also, constipation in elderly persons and patients with coronary thrombosis and cardiac failure.

Dosage: adults, 1 to 3 capsules or 5–15ml suspension taken at night. Children over 6 years of age, 1 capsule or 5ml suspension taken at night.

Special care: pregnancy, breast-feeding.

Avoid use: children under 6 years, patients with intestinal obstruction.

Side effects: red discoloration of urine and skin with which urine may come into contact.

Manufacturer: non-proprietary, available from Evans as **Normax**.

Co-Dydramol

Description: a compound opiate analgesic preparation combining 10mg dihydrocodeine tartrate with 500mg paracetamol in the form of tablets.

Used for: relief of mild to moderate pain.
Dosage: adults, 1 to 2 tablets every 4 to 6 hours with a maximum of 8 daily.
Special care: pregnant women, elderly persons, patients with allergies, underactive thyroid, liver or kidney disease.
Avoid use: children, patients with obstructive airways disease or respiratory depression.
Possible interaction: CNS sedatives, alcohol.
Side effects: headaches, constipation, nausea.
Manufacturer: Non-proprietary, available from several companies.

Co-Proxamol
Description: a compound opiate analgesic preparation combining 32.5mg dextropropoxyphene hydrochloride and 325mg paracetamol in tablet form.
Used for: relief of mild to moderate pain.
Dosage: adults, 2 tablets 3 or 4 times each day.
Special care: pregnant women, elderly persons, patients with liver or kidney disease.
Avoid use: children.
Possible interaction: CNS sedatives, alcohol, anticonvulsant and anticoagulant drugs.
Side effects: risk of dependence and tolerance, dizziness, rash, nausea, constipation, drowsiness.
Manufacturer: non-proprietary, available from several companies.

Cobadex
Description: a mildly potent topical corticosteroid preparation produced in the form of a cream containing 1% hydrocortisone and 20% dimethicone.
Used for: mild inflammatory skin conditions such as eczema which are responsive to steroids. Also, anal and vulval pruritis (itching).
Dosage: apply thinly 2 or 3 times daily to affected area.
Special care: use in children or on face should be limited to a maximum period of 5 days. Should be gradually withdrawn after prolonged use.
Avoid use: various skin conditions including acne, leg ulcers, scabies, viral skin disease, ringworm, tuberculosis, untreated bacterial or fungal infections. Continuous use or long-term use in pregnancy.
Side effects: thinning of skin, suppression of adrenal glands, hair growth.
Manufacturer: Cox.

Cobalin-H
Description: a preparation of vitamin B_{12} produced in ampoules for injection containing 1000µg hydroxocobalamin per ml.

Used for: B_{12} responsive macrocytic anaemia (a disorder of the blood characterized by reduced production of red blood cells and the presence of large, fragile red blood cells), megaloblastic anaemia, tobacco amblyopia (an eye disorder).
Dosage: for anaemias, 250–1000µg by intramuscular injection on alternate days for 1 to 2 weeks. Afterwards, 250µg once a week until normal blood count is achieved. Maintenance dose is 1000µg every 2 to 3 months.
Special care: should only be given when cause of anaemia (either lack of vitamin B_{12} or of folate) has been established.
Manufacturer: Link.

Codafen Continus
Description: a combined opiate analgesic and NSAID produced in the form of pink/white tablets containing 20mg codeine phosphate and 300mg of sustained-release ibuprofen.
Used for: relief of pain including postoperative, dental and period pain.
Dosage: adults, 2 tablets every 12 hours at first increasing to 3 tablets every 12 hours if needed. Maintenance dose is 1 to 3 tablets each 12 hours.
Special care: Pregnancy, elderly, allergy to anti-inflammatory drugs or aspirin. Those with liver or kidney disease, heart failure, hypotension, hypo-thyroidism, head injury, history of bronchospasm.
Avoid use: children, patients with peptic ulcer or history of peptic ulcer, respiratory depression, breathing disorders.
Possible interaction: CNS sedatives, anticoagulants taken by mouth, thiazides, MAOIs, quinolones.
Side effects: dizziness, blurring of vision, headache, gastrointestinal upset and bleeding, peptic ulcer, drowsiness. Rarely, disturbance of liver and kidney function, thrombocytopenia, agranulocytosis (abnormal blood disorder in which there is a reduction in the number of certain white blood cells).
Manufacturer: NAPP.

Codalax
Description: a preparation which combines a stimulant laxative and faecal softener produced in the form of a solution of 2 different strengths. It contains 200mg Poloxamer '188' and 25mg danthron per 5ml. **Codalax Forte** contains 1g Poloxamer '188' and 75mg danthron per 5ml.
Used for: treatment and prevention of constipation in terminally ill persons (which has been caused by analgesic drugs). Also, constipation in elderly persons and patients with coronary thrombosis or cardiac failure.

Dosage: adults, Codalax, 5–10ml taken at night; Codalax Forte, 5ml taken at night. Children, Codalax only, 2.5–5ml taken at night.
Special care: pregnancy, incontinence.
Avoid use: babies in nappies, patients suffering from severe painful conditions of the abdomen or intestinal blockage.
Side effects: red discoloration of urine and skin with which urine comes into contact.
Manufacturer: Napp.

Codeine Phosphate

Description: an opiate analgesic preparation which additionally acts as a cough suppressant, and is available in the form of tablets and as a solution. The tablets are available in 3 strengths of 15mg, 30mg and 60mg codeine phosphate. The solution contains 25mg codeine phosphate per 5ml.
Used for: relief of mild to moderate pain.
Dosage: adults, 10–60mg every 4 hours with a maximum dose of 200mg each day. Children, 1 to 12 years, 3mg per kg of body weight, in divided doses, each day.
Special care: elderly persons, women in labour, patients with hyperthyroidism or serious liver disease.
Avoid use: children under 1 year of age, patients with obstructive airways disease or respiratory depression.
Possible interaction: central nervous system sedatives, MAOIs.
Side effects: blurred vision, drowsiness, dry mouth, dependence and tolerance, constipation.
Manufacturer: non-proprietary.

Cogentin

Description: an anticholinergic preparation produced as tablets and in ampoules for injection. White, scored tablets, contain 2mg benztropine mesylate and are coded MSD 60. **Cogentin Injection** contains 1mg per ml in 2ml ampoules.
Used for: treatment of Parkinson's disease including drug-induced symptoms of tremor and involuntary muscle movements (dyskinesia).
Dosage: tablets 0.5mg each day at first increasing gradually as required by 0.5mg every 5 or 6 days. Maximum dose is 6mg daily. Children over 3 years consult manufacturer. Adults, injection (for emergency treatment), 1–2mg given intramuscularly or intravenously.
Special care: narrow angle glaucoma, tachycardia, enlarged prostate gland, gastrointestinal blockage. Drug should be withdrawn slowly.
Avoid use: patients with movement disorder (tardive dyskinesia) or children under 3 years.

Possible interaction: antidepressants, phenothiazines, antidopaminergic drugs.
Side effects: agitation and confusion, anticholinergic effects; with higher doses, rash.
Manufacturer: MSD.

Colestid

Description: a form of a resin which is a bile acid sequestrant acting as a lipid-lowering agent. Colestid is available as 5g yellow granules in sachets containing colestipol hydrochloride. Also, **Colestid Orange** granules consisting of 5g orange-flavoured powder containing colestipol hydro-chloride with aspartame.
Used for: hyperlipidaemias (high fat levels in blood) particularly type IIa.
Dosage: adults, 5–30g each day in 1 or 2 divided doses taken with liquid. Children, consult manufacturer.
Special care: pregnancy, nursing mothers, additional vitamins A, D and K may be needed.
Avoid use: complete biliary blockage (total obstruction of bile duct).
Possible interaction: diuretics, digitalis, antibiotics. Any drug should be taken 1 hour before or 4 hours after Colestid as there may be intereference with absorption.
Side effects: constipation.
Manufacturer: Upjohn.

Colifoam

Description: a corticosteroid produced in the form of an aerosol foam containing 10% hydrocortisone acetate in mucoadherent foam.
Used for: ulcerative colitis and inflammation of the bowel.
Dosage: adults, 1 applicatorful into rectum once or twice each day for 2 or 3 weeks. Afterwards the same dosage every second day.
Special care: pregnant women, patients with severe ulcerative disease. Avoid use for prolonged periods.
Avoid use: children, patients with intestinal obstruction, abscess, perforation, peritonitis. Also, patients with recent anastomoses within the intestine, or extensive fistulas. Patients suffering from fungal or viral infections or tuberculosis.
Side effects: systemic corticosteroid effects including mood changes, thinning of bones, mood swings, elevated blood sugar levels.
Manufacturer: Stafford-Miller.

Colofac

Description: an anticholinergic, antispasmodic preparation produced in the form of tablets and as a liquid. White, sugar-coated tablets contain 135mg mebeverine hydrochloride. Yellow banana-flavoured, sugar-free **Colofac Suspension** contains mebeverine pamoate (equivalent to 50mg mebeverine hydrochloride per 5ml).

Used for: bowel spasm and gastrointestinal spasm in irritable bowel syndrome and gastrointestinal disorders.

Dosage: adults, 1 tablet or 15ml suspension 20 minutes before a meal 3 times each day. Children over 10 years, same as adult dose.

Avoid use: children under 10 years.

Manufacturer: Duphar.

Colomycin

Description: a polymyxin antibiotic preparation produced in the form of powder in vials for reconstitution with water and injection, syrup, tablets and as a powder for topical application. Colomycin powder for injection consists of 500,000 units colistin sulphomethate sodium or 1 million units colistin sulphomethate sodium in vials. **Colomycin Syrup** contains 250,000 units colistin sulphate per 5ml. **Colomycin Tablets** are quarter-scored and white containing 1.5 million units colistin sulphate and are marked with P inside a hexagon. **Colomycin Powder** for topical application contains 1g colistin sulphate in vial.

Used for: burns and wounds, surgery, skin infections, ENT infections, gram negative infections, aerosol therapy.

Dosage: adults (over 60kg body weight), injection, 2 mega units every 8 hours; children 50,000 units/kg body weight each day 8-hourly. Adults, tablets, 1 to 2 8-hourly; children, syrup, up to 15kg body weight, 5–10ml; 15–30kg, 15–30ml; over 30kg same as adult. All taken 8-hourly.

Special care: patients with kidney disease, porphyria.

Avoid use: pregnancy, breast-feeding, myasthenia gravis.

Possible interaction: muscle relaxant drugs, other antibiotic drugs, anticoagulants, cytotoxics, cholinergics, diuretics, bisophonates, cyclosporin.

Side effects: paruesthesia ('pins and needles'), vertigo, muscle weakness, apnoea (temporary halt in breathing), toxic effects on kidneys. Rarely, confusion, slurred speech, psychosis, bronchospasm (on inhalation).

Manufacturer: Pharmax.

Combantrin

Description: a broad-acting antihelmintic preparation produced in the form of orange tablets containing 125mg pyrantel embonate.

Used for: to treat infestations of hookworm, roundworm, threadworm and trichostrongyliasis.

Dosage: adults and children over 6 months of age, 10mg per kg of body weight as a single dose.

Special care: patients with liver disorders.

Side effects: central nervous system effects, rash, gastrointestinal upset.

Manufacturer: Pfizer.

Combidol

Description: a bile acid preparation available in the form of white, film-coated tablets containing 125mg chenodeoxycholic acid marked COMBIDOL 60.

Used for: to dissolve small or medium sized radiolucent gallstones in patients who have slight symptoms and unimpaired gall bladder function.

Dosage: adults, 2 or 3 tablets each day (5mg per kg of body weight) either as single night time dose, or in divided doses after meals with final dose taken before bedtime. If patient is 120% or more above ideal body weight, 6 tablets (7.5mg per kg of body weight) should be taken daily.

Avoid use: children, pregnancy, breast-feeding, women who are not using contraception, patients with non-functioning or impaired gall bladder, those with inflammatory diseases of colon and small intestine, peptic ulcer, chronic liver disease.

Possible interaction: bile acid sequestrants, antacids, oestrogens, oral contraceptives, other drugs which influence cholesterol levels.

Side effects: minor effects on liver and a rise in serum levels of transaminases (enzymes), diarrhoea, pruritis (itching), gallstones may become opaque.

Manufacturer: CP Pharmaceuticals.

Concordin

Description: a TCAD preparation available as pink film-coated tablets containing 5mg protryptyline hydrochloride and marked MSD 26, and white, film-coated tablets contain 10mg and marked MSD 47.

Used for: depression.

Dosage: adults, 15–60mg each day in divided doses. Reduced dose of 5mg 3 times each day in elderly persons.

Special care: breast-feeding, liver or kidney disease, epilepsy, heart and circulatory diseases, diabetes, hyperthyroidism, tumours of adrenal gland, retention of urine, glaucoma. Also, certain psychiatric conditions, suicidal tendencies and psychoses.

Avoid use: pregnant women, children, patients with serious liver disease, heart atack or heart block.

Possible interaction: alcohol, barbiturates, other

antidepressant drugs, antihypertensives, cimetidine, oestrogens, local anaesthetics containing adrenaline or noradrenaline, anticholinergic drugs.

Side effects: nervousness, drowsiness, dizziness, sweating, tremor, weariness, gastrointestinal upset, insomnia, hypotension. Anticholinergic effects including constipation, urine retention, blurring of vision, dry mouth. Allergic skin rashes, blood changes, jaundice, heart arrhythmias, weight gain or loss, changes in libido, enlargement of breasts, production of milk, blood sugar changes. Mania and schizophrenic symptoms may be activated, especially in elderly persons.

Manufacturer: MSD.

Condyline

Description: a preparation available in the form of a solution with applicators containing 0.5% podophyllotoxin in alcoholic base.

Used for: genital warts.

Dosage: adults, apply solution twice each day for 3 days directly on to warts. Repeat at 4 day intervals if required for a maximum of 5 weeks.

Avoid use: children, open wounds.

Side effects: irritation at site of application.

Manufacturer: Yamanouchi.

Conova 30

Description: a combined oestrogen/progestogen oral contraceptive produced in the form of white film-coated tablets containing 30μg of ethinyloestradiol and 2mg ethynodiol diacetate, marked with the maker's name and 930.

Used for: oral contraception.

Dosage: 1 daily for 21 days starting on fifth day of period followed by 7 tablet-free days.

Special care: patients with asthma, varicose veins, hypertension, diabetes, severe kidney disease or kidney dialysis, Raynaud's disease, hyperprolactinaemia (elevated levels of the hormone, prolactin, in the blood), depressive illness. Blood pressure should be checked and pelvic organs and breasts examined regularly before and during the period the drug is being taken. Risk of thrombosis increases with age, smoking and obesity.

Avoid use: pregnant women, patients with heart or circulatory disease, heart valve disease, history of or at risk of thrombosis, hypertension, hormone-dependent cancers. Also, those with various liver diseases and disorders including liver tumour (adenoma), porphyria, Dublin-Johnson syndrome and Rotor syndrome, abnormal liver function tests. Patients with recent trophoblastic disease, chorea, sickle cell anaemia, undiagnosed vaginal bleeding,

ostosclerosis.

Possible interaction: barbiturates, tetracyclines, rifampicin, phenytoin, griseofulvin, carbamazepine, chloral hydrate, glutethimide, ethosuximide dichloralphenazone.

Side effects: cervical erosion and vaginal discharge, pains and leg cramps, loss of libido, feeling of bloatedness due to fluid retention, weight gain, enlargement of breasts, depression, nausea, headaches, breakthrough bleeding.

Manufacturer: Gold Cross.

Convulex

Description: an anticonvulsant carboxylic acid preparation produced in the form of soft enteric-coated gelatin capsules of 3 different strengths containing 150mg, 300mg and 500mg of valproic acid.

Used for: epilepsy.

Dosage: adults and children, 15mg per kg of body weight at first in divided doses, gradually increasing by 5–10mg/kg body weight each day as required.

Special care: pregnant women, coagulation tests and liver function tests should be carried out before starting therapy or increasing dose and also at 2-monthly intervals. Urine tests give false positives for ketones.

Avoid use: patients with liver disease.

Possible interaction: alcohol, barbiturates, antidepressants, other antiepileptic drugs, anti-coagulants, neuroleptic drugs.

Side effects: gastrointestinal upset, central nervous system effects, toxic effects on liver coagulation. Rarely, there may be short-lived hair loss, pancreatitis.

Manufacturer: Pharmacia.

Coracten

Description: an antianginal and antihypertensive preparation which is a class II calcium antagonist available as sustained-release capsules of 2 different strengths. Grey/pink capsules contain 10mg nifedipine and pink/brown capsules contain 20mg nifedipine. Both are marked with the strength and name.

Used for: prevention of angina, hypertension.

Dosage: adults, 20mg every 12 hours, adjusted according to response within the range of 10–40mg each 12 hours.

Special care: patients with weak hearts, diabetes, liver disease, hypotension, hypovolaemia (an abnormally low volume of circulating blood).

Avoid use: children, pregnant women, patients with cardiogenic (heart) shock.

Possible interaction: cimetidine, quinidine, antihypertensive drugs.

Side effects: flushing, headache, dizziness, oedema, lethargy, nausea, rash, pain in eyes, frequency of urination, gum hyperplasia (increase in number of cells); rarely, allergic-type jaundice.
Manufacturer: Evans.

Cordarone X

Description: a proprietary class III antiarrhythmic preparation produced in the form of tablets of 2 different strengths. White, scored tablets, marked with strength and action potential symbol contain 100mg or 200mg of amiodarone hydrochloride. Also, **Cordarone X** intravenous injection comprising 50mg per ml of solution in ampoules for injection.
Used for: various heart rhythm disorders especially those which do not respond to other drugs. Tachycardia associated with Wolfe-Parkinson-White syndrome.
Dosage: adults, 200mg 3 times each day for first week then 200mg twice each day for the following week. Maintenance dose is usually in the order of 200mg each day and the minimum necessary should be used. Children, manufacturer should be consulted.
Special care: pregnancy, heart failure, elderly, liver or kidney disease, enlargement of prostate gland, glaucoma, sensitivity to iodine. Liver, kidney and thyroid function should be tested throughout the course of treatment. Eyes should also be monitored and therapy started under hospital supervision.
Avoid use: breast-feeding, patients with heart block, shock, history of thyroid disease, serious bradycardia.
Possible interaction: other antiarrhythmic drugs, ß-blockers, diuretics, digoxin, phenytoin, calcium antagonists, anti-coagulants taken by mouth, anaesthetics.
Side effects: micro-deposits on cornea of eyes, sensitivity to light, effects on eyes, heart, thyroid, liver and nervous system, pulmonary fibrosis or alveolitis (inflammation of alveoli of lungs).
Manufacturer: Sanofi Winthrop.

Cordilox

Description: an antihypertensive and antiarrhythmic preparation which is a class I calcium antagonist produced as tablets of 3 different strengths and as a solution for intravenous injection. Yellow, film-coated tablets, marked with the name and strength, contain 40mg, 80mg and 120mg of verapamil hydrochloride. **Cordilox Intravenous** contains 2.5mg verapamil hydrochloride per ml in ampoules for injection.

Used for: supraventricular heart arrhythmias, hypertension, angina.
Dosage: adults, heart arrhythmias, 40–120mg 3 times each day; children under 2 years, 20mg 2 or 3 times daily; over 2 years, 40–120mg 2 or 3 times each day. Adults, hypertension, 240–480mg each day in 2 to 3 divided doses. Adults, angina, 8–120mg 3 times each day.
Special care: patients with weak heart should take digitalis and diuretics; persons with first degree heart block, kidney or liver disease, heart attack, heart conduction disorders, bradycardia, hypotension.
Avoid use: severe bradycardia, second or third degree heart block, heart failure, heart shock, sick sinus syndrome.
Possible interaction: ß-blockers, digoxin, quinidine.
Side effects: flushes and constipation.
Manufacturer: Baker Norton.

Corguard

Description: an antihypertensive, non-cardioselective ß-blocker produced in the form of pale blue tablets of 2 different strengths containing either 40 or 80mg of nadolol and marked SQUIBB 207 or SQUIBB 241 respectively.
Used for: heart arrythmias, angina, hypertension, additional therapy in thyroid gland disease (thyrotoxicosis), prevention of migraine.
Dosage: heart arrhythmias, 40mg each day at first increasing as required to maximum of 160mg; angina, 40mg each day at first increasing as required with usual daily dose in the order of 40–240mg; hypotension, 80mg each day at first increasing as needed with usual daily dose in the order of 80–240mg; thyrotoxicosis, 80–160mg once each day; prevention of migraine, 40mg each day at first increasing if necessary to a usual daily dose in the order of 80–160mg.
Special care: pregnancy, breast-feeding, patients with weak hearts should receive diuretics and digitalis, liver or kidney disease, diabetes, metabolic acidosis. Persons undergoing general anaesthesia may need to be withdrawn before planned surgery. Withdraw drug gradually.
Avoid use: children, patients with obstructive airways disease or history of bronchospasm (asthma), various heart disorders including heart block, heart shock, heart failure, sick sinus syndrome, serious peripheral arterial disease, sinus bradycardia.
Possible interaction: cardiac depressant anaesthetics, antihypertensives, ergotamine, sympathomimetics, verapamil, clonidine withdrawal, CNS depressants,

class I antiarrhythmic drugs, cimetidine, reserpine, indomethacin, hypoglycaemics.

Side effects: bradycardia, fatigue on exercise, cold hands and feet, disturbance of sleep, gastrointestinal upset, bronchospasm, heart failure. Withdraw drug gradually if dry eyes or skin rash occur.

Manufacturer: Sanofi Winthrop.

Corgaretic 40

Description: a combined antihypertensive, non-cardioselective ß-blocker and thiazide diuretic produced in the form of white, mottled, scored tablets, marked SQUIBB 283, and containing 40mg nadolol and 5mg bendrofluazide. Also, **Corgaretic 80**, white, mottled, scored tablets marked SQUIBB 284, and containing 80mg nadolol and 5mg bendrofluazide.

Used for: hypertension.

Dosage: adults, 1 to 2 tablets a day (Cor-garetic 40), increasing if required to a maximum dose of 2 Corgaretic 80 tablets.

Special care: pregnancy, breast-feeding, weak hearts (should receive digitalis and diuretics), liver or kidney disease, diabetes, metabolic acidosis, gout. Persons undergoing general anaesthesia, may require to be withdrawn before planned surgery. Electrolyte levels should be monitored.

Avoid use: children, patients with obstructive airways disease or history of bronchospasm (asthma), various heart disorders including heart block, heart shock, heart failure, sick sinus syndrome, serious peripheral arterial disease, sinus bradycardia. Severe or progressive kidney failure, anuria.

Possible interaction: cardiac depressant anaesthetics, antihypertensives, ergotamine, sympathomimetics, verapamil, clonidine with-drawal, central nervous system depressants, class I antiarrhythmic drugs, cimetidine, reserpine, indomethacin, hypo-glycaemics, lithium, digitalis.

Side effects: bradycardia, fatigue on exercise, cold hands and feet, disturbance of sleep, gastrointestinal upset, bronchospasm, heart failure, blood changes, sensitivity to light, gout. Withdraw drug gradually if skin rash or dry eyes occur.

Manufacturer: Sanofi Winthrop.

Corlan

Description: a corticosteroid available as pellets marked CORLAN and GLAXO containing 2.5mg of hydrocortisone (as sodium succinate).

Used for: mouth ulcers.

Dosage: a pellet held in mouth in contact with ulcer and allowed to dissolve.

Special care: pregnant women.

Avoid use: patients with untreated mouth infections.

Manufacturer: Evans.

Cortistab

Description: a glucocorticoid-mineralocorticoid (corticosteroid) preparation (corticosteroid hormones are produced by the cortex region of the adrenal glands) available as white, scored tablets containing either 5mg or 25mg of cortisone acetate.

Used for: inflammatory and allergic disorders, rheumatic conditions and collagen diseases, hormonal replacement therapy when adrenal glands have been removed.

Dosage: adults, 12.5–50mg each day, children 5–25mg each day in divided doses.

Special care: pregnancy, liver cirrhosis, glaucoma, epilepsy, diabetes, hypertension, acute glomerulonephritis (inflammation of part of the kidney tubules), peptic ulcer, active infections, tuberculosis, fungal and viral infections. Patients with osteoporosis, recent intestinal anastomoses, thrombophlebitis, nephritis, secondary cancers, infectious diseases which cause skin spots or rash. Patients should avoid contact with chicken pox or *Herpes zoster* virus while receiving therapy and for 3 months after treatment. In the event of contact or contracting chicken pox, further specialist treatment should be given. Withdraw drug gradually.

Possible interaction: hypoglycaemics, NSAIDs, anticoagulants taken by mouth, anticholinesterases, diuretics, cardiac glycosides, ephedrine, phenytoin, rifampicin, phenobarbitone.

Side effects: hypertension, skin changes, fluid retention, hyperglycaemia, loss of potassium, osteoporosis in elderly patients, peptic ulcer, mood changes—euphoria and depression and possibly confusion.

Manufacturer: Boots.

Cortisyl

Description: a glucocorticoid-mineralocorticoid (corticosteroid) preparation produced in the form of white, scored tablets containing 25mg of cortisone acetate.

Used for: replacement therapy following removal of adrenal glands and in Addison's disease (a failure of the cortex of the adrenal glands to produce their hormones).

Dosage: adults, acute attacks, up to 300mg each day with usual maintenance in the order of 12.5mg to 37.5mg daily.

Special care: pregnancy, liver cirrhosis, glaucoma, epilepsy, diabetes, hypertension, acute glomerulonephritis (inflammation of part of the kidney tubules), peptic ulcer, active infections, tuberculosis, fungal and viral infections. Patients with osteoporosis, recent intestinal anastomoses, thrombophlebitis, nephritis, secondary cancers, infectious diseases which cause skin spots or rash. Patients should avoid contact with chicken pox or *Herpes zoster* virus while receiving therapy and for 3 months after treatment. In the event of contact or contracting chicken pox, further specialist treatment should be given. Withdraw drug gradually.

Avoid use: children.

Possible interaction: hypoglycaemics, NSAIDs, anticoagulants taken by mouth, anticholinesterases, diuretics, cardiac glycosides, ephedrine, phenytoin, rifampicin, phenobarbitone.

Side effects: hypertension, skin changes, fluid retention, hyperglycaemia, loss of potassium, osteoporosis, peptic ulcer, mood changes—euphoria and depression.

Manufacturer: Roussel.

Corwin

Description: a sympathomimetic heart muscle stimulant which is a partial ß1-agonist, produced in the form of yellow, film-coated tablets containing 200mg of xamoterol (as fumerate) marked with symbol and CORWIN.

Used for: chronic mild heart failure.

Dosage: adults, start treatment in hsopital with 1 tablet daily in first instance, increasing to 1 tablet twice daily if there is a favourable response.

Special care: withdraw drug if there is a deterioration in the progress of the disease. Patients with obstructive airways disease, disease of heart muscle and a heart valve (aortic stenosis), kidney disease.

Avoid use: children, pregnancy, breast-feeding, more severe forms of heart failure, fatigue when resting and breathlessness, hypotension, tachycardia. Patients with fluid in lungs (pulmonary oedema) or other fluid retention. Those needing ACE inhibitor drugs or taking higher doses of loop diuretics (equivalent to 40mg frusemide).

Side effects: muscle cramps, rash, gastrointestinal upset, headache, dizziness, palpitations.

Manufacturer: Stuart.

Cosmegen Lyovac

Description: a cytotoxic antibiotic drug produced in the form of a powder in vials for reconstitution and injection, containing 0.5mg actinomycin D.

Used for: cancers in children e.g. leukaemia.

Dosage: fast running intravenous infusion at 3 week intervals or as directed by cancer specialist.

Side effects: leakage at injection site causes severe tissue death and damage, vomiting, nausea, baldness, suppression of bone marrow, inflammation of mucous membranes, e.g. in nose and throat.

Manufacturer: M.S.D.

Coversyl

Description: an antihypertensive preparation which is an ACE inhibitor and is produced as tablets of 2 different strengths. White tablets contain 2mg perindopril tert-butylamine and white, scored oblong tablets contain 4mg.

Used for: additional therapy with digitalis and/or diuretics in congestive heart failure, hypertension.

Dosage: adults, heart failure, treatment should start in hospital under close supervision with 2mg once daily taken in the morning increasing to 4mg once each day. Any diuretic should be withdrawn 3 days before the start of treatment. Hypertension, 2mg once each day before food increasing to daily maintenance dose of 4mg (8mg a day is maximum dose). Elderly persons should take a reduced dose of 2mg each day under close medical supervision. Any diuretic should be withdrawn 3 days before start of treatment.

Special care: patients with kidney disorders or receiving dialysis. Kidney function should be monitored before and during treatment; patients undergoing anaesthesia and surgery.

Avoid use: children, pregnancy, breast-feeding.

Possible interaction: antidepressants, other antihypertensives, lithium, potassium supplements, potassium-sparing diuretics.

Side effects: hypotension, skin rashes and itching, flushing, loss of sense of taste, oedema, headache, malaise, fatigue, nausea, pain in abdomen, weakness, slight cough, blood changes, protein in urine.

Manufacturer: Servier.

Cromogen

Description: an anti-inflammatory, non-steroidal, bronchodilator produced in the form of an aerosol for inhalation containing 5mg of sodium cromoglycate per metered dose aerosol. Also, **Cromogen Steri-Neb**, a preservative-free solution containing 10mg sodium cromoglycate per ml, available as a single dose for use with nebulizer.

Used for: prevention of asthma.

Dosage: adults and children, 2 puffs 4 times each day in first instance with a maintenance dose of 1 puff 4 times daily. Cromogen Steri-Neb, 20mg with power-operated nebulizer 4 times each day at 3 to 6 hourly intervals. If necessary frequency can be increased to 5 or 6 times each day and, to be effective, therapy must be continuous.

Side effects: irritation of throat and short-lived cough (due to inhalation of powder). Rarely, short-lived bronchospasm.

Manufacturer: Baker-Norton.

Crystapen

Description: a preparation of benzylpenicillin or penicillin G, an antibiotic which is inactivated by the penicillinase enzymes produced by certain bacteria. It is inactivated by stomach (gastric) juices and poorly absorbed from the gut and hence is produced as a solution for intravenous or intramuscular injection. Crystapen 600mg benzylpenicillin sodium (unbuffered) as powder in vials for reconstitution and injection.

Used for: gonorrhoea, septicaemia, endocarditis, osteomyelitis, meningitis, respiratory tract, ear, nose and throat, skin and soft tissue infections.

Dosage: adults, 600–1200mg by intravenous or intramuscular injection each day in 2, 3 or 4 divided doses. (For meningitis, up to 14.4g daily in divided doses may be needed). Children, newborns, 30mg per kg of body weight in 2, 3 or 4 divided doses; 1 month to 12 years, 10–20mg per kg each day in 2, 3 or 4 divided doses. For meningitis, age 1 week and under, 60–90mg per kg, in 2 divided doses; 1 week to 1 month, 90–120mg per kg each day in 3 divided doses; 1 month to 12 years, 150–300mg per kg each day in 4, 5 or 6 divided doses. All doses are delivered by intravenous or intramuscular injection.

Special care: history of penicillin allergy or kidney disease.

Avoid use: allergy to penicillin.

Side effects: allergic responses including rash, joint pains, fever, blood changes and anaphylactic shock in hypersensitive persons.

Manufacturer: Britannia.

Cyclimorph^{CD}

Description: a strong analgesic preparation which combines an opiate with an anti-emetic and is available as solutions of 2 different strengths in 1ml ampoules for injection. Cyclimorph 10 contains 10mg morphine tartrate and 50mg cyclizine tartrate per ml; **Cyclimorph 15** contains 15mg morphine tartrate and 50mg cyclizine tartrate per ml.

Used for: acute and chronic intractable pain.

Dosage: adults, Cyclimorph 10, 1ml by subcutaneous, intravenous or intramuscular injection which can be repeated after 4 hours but

maximum dose is 3ml in 24 hours. Children, age 1 to 5 years, 0.25–0.5ml as 1 single dose; 6 to 12 years, 0.5–1ml as 1 single dose. Adults, Cyclimorph 15, 1ml by subcutaneous, intravenous or intramuscular injection which may be repeated after 4 hours but maximum dose is 3ml in 24 hours.

Special care: women in labour, elderly, liver disease or hypothyroidism.

Avoid use: children under 1 year, patients with blocked airways or respiratory depression.

Possible interaction: central nervous system sedatives, MAOIs.

Side effects: drug dependence and tolerance may develop and Chief Medical Officer should be notified in cases of addiction. Rash, constipation, dizziness, nausea.

Manufacturer: Wellcome.

Cyclo-Progynova

Description: a combined oestrogen/progestogen hormonal preparation available as tablets in 2 different strengths. Cyclo-Progynova 1mg consists of a course of sugar-coated tablets; 11 beige ones contain 1mg oestradiol valerate and 10 brown ones contain 1mg oestradiol valerate and 0.25mg levonorgestrel.

Cyclo-Progynova 2mg consists of a course of sugar-coated tablets; 11 white ones contain 2mg oestradiol valerate and 10 brown ones contain 2mg oestradiol valerate and 0.5mg norgestrel (= 0.25mg levonorgestrel).

Used for: menopausal symptoms including the prevention of osteoporosis.

Dosage: 1 oestradiol tablet each day for 11 days (beginning on fifth day of period, if present), followed by 1 combined oestradiol/levonorgestrel tablet for 10 days. Then there are 7 tablet-free days before course is repeated. The lower strength preparation should be tried first.

Special care: women at any risk of thrombosis and those with liver disease. Liver function should be monitored every 2 to 3 months during treatment. Patients with diabetes, porphyria, migraine, epilepsy, hypertension, fibroids in the uterus, multiple sclerosis, ostosclerosis, gallstones, tetany. These persons should be closely monitored. Also, women with a family history of breast cancer or fibrocystic disease of the breast should be carefully monitored. Breasts and pelvic organs should be examined and blood pressure checked regularly before and during the period of treatment.

Avoid use: pregnancy, breast-feeding, endometriosis, undiagnosed vaginal bleeding, hormone-dependent cancers, breast cancer, serious heart, liver or kidney

disease, thromboembolism. Also, women with kidney, liver or heart disease and Rotor or Dublin-Johnson syndromes. Drug should be stopped 6 weeks before planned surgery and during any condition which makes thrombosis more likely.
Possible interaction: drugs which induce liver enzymes.
Side effects: breakthrough bleeding, weight gain, tenderness in breasts, gastrointestinal upset, dizziness, nausea, headache, vomiting. Drug should be stopped immediately in the event of frequent severe headaches, migraine, disturbance of vision, thromboembolism or thrombophlebitis, jaundice or sudden blood pressure rise, pregnancy.
Manufacturer: Schering HC.

Cyclocaps

Description: an anti-inflammatory, bronchodilator which is a selective ß2-agonist produced as a powder in capsules of 2 strengths for inhalation by means of a cyclohaler. Clear/light green capsules, marked with Greek letters and 935, contain 200µg salbutamol (as sulphate). Clear/dark green capsules marked with Greek letters and 945, contain 400µg.
Used for: treatment and prevention of asthma.
Dosage: acute attack, 200 or 400µg as a single dose. Prevention, 400µg as a single dose repeated 3 to 4 times each day. Children, acute attack, 200µg as a single dose. Prevention, 200µg as a single dose repeated 3 or 4 times each day.
Special care: pregnancy, hypertension, angina, weak hearts, heart arrhythmias, hyperthyroidism.
Possible interaction: sympathomimetics.
Side effects: headache, tremor in muscles, dilation of blood vessels in skin.
Manufacturer: DuPont

Cyclogest

Description: a hormonal preparation in the form of suppositories containing either 200mg or 400mg of progesterone.
Used for: premenstrual syndrome, depression following childbirth (but effectiveness is controversial and subject to debate).
Dosage: adults, 200 or 400mg via rectum or vagina once or twice each day from the twelfth or fourteenth day of monthly cycle until period begins.
Special care: use rectally if barrier contraceptives are being used or if patient has thrush infection. Breast-feeding mothers and women with liver, kidney, heart disease, diabetes, hypertension.
Avoid use: women with abnormal and undiagnosed vaginal bleeding or who have a history of, or are at risk from, thromboembolic disorders. Also, those

suffering from breast cancer, porphyria, serious arterial disease.
Possible interaction: cyclosporins.
Side effects: gastrointestinal upset, weight changes, breast tenderness, change in libido, alteration in menstrual cycle, rash, acne.
Manufacturer: Hoechst.

Cyklokapron

Description: an antifibrinolytic preparation produced in the form of tablets, syrup and as a solution for injection. White, oblong, film-coated scored tablets, marked C-Y, contain 500mg tranexamic acid. **Cyklokapron Syrup** contains 500mg tranexamic acid per 5ml; also **Cyklokapron Injection** contains 100mg tranexamic acid per ml in ampoules for injection.
Used for: local or general fibrinolytic disorders, i.e. those characterized by haemorrhage; menorrhagia (abnormally heavy menstrual bleeding or prolonged periods).
Dosage: local fibrinolysis, 15–25mg per kg of body weight 2 or 3 times each day. (For more general fibrinolytic states, as directed by physician). Children, 25mg per kg of body weight 2 or 3 times each day. Adults, menorrhagia, 1 to 1½g 3 or 4 times each day for up to 4 days.
Special care: patients with kidney disorders, haematuria (blood in urine), especially associated with haemophilia. Patients suffering from angioneurotic oedema require eye and liver function tests during the course of long-term treatment.
Avoid use: history of thrombosis.
Side effects: gastrointestinal upset. If disturbance in colour vision occurs, drug should be withdrawn.
Manufacturer: Pharmacia.

Cymevene

Description: an antiviral preparation available as a powder in vials for reconstitution and injection containing 500mg ganciclovir.
Used for: life-threatening viral infections or those which threaten sight, caused by cytomegalovirus in patients with reduced immunity.
Dosage: adults and children, 5mg per kg of body weight given by intravenous infusion over a period of 1-hour every 12 hours for a period of 14 to 21 days. 6mg per kg of body weight may be required for patients who have sight-threatening infection.
Special care: polythene gloves and safety glasses must be worn while handing the preparation and accidental splashes on skin should be washed off immediately with soap and water. Regular blood counts required due to toxic effects on blood;

potential carcinogen. Patients with kidney disease. Should be administered carefully into veins with good bloodflow and patient's fluid level should be maintained after infusion.

Avoid use: pregnant women, lactating mothers should not breastfeed until 72 hours have elapsed since last dose, allergy to ganciclovir or acyclovir. Patients with abnormally low neutrophil (a type of white blood cell) counts.

Possible interaction: other antiviral drugs, zidovudine.

Side effects: effects on blood including anaemia and severe reduction in levels of white blood cells, elevated levels of serum creatinine and blood urea nitrogen. Effects on all body systems and functions, fever, rash, malaise.

Manufacturer: Syntex.

Cyprostat

Description: an anti-androgen preparation used to treat prostate cancer, a type which is hormone-dependent and develops under the influence of the male sex hormone, androgen. The drug blocks androgens produced by the adrenal glands and testes. Cyprostat is available in the form of tablets of 2 strengths; white scored tablets, marked BV within a hexagon, contain 50mg cyproterone acetate. White scored tablets, marked LA within a hexagon, contain 100mg cyproterone acetate.

Used for: cancer of the prostate.

Dosage: 300mg each day in 2 or 3 divided doses after food.

Special care: diabetes, liver disease, history of thrombosis, severe depression.

Side effects: weariness, infertility, liver disorders, breast enlargement, anaemia.

Manufacturer: Schering HC.

Cystrin

Description: an anticholinergic and antispasmodic preparation available as white tablets containing 3mg oxybutynin hydrochloride and white scored tablets, marked L11, containing 5mg oxybutynin hydrochloride.

Used for: incontinence, urgency and frequency of urination and night-time bed-wetting in children.

Dosage: 5mg 2 or 3 times each day (with a maximum daily dose of 20mg), in divided doses. Elderly persons, 3mg twice each day adjusted according to response. Children, 5 years and over, 3mg twice each day in first instance, adjusted according to response to usual dose in the order of 5mg 2 or 3 times daily. For night-time bed-wetting, last dose should be taken at bedtime.

Special care: pregnant women, disease of the autonomic nervous system, liver or kidney disease, heart arrhythmias, heart failure, enlarged prostate, tachycardia, hyperthyroidism, hiatus hernia.

Avoid use: breast-feeding, blocked gastrointestinal tract or bladder, other intestinal diseases, glaucoma, myasthenia gravis, severe ulcerative colitis.

Possible interaction: other anticholinergics, TCADs, digoxin, levodopa, amantadine, phenothiazines, butyrophenones.

Side effects: facial flushing, anticholinergic effects.

Cytamen

Description: a proprietary vitamin B12 preparation produced as a solution in 1ml ampoules for injection containing 1000µg cyanocobalamin per ml.

Used for: vitamin B12 responsive macrocytic anaemias (characterized by the presence of fragile and enlarged red blood cells), megaloblastic anaemia.

Dosage: adults and children, 250–1000µg by intramuscular injection every other day for 1 or 2 weeks and then 250µg once a week until normal blood count is achieved. Usual maintenance dose is 1000µg each month.

Possible interaction: oral contraceptives, chloramphenicol.

Side effects: rarely, allergic reactions.

Manufacturer: Evans

Cytosar

Description: a powerful cytotoxic antimetabolite produced as a powder in vials for reconstitution and injection, containing 100mg or 500mg cytarabine.

Used for: to induce remission in acute myeloblastic anaemia.

Dosage: given subcutaneously or intravenously, as directed by physician skilled in cancer chemotherapy.

Special care: requires careful monitoring of blood counts.

Side effects: severe myelosuppression (bone marrow suppression), loss of hair, nausea and vomiting; early menopause in women and sterility in men if therapy is prolonged, local tissue death if there is leakage at the injection site.

Manufacturer: Upjohn.

Cytotec

Description: a synthetic form of prostaglandin (a naturally occurring hormone-like substance present in many body tissues) which inhibits the seretion of gastric juice and promotes the healing of ulcers. It is produced in the form of white, hexagonal tablets, containing 200µg misoprostol, and marked SEARLE 1461.

Used for: stomach and duodenal ulcers, ulceration caused by NSAIDs, prevention of NSAID ulceration.

Dosage: adults, 4 tablets each day with meals, in divided doses, with last taken at bedtime for 1 to 2 months. Prevention of ulcers, 1 tablet 2, 3 or 4 times each day during the period that NSAID is being taken.

Special care: women should use effective contraception, patients with circulatory diseases including peripheral or coronary vascular disease and cerebrovascular disease.

Avoid use: children, pregnancy, women planning pregnancy, breast-feeding.

Side effects: gastrointestinal upset, diarrhoea, pain in abdomen, vaginal bleeding and disturbance of menstrual cycle, dizziness, rash.

Manufacturer: Searle.

D

Daktacort

Description: an antifungal/antibacterial agent with mild steroid, comprising miconazole nitrate (2%) and hydrocortisone (1%). Available as cream and ointment.

Used for: fungal and bacterial (Gram-positive) infections where there is associated inflammation.

Dosage: to be applied 2 or 3 times daily.

Special care: use on face or for children should be limited to 5 days maximum. Withdraw gradually after prolonged use.

Avoid use: on acne, leg ulcers, tuberculous, ringworm or viral skin disease, perioral dermatitis, untreated infections whether fungal or bacterial. Extensive or prolonged use during pregnancy.

Side effects: skin atrophy, striae and telangiectasia (permanent widening of superficial blood vessels), suppression of adrenal glands, Cushingoid changes (see Cushing's syndrome).

Manufacturer: Janssen.

Dalacin Cream

Description: an antibacterial cream (clindamycin phosphate) available as a 2% cream.

Used for: bacterial vaginosis.

Dosage: 1 applicatorful intravaginally each night for 7 days.

Special care: less effectiveness from barrier contraceptives.

Avoid use: in cases of lincomycin sensitivity.

Side effects: vaginal irritation, gastrointestinal upset. Discontinue with colitis or diarrhoea.

Manufacturer: Upjohn.

Dalacin C

Description: a lincosamide, clindamycin hydrochloride as 75mg (lavender) and 150mg maroon/lavender capsules. Also **Dalacin Paediatric**, clindamycin palmitate, containing 75mg per 5ml available as 100mg powder.

Used for: serious infections sensitive to clindamycin.

Dosage: 150–450mg every 6 hours. Children under 12 months, 2.5ml every 6 or 8 hours; 1 to 3 years, 2.5–5ml; 4 to 7 years, 5–7.5ml; 8 to 12 years, 7.5–10ml, all every 6 hours.

Also **Dalacin Phosphate**, available as ampoules, 150mg/ml, of clindamycin phosphate.

Dosage: 600mg–2.7g in divided doses each day, by intramuscular injection or intravenous infusion. Children over 1 month, 15–40mg/kg daily in divided doses.

Special care: kidney or liver disease, cease use should colitis or diarrhoea occur.

Avoid use: in cases of lincomycin sensitivity.

Possible interaction: neuromuscular blocking agents.

Side effects: jaundice and blood disorders, gastrointestinal upsets.

Manufacturer: Upjohn.

Dalacin T

Description: antibiotic clindomycin phosphate in a 10mg/ml solution. Also, **Dalacin T Lotion** available as an aqueous solution in a roll-on bottle.

Used for: moderate to severe acne vulgaris.

Dosage: apply twice daily.

Special care: avoid eyes and mucous membranes.

Avoid use: in cases of lincomycin sensitivity.

Possible interaction: keratolytics (applies to the solution).

Side effects: dermatitis, dry skin, folliculitis (solution). Discontinue should colitis or diarrhoea occur.

Manufacturer: Upjohn.

Dalmane

Description: a long-acting benzodiazepine (hypnotic) prepared as flurazepam hydrochloride in strengths of 15mg (grey/yellow capsules) and 30mg (black/grey capsules) marked with ROCHE and strength.

Used for: short-term treatment of severe or disabling insomnia.

Dosage: 15–30mg at bedtime (elderly, 15mg).

Special care: chronic liver, kidney or lung disease, the elderly. Also during pregnancy, labour or lactation. To be withdrawn gradually. May impair judgement.

Avoid use: acute lung disease, depression of the respiration, obsessional states, chronic psychosis. Not for children.

Possible interaction: anticonvulsants, CNS depressants, alcohol.

Side effects: confusion, vertigo, drowsiness, ataxia, light-headedness, gastrointestinal upsets, skin rashes, hypotension, disturbance in vision. Urine retention, changes in libido. Dependence is possible.

Manufacturer: Roche.

Danol

Description: a gonadotrophin release inhibitor, danazol, available in capsules of 100mg (white/grey) and 200mg (white/pink), marked with name and strength.

Used for: menorrhagia (long or heavy menstruation).

Dosage: 200mg daily for 3 months starting on the first day of menstruation.

Also used for: endometriosis and as a pre-operative preparation for endometrial ablation.

Dosage: 400mg daily for 6 to 9 months. 400–800mg daily for 3 to 6 weeks before ablation.

Also used for: severe mastalgia, benign breast cysts, gynaecomastia.

Dosage: 200–400mg daily for up to 6 months depending upon the condition.

Special care: migraine, epilepsy, hypertension, other cardiovascular diseases, diabetes, polycythaemia (increase in blood erythrocytes), conditions adversely affected by fluid retention.

Avoid use: pregnancy, lactation, porphyria, severe kidney, heart or liver disease, vaginal bleeding, androgen-dependent tumour, thromboembolic disease.

Possible interaction: steroids, anticonvulsants, anticoagulants, cyclosporin, antihypertensives, hypoglycaemics.

Side effects: backache, flushes, muscle spasms, nausea, rashes, male hormone effects, fluid retention, menstrual disturbances, headache, emotional disturbance, cholestatic jaundice (due to blockage of bile flow through any part of the biliary system).

Manufacturer: Sanofi Winthrop.

Dantrium

Description: a muscle relaxant, dantrolene sodium, available in capsules (orange with light brown cap) of strength 25mg and 100mg, marked 0030 and 0033 respectively.

Used for: severe or chronic spasticity of skeletal muscle.

Dosage: 25mg daily to start, increasing to a maximum of 100mg 4 times per day.

Special care: lung or heart disease, pregnancy. Liver to be checked before and 6 weeks after the start of treatment.

Avoid use: liver disease, where spasticity is useful for movement.

Possible interaction: CNS depressants, alcohol.

Side effects: diarrhoea, drowsiness, weakness, fatigue.

Manufacturer: Procter & Gamble Pharmaceuticals.

Daonil

Description: a sulphonylurea, glibenclamide, available as white oblong tablets (5mg) marked LDI with symbol. Also **Semi-Daonil** (2.5mg white tablet).

Used for: maturity-onset diabetes (non-insulin-dependent diabetes mellitus).

Dosage: 5mg daily at breakfast increasing by 2.5–5mg weekly to a maximum of 15mg.

Special care: kidney failure, the elderly.

Avoid use: juvenile, growth-onset or unstable brittle diabetes (all now called insulin-dependent diabetes mellitus), severe liver or kidney disease, ketoacidosis, stress, infections, surgery, endocrine disorders. Pregnancy or lactation.

Possible interaction: MAOIs, corticosteroids, corticotrophin, oral contraceptives, alcohol, ß-blockers. Also glucagon, chloramphenicol, rifampicin, sulphonamides, aspirin, phenylbutazone, cyclophosphamide, oral anticoagulants, clofibrate, benzafibrate.

Side effects: sensitivity including skin rash.

Manufacturer: Hoechst.

Daranide

Description: a preparation of dichlorphenamide in yellow tablet form (50mg, marked MSD 49) which is a weak diuretic, reducing fluid in the aqueous humour of the eye.

Used for: treatment of glaucoma.

Dosage: 2 to 4 tablets initially then 2 every 12 hours. Thereafter $^1/_2$ to 1 tablet up to 3 times daily.

Avoid use: with children or with patients suffering from kidney or liver disease, pulmonary obstruction, low sodium or potassium levels. During pregnancy.

Possible interaction: with steroids, local anaesthetics, anticoagulants, anticonvulsants, antidiabetics, salicylates, digitalis, hypoglycaemics and ACTH (adrenocorticotrophic hormone).

Side effects: gastrointestinal upsets, weight loss, frequent urination, headache, lassitude, itching, abnormal blood condition (dyscrasia).

Manufacturer: Merck, Sharp and Dohme.

DDAVP

Description: The acetate of desmopressin, an analogue of the hormone vasopressin and an antidiuretic compound.

Used for: it is administered as nose drops for the treatment of diabetes insipidus and enuresis (bed-wetting, the involuntary passing of urine).

Dosage: adults, 0.1–0.2ml once or twice daily. Children, 0.05–0.2ml at the same rate. (Lower dosage for infants). Also available as white tablets: 0.2–0.4mg at bedtime for adults and children over 5 with enuresin; 0.1mg thrice daily for diabetes insipidus. Injection also available.

Avoid use: in pregnancy and for patients with epilepsy, migraine, asthma or chronic kidney disease.

Side effects: may cause fluid retention, headache, nausea and vomiting.

Manufacturer: Ferring.

Deca-Durabolin

Description: a form of the anabolic steroid nandrolone, in ampoules or syringes.

Used for: its protein-building properties (in conjunction with a nourishing diet), particularly after major surgery or debilitating disease. It was administered for osteoporosis but is no longer advocated as its value is dubious. It may be used to treat cancers linked to sex hormones.

Dosage: 50mg every 3 weeks, by intramuscular injection.

Special care: in case of heart, liver or kidney impairment, hypertension, migraine, epilepsy and diabetes.

Possible interaction: with anticoagulants, hypoglycaemics.

Side effects: oedema, hypercalcaemia, some virilization in women (i.e. appearance of male features such as deepening of the voice, growth of body hair and increase in musculature).

Manufacturer: Organon.

Deca-Durabolin 100

Description: The same form of the anabolic steroid nandrolene as is found in Deca-Durabolin.

Used for: the treatment of some forms of anaemia, e.g. aplastic anaemia, also post-cytotoxic therapy anaemia, and anaemia associated with chronic kidney failure.

Dosage: all administered by intramuscular injection: 50–150mg weekly (aplastic); 200mg per week from 2 weeks before cytotoxic therapy until the blood returns to normal; 100mg (females) or 200mg (males) weekly for kidney failure.

Special care: in cases of heart, liver or kidney impairment, hypertension, migraine, epilepsy and diabetes.

Avoid use: in pregnancy, also where there is a known or suspected prostate or mammary cancer in males.

Possible interaction: with anticoagulants, hypoglycaemics.

Side effects: oedema, hypercalcaemia, some virilization in women (i.e. appearance of male features such as deepening of the voice, growth of body hair and increase in musculature).

Manufacturer: Organon.

Decadron

Description: a corticosteroid preparation available as white (0.5mg) tablets marked MSD 41, or injection.

Used for: treatment of inflammation, particularly in allergic or rheumatic conditions.

Dosage: often a daily dose; magnitude varies with the case.

Special care: to be taken in numerous conditions including nephritis, osteoporosis, peptic ulcer and metastatic carcinoma. Also viral/fungal infections, tuberculosis, hypertension, glaucoma, epilepsy, diabetes, cirrhosis and hypothyroidism. Also pregnancy and stress. To be withdrawn gradually.

Possible interaction: NSAIDs, diuretics, hypoglycaemics, oral anticoagulants, phenobarbitone, ephedrine, phenytoin, anticholinesterases and others.

Side effects: osteoporosis, depression, hyperglycaemia, euphoria, peptic ulceration.

Manufacturer: Merck, Sharp and Dohme.

Decaserpyl

Description: an alkaloid (methoserpidine) compound originally derived from the dried root of the shrub *Rauwolfia serpentina*. It is available in tablet form, 5mg (white) and 10mg (pink), marked D/5 and D/10 respectively, both with RL on reverse.

Used for: treatment of high blood pressure.

Dosage: 10mg 3 times per day initially. This can be increased by 5–10mg daily on a weekly basis up to a maximum of 50mg per dose.

Special care: during pregnancy or lactation.

Avoid use: in patients with a history of mental depression; peptic ulcer, ulcerative colitis or severe kidney disease; Parkinson's disease. It should not be given to children.

Possible interaction: anticonvulsants.

Side effects: vertigo, tremor, lethargy, nasal congestion, and gastrointestinal upset.

Manufacturer: Roussel.

Declinax

Description: The sulphate of debrisoquine available in (white) tablet form marked ROCHE 10 at 10mg strength, and used for moderate to severe hypertension.

Used for: treatment of high blood pressure.

Dosage: 10–20mg once or twice daily to begin with. This may be increased to a daily dose of 120mg.

Special care: with cases of kidney disease.

Avoid use: in cases of recent heart attack; phaeochromocytoma. Not to be used for children.

Possible interaction: sympathomimetics (drugs that stimulate the sympathetic nervous system and whose action resembles noradrenaline), some antidepressants.

Side effects: headache, general malaise, postural hypotension (i.e. low blood pressure on standing) and failure to ejaculate.

Manufacturer: Roche.

Decortisyl

Description: a corticosteroid containing prednisone, a glucocorticoid steroid. It is available as white tablets (5mg).

Used for: rheumatic and allergic conditions.

Dosage: a divided daily dose of 20–40mg reducing by 2.5/5mg every 3 to 4 days to achieve maintenance daily dosage of 5–20mg. Children 1 to 7 years, quarter to half dose; 7 to 12 years, half to three-quarters dose.

Special care: with numerous conditions including nephritis, osteoporosis, peptic ulcer and metastatic carcinoma. Also viral/fungal infections, tuberculosis, hypertension, glaucoma, epilepsy, diabetes, cirrhosis and hypothyroidism. Also pregnancy and stress. Not to be given to children under 12 months. To be withdrawn gradually.

Possible interaction: NSAIDs, diuretics, hypoglycaemics, oral anticoagulants, phenobarbitone, ephedrine, phenytoin, anticholinesterases and others.

Side effects: osteoporosis, depression, hyperglycaemia, euphoria, peptic ulceration.

Manufacturer: Roussel.

Deltacortil

Description: a corticosteroid preparation containing the glucocorticoid steroid, prednisolone. It is available as 2 enteric-coated tablets, brown (2.5mg) and red (5mg) marked Pfizer.

Used for: allergic conditions, collagen disorders or inflammation.

Dosage: 5–60mg daily, reducing to a minimum for maintenance.

Special care: with numerous conditions including nephritis, osteoporosis, peptic ulcer and metastatic carcinoma. Also viral/fungal infections, tuberculosis, hypertension, glaucoma, epilepsy, diabetes, cirrhosis and hypothyroidism. Also pregnancy and stress. To be withdrawn gradually. Not to be given to children under 12 months.

Possible interaction: NSAIDs, diuretics, hypoglycaemics, oral anticoagulants, phenobarbitone, ephedrine, phenytoin, anticholinesterases and others.

Side effects: osteoporosis, depression, hyperglycaemia, euphoria, peptic ulceration.

Manufacturer: Pfizer.

Deltastab

Description: a corticosteroid preparation containing prednisolone acetate, a glucocorticoid steroid. Available as white tablets (1mg and 5mg) and ampoules of an aqueous solution (25mg/ml).

Used for: (tablets) treatment of inflammation associated with rheumatic and allergic conditions and collagen disorders. Solution injected into joints for rheumatic conditions and intramuscularly for systemic therapy.

Dosage: tablets initially 10–20mg daily (up to 60mg for severe cases), reducing as soon as possible to a maintenance daily dose of 2.5–15mg. Injection of solution in range 5–25mg depending on joint size up to 3 times daily. Intramuscular injection 25–100mg once or twice weekly. Children should receive only minimal doses and for the shortest possible time and even then only when specifically indicated.

Special care: with numerous conditions including nephritis, osteoporosis, peptic ulcer and metastatic carcinoma. Also viral/fungal infections, tuberculosis, hypertension, glaucoma, epilepsy, diabetes, cirrhosis and hypothyroidism. Also pregnancy and stress. To be withdrawn gradually. Not to be given to children under 12 months.

Possible interaction: NSAIDs, diuretics, hypoglycaemics, oral anticoagulants, phenobarbitone, ephedrine, phenytoin, anticholinesterases and others.

Side effects: osteoporosis, depression, hyperglycaemia, euphoria, peptic ulceration.

Manufacturer: Pfizer.

Dentomycin

Description: an antibacterial available as a 2% gel of minocycline hydrochloride.

Used for: periodontitis (disease causing formation of spaces 'pockets' between gums and teeth and loss of bone and connective fibres) where pockets are 5mm or more.

Dosage: using the applicator, the gel is put into the pockets 2 or 3 times at 14-day intervals. After completion of treatment, not to be repeated within 6 months.

Special care: in cases of liver or kidney impairment. Pregnancy, nursing mothers. No intake of food or drink and no rinsing of mouth (including cleaning of teeth) for 2 hours after treatment.

Avoid use: not suitable for children.

Possible interaction: anticoagulants.

Side effects: local irritation.

Manufacturer: Lederle.

Depixol

Description: a thioxanthene antipsychotic drug available in several forms. Yellow tablets (marked LUNDBECK) contain 3mg flupenthixol dihydrochloride. **Depixol Injection** is available as the decanoate of flupenthixol in ampoules, vials and syringes (20mg/ml). **Depixol Conc.** and **Depixol Low Volume** are concentrated forms of the decanoate (100mg/ml and 200mg/ml respectively), for injection.

Used for: schizophrenia and other mental disorders, especially for apathetic and withdrawn patients.

Dosage: Depixol—1 to 3 tablets twice daily (6 maximum); Depixol injection—deep intramuscular injection of 20–40mg every 2 to 4 weeks; Depixol Conc. and Depixol Low Volume—50mg 4-weekly up to 300mg every 2 weeks by deep intramuscular injection.

Special care: with the elderly, sufferers of Parkinson's disease or kidney, liver, respiratory or cardiovascular disease and anyone with an intolerance to neuroleptic drugs taken orally.

Avoid use: in pregnancy and lactation. Patients who are comatose, excitable or overactive. Not for children.

Possible interaction: alcohol, analgesics and central nervous system depressants. Also anticonvulsants, antidiabetics, levodopa and antihypertensives.

Side effects: muscular spasms, rigidity and tremor, dry mouth and nasal stuffiness, urine retention, increased heart rate, constipation, weight gain, drowsiness, lethargy, fatigue, blood and skin changes, menstrual changes and galactorrhoea.

Manufacturer: Lundbeck.

Depo-Medrone

Description: a corticosteroid preparation containing the glucocorticoid steroid methylprednisolone acetate as vials of 40mg/ml. Also, **Depo-Medrone with Lidocaine,** which in addition contains 10mg/ml lignocaine hydrochloride local anaesthetic.

Used for: severe allergic rhinitis, asthma, osteo- and rheumatoid arthritis, collagen disorders and skin diseases (Depo-Medrone). Local use for rheumatic or inflammatory conditions (Depo-Medrone with Lidocaine).

Dosage: by injection into joints or soft tisue, 4–80mg (according to joint size or amount of tissue) repeated 1–5 weekly depending upon response.

Special care: with numerous conditions including nephritis, osteoporosis, peptic ulcer and metastatic carcinoma. Also viral/fungal infections, tuberculosis, hypertension, glaucoma, epilepsy, diabetes, cirrhosis and hypothyroidism. Also pregnancy and stress. To be withdrawn gradually. Not to be given to children under 12 months.

Possible interaction: NSAIDs, diuretics, hypoglycaemics, oral anticoagulants, phenobarbitone, ephedrine, phenytoin, anticholinesterases and others.

Side effects: osteoporosis, depression, hyperglycaemia, euphoria, peptic ulceration.

Manufacturer: Upjohn.

Depo-Provera

Description: a depot-injectable preparation of the progestogen medroxyprogesterone acetate available in vials as a suspension of 150mg/ml and 50mg/ml.

Used for: contraception for women who cannot use other methods and endometriosis. (Also used in treatment of certain types of carcinoma.)

Dosage: for contraception: 50mg by deep intramuscular injection during the first 5 days of the cycle or within 5 weeks of giving birth, repeated 3-monthly; for endometriosis: 50mg weekly or 100mg 2-weekly by intramuscular injection over 6 months and longer if necessary.

Special care: undiagnosed abnormal vaginal bleeding, diabetes or severe depressison. Also, wait 6 weeks after birth if lactating; not for genital malignancy.

Avoid use: pregnancy. Also hormone-dependent carcinoma.

Side effects: temporary fertility with continuous treatment, irregular or heavy vaginal bleeding during early cycles, weight gain, back pain and fluid retention.

Manufacturer: Upjohn.

Depostat

Description: a depot progestogen available as 2ml ampoules of gestronol hexanoate (100mg/ml).

Used for: benign hyperplasia of the prostate and endometrial cancer.

Dosage: 200–400mg by intramuscular injection every 5 to 7 days for both conditions.

Special care: migraine, epilepsy, asthma and diabetes, kidney disease.

Avoid use: liver disease, severe arterial disease, carcinoma of the breast or genital tract.

Side effects: nausea, fluid retention, weight gain.

Manufacturer: Schering H.C.

Dermovate

Description: a potent steroid, clobetasol proprionate, available as 0.05% cream and ointment. Also available as **Dermovate Scalp Application** (solution), and **Dermovate-NN** which is also an antifungal/antibacterial agent containing, in addition, 0.5% neomycin sulphate and 100,000 units/g nystatin.

Used for: psoriasis, eczemas that are hard to control, inflammatory skin diseases. Dermovate-NN is for such conditions when infection is present or suspected.

Dosage: to be applied sparingly once or twice daily for a maximum of 4 weeks (maximum of 50g weekly for Dermovate-NN), then review.

Special care: limit use of face to 5 days. Withdraw gradually.

Avoid use: on acne, scabies, leg ulcers or prolonged use in pregnancy. Not for children.

Side effects: Cushingoid (see Cushing's syndrome) changes, skin atrophy, telangiectasia (multiple telangiectases, collections of distended blood capillaries).

Manufacturer: Glaxo.

Deseril

Description: The maleate of methysergide which acts as a serotonin antagonist. Serotonin is active in inflammation (similar to histamine) and also acts as a neurotransmitter and is released by the liver and certain tumours. Available as white tablets of 1mg strength marked DSL.

Used for: diarrhoea associated with carcinoid disease, i.e. a tumour in certain glands in the intestine. For relief of recurring severe migraine, histamine (cluster) headaches and headaches where other treatments have failed.

Dosage: for diarrhoea: 12 to twenty daily with meals, in divided doses. For migraine: 1 or 2 tablets 3 times per day with meals.

Special care: anyone with a history of peptic ulcer. In treating migraine, 6 months of therapy should be followed by a month's interval and the dosage reduced 2 to 3 weeks before withdrawal. Patient should be monitored regularly.

Avoid use: pregnancy or lactation; coronary, peripheral or occlusive vascular disorders; heart or

lung disease; severe hypertension; liver or kidney impairment; disease of the urinary tract; poor health, weakness and malnutrition (cachexia); sepsis; phlebitis or cellulitis (skin infection leading to abscess and tissue destruction) of the lower extremities. Not recommended for children.

Possible interaction: vasopressors and vasoconstrictors; ergot alkaloids (alkaloids derived from the fungus *Laviceps purpurea*).

Side effects: dizziness, nausea, oedema, lassitude, leg cramps, drowsiness, weight gain, rashes, hair loss, CNS disturbances, abdominal discomfort, arterial spasm. Discontinue in the event of inflammatory fibrosis.

Manufacturer: Sandoz.

Desferal

Description: desferrioxamine mesylate as 500mg powder in a vial for reconstitution and injection. Desferal acts as a chelating agent with the iron, i.e. it locks up the iron chemically, enabling it to be removed from the system.

Used for: iron poisoning, haemochromatoses (excess deposits of iron in the body due to faulty iron metabolism), excess aluminium in dialysis patients.

Dosage: depending upon condition and circumstances—by mouth, intramuscular injection or intravenous infusion.

Special care: kidney dysfunction; pregnancy and lactation; patients with aluminium-related encephalopathy may have seizures (treat first with Clonazepam).

Possible interaction: erythropoietin, prochlorperazine.

Side effects: hypotension if given too rapidly intravenously; cardiovascular, gastrointestinal and neurological disturbances; changes in lens and retina; urine has red colouration; leg cramps; liver and kidney dysfunction; blood conditions, e.g. anaemia.

Manufacturer: Ciba.

Destolit

Description: a bile acid, visodeoxycholic acid, available as white tablets (150mg) marked DESTOLIT.

Used for: dissolution of small cholesterol gallstones.

Dosage: 3 to 4 daily in 2 doses after meals, 1 after an evening meal. To be continued for 3 to 4 months after stones have been dissolved.

Avoid use: active gastric or duodenal ulcer; liver and intestine conditions affecting recycling of bile between intestine and liver; if gall bladder not functioning; women if not using contraception (non-hormonal methods ideally). Not for children.

Possible interaction: oestrogens; oral contraceptives; agents lowering cholesterol levels.

Manufacturer: Merrell Dow.

Deteclo

Description: a compound tetracycline preparation containing chlortetracycline hydrochloride (115.4mg), tetracycline hydrochloride (115.4mg) and demeclocycline hydrochloride (69.2mg) in blue film-coated tablets, marked LL, and 5422 on the reverse.

Used for: ear, nose and throat infections; infection of respiratory, gastrointestinal and urinary tracts and soft tissues; severe cases of acne vulgaris.

Dosage: 1 tablet 12-hourly.

Special care: impaired liver.

Avoid use: during pregnancy and lactation; kidney impairment; SLE.

Possible interaction: penicillins; anticoagulants; oral contraceptives; milk, antacids or mineral supplements.

Side effects: allergic reactions; gastrointestinal upsets; superinfection (i.e. one infection arising during the course of another); withdraw in the case of intracranial hypertension.

Manufacturer: Lederle.

Dexa-Rhinaspray

Description: a metered dose aersol for nasal inhalation consisting of a corticosteroid (dexamethasone-21 isonicotinate, 20mg per dose), antibiotic (neomycin sulphate, 100mg) and the sympathomimetic (i.e. something that mimics the effects of organ stimulation by the sympathetic nervous system) tramazoline hydrochloride (120mg).

Used for: allergic rhinitis (e.g. hay fever).

Dosage: 1 dose per nostril up to 6 times per 24 hours. One dose twice daily for children 5 to 12 years. Not recommended for children under 5 years.

Special care: not to be used over a prolonged period.

Side effects: nasal irritation.

Manufacturer: Boehringer Ingelheim.

Dexedrine^{CD}

Description: a sympathomimetic, dexamphetamine sulphate, available as a white tablet (5mg strength), marked EVANS DB5.

Used for: narcolepsy, untreatable hyperactivity in children.

Dosage: 1 tablet twice daily increasing weekly by 10mg to a maximum of 60mg daily. For the elderly, 5mg daily increasing by 5mg every week. Not recommended for children under 3 years; 2.5mg daily increasing by 2.5mg every week for children aged 3 to 5 and 5–10mg daily for children aged 6 to 12 years, increasing at weekly intervals by 5mg. A maximum of 20mg daily is customary.

Special care: pregnancy.

Avoid use: glaucoma; hypertension; hyperexcitability; hyperthyroidism; in cases of cardiovascular disease; where there is a history of drug abuse.

Possible interaction: guanethidine, MAOIs.

Side effects: restlessness and insomnia; retarded growth; euphoria; dry mouth; sweating, palpitations; tachycardia; disturbances of the central nervous system and stomach; raised blood pressure. Also, possible dependence.

Manufacturer: Evans.

Dextropropoxyphene

Description: an opiate and weak analgesic, dextropropoxyphene napsylate, available as capsules (60mg strength).

Used for: mild to moderate pain anywhere in the body.

Dosage: 3 to 4 capsules per day.

Special care: pregnancy, elderly; liver or kidney impairment.

Avoid use: in children.

Possible interaction: anticoagulants; anti-convulsants; alcohol or depressants of the central nervous system.

Side effects: constipation; rash; nausea and dizziness; drowsiness. May develop tolerance and dependence.

Manufacturer: Lilly.

DHC Continus

Description: an opiate, dihydrocodeine tartrate, available as white capsules for sustained (prolonged) release and in strengths of 60, 90 and 120mg, marked with DHC and strength.

Used for: chronic severe pain e.g. as associated with cancer.

Dosage: 60-120mg 12-hourly.

Special care: chronic liver disease; kidney impairment; in pregnancy or the elderly; allergies; hypothyroidism; raised intracranial pressure.

Avoid use: depression of respiration; disease causing obstruction of the airways.

Possible interaction: MAOIs, alcohol and central nervous system depressants.

Side effects: headache; vertigo; nausea; constipation.

Manufacturer: Napp.

Diabinese

Description: a sulphonylurea, and hypoglycaemic agent containing chlorpropamide and available as white tablets of strength 100 and 250mg. Marked with DIA, strength and Pfizer.

Used for: type II non-insulin dependent diabetes, adult-onset diabetes mellitus (when the pancreas is still active to some extent).

Dosage: usually 100–250mg daily with breakfast, maximum 500mg.

Special care: the elderly or patients with kidney failure.

Avoid use: during pregnancy or lactation; juvenile, growth-onset or unstable brittle diabetes (insulin-dependent diabetes mellitus); ketoacidosis; severe kidney or liver disorders; stress, infections or surgery; endocrine disorders.

Possible interaction: MAOIs, corticosteroids, ß-blockers, diuretics, corticotrophin (ACTH), oral contraceptives, alcohol. Also aspirin, oral anticoagulants, bezafibrate, clofibrate, phenylbutazone, cyclophosphamide, rifampicin, sulphonamides and chloramphenicol. Also glucagon.

Side effects: skin rash and other sensitivity reactions. Other conditions tend to be rare, e.g. hyponatraemia (low blood sodium concentration) or aplastic anaemia.

Manufacturer: Pfizer.

Diamicron

Description: a sulphonylurea, and hypoglycaemic agent, containing gliclazide and available as white tablets (80mg strength).

Used for: type II non-insulin-dependent diabetes, adult-onset diabetes mellitus (when the pancreas is still active to some extent).

Dosage: half to 1 daily up to a maximum of 4 (2 divided doses if above 2 tablets).

Special care: the elderly or patients with kidney failure.

Avoid use: during pregnancy or lactation; juvenile, growth-onset or unstable brittle diabetes (insulin-dependent diabetes mellitus); ketoacidosis; severe kidney or liver disorders; stress, infections or surgery; endocrine disorders.

Possible interaction: MAOIs, corticosteroids, ß-blockers, diuretics, corticotrophin (ACTH), oral contraceptives, alcohol. Also aspirin, oral anticoagulants, and the generic drugs bezafibrate, clofibrate, phenylbutazone, cyclophosphamide, rifampicin, sulphonamides and chloramphenicol. Also glucagon.

Side effects: skin rash and other sensitivity reactions. Other conditions tend to be rare, e.g. hyponatraemia (low blood sodium concentration) or aplastic anaemia.

Manufacturer: Servier.

Diamox

Description: a carbonic anhydrase inhibitor, acetazolamide, available as white tablets (250mg strength) marked LEDERLE 4395.

Used for: congestive heart failure and oedema; epilepsy; glaucoma.

Dosage: for heart failure, oedema: 250–375mg to start, each morning or on alternate days. For premenstrual oedema, 125–375mg in 1 dose 5 to 10 days before menstruation. For epilepsy: 250–1000mg each day. Children under 24 months 125mg daily; 2 to 12 years 125–750mg daily. For glaucoma: 250–1000mg daily. Children, 125–750mg daily; infants, 125mg daily. All in divided doses.

Also **Diamox SR**

Description: as for Diamox, but available as 250mg strength sustained-release orange capsule.

Used for: glaucoma.

Dosage: 1 to 2 daily.

Also **Diamox Parenteral**

Description: as for Diamox, but available as powder in a vial, 500mg strength.

Used for: congestive heart failure and oedema; epilepsy; glaucoma.

Dosage: intravenous or intramuscular injection of equivalent oral dose.

Special care: diabetes, lactation, gout, potassium supplements may be required. Monitor blood, electrolytes and fluid. Also for glaucoma treatment: emphysema and pulmonary obstruction, any unusual rashes to be reported.

Avoid use: pregnancy, certain kidney conditions, chronic closed angle glaucoma, adrenal insufficiency, hypersensitivity to sulphonamides, depletion of sodium or potassium. Also for glaucoma—liver impairment.

Possible interaction: oral anticoagulants, hypoglycaemics, folic acid antagonists.

Side effects: headache, drowsiness, thirst, flushing, polyuria, blood dyscrasias, rash, excitability, paraesthesia (tingling, 'pins and needles').

Manufacturer: Storz.

Dianette

Description: the oestrogen/anti-androgen ethinyl-oestradiol (35µg) with 2mg cyproterone acetate, available as beige tablets.

Used for: severe acne in women; for prolonged oral antibiotic therapy; idiopathic hirsutism.

Dosage: 1 daily for 3 weeks starting on first day of cycle (then 7 days without).

Special care: diabetes, varicose veins, hypertension, Raynaud's disease (numbness in the fingers due to spasm of arteries), asthma, chronic kidney disease (or dialysis), severe depression, multiple sclerosis.

Avoid use: not recommended for children. Also with cardiovascular conditions such as angina, ischaemia, heart valve disease, sickle cell anaemia, those at risk of and with a history of thrombosis. Patients with liver disorders; hormone-dependent carcinoma, undiagnosed vaginal bleeding, pregnancy, chorea, otosclerosis (bone overgrowth in the inner ear causing deafness), haemolytic uraemic syndrome (sudden destruction of red blood cells causing acute kidney failure).

Possible interaction: tetracyclines, barbiturates, phenytoin, griseofulvin, primidone, carbamazepine, rifampicin, chloral hydrate, ethosuximide, glutethimide, dichloralphenazone.

Side effects: leg pains and cramps, depression, enlargement of breasts, fluid retention, headaches, nausea, weight gain, loss of libido, vaginal discharge.

Manufacturer: Schering H.C.

Diaphine^{CD}

Description: The analgesic opiate, diamorphine hydrochloride available as powder in ampoules in strengths of 5, 10, 30, 100 and 500mg.

Used for: severe pain.

Dosage: 5–10mg subcutaneously or intramuscularly, to be varied according to patient response.

Special care: liver or kidney impairment, hypotension, hypothyroidism, myxoedema, reduced respiratory capacity, depression of the CNS, toxic psychoses, prostatic hypertrophy, stricture of the urethra, acute alcoholism, delirium tremens, severe diarrhoea, the elderly.

Avoid use: in children. With head injuries, raised intracranial pressure, acute liver disease, acute respiratory depression, diseases causing obstruction of the airways.

Possible interaction: depressants of the central nervous system, MAOIs.

Side effects: shock, cardiac arrest, vomiting, nausea, constipation, depression of respiration. Possible tolerance and dependence.

Manufacturer: Napp.

Diarrest

Description: a combined opiate, antispasmodic and electrolyte containing 5mg codeine phosphate, 2.5mg dicyclomine hydrochloride, 40mg potassium chloride, 50mg sodium chloride, 50mg sodium citrate per 5ml. Available in 200ml bottles.

Used for: diarrhoea and to maintain levels of electrolytes during attacks.

Dosage: 20ml 4 times per day with water. Children, at the same frequency: 10 to 13 years, 15ml; 6 to 9 years, 10ml; 4 to 5 years, 5ml; under 4 years, contact the manufacturer.

Special care: cardiac failure, liver or kidney malfunction, glaucoma, thyrotoxicosis, ulcerative colitis.

Avoid use: diverticular disease, pseudomembranous colitis (severe colitis occurring in debilitated patients taking broad-spectrum antibiotics).

Possible interaction: MAOIs.

Side effects: sedation.

Manufacturer: Galen.

Diazemuls

Description: a long-acting anxiolytic, benzodiazepine, available as an emulsion of 10mg in 2ml.

Used for: severe acute anxiety, delirium tremens; acute muscle spasms; anticonvulsant for status epilepticus (continual seizures resulting in brain damage if not stopped); and as a premedication.

Dosage: 10mg (5mg for elderly) by infusion or intravenous injection at 4-hourly intervals; 0.2mg/kg for children by the same means. As an anticonvulsant, 0.15–0.25mg/kg by intravenous injection, repeated after half to one hour and then up to 3mg/kg over 24 hours by intravenous infusion. For premedication, 0.1–0.2mg/kg by intravenous injection.

Special care: chronic lung insufficiency, chronic liver or kidney disease, the elderly, pregnant, during labour or lactation. Judgement and dexterity may be affected, long-term use is to be avoided. To be withdrawn gradually.

Avoid use: acute lung insufficiency, depression of respiration (escept in cases of acute muscle spasms). Also when treating anxiety, obsessional states or chronic psychosis.

Possible interaction: alcohol and other CNS depressants, anticonvulsants.

Side effects: vertigo, gastrointestinal upsets, confusion, ataxia, drowsiness, light-headedness, hypotension, disturbance of vision, skin rashes. Also urine retention, changes in libido. Dependence a potential problem.

Manufacturer: Dumex.

Diazepam

Description: an anxiolytic, long-acting benzodiazepine, available as 2, 5 and 10mg tablets and as **Diazepam Elixir** (2mg/5ml).

Used for: severe anxiety in the short term, acute alcohol withdrawal, night terrors and sleepwalking in children.

Dosage: 6–30mg daily (elderly 3–15mg); children 1–5mg at bedtime.

Special care: chronic lung insufficiency, chronic liver or kidney disease, the elderly, pregnant, during labour or lactation. Judgement and dexterity may be affected, long-term use is to be avoided. To be withdrawn gradually.

Avoid use: acute lung insufficiency, depression of respiration, obsessional states or chronic psychosis.

Possible interaction: alcohol, other CNS depressants, anticonvulsants.

Side effects: vertigo, gastrointestinal upsets, confusion, ataxia, drowsiness, light-headedness, hypotension, disturbance of vision, skin rashes. Also urine retention, changes in libido. Dependence a potential problem.

Manufacturer: non-proprietary.

Dibenyline

Description: an anti-adrenaline antihypertensive, phenoxybenzamine hydrochloride, available as 10mg red and white capsules marked SKF. Also as **Dibenyline Injection** (50mg/ml) in 2ml doses.

Used for: vasodilation to treat high blood pressure associated with phaeochromocytoma.

Dosage: 1 capsule daily increasing by 1 each day to achieve control. Children, 1–2mg/kg daily in divided doses.

Special care: the elderly, kidney disease, cardiovascular or cerebrovascular disease, congestive heart failure.

Avoid use: after myocardial infarction, cerebrovascular accident (i.e. heart attack or stroke).

Side effects: dizziness, tachycardia, low blood pressure on standing, failure to ejaculate, pinpoint pupils (miosis).

Manufacturer: Forley.

Diclomax Retard

Description: White, sustained-release capsules containing diclofenac sodium (100mg).

Used for: osteoarthritis, rheumatoid arthritis, ankylosing spondylitis, musculoskeletal disorders such as sprains and strains, back pains. Acute gout.

Dosage: 1 tablet daily with food.

Special care: kidney, liver or heart disorders, pregnancy or lactation, the elderly, blood disorders, hepatic porphyria (production of excess porphyrins in the liver producing abdominal pain, neuropathy and photosensitivity), and those with a history of gastrointestinal lesions. Patients on long-term treatment should be monitored.

Avoid use: active peptic ulcer, asthma, aspirin or anti-inflammatory drug-induced allergy, during last 3 months of pregnancy. Not recommended for children.

Possible interaction: steroids, NSAIDs, anticoagulants, antidiabetics, quinolones, diuretics, salicylates, lithium, digoxin, methotrexate, cyclosporin.

Side effects: headache, oedema, gastrointestinal upsets, peptic ulcer, liver and kidney malfunction, skin reactions.

Manufacturer: Parke-Davis.

Diconal[CD]

Description: an opiate and antiemetic containing cyclizine hydrochloride (30mg) and dipipanone hydrochloride (10mg) and available as a pink tablet, coded WELLCOME F3A.

Used for: moderate to severe pain.

Dosage: 1 initially, then as advised.

Special care: in pregnancy or with severe liver or kidney diseases.

Avoid use: respiratory depression, diseases causing obstruction of the airways. Not suitable for children.

Possible interaction: alcohol, depressants of the central nervous system, MAOIs.

Side effects: dry mouth, drowsiness, blurred vision. Tolerance and dependence may occur.

Manufacturer: Wellcome.

Dicynene

Description: a haemostatic drug and preparation of ethamsylate, available as ampoules (250mg/2ml) and 500mg white capsules.

Used for: prevention and treatment of periventricular bleeding in low birth weight infants. Also menorrhagia (abnormally heavy menstrual bleeding).

Dosage: for the newly born, 12.5mg/kg body weight 6 hourly within 2 hours of birth given intravenously or intramuscularly, continuing for 4 days. For menorrhagia, one 500mg capsule 4 times per day from the start of bleeding to the end of menstruation.

Side effects: headache, nausea, rash.

Manufacturer: Delandale.

Didronel PMO

Description: a diphosphonate/calcium supplement available as white capsule-shaped tablets containing 400mg etidronate disodium marked NE and 406; with 1250mg calcium carbonate (Cacit) as pink effervescent tablets with an orange taste.

Used for: vertebral osteoporosis.

Dosage: 1 tablet daily for 14 days taken with water in the middle of a 4-hour fast, followed by 1 Cacit tablet daily in water for 76 days. The 90-day cycle is repeated for 3 years.

Also **Didronel Injection**

Description: ampoules of 50mg/ml etidronate disodium.

Used for: hypercalcaemia associated with malignant tumours.

Dosage: slow intravenous infusion of 7.5mg/kg daily for 3 days. Interval of 7 days thereafter.

Also **Didronel Tablets**

Description: 200mg of etidronate disodium in white rectangular tablets.

Used for: Paget's disease after treatment for hypercalcaemia of malignancy.

Dosage: 5mg/kg daily taken in the middle of a 4-hour fast over 6 months maximum (for Paget's disease). For hypercalcaemia, 20mg/kg for 30 days.

Special care: pregnancy, lactation, enterocolitis (inflammation of the colon and small intestine). Monitor kidney function and ensure adequate intake of calcium and vitamin D.

Avoid use: severe kidney disease. Not recommended for children.

Side effects: diarrhoea, nausea.

Manufacturer: Procter & Gamble Pharmaceuticals.

Diflucan

Description: a triazole, fluconazole, available as blue and white (50mg), purple and white (200mg) capsules and **Diflucan Suspension** (50mg and 200mg/5ml) and **Diflucan Infusion** (bottles with 2mg/ml). Both capsules marked with FLU, strength and PFIZER.

Used for: candidiasis (thrush) whether oral or vaginal, systemic candidiasis, cryptococcosis (infection, with *Cryptococcus*, of the lungs and possibly the brains and CNS), oral/oropharyngeal candidosis, prevention of fungal infections following cytotoxic radio- or chemotherapy, for maintenance in AIDS sufferers to prevent relapse of cryptococcal meningitis.

Dosage: oral/vaginal candidiasis, 50–100mg daily for 14 to 30 days. Systemic candidiasis, 400mg on first day, and 200–400mg daily thereafter. Oropharyngeal, 50–100mg daily for 7 to 14 days. Maintenance against meningitis, 100–100mg daily. Prevention of fungal infections, 50–100mg daily. Doses delivered orally or by intravenous infusion. For children over 1 year, only in the case of life-threatening infections, 3–6mg/kg daily.

Special care: kidney damage with multiple doses.

Avoid use: during pregnancy or lactation.

Possible interaction: oral sulphonylureas, phenytoin, cyclosporin, rifampicin, theophylline, anticoagulants.

Side effects: gastrointestinal upsets.

Manufacturer: Pfizer.

Digibind

Description: an antidote for digoxin comprising 40mg of antibody fragments in a vial for reconstitution.

Used for: digoxin overdose.

Dosage: seek advice.

Special care: kidney disease.

Avoid use: allergy to ovine protein.

Side effects: hypokalaemia.

Manufacturer: Wellcome.

Dihydrocodeine

Description: an analgesic opiate, dihydrocodeine tartrate, available as tablets (30mg strength). Also as **Dihydrocodeine Oral Solution**, a syrup containing 10mg per 5ml.

Used for: moderate to severe pain.

Dosage: 1 tablet or 5–15ml 4 to 6-hourly, after food and as required. Children, 4 to 12 years, 0.5–1mg/kg body weight, 4 to 6-hourly. Not suitable for children under 4 years.

Also **Dihydrocodeine Injection** as 50mg/ml in ampoules.

Dosage: up to 50mg by deep subcutaneous or intramuscular injection. Children, same details as for dihydrocodeine/oral solution.

Special care: kidney disease or chronic liver disease, allergies, hypothyroidism. The elderly or pregnant.

Avoid use: respiratory depression, or diseases that cause obstruction of the airways.

Possible interaction: MAOIs, alcohol, depressants of the CNS.

Side effects: nausea, headache, vertigo, constipation.

Manufacturer: Knapp.

Dilzem SR

Description: an antihypertensive/antianginal calcium ion antagonist prepared as diltiazem hydrochloride. Available as beige sustained-release capsules of strengths 60, 90 or 120mg, marked with strength.

Used for: angina, mild to moderate hypertension.

Dosage: 90mg twice daily initially increasing to 180mg if required. For the elderly 60mg twice daily.

Also **Dilzem XL**, white capsules of diltiazem hydrochloride available as 120, 180 or 240mg strengths.

Dosage: 180mg daily increasing to 360mg. For the elderly, 120mg daily.

Special care: diabetes, mild bradycardia, impaired left ventricular function, 1st degree AV block or prolonged P-R interval.

Avoid use: pregnancy or lactation, 2nd or 3rd degree AV block, left ventricular failure, bradycardia, liver or kidney disease, sick sinus syndrome (syndromes associated with dysfunction of the sinus (sinoatrial) node, the heart tissue that generates the cardiac electrical impulse).

Possible interaction: infusion of dantrolene, other cardiac depressants or hypertensives, also cyclosporin, digoxin, lithium, diazepam, cimetidine, theophylline, carbamazepine.

Side effects: ankle oedema, nausea, rash, headache, flushes, gastrointestinal upset, SA or AV block.

Manufacturer: Elan.

Dimetriose

Description: a gonadotrophin release inhibitor, gestrinone, in white capsules (2–5mg).

Used for: endometriosis.

Dosage: 1 twice weekly on the first and fourth day of the cycle, then on the same days of the week throughout the treatment.

Special care: diabetes, hyperlipidaemia.

Avoid use: in pregnancy, lactation. Severe heart, kidney or liver disease, metabolic or vascular disorders.

Possible interaction: rifampicin, oral contraceptives, anticonvulsants.

Side effects: gastrointestinal upsets, cramp, hirsutism, depression, voice changes, acne, weight gain.

Manufacturer: Roussel.

Dindevan

Description: an anticoagulant, phenindione, of strengths 10 (white, marked D10), 25 (green, marked D25) and 50mg (white, marked D50).

Used for: thromboembolic conditions.

Dosage: 200mg to start, then 100mg the following day and subsequent daily maintenance dose of 50–150mg.

Special care: the elderly, acute illness, vitamin K deficiency. Hypertension, weight changes, kidney disease.

Avoid use: severe liver or kidney disease, haemorrhagic conditions, within 24 hours of surgery or labour. Pregnancy or lactation.

Possible interaction: corticosteroids, NSAIDs, sulphonamides, oral hypoglycaemics, quinidine, antibiotics, phenformin, drugs affecting liver enzymes, cimetidine.

Side effects: diarrhoea, hepatitis, kidney damage, urine discoloured, fever, rash, leucopenia, agranulocytosis (abnormal blood condition involving a reduction in the number of granulocytes).

Manufacturer: Goldshield.

Dioderm

Description: a topical steroid, hydrocortisone, available as a 0.1% cream.

Used for: allergic, pruritic or inflammatory skin conditions.

Dosage: to be applied sparingly. Rub in well twice daily.

Special care: maximum 5 days use on face or for children. Withdraw gradually after prolonged use.

Avoid use: acne (and rosacea), scabies, leg ulcers, peri-oral dermatitis, untreated fungal or viral infections, tuberculous, ringworm or viral skin disease. Extensively or for prolonged period in pregnancy.

Side effects: skin atrophy, striae, telangiectasia (multiple telangiectases, which are collections of distended blood capillaries), Cushingoid changes (see Cushing's syndrome).

Manufacturer: Dermal.

Dipentum

Description: a salicylate, olsalazine sodium, available as a 250mg caramel capsule.

Used for: acute mild ulcerative colitis.

Dosage: 4 daily with food to begin, maximum 12 daily (all in divided doses). For maintenance, 2 twice daily with food. Not recommended for children.

Avoid use: pregnancy, severe kidney disease, hypersensitivity to salicylates.

Side effects: headache, rash, arthralgia (joint pain), gastrointestinal upset.

Manufacturer: Kabi Pharmacia.

Diprivan

Description: a general anaesthetic, propofol, containing 10mg/ml as an emulsion in vials and ampoules. Associated with rapid recovery without a hangover effect.

Used for: general anaesthesia at the start of surgery, and its maintenance.

Dosage: by intravenous injection, 2–2.5mg/kg (less in the elderly) at 20–40mg per 10 seconds; adjusted for children. Maintenance, 4–12mg/kg/hour.

Side effects: occasionally convulsions and brachycardia.

Manufacturer: Zeneca.

Diprosalic

Description: a potent steroid and keratolytic (causing shedding of outer skin layer) ointment, containing betamethasone dipropionate (0.05%) and salicylic acid (3%).

Used for hard skin and dry skin disorders.

Dosage: apply thinly once or twice per day.

Also **Diprosalic Scalp Application** comprising betamethasone dipropionate (0.05%), salicylic acid (2%) in solution.

Dosage: apply a few drops to the scalp and rub in, twice daily.

Special care: limit use on face to 5 days. Withdraw gradually after prolonged use.

Avoid use: leg ulcers, scabies, peri-oral dermatitis, untreated fungal or viral infections, tuberculous, ringworm or viral skin diseases, acne. Lengthy or extensive use in pregnancy. Not for children.

Side effects: skin striae and atrophy, telangiectasia (multiple telangiectases, which are collections of distended blood capillaries), Cushingoid changes (see Cushing's syndrome), adrenal gland suppression.

Manufacturer: Schering-Plough.

Diprosone

Description: a potent steroid, betamethasone dipropionate, as 0.05% cream and ointment.

Used for: skin diseases that respond to steroid treatment.

Dosage: apply sparingly once or twice per day.

Also **Diprosone Lotion**, 0.05% betamethasone dipropionate in alcoholic solution.

Used for: scalp skin diseases

Dosage: apply a few drops twice daily

Special care: limit use on face to 5 days. Withdraw gradually after prolonged use.

Avoid use: leg ulcers, scabies, peri-oral dermatitis, untreated fungal or viral infections, tuberculous, ringworm or viral skin diseases, acne. Lengthy or extensive use in pregnancy. Not for children.

Side effects: skin striae and atrophy, telangiectasia (multiple telangiectases, which are collections of distended blood capillaries), Cushingoid changes (see Cushing's syndrome), adrenal gland suppression.

Manufacturer: Schering-Plough.

Dirythmin SA

Description: an antiarrhythmic, disopyramide phosphate, available as a white 150mg film-coated sustained-release tablet, marked A over DR.

Used for: heart arrhythmias.

Dosage: 2 every 12 hours, maximum 5 per day.

Special care: kidney and liver failure, pregnancy, prostatic hypertrophy, glaucoma, urine retention, hypokalaemia, 1st degree AV block.

Avoid use: cardiomyopathy, cardiogenic shock (low cardiac output), disease of the sinoatrial node when there is no pacemaker, 2nd or 3rd degree AV block. Not recommended for children.

Possible interaction: ß-blockers, other anti-arrhythmics in the same class, erythromycin, agents causing potassium reduction, anticholinergics (inhibiting the action of acetylcholine).

Side effects: anticholinergic effects.

Manufacturer. Astra.

Disipal

Description: an anticholinergic, orphenadrine hydrochloride, available in yellow, sugar-coated tablets, strength 50mg, marked DISIPAL.

Used for: Parkinson's disease.

Dosage: 50mg 3 times per day initially, increased by 50mg every 2 to 3 days. Maintenance 100–300mg per day. Maximum 400mg daily.

Special care: heart disorders, gastrointestinal obstructions. Withdraw slowly.

Avoid use: prostatic hypertrophy (enlarged prostate), glaucoma, tardive dyskinesia (repetitive muscular movements of the limbs, face or trunk).

Possible interaction: antihistamines, anti-depressants, phenothiazines.

Side effects: confusion, agitation, rashes with high dosages, euphoria, anticholinergic effects.

Manufacturer: Brocades.

Distaclor MR

Description: a cephalosporin, cefaclor, available as a blue sustained-release tablet (375mg strength) marked with name and strength.

Used for: infections of the skin, soft tissue and respiratory tract, otitis media, infections of the urinary tract.

Dosage: 1 twice daily or 2 twice daily for the treatment of pneumonia. Not recommended for children.

Also **Distaclor Capsules** available in white/violet (250mg), violet/grey (500mg) capsules; and Distaclor Suspension (125, 250mg/5ml.)

Dosage: 250mg every 8 hours up to a maximum of 4g per day. Children from 1 month–1 year, 62.5mg; 1 to 5 years, 125mg; over 5 years, 250mg. All 3 times per day to a maximum of 1g.

Special care: pregnancy or lactation. Kidney disease, hypersensitivity to penicillins.

Possible interaction: anticoagulants.

Side effects: gastrointestinal upsets, hypersensitivity

reactions, pseudomembranous colitis (a severe form of colitis).
Manufacturer: Lilly.

Distalgesic
Description: an analgesic and compound opiate containing dextropropoxyphene hydrochloride (32.5mg) and paracetamol (325mg), available in white oblong film-coated tablets marked DG.
Used for: mild to moderate pain.
Dosage: 2, 3 or 4 times per day. Not recommended for children.
Special care: kidney or liver disease, pregnancy or the elderly.
Possible interaction: anticonvulsants, anticoagulants, alcohol, depressants of the central nervous system.
Side effects: constipation, drowsiness, dizziness, nausea, rash, tolerance and dependence.
Manufacturer: Dista.

Distamine
Description: a penicillin derivative penicillamine, available as white tablets of strengths 50, 125 (marked DS and 125) and 250mg (marked DM and 250).
Used for: severe active rheumatoid arthritis, heavy metal poisoning, chronic hepatitis, cystinuria (abnormal occurrence of cystine, an amino acid, in the urine), Wilson's disease (a defect in copper metabolism causing deposition of copper in the liver or brain, producing jaundice and cirrhosis, and mental retardation respectively).
Dosage: 125–250mg daily for 4 weeks increasing by 125–2500 mg at intervals of 4 to 12 weeks. Maximum daily dose 1.5g. Maintenance dose 500–750mg.. For the elderly, 50–125mg daily increasing to 500–750mg and a maximum of 1g per day.Children, 50mg per day for 1 month increasing 4-weekly. Maintenance 15–20mg/kg of body weight per day.
Special care: kidney disease, sensitivity to penicillin, blood, urine and functioning of kidneys should be monitored during treatment.
Avoid use: pregnancy, lactation, agranulocytosis (abnormal blood condition involving a reduction in the number of granulocytes), thrombocytopenia, lupus erythematosus (an inflammatory disease affecting the skin and some internal organs, regarded as an autoimmune disease).
Possible interaction: antacids, gold, zinc or iron salts, cytotoxic or antimalarial drugs, phenylbutazone.
Side effects: fever, rash, anorexia, nausea, blood

disorders, loss of taste, proteinuria, myasthenia gravis, haematuria, SLE, nephrotic syndrome.
Manufacturer: Dista.

Ditropan
Description: an anticholinergic/antispasmodic, oxybutynin hydrochloride, available as blue tablets in strengths 2.5mg and 5mg. All marked with tablet name, strength and company initials.
Also **Ditropan Elixir** as 2.5mg/5ml.
Used for: nocturnal enuresis (involuntary urination/ bed-wetting), urinary frequency and incontinence, neurogenic bladder instability (often relating to the detrusor muscle of the bladder).
Dosage: 5mg 2 or 3 times per day to a daily maximum of 20g. 5mg twice daily for the elderly. Not recommended for children under 5; 5mg 2 or 3 times per day for children over 5. Last dose to be given at bedtime for nocturnal enuresis.
Special care: liver or kidney disease, hyperthyroidism, congestive heart failure, coronary artery disease, cardiac arrhythmias, tachycardia, hiatus hernia, prostatic hypertrophy, autonomic neuropathy. The frail, elderly or in pregnancy.
Avoid use: bladder or bowel obstruction, severe ulcerative colitis, glaucoma, lactation, myasthenia gravis, intestinal atony (weak), toxic megacolon (a serious complication of ulcerative colitis, involving massive dilatation of the colon).
Possible interaction: levodopa, digoxin, butyrophenones, amantadine, phenothiazines, tricyclic antidepressants, anticholinergics.
Side effects: facial flushes, anticholinergic effects (limit transmission of parasympathetic nerve impulses).
Manufacturer: Smith & Nephew Pharmaceuticals.

Diumide-K Continus
Description: a loop diuretic (a powerful, short-duration drug that acts on the loop of Henle in the kidney) and potassium ion supplement, available as frusemide (40mg) and sustained-release potassium chloride (600mg) in white and orange film-coated tablets marked DK.
Used for: kidney and liver disease where a potassium supplement is required, oedema including that associated with congestive heart failure.
Dosage: 1 tablet per day, taken in the morning.
Special care: diabetes, pregnancy, lactation. Gout, prostatic hypertrophy, liver or kidney disease, impaired urination.
Avoid use: hyperkalaemia, Addison's disease, precomatose states in cases of liver cirrhosis.
Possible interaction: NSAIDs, cephalosporins,

antihypertensives, lithium, digitalis, amino-glycosides, potassium-sparing diuretics.
Side effects: gout. To be discontinued if small bowel appears to be ulcerated or obstructed.
Manufacturer: ASTA Medica.

Diurexan

Description: a thiazide-like diuretic, xipamide, available as 20mg, white tablets, marked A.
Used for: oedema, hypertension, congestive heart failure.
Dosage: 1 each morning for hypertension; 2 each morning for oedema initially, then 1 to 4 daily as required. Not recommended for children.
Special care: liver or kidney disease, liver cirrhosis, diabetes, SLE, gout. The elderly, during pregnancy or lactation. Monitor fluid glucose and electrolytes.
Avoid use: severe liver or kidney failure, hypercalcaemia, sensitivity to sulphonamides, Addison's disease.
Possible interaction: NSAIDs, corticosteroids, carbenoxolone, tubocurarine, antidiabetic agents, alcohol, barbiturates, opioids, lithium, cardiac glycosides.
Side effects: gastrointestinal upset, photosensitivity, rash, blood disorders, pancreatitis, dizziness, impotence, electrolyte and metabolic disturbance.
Manufacturer: ASTA Medica.

Dobutrex

Description: a ß₁-antagonist (acts on beta₁ receptors in cardiac muscle) dobutamine hydrochloride available in vials, as a solution of 12.5mg/ml.
Used for: cardiac surgery, cardiomyopathies, septic and cardiogenic shock (low cardiac output with acute myocardial infarction and congestive heart failure), inotropic (i.e. affecting heart muscle contraction) support in infarction.
Dosage: intravenous infusion of 2.5–10mg/kg/minute varying with response.
Special care: severe hypotension complicating cardiogenic shock.
Side effects: tachycardia, increase in systolic blood pressure indicating overdosage.
Manufacturer: Lilly.

Dolmatil

Description: a substitute benzamide, sulpiride, available as white tablets (200mg) marked D200.
Used for: chronic schizophrenia.
Dosage: over 14 years, 400–800mg initially per day in divided doses then 200–1200mg twice daily varying with required result. Not recommended for children under 14 years.

Special care: epilepsy, pregnancy, kidney disease, hypomania (a mental state of hyperactivity and irritability).
Avoid use: phaeochromocytoma.
Possible interaction: alcohol, analgesics, depressants of the CNS, antidepressants, antdiabetics, levodopa, anticonvulsants, antihypertensives.
Side effects: muscle spasms, restlessness, rigidity and tremor, urine retention, tachycardia, constipation, dry mouth, hypotension, blurred vision, impotence, weight gain, galactorrhea, hypothermia, amenorrhoea, blood and skin disorders, lethargy, jaundice.
Manufacturer: Delandale.

Dolobid

Description: a salicylate analgesic and anti-inflammatory drug containing diflurisal and available as peach (250mg) and orange (500mg) film-coated tablets, marked DOLOBID.
Used for: acute and chronic pain; rheumatoid arthritis and osteoarthritis.
Dosage: 500mg twice daily then 250–500mg twice daily for maintenance. For arthritis, 500–1000mg daily, in 1 or 2 doses and varying according to the response. Not recommended for children.
Special care: kidney or liver disease, heart failure, the elderly, a history of gastrointestinal ulcers or haemorrhage. Kidneys and liver to be monitored during long-term treatment.
Avoid use: pregnancy, lactation, active peptic ulcer, aspirin or anti-inflammatory-induced allergy or asthma.
Possible interaction: anticoagulants, indomethacin.
Side effects: diarrhoea, dyspepsia, headache, rash, tinnitus, dizziness, gastrointestinal pain.
Manufacturer: Morson.

Doloxene

Description: an opiate, dextropropoxyphene napsylate, available as pink capsules (60mg) marked LILLY H64.
Used for: mild to moderate pain.
Dosage: 1, 3 or 4 times per day.
Special care: pregnancy, the elderly, kidney or liver disease.
Possible interaction: anticonvulsants, anticoagulants, alcohol, CNS depressants.
Side effects: drowsiness, constipation, nausea, dizziness, rash. Also tolerance and dependence.
Manufacturer: Lilly.

Doloxene CO

Description: an analgesic comprising an opiate,

salicylate and xanthine containing dextro-propoxyphene napsylate (100mg), aspirin (375mg) and caffeine (30mg) and available as red and grey capsules marked H91.
Used for: mild to moderate pain.
Dosage: 1, 3 to 4 times per day.
Special care: kidney or liver disease (monitor during long-term treatment), heart failure, the elderly, anti-inflammatory induced allergies or a history of bronchospasm.
Avoid use: haemophilia, active peptic ulcer, hypoprothrombinaemia (lack of prothrombin in the blood, upsetting clotting function).
Possible interaction: alcohol, CNS depressants, anticonvulsants, anticoagulants, hypoglycaemics, uricosurics (drugs for elimination of uric acid or relief of pain due to gout).
Side effects: nausea, rash, drowsiness, constipation, dizziness. Also tolerance and dependence.
Manufacturer: Lilly.

Dopacard

Description: a catecholamine, dopexamine hydrochloride, available in ampoules as a solution (50mg/5ml).
Used for: inotropic (i.e. affecting heart muscle contraction) support and vasodilation in heart failure during cardiac surgery.
Dosage: 0.5mg/kg/minute by intravenous infusion which may be increased to 6mg/kg/minute.
Special care: myocardial infarction, recent angina, hyperglycaemia, hypokalaemia. Monitor pulse, blood pressure etc.
Avoid use: thrombocytopenia, phaeochromocytoma, obstruction of the left ventricular outlet.
Side effects: increased heart rate, nausea, vomiting, tremor, anginal pain.
Manufacturer: Porton.

Dopram

Description: a respiratory stimulant, doxapram hydrochloride, available in 5ml ampoules (20mg/ml). Also **Dopram Infusion** (2mg/ml).
Used for: ventilatory failure in cases of chronic obstructive airways disease.
Dosage: 1.5–4mg per minute by intravenous infusion, varying according to patient's condition and response.
Special care: epilepsy, liver impairment; used only under precise, expert supervision in hospital.
Avoid use: coronary artery disease, severe hypertension, thyrotoxicosis, status asthmaticus (i.e. an asthma attack which lasts over a period of 24 hours).

Possible interaction: sympathomimetics, theophylline.
Side effects: dizziness, increase in heart rate and blood pressure.
Manufacturer: Wyeth.

Doralese

Description: a selective a₁ blocker, indoramin, available as pale yellow triangular film-coated tablets (20mg strength).
Used for: obstruction of urine outflow due to benign prostatic hypertrophy.
Dosage: 1 tablet twice daily.
Special care: liver or kidney disease, patients with poor heart function, epilepsy, depression, Parkinson's disease.
Avoid use: in cases of heart failure.
Possible interaction: antihypertensives, MAOIs.
Side effects: drowsiness, dry mouth, blocked nose, ejaculation failure, weight gain.
Manufacturer: Bencard.

Dovonex

Description: an ointment and vitamin D analogue, containing 0.005% calcipotriol, also available as **Doveonex Cream**.
Used for: mild to moderate psoriasis.
Dosage: to be applied twice daily up to a maximum of 100g per week.
Special care: during pregnancy and lactation. Avoid the face.
Avoid use: calcium metabolism disorders.
Side effects: temporary irritation, facial (including peri-oral) dermatitis.
Manufacturer: Leo.

Dozic

Description: an antipsychotic drug, butyrophenone available as a liquid preparation of haloperidol in 2 strengths, 1 and 2mg/ml.
Used for: mania, schizophrenia, psychoses, delirium tremens, alcohol withdrawal syndrome, childhood behavioural disorders.
Dosage: psychosis in the elderly: 0.5 0 2mg initially, others 0.5–5mg, both 2 to 3 times per day, increasing as required to a daily maximum of 200mg. This is reduced when control is gained, to a daily dose of 5–10mg. For anxiety, 0.5mg twice daily. For children, 0.05mg/kg daily in 2 divided doses.
Special care: liver or kidney failure, epilepsy, Parkinson's disease, pregnancy, thyrotoxicosis and severe cardiovascular disease.
Avoid use: if patient is unconscious.

Possible interaction: alcohol, analgesics, CNS depressants, anticonvulsants, antidiabetics, antidepressants, antihypertensives, levodopa.

Side effects: spasms of eye, face, neck and back muscles, dry mouth, blocked nose, restlessness, tremor and rigidity, tardive dyskinesia (involuntary, repetitious muscle movements), urine retention, tachycardia, constipation, blurred vision, weight gain, impotence, hypothermia, menstrual changes, skin and blood changes, drowsiness, lethargy, sometimes fits.

Manufacturer: R.P. Drugs.

Driclor

Description: a 20% solution of aluminium chloride hexahydrate in roll-on bottle.

Used for: very heavy sweating (hyperhidiosis) of hands, feet and armpits.

Dosage: apply at night and wash off in the morning. Reduce applications as sweating lessens. Use only on feet for children.

Special care: area to be treated should be dry and not shaved. Contact with clothes and jewellery to be avoided.

Avoid use: on broken or inflamed skin.

Side effects: skin irritation.

Manufacturer: Stiefel.

Drogenil

Description: an anti-androgen and form of flutamide available as a 250mg yellow tablet.

Used for: advanced prostatic cancer.

Dosage: 1 tablet 3 times per day.

Special care: fluid retention in patients with heart disease. Liver function tests should be performed periodically.

Possible interaction: warfarin.

Side effects: gynaecomastia, breast tenderness, gastrointestinal upsets, galactorrhea. Increased appetite, tiredness and insomnia.

Manufacturer: Schering-Plough.

Droleptan

Description: a butyrophenone, droperidol, available as a 10mg yellow tablet marked JANSSEN and D10. Also **Droleptan Liquid** as 1mg/ml of droperidol.

Used for: the rapid soothing of manic, agitated patients.

Dosage: 5–20mg every 4 to 8 hours. Children 0.5–1mg daily. Adjusted to match response.

Also **Droleptan Injection** available as 2ml ampoules (5mg/ml).

Dosage: 5–15mg intravenously or up to 10mg intramuscularly every 4 to 6 hours. Children 0.5–1mg daily, intramuscularly. Adjust to match response.

Also available as 2ml ampoules containing 5mg/ml.

Used for: postoperative or chemotherapy-induced nausea.

Dosage: 5mg intravenously or intramuscularly postoperatively. 1–10mg by the same means 30 minutes before chemotherapy then 1–3mg/hr by continuous intravenous infusion or 1–5mg intramuscularly or intravenously every 1 to 6 hours. Children 0.02–0.075mg/kg by the same means.

Special care: Parkinson's disease, epilepsy, pregnancy, lactation, severe liver disease.

Avoid use: severe depression or comatose states.

Possible interaction: alcohol, analgesics, depressants of the CNS, anticonvulsants, antidiabetics, antidepressants, antihypertensives, levodopa.

Side effects: spasms of eye, face, neck and back muscles, dry mouth, blocked nose, restlessness, tremor and rigidity, tardive dyskinesia (involuntary, repetitious muscle movements), urine retention, tachycardia, constipation, blurred vision, weight gain, impotence, hypothermia, menstrual changes, skin and blood changes, drowsiness, lethargy, sometimes fits.

Manufacturer: Janssen.

DTIC-Dome

Description: a cytotoxic drug and preparation of dacarbazine available as powder in vials for reconstitution (100 and 200mg).

Used for: soft tissue sarcomas and in combination for Hodgkin's disease.

Dosage: by intravenous injection.

Special care: an anti-emetic should be given simultaneously to lessen the risk of nausea and vomiting. Kidney function and hearing should be monitored.

Avoid use: again within 4 weeks.

Side effects: severe nausea and vomiting, alopecia, bone marrow suppression (necessitating blood counts), skin irritation.

Manufacturer: Bayer.

Duovent

Description: a ß2 agonist and anticholinergic consisting of 100µg ipratropium bromide in a metered dose aerosol. Also **Duovent Autohaler**.

Used for: obstruction to airways; for bronchodilation.

Dosage: 1 or 2 puffs 3 to 4 times daily. Children over 6, 1 puff 3 times per day. Not recommended for children under 6.

Also **Duovent UDVS**, 1.25mg fenoterol hydrobromide and 500µg ipratropium bromide per 4ml of solution, in vials.

Used for: acute severe asthma.

Dosage: over 14 years, 1 vial nebulized immediately. Repeat under supervision. Maximum of 4 vials in 24 hours.

Special care: angina, arrhythmias, hyperthyroidism, heart muscle disease, hypertension, glaucoma, prostatic hypertrophy.

Possible interaction: sympathomimetics.

Side effects: headache, dry mouth, peripheral dilatation.

Manufacturer: Boehringer Ingelheim.

Duphaston

Description: a progestogen, dydrogesterone, available as a white tablet (10mg strength) marked DUPHAR 155.

Used for: dysmenorrhoea (painful menstruation), dysfunctional (abnormal) bleeding, endometriosis, premenstrual syndrome (PMS), as part of hormone replacement therapy (HRT), habitual and threatened abortion.

Dosage: 1 twice daily from day 5 to 25 of the cycle (dysmenorrhoea); 1 tablet 2 or 3 times per day from days 5 to 25 or continuously (endometriosis); 1 twice daily from days 12 to 26 (PMS), 1 twice daily for the first 12 to 14 days of the month (HRT).

Special care: high blood pressure, tendency to thrombosis, liver abnormalities, ovarian cysts, migraine, diabetes.

Avoid use: pregnancy, severe heart or kidney disease, previous ectopic pregnancy, benign liver tumours, undiagnosed vaginal bleeding.

Possible interaction: cyclosporin.

Side effects: breast tenderness, irregular menstruation, acne, fluid retention and weight gain.

Manufacturer: Duphar.

Duromine^CD

Desription: a CNS stimulant, phentermine, available as sustained-release capsules, 15mg (green/grey) and 30mg (maroon/grey), both marked with name and strength.

Used for: obesity.

Dosage: 15–30mg daily, at breakfast.

Special care: angina, arrhythmias, hypertension.

Avoid use: pregnancy, lactation, arteriosclerosis, hyperthyroidism, severe hypertension, drug/alcohol abuse, past psychiatric illness.

Possible interaction: antihypertensives, sympathomimetics, MAOIs, psychotropics (mood-affecting drugs).

Side effects: oedema, tachycardia, raised blood pressure, restlessness, hallucinations. Possible tolerance, dependence, psychoses—avoid prolonged use.

Manufacturer: 3M Health Care.

Dyazide

Description: a potassium-sparing thiazide diuretic, consisting of 50mg triamterene and 25mg hydrochlorothiazide in peach tablets coded SKF E93.

Used for: oedema, mild to moderate hypertension.

Dosage: 1 twice daily after meals, falling to 1 daily (oedema), daily maximum of 4. Initially 1 daily for hypertension.

Special care: diabetes, acidosis, gout, pregnancy, lactation, pancreatitis, liver or kidney disease.

Avoid use: Addison's disease, hypercalcaemia, hyperkalaemia, severe liver or kidney failure.

Possible interaction: potassium supplements, potassium-sparing diuretics, lithium, digitalis, NSAIDs, ACE inhibitors, antihypertensives.

Side effects: diarrhoea, nausea, vomiting, headache, dry mouth, weakness, cramps, rash, hypercalcaemia, hyperglycaemia, low blood pressure.

Manufacturer: Smith, Kline & French.

Dyspamet

Description: a form of cimetidine in white square chewable tablets (200mg). Also, **Dyspamet Suspension** (200mg/5ml).

Used for: persistent acid-related dyspeptic conditions.

Dosage: 2 chewed thoroughly (or 10ml) twice daily, at breakfast and bedtime. Minimum recommended course, 4 weeks.

Special care: exclude malignancy first; pregnancy, lactation, impaired kidneys, monitor for long-term treatment.

Possible interaction: phenytoin, theophylline, oral anticoagulants.

Side effects: tiredness, dizziness, rash, diarrhoea, gynaecomastia, confusion.

Manufacturer: Smith, Kline & French.

Dysport

Description: a bacterial, botulinum, toxin, type A-haemagglutinin complex (500 units as pellets in vial).

Used for: eyelid and hemifacial spasm.

Dosage: 120 units for affected eye, by subcutaneous injection, spread over 4 sites around the eye (see accompanying literature). Repeat as necessary or every 8 weeks.

Special care: pregnancy, lactation, caution to inject accurately.

Side effects: minor bruising and eyelid swelling, paralysis of mid-facial muscles, reduced blinking giving dry eyes and keratitis (inflammation of the cornea), double vision, eyelid droop (ptosis).

Manufacturer: Porton.

Dytac

Description: a potassium-sparing diuretic, triamterene, available as 50mg capsules marked SKF.

Used for: oedema in congestive heart failure, liver or kidney disease.

Dosage: 3 to 5 per day in divided doses. Use on alternate days after first week.

Special care: elderly, gout, pregnancy, lactation, liver or kidney disease, acidosis, diabetic nephropathy (kidney disease related to diabetes).

Avoid use: Addison's disease, hyperkalaemia, progessive kidney or liver disease.

Possible interaction: potassium supplements, potassium-sparing diuretics, ACE inhibitors, antihypertensives, indomethacin.

Side effects: weakness, headache, cramps, nausea, diarrhoea, dry mouth, rash, blood dyscrasias (abnormal blood or bone marrow condition e.g. leukaemia), metabolic disturbances.

Manufacturer: Pharmark.

Dytide

Description: a potassium-sparing thyazide diuretic comprising 50mg triamterene and 25mg benzthiazide in capsules (clear/maroon) marked SKF.

Used for: oedema.

Dosage: 2 after breakfast and 1 after lunch to begin with, then 1 or 2 on alternate days for maintenance.

Special care: liver or kidney disease, gout, elderly, pregnancy, lactation, diabetes.

Avoid use: severe kidney failure or progressive liver or kidney disease, Addison's disease, hyper-calcaemia, diabetic ketoacidosis (acute side effects of uncontrolled diabetes mellitus with electrolyte imbalance, very high blood glucose and acidosis).

Possible interaction: potassium supplements, potassium-sparing diuretics, indomethasin, ACE inhibitors, antihypertensives, digitalis, lithium.

Side effects: weakness, headache, nausea, cramps, diarrhoea, rash, dry mouth, blood dyscrasias (abnormal blood or bone marrow conditions, e.g. leukaemia), metabolic disturbances.

Manufacturer: Pharmark.

E

Econacort

Description: a combined topical steroid and antifungal antibacterial preparation produced in the form of a cream containing 1% hydrocortisone and 1% econazole nitrate.

Used for: Gram-positive bacterial and fungal skin infections with inflammation.

Dosage: massage into affected skin morning and night.

Special care: use in children or on face should be limited to a period of 5 days; short-term use only and withdraw gradually.

Avoid use: continuous or prolonged use especially in pregnant women, untreated bacterial or fungal infections, infections caused by tuberculosis, viruses or ringworm, acne, leg ulcers, scabies, peri-oral dermatitis.

Side effects: adrenal gland suppression, thinning of skin, fluid retention.

Manufacturer: Squibb.

Edecrin

Description: a proprietary loop diuretic (one which acts on part of the loops of Henle of the kidney tubules), in the form of white scored tablets, marked MSD 90, containing 50mg ethacrynic acid. Also **Edecrin Injection** containing sodium ethacrynate equivalent to 50mg ethacrynic acid as powder in vial for reconstitution.

Used for: oedema including that which accompanies liver and kidney diseases and congestive heart failure.

Dosage: adults, 1 tablet daily after breakfast in first instance increasing by half to 1 each day as required. Usual dose is in the order of 1 to 3 tablets daily with maximum of 8 in divided doses. Injection: 50mg given intravenously. Children, 2 to 12 years, half tablet each day after breakfast, increasing by half tablet to the minimum effective dose required.

Special care: pregnancy, gout, enlarged prostate gland, liver disease, diabetes, impaired urination. Electrolyte levels should be monitored and potassium supplements may be needed.

Avoid use: children under 2 years, breast-feeding mothers, patients suffering from anuria, liver cirrhosis, serious kidney failure.

Possible interaction: antihypertensives, corticosteroids, digitalis, lithium, warfarin, aminoglycosides.

Side effects: blood changes, gastrointestinal upset, jaundice, gout.

Manufacturer: M.S.D.

Efalith

Description: a proprietary anti-inflammatory preparation produced as an ointment containing 8% lithium succinate and 0.05% zinc sulphate.

Used for: seborrhoeic dermatitis.

Dosage: apply thinly to affected skin and rub in, twice each day in the morning and at night.

Special care: patients with psoriasis; avoid eyes and mucous membranes.

Avoid use: children.

Side effects: local irritation at site of application.

Manufacturer: Searle.

Efamast

Description: a fatty acid preparation in soft gelatin, oblong-shaped capsules containing 40mg gamolenic acid.

Used for: mastalgia (breast pain).

Dosage: adults, 3 to 4 capsules twice each day.

Special care: patients suffering from epilepsy. Possibility of breast cancer should be eliminated before treatment begins.

Side effects: headache, nausea.

Manufacturer: Searle.

Efcortelan

Description: a topical corticosteroid preparation produced as cream and ointment of different strengths containing 0.5%, 1% or 2.5% hydrocortisone. Mildly potent.

Used for: dermatitis, inflammation and itching in anal and urinongenital areas, neurodermatitis (an itching skin disorder seen in nervous, anxious persons).

Dosage: rub into affected areas 2 or 3 times each day.

Special care: use in children or on face should be limited to 5 days. Short-term use and withdraw gradually.

Avoid use: long-term or extensive use, especially in pregnant women. Untreated fungus or bacterial skin infections or those which are viral or tuberculous in origin, ringworm, acne, leg ulcers, scabies.

Side effects: thinning of skin, adrenal gland suppression, hair growth.

Manufacturer: Glaxo.

Efcoertelan Soluble

Description: a glucocorticoid-mineralocorticoid preparation produced as a powder in vials for reconstitution and injection and containing 100mg hydrocortisone (as sodium succinate).

Used for: severe shock, adrenal gland failure, status asthmaticus (very severe and prolonged asthma attack which may prove life-threatening).

Dosage: adults, 100–500mg by slow intravenous injection repeated according to patient's response. Children up to 1 year, 25mg; 1 to 5 years, 50mg; 6 to 12 years, 100mg, all given by slow intravenous injection.

Special care: pregnancy, hypertension, various inflammatory kidney disorders (nephritis, glomerulonephritis), diabetes, osteoporosis, epilepsy, secondary cancers, recent intestinal anastomoses, liver cirrhosis, thrombophlebitis, peptic ulcer, exanthematous diseases (characterized by rash). Also, stress or psychoses. Contact with chicken pox should be avoided (and specialist care is required for those contracting this disease). Drug should be withdrawn gradually.

Possible interaction: NSAIDs, anticholinesterases, diuretics, anticoagulants taken by mouth, cardiac glycosides, phenobarbitone, phenytoin, rifampicin, ephedrine.

Side effects: hypertension, weakness, depression and euphoria, hyperglycaemia, peptic ulcer, potassium loss, fluid retention, Cushingoid changes (as in Cushing's Syndrome).

Manufacturer: Glaxo.

Efcortesol

Description: a glucocorticoid-mineralocorticoid preparation produced as a solution in ampoules for injection, containing 100mg hydrocortisone (as sodium phosphate) per ml. Efcortesol is available in 1ml and 5ml ampoules.

Used for: severe shock, adrenal gland failure, status asthmaticus (very severe and prolonged asthma attack which may prove life-threatening).

Dosage: adults, 100–500mg by slow intravenous injection repeated according to patient's response. Children, up to 1 year, 25mg; 1 to 5 years, 50mg; 6 to 12 years, 100mg, all given by slow intravenous injection.

Special care: pregnancy, hypertension, various inflammatory kidney disorders (nephritis, glomerulonephritis), diabetes, osteoporosis, epilepsy, secondary cancers, recent intestinal anastomoses, liver cirrhosis, thrombophlebitis, peptic ulcer, exanthematous diseases (characterized by rash). Also, patients suffering from stress or psychoses. Contact with chicken pox should be avoided (and specialist care is required for those contracting this disease). Drug should be withdrawn gradually.,

Possible interaction: NSAIDs, anticholin-esterases, diuretics, anticoagulants taken by mouth, cardiac glycosides, phenobarbitone, phenytoin, rifampicin, ephedrine.

Side effects: hypertension, weakness, depression and euphoria, hyperglycaemia, peptic ulcer, potassium loss, fluid retention, Cushingoid changes (as in Cushing's Syndrome).

Manufacturer: Glaxo.

Eldepryl

Description: a proprietary preparation of an anti-Parkinson's disease drug which is a monoamine oxidase-B inhibitor (monoamine oxidase B is an enzyme which breaks down dopamine). A deficiency in dopamine accompanies Parkinson's disease and the drug prolongs dopaminergic function in the brain. Eldepryl is produced as white, scored tablets of 2 strengths containing 5mg and 10mg selegiline hydrochloride.

Used for: Parkinson's disease; (sometimes given along with levodopa).

Dosage: adults, 10mg daily either as a single morning dose, or in divided doses in the morning and middle of the day; taken with meals.

Special care: if taken with levodopa, side effects of this may be increased and the dosage of levodopa may need to be reduced.

Side effects: nausea, confusion, agitation, vomiting, hypotension.

Manufacturer: Britannia.

Eldisine

Description: a cytotoxic drug which is a vinca alkaloid produced in the form of a powder in vials for reconstitution and injection. Eldisine contains 5mg vindesine sulphate in vial and in addition, 5ml diluent.

Used for: leukaemia, lymphomas and some other

forms of solid tumour, e.g. those which may affect the lung or breast.

Dosage: as directed by physician skilled in cancer chemotherapy.

Special care: precautions must be observed in handling. Powder should be reconstituted by skilled staff wearing protective clothing and gloves under controlled conditions. Contact with skin and eyes should be avoided.

Side effects: vomiting, hair loss, bone marrow suppression, possible early menopause in women, sterility in men.

Manufacturer: Lilly.

Elocon

Description: a topical and potent steroid produced as an ointment and cream containing 0.1% mometasone furoate. Also **Elocon Lotion** (same strength).

Used for: atopic dermatitis (extremely itchy, damaged skin (caused by scratching in allergic individuals), psoriasis including that of the scalp, seborrhoeic dermatitis.

Dosage: apply thinly once each day.

Special care: pregnancy, hypertension, various inflammatory kidney disorders (nephritis, glomerulonephritis), diabetes, osteoporosis, epilepsy, secondary cancers, recent intestinal anastomoses, liver cirrhosis, thrombophlebitis, peptic ulcer, exanthematous diseases (characterized by rash). Also, stress or psychoses. Contact with chicken pox should be avoided (and specialist care is required for those contracting this disease). Drug should be withdrawn gradually.

Possible interaction: NSAIDs, diuretics, anticholinesterases, anticoagulants taken by mouth, cardiac glycosides, phenobarbitone, phenytoin, rifampicin, ephedrine.

Side effects: hypertension, weakness, depression and euphoria, hyperglycaemia, peptic ulcer, potassium loss, fluid retention, Cushingoid changes (as in Cushing's Syndrome). Any adverse reactions should be reported to Committee on Safety of Medicines.

Manufacturer: Schering-Plough.

Eltroxin

Description: a preparation of thyroid hormone, thyroxine sodium, produced in the form of tablets of 2 strengths: 50 µg (white, scored) and 100µg (white) both marked with name and strength.

Used for: hypothyroidism in children and adults, including cretinism and myxoedema.

Dosage: adults, 50–100µg each day in first instance

increasing every 3 to 4 weeks by 50µg according to response until optimum dose is achieved. Maximum dose is 100–100µg each day. Children 25µg each day in first instance, increasing every 2 to 4 weeks by 25µg according to response. Dose should then be slightly reduced.

Special care: pregnancy, breast-feeding, elderly, patients with weak hearts or with reduced adrenal gland function.

Possible interaction: anticonvulsants, sympathomimetics, antidiabetics, tricyclics, cardiac glycosides, anticoagulants.

Side effects: tachycardia, muscular cramps, chest pains, sweating, flushing, arrhythmias, severe weight loss.

Manufacturer: Goldshield.

Elyzol

Description: an antibacterial preparation produced in the form of a gel with applicator containing 25% metronidazole.

Used for: additional therapy in severe periodontal disease.

Dosage: apply gel to affected area and repeat after 1 week.

Special care: pregnant women.

Avoid use: do not repeat therapy until 6 months have elapsed. Not for children.

Possible interaction: alcohol, disulfiram, anticoagulants taken orally.

Side effects: local inflammation, headache.

Manufacturer: Dumex.

Emcor

Description: an antianginal and anti-hypertensive preparation, which is a cardioselective ß-blocker, produced in the form of heart-shaped, orange, film-coated tablets containing 10mg bisoprolol fumerate. Also, **Emcor LS** (5mg) which are yellow, scored, film-coated tablets.

Used for: angina, hypertension.

Dosage: 10mg once each day with a maximum daily dose of 20mg.

Special care: pregnancy, breast-feeding, liver or kidney disease, diabetes, metabolic acidosis, general anaesthesia. May require to be withdrawn before planned surgery and should be stopped gradually. Patients with weak heart should receive diuretics and digitalis.

Avoid use: children, patients with obstructive airways disease or history of bronchospasm, heart and circulatory diseases including heart block, heart failure, heart shock, sick sinus syndrome, sinus bradycardia and peripheral arterial disease.

Possible interaction: CNS depressants, cardiac-depressant anaesthetics, ergotamine, indomethacin, reserpine, sympathomimetics, some other anti-hypertensives, clonidine withdrawal, cimetidine, hypoglycaemic, verapamil, class I antiarrhythmics.
Side effects: cold feet and hands, fatigue on exertion, disturbance of sleep, gastrointestinal upset, bradycardia, bronchospasm, heart failure. Withdraw gradually if dry eyes or skin rash appear.
Manufacturer: Merck.

Emeside

Description: an anticonvulsant preparation produced as capsules and as a flavoured syrup. Orange capsules contain 250mg ethosuximide and blackcurrant or orange-flavoured **Emeside Syrup** contains 250mg per 5ml.
Used for: epilepsy.
Dosage: adults, 500mg each day in first instance increasing by 250mg at 5 to 7-day intervals until condition is controlled. Maximum daily dose is 2g. Children under 6 years, 250mg each day in first instance adjusted every few days by small amounts until condition is controlled. Maximum daily dose is 1g. Children over 6 years receive adult dose.
Special care: pregnancy, breast-feeding; liver or kidney disease. Drug should be withdrawn gradually.
Side effects: blood changes, central nervous system effects, gastrointestinal upset, SLE, skin rashes.
Manufacturer: L.A.B.

Emflex

Description: an NSAID which is a form of indomethacin and is produced as orange/yellow capsules containing 60mg acemetacin.
Used for: osteoarthritis, rheumatoid arthritis, pain and inflammation following surgery and lower back pain.
Dosage: adults, 2 capsules daily in divided doses, taken with food, a glass of milk, or with an antacid preparation. The maximum daily dosage is 3 capsules.
Special care: liver or kidney disease, congestive heart failure, elderly persons, septic infections, epilepsy, Parkinson's disease, psychiatric illness, imbalance in fluid or electrolyte levels. Patients on long-term treatment should receive checks on liver and kidney function, blood count and eyes.
Avoid use: children, pregnancy, breast-feeding, certain gastrointestinal disorders, peptic ulcer, angioneurotic oedema. Also, allergy to NSAID or aspirin.
Possible interaction: thiazides, salcylates, lithium,

anticoagulants, frusemide, probenecid, ACE inhibitors, methotrexate, ß-blockers, triamterene haloperidol, quinolones.
Side effects: blood changes, dizziness, blurring of vision, headache, tinnitus, gastrointestinal upset, oedema.
Manufacturer: Merck.

Eminase

Description: a fibrinolytic preparation produced in the form of a powder in vials for reconstitution and injection, containing 30 units anistreplase.
Used for: myocardial infarction.
Dosage: adults, one 30-unit dose within 6 hours of myocardial infarction, given over a period of 4 to 5 minutes by slow intravenous injection.
Special care: pregnancy, breast-feeding, heart arrhythmias, risk of bleeding, increased risk of thrombi or emboli.
Avoid use: children, treatment should not be repeated after first 5 days for 12 months, patients who have had surgery within past 10 days, those with menorrhagia, aneurysm, serious hypertension, peptic ulcer, CVA.
Side effects: vomiting, fever, nausea, allergic responses, flushing, hypotension, bleeding, bradycardia.
Manufacturer: Beecham.

Emla

Description: a local anaesthetic preparation produced in the form of a cream containing 25mg lignocaine, 25mg prilocaine per g.
Used for: local anaesthesia of skin and genital area (removal of genital warts).
Dosage: adults and children, minor surgery, 2g applied to affected area for a minimum of 1 hour and a maximum of 5 hours. For larger areas, 1.5–3g per 10cm^2 of skin for minimum of 2 hours and maximum of 5 hours. (Cream is applied as a thick layer under a dressing). Genital warts, 10g applied for 5 to 10 minutes before surgical removal.
Avoid use: infants, patients with atopic dermatitis, on wounds or mucous membranes.
Side effects: local slight skin reactions.
Manufacturer: Astra.

Endobulin

Description: a preparation of human normal immunoglobin (HNIG) available as a concentrate which is freeze-dried plus diluent, for reconstitution and intravenous infusion.
Used for: replacement therapy in patients with deficient immunoglobulins (gamma globulins) which are antibodies present in blood serum.

Dosage: depending upon particular syndrome or disease being treated, in the order of 0.4g to 1g/kg body weight by intravenous infusion for 4 or 5 days, or within first 2 weeks. Some conditions require maintenance doses in the order of 0.1–0.6g/kg body weight each month in 1 or 2 doses.

Special care: pregnant women, patients with diabetes. Monitor closely during infusion for signs of anaphylaxis. Special care in patients with selective immunoglobulin A deficiency who are sensitized and carry antibodies to IGA.

Avoid use: patients known to have certain types of antibody to immunoglobulin.

Possible interaction: live vaccines.

Side effects: fever, chills, headache, fatigue; rarely, anaphylaxis.

Manufacturer: Immuno.

Endoxana

Description: an alkylating cytotoxic drug produced as a powder in vials containing 100mg, 200mg, 500mg or 1g of cyclophosphamide, for reconstitution and injection. It is also available as white sugar-coated tablets (50mg).

Used for: malignant diseases e.g. lymphoma, leukaemia and some solid tumours.

Dosage: adults, taken with Uromitexan as directed by physician skilled in cancer chemotherapy.

Special care: patients with diabetes, elderly or debilitated persons.

Avoid use: children.

Possible interaction: sulphonylureas, radiotherapy, doxorubicin.

Side effects: vomiting, hair loss, nausea, bone marrow suppression and suppression of the reticulo-endothelial system, toxic effects on heart and urinary tract, haematuria, male sterility (Azoospermia—a lack of spermaztozoa in the semen), amenorrhoea.

Manufacturer: ASTA Medica.

Engerix B

Description: a genetically derived suspension of hepatitis B surface antigen (from yeast cells) containing 20 micrograms per ml adsorbed onto aluminium hydroxide, in vials or pre-filled syringes.

Used for: immunization against the Hepatitis B virus.

Dosage: adults, first dose 1ml by intramuscular injection into the deltoid muscle (upper arm) repeated after an interval of 1 month and 6 months. Children, first dose of 0.5ml by intramuscular injection into the thigh repeated after an interval of 1 month and 6 months.

Special care: pregnant women, patients receiving kidney dialysis or who have a deficient immune system may need to receive additional doses.

Avoid use: severe infections accompanied by fever.

Side effects: slight short-lived soreness at injection site, with inflammation and hardening, dizziness, feverishness, nausea, malaise.

Manufacturer: S.K. & F.

Epanutin

Description: an anticonvulsant available as capsules and suspension, which belongs to a group called hydantoins which are similar in composition to barbiturates. White/purple, white/pink and white/orange capsules contain 25mg, 50mg and 100mg of phenytoin sodium respectively. All marked with capsule name and strength. Also, **Epanutin Suspension** containing 30mg phenytoin per 5ml and **Epanutin Infatabs** containing 50mg phenytoin in the form of triangular, scored, yellow, chewable tablets.

Used for: prevention and treatment of grand mal (tonic clonic) epileptic seizures, partial (focal) epileptic seizures and seizures which may follow trauma to the brain due to neurosurgery or head injury. Also, trigeminal neuralgia.

Dosage: adults, capsules, 3–4mg/kg body weight in first instance each day, gradually increasing until condition is controlled. Maintenance dose is in the order of 200–500mg in divided doses each day. Suspension: 15ml 3 times each day. Infatabs: 2 tablets 2, 3 or 4 times each day. Children, capsules, (all except newborn babies), 5mg/kg body weight in 2 divided doses, with a maintenance dose in the order of 4–8mg/kg body weight each day. Suspension, under 6 years of age, 5ml twice each day increasing to 5ml 3 or 4 times each day if needed; 6 to 12 years, adult dose. Infatabs: under 6 years of age, half of 1 tablet 2, 3 or 4 times each day; 7 to 12 years, 1 tablet 2, 3 or 4 times each day.

Special care: pregnancy, breast-feeding, liver disease. Adequate intake of vitamin D is necessary and drug should be stopped gradually.

Possible interaction: isoniazid, sulthiame, anticoagulants of the coumarin group, chloramphenicol, oral contraceptives, doxycycline.

Side effects: upset stomach, lack of sleep, allergic effects, blood changes, unsteadiness, swelling of gums and lymph glands; in young persons there may be unusual growth of hair (hirsutism) and motor activity. Rapid abnormal eye movements (nystagmus) may occur and drug should be withdrawn in the event of skin rash.

Manufacturer: Parke-Davis.

Epanutin Parenteral

Description: an anticonvulsant and class I anti-arrhythmic preparation available in ampoules for injection containing 50mg phenytoin sodium per ml.
Used for: status epilepticus (an emergency situation in which a patient suffers continuous epileptic seizures without regaining consciousness in between. If the convulsions are not halted, the person suffers irreversible brain damage and may die). Also used for prevention of seizures during neurosurgical operations and for heart arrhythmias, particularly those caused by digitalis.
Dosage: adults, status epilepticus, 150–250mg by slow intravenous injection followed by 100–150mg after half an hour if needed. Heart arrhythmias, 3.5–5mg/kg body weight in first instance, by intravenous injection, the rate of which should not be greater than 50mg per minute. This can be repeated once if required. Children for status epilepticus only, dose in proportion to that for a 70kg adult, reduced accordingly.
Special care: pregnant women, breast-feeding mothers, ECG and close monitoring needed; resuscitation equipment should be on hand.
Avoid use: patients with heart block.
Possible interaction: isoniazid, sulthiame, anticoagulants of the coumarin group, chloramphenicol, oral contraceptives, doxycycline.
Side effects: upset stomach, lack of sleep, allergic effects, blood changes, unsteadiness, swelling of gums and lymph glands; in young persons there may be unusual growth of hair (hirsutism) and motor activity. Rapid abnormal eye movements (nystagmus) may occur and drug should be withdrawn in the event of skin rash.
Manufacturer: Parke-Davis.

Epifoam

Description: a combined corticosteroid and local anaesthetic produced as a foam in an aerosol. Epifoam contains 1% hydrocortisone acetate and 1% paramoxine hydrochloride.
Used for: injury to the perineum including pain following episiotomy.
Dosage: adults, apply 3 to 4 times each day on non-absorbent sterile dressing for a period not exceeding 7 days.
Avoid use: children, infected skin conditions.
Manufacturer: Stafford-Miller.

Epilim

Description: an anticonvulsant and carboxylic acid derivative, sodium valproate, available as lilac, enteric-coated tablets containing 200mg or 500mg.

Epilim Crushable white, scored tablets(100mg); **Epilim Syrup** (red) contains 200mg per 5ml; **Epilim Liquid** (sugar-free, red) contains 200mg per 5ml; **Epilim Chrono** sustained-release tablets are lilac-coloured and contain 200mg, 300mg and 500mg as valproate and valproic acid. **Epilim Intravenous** contains 400mg powder in vial for reconstitution and injection.
Dosage: adults, 600mg each day in 2 divided doses in first instance, then gradually increasing after intervals of 3 days by 200mg until optimum control dose is achieved. Usual maintenance dose is in the order of 1–2g each day with a maximum of 2.5g. Children, less than 20kg body weight, 20mg/kg each day at first; over 20kg, 400mg each day at first. Both in divided doses and both gradually increased until optimum control dose is achieved. Epilim Intravenous (for patients not able to take the oral preparations), adults, 400–800mg each day by slow intravenous injection or infusion with a maximum dose of 2.5g. Children, 20–30mg/kg body weight by slow intravenous injection or infusion.
Special care: pregnant women, children with brain damage, mental retardation or congenital metabolic disorders accompanying severe epilepsy. Patients should be monitored for signs of liver failure and liver function tests should be carried out. Patients having urine tests for diabetes may show false positives for ketones.
Avoid use: patients with liver disorders.
Possible interaction: other anticonvulsant drugs, anticoagulants, antidepressants.
Side effects: liver failure, oedema, pancreatitis, gain in weight, loss of hair, blood changes, effects on nervous system.
Manufacturer: Sanofi Winthrop.

Epogam

Description: a fatty acid preparation in the form of gelatin caspsules containing 40mg gamolenic acid and marked Epogam 240. Also, **Epogam Paediatric**, gelatin capsules containing 80mg and marked EPOGAM 60.
Used for: relief of eczema.
Dosage: Capsules are snipped open and contents poured onto food, in drink, or swallowed directly. Adults 4 to 6 capsules twice each day. Epogram paediatric, 2 to 3 capsules each day. Children, over 1 year, 2 to 4 Epogram 240 capsules or 1 to 2 Epogram Paediatric capsules, both twice each day.
Special care: patients with epilepsy.
Avoid use: children under 1 year.
Side effects: headache, nausea.
Manufacturer: Searle.

Eppy

Description: a sympathomimetic preparation available in the form of eye drops containing 1% adrenaline.
Used for: glaucoma (primary open angle and secondary).
Dosage: adults, 1 drop once or twice each day.
Avoid use: children, patients with narrow angle glaucoma or aphakia (absence of all or part of the lens of the eye, usually because it has been surgically removed, e.g. to treat cataracts).
Possible interaction: TCADs, MAOIs.
Side effects: headache, pain in region of eyes and redness due to increased blood flow (hyperaemia), melanosis; rarely, systemic effects.
Manufacturer: Chauvin.

Eprex

Description: a preparation of synthesised human erythropoietin, a glycoprotein hormone, produced by some kidney cells and released into the blood in conditions in which there is a lack of oxygen reaching the tissues. This increases the rate of production of red blood cells (erythropoiesis) which are responsible for transporting oxygen in the circulation. Eprex is produced in vials or pre-filled syringes as a medium for injection and containing epoetin alfa solution.
Used for: anaemia which accompanies chronic renal failure in both dialysis and non-dialysis patients.
Dosage: adults, dialysis patients, (following dialysis), 50iu/kg body weight 3 times each week at first by intravenous or subcutaneous injection. Non-dialysis patients, same dose by subcutaneous injection. Dose increased and adjusted depending upon response and haemoglobin level required. Children, 50µ/kg body weight 3 times each week after dialysis, in first instance. Dose is then adjusted according to patient's condition.
Special care: pregnancy, liver failure, hypertension, ischaemic vascular disease, history of epilepsy. Haemoglobin levels, blood pressure, electrolyte levels and blood count require consistent monitoring. Iron supplements may be needed and treatment for any other causes of anaemia; diet and dialysis treatment may need to be altered.
Avoid use: hypertension which is uncontrolled.
Possible interaction: cyclosporin.
Side effects: headache, rise in blood pressure, feverish flu-like symptoms, skin reactions, seizures, thrombosis.
Manufacturer: Cilag.

Equagesic[CD]

Description: a compound analgesic preparation which is a controlled drug and combines an opiate, muscle relaxant and salicylate. Three layered pink, white, yellow tablets contain 75mg ethoheptazine citrate, 150mg meprobamate and 250mg aspirin and are marked WYETH on the yellow surface.
Used for: relief of severe muscle and bone pain.
Dosage: adults, 2 tablets 3 or 4 times each day.
Special care: for short-term use only; special care in elderly persons, those suffering from depression or at risk of suicide. Patients with heart failure, liver disease, history of epilepsy.
Avoid use: pregnancy, breast-feeding, children, kidney disease, porphyria, peptic ulcer, alcoholism, haemophilia, allergy to aspirin or other anti-inflammatory drugs.
Possible interaction: anticoagulants, antidiabetic drugs, alcohol, central nervous system sedatives, uricosurics (drugs which lower uric acid levels).
Side efects: blood changes, giddiness, nausea, sleepiness, rash, ataxia.
Manufacturer: Wyeth.

Equanil[CD]

Description: a carbamate tranquillizer which acts as an anxiolytic and a controlled drug. It is available in the form of white, scored tablets of 2 different strengths containing 200mg or 400mg of meprobamate. Both are marked E and WYETH.
Used for: short-term relief of anxiety and muscular tension.
Dosage: adults, 400mg 3 times each day at at night; elderly persons, 200mg 3 times each day.
Special care: pregnancy, breast-feeding, liver or kidney disease, history of depression, epilepsy. Drug should be stopped gradually.
Avoid use: children, patients suffering from alcoholism or acute intermittent porphyria.
Possible interaction: CNS depressants, phenytoin, TCADs, rifampicin, alcohol, anticoagulants of the coumarin type, phenothiazines, griseofulvin, oral contraceptives.
Side effects: addiction may occur and ability to perform skilled tasks such as driving impaired. Gastrointestinal upset, hypotension, disturbance to central nervous system and excitement, feeling of 'pins and needles' (paraesthesia), blood disorders, low blood pressure, allergic reactions.
Manufacturer: Wyeth.

Eradacin

Description: a 4-quinolone antibiotic preparation produced in the form of yellow/red capsules containing 150mg acrosoxacin.
Used for: treatment of acute gonorrhoea.

Dosage: adults, 1 dose of 2 tablets each day.
Special care: pregnant women, patients with liver or kidney disease.
Avoid use: children.
Side effects: drowsiness, headaches, giddiness, gastrointestinal upset.
Manufacturer: Sanofi Winthrop.

Ervevax

Description: a form of live attenuated virus of Wistar RA27/3 used as a vaccine against Rubella (German measles). It is produced as pink pellets in vials, along with diluent, for reconstitution and injection.
Used for: immunization against Rubella.
Dosage: 0.5ml by intravenous, intramuscular or subcutaneous injection.
Avoid use: pregnancy, severe fever, altered immunity due to malignant diseases including leukaemia and lymphoma.
Possible interaction: other live vaccines (with the exception of polio vaccine taken by mouth), transfusions, cytotoxic drugs, immunoglobulins, corticosteroids, irradiation.
Side effects: pains in joints, rash, feverishness, lymphadenopathy (a disease of lymph vessels and nodes).
Manufacturer: S.K. & F.

Erymax

Description: an antibiotic preparation of the macrolide, erythromycin, produced as small enteric-coated pellets contained in clear/orange capsules (250mg strength).
Used for: infections sensitive to erythromycin especially in patients with penicillin hypersensitivity. These include legionnaire's disease, campylobacter enteritis, syphilis, chronic prostatitis, pneumonia, non-gonococcal urethritis and acne. Also used as a preventative against whooping cough and diphtheria.
Dosage: adults, for most infections, 250mg at 6-hour intervals or 500mg every 12 hours taken before or with food. For acne, 1 tablet twice each day for 1 month, then 1 tablet daily as maintenance dose. Children, infections, 30–50mg/kg body weight each day in divided doses at 6-hour intervals or twice daily.
Special care: patients with liver disease.
Possible interaction: digoxin, astemizole, anticoagulants taken by mouth, terfenadine, carbamazepine, theophylline.
Side effects: allergic reactions, gastrointestinal upset, cholestatic jaundice.
Manufacturer: Elan.

Erythrocin

Description: an antibiotic preparation of the macrolide, erythromycin, produced in the form of oblong, white, film-coated tablets, containing 250mg and 500mg (as stearate), all marked with company symbol.
Used for: infections sensitive to erythromycin especially in patients with penicillin hypersensitivity. Acne.
Dosage: adults, 1–2g each day in divided doses.
Special care: patients with liver disease.
Avoid use: children.
Possible interaction: digoxin, anticoagulants taken by mouth, astemizole, theophylline, terfenadine, carbamazepine.
Side effects: allergic reactions, gastrointestinal upset, cholestatic jaundice.
Manufacturer: Abbott.

Erythromid

Description: an antibiotic preparation of the macrolide, erythromycin, in the form of enteric-coated and film-coated orange tablets containing 250mg. Also, **Erythromid DS®** enteric-coated and film-coated orange tablets containing 500mg.
Used for: infections sensitive to erythromycin especially in patients with penicillin hypersensitivity. Acne.
Dosage: adults, 1–2g each day in divided doses with a maximum of 4g in exceptionally severe cases of infection. Children over 8 years, same as adult dose.
Special care: patients with liver disease.
Avoid use: children under 8 years of age.
Possible interaction: digoxin, oral anticoagulants, astemizole, theophylline, terfenadine, carbamazepine.
Side effects: allergic reactions, gastrointestinal upset, cholestatic jaundice.
Manufacturer: Abbott.

Erythroped A

Description: an antibiotic preparation of the macrolide, erythromycin (as ethyl succinate), produced as oval, film-coated yellow tablets (500mg); **Erythroped A** sachets contain 1g in the form of granules. **Erythroped Sachets** contain 250mg; **Erythroped Suspension** contains 250mg per 5ml solution. **Erythroped Sugar-Free Suspension** contains 125mg per 5ml. **Erythroped Forte** available as 500mg per 5ml suspension or as granules in sachet. **Erythroped P.I. Sugar-Free Suspension** contains 125mg per 5ml solution.
Used for: infections sensitive to erythromycin especially in patients with penicillin hypersensitivity. Acne.

Dosage: adults, 1g twice each day. Children under 2 years, 250mg; 2 to 8 years, 500mg; over 8 years, 1g. All twice daily.

Special care: patients with liver disease.

Possible interaction: digoxin, oral anticoagulants, astemizole, theophylline, terfenadine, carbamazepine.

Side effects: allergic reactions, gastrointestinal upset, cholestatic jaundice.

Manufacturer: Abbott.

Esidrex

Description: a proprietary thiazide diuretic preparation produced in the form of white scored tablets containing 25mg and 50mg of hydrochlorthiazide, and marked CIBA and UT.

Used for: oedema and hypertension.

Dosage: 25–100mg each morning after breakfast as a single dose, in first instance. Dose is then reduced to 25–50mg taken on alternate days.

Special care: pregnancy, breast-feeding, elderly persons, diabetes, kidney or liver disease, gout, cirrhosis of the liver, SLE. Monitoring of electrolytes, glucose and fluid levels should be carried out.

Avoid use: patients with serious kidney or liver failure, sensitivity to sulphonamide drugs, Addison's disease, hypercalcaemia.

Possible interaction: NSAIDs, alcohol, opioid and barbiturate drugs, antidiabetic preparations, corticosteroids, cardiac glycosides, lithium, carbenoxolone, tubocurarine.

Side effects: disturbance of metabolism and electrolyte levels, sensitivity to light, blood changes, rash, gastrointestinal upset, pancreatitis, anorexia, giddiness, impotence.

Manufacturer: CIBA.

Eskazole

Description: an anthelmintic preparation designed to act against the larval stages of 2 species of small parasitic tapeworms, *Echinococcus granulosus* and *Echinococcus multilocularis*. It is produced in the form of oblong, orange, scored tablets marked SKF, containing 400mg algendazole.

Used for: hydatid cysts.

Dosage: adults over 60kg body weight 800mg each day for 28 days in divided doses, followed by 14 tablet-free days. There should be a maximum of 3 cycles of treatment.

Special care: blood counts and liver function tests should be carried out.

Avoid use: children, adults under 60kg bodyweight, women should use non-hormonal methods of contraception during treatment and for 1 month afterwards.

Possible interaction: oral contraceptives, theophylline, anticoagulants, hypoglycaemics taken orally.

Side effects: changes in blood and liver enzymes, headache, rash, giddiness, fever, hair loss. Any advere side effects should be reported.

Manufacturer: Smith-Kline.

Estracombi

Description: a combined oestrogen, progestogen preparation in the form of patches containing either 50μg oestradiol per 24 hours, or 50μg oestradiol and 250μg norethisterone acetate per 24 hours, marked CGDWD and CGFNF respectively.

Used for: hormone replacement therapy for menopausal women. Prevention of osteoporosis after the menopause.

Dosage: oestradiol only patch is applied to hairless skin below waist twice each week for 2 weeks, followed by the combined patch twice weekly for 2 weeks. The patches are changed every 3 to 4 days and placed on a different area of skin each time.

Special care: patients with a history, or considered to be at risk, of thrombosis, those with liver disease. Liver function should be monitored and breasts and pelvic organs examined periodically during the period of therapy. Women with any of the following require particularly careful monitoring: diabetes, fibroids in uterus, multiple sclerosis, hypertension, tetany, epilepsy, porphyria, gallstones, migraine, otosclerosis, history of breast cancer.

Avoid use: pregnancy, breast-feeding, thrombosis or thromboembolic disorders, serious heart, kidney or liver disease, endometriosis or vaginal bleeding which is undiagnosed, hormone-dependent cancers such as breast or uterine carcinoma, Dublin-Johnson or Rotor syndrome.

Possible interaction: drugs which induce liver enzymes.

Side effects: enlargement of and soreness in breasts, breakthrough bleeding, vomiting, nausea, gastro-intestinal disturbance, gain in weight, dizziness, headache. Withdraw immediately if frequent severe headaches or migraines occur, disordered vision, pregnancy, rise in blood pressure, signs of thrombo-embolism, jaundice. Stop before planned surgery.

Manufacturer: CIBA.

Estracyt

Description: a preparation of a sex hormone used to treat cancer, which is an oestrogenic alkylating agent, produced in the form of off-white capsules containing 140mg estramustine phosphate (as disodium salt).

Used for: prostatic cancer.

Dosage: adults, 4 capsules each day in divided doses taken 1 hour before meals or 2 hours afterwards, in first instance. Dose is then adjusted according to response of patient's conditioin with an average between 1 and 10 capsules each day. Capsules must not be taken with milk or dairy products.

Special care: bone marrow disorder.

Avoid use: patients with serious heart or liver disease or peptic ulcer.

Possible interaction: milk and dairy products.

Side effects: enlargement of breasts, toxic effects on heart, disturbance of liver function, gastrointestinal upset.

Manufacturer: Pharmacia.

Estraderm

Description: an oestrogen patch containing either 25, 50 or 100µg oestradiol.

Used for: hormone replacement therapy in menopausal women. Prevention of osteoporosis following menopause.

Dosage: for oestrogen replacement; 1 patch is applied to hairless skin below waist and replaced every 3 or 4 days at a different site. The 50µg patch is used for prevention of osteoporosis.

Special care: patients with a history, or at risk, of thrombosis, those with liver disease. Liver function should be monitored and breasts and pelvic organs examined periodically during the period of therapy. Women with any of the following require particularly careful monitoring: diabetes, fibroids in uterus, multiple sclerosis, hypertension, tetany, epilepsy, porphyria, gallstones, migraine, otosclerosis (an hereditary rare disorder of the inner ear), history of breast cancer.

Avoid use: pregnant women, breast-feeding mothers, thrombosis or thromboembolic disorders, serious heart, kidney or liver disease, endometriosis or vaginal bleeding which is undiagnosed, hormone-dependent cancers such as breast or uterine carcinoma, Dublin-Johnson syndrome or Rotor syndrome.

Possible interaction: drugs which induce liver enzymes.

Side effects: enlargement of and soreness in breasts, breakthrough bleeding, vomiting, nausea, gastrointestinal disturbance, gain in weight, dizziness, headache. Withdraw immediately if frequent, severe headaches or migraines occur, disordered vision, pregnancy, rise in blood pressure, signs of thromboembolism, jaundice. Stop before planned surgery.

Manufacturer: CIBA.

Estradurin

Description: a preparation of a sex hormone used to treat cancer and local anaesthetic. It is produced as a powder in vials for reconstitution and injection and contains 80mg polyoestradiol phosphate and 5mg mepivacaine.

Used for: prostate cancer.

Dosage: adults, 80–160mg every 4 weeks given by deep intramuscular injection. Maintenance dose in order of 40–80mg.

Side effects: enlargement of breasts, impotence, oedema, heart disease and thromboembolism, jaundice, nausea.

Manufacturer: Pharmacia.

Estrapak

Description: a combined oestrogen/progestogen preparation available as a patch containing 50µg oestradiol per 24 hours, and as red tablets, marked DG and LK, containing 1mg norethisterone acetate.

Used for: hormone replacement therapy for menopausal women. Prevention of osteoporosis after the menopause.

Dosage: apply patch to hairless skin below waist and replace with new patch in different site every 3 to 4 days. Take 1 tablet each day starting on 15th day through to 26th day of each period of 28 days of oestrogen replacement therapy. Therapy should begin within 5 days of the start of the period if this is present.

Special care: patients with a history, or considered to be at risk, of thrombosis, those with liver disease. Liver function should be monitored and breasts and pelvic organs examined periodically during the period of therapy. Women with any of the following require particularly careful monitoring: diabetes, fibroids in uterus, multiple sclerosis, hypertension, tetany, epilepsy, porphyria, gallstones, migraine, otosclerosis, history of breast cancer.

Avoid use: pregnancy, breast-feeding, thrombosis or thromboembolic disorders, serious heart, kidney or liver disease, endometriosis or vaginal bleeding which is undiagnosed, hormone-dependent cancers such as breast or uterine carcinoma, Dublin-Johnson or Rotor syndrome.

Possible interaction: drugs which induce liver enzymes.

Side effects: enlargement of and soreness in breasts, breakthrough bleeding, vomiting, nausea, gastrointestinal disturbance, gain in weight, dizziness, headache. Withdraw immediately if frequent, severe headaches or migraines occur, disordered vision, pregnancy, rise in blood pressure, signs of thromboembolism, jaundice. Stop before planned surgery.

Manufacturer: CIBA.

Ethmozine

Description: a class I antiarrhythmic preparation, moracizine hydrochloride, available in the form of white, film-coated tablets of different strengths. Round tablets contain 200mg; oval tablets contain 250mg and capsule-shaped tablets contain 300mg. All are marked ROBERTS and with name and strength.

Used for: ventricular arrhythmias (arising in the ventricles of the heart).

Dosage: adults, 200–300mg at 8-hour intervals which may be increased, if required, by 150mg per day every 3 days to a maximum daily dose of 900mg.

Special care: pregnancy, liver or kidney disease, congestive heart failure, sick sinus syndrome. Therapy should be started in hospital and electrolyte levels stabilised before beginning. ECG should be monitored.

Avoid use: breast-feeding, children, patients with heart block, heart shock, recent myocardial infarction.

Possible interaction: cimetidine, theophylline, digoxin.

Side effects: gastrointestinal upset, chest, muscle and bone pains, disturbance of sleep, blurring of vision, sweating, dry mouth, nervousness, giddiness. If unexplained liver disorder, withdraw drug.

Manufacturer: Monmouth.

Eudemine

Description: an antihypertensive (vasodilator) and hyperglycaemic produced in ampoules for injection to treat hypertension and as tablets for hypoglycaemia. Ampoules contain 15mg diazoxide/ml and white, sugar-coated tablets contain 50mg diazoxide.

Used for: serious hypertension, especially arising from kidney disease, hypertensive crisis, intractable hypoglycaemia.

Dosage: adults, for hypertension, 300mg by fast, intravenous injection while patient is lying down. Children, 5mg/kg body weight by fast intravenous injection. Adults and children, for hypoglycaemia, 5mg/kg body weight each day at first in 2 or 3 divided doses. Afterwards, adjust according to response.

Special care: pregnancy, serious kidney, heart or cerebral disease, kidney failure, low blood protein levels. Regular checks on blood count, blood pressure, blood glucose levels are required and also monitoring of development and growth in children.

Possible interaction: anticoagulants of coumarin type, other antihypertensives, diuretics.

Side effects: hyperglycaemia, nausea, imbalance electrolyte and fluid levels, tachycardia, vomiting, arrhythmias, orthostatic hypotension (low blood pressure when person is standing), delay in onset of labour, possible coma.

Manufacutrer: Link.

Euglucon

Description: an oral hypoglycaemic preparation, glibenclamide, in the form of white tablets of 2 strengths. Tablets marked EU and 2.5 contain 2.5mg and scored, oblong tablets, marked EU-BM, contain 5mg. Glibenclamide belongs to a group of antidiabetic agents called sulphonylureas which enhance the effects of insulin and stimulate its secretion from cells in the pancreas.

Used for: diabetes which develops in adults (maturity-onset or non-insulin dependent type II diabetes).

Dosage: adults, 5mg each day at first, taken at breakfast time, increasing if required by 2.5mg each day at intervals of 1 week. The maximum daily dose is 15mg.

Special care: elderly persons or patients with kidney failure.

Avoid use: pregnancy, breast-feeding, some other types of diabetes (including juvenile, unstable-brittle and growth-onset), patients with infections, hormonal disorders, serious kidney or liver disease, stress, undergoing surgery, ketoacidosis (accumulation of ketones in the body characterized by 'pear drops' smell on breath and resulting from diabetes mellitus).

Possible interaction: chloramphenicol, diuretics, anticoagulants taken by mouth, glucagon, chlorpropamide, metiformin, aspirin, MAOIs, oral contraceptives, corticotrophin, corticosteroids, alcohol, phenylbutazone, cyclophosphamide, rifampicin, bezafibrate, diuretics, anticoagulants taken orally.

Side effects: allergic reactions including skin rash.

Manufacturer: Roussel.

Eugynon 30

Description: a combined oestrogen/progestogen and contraceptive produced in the form of white, sugar-coated tablets containing 30µg ethinyloestradiol and 250µg levonorgestrel.

Used for: oral contraception.

Dosage: 1 tablet each day for 21 days starting on first day of period followed by 7 tablet-free days.

Special care: hypertension, severe kidney disease, dialysis, Raynaud's disease, diabetes, multiple sclerosis, asthma, varicose veins, elevated levels of prolactin (a hormone) in the blood (hyperprolactaemia). Risk of thrombosis increases with smoking, age and obesity. Blood pressure, breasts and pelvic organs should be checked during period of treatment.

Avoid use: pregnancy, heart and circulatory diseases, angina, sickle cell anaemia, pulmonary hypertension. Also hormone-dependent cancers, otosclerosis, undiagnosed vaginal bleeding, chorea, liver disease, history of cholestatic jaundice of pregnancy, infectious hepatitis, Dublin-Johnson syndrome, Rotor syndrome, recent trophoblastic disease.

Possible interaction: phenytoin, carbamazepine, tetracyclines, primidone, chloral hydrate, glutehimide, rifampicin, griseofulvin, dichloralphenazone, ethosuximide, barbiturates.

Side effects: feeling of bloatedness due to fluid retention, leg pains, breast enlargement, muscular cramps, weight gain, breakthrough bleeding, depression, vaginal discharge, loss of libido, nausea, brown patches on skin (chloasma). Stop drug immediately if frequent, severe headaches occur or signs of thromboses, rise in blood pressure. Drug should be discontinued before major planned surgery.

Manufacturer: Schering H.C.

Eumovate

Description: a moderately potent topical steroid in the form of cream and ointment containing 0.05% clobetasone butyrate.

Used for: dermatitis, eczema and skin conditions responsive to steroids.

Dosage: apply thinly to affected area up to 4 times each day.

Special care: should not be used on face or on children for more than 5 days. Should be stopped gradually.

Avoid use: prolonged or extensive use especially pregnant women or continual use as a preventative. Should not be used to treat acne, leg ulcers, scabies, peri-oral dermatitis, tuberculous skin conditions, skin disorders caused by viruses, ringworm, any untreated bacterial or fungal skin infections.

Side effects: thinning of skin, adrenal gland suppression, hair growth, Cushingoid type symptoms (Cushing's syndrome).

Manufacturer: Glaxo.

Eumovate Eyedrops

Description: Moderately potent steroid eyedrops containing 0.1% clobetasone butyrate. Also **Eumovate-N** which additionally contains an antibiotic (0.5% neomycin sulphate as eyedrops).

Used for: drops containing clobetasone butyrate only are used for non-infected inflammatory conditions of the eye. Eumovate-N drops are used for infected inflammatory conditions of the eye.

Dosage: 1 or 2 drops 4 times each day with more severe infections requiring more frequent application every 1 or 2 hours.

Special care: do not use for prolonged periods especially pregnant women and young children.

Avoid use: patients with soft contact lenses, those with tuberculous, fungal or viral infections, glaucoma, dendritic ulcer, infections containing pus.

Side effects: thinning of cornea, cataracts, rise in pressure within eye, fungal infection, sensitization (patient becomes hypersensitive to drug).

Manufacturer: Cusi.

Evorel

Description: an oestrogen patch containing 50µg oestradiol per 24 hours.

Used for: hormone replacement therapy in menopausal women.

Dosage: apply patch to hairless area of skin below waist and change for a new patch in a different site after 3 or 4 days. Women who have not had a hysterectomy should also receive a progestogen preparation for 12 out of each 28 day period of treatment.

Special care: patients with history of or considered to be at risk of thrombosis, those with liver disease. Careful monitoring of women with any of the following is required: fibroids in uterus, otosclerosis, porphyria, tetany, epilepsy, gallstones, migraine, multiple sclerosis, hypertension, diabetes. Regular examination of pelvic organs and breasts required during course of therapy, especially in women with family history of breast cancer.

Avoid use: pregnancy, breast-feeding, women with breast cancer or other cancers which are hormone-dependent, e.g. of genital tract; serious heart, liver or kidney disease, endometriosis, thrombosis, Dublin-Johnson or Rotor syndrome, undiagnosed vaginal bleeding.

Possible interaction: drugs which induce liver enzymes.

Side effects: enlargement and tenderness of breasts, nausea and vomiting, weight gain, breakthrough bleeding, gastrointestinal upset, headache, giddiness. Withdraw drug immediately if any sign of thrombosis, rise in blood pressure, severe and frequent headaches, migraines, disturbance of vision, jaundice, pregnancy. Stop before planned surgery.

Manufacturer: Ortho.

Exelderm

Description: an antifungal preparation, an imidazole, produced in the form of a cream containing 1% sulconazole nitrate.

Used for: fungal skin and nail infections.

Dosage: massage in twice each day and continue for 2 to 3 weeks after symptoms have disappeared.

Avoid use: contact with eyes.

Side effects: skin irritation—stop use.

Manufacturer: Zeneca.

Exirel

Description: a bronchodilator selective ß2-agonist produced in the form of capsules. Olive/turquoise capsules contain 10mg pirbuterol (as hydrochloride) and beige/turquoise capsules contain 15mg. All are marked with strength, 3M and MXR. Also, **Exirel Inhaler** containing 0.2mg pirbuterol (as acetate) per metered dose delivered by aerosol inhaler.

Used for: bronchial spasm in asthma, emphysema and bronchitis.

Dosage: adults, tablets, 10–15mg 3 or 4 times each day with a maximum dose of 60mg. Inhaler, relief of acute attack, 1 or 2 puffs in 1 dose; prevention, 2 puffs 3 or 4 times each day with a maximum of 12 puffs in 24 hours.

Special care: pregnant women, patients with weak hearts, heart arrhythmias, hypertension, angina, hyperthyroidism.

Avoid use: children.

Possible interaction: sympathomimetics.

Side effects: dilation of peripheral blood vessels, headache, nervousness, tremor.

Manufacturer: 3M Health Care.

Exocin

Description: a 4-quinolone antibiotic preparation produced in the form of eyedrops containing 0.3% olfloxacin.

Used for: bacterial eye infections.

Dosage: 1 or 2 drops every 2 to 4 hours into eye during first 2 days of treatment. Then reduce to 1 or 2 drops 4 times daily. Use for a maximum period of 10 days.

Special care: pregnancy, breast-feeding.

Avoid use: patients with soft contact lenses.

Side effects: short-lived eye irritation, rarely headache, dizzines, nausea, numbness.

Manufacturer: Allergan.

Exosurf Neonatal

Description: a preparation which acts as a lung surfactant produced as a powder in vials (with diluent) for reconstitution. The powder contains 108mg colfosceril palmitate.

Used for: newborn babies suffering from respiratory distress syndrome who are receiving mechanical ventilation.

Dosage: 67.5mg/kg body weight by means of endotracheal tube; may be repeated after 12 hours.

Special care: for use in babies of a weight greater than 700g; must be continually monitored due to risk of too much oxygen entering blood.

Side effects: tube may become blocked by mucous secretions; risk of pulmonary haemorrhage.

Manufacturer: Wellcome.

Eye-Crom

Description: an anti-inflammatory preparation in the form of eye drops containing 2% sodium cromoglycate.

Used for: allergic conjunctivitis.

Dosage: 1 or 2 drops into eye up to 4 times each day continuing after symptoms have disappeared.

Avoid use: patients with soft contact lenses.

Side effects: passing stinging or burning in eye.

Manufacturer: Norton.

F

Fabrol

Description: a mucolytic preparation produced in the form of granules in sachets for dissolving in water containing 200mg acetylcysteine. It is for cystic fibrosis patients with accompanying abdominal complications.

Used for: bronchitis and infections of the respiratory tract in which a lot of mucus is produced; abdominal problems in cystic fibrosis.

Dosage: respiratory diseases, 3 sachets daily in divided doses; cystic fibrosis, normally 1 or 2 sachets 3 times each day. Children, respiratory diseases, under 2 years, 1 sachet each day; 2 to 6 years, 1 sachet twice each day; over 6 years, as adult dose. Cystic fibrosis, under 2 years, half to 1 sachet 3 times each day; 2 to 6 years, 1 or 2 sachets 3 times each day.

Special care: patients with diabetes.

Side effects: headache, skin rash, vomiting and nausea, gastrointestinal upset, tinnitus; rarely bronchospasm, anaphylactic reactions (notify Committee on Safety of Medicines).

Manufacturer: Zyma.

Famvir

Description: a preparation which interferes with the manufacture of DNA within cells infected by a virus and is a nucleoside analogue produced in the form of white, film-coated tablets containing 250mg famciclovir. The tablets are marked with the strength and name.

Used for: infections caused by herpes zoster virus.

Dosage: adults, 1 tablet 3 times each day for 1 week.

Special care: kidney disease.

Avoid use: children, pregnancy breast-feeding mothers.

Side effects: nausea, headache.

Manufacturer: Smith Kline Beecham.

Fansidar

Description: a compound antimalarial preparation, combining a sulphonamide with a diaminopyrimidine drug, produced in the form of quarter-scored white tablets containing 500mg sulfadoxine and 25mg pyrimethamine. The tablets are marked with a hexagon and ROCHE.

Used for: treatment and prevention of malaria (caused by *Plasmodium falciparum*), especially where the disease does not respond to chloroquine.

Dosage: for prevention, adults and children over fourteen years, 1 tablet taken weekly; for treatment, adults and children over fourteen years, 2 to 3 tablets as a single dose. Children, for prevention, under 4 years of age quarter of adult dose; 4 to 8 years, half adult dose; 9 to fourteen years threequarters adult dose. For treatment, under 4 years of age, half tablet; 4 to 6 years, 1 tablet; 7 to 9 years, 1 and a half tablets; 10 to fourteen years, 2 tablets. All ages take tablets as a single dose.

Special care: patients should avoid being out in the sun and regular blood checks are required during long-term preventative treatment.

Avoid use: pregnancy, breast-feeding, newborn babies, patients with serious kidney or liver disease, blood changes or a sensitivity to sulphonamide drugs.

Possible interaction: folate inhibitors.

Side effects: discontinue therapy if pharyngitis (inflammation of pharynx) or pruritis occur. Gastrointestinal upset, blood changes, skin rash. More rarely, allergic skin conditions.

Manufacturer: Roche.

Farlutal

Description: an anticancer drug which is a synthetic version of the female sex hormone, progestogen. It is produced in the form of a suspension in vials for injection, containing 200mg medroxyprogesterone acetate per ml and also in tablets of 3 strengths. White tablets contain 100mg; white scored tablets contain 250mg. Both are marked with tablet strength. White, scored, elongated tablets contain 500mg and are marked FCE 500.

Used for: cancer of breast, endometrium (womb), kidney cells and prostate gland.

Dosage: adults, tablets, breast cancer, 1–1.5g each day; kidney or prostate cancer, 100 -500mg each day.

Special care: patients suffering from epilepsy, diabetes, kidney or heart disease, asthma, migraine.
Avoid use: children, pregnant women, patients with thromboembolism, liver disease, thrombophlebitis (inflamed veins), hypercalcaemia.
Side effects: abnormal menstruation, abnormal production of breast milk, corticoid symptoms.
Manufacturer: Pharmacia.

Fasigyn

Description: an antibacterial preparation which is a nitroimidazole drug effective against certain anaerobic bacteria. It is produced in the form of white, film-coated tablets containing 500mg tinidazole.
Used for: treatment of infections caused by anaerobic bacteria and prevention of such during surgery. Particular sites of such infections are the mouth, gut and vagina (purulent gingivitis, pelvic inflammatory disease, non-specific vaginitis).
Dosage: adults, prevention of infection, 4 tablets taken as 1 dose; treatment, 4 tablets taken as 1 dose at first followed by 2 each day for 5 to 6 days.
Special care: pregnancy, breast-feeding.
Avoid use: children, patients with blood changes or neurological disorders.
Possible interaction: alcohol.
Side effects: unpleasant taste in mouth and furring of tongue, gastrointestinal upset, nettle rash (urticaria), disturbance of central nervous system, dark-coloured urine, angioneurotic oedema. Rarely, nerve damage and leucopenia if drug is taken long-term.
Manufacturer: Pfizer

Faverin

Description: an antidepressant drug, fluvoxamine, of a type known as 5HT reuptake inhibitors. Faverin is produced in the form of yellow, enteric-coated tablets of 2 strengths containing 50mg, marked DUPHAR and 291, or 100g, marked DUPHAR and 313.
Used for: depression.
Dosage: adults, 100mg taken at night in first instance with a normal maintenance dose in the order of 100–200mg each day in divided doses. The maximum dose is 300mg each day.
Special care: pregnancy, breast-feeding, kidney or liver disease or history of epilepsy.
Avoid use: children.
Possible interaction: alcohol, benzodiazepines, tryptophan, MAOIs, lithium, carbamazepine, propanolol, phenytoin, theophylline, tricyclic antidepressants.
Side effects: gastrointestinal upset, nausea,

diarrhoea, vomiting, nervousness, sleepiness, anorexia, convulsions, tremor.
Manufacturer: Duphar.

Feldene

Description: a proprietary NSAID and oxicam, piroxicam, which is produced in a number of different forms. Feldene Capsules: blue/maroon capsules, marked FEL 10 and Pfizer, contain 10mg; maroon capsules, marked FEL 20 and Pfizer, contain 20mg. **Feldene Dispersible**: scored, white tablets containing either 10mg or 20mg and marked FEL 10 and Pfizer or FEL 20 and Pfizer respectively. Higher strength tablets are oblong in shape. **Feldene Melt**: fast dissolving, off-white coloured tablets containing 20mg; **Feldene Suppositories** contain 20mg; **Feldene Intramuscular Injection**: solution in ampoules containing 20mg per ml. **Feldene Gel:** a topical gel containing 0.5% piroxicam.
Used for: arthritic diseases including juvenile arthritis, gout, rheumatoid arthritis, ankylosing spondylitis, osteoarthritis and other skeletal and muscle diosrders.
Dosage: adults, preparations taken by mouth or suppositories depending upon condition being treated, but about 20–40mg each day (Melt tablets are dissolved on tongue and dispersible tablets dissolved in water or swallowed whole). Injection, used for acute attacks, 1 dose of 20–40mg by deep intramuscular injection into buttock. Then tablets should be taken for maintenance. Feldene Gel is for use by adults only in patients with tendinitis, musculoskeletal injuries or joint problems. 3cm gel is applied to affected area 3 or 4 times each day for 4 weeks. Children over 6 years of age, for juvenile arthritis only, usually dispersible tablets, under 15kg of body weight, 5mg; 16–25kg of body weight, 10mg; 26–45kg body weight, 15mg; over 45kg body weight, 20mg. All are daily doses. Injection and gel are not for use in children.
Special care: eldery, heart failure, liver or kidney disease. Feldene gel should not be applied to broken or infected skin or eyes, and mucous membranes should be avoided.
Avoid use: pregnancy, breast-feeding, patients with allergy to NSAID or aspirin, peptic ulcers, history of ulcers, anal inflammation (use suppositories).
Possible interaction: other NSAIDs, lithium, anticoagulants, hypoglycaemics.
Side effects: gastrointestinal upset, oedema, central nervous system disturbance, malaise, tinnitus, inflammation at injection site. Gel may cause skin irritation, rash and itching.
Manufacturer: Pfizer.

Femodene

Description: a combined oestrogen/progestogen hormonal oral contraceptive in the form of white, sugar-coated tablets containing 30µg ethinyloestradiol and 75µg gestodene.

Used for: oral contraception.

Dosage: 1 tablet daily, beginning on day 1 of period, for 21 days followed by 7 tablet-free days.

Special care: hypertension, severe kidney disease receiving dialysis, Raynaud's disease, diabetes, multiple sclerosis, asthma, varicose veins, elevated levels of prolactin (a hormone) in the blood (hyperprolactaemia). Risk of thrombosis increases with smoking, age and obesity. Blood pressure, breasts and pelvic organs should be checked during period of treatment.

Avoid use: pregnancy, heart and circulatory diseases, angina, sickle cell anaemia, pulmonary hypertension. Also hormone-dependent cancers, undiagnosed vaginal bleeding, chorea, liver disease, history of cholestatic jaundice of pregnancy, infectious hepatitis, Dublin-Johnson syndrome, Rotor syndrome, recent trophoblasic disease.

Possible interaction: phenytoin, carbamazepine, tetracyclines, primidone, chloral hydrate, glutehimide, rifampicin, griseofulvin, dichloralphenazone, ethosuximide, barbiturates.

Side effects: feeling of bloatedness due to fluid retention, leg pains, breast enlargement, muscular cramps, weight gain, breakthrough bleeding, depression, vaginal discharge, loss of libido, nausea, brown patches on skin (chloasma). Stop drug immediately if frequent, severe headaches occur or signs of thromboses, rise in blood pressure. Drug should be discontinued before major planned surgery.

Manufacturer: Schering H.C.

Femodene E.D.

Description: a combined oestrogen/progestogen hormonal oral contraceptive preparation consisting of 21 white, sugar-coated tablets containing 30µg ethinyloestradiol and 75µg gestodene and 7 white, sugar-coated placebo tablets containing lactose.

Used for: oral contraception.

Dosage: 1 tablet daily starting on first day of period with numbered tablet from red part of pack. Tablets are taken each day without a break, either hormonal or placebo depending upon the time in the cycle.

Special care: hypertension, severe kidney disease receiving dialysis, Raynaud's disease, diabetes, multiple sclerosis, asthma, varicose veins, elevated levels of prolactin (a hormone) in the blood (hyperprolactaemia). Risk of thrombosis increases with smoking, age and obesity. Blood pressure, breasts and pelvic organs should be checked during period of treatment.

Avoid use: pregnancy, heart and circulatory diseases, angina, sickle cell anaemia, pulmonary hypertension. Also hormone-dependent cancers, otosclerosis, undiagnosed vaginal bleeding, chorea, liver disease, history of cholestatic jaundice of pregnancy, infectious hepatitis, Dublin-Johnson syndrome, Rotor syndrome, recent trophoblasic disease.

Possible interaction: phenytoin, carbamazepine, tetracyclines, primidone, chloral hydrate, glutehimide, rifampicin, griseofulvin, dichloralphenazone, ethosuximide, barbiturates.

Side effects: feeling of bloatedness due to fluid retention, leg pains, breast enlargement, muscular cramps, weight gain, breakthrough bleeding, depression, vaginal discharge, loss of libido, nausea, brown patches on skin (chloasma). Stop drug immediately if frequent, severe headaches occur or signs of thromboses, rise in blood pressure. Drug should be discontinued before major planned surgery.

Manufacturer: Schering H.C.

Femulen

Description: a hormonal preparation which is a progestogen only contraceptive in the form of white tablets containing 500µg ethinodiol diacetate marked with manufacturer's name.

Used for: oral contraception.

Dosage: 1 tablet at same time each day starting on first day of period and continuing without a break.

Special care: patients with history of, or considered to be at risk of thrombosis, hypertension, cysts on ovaries, hormone dependent cancer, liver disease. Blood pressure, breasts and pelvic organs should be checked regularly during the course of treatment.

Avoid use: pregnancy, previous ectopic pregnancy, history of heart or arterial disease or stroke, liver tumour, recent trophoblastic cancer, undiagnosed vaginal bleeding.

Possible interaction: meprobamate, chloral hydrate, ethosuximide, barbiturates, carbamazepine, chlorpromazine, griseofulvin, dichloralphenazone, pyrimidone, rifampicin, phenytoin, glutethimide.

Side effects: headache, breast tenderness, ovarian cysts, acne, disruption to normal pattern of menstrual bleeding, acne. Discontinue immediately if jaundice, signs of thrombosis or thrombophlebitis occur.

Manufacturer: Gold Cross.

Fenbid Spansule

Description: a proprietary NSAID which is a propionic acid produced in the form of sustained-release spansules. Maroon/pink capsules contain off-white pellets consisting of 300mg ibuprofen.

Used for: pain and arthritic conditions including ankylosing spondylitis, rheumatoid arthritis, osteoarthritis and other disorders of the skeleton and joints.

Dosage: 2 capsules twice each day at first increasing to 3 capsules twice daily if required. The maintenance dose is in the order of 1 or 2 capsules twice each day.

Special care: pregnancy, breast-feeding, elderly, asthma, disease of the gastrointestinal tract, heart, liver or kidney disorders. Patients taking the drug long-term require careful monitoring.

Avoid use: children, patients with allergy to aspirin or other anti-inflammatory drugs, peptic ulcer.

Possible interaction: thiazide diuretics, quinolones, anticoagulant drugs.

Side effects: rash, gastrointestinal upset and possibly bleeding, thrombocytopenia (If a patient contracts aseptic meningitis, it must be reported to the Committee on the Safety of Medicines).

Manufacturer: Goldshield.

Fenopron

Description: a proprietary NSAID and propionic acid, fenoprofen (as calcium salt), produced in the form of tablets of 2 different strengths. Oval-shaped, orange tablets, coded DISTA 4019, contain 300mg ; oblong-shaped orange tablets coded DISTA 4021, contain 600mg.

Used for: pain and arthritic conditions including ankylosing spondylitis, rheumatoid arthritis and osteoarthritis.

Dosage: 300–600mg 3 to 4 times daily with a maximum daily dose of 3g.

Special care: pregnancy, breast-feeding, elderly, liver or kidney disease, heart failure, asthma, a history of disorders involving gastrointestinal bleeding. Patients taking the drug long-term should receive careful monitoring.

Avoid use: children, patients with ulcers, allergy to aspirin or anti-inflammatory drugs, serious kidney disorders.

Possible interaction: aspirin, quinolones, loop diuretics, anticoagulants, hydantoins, phenobarbitone, sulphonylureas.

Side effects: allergic responses, intolerance of gastrointestinal tract, blood changes, kidney and liver disorders.

Manufacturers: Dista.

Fentazin

Description: a potent antipsychotic preparation and group III phenothiazine (a piperazine), produced as tablets of 2 strengths. White, sugar-coated tablets, coded 1C, contain 2mg perphenazine; white, sugar-coated tablets coded 2C contain 4mg.

Used for: various serious psychiatric disorders including schizophrenia, psychoses, anxiety, nervous stress, vomiting and nausea.

Dosage: adults, 12mg each day in divided doses with a maximum of 24mg daily; elderly persons, quarter to half the full dose.

Special care: pregnancy, breast-feeding, epilepsy, glaucoma, Parkinson's disease, liver disease, hypothyroidism, myasthenia gravis, cardiovascular disease, phaeochromocytoma, enlarged prostate gland.

Avoid use: children, patients with depressed bone marrow or in comatose states.

Possible interaction: alcohol, anti-arrhythmic drugs, anaesthetics, antidepressants, antacids, rifampicin, sulphonylureas, antihypertensives, antiepileptic and antidiabetic drugs.

Side effects: allergic responses, effects on liver and jaundice, changes in menstruation, breasts, weight gain, impotence, effects on heart rhythm (tachycardia), blurred vision, dry mouth, difficulty with urination, blocked nose, constipation, drowsiness, pallor, apathy, insomnia, hypotension, convulsions, effects on eyes and skin colouration with higher doses.

Manufacturer: Forley.

Ferfolic SV

Description: a combined mineral and vitamin preparation with a haematinic (iron) and vitamin B component. It is produced in the form of pink, sugar-coated tablets containing 4mg folic acid, 250mg ferrous gluconate and 10mg ascorbic acid.

Used for: anaemias and conditions characterized by deficiency of iron and folic acid. Also used as a preventative to reduce the risk of neural tube defects in a foetus, when a mother known to be at risk is planning a pregnancy.

Dosage: adults, for deficiency, 1 tablet 3 times each day. Prevention of neural tube defects, 1 tablet each day when conception is planned and continuing during first 3 months of pregnancy.

Avoid use: children, patients with megaloblastic anaemia.

Possible interaction: tetracycline antibiotics.

Side effects: constipation, nausea.

Manufacturer: Sinclair.

Fertiral

Description: a hormonal preparation of

gonadotrophin-releasing hormone, produced in the form of a solution in ampoules for infusion containing 500 micrograms gonadorelin per ml.

Used for: amenorrhoea and certain types of infertility in women.

Dosage: determined individually.

Special care: maximum period of treatment is 6 months and should be discontinued in the event of pregnancy.

Avoid use: patients with cysts in the ovaries or lining of the womb.

Side effects: headache, nausea, abdominal pain, pain at infusion site, menorrhagia (abnormally long or heavy menstrual periods).

Manufacturer: Hoechst.

Filair

Description: an anti-inflammatory corticosteroid preparation containing 50 or 100µg beclomethasone dipropionate delivered by metered dose aerosol. Also, **Filair Forte** containing 250µg.

Used for: reversible obstructive airways disease (asthma).

Dosage: adults, 100µg, 3 or 4 times each day or 200µg twice each day. In extremely severe conditions 600–800µg in divided doses, with a maximum of 1mg, may be taken. Filair Forte, 500µg twice each day or 250µg 4 times each day. Children, Filair only, 50–100µg 2, 3 or 4 times each day.

Special care: pregnancy, history of or active pulmonary tuberculosis, those transferring from other (systemic) steroid drugs.

Side effects: hoarse voice, candidiasis (yeast-like fungal infection) of throat and mouth.

Manufacturer: 3M Health Care.

Flagyl

Description: an antibacterial preparation and nitroimidazoles, which is effective against anaerobic bacteria and certain other infective organisms. It is produced in a variety of forms: Flagyl tablets, off-white, film-coated tablets contain 200mg and 400mg metronidazole, the higher strength being capsule-shaped. Both are marked with strength and tablet name. **Flagyl-S Suspension** contains 200mg metronidazole (as benzoate) per 5ml liquid. **Flagyl Suppositories** contain 500mg and 1g metronidazole. **Flagyl Compak** consists of fourteen off-white, film-coated, capsule-shaped tablets containing 400mg metronidazole, marked with name and strength and also fourteen pale yellow coloured pessaries containing 100,000 units nystatin. **Flagyl Intravenous Infusion** contains 5mg metronidazole per ml in ampoules for intravenous infusion.

Used for: infections caused by anaerobic bacteria, amoebic dysentery, abscess of liver, trichomoniasis (of urogenital tract), vaginosis of bacterial origin, dental infections and severe ulcerative gingivitis. Prevention of infection before surgery.

Dosage: depending upon condition being treated, adults, in the order of 400mg–1g every 8 hours in first instance, then reduced doses. Period of treatment is usually 1 week. Children receive reduced doses usually in the order of 7.5mg/kg body weight. In cases of vaginosis, sexual partner should also receive therapy at same time.

Special care: pregnancy, breast-feeding, patients with disorders of central nervous system, hepatic encephalopathy (a liver disease in which toxic substances normally removed by the liver interfere with the function of the brain).

Possible interaction: phenobarbitone, alcohol, lithium, anticoagulant drugs taken orally.

Side effects: central nervous system effects, dark coloured urine, unpleasant taste in mouth and furring of tongue, gastrointestinal upset, rash, angioneurotic oedema, leucopenia. Long-term therapy may cause neuropathy (nerve disorders) and epileptic-type fits.

Manufacturer: Theraplix.

Flamazine

Description: an antibacterial cream containing 1% silver sulphadiazine.

Used for: burns, skin wounds, pressure sores, infected leg ulcers, areas where skin has been removed for grafting.

Dosage: apply a layer of cream 3–5mm thick beneath dressing which should be changed daily for burns and 3 times each week for ulcers.

Special care: patients with liver or kidney disorders.

Avoid use: pregnancy, newborn babies.

Possible interaction: wound-cleaning agents with enzyme action, phenytoin, hypoglycaemic drugs taken orally, sulphonamides.

Manufacturer: S.N.P.

Flaxedil

Description: a muscle relaxant produced as a solution in ampoules for injection, containing 40mg gallamine triethiodide per ml.

Used for: to produce paralysis during surgical operations after the patient has become unconscious and for seriously ill patients receiving prolonged artificial ventilation in intensive care.

Dosage: given by intravenous injection. Adults, 80–120mg and then 20–40mg as needed. Child, 1.5mg/kg body weight; newborn baby, 600µg/kg body weight.

Special care: kidney disorder.

Avoid use: serious kidney disease.

Possible interaction: some antiarrhythmic drugs, some antibacterial drugs, propranolol, verapamil, nifedipine, some cholinergics, magnesium salts, lithium.

Side effects: tachycardia.

Manufacturer: Rhône-Poulenc Rorer.

Flemoxin

Description: an antibiotic preparation which is a broad-spectrum penicillin. Flemoxin is produced as white, scored, dissolvable tablets of 2 strengths containing 375mg (marked gbr 183) and 750mg (marked gbr 185) amoxicillin (as trihydrate).

Used for: soft tissue, respiratory tract, urinary tract and ear, nose and throat infections.

Dosage: depending upon type of infection; adults in the order of 375mg–3g, usually twice each day. Tablets may be dissolved in water or swallowed whole. Children, 2–5 years of age, 750mg twice each day; 5 to 10 years, half adult dose; over 10 years, adult dose.

Special care: patients with lymphatic leukaemia, glandular fever.

Side effects: allergic reactions, rash, gastrointestinal upset.

Manufacturer: Paines and Byrne.

Flexin Continus

Description: a NSAID available as continuous-release tablets of thee strengths, all of which are capsule-shaped and marked with strength and 1C. Green, red and yellow tablets contain 25mg, 50mg and 75mg indomethacin respectively.

Used for: arthritic disorders of joints and skeleton including osteoarthritis, ankylosing spondylitis, rheumatoid arthritis, degenerative disease of the hip joint, other musculoskeletal and back disorders which cause pain, dysmenorrhoea (period pain).

Dosage: adults, 25–200mg each day in 1 or 2 divided doses taken with food, milk or antacid preparation.

Special care: elderly persons, patients with heart failure, liver or kidney disease, disorders of the central nervous system. Those taking the drug long-term require careful monitoring and eye tests.

Avoid use: pregnancy, breast-feeding, allergy to aspirin or anti-inflammatory drug, defects in blood coagulation, stomach ulcer or ulcer of gastrointestinal lesions.

Possible interaction: corticosteroids, ß-blockers, quinolones, diuretics, methotrexate, salicylates, lithium, probenecid, anticoagulants.

Side effects: rash, blood changes, effects on central nervous system, giddiness, visual disturbance, corneal deposits, blood in urine, adverse kidney effects (nephrotoxicity), tinnitus, inflammation of small blood vessels (angitis). Drug should be discontinued if recurring headaches or gastrointestinal bleeding occur.

Manufacturer: Napp.

Flixonase

Description: a corticosteroid nasal spray 50 µg fluticasone propionate per metered dose.

Used for: prevention and treatment of allergic rhinitis (hay fever), nasal congestion.

Dosage: adults, 2 sprays into each nostril in the morning, with a maximum of 4 sprays into both nostrils daily. Children, over 4 years of age, 1 spray (maximum of 2) into each nostril daily.

Special care: pregnancy, breast-feeding, transferring from other (systemic) steroid drugs taken orally.

Avoid use: children under 4 years of age.

Side effects: nosebleed, irritation of nose, interference with sense of taste and smell.

Manufacturer: A & H.

Flixotide

Description: a corticosteroid preparation containing fluticasone propionate for use with diskhaler and inhaler. 50, 100, 250 and 500µg fluticasone propionate disks are for use with breath-operated diskhaler delivery system. Also, 25, 50, 125 and 250µg fluticasone propionate per dose are for use with metered dose aerosol delivery system.

Used for: prevention of bronchial asthma.

Dosage: adults, 100–1000µg twice each day; children over 4 years of age, 50–100µg twice each day.

Special care: pregnancy, transferring from other (systemic) steroid drugs taken orally, those with history of or with active tuberculosis.

Avoid use: children under 4 years of age.

Side effects: candidiasis (a yeast-like fungal infection) of throat and mouth, hoarseness, occasional unexplained bronchospasm.

Manufacturer: A & H.

Flolan

Description: an anticoagulant prostaglandin preparation produced in the form of a powder containing 500µg epoprostenol (as sodium salt) with a diluent for reconstitution and infusion.

Used for: prevention of blood clotting during and following heart surgery; kidney dialysis (with heparin).

Dosage: according to manufacturer's literature.

Special care: if being given with heparin in kidney dialysis, anticoagulant monitoring must be carried out. Must be given by continuous intravenous infusion.
Side effects: vasodilation, flushing, hypotension, headache, pallor, bradycardia, sweating.
Manufacturer: Wellcome.

Florinef

Description: a corticosteroid mineralocorticoid preparation produced in the form of scored, pink tablets coded 429 and marked SQUIBB, containing 0.1mg fludrocortisone acetate. Mineralocorticoids regulate the salt/water balance in the body.
Used for: treatment of salt-losing adrenogenital syndrome and to partially replace hormones in Addison's disease.
Dosage: adults, 0.05–3mg each day; children, according to body weight, age and condition being treated.
Special care: pregnancy, hypertension, epilepsy, kidney inflammation (nephritis, glomerulonephritis), diabetes, inflamed veins, stomach ulcer. Patients with glaucoma, secondary cancers, osteoporosis, liver cirrhosis, tuberculosis and other bacterial, viral or fungal infections, recent surgical bowel anastomoses, those suffering from psychoses or stress. Contact wtht chicken pox should be avoided and medical advice sought in the event of this occurring. Withdraw drug gradually.
Possible interaction: anticoagulants taken orally, diuretics, ephedrine, phenytoin, cardiac glycosides, NSAIDs, phenobarbitone, hypoglycaemics, rifampicin, anticholinesterases.
Side effects: fluid retention, hypertension, weakness in muscles, loss of potassium, Cushingoid changes (as in Cushing's syndrome).
Manufacturer: Squibb.

Floxapen

Description: a penicillinase-resistant form of penicillin. (Penicillinase is an enzyme produced by some bacteria that renders penicillin inactive, hence the infection being treated will be resistant to the antibiotic). Floxapen is produced in several forms: black/caramel-coloured capsules of 2 strengths containing 250mg and 500mg flucloxacillin sodium, each marked with strength and name. **Floxapen Syrup** contains 125mg flucloxacillin (as magnesium salt) per 5ml, supplied as powder for reconstitution with water to make 100ml. **Floxapen Syrup Forte** contains 250mg per 5ml, supplied as powder to make 100ml. **Floxapen Injection** is supplied as powder in vials for reconstitution at strengths of 250mg, 500mg and 1g flucloxacillin (as sodium salt).
Used for: ear, nose, throat, soft tisssue, skin infections and other infections including those caused by staphylococci bacteria resistant to penicillin.
Dosage: capsules and syrup, 250mg 4 times each day taken 1 hour to half an hour before meals. Injection, 250mg–1g given intravenously 4 times each day. Children, capsules, syrup and injection, age 2 years and under, quarter of adult dose; age 2 to 10 years, half adult dose; over 10 years, adult dose.
Avoid use: allergy to penicillin.
Side effects: gastrointestinal upset, allergic responses, rarely cholestatic jaundice.
Manufacturer: Beecham.

Fluanxol

Description: an antidepressant preparation and a thioxanthene, available as red, sugar-coated tablets of 2 strengths, containing 0.5mg and 1mg of flupenthixol (as dihydrochloride), both marked LUNDBECK.
Used for: short-term treatment of depression which may be accompanied by symptoms of anxiety.
Dosage: adults, 1–2mg as a single dose taken in the morning with a maximum daily amount of 3mg in divided doses. Elderly persons, 0.5mg as a single morning dose with a daily maximum of 2g in divided doses.
Special care: patients with serious heart, circulatory, liver or kidney disease, arteriosclerosis, Parkinson's disease, elderly persons in confused states.
Avoid use: children, overactive, excitable persons, those with very severe depression.
Possible interaction: other antidepressants, central nervous system sedatives, antihypertensives, anticonvulsants, levodopa, alcohol, antidiabetic drugs.
Side effects: dry mouth, blocked nose, visual disturbances, muscular spasms and Parkinson's disease-like symptoms, hypotension, tiredness and lethargy. Weight gain, sleepiness, constipation, difficulty passing urine, enlargement of breasts and abnormal production of milk, dermatitis, blood changes, tachycardia and effects on ECG, jaundice, fits.
Manufacturer: Lundbeck.

Fluvirin

Description: a vaccine against influenza containing inactivated surface antigens of 3 strains of influenza virus produced in the form of 15 μs of each strain per 0.5ml solution in pre-filled syringes.

Used for: immunization against influenza.

Dosage: adults, 0.5ml by intramuscular or deep subcutaneous injection. Children over 4 years of age, 0.5ml followed by a further 0.5ml after 1 month to 6 weeks.

Special care: pregnant women.

Avoid use: children under 4 years of age, patients with allergy to chicken or egg protein (as vaccines are cultivated on these).

Side effects: feverishness, headache, malaise, soreness at injection site, all uncommon and transient.

Manufacturer: Evans.

Fluzone

Description: a vaccine against influenza containing inactivated split virion of 3 strains of influenza virus. Produced in the form of pre-filled syringes containing 15 μs of each strain per 0.5ml.

Used for: immunization against influenza.

Dosage: adults, 0.5ml by subcutaneous or intramuscular injection; children 6 months to 3 years, 0.25ml followed by further 0.25ml afer 1 month; 3 years to 12 years, 0.5ml followed by further 0.5ml after 1 month; over thirteen years as adult.

Avoid use: patients with feverish illness, those with allergy to egg protein.

Side effects: feverishness, headache, malaise, soreness at injection site (of transient nature).

Manufacturer: Servier.

FML

Description: an anti-inflammatory corticosteroid in the form of eyedrops containing 0.1% fluorometholone. Also **FML-Neo** corticosteroid and aminoglycoside eyedrops containing 0.1% fluorometholone and 0.5% neomycin sulphate.

Used for: FML—eye inflammation in which there is an absence of infection. FML Neo—eye inflammation in which infection is present.

Dosage: adults, 1 to 2 drops 2, 3 or 4 times daily directly into eye; children over 2 years of age, as adult dose.

Special care: glaucoma; prolonged use in young children or pregnant women.

Avoid use: infections with tuberculous, viral or fungal origin and those in which pus is present; soft contact lenses.

Side effects: rise in pressure within eye, thinning of cornea, secondary fungal infection, cataract.

Manufacturer: Allergan.

Folicin

Description: a haematinic and mineral supplement available in the form of white, sugar-coated tablets containing 2.5mg folic acid, 2.5mg manganese sulphate and 200mg dried ferrous sulphate (equivalent to 60mg iron).

Used for: prevention and treatment of anaemia in pregnant women.

Dosage: adults, 1 to 2 tablets each day.

Avoid use: patients with megaloblastic anaemia.

Possible interaction: levodopa, tetracyclines.

Side effects: constipation, nausea.

Manufacturer: Link.

Forceval

Description: a preparation containing minerals, trace elements and vitamins produced in the form of brown/red gelatin capsules marked 6377 and FORCEVAL. Also, **Forceval Junior** available as oval brown gelatin capsules marked 571 and FORCEVAL.

Used for: a dietary supplement to prevent and treat mineral and vitamin deficiencies in patients unable to obtain adequate amounts from food alone. May be used, for example, in patients recuperating from serious illness or surgery, and those on special controlled diets or who have intolerance to foods.

Dosage: 1 capsule daily; children, Forceval Junior only, over 5 years of age, 2 capsules each day.

Avoid use: children under 5 years, patients with disorders of iron absorption and storage (haemochromatosis) or with hypercalcaemia.

Possible interaction: tetracyclines, anticoagulant drugs, phenytoin.

Manufacturer: Unigreg.

Fortagesic^{CD}

Description: a controlled drug combining a narcotic analgesic with paracetamol, which has analgesic and antipyretic properties (reduces fever). It is produced in the form of white tablets, marked with name and symbol, containing 15mg pentazocine (as hydrochloride) and 500mg paracetamol. Pentazocine is a moderately potent analgesic and is less likely to cause addiction than some other narcotic drugs.

Used for: pain caused by disorders of bone and muscle.

Dosage: 2 tablets up to 4 times each day; children over 7 years, 1 tablet every 3 to 4 hours with a maximum of 4 in 24 hours.

Special care: pregnancy, liver, kidney or respiratory diseases, porphyria.

Avoid use: patients with brain injury or disease, raised intracranial pressure or who are narcotic dependent.

Possible interaction: alcohol, other narcotic drugs, MAOIs.
Side effects: nausea, dizziness, sedation, drug-induced symptoms of psychosis.
Manufacturer: Sanofi Winthrop.

Fortral^{CD}

Description: a narcotic antagonist and controlled drug, produced in a variety of forms. White, film-coated tablets contain 25mg pentazocine hydrochloride, marked with symbol and name. **Fortral Capsules** marked FORTRAL 50 and coloured yellow/grey, contain 50mg. **Fortral Injection** contain 30mg pentazocine (as acetate) per ml in ampoules. **Fortral Suppositories** contain 50mg.
Used for: relief of pain.
Dosage: adults, tablets or capsules, 25–100mg after meals every 3 to 4 hours; injection, 30–60mg by intravenous, intramuscular or subcutaneous injection every 3 to 4 hours; suppositories, 1 when required with a maximum of 4 in 24 hours. Children, tablets or capsules, 6 to 12 years, 25mg every 3 to 4 hours. Injection, children 1 to 12 years, either a maximum of 1mg/kg body weight as single dose by subcutaneous or intramuscular injection, or 0.5mg/kg body weight given intravenously as single dose.
Special care: pregnancy, liver, kidney or respiratory diseases.
Avoid use: children under 1 year of age, patients with brain injury or disease, raised intracranial pressure, narcotic dependent or who have porphyria.
Possible interaction: other narcotic drugs, alcohol, MAOIs.
Side effects: nausea, dizziness, sedation, drug-induced symptoms of psychosis.
Manufacturer: Sterwin.

Fortrum

Description: a cephalosporin antibiotic preparation produced in the form of powder in vials for reconstitution and injection, containing 250mg 500mg, 1g, 2g and 3g ceftazidime (as pentahydrate).
Used for: urinary and gastrointestinal tract infections, infections of ear, nose and throat, joints, bones, soft tissues, skin, meningitis, septicaemia and infections in patients who are immunocompromised.
Dosage: adults, 1g every 8 hours or 2g at 12 hour intervals. If infection is extremely severe, 2g every 8 to 12 hours. Single doses above 1g should be given intravenously, lower doses by intravenous injection or infusion or intramuscularly. Children, 2 months

and under, 25–60mg/kg body weight in 2 divided doses each day; over 2 months, 30–100mg/kg body weight each day in 2 or 3 divided doses. A dose of up to 150mg/kg body weight may be given in cases of meningitis or if immunocompromised. In children, the intravenous route should be used. Elderly persons, a maximum dose of 3g each day depending upon type and severity of infection.
Special care: pregnant women, patients with allergy to penicillin (about 10% of whom are also allergic to cephalosporins), kidney disease.
Possible interaction: loop diuretics, aminoglycosides.
Side effects: gastrointestinal upset, pain at injection site, blood changes involving white blood cells, candidiasis (infection caused by yeast-like fungus), allergic reactions, positive Coombs test, rise in level of blood urea and liver enzymes.
Manufacturer: Glaxo.

Foscavir

Description: an antiviral preparation containing 24mg foscarnet sodium hexahydrate per ml produced as bottles of isotonic infusion.
Used for: life-threatening infections of viral origin particularly those of the eyes in patients with AIDS (cytomegalovirus retinitis).
Dosage: adults, 20mg/kg body weight by intravenous infusion over half an hour, then 21–200mg/kg body weight each day for 2 to 3 weeks. (Dose depending upon kidney function).
Special care: patients with kidney disease, hypocalcaemia. Blood tests are required during therapy and patient should receive adequate fluids.
Avoid use: patients with severe kidney disease, pregnancy, breast-feeding.
Side effects: rash, nausea, headache, vomiting, tiredness, disturbance of kidney function including kidney failure, decreased haemoglobin and calcium levels. Rarely, convulsions, inflamed veins, hypoglycaemia.
Manufacturer: Astra.

Fragmin

Description: an anticoagulant preparation which is a low molecular weight heparin produced as a solution in ampoules for injection and which contain 2500 units or 10,000 units dalteparin sodium per ml. **Fragmin Pre-Filled Syringes** contain 2500 units or 5000 units dalteparin sodium per 0.2ml.
Used for: prevention of thrombosis during and after surgery and clotting in extracorporeal circulation during dialysis treatment.
Dosage: dependent upon condition being treated

(i.e. surgery or dialysis) and if patient is at high or low risk of bleeding (dialysis).

Special care: pregnancy, breast-feeding, liver disease, those at high risk of bleeding or in whom therapeutic effects of drug occur in narrow dose range. Careful monitoring and blood checks required.

Possible interaction: cardiac glycosides, other anticoagulant and antiplatelet drugs, indomethacin, tetracyclines, probencid, antihistamines, dextran, sulphinpyrazone, aspirin, ethacrynic acid, vitamin K antagonists, cytostatics, dipyradamole, cardiac glycosides.

Side effects: bleeding if dose is high.

Manufacturer: Pharmacia.

Frisium

Description: an anxiolytic and anticonvulsant which is a long-acting benzodiazepine produced in the form of blue capsules containing 10mg clobazum and marked FRISIUM.

Used for: anxiety and tense and agitated states; additional therapy in the treatment of epilepsy.

Dosage: adults, 20–30mg each day in divided dose or as single bedtime dose with a maximum of 60mg daily. Elderly persons, 20 mg each day. Children, age 3 to 12 years, half adult dose.

Special care: pregnancy, women in labour, breast-feeding, elderl, liver or kidney disease. Short-term use and withdraw gradually.

Avoid use: patients with breathing difficulties, lung diseases and respiratory depression, those suffering from phobic, psychotic or obsessional psychiatric illnesses. Children under 3 years.

Possible interaction: other central nervous system depressant drugs, anticonvulsants, alcohol.

Side effects: gastrointestinal upset, light-headedness, disturbance of vision, vertigo, sleepiness, hypotension, confusion, rash, urine retention, reduced libido, ataxia. Rarely there may be blood changes and jaundice. Performance of skilled tasks and judgement is impaired, risk of dependence with higher doses and longer term therapy.

Manufacturer: Hoechst.

Froben

Description: an analgesic preparation which is a proprionic acid produced in the form of tablets of 2 strengths. Yellow, sugar-coated tablets contain 50mg and 100mg flurbiprofen, marked F50 and F100 respectively. Also **Froben SR** which are yellow, sustained-release capsules marked FSR containing 200mg flurbiprofen. **Froben Suppositories** contain 100mg flurbiprofen

Used for: pain including dysmenorrhoea (period pain) (Froben tablets); musculoskeletal diseases, osteoarthritis and ankylosing spondylitis (Froben SR and Suppositories).

Dosage: adults, tablets, 100–200mg each day in divided doses with a maximum daily dose of 300mg. SR Capsules, 1 each day after evening meal. Suppositories, 150mg—200mg each day as divided doses with a daily maximum of 300mg.

Special care: pregnancy, breast-feeding, elderly, liver or kidney disease, heart failure, asthma. Those taking the drug long-term require careful monitoring.

Avoid use: children, patients with allergy to aspirin or anti-inflammatory drugs, those with stomach ulcer or gastrointestinal bleeding.

Possible interaction: anticoagulant drugs, frusemide, quinolones.

Side effects: rash, intolerance of gastrointestinal system, rarely thrombocytopenia, jaundice.

Manufacturer: Boots.

Fru-Co

Description: a potassium-sparing and loop diuretic produced in the form of scored, orange tablets containing 40mg frusemide amd 5mg amiloride hydrochloride (co-amilofuse), marked FRO-CO.

Used for: oedema accompanying kidney or liver disease, heart failure.

Dosage: adults, 1 or 2 tablets taken in the morning.

Special care: pregnancy, breast-feeding, elderly, liver or kidney disease, enlarged prostate gland, difficulty in urination, gout, diabetes, acidosis.

Avoid use: children, hyperkalaemia, coma resulting from cirrhosis of the liver, progressive kidney failure.

Possible interaction: other potassium-sparing diuretics and potassium supplements, hypo-glycaemics, aminoglycosides, cephalosporins, lithium, antihypertensives, digitalis, NSAIDs, non-depolarizing muscle relaxants (anaesthetics), ACE inhibitors.

Side effects: rash, gastrointestinal upset, malaise; rarely, blood changes.

Manufacturer: Baker Norton.

Frumil

Description: a preparation which is a loop and potassium-sparing diuretic produced in the form of scored, orange tablets containing 40mg frusemide and 5mg amiloride hydrochloride (co-amilofruse) marked FRUMIL. Also **Frumil LS**, orange tablets containing 20mg frusemide and 2.5mg amiloride hydrochloride, marked LS. **Frumil Forte**, orange scored tablets containing 80mg frusemide and 10mg amiloride hydrochloride, marked DS.

Used for: oedema accompanying kidney or liver disease and heart failure.

Dosage: adults, Frumil tablets, 1 or 2 taken in morning; Frumil LS and Frumil Forte, 1 tablet taken in morning.

Special care: elderly, liver or kidney disease, enlarged prostate gland, difficulty in urination, gout, diabetes, acidosis.

Avoid use: children, pregnancy, breast-feeding, hyperkalaemia, coma resulting from cirrhosis of the liver, progressive kidney failure.

Possible interaction: other potassium-sparing diuretics and potassium supplements, ACE inhibitors, hypoglycaemics, antihypertensives, non-depolarizing muscle relaxants (anaesthetics), cardiac glycosides, NSAIDs, aminoglycosides, lithium, cephalosporins.

Side effects: rash, gastrointestinal upset, malaise; rarely, blood changes.

Manufacturer: Theraplix.

Frusene

Description: a potassium-sparing and loop diuretic produced in the form of scored yellow tablets containing 40mg frusemide and 50mg triamterene.

Used for: oedema accompanying liver or heart disease, congestive heart failure.

Dosage: adults, half to 2 tablets each day with a daily maximum of 6 (in divided doses).

Special care: pregnancy, breast-feeding mothers, gout, enlarged prostate gland, difficulty in urination, acidosis, liver or kidney disease, diabetes.

Avoid use: children, patients with coma resulting from liver cirrhosis, hyperkalaemia, progressive kidney failure.

Possible interaction: other potassium-sparing diuretics and potassium supplements, amino-glycosides, cardiac glycosides, neuromuscular blocking drugs, lithium, theophylline, NSAIDs, cephalosporins.

Side effects: rash, gastrointestinal upset, malaise; rarely, blood changes.

Manufacturer: Fisons.

Fucibet

Description: a potent steroid and antibacterial agent in the form of a cream containing 0.1% betmethasone valerate and 2% fusidic acid.

Used for: eczema in which bacterial infection is likely to be present.

Dosage: apply thinly 2 or 3 times each day to affected skin; reduce dose when condition improves.

Special care: short-term use only (maximum of few weeks when lower potency substitute should be tried, if needed), withdraw gradually.

Avoid use: children, extensive or longer-term use in pregnant women, infections due to ringworm, virus, tuberculosis, untreated bacterial and fungal infections, leg ulcers, scabies, acne.

Side effects: adrenal gland suppression, skin thinning, abnormal hair growth, skin changes as in Cushing's syndrome.

Manufacturer: Leo.

Fucidin H

Description: an antibacterial agent and mildly potent corticosteroid. It is available as ointment, cream or gel, all containing 2% sodium fusidate and 1% hydrocortisone.

Used for: dermatitis in which bacterial infection is likely to be present.

Dosage: apply thinly 2 or 3 times each day to affected skin and reduce dose when condition improves.

Special care: limit use in children or on face to a maximum period of 5 days.

Avoid use: extensive or long-term use especially in pregnant women, infections due to ringworm, virus, tuberculosis, untreated bacterial and fungal infections, leg ulcers, scabies, acne.

Side effects: adrenal gland suppression, skin thinning, abnormal hair growth, skin changes as in Cushing's syndrome.

Manufacturer: Leo.

Fucithalmic

Description: an antibacterial preparation produced in the form of an eye gel which becomes liquid when in contact with eye, containing 1% fusidic acid.

Used for: conjunctivitis where bacteria, especially staphylococci, are cause of infection.

Dosage: apply 1 drop into eye twice each day.

Side effects: allergic reaction, local irritation of short-lived nature.

Manufacturer: Leo.

Fulcin

Description: an antifungal preparation produced in the form of tablets of 2 strengths and as a solution. Scored, white tablets, marked ICI, contain 125mg and 500mg griseofulvin. **Fulcin Suspension** contains 125mg griseofulvin per 5ml of suspension.

Used for: fungal infections of scalp, skin and nails where ointments and creams have been ineffective or are not considered to be appropriate.

Dosage: adults, 125mg 4 times each day or a single

dose of 500mg. Children, 10mg/kg body weight in divided doses or as a single dose.

Avoid use: pregnancy, serious liver disease or porphyria.

Possible interaction: oral contraceptives, alcohol, barbiturates, anticoagulants of the coumarin group.

Side effects: allergic responses and rash, sensitivity to light, headache, stomach upset, blood changes involving white blood cells; rarely, a collagen disease.

Manufacturer: ICI.

Fungilin

Description: an antifungal preparation and polyene antibiotic, amphotericin, effective against filamentous and yeast-like fungi and which does not produce drug resistance. Fungilin is produced in the form of scored brown tablets containing 100mg and marked SQUIBB 430. **Fungilin Suspension** coloured yellow and containing 100mg per ml of solution. **Fungilin Lozenges** coloured yellow containing 10mg and marked SQUIBB 929.

Used for: candidiasis of the intestine, vagina and skin (thrush) and prevention of infection. Lozenges are used for mouth infections.

Dosage: adults, 1 to 2 tablets or 1–2ml suspension each day; lozenges, 1 dissolved slowly in mouth 4 to 8 times each day. Children, suspension, 1ml 4 times each day.

Side effects: gastrointestinal upset if dose is high.

Manufacturer: Squibb.

Fungizone

Description: an antifungal preparation and polyene antibiotic, effective against filamentous and yeast-like fungi and which does not produce drug resistance. It is produced as a powder in vials for reconstitution and injection containing 50mg amphotericin sodium desoxycholate complex.

Used for: serious, life-threatening systemic fungal infections.

Dosage: by intravenous infusion, 250 µs/kg body weight each day increasing to 1mg in cases of severe infection, if drug is tolerated. Maximum dose is 1.5mg/kg body weight each day or every other day.

Special care: produces toxic side effects when given in this way, hence patients require close monitoring of liver and kidney function, blood counts, electrolyte levels in blood plasma.

Special care: pregnancy, breast-feeding. Change injection site frequently.

Side effects: irritation at injection site, rash, vomiting, diarrhoea, nausea, headache, abdominal pain, anorexia, pain in muscles and joints, fever, adverse effects on liver, kidneys, heart, nerves,

convulsions, loss of hearing, anaphylactic-type allergic reactions.

Manufacturer: Squibb.

Furadantin

Description: an antibacterial preparation which is of a type known as nitofurans (synthetic antibiotic drugs). It is produced in the form of scored, yellow pentagonal-shaped tablets of 2 strengths containing 50mg and 100mg nitrofurantoin both marked with strength and name. Also **Furadantin Suspension** containing 25mg nitrofurantoin per 5ml suspension.

Used for: treatment and prevention of genital and urinary tract infections, (e.g. in patient undergoing surgery or exploratory procedure), pyelitis.

Dosage: adults, depending upon condition being treated, in the order of 50–100mg 4 times each day for 1 week (or once a day at bedtime if for prevention of infection on longer term basis). Children, age 3 months to 10 years, in the order of 3mg/kg body weight 4 times each day for 1 week or 1mg/kg once daily if for prevention. Over 10 years, same as adult.

Special care: children under 3 months, breast-feeding, elderly, patients with diabetes, vitamin B deficiency or who are debilitated, anaemia, imbalance of electrolyte (salt) levels. Patients should receive monitoring of liver and lung function if undergoing long-term treatment.

Avoid use: women at end of pregnancy, kidney disorder, anuria or oliguria.

Possible interaction: probenecid, quinolones, magnesium trisilicate, sulphinpyrazone.

Side effects: gastrointestinal upset, blood changes, allergic reactions. Drug should be stopped immediately if signs of peripheral nerve damage, lung disorder, breakdown of red blood cells (haemolysis), hepatitis occur.

Manufacturer: P. & G.P.

Fybogel Mebervine

Description: a bulking agent and antispasmodic preparation, produced in the form of effervescent granules in sachets for dissolving in water, containing 135mg mebeverine hydrochloride, 3.5g ispaghula husk.

Used for: irritable bowel syndrome, diverticular disease, constipation due to insufficient dietary fibre.

Dosage: adults, 1 sachet every morning and evening half an hour before meals in water. Additional sachet before midday meal may also be taken.

Avoid use: patients with intestinal obstruction, serious heart, circulatory and kidney disorders.

Manufacturer: Reckitt and Colman.

G

Galenamet

Description: a preparation that is an H$_2$-receptor antagonist which acts to reduce the secretion of stomach acid, thereby promoting the healing of ulcers. It is available in tablets of 3 strengths containing 200mg, 400mg and 800mg cimetidine.

Used for: gastrointestinal ulcers, Zollinger-Ellison syndrome, reflux oesophagitis.

Dosage: for ulcers, 400mg twice each day morning and night, or 800mg taken at night; occasionally, 400mg 4 times each day may be required with an absolute maximum of 2.4g daily in divided doses (in rare cases of stress ulceration). Zollinger-Ellison syndrome and reflux oesophagitis 400mg 4 times each day. Children, 20–30mg/kg body weight each day in divided doses.

Special care: pregnancy, breast-feeding, liver or kidney disease.

Possible interaction: phenytoin, warfarin, theophylline, some antidepressants, sulphonylureas, carbamazepine, some antifungal drugs, quinine, chloroquine, some antipsychotic drugs, benzodiazepines, ß-blockers, calcium channel blockers, cyclosporin, fluorouracil, flosequinan.

Side effects: rash, dizziness, fatigue, headache, confusion, change in bowel habit, lowered blood count, liver effects, allergic responses, bradycardia, pancreatitis, nephritis (inflammation in kidney), gynaecomastia, heart block. All are rare, but have been reported and may be more likely with higher doses.

Manufacturer: Galen.

Galenamox

Description: an antibiotic preparation of amoxycillin, a broad-spectrum penicillin but one which is inactivated by the penicillinase enzymes produced by some bacteria. Hence some infections do not respond as the bacteria causing them are resistant. Galenamox is available in the form of capsules of 2 strengths containing 250mg and 500mg amoxycillin (as trihydrate). Also as **Galenamox Suspension** containing 125mg or 250mg per 5ml solution.

Used for: middle ear infections, secondary infections in chronic bronchitis, urinary tract infections, gonorrhoea, typhoid fever, prevention of endocarditis.

Dosage: depending upon type of infection but in the order of 250mg–500mg every 8 hours with higher doses of 3g every 12 hours sometimes being required. Children, depending upon condition being treated but in the order of 125mg–250mg every 8 hours (up to 10 years of age). Higher doses may sometimes be needed.

Manufacturer: Galen.

Gamanil

Description: a TCAD preparation available as scored, maroon-coloured, film-coated tablets containing 70mg lofepramine (as hydrochloride).

Used for: depression.

Dosage: adults, 1 tablet in morning and either 1 or 2 at night. Reduced doses for elderly patients.

Special care: elderly, breast-feeding, glaucoma, urinary retention, hyperthyroidism, diabetes, adrenal gland tumour, epilepsy, certain psychiatric disorders or at risk of suicide. Regular blood tests should be carried out.

Avoid use: pregnancy, heart block, heart attack, serious liver disease.

Possible interaction: other antidepressants, antihypertensives, barbiturates, alcohol, MAOIs, cimetidine, local anaesthetics containing noradrenaline or adrenaline, oestrogens.

Side effects: blurred vision, hypotension, sweating, anxiety, dizziness, sleeplessness, ataxia, muscle weakness, drowsiness, palpitations, dry mouth, tachycardia, constipation, gastrointestinal upset, weight changes, allergic responses including skin rash, blood changes, loss of libido or impotence, enlargement of breasts, abnormal milk production, jaundice. Also psychiatric effects especailly in the elderly.

Manufacturer: Merck.

Gammabulin

Description: a preparation of 16% human normal

immunoglobulin (HNIG) as a solution for intramuscular injection.

Used for: immunization against hepatitis A, measles, rubella in pregnant women, antibody deficiency syndrome.

Dosage: prevention of hepatitis A, adults and children, 0.02–0.04ml/kg body weight and possibly 0.06–0.12ml/kg body weight if risk is great. Prevention of measles, 0.2ml/kg body weight. Prevention of rubella in pregnant women, 20ml. All given by intramuscular injection.

Possible interaction: live vaccines.

Manufacturer: Immuno.

Ganda

Description: an adrenergic neurone blocker with a sympathomimetic produced in the form of drops to reduce pressure within the eye. It is available in 2 strengths: **Ganda 1 + 0.2** contains 1% guanethidine monosulphate and 0.2% adrenaline; **Ganda 3 + 0.5** contains 3% guanethidine monosulphate and 0.5% adrenaline.

Used for: glaucoma.

Dosage: 1 drop into eye once or twice each day.

Special care: examination of eye for signs of damage to cornea and conjunctiva is required during long-term therapy, and drops should be withdrawn if this occurs.

Avoid use: narrow angle glaucoma, aphakia (a condition in which all or part of the lens of the eye is absent, usually due to surgical removal of a cataract).

Possible interaction: MAOIs.

Side effects: headache, discomfort in eye, skin reactions, melanosis (overproduction of the pigment melanin), initial rise in pressure within eye; rarely, other whole body (systemic) effects.

Manufacturer: Chauvin.

Garamycin

Description: an antibiotic preparation available in the form of drops containing 0.3% gentamicin (as sulphate).

Used for: external ear and eye infections.

Dosage: 3 to 4 drops 3 to 4 times each day.

Special care: patients with perforated ear drum (if being used to treat ear infections).

Avoid use: infections of viral, tuberculous or fungal origin or in which pus is present.

Side effects: superinfection, possible mild irritation of short-lived duration, blurred vision (eye infections).

Manufacturer: Schering-Plough.

Gastrobid Continus

Description: an antidopaminergic preparation used to treat gastrointestinal upset and available as white, sustained-release tablets containing 15mg metoclopramide hydrochloride marked with strength and NAPP.

Used for: hiatus hernia, reflux oesophagitis (where there is a backflow of acid stomach juice) duodenitis and gastritis (inflammation of duodenum and stomach), dyspepsia. Also, nausea and vomiting including that which may result from chemotherapy for cancer.

Dosage: adults over 20 years of age, 1 tablet twice each day.

Special care: pregnancy, breast-feeding, kidney disease.

Avoid use: children and young adults under 20 years, recent surgery of gastrointestinal tract, those with breast cancer which is prolactin-dependent or phaeochromocytoma.

Possible interaction: anticholinergic drugs, butyrophenones, phenothiazines.

Side effects: elevated prolactin levels in blood, extrapyramidal responses (concerned with reflex muscle movements of a stereotyped nature, e.g. knee jerk).

Manufacturer: Napp.

Gastromax

Description: an antidopaminergic preparation used to treat gastrointestinal upset and available as yellow/orange sustained-release capsules containing 30mg metoclopramide hydrochloride.

Used for: gastrointestinal disturbance and upset, nausea and vomiting including that which may be drug-induced (cancer chemotherapy).

Dosage: adults over 20 years of age and elderly persons, 1 tablet each day taken before a meal.

Special care: elderly persons and patients with kidney disease.

Avoid use: children and young adults under 20 years of age, pregnancy, breast-feeding, phaeochromo-cytoma.

Possible interaction: anticholinergic drugs, butyrophenones, phenothiazines.

Side effects: raised prolactin levels in blood, extrapyramidal responses (concerned with reflex muscle movements of a stereotyped nature, e.g. knee jerk).

Manufacturer: Pharmacia.

Gasrozepin

Description: an anticholinergic preparation (a selective antimuscarine drug) which acts to reduce the production and secretion of acid stomach juices. It is produced in the form of scored white tablets containing 50mg pirenzepine marked G over 50 and with manufacturer's logo.

Used for: stomach and duodenal ulcers.

Dosage: adults, 1 tablet twice each day taken thirty minutes before meals for a period of 1 month to 6 weeks. Maximum of 3 tablets each day in divided doses.

Special care: kidney disease.

Avoid use: children, pregnancy, closed angle glaucoma, enlarged prostate gland, paralytic ileus (a condition in which there is a reduction or absence of movement along the gastrointestinal tract, which may result from a number of different causes), pyloric stenosis.

Side effects: disturbance of vision and dry mouth; rarely, blood changes.

Manufacturer: Boots.

Genotropin

Description: a preparation of the synthetic human growth hormone, somatotropin, produced as a powder containing 4 units in vials (along with ampoules of solution for reconstitution). Various other preparations are available, e.g. **Genotropin Multidose, Genotropin Cartridges, Genotropin Kabivial Multidose** and **Genotropin Kabiquick**.

Used for: children in whom growth is stunted due to absence or reduced amount of pituitary growth hormone, Turner's syndrome.

Dosage: growth hormone deficiency, usual dose in the order of 0.5–0.7 units/kg body weight each week by subcutaneous injection. Turner's syndrome, 1 unit/kg body weight each week by subcutaneous injection.

Special care: patients with diabetes mellitus.

Avoid use: patients with closed epiphyses.

Manufacturer: Pharmacia.

Genticin

Description: an antibiotic and aminoglycoside preparation in the form of drops containing 0.3% gentamicin (as sulphate).

Used for: ear and eye bacterial infections.

Dosage: ear, 2, 3 or 4 drops 3 or 4 times each day; eye, 1 to 3 drops 3 or 4 times each day.

Special care: with ear infections in patients with perforated eardrum.

Side effects: superinfection (secondary infection); eye infections, slight irritation of eye which is short-lived, blurring of vision.

Manufacturer: Roche.

Gentisone HC

Description: a compound antibiotic and

corticosteroid in the form of eardrops containing 0.3% gentamicin (as sulphate) and 1% hydrocortisone acetate.

Used for: external and middle ear infections.

Dosage: 2 to 4 drops placed in ear 3 or 4 times each day and at bedtime. As an alternative, wicks dipped in the solution may be placed in the ear to deliver the dose.

Special care: pregnancy, limit use in young children, patients with perforated eardrum.

Side effects: superinfection (secondary infection).

Manufacturer: Roche.

Gestanin

Description: a hormonal preparation of a progestogen produced in the form of white tablets containing 5mg allyloestrenol and coded ORGANON and GK4.

Used for: recurrent or threatened miscarriage, threatened premature labour.

Dosage: recurrent miscarriage, 1 tablet 3 times each day as soon as there is confirmation of the pregnancy continuing until 1 month beyond the end of the risk period; threatened premature labour, up to 8 tablets each day according to response.

Avoid use: patients with liver disease.

Side effects: nausea.

Manufacturer: Organon.

Gestone

Description: a hormonal preparation of a progestogen produced in ampoules for injection in 2 strengths, containing 25mg and 50mg progesterone/ml. Also, as 2ml ampoules containing 100mg progesterone.

Used for: maintenace of pregnancy in early stages in women with history of spontaneous abortion.

Dosage: adults, 25–100mg each day by deep intramuscular injection from fifteenth day of pregnancy to eighth to sixteenth week.

Special care: patients with migraine, epilepsy, diabetes.

Avoid use: patients with breast cancer, history of thrombosis, liver disease, vaginal bleeding which is undiagnosed.

Manufacturer: Paines and Byrne.

Glaucol

Description: a ß-blocker produced in the form of an eye solution in single dose vials of 2 strengths containing 0.25% and 0.5% timolol (as maleate).

Used for: open angle glaucoma, secondary glaucoma, hypertension within the eye.

Dosage: adults, 1 drop of lower strength solution

twice each day increasing to higher strength if necessary.

Special care: pregnancy, breast-feeding, elderly. Withdraw drops gradually.

Avoid use: patients with heart block, bradycardia, asthma, history of obstructive lung disease.

Possible interaction: antihypertensive drugs, adrenaline, verapamil.

Side effects: irritation of eye, absorption into blood may cause other systemic (whole body) ß-blocker side effects, e.g. disturbance of sleep, cold hands and feet, fatigue on exercise, bradycardia, gastrointestinal upset, heart failure, bronchospasm.

Manufacturer: Baker Norton.

Glibenese

Description: a sulphonylurea drug produced in the form of scored, oblong, white tablets containing 5mg glipizide and marked Pfizer and GBS/5.

Used for: maturity-onset diabetes.

Dosage: adults, 2.5mg–5mg each day taken either before breakfast or lunch. Dose may be increased if required by 2.5–5mg daily every third, fourth or fifth day with a maximum of 40mg each day. Doses in excess of 15mg daily should be taken before meals as divided doses. Usual maintenance dose is in the order of 2.5–30mg depending upon response.

Special care: elderly, kidney failure.

Avoid use: children, pregnancy, breast-feeding, other forms of diabetes including unstable brittle diabetes, growth-onset diabetes, juvenile diabetes, ketoacidosis (an accumulation of ketones within the body due to diabetes), infections, serious kidney or liver disease. Also, patients suffering from stress, infections or undergoing suregery.

Possible interaction: sulphonamides, anticoagulants taken orally, corticotrophin, corticosteroids, aspirin, rifampicin, glucagon, oral contraceptives, MAOIs, alcohol, chloramphenicol, ß-blockers, clofibrate, bezafibrate, diuretics, chloro-propamide, metformin, acetohexamide.

Side effects: allergic reactions, skin rash.

Manufacturer: Pfizer.

Glucagon

Description: a hyperglycaemic preparation produced as a powder in vials along with diluent for reconstitution and injection. Glucagon is produced by Lilly as 1.09mg glucagon hydrochloride and by Novo as 1mg glucagon hydrochloride.

Used for: patients in whom blood sugar level has fallen to seriously low levels (e.g. diabetics taking insulin) and who have become unconscious.

Dosage: 0.5mg–1mg by intravenous, intramuscular or subcutaneous injection in patients who cannot be roused enough to take glucose or sucrose by mouth. If patient still does not wake up, an intravenous dose of glucose should be given.

Special care: pregnancy, breast-feeding.

Avoid use: phaeochromocytoma, pancreatic tumours (glucagonoma or insulinoma).

Possible interaction: warfarin.

Side effects: gastrointestinal upset, diarrhoea, nausea, vomiting, allergic responses, hypokalaemia.

Manufacturer: Lilly and Novo.

Glucobay

Description: an oral hypoglycaemic preparation which acts to inhibit the activity of the digestive enzyme, alpha-glucosidase, which breaks down carbohydrates. It is produced in the form of off-white tablets of 2 strengths containing 50mg and 100mg acarbose and marked G50 or G100 respectively and with Bayer logo.

Used for: additional therapy (or on its own) in diabetes which is non-insulin dependent and is not completely controlled by diet or oral hypoglycaemics.

Dosage: adults, 50mg 3 times each day at first for 6 to 8 weeks increasing to 100mg 3 times daily if required. The maximum dose is 200mg 3 times each day.

Special care: with maximum dose, the level of liver enzyme, hepatic transaminase, should be carefully monitored. Also monitor patients receiving hypoglycaemics.

Avoid use: pregnancy, breast-feeding, various disorders of the gastrointestinal tract including inflammation of the bowel, obstruction of intestine, ulceration of colon, disorders of absorption.

Possible interaction: pancreatic enzymes, adsorbent agents, cholestyramine, neomycin.

Side effects: flatulence, feeling of bloatedness, diarrhoea, pain in abdomen.

Manufacturer: Bayer.

Glucophage

Description: a biguanide antidiabetic drug available as white, film-coated tablets of 2 strengths containing 500mg and 850mg of metformin hydrochloride and marked with strength and GL.

Used for: additional therapy with sulphonylureas in maturity-onset diabetes, or on its own. Also, as additional therapy in insulin-dependent diabetes, particularly in overweight patients.

Dosage: 500mg twice each day in first instance or 850mg taken with meals. Dose may be gradually increased if needed to a daily maximum of 3g and then should be reduced for maintenance. Normal maintenance dose is in the order of three 500mg or two 850mg doses each day.

Special care: elderly, kidney failure.

Avoid use: pregnancy, breast-feeding, other forms of diabetes including growth-onset, juvenile, unstable brittle diabetes, ketoacidosis (excess amount of ketones in body), infections, hormonal disorders, stress, serious kidney or liver disease, patients undergoing surgery.

Possible interaction: MAOIs, sulphonamides, anticoagulants taken by mouth, corticotrophin, corticosteroids, aspirin, rifampicin, glucagon, oral contraceptives, alcohol, chloramphenicol, ß-blockers, clofibrate, bezafibrate, diuretics, chloropropamide, metformin, acetohexamide.

Side effects: allergic reactions, skin rash.

Manufacturer: Lipha.

Glurenorm

Description: sulphonylurea available as scored, white tablets containing 30mg gliquidone and marked G.

Used for: maturity-onset diabetes.

Dosage: in the order of 45–600mg each day in divided doses before meals. Maximum dose is 180mg each day.

Special care: elderly persons, patients with kidney failure.

Avoid use: pregnancy, breast-feeding, other forms of diabetes including growth-onset, juvenile, unstable brittle diabetes, ketoacidosis (excess amount of ketones in body as a result of diabetes detected by smell of acetone on breath), infections, hormonal disorders, stress, serious kidney or liver disease, patients undergoing surgery.

Possible interaction: MAOIs, sulphonamides, anticoagulants taken by mouth, corticotrophin, corticosteroids, aspirin, rifampicin, glucagon, oral contraceptives, alcohol, chloramphenicol, ß-blockers, clofibrate, bezafibrate, diuretics, chloropropamide, metformin, acetohexamide.

Side effects: allergic reactions, skin rash.

Manufacturer: Sanofi Winthrop.

Glypressin

Description: a vasopressin analogue, produced as a powder in vials containing 1mg terlipressin, along with diluent for reconstitution and injection.

Used for: bleeding varicose veins in the oesophagus.

Dosage: adults, 2mg given by intravenous bolus injection (a dose given all at once) followed by further 1 or 2mg doses 4, 5 or 6 hours later for a maximum period of 72 hours.

Special care: patients with various heart conditions including weak heart, arrhythmias, and also serious atherosclerosis or hypertension. Blood levels of electrolytes (salts), fluid balance and blood pressure require careful monitoring.

Avoid use: pregnancy.

Side effects: hypertension, paleness, headache, cramps in abdomen.

Manufacturer: Ferring.

Gonadotrophin L.H.

Description: a hormonal preparation available as a powder in ampoules, with solvent for reconstitution and injection. It is available at various strengths containing 500 units, 1000 units and 5000 units of chorionic gonadotrophin.

Used for: in males, delayed puberty, failure of the testes to descend into the scrotum (cryptorchidism), a reduced amount of spermatozoa in the semen (oligospermia), a cause of infertility. In females, infertility caused by a lack of ovulation.

Dosage: boys, 7 to 10 years, 500 units 3 times each week given by injection for a period of 6 to 10 weeks. Adults, as directed by physician. Women, 10,000 units by injection in middle of monthly cycle following therapy to stimulate maturation of ovarian follicles.

Special care: heart or kidney disease, asthma, migraine or epilepsy.

Side effects: fatigue, headache, oedema, allergic reactions; young boys may become sexually precocious.

Manufacturer: Paines and Byrne.

Gopten

Description: an antihypertensive preparation and ACE inhibitor available as capsules of 3 strengths. Yellow/red, orange/red and red/red capsules contain 0.5mg, 1mg and 2mg trandolapril respectively.

Used for: hypertension.

Dosage: adults, 0.5mg once each day in first instance, then doubling at 2 to 4 week intervals. The maximum single dose is 4mg each day with a maintenance dose of 1–2mg once daily.

Special care: any diuretics should be stopped 2 or 3 days before treatment begins. Special care in patients undergoing anaesthesia or surgery, those with congestive heart failure, liver or kidney disease, having kidney dialysis. Kidney function should be monitored before starting and during therapy.

Avoid use: children, pregnancy, breast-feeding, obstruction of heart outflow or aortic stenosis. Those with angioneurotic oedema, caused by previous treatment with ACE inhibitors.

Possible interaction: NSAIDs, potassium-sparing diuretics.

Side effects: headache, cough, rash, giddiness, weakness, palpitations, hypotension. Rarely there may be depression of bone marrow, blood changes (agranulocytosis—characterized by serious deficiency of certain white blood cells), angioneurotic oedema.

Manufacturer: Knoll.

Graneodin

Description: a broad-spectrum aminoglycoside antibiotic preparation available as an ointment containing 0.25% neomycin sulphate and 0.025% gramicidin.

Used for: minor bacterial infections of the skin and prevention of infection during minor surgery.

Dosage: apply ointment to affected area 2, 3 or 4 times daily.

Special care: dressings should not be used and ointment is not suitable for large areas of damaged skin.

Avoid use: persistent, more deep-rooted infections.

Side effects: toxic effects on tissues and organs, sensitization.

Manufacturer: Squibb.

Granocyte

Description: a drug containing recombinant granulocyte stimulating factor produced as a powder in vials, along with solution, for reconstitution and injection. It contains 263 µg lenograstim (recombinant human granulocyte-colony stimulating factor).

Used for: neutropenia in patients who have had bone marrow transplants, or cytotoxic cancer chemotherapy.

Dosage: adults, bone marrow transplant patients, 150 micrograms/m² body surface by subcutaenous infusion over half-hour period each day. Therapy should begin the day after transplantation and continue until conditon improves, for a maximum period of 28 days. Cancer therapy, 150 micrograms/m² body surface each day by subcutaneous injection, starting the day after chemotherapy has finished. Continue until condition improves for a maximum period of 28 days. Children over 2 years, same as adult dose.

Special care: pregnancy, breast-feeding, precancerous myeloid (bone marrow) conditions, serious kidney or liver disease. Regular blood counts and checks should be carried out.

Avoid use: children under 2 years of age, patients with myeloid growths.

Side effects: pain at injection site and in bones.

Manufacturer: Chugai Pharma UK Limted/Rhône-Poulenc Rorer Limited.

Gregoderm

Description: an antibacterial, antifungal and mildly potent steroid preparation available in the form of an ointment containing 2,720 units neomycin sulphate, 100,000 units nystatin, 100,000 units polymixin B sulphate and 10mg hydrocortisone/g.

Used for: inflammation of the skin where infection is also present, psoriasis, itching in anal and urogenital areas.

Dosage: apply ointment 2 or 3 times each day to affected area.

Special care: use should be limited in children, infants and on face to a maximum period of 5 days. Should be gradually withdrawn after longer-term use.

Avoid use: extensive or long-term use in pregnancy or for prevention of skin conditions. Patients with acne, or skin infections with tuberculous or viral origin, leg ulcers, ringworm, scabies, dermatitis in region of mouth, any untreated bacterial or fungal infections.

Side effects: skin thinning, suppression of adrenal glands, abnorml hair growth, changes as in Cushing's syndrome.

Manufacturer: Unigreg.

Grisovin

Description: an antifungal preparation available in the form of white, film-coated tablets of 2 strengths containing 125mg and 500mg griseofulvin both marked with name, strength and manufacturer's name.

Used for: fungal infections of nails, skin and scalp, especially those not suitable for treatment with topical preparations.

Dosage: adults, 500mg–1g each day in divided doses after meals. Dose should not fall below 10mg/kg body weight. Children, 10mg/kg body weight each day as divided doses.

Special care: pregnancy, long-term use.

Avoid use: patients with serious liver disease, porphyria, systemic lupus erythematosus (SLE), a rare collagen disease.

Possible interaction: anticoagulants of the coumarin type, oral contraceptives, alcohol, barbiturates.

Manufacturer: Glaxo.

Gyno-Daktarin 1

Description: an antifungal and antibacterial preparation, micronazole nitrate, produced in a variety of forms: white, soft vaginal capsules

contain 1200mg; **Gyno-Daktarin Pessaries** contain 100mg per pessary; **Gyno-Daktarin Combipak** consists of 14 pessaries plus cream; **Gyno-Daktarin Cream** contains 2% per 78g with applicator.
Used for: candidiasis (thrush) of the vagina or vulva.
Dosage: adults, capsules, 1 at night, inserted into vagina as single dose. Pessaries, 1 inserted twice each day for 7 days. Combipak, 1 pessary and 1 application of cream inserted twice each day. Cream, 1 applicatorful of cream inserted twice each day for 7 days. Male sexual partner should also apply cream twice daily for 7 days.
Side effects: slight burning or discomfort of short-lived nature.
Manufacturer: Janssen.

Gyno-Pevaryl 1
Description: an antifungal preparation available as vaginal pessaries or cream or as a combination of both, all containing econazole nitrate. **Gyno-Pevaryl Pessaries** contain 150mg; **Gyno-Pevaryl Cream** contains 1% in 15g. Also available, **Gyno-Pevaryl 1 Combipak** (1 pessary and 15g cream); **Gyno-Pevaryl Combipak** (3 pessaries, 15g cream).
Used for: vulvitis (inflammation of vulva), vaginitis (inflammation of vagina), treatment of sexual partner in order to prevent reinfection.
Dosage: adults, pessaries, 1 inserted at night as single dose or for 3 consecutive nights; cream, apply twice each day for 2 weeks.
Side effects: slight burning or discomfort of short-lived nature.
Manufacturer: Cilag.

H

Haelan

Description: a moderately potent steroid preparation available as cream and ointment containing 0.0125% flurandrenolone. Also, **Haelan C** (combining the steroid with an antibacterial/antifungal agent), which also contains 3% clioquinol as cream and ointment. **Haelan Tape** is a clear, adhesive polythene film impregnated with 4 μg/cm².

Used for: inflammatory skin conditions which are responsive to steroids. Haelan C is used when infection is present.

Dosage: cream or ointment, apply 2 or 3 times each day to clean skin. Tape, apply to affected area and leave in place for 12 hours.

Special care: Haelan C may stain clothing and skin; use in children or on face should be limited to a maximum period of 5 days. Short-term use and withdraw slowly if use has been more prolonged.

Avoid use: extensive or prolonged use in pregnancy or continuous use as preventative measure, patients with untreated bacterial or fungal infections, acne, leg ulcers, scabies, skin disease of tuberculous or viral origin, ringworm, dermatitis in area of mouth. (Haelan C is, however, used for some infected conditions).

Side effects: adrenal gland suppression, skin thinning, abnormal hair growth, skin changes as in Cushing's syndrome.

Manufacturer: Dista.

Halciderm

Description: a very potent topical steroid preparation available in the form of a cream containing 0.1% halcinomide.

Used for: inflammatory skin conditions responsive to steroids.

Dosage: apply to affected area 2 or 3 times each day.

Special care: should not be used for more than 5 days, short-term use only and a milder substitute should be tried as soon as possible.

Avoid use: children, extensive or prolonged use, especially in pregnancy or as a preventative measure. Avoid use in patients with untreated bacterial or fungal infections, acne, leg ulcers, scabies, skin disease of tuberculous or viral origin, ringworm, dermatitis in area of mouth.

Side effects: adrenal gland suppression, skin thinning, abnormal hair growth, skin changes as in Cushing's syndrome.

Manufacturer: Dista.

Haldol Decanoate

Description: an antipsychotic drug, haloperidol (as decanoate), which is a depot butyrophenone available in ampoules for injection at 2 strengths containing 50mg/ml and 100mg/ml. Also, **Haldol Tablets** of 2 strengths, blue, coded H5, containing 5mg and yellow, coded H10, containing 10mg. Both are marked Janssen and also scored. **Haldol Oral Liquid** containing 2mg/ml and 10mg/ml and **Haldol Injection** containing 5mg/ml.

Used for: Haldol decanoate, long-term sedative treatment for various forms of psychiatric illness including psychoses, schizophrenia, disturbed behaviour. Other preparations: mania, schizophrenia, psychoses, symptoms precipitated by alcohol withdrawal; delirium tremens. Also used as pre-anaesthetic sedative for anxiety, vomiting and nausea and disturbed behaviour in children.

Dosage: Haldol decanoate, adults only, usual dose in order of 50mg–300mg by deep intramuscular injection once each month. Other oral preparations, adults, 0.5mg–5mg 2 or 3 times each day depending upon condition being treated. Dose may be gradually increased if needed to a daily maximum of 200mg and then should be reduced for maintenance. Haldol injection, for psychoses, 2–30mg by intramuscular injection followed by further dose of 5mg at 1 to 8 hour intervals until condition improves. Children, oral preparations, 0.05mg/kg body weight each day in 2 divided doses.

Special care: pregnancy, breast-feeding, serious heart and circulatory disease, kidney or liver failure, Parkinson's disease, epilepsy.

Avoid use: patients in states of coma.

Possible interaction: rifampicin, carbamazepine, lithium, alcohol.

Side effects: hypotension, pallor, drowsiness, tachycardia, palpitations, nightmares, hypothermia, disturbance of sleep, depression, dry mouth, blocked nose, difficulty in urination, blurring of vision, changes in menstruation, breasts and weight, blood changes, ECG and EEG changes, jaundice, skin reactions.
Manufacturer: Janssen.

Halfan

Description: an antimalarial preparation which is a phenanthrene drug, produced in the form of scored, capsule-shaped, white tablets, marked HALFAN, containing 250mg halofantrine hydrochloride.
Used for: treatment of malaria caused by *Pllasmodium vivax* and *Plasmodium falciparum*.
Dosage: adults, 6 tablets taken at 6 hour intervals in 3 divided doses. The dose is repeated 1 week later in patients who are not immune. Tablets should not be taken with meals. Children, over 37kg in weight, same as adult.
Special care: women who may become pregnant, patients with malarial complications or malaria affecting the brain.
Avoid use: pregnancy, breast-feeding, children under 37kg in weight, patients with some forms of heart disease. Not to be used as a preventative for malaria.
Possible interaction: TCADs, antiarrhythmic drugs, astemizole, neuroleptic drugs, terfenadine, chloroquine, quinine, mefloquine.
Side effects: heart arrhythmia, pain in abdomen, gastrointestinal upset, a short-lived rise in transaminase enzymes in the blood.
Manufacturer: S.K. & F.

Hamarin

Description: a xanthine oxidase inhibitor produced in the form of scored, white tablets containing 300mg allopurinol and marked with name, strength and triangle symbol. Allopurinol acts on the enzyme xanthine oxidase which converts the substances xanthine and hypoxanthine into uric acid. Hence the levels of uric acid in the blood are reduced and there is less likelihood of an attack of gout.
Used for: treatment of gout, prevention of stones formed from uric acid or calcium oxalate.
Dosage: adults, usual single dose in the order of 100mg–300mg each day increasing for prevention to a maintenance dose in the range 200–600mg daily.
Special care: pregnancy, elderly, liver or kidney disease. When treatment starts, an anti-inflammatory drug or colchicine should be taken for

4 weeks and the patient should drink plenty of fluids.
Avoid use: children, acute gout.
Possible interaction: chloropamide, azanthioprine, mercatopurine, anticoagulant drugs.
Side effects: acute gout, nausea, drug should be stopped in the event of skin rash occurring.
Manufacturer: Roche.

Harmogen

Description: a hormonal oestrogen preparation produced in the form of long, peach-coloured, scored tablets containing 1.5mg piperazine oestrone sulphate and marked LV.
Used for: hormonal replacement therapy in menopausal women and prevention of osteoporosis following menopause.
Dosage: adults, 1 to 2 tablets each day, along with a progestogen preparation for the last 10 to 13 days of each 28 day cycle in women who have not had a hysterectomy.
Special care: patients considered to be at risk of thrombosis or with liver disease. Women with any of the following disorders should be carefully monitored: fibroids in the womb, multiple sclerosis, diabetes, tetany, porphyria, epilepsy, liver disease, hypertension, migraine, otosclerosis, gallstones. Breasts, pelvic organs and blood pressure should be checked at regular intervals during the course of treatment.
Avoid use: pregnancy, breast-feeding, women with conditions which might lead to thrombosis, thrombophlebitis, serious heart, kidney or liver disease, breast cancer, oestrogen-dependent cancers including those of reproductive system, endometriosis, vaginal bleeding which is undiagnosed.
Possible interaction: drugs which induce liver enzymes.
Side effects: tenderness and enlargement of breasts, weight gain, breakthrough bleeding, giddiness, vomiting and nausea, gastrointestinal upset. Treatment should be halted immediately if severe headaches occur, disturbance of vision, hypertension or any indications of thrombosis, jaundice. Also, in the event of pregnancy and 6 weeks before planned surgery.
Manufacturer: Upjohn.

Havrix Monodose

Description: a preparation of inactivated hepatitis A virus HM available in pre-filled syringes containing 1440 ELISA units/ml adsorbed on aluminium hydroxide. **Havrix Original**, pre-filled 1ml syringes containing 720 ELISA units/ml of hepatitis A virus HM 175 strain adsorbed on aluminium hydroxide. Also, **Havrix Junior**, pre-filled 0.5ml syringes containing 720 ELISA units/ml of hepatitis A virus HM 175 strain adsorbed on aluminium hydroxide.

Used for: immunization against hepatitis A virus.

Dosage: adults and children age 16 and over, Havrix Monodose, primary immunization, 1 intramuscular injection of 1ml followed by repeated dose 6 to 12 months later. Havrix original, primary immunization, 1 intramuscular injection of 1ml followed by repeated doses after 2 to 4 weeks and 6 to 12 months. Children under 16 years, Havrix junior only, age 1 to 15 years, primary immunization, 0.5ml by intramuscular injection followed by repeated doses 2 to 4 weeks and 6 to 12 months later.

Special care: pregnancy, breast-feeding, infections, dialysis or with lowered immunity. Patients with bleeding disorders may need subcutaneous injection.

Avoid use: patients with severe fever, children under 1 year.

Possible interaction: nausea, fatigue, malaise, soreness and skin reactions at injection site, appetite loss.

Manufacturer: Smith Kline Beecham.

Hemabate

Description: a prostaglandin preparation produced in ampoules for injection containing 250µg carboprost as trometamol salt/ml.

Used for: haemorrhage following childbirth in patients who have not responded to other drugs (oxytocin and ergometrine).

Dosage: 1 deep intramuscular injection of 250 micrograms which may be repeated after 1 ½ hours. If the condition is very severe, repeat dose can be given after 15 minutes. Maximum total dose is 12mg.

Special care: patients with hypertension, hypotension, history of glaucoma or hypertension in eye, diabetes, asthma, jaundice, epilepsy, previous uterine injury (high doses may cause rupture of uterus).

Avoid use: patients with heart, liver, kidney or lung disease, pelvic inflammatory disease.

Side effects: gastrointestinal upset, vomiting, nausea, diarrhoea, flushing, high temperature (hyperthermia), bronchospasm. Rarely, chills, headache, fluid in lungs, sweating, giddiness, pain and skin changes at injection site.

Manufacturer: Upjohn.

Heminevrin

Description: a hypnotic, sedative preparation produced in the form of capsules and as a syrup. Grey-brown capsules contain 192mg chlormethiazole in miglyol, 1 capsule being equivalent to 5ml of syrup. Syrup contains 250mg chlormethiazole edisylate/5ml.

Used for: insomnia in elderly persons, short-lived therapy only. Sedation in elderly patients with senile psychosis, anxiety, confusion, disturbance of sleep, tension, alcohol withdrawal.

Dosage: adults, capsules, 2 at bedtime or 1 three times each day for sedation. Syrup, 10ml in drink at bedtime or three 5ml doses through day for sedation. For alcohol withdrawal symptoms, 3 capsules 4 times each day reducing over 6 days to nil.

Special care: lung, liver or kidney disease.

Avoid use: breast-feeding, children, serious lung disease.

Possible interaction: other central nervous system sedatives, alcohol.

Side effects: blocked and sore nose, sore eyes, gastrointestinal upset, sedation, judgement and performance of skilled tasks (e.g. driving) is impaired, confusion, agitation, anaphylactic type allergic reactions.

Manufacturer: Astra.

Heminevrin I-V Infusion

Description: an anticonvulsant sedative preparation available as a solution for infusion containing 8mg chlormethiazole edisylate/ml.

Used for: status epilepticus (a life-threatening condition characterized by continuous convulsions which can cause irreversible brain damage and a dangerous imbalance in the level of salts in the body), pre-eclamptic toxaemia (an abnormal condition which may arise in pregnancy).

Dosage: adults, 60 drops per minute until patient is sedated and then 10–15 drops per minute. Status epilepticus, 40–100ml over a period of 5 to 10 minutes, all by rapid infusion. Children, status epilepticus, 80 µg/kg body weight (0.01ml) per minute at first, with increase if required every 2 to 4 hours until condition is under control. Then dose is gradually reduced unless seizures recur.

Special care: patients with lung disorder or history of obstructive lung disease.

Avoid use: breast-feeding, patients with severe lung disorders.

Possible interaction: central nervous system, sedatives, alcohol.

Side effects: blocked and sore nose, sore eyes,

sedation, confusion, agitation, gastrointestinal upset. Judgement and the ability to perform skilled tasks is impaired.
Manufacturer: Astra.

Herpid

Description: an antiviral preparation available as a solution containing 5% idoxuridine in dimethyl sulphoxide.
Used for: skin infections caused by *herpes zoster* and *herpes simplex*.
Dosage: adults, apply solution (with applicator brush) 4 times each day for a period of 4 days.
Avoid use: pregnancy, breast-feeding.
Manufacturer: Yamanouchi.

Hibtiter

Description: a preparation of inactivated surface antigen consisting of polysaccharide from the capsule of *H. influenzae* type B joined to diphtheria protein.
Used for: immunization against meningitis, epiglottitis and other diseases caused by *H. influenzae* type B.
Dosage: children only, aged 2 months to 1 year, 3 intramuscular injections of 0.5ml at 4 week intervals, normally along with diphtheria, tetanus, polio immunization.
Special care: same vaccine must be used throughout course of immunization.
Avoid use: children with acute infections.
Side effects: possible skin reaction (reddening) at injection site.
Manufacturer: Lederle.

Honvan

Description: a hormonal oestrogen preparation available in ampoules for injection and also in the form of tablets, both containing tetrasodium fosfesterol which is converted to stilboestrol by enzyme activity. The ampoules contain 276mg tetrasodium fosfesterol/5ml and white tablets contain 100mg.
Used for: cancer of the prostate gland.
Dosage: adults, injection, 552–1104mg by slow intravenous injection daily for a minimum of 5 days. Then 276mg 1 to 4 times each week for maintenance. Tablets, for maintenance, 100–200mg 3 times each day then reducing to 100–300mg in divided doses as daily dose.
Special care: patients with liver disease.
Side effects: thrombosis, oedema, nausea, gynaecomastia, impotence, pain in perineal area.
Manufacturer: ASTA Medica.

Hormonin

Description: a hormonal oestrogen preparation available in the form of scored, pink tablets containing 0.27mg oestriol, 1.4mg oestrone and 0.6mg oestradiol.
Used for: hormone replacement therapy in women with menopausal symptoms, prevention of osteoporosis after menopause.
Dosage: 1 to 2 tablets each day, with a progestogen for last 12 or 13 days of 28 day cycle unless patient has had a hysterectomy.
Special care: women at risk of thrombosis or with liver disorder—liver function should be monitored. Women with any of the following should also receive careful monitoring: otosclerosis, porphyria, fibroids in the uterus, epilepsy, migraine, multiple sclerosis, diabetes, hypertension, tetany, gallstones. Blood pressure, pelvic organs and breasts should be checked regularly during the course of treatment.
Avoid use: pregnancy, breast-feeding, breast cancer, cancer of reproductive system or any hormone-dependent cancer, serious heart, liver or kidney disease, any conditions likely to lead to thrombosis, Rotor or Dublin-Johnson syndrome, endometriosis or vaginal bleeding of unknown cause.
Possible interaction: drugs which induce liver enzymes.
Side effects: breast enlargement and soreness, weight gain, nausea, vomiting, gastrointestinal upset, headache, giddiness, breakthrough bleeding.
Manufacturer: Shire.

Humatrope

Description: a synthetic growth hormone available as powder in ampoules, with diluent for reconstitution and injection, containing 4 units or 16 units of somatropin (rbe).
Used for: failure of growth in children due to lack of growth hormone, Turner's syndrome.
Dosage: children, deficiency of growth hormone, either 0.07 units/kg body-weight each day or 0.16 units/kg body-weight 3 times each week, all by intramuscular or subcutaneous injection. Turner's syndrome, 0.8–0.9 units/kg body-weight each week in 6 or 7 doses given by intramuscular or subcutaneous injection.
Special care: children with diabetes, intracranial lesion (damaged tissue within cranium), a deficiency of ACTH (adrenocorticotrophic hormone—an adrenal gland hormone). Thyroid function should be monitored during the course of therapy.
Avoid use: patients with tumour, fused epiphyses, pregnancy, breast-feeding.
Manufacturer: Lilly.

Humegon

Description: a combined preparation of human menopausal gonadotrophins (HMG) available as powder in ampoules with solvent in 2 strengths. 75 units HMG (equivalent to 75 units of follicle-stimulating hormone (FSH) and 75 units luteinizing hormone (LH)) and 150 units HMG (equivalent to 150 units FSH and 150 units LH).

Used for: male and female infertility due to a lack of gonadotrophin resulting in insufficient stimulation of the gonads (sex organs). Also, for stimulation of ovaries to produce excess eggs for IVF (*in vitro* fertilization).

Dosage: males and females, by intramus-cular injection, according to individual's requirements as directed by physician.

Special care: males and females, exclude all other causes of infertility. Females, monitor size of ovaries and levels of oestrogen during the course of therapy.

Avoid use: tumours of the pituitary gland, testes and ovaries.

Side effects: skin rashes, risk of miscarriage and multiple pregnancy.

Manufacturer: Organon.

Hydergine

Description: a cerebral activator-ergot alkaloid available as scored, white tablets containing 1.5mg or 4.5mg codergocrine mesylate both marked with strength and name.

Used for: additional therapy in the treatment of moderate dementia in elderly persons.

Dosage: adults, 4.5mg each day.

Special care: severe bradycardia.

Avoid use: children.

Side effects: blocked nose, rash, flushing, headache, pain in abdomen, giddiness, hypotension, when rising from lying down (postural hypotension).

Manufacturer: Sandoz.

Hydrea

Description: a DNA reactive cytotoxic drug available as pink/green capsules containing 500mg hydroxyurea marked SQUIBB and 830.

Used for: treatment of chronic myeloid leukaemia.

Dosage: 20–30mg/kg body weight each day or 80mg/kg body weight every third day.

Side effects: nausea, vomiting, skin rashes, bone marrow suppression.

Manufacturer: Squibb.

Hydrenox

Description: a thiazide diuretic preparation available as scored white tablets containing 50mg hydroflumethazide marked H inside a hexagon shape.

Used for: hypertension, oedema.

Dosage: adults, for oedema, 50–200mg as a single dose taken in the morning, in first instance, then reducing to a 25mg–50mg maintenance dose taken on alternate days. For hypertension, 25mg–50mg each day. Children, 1mg/kg body weight each day.

Special care: pregnancy, breast-feeding, elderly, kidney or liver disease, liver cirrhosis, SLE, diabetes, gout. Glucose, fluid and electrolyte (salt) levels should be monitored during the course of therapy.

Avoid use: patients with hypercalcaemia, serious kidney or liver disease, a sensitivity to sulphonamide drugs, Addison's disease.

Possible interaction: NSAIDs, barbiturates, alcohol, opiod drugs. Cardiac glycosides, lithium, carbenoxolone, corticosteroids, tubocurarine.

Side effects: gastrointestinal upset, blood changes, sensitivity to light, disturbance of electrolyte balance and metabolism, skin rash, pancreatitis, anorexia, dizziness, impotence.

Manufacturer: Boots.

Hyrocal

Description: a topical, mildly potent corticosteroid preparation available as cream or ointment containing 1% hydrocortisone acetate and calamine.

Used for: irritated skin conditions responsive to steroids.

Dosage: apply to affected skin 2 or 3 times each day.

Special care: use in children or on face should be limited to a period not exceeding 5 days. Stop gradually if preparation has been used for a long period.

Avoid use: extensive or long-term use, especially in pregnant women or for prevention of skin conditions. Patients with bacterial or fungal infections which are untreated. Skin disease of viral or tuberculous origin or due to ringworm, acne, dermatitis in mouth area, leg ulcers, scabies.

Side effects: thinning of skin, suppression of adrenal glands, abnormal hair growth, skin changes as in Cushing's syndrome.

Manufacturer: Bioglan.

Hydrocortistab Cream

Description: a mildly potent topical steroid preparation available as cream or ointment containing 1% hydrocortisone acetate.

Used for: irritated skin conditions responsive to steroids.

Dosage: apply thinly to affected skin 2 or 3 times each day.

Special care: use in children or on face should be limited to a period not exceeding 5 days. Stop gradually if preparation has been used for a long period.

Avoid use: extensive or long-term use, especially in pregnant women or for prevention of skin conditions. Patients with bacterial or fungal infections which are untreated. Skin disease of viral or tuberculous origin or due to ringworm, acne, dermatitis in mouth area, leg ulcers, scabies.

Side effects: thinning of skin, suppression of adrenal glands, abnormal hair growth, skin changes as in Cushing's syndrome.

Manufacturer: Boots.

Hydrocortistab Tablets

Description: a corticosteroid (glucocorticoid and mineralocorticosteroid) preparation available as scored, white tablets containing 20mg hydrocortisone. Also **Hydrocortistab Injection** available in ampoules containing 25mg hydrocortisone acetate/ml.

Used for: tablets, hormone replacement therapy, emergency treatment or asthma attack, anaphylaxis, allergic drug response, serum sickness, angioneurotic oedema. Injection, directly into joints in rheumatic diseases and soft tissue injuries.

Dosage: adults, tablets, replacement therapy, 20–30mg each day; emergency treatment, as directed by a physician according to patient's condition. Injection, 5–50mg each day directly into joint with a maximum of 3 injections daily. Children, tablets, replacement therapy, 10–30mg each day in divided doses; emergency treatment as directed by physician according to patient's condition. Injection, 5–30mg each day directly into joint with a maximum of 3 injections daily.

Special care: pregnancy, hyperthyroidism, liver cirrhosis, inflammation in kidneys (glomerulonephritis, nephritis), inflammation of veins, peptic ulcer, hypertension. Also, diabetes, recent surgical anastomoses of gastrointestinal tract, epilepsy, osteoporosis, infectious diseases characterized by skin rash, other infections, tuberculosis, those of fungal or viral origin. Patients with psychoses or suffering from stress. Drug should be gradually withdrawn and patients in contact with *Herpes zoster* virus or chicken pox should seek medical advice and treatment.

Possible interaction: anticoagulants taken orally, diuretics, NSAIDs, cardiac glycosides, anticholinesterases, rifampicin, hypoglycaemics, phenytoin, ephedrine, phenobarbitone.

Side effects: peptic ulcer, skin changes, osteoporosis, depression and euphoria, hyper-glycaemia.

Manufacturer: Boots.

Hydrocortisyl

Description: a mildly potent topical steroid preparation available as cream or ointment containing 1% hydrocortisone acetate.

Used for: irritated skin conditions responsive to steroids.

Dosage: apply thinly to affected skin 2 or 3 times each day.

Special care: use in children or on face should be limited to a period not exceeding 5 days. Stop gradually if preparation has been used for a long period.

Avoid use: extensive or long-term use, especially in pregnant women or for prevention of skin conditions. Patients with bacterial or fungal infections which are untreated. Skin disease of viral or tuberculous origin or due to ringworm, acne, dermatitis in mouth area, leg ulcers, scabies.

Side effects: thinning of skin, suppression of adrenal glands, abnormal hair growth, skin changes as in Cushing's syndrome.

Manufacturer: Roussel.

Hydrocortone

Description: a corticosteroid (glucocorticoid and mineralocorticoid) available as quarter-scored, white tablets containing 10mg or 20mg hydrocortisone and coded MSD 619, MSD 625 respectively.

Used for: hormone replacement therapy due to reduced production of hormones from the adrenal cortex (adrenal glands).

Dosage: 20–30mg each day in divided doses or as directed by physician.

Special care: pregnancy, hyperthyroidism, liver cirrhosis, inflammation in kidneys (glomerulonephritis, nephritis), thrombophlebitis, peptic ulcer, hypertension. Also, diabetes, recent surgical anastomoses of gastrointestinal tract, epilepsy, osteoporosis, infectious diseases characterized by skin rash, other infections, tuberculosis, those of fungal or viral origin. Patients with psychoses or suffering from stress. Drug should be gradually withdrawn and patients in contact with *Herpes zoster* virus or chicken pox should seek medical advice and treatment.

Possible interaction: anticoagulants taken orally, diuretics, NSAIDs, cardiac glycosides, anticholinesterases, rifampicin, hypoglycaemics, phenytoin, ephedrine, phenobarbitone.

Side effects: peptic ulcer, skin changes as in Cushing's syndrome, osteoporosis, depression and euphoria, hyperglycaemia.
Manufacturer: M.S.D.

Hydromet
Description: a compound antihypertensive preparation combining a central alpha-agonist and thiazide diuretic. It is available as pink, film-coated tablets containing 250mg methydopa and 15mg hydrochlorothiazide, marked MSD 423.
Used for: hypertension.
Dosage: adults, 1 tablet twice each day at first gradually increasing at intervals of 2 days. The maximum daily dose is 12 tablets.
Special care: pregnancy, breast-feeding, diabetes, kidney or liver disease, gout, history of liver disease, haemolytic anaemia, undergoing anaesthesia. A potassium supplement may be needed.
Avoid use: patients with serious liver disease, severe kidney failure, phaeochromocytoma, depression.
Possible interaction: antidiabetic substances, TCADs, ACTH (adreno-corticotrophic hormone), corticosteroids, MAOIs, tubocurarine, sympathomimetics, phenothiazines, digitalis, lithium.
Side effects: blocked nose, dry mouth, gastro-intestinal upset, headache, blood changes, sedation, depression, weakness, bradycardia.
Manufacturer: M.S.D.

Hydrosaluric
Description: a thiazide diuretic preparation available as scored, white tablets of 2 strengths containing 25mg and 50mg of hydrochlorthiazide and marked MSD 42 and MSD 105 respectively.
Used for: hypertension, oedema.
Dosage: adults, oedema, 25mg–100mg once or twice each day or when needed with a maximum daily dose of 200mg. Hypertension, 25–50mg as a single or divided dose each day at first, then adjusting but with a maximum daily dose of 100mg. Children, 6 months and under, 3.5mg/kg body weight each day; 6 months to 2 years, 12.5–37.5mg each day; 2 to 12 years, 27.5–100mg each day. All are in 2 divided doses.
Special care: pregnancy, liver or kidney disease, gout, electrolyte (salts) imbalance, SLE, diabetes. Patients may also require a potassium supplement.
Avoid use: breast-feeding mothers, patients with serious liver or kidney disease, anuria, hypercalcaemia, Addison's disease.
Possible interaction: NSAIDs, anti-hypertensives,

central nervous system depressants, muscle relaxants, corticosteroids, ACE inhibitors, digitalis, lithium.
Side effects: blood changes, fatigue, sensitivity to light, gout, hypokalaemia.
Manufacturer: M.S.D.

Hygroton
Description: a proprietary, thiazide-like diuretic preparation produced in the form of scored, pale yellow tablets containing 50mg chlorthalidone marked GEIGY and coded ZA.
Used for: hypertension, oedema.
Dosage: adults, hypertension, 25mg–50mg each day as a single dose with breakfast. Oedema, 50mg each day or 100–200mg every other day reducing to a maintenance dose in the order of 50–100mg 3 times each week. Children, up to 2mg/kg body weight each day.
Special care: pregnancy, breast-feeding, elderly, kidney or liver disease, liver cirrhosis, SLE, gout, diabetes. Glucose, fluid and electrolyte (salts) levels should be carefully monitored during the course of therapy.
Avoid use: patients with serious kidney or liver failure, sensitivity to sulphonamide drugs, hypercalcaemia, Addison's disease.
Possible interaction: NSAIDs, barbiturates, antidiabetic substances, corticosteroids, alcohol, tubocurarine, opiods, carbenoxolone, lithium, cardiac glycosides.
Side effects: gastrointestinal upset, blood changes, skin rash, upset of electrolyte balance and metabolism, sensitivity to light, anorexia, impotence, disturbance of vision, pancreatitis, dizziness.
Manufacturer: Geigy.

Hypnomidate
Description: a reparation which induces general anaesthesia produced in ampoules for injection containing 2mg etomidate/ml. Also, **Hypnomidate Concentrate** containing 125mg etomidate/ml (diluted before use).
Used for: induction of general anaesthesia.
Dosage: by slow intravenous injection, 100–300µg/kg body weight/minute, dose depending upon patient's condition.
Special care: best used following premedication.
Avoid use: porphyria.
Possible interaction: anxiolytics, hypnotics, antidepressants, anti-hypertensives, antipsychotics, calcium-channel blockers, ß-blockers.
Side effects: muscle movement and pain with

injection (lessened with pre-medication). Repeated doses may cause adrenal gland suppression.

Manufacturer: Janssen.

Hypnovel

Description: a benzodiazepine drug which has hypnotic, anxiolytic effects, available as a solution in ampoules for injection containing 10mg midazolam/ml.

Used for: sedation in patients undergoing minor surgery, those in intensive care, premedication in patients who are to receive general anaesthesia, induction of anaesthesia.

Dosage: adults, for sedation, 2mg (1–1.5mg in elderly persons) given by intravenous injection over thirty seconds. Then 0.5–1mg at 2 minute intervals if needed. Usual dose range is in the order of 2.5–7.5mg (1–2mg in elderly persons). Sedation of intensive care patients, 30–300µg/kg body weight by intravenous infusion over 5 minutes followed by 30–200µg/kg body weight every hour. Reduced doses may be indicated, especially if another drug (opioid analgesic) is also being given. Premedication, 70–100µg/kg body weight 1 hour to half an hour before general anaesthetic, given by intramuscular injection. Usual dose is in the order of 5mg (2.5mg in elderly persons).

Special care: breast-feeding, elderly, liver or kidney disease, lung disorders, myasthenia gravis, personality disorder. If use has been prolonged (as with intensive care patients) the drug should be gradually withdrawn.

Avoid use: patients with serious lung disorders, depressed respiration or in the last 3 months of pregnancy.

Possible interaction: central nervous system depressants, cimetidine, alcohol, erythromycin, anticonvulsant drugs.

Side effects: pain at injection site, dizziness, headache, circulatory changes, temporary halt in breathing (apnoea), hiccoughs.

Manufacturer: Roche.

Hypovase

Description: an antihypertensive preparation which is a selective alpha₁-blocker. It is produced as tablets of various strengths all containing prazosin hydrochloride. White 500µg tablets marked Pfizer; scored, orange 1mg tablets marked HYP/1; scored,

white 2mg tablets marked HYP/2; scored, white 5mg tablets marked HYP/5 and Pfizer.

Used for: congestive heart failure, hypertension, Raynaud's disease, additional therapy in the treatment of urinary tract obstruction when the cause is benign enlargement of the prostate gland.

Dosage: adults, congestive heart failure, 500µg in first instance increasing to 1mg 3 or 4 times each day. Then a usual maintenance dose in the order of 4–20mg in divided doses. Hypertension, 500µg as evening dose at first, followed by 500µg 2 or 3 times each day for a period of 3 days to 1 week. Then, 1mg 2 or 3 times each day for 3 days to 1 week. The dose may be further increased gradually as required with a daily maximum of 20mg. Raynaud's disease, 500µg twice each day at first, then a maintenance dose of 1 or 2mg twice each day. Additional therapy in urine obstruction, 500µg twice each day at first increasing to a maintenance dose of 2mg twice each day.

Special care: heart failure, patients suffering from congestive heart failure caused by stenosis; urinary tract obstruction, patients liable to fainting during urination.

Possible interaction: other anti-hypertensive drugs.

Side effects: dry mouth, dizziness on rising from lying down, sudden short-lived loss of consciousness, weariness, skin rash, blurring of vision.

Manufacturer: Invicta.

Hytrin and Hytrin BPH

Description: an antihypertensive preparation which is a selective alpha₁-blocker produced as tablets of 4 different strengths, all containing terazosin (as hydrochloride). White 1mg, yellow 2mg, brown 5mg and blue 10mg tablets are all marked with triangle-shaped symbols and logo.

Used for: hypertension, urine obstruction caused by benign enlargement of prostate gland.

Dosage: 1mg taken at bedtime at first then gradually increased at weekly intervals. The usual maintenance dose is in the order of 2–10mg taken once each day.

Special care: in patients liable to fainting.

Possible interaction: other anti-hypertensive drugs.

Side effects: initial dose may cause fainting, hypotension on rising from lying down, dizziness, weariness, fluid retention and swelling of lower limbs.

Manufacturer: Abbott.

I

Idoxene

Description: an antiviral preparation available as an eye ointment containing 0.5% idoxuridine.
Used for: herpetic keratitis (an inflammation and infection of the cornea caused by *Herpes simplex* virus).
Dosage: apply 4 times each day and at bedtime and continue for 3 to 5 days after condition has cleared. Maximum period of treatment is 3 weeks.
Special care: pregnancy.
Possible interaction: boric acid, corticosteroids.
Side effects: local irritation in eye and pain, swelling due to oedema.
Manufacturer: Spodefell.

Iduridin

Description: an antiviral skin preparation available as a solution with applicator in 2 strengths, containing 5% and 40% idoxuridine, both in dimethyl sulphoxide.
Used for: viral skin infections caused by *Herpes zoster* and *Herpes simplex*.
Dosage: adults and children over 12 years, apply 5% solution to infected area 4 times daily for 4 days. For severe *Herpes zoster* infections (shingles) only, the 40% solution should be used, applied on lint and changed every 24 hours, for a period of 4 days.
Special care: preparation may stain clothing.
Avoid use: children under 12 years, pregnancy, breast-feeding.
Manufacturer: Ferring.

Ilosone

Description: a macrolide antibiotic preparation available as red/ivory capsules containing 250mg erythromycin estolate and marked DISTA. Also **Ilosone Tablets**, oblong, pink, containing 500mg; **Ilosone Suspension** contains 125mg erythromycin estolate/5ml; **Ilosone Suspension Forte** contains 250mg/5ml.
Used for: respiratory and urinary tract infections, soft tissue, skin, dental infections, infections of the middle ear, acne.
Dosage: adults, 250mg every 6 hours with a maximum of 4g each day. Children 20–50mg/kg body weight each day in divided doses.
Avoid use: patients with liver disease or disorder, history of jaundice.
Possible interaction: anticoagulants taken orally, probenecid, carbamazepine, ergotamine, cyclosporin, lincomycin, theophylline, dihydroergotamine, alfentanil, clindamycin, triazolam, bromocriptine, digoxin.
Side effects: gastrointestinal upset, allergic responses, cholestatic jaundice.
Manufacturer: Dista.

Ilube

Description: a lubricant eye preparation available in the form of drops containing 5% acetylcysteine and 0.35% hypromellose.
Used for: dry eyes caused by insufficient secretion of tears or abnormal mucus production.
Dosage: 1 or 2 drops into affected eye 3 or 4 times each day.
Avoid use: patients with soft contact lenses.
Manufacturer: Cusi.

Imdur

Description: an antianginal nitrate preparation available in the form of scored oval, yellow, film-coated, sustained-release tablets containing 60mg isosorbide mononitrate marked A/ID.
Used for: prevention of angina.
Dosage: adults, 1 tablet each day taken in the morning increasing to 2 daily if necessary, as a single dose. If headache occurs, reduce to half a tablet each day.
Avoid use: children.
Side effects: nausea, headache, dizziness.
Manufacturer: Astra.

Imigran

Description: a preparation which is a seratonin agonist available as capsule-shaped, white, film-coated tablets containing 100mg sumatriptan (as succinate), marked with name and company. Also, **Imigran Subject Injection**, pre-filled syringes containing 6mg sumatriptan/0.5ml with auto-injector.

Used for: acute attacks of migraine which may be accompanied by aura.

Dosage: tablets, 1 tablet as soon as possible after attack starts which may be repeated if condition improves, but should not exceed 3 tablets in 24 hours. If migraine does not respond in first instance, a repeat dose should not be taken. Injection, 6mg by subcutaneous injection as soon as possible after attack begins which may be repeated after 1 hour if condition improves. The maximum dose is 12mg in 24 hours.

Special care: pregnancy, breast-feeding, liver, kidney or heart disease, indications of coronary artery disease; persons who have misused other migraine preparations. Patients should exercise care if driving or operating machinery.

Avoid use: children, elderly persons, patients with history of heart attack, heart spasm, uncontrolled hypertension, heart disease, Prinzmetal's angina.

Possible interaction: ergotamine, 5-HT re-uptake inhibitors (an antidepressant group), lithium, MAOIs.

Side effects: blood pressure rise, pain at injection site, tiredness, feeling of heaviness and pressure, dizziness, sleepiness, slight disturbance of liver function. Drug should be withdrawn if there is pain in chest or throat and cause investigated.

Manufacturer: Glaxo.

Immukin

Description: a preparation of recombinant human interferon gamma-Ib available as a solution in vials for injection at a strength of 200 micrograms/ml.

Used for: additional treatment (with antibiotics) to lessen the incidence of serious infections acquired by patients with chronic granulomatous disease (any 1 of a number of diseases giving rise to masses of granulation tissue, known as granulomata, e.g. tuberculosis and leprosy).

Dosage: adults and children with body surface area exceeding 0.5m^2, 50 µg/m^2 by subcutaneous injection 3 times each week. Children with body surface area less than 0.5m^2, 1.5 µg/kg body weight 3 times each week.

Special care: patients with serious liver or kidney disease, heart disease (congestive heart failure, arrhythmia, ischaemic heart disease), seizures, central nervous system disorders. Blood, liver and kidney function tests and urine analysis must be carried out during the course of therapy.

Avoid use: children under 6 months.

Possible interaction: alcohol.

Side effects: headache, chills, pain, fever, rash, nausea and vomiting, pain at injection site, ability to perform skilled tasks, e.g. driving and operating machinery may be impaired.

Manufacturer: Boehringer-Ingelheim.

Imunovir

Description: an antiviral preparation and immunopotentiator produced in the form of white tablets containing 500mg inosine pranobex.

Used for: infections of mucous membranes and skin caused by *Herpes simplex* virus, (type I and/or II) e.g. genital warts, subacute inflammation of the brain.

Dosage: *Herpes simplex* infections, 1g 4 times each day for 1 to 2 weeks; inflammation of the brain, 50–100mg/kg body weight each day in divided doses.

Special care: patients with abnormally high blood levels of uric acid (hyperuricaemia), gout, kidney disease.

Avoid use: children.

Side effects: raised uric acid levels.

Manufacturer: Leo.

Imuran

Description: a cytotoxic immunosuppressant preparation, azathioprine, produced in the form of film-coated tablets of 2 strengths. Orange tablets (25mg) are marked Imuran 25; yellow tablets (50mg) are marked Imuran 50. Also, **Imuran Injection** containing 50mg azathioprine (as sodium salt) produced as powder in vials for reconstitution.

Used for: to suppress organ or tissue rejection following transplant operations; some diseases of the autoimmune system especially when treatment with corticosteroids alone has proved to be inadequate.

Dosage: tablets and/or injection, prevention of rejection of transplant, usually up to 5mg/kg body weight at first and then a maintenance dose in the order of 1–4mg/kg body weight each day. Autoimmune diseases, up to 3mg/kg body weight each day at first reducing to 1–3mg/kg body weight daily as maintenance dose.

Special care: the injection is an irritant and hence should only be used if tablets cannot be taken. Special care in pregnant women, patients should avoid excessive exposure to sun, persons with kidney or liver disease or suffering from infections. Blood counts and other monitoring for toxic effects should be carried out.

Possible interaction: skin rashes, bone marrow suppression, gastrointestinal upset, toxic effects on liver.

Manufacturer: Wellcome.

Inderal

Description: a preparation which is a non-cardioselective ß-blocker, produced as pink, film-coated tablets containing 10mg, 40mg and 80mg propanolol hydrochloride all marked with name, strength and ICI. Also, **Inderal Injection** containing 1mg/ml in ampoules for injection.

Used for: heart arrhythmias, in the prevention of a second heart attack, angina pectoris, hypertension, enlarged and weakened heart muscle. Fallot's tetralogy (a congenital defect of the heart), phaeochromocytoma, situational and generalized anxiety.

Dosage: heart attack, 40mg 4 times each day for 2 or 3 days starting from 5 to twenty-1 days after first attack. Then a maintenance dose of 80mg twice each day. Arrhythmias, 10–40mg 3 or 4 times each day. Angina, 40mg 2 or 3 times each day at first increasing at weekly intervals if required to a usual dose in the order of 120–240mg daily. Hypertension, 80mg twice each day at first increasing at weekly intervals if required to usual dose in the order of 160–320mg daily. Phaeochromocytoma, 60mg each day taken along with an alpha-blocker for 3 days before operation for removal. If tumour is inoperable, a 30mg daily dose should be taken. Situational anxiety, 40mg twice each day, generalised anxiety, the same dose by increasing to 3 times each day if needed. Children, arrhythmias, 0.25–0.5mg/kg body weight 3 to 4 times each day. Fallot's tetralogy, up to 1mg/kg body weight 3 or 4 times each day. Phaeochromocytoma, 0.25–0.5mg/kg body weight 3 or 4 times each day.

Special care: pregnancy, breast-feeding, patients underoing planned surgery, those with liver or kidney disease, diabetes, metabolic acidosis. Patients with weak hearts may require diuretics and digitalis. Drug should be gradually withdrawn.

Avoid use: patients with history of bronchospasm, obstructive airways disease, heart block, heart shock, disease of peripheral arteries, sinus bradycardia, uncompensated heart failure.

Possible interaction: sympathomimetics, cimetidine, heart depressant anaesthetics, indomethacin, clonidine withdrawal, hypoglycaemics, class I antiarrhythmics, ergotamine, verapamil, reserpine, antihypertensives.

Side effects: bradycardia, cold hands and feet, tiredness with exercise, gastrointestinal upset, disturbance of sleep, bronchospasm, heart failure. Drug should be gradually withdrawn if skin rash or dry eyes occur.

Manufacturer: Zeneca.

Inderal LA

Description: an antianginal, antihypertensive and anxiolytic preparation which is a non-cardioselective ß-blocker. It is produced as pink/purple sustained-release capsules containing 160mg propanolol hydrochloride marked ICI and INDERAL LA. Also, **Half-Inderal LA**, pink/purple sustained-release capsules containing 80mg propanolol hydrochloride marked ICI and HALF-INDERAL LA.

Used for: angina, hypertension, additional therapy in thyrotoxicosis, also treatment of symptoms of anxiety.

Dosage: angina, 80mg or 160mg each day with a maximum daily dose of 240mg. Hypertension, 160mg each day at first increasing by 80mg gradually if needed until condition is controlled. Thyrotoxicosis, 80mg or 160mg each day with a maximum daily dose of 240mg. Situational anxiety, 80mg each day, generalised anxiety, 80–160mg each day.

Special care: pregnancy, breast-feeding, patients undergoing planned surgery, liver or kidney disease, diabetes, metabolic acidosis. Patients with weak hearts may require diuretics and digitalis. Drug should be gradually withdrawn.

Avoid use: children, patients with history of bronchospasm, obstructive airways disease, heart block, heart shock, disease of peripheral arteries, sinus bradycardia, uncompensated heart failure.

Possible interaction: sympathomimetics, cimetidine, heart depressant anaesthetics, indomethacin, clonidine withdrawal, hypoglycaemics, class I antiarrhythmics, ergotamine, verapamil, reserpine, antihypertensives.

Side effects: bradycardia, cold hands and feet, tiredness with exercise, gastrointestinal upset, disturbance of sleep, bronchospasm, heart failure. Drug should be gradually withdrawn if skin rash or dry eyes occur.

Manufacturer: Zeneca.

Inderetic

Description: an antihypertensive preparation combining a non-cardioselective ß-blocker and thiazide diuretic, available as white capsules containing 80mg propanolol hydrochloride and 2.5mg bendrofluazide.

Used for: hypertension.

Dosage: adults, 1 tablet twice each day.

Special care: pregnancy, breast-feeding, patients undergoing general anaesthesia or planned surgery, liver or kidney disease, gout, diabetes, metabolic acidosis. Patients with weak hearts may require diuretics and digitalis. Potassium supplements may be needed and patient's electrolyte levels should be monitored.

Avoid use: children, patients with heart block, heart shock, sinus bradycardia, peripheral disease of the arteries, sick sinus syndrome, uncompensated heart failure, obstruction of heart outflow, aortic stenosis (narrrowing of aorta). Those with history of breathing difficulties, bronchospasm, obstructive airways disease.

Possible interaction: sympathomimetics, class I antiarrhythmics, indomethacin, cimetidine, clonidine withdrawal, antihypertensives, ergot alkaloids, heart depressant anaesthetics, depressants, reserpine, hypoglycaemics. Digitalis, potassium-sparing diuretics, potassium supplements, lithium.

Side effects: bradycardia, cold hands and feet, fatigue on exertion, disturbance of sleep, gastrointestinal upset, heart failure, bronchospasm. Blood changes, sensitivity to light, gout, muscular weakness.

Manufacturer: Zeneca.

Inderex

Description: an antihypertensive preparation which combines a non-cardioselective ß-blocker and thiazide diuretic. It is available as grey/pink sustained-release capsules containing 160mg propanolol and 80mg bendrofluazide marked ICI and Inderex.

Used for: hypertension.

Dosage: adults, 1 twice each day.

Special care: pregnancy, breast-feeding, patients undergoing general anaesthesia or planned surgery, liver or kidney disease, gout, diabetes, metabolic acidosis. Patients with weak hearts may require diuretics and digitalis. Potassium supplements may be needed and patient's electrolyte levels should be monitored.

Avoid use: children, patients with heart block, heart shock, sinus bradycardia, peripheral disease of the arteries, sick sinus syndrome, uncompensated heart failure, obstruction of heart outflow, aortic stenosis (narrrowing of aorta). Those with history of breathing difficulties, bronchospasm, obstructive airways disease.

Possible interaction: sympathomimetics, class I antiarrhythmics, indomethacin, cimetidine, clonidine withdrawal, antihypertensives, ergot alkaloids, heart depressant anaesthetics, central nervous system depressants, reserpine, hypoglycaemics. Digitalis, potassium-sparing diuretics, potassium supplements, lithium.

Side effects: bradycardia, cold hands and feet, fatigue on exertion, disturbance of sleep, gastrointestinal upset, heart failure, bronchospasm. Blood changes, sensitivity to light, gout, muscular weakness.

Manufacturer: Zeneca.

Indocid

Description: an NSAID and indole available in a variety of forms: capsules are ivory-coloured and contain 25mg and 50mg indomethacin both marked with name and strength. **Indocid Suspension** contains 25mg/5ml; **Indocid Suppositories** contain 100mg indomethacin. **Indocid-R** are blue/yellow sustained-release capsules containing 75mg indomethacin marked INDOCID-R 693.

Used for: diseases of skeleton and joints including ankylosing spondylitis, osteoarthritis, lumbago, rheumatoid arthritis, degenerative disease of hip joint, acute joint disorders, acute gout (except Indocid-R). Also, dysmenorrhoea.

Dosage: adults, capsules and suspension, 50–200mg each day in divided doses with meals. Indocid-R, 1 tablet once or twice each day, suppositories, 1 at night and 1 in the morning if needed.

Special care: elderly persons, patients with heart failure, disorders of central nervous system, liver or kidney disease. Patients taking drug long-term should receive careful monitoring.

Avoid use: children, pregnancy, breast-feeding, history of gastrointestinal ulcer or peptic ulcer, allergy to anti-inflammatory drug or aspirin, angioneurotic oedema, recent proctitis (inflammation of the rectum and anus).

Possible interaction: methotrexate, anticoagulants, corticosteroids, quinolones, probenecid, aminoglycosides, salicylates, ß-blockers, lithium, diuretics.

Side effects: blood changes, effects on central nervous system, gastrointestinal intolerance, disturbance of vision and corneal deposits. If recurring headaches or gastrointestinal bleeding occur, drug should be withdrawn. Eye tests should be carried out during the course of long-term therapy.

Manufacturer: Morson.

Indocid PDA

Description: a prostaglandin synthetase inhibitor produced as a powder in vials for reconstitution and injection containing 1mg indomethacin (as sodium trihydrate).

Used for: patent ductus arteriosus (PDA) in premature babies (a condition in which there is a connection between the aorta and pulmonary artery, the ductus arteriosus, which normally closes after birth).

Dosage: 3 intravenous injections, at intervals of 12 to 24 hours depending upon baby's age, condition and urinary output.

Special care: kidney function and plasma levels of electrolytes should be monitored.

Avoid use: babies with serious kidney disorders, untreated infection, bleeding, disorders of blood coagulation.

Possible interaction: frusemide, aminoglycosides, digitalis.

Side effects: bleeding, disturbance in urine production, elevated creatine levels in blood, imbalance in electrolyte (salts) levels. If liver disease develops, drug should be withdrawn.

Manufacturer: Morson.

Indomod

Description: an NSAID Indole preparation available in the form of capsules of 2 strengths containing enteric-coated, continuous-release pellets. Orange capsules, marked AB27, contain 25mg and brown capsules, marked AB26, contain 75mg indomethacin respectively.

Used for: joint and bone disorders, including ankylosing spondylitis, rheumatoid arthritis, osteoarthritis, tenosynovitis, tendinitis, bursitis, gout.

Dosage: adults, 50–75mg as single or 2 doses each day increasing once a week by 25 or 50mg to a maximum daily dose of 200mg.

Special care: elderly persons, patients with heart failure, liver or kidney disease, disorders of central nervous systen. Patients taking drug long-term require careful monitoring and eye tests.

Avoid use: pregnancy, breast-feeding, history of ulcers or active ulcer, allergy to NSAID or aspirin.

Possible interaction: salicylates, probenecid, ß-blockers, corticosteroids, lithium, diuretics, quinolones, anticoagulants.

Side effects: disturbance of vision, deposits in cornea; if recurrent headaches or gastrointestinal bleeding occur, drug should be withdrawn.

Manufacturer: Indomod.

Influvac

Description: a preparation of inactivated surface antigen obtained from 4 strains of influenza virus. It is produced in pre-filled syringes containing 15µg of each strain of influenza virus/0.5ml suspension.

Dosage: adults, 0.5ml by deep subcutaneous or intramuscular injection. Children, aged 4 to 13

years, 0.5ml then repeated dose 4 to 6 weeks later.

Avoid use: children under 4 years, patients with allergy to poultry, eggs or feathers, (chick embryos used to culture virus strains). Patients with feverish conditions.

Side effects: tiredness, headache, feverishness, pain at injection site.

Manufacturer: Duphar.

Innohep

Description: an anticoagulant preparation which is a low molecular weight heparin produced as solutions in ampoules or pre-filled syringes for injection. Syringes contain 3500 units activity of anti-factor Xa tinzaparin/0.3ml. Ampoules contain 5000 units activity of anti-factor Xa tinzaparin/0.5ml.

Used for: prevention of thrombosis in patients having orthopaedic or general surgical operations.

Dosage: orthopaedic surgery, 50 units/kg body weight 2 hours before operation by subcutaneous injection then same dose once each day for next 7 to 10 days. General surgery, 3500 units 2 hours before operation by subcutaneous injection then same dose once each day for next 7 to 10 days.

Special care: pregnancy, breast-feeding, asthma, severe liver or kidney disease.

Avoid use: children, patients liable to bleeding, active peptic ulcer, serious hypertension which is uncontrolled, septic endocarditis.

Possible interaction: drugs which affect blood coagulation or platelets.

Side effects: risk of haemorrhage, slight bruising, skin rash, blood changes, short-lived rise in liver enzymes.

Manufacturer: Leo.

Innovace

Description: an antihypertensive preparation which is an ACE inhibitor produced as tablets of different strengths, all marked INNOVACE and containing enalapril maleate: white, round 2.5mg tablets; white, scored 5mg tablets; red, triangular 10mg tablets; peach, triangular 20mg tablets.

Used for: congestive heart failure, with digitalis and potassium-sparing diuretics. Prevention of heart attack and progression of disease in left ventricle of heart.

Dosage: adults, 2.5mg once each day at first increasing to a usual maintenance dose in the order of 20mg, maximum is 40mg. Treatment should normally begin in hospital and diuretics discontinued or reduced before therapy starts.

Special care: breast-feeding, patients undergoing anaesthesia, those with kidney disease and hypertension associated with this, patients have kidney dialysis, serious congestive heart failure. Kidney function should be monitored during course of therapy.

Avoid use: children, pregnancy, patients with obstruction to outflow of heart or aortic stenosis (narrowing of aorta).

Possible interaction: potassium supplements or potassium-sparing diuretics, other anti-hypertensives, lithium.

Side effects: tiredness, headache, dizziness, cough, gastrointestinal upset, oedema, hypotension.

Manufacturer: M.S.D.

Innozide

Description: an antihypertensive preparation combining an ACE inhibitor and thiazide diuretic produced in the form of scored, yellow tablets containing 20mg enalapril maleate and 12.5mg hydrochlorthiazide marked MSD 718.

Used for: mild to moderate hypotension in patients who have become accustomed to the same components taken individually.

Dosage: adults, 1 tablet each day with a maximum of 2 if needed.

Special care: breast-feeding, imbalance in levels of electrolytes (salts) or fluid, kidney or liver disease, heart disease or disease of the blood vessels of the brain. Patients receiving kidney dialysis, suffering from gout, diabetes or undergoing anaesthesia.

Avoid use: children, pregnancy, angio-neurotic oedema resulting from previous treatment with ACE inhibitor, anuria.

Possible interaction: hypoglycaemics, tubocurarine, corticosteroids, potassium supplements, potassium-sparing diuretics, NSAIDs, central nervous system depressants, lithium.

Side effects: cough, tiredness, headache, skin rash, hypotension, pain in chest, dizziness, weakness, kidney failure, impotence, angioneurotic oedema.

Manufacturer: M.S.D.

Instillagel

Description: a preparation which has disinfectant and local anaesthetic properties produced in the form of a gel in disposable syringes. It contains 2% lignocaine hydrochloride, 0.25% chlorhexidine gluconate, 0.06% methyl hydroxybenzoate, 0.025% propyl hydroxybenzoate.

Used for: to disinfect and lubricate catheters during insertion and as local anaesthetic.

Dosage: 6–11ml into urethra.

Special care: patients with serious, local haemorrhage.

Manufacturer: CliniMed.

Intal Syncroner

Description: a bronchodilator and NSAID, sodium cromoglycate, produced in a variety of different forms: **Intal Metered Dose Aerosol** with spacer device, delivers 5mg/dose. **Intal Inhaler** also delivers 53mg/dose and is a metered dose aerosol. **Intal Spincap**, clear yellow spincaps contain 20mg and are marked INTAL P and FISONS. **Intal Nebuliser Solution** contains 10mg/2ml in ampoules for use with nebulizer. **Intal Fisonaire**, a metered dose aerosol with spacer device within chamber delivering 5mg/dose.

Used for: prevention of bronchial asthma.

Dosage: adults and children, inhaler, 2 puffs 4 times each day reducing to 1 puff for maintenance. Spincaps, 4 each day in spinhaler taken at regular times. Nebuliser, 20mg 4 to 6 times each day continuously.

Side effects: irritated throat, short-lived cough; rarely, bronchospasm.

Manufacturer: Fisons.

Intraval Sodium

Description: a general anaesthetic preparation produced as a powder for reconstitution containing 0.5 and 2.5g thiopentone sodium.

Used for: induction of general anaesthesia.

Dosage: (in fit persons who have received premedication), 100–150mg over 10 to 15 seconds by intravenous injection; may be repeated after half a minute if required. Or, up to 4mg/kg body weight may be given. Children, 2–7mg/kg body weight.

Special care: depression of respiration and heart may occur if dose is too high.

Possible interaction: alcohol.

Side effects: sedative effects and slow metabolism for up to 24 hours. Ability to perform skilled tasks, e.g. driving, may be impaired.

Manufacturer: Theraplix.

Intron A

Description: a single-subtype recombinant interferon preparation produced as a powder in vials with solution for reconstitution and injection, in different strengths of 1, 3, 5, 10, 25 and 30 megaunits interferon alfa-2b (rbe).

Used for: leukaemia, maintenance of remission in multiple myeloma, non-Hodgkins lymphoma, AIDS-related Kaposi's sarcoma.

Dosage: according to individual need as directed by physician.

Avoid use: pregnant women.

Possible interaction: theophylline.

Side effects: weariness, depression, influenza-like

symptoms, bone marrow suppression, rash; seizures and coma (with higher doses especially in elderly persons).
Manufacturer: Schering-Plough.

Intropin
Description: a potent sympathomimetic drug which is an intropic agent produced in ampoules for injection containing 40mg dopamine hydrochloride/ml.
Used for: cardiogenic shock following heart attack and heart failure in cardiac surgery.
Dosage: 2–5 µg/kg body-weight/minute by intravenous infusion but dose is critical.
Special care: hypovalaemia (abnormally low volume of circulating blood) should be corrected.
Avoid use: patients with phaeochromocytoma, fast arrhythmia.
Possible interaction: antidepressants.
Side effects: tachycardia, hypo and hypertension, constriction of peripheral blood vessels, vomiting and nausea.
Manufacturer: DuPont.

Iodoflex
Description: a preparation which is absorbent and antibacterial available as a paste with removable gauze, containing cadexomer iodine.
Used for: chronic leg ulcers.
Dosage: adults and children over 2 years, apply up to 50g to ulcer and cover with additional dressing; renew when dressing is saturated or 3 times each week. Dose should not exceed 150g in any week and use should be restricted to a period of 3 months.
Special care: patients with disorders of the thyroid gland.
Avoid use: children under 2 years, pregnancy, breast-feeding, patients with thyroid disorders (Grave's disease, Hashimoto's thyroiditis, non-toxic nodular goitre).
Possible interaction: sulphafurazoles, lithium, sulphonylureas.
Manufacturer: Perstop.

Iodosorb
Description: an adsorbent and antibacterial available as a powder in sachets containing cadexomer iodine. Also **Iodosorb Ointment** containing cadexomer iodine.
Used for: leg ulcers, bedsores and moist wounds.
Dosage: adults, apply a layer at least 3mm thick and cover with sterile dressing. Change when dressing is saturated. Ointment, (for chronic leg ulcers), as above but no more than 150g should be used in any

1 week and course of therapy should not exceed 3 months.
Special care: patients with disorders of the thyroid gland.
Avoid use: children, pregnancy, breast-feeding, patients with thyroid disorders (Grave's disease, Hashimoto's thyroiditis, non-toxic nodular goitre).
Possible interaction: sulphafurazoles, lithium, sulphonylureas.
Manufacturer: Perstop.

Ionamin[CD]
Description: a central nervous system stimulant which acts as an appetite-suppressant. It is available as sustained-release capsules of 2 strengths: yellow/grey containing 15mg phentermine as resin complex and yellow, containing 30mg phentermine as resin complex. Both are marked with name and strength.
Used for: obesity.
Dosage: adults, 15–30mg each day before breakfast.
Special care: angina, hypertension, heart arrhythmias. For short-term use only.
Avoid use: children, pregnancy, breast-feeding, hyperthyroidism, severe hypertension, arteriosclerosis. Those with history of drug or alcohol abuse or psychiatric illnesses.
Possible interaction: methyldopa, sympathomimetics, guanethidine, MAOIs, psychotropic drugs.
Side effects: drug dependence and tolerance, dry mouth, rise in blood pressure, agitation and nervousness, palpitations, psychiatric disturbances.
Manufacturer: Lipha.

Iodipine
Description: an eye solution which is an alpha$_2$-agonist available in single dose (0.25ml) ampoules containing 1.15% apraclonidine hydrochloride.
Used for: control and prevention of any rise in pressure within the eye following anterior segment laser surgery.
Dosage: 1 drop into eye 1 hour before laser treatment and 1 drop immediately after surgery is completed.
Special care: pregnancy, breast-feeding, serious heart and circulatory disease, hypertension, history of fainting. If there is a great reduction in the pressure within the eye, this should receive careful monitoring.
Avoid use: children.
Possible interaction: MAOIs, sympathomimetics, TCADs.
Side effects: blanching of conjunctiva of eye and retraction of eyelids, dilation of pupil. Possible

effects on heart and circulation due to absorption of drug.
Manufacturer: Alcon.

Ipral

Description: a sulphonamide antibiotic preparation which is a folic acid inhibitor available as white tablets containing 100mg and 200mg trimethoprim, marked SQUIBB 513 and SQUIBB 514 respectively.
Used for: prevention and treatment of infections of the urinary tract; treatment of respiratory tract infections.
Dosage: adults, treatment, 200mg twice each day; prevention of urinary tract infections, 100mg taken at night. Children, over 6 years of age, 100mg twice each day.
Special care: patients with kidney disorder or folate deficiency. Regular blood tests are required during long-term treatment.
Avoid use: children under 6 years, pregnancy, serious kidney disease.
Side effects: gastrointestinal upset, skin reactions, folate deficiency if drug is taken long-term.
Manufacutrer: Squibb.

Ismelin

Description: an antihypertensive preparation, guanethidine sulphate, which is an adrenergic neurone blocker, available as white tablets containing 10mg and pink tablets containing 25mg. Both are marked with strength and name. Also **Ismelin Injection** containing 10mg/ml in ampoules.
Used for: hypertension.
Dosage: adults, 10mg each day at first increasing by 10mg once a week if needed to a usual dose in the order of 25–50mg.
Special care: pregnancy, kidney disease, asthma, peptic ulcer, arteriosclerosis, anaesthesia.
Avoid use: patients with heart or kidney failure, phaeochromocytoma.
Possible interaction: sympathomimetics, MAOIs, hypoglycaemics, digitalis, contraceptive pill, TCADs, antiarrhythmics, antipsychotics, other anti-hypertensives.
Side effects: blocked nose, blood changes, oedema, failure to reach sexual climax (males), bradycardia, diarrhoea, hypotension when rising from lying down.
Manufacturer: Ciba.

Isopto Atropine

Description: lubricant and anticholinergic eyedrops containing 1% atropine sulphate and 0.5% hypromellose.

Used for: to produce long-lasting mydriasis (the drug is mydriatic)—fixed dilation of the pupil of the eye, and cycloplegia (cycloplegic)—paralysis of the ciliary muscles. This is in order to allow detailed examination of the eye to be carried out.
Dosage: adults, for uveitis (inflammation of the uveal tract), 1 drop 3 times each day; for refraction, 1 to 2 drops 1 hour before eye is examined. Children, uveitis, 1 drop 3 times each day; refraction, 1 drop twice each day for 1 to 2 days before eye is examined.
Special care: infants, pressure should be applied over lachrymal (tear) sac for 1 minute.
Avoid use: patients with soft contact lenses, narrow angle glaucoma.
Side effects: dry mouth, sensitivity to light, stinging in eye, blurring of vision, headache, tachycardia. Also changes in behaviour and psychotic responses.
Manufacturer: Alcon.

Isopto Carbachol

Description: lubricant and cholinergic eyedrops containing 3% carbachol and 1% hypromellose.
Used for: glaucoma.
Dosage: adults, 2 drops 3 times each day.
Avoid use: children, patients with severe iritis (inflammation of the iris), abrasion of the cornea, wearing soft contact lenses.
Manufacturer: Alcon.

Isopto Carpine

Description: lubricant and cholinergic eyedrops available at different strengths containing 0.5%, 1%, 2%, 3% and 4% pilocarpine all with 0.5% hypromellose.
Used for: glaucoma.
Dosage: adults, 2 drops 3 times each day.
Avoid use: children, patients with severe iritis (inflammation of the iris), wearing soft contact lenses.
Manufacturer: Alcon.

Isotrex

Description: a topical preparation of vitamin A derivative available as a gel containing 0.05% isotretinoin.
Used for: acne vulgaris.
Dosage: apply thinly once or twice each day for at least 6 to 8 weeks.
Special care: avoid mucous membranes, mouth, angles of nose, eyes, damaged or sunburnt areas. Ultraviolet light should be avoided.
Avoid use: pregnancy, breast-feeding, family history or history of epithelioma of skin (abnormal growth which may or may not be malignant).

Possible interaction: keratolytics.
Side effects: local skin irritation.
Manufacturer: Stiefel.

Istin

Description: an antianginal and antihypertensive preparation which is a class II calcium antagonist. It is available as 5mg and 10mg white tablets containing amlodipine besylate, marked Pfizer and ITN 5 and ITN 10 respectively.

Used for: angina in myocardial ischaemia, hypertension.
Dosage: adults, 5mg once each day; maximum dose, 10mg daily.
Special care: pregnancy, breast-feeding, children, liver disease.
Side effects: oedema, headache, dizziness, tiredness, nausea, flushing.
Manufacturer: Pfizer.

J

Jectofer

Description: a haematinic compound available in ampoules for injection containing iron sorbitol and citric acid (equivalent to 50mg of iron/ml).

Used for: anaemia caused by iron deficiency.

Dosage: adults and children over 3kg in weight by intramuscular injection as a single dose. The maximum dose for each injection is 100mg.

Avoid use: patients with certain other types of anaemia (hypoplastic or aplastic), seriously damaged kidney or liver, acute leukaemia.

Side effects: heart arrhythmias.

Manufacturer: Astra.

Jexin

Description: a non-depolarizing (or competitive) muscle relaxant preparation used in anaesthesia produced in ampoules for injection containing 10mg tubocurarine chloride/ml.

Used for: production of muscle relaxation during surgery and for patients in intensive care units receiving long-term assisted ventilation.

Dosage: adults, 15–30mg by intravenous injection at first then 5–10mg as needed. Children, 300–500µg/kg body weight at first, then 60–100µg/kg, as needed. Newborn babies, 200–250µg/kg body weight at first then 40–50µg/kg, as needed.

Special care: kidney disease or damage, those in whom hypotension would be undesirable.

Avoid use: patients with myasthenia gravis.

Possible interaction: aminoglycosides, clindamycin, azlocillin, colistin, verapamil, nifedipine, cholinergics, magnesium salts.

Side effects: short-lived hypotension, skin rash.

Manufacturer: Evans.

Junifen

Description: an NSAID produced as a sugar-free, orange-flavoured suspension containing 100mg ibuprofen/5ml.

Used for: relief of pain and reduction of fever in children.

Dosage: children, 1 to 2 years, 2.5ml; 3 to 7 years, 5ml; 8 to 12 years, 10ml. All given 3 to 4 times each day.

Special care: pregnancy, breast-feeding, patients with liver, kidney or heart disease or damage, asthma, gastrointestinal disease, patients receiving long-term therapy require careful monitoring.

Avoid use: children under 1 year and those less than 7kg body weight, allergy to aspirin or NSAID, peptic ulcer.

Possible interaction: thiazide diuretics, anticoagulants, quinolones.

Side effects: rash, thrombocytopenia, gastrointestinal upset or haemorrhage.

Manufacturer: Boots.

K

Kabiglobulin

Description: a preparation of human normal immunoglobulin (HNIG) available as a 16% solution in ampoules for injection.

Used for: prevention of hepatitis A infection, prevention of measles, prevention of rubella in pregnancy, burns, antibody deficiency conditions.

Dosage: prevention of hepatitis A, adults and children, usual dose 0.02ml 0 0.04ml/kg body weight or 0.06–0.12 ml if risk is greater. Prevention of measles, 0.02ml/kg body weight or 0.04ml/kg body weight to allow mild attack. Rubella in pregnancy, adults, 20ml to prevent clinical attack. All doses given by intramuscular injection.

Possible interaction: live vaccines.

Manufacturer: Pharmacia.

Kabikinase

Description: a fibrinolytic preparation available as a powder in vials for reconstitution and injection in 3 strengths, containing 250,000 units, 750,000 units and 1.5 million units streptokinase.

Used for: to disperse blood clots in life-threatening conditions as in pulmonary embolism, heart atack, deep vein thrombosis, arterial thromboembolism, clots during haemodialysis (kidney dialysis).

Dosage: adults, up to 600,000 units given over thirty minutes by intravascular route (into blood vessel), in first instance. Maintenance dose, 100,000 units every hour for 3 to 6 days. Heart attack, 1.5 million units by intravenous infusion over 1 hour then 150mg of aspirin each day for a minimum of 4 weeks. Children, 1300–1400 units/kg body weight each hour for 3 to 6 days. Other conditions may require different doses.

Special care: patients with pancreatitis, ensure no pre-existing clot which on dissolution might cause embolism. Special care with follow-on anti-coagulant therapy.

Avoid use: pregnancy, patients with recent haemorrhage, surgery or injury, bleeding disorders. Also coagulation disorders, serious hypertension, streptococcal infections, serious liver or kidney damage or disease, peptic ulcer, endocarditis caused by bacteria. Patients with known allergy to streptokinase or who have received treatment with this or anistreplase during the previous 5 days to 6 months.

Possible interaction: drugs acting on blood platelets, anticoagulants.

Side effects: haemorrhage, fever, hypotension, heart arrhythmias; rarely, anaphylaxis (shock).

Manufacturer: Pharmacia.

Kalspare

Description: a compound diuretic preparation with thiazide-like activity and also potassium-sparing, available in the form of film-coated orange tablets, containing 50mg chlorthalidone and 50mg triamterene, scored on 1 side and marked A on the other.

Used for: hypertension, oedema.

Dosage: adults, hypertension, 1 tablet every morning increasing to 2 as single daily dose if required. Oedema, 1 tablet every morning increasing to 2 daily as single dose if condition has not improved after 7 days.

Special care: pregnancy, breast-feeding, liver or kidney disease or damage, diabetes, gout, acidosis.

Avoid use: patients with serious or worsening kidney failure, anuria, hyperkalaemia.

Possible interaction: potassium-sparing diuretics, potassium supplements, ACE inhibitors, lithium, antihypertensives, digitalis.

Side effects: sensitivity to light, cramps, skin rash, blood changes, gout.

Manufacturer: Cusi.

Kalten

Description: a compound hypertensive preparation combining a cardio-selective ß-blocker, thiazide and potassium-sparing diuretic. It is available as cream/red capsules containing 50mg atenolol, 25mg hydrochlorothiazide and 2.5mg amiloride hydrochloride marked with logo and KALTEN.

Used for: hypertension.

Dosage: adults, 1 tablet each day.

Special care: pregnancy, breast-feeding, general

anaesthesia, liver or kidney disease, diabetes, gout, metabolic acidosis. Patients with weak hearts may require treatment with diuretics and digitalis.

Avoid use: obstructive airways disease or history of bronchospasm, heart block, heart shock, heart failure, disease of peripheral arteries, sick sinus syndrome, serious or worsening kidney failure, anuria.

Possible interaction: sympathomimetics, heart depressant anaesthetics, central nervous system depressants, ergotamine, class I antiarrhythmics, indomethacin, verapamil, hypoglycaemics, clonidine withdrawal, reserpine, cimetidine, clonidine withdrawal. Potassium supplements, potassium-sparing diuretics, digitalis, lithium.

Side effects: gastrointestinal upset, cold hands and feet, disturbance of sleep, fatigue on exertion, bronchospasm, bradycardia. Sensitivity to light, gout, blood changes, muscle weakness. If unexplained skin rash or dry eyes occur, therapy should be stopped. Withdraw drug gradually.

Manufacturer: Stuart.

Kannasyn

Description: a broad-spectrum aminoglycoside antibiotic preparation available as a powder in vials for reconstitution and injection containing 1g kanamycin (as acid sulphate).

Used for: serious infections such as meningitis and septicaemia, especially where there is resistance to other antibiotics.

Dosage: adults, 1g by intramuscular injections each day in 2, 3 or 4 divided doses for a maximum period of 6 days. Children, 15mg/kg body weight by intramuscular injections in 2, 3 or 4 divided doses each day for a maximum period of 6 days.

Special care: patients with kidney disorders, Parkinson's disease, myasthenia gravis; careful control of blood levels and dosage is required.

Avoid use: pregnancy, breast-feeding.

Possible interaction: anaesthetics, frusemide, neuromuscular blocking drugs, ethacrynic acid.

Side effects: damage to hearing and balance, harmful effects on kidneys.

Manufacturer: Sanofi Swinthrop.

Kapake

Description: a compound analgesic preparation available in the form of scored, white oval tablets containing 500mg paracetamol and 30mg codeine phosphate, marked KAPAKE.

Used for: severe pain.

Dosage: adults, 1 or 2 tablets every 4 hours with a maximum of 8 in 24 hours.

Special care: elderly, kidney or liver disease, inflammation or obstruction of the bowel, enlargement of the prostate gland, Addison's disease, hypothyroidism.

Avoid use: children, pregnancy, breast-feeding, breathing difficulties, obstructive airways disease, raised pressure inside cranium, alcoholism.

Possible interaction: MAOIs, central nervous system depressants.

Side effects: drug dependence and tolerance, dry mouth, dizziness, nausea, blurring of vision, constipation, nausea, sleepiness.

Manufacturer: Galen.

Kefadol

Description: a cephalosporin antibiotic preparation available as a powder in vials for reconstitution and injection containing 1g cefamandole (as nafate).

Used for: life-threatening, severe infections.

Dosage: adults, 500mg–2g given by intramuscular or intravenous injection every 4 to 8 hours with a maximum dose of 12g every 24 hours. Children over 1 month, 50—100mg/kg body weight each day every 4 to 8 hours, with a maximum dose of 150mg/kg body weight daily.

Special care: patients with kidney disease or sensitivity to penicillin.

Avoid use: children under 1 month.

Possible interaction: aminoglycosides, loop diuretics.

Side effects: gastrointestinal upset, blood changes (reduction in levels of white blood cells), thrombocytopenia. Also, allergic reactions, rise in level of blood urea and liver enzymes, cholestatic jaundice, short-lived hepatitis, positive Coomb's test (a test for rhesus antibodies).

Manufacturer: Dista.

Keflex

Description: a cephalosporin antibiotic preparation, cephalexin monohydrate, produced in a number of different forms. White/dark green capsules contain 250mg , and dark green/pale green capsules contain 500mg coded LILLY H69 and LILLY H71 respectively. **Keflex Tablets**, peach-coloured containing 250mg coded LILLY U57 and peach, oval tablets containing 500mg coded LILLY U49. Also, **Keflex Suspension** in 2 strengths containing 125mg and 250mg/5ml solution.

Used for: urinary tract infections, inflammation of middle ear, infections of respiratory tract, skin, bone, soft tissue. Also dental infections.

Dosage: adults, 1–4g each day in divided doses. Children, 25–50mg/kg body weight each day in divided doses.

Special care: patients with kidney disorder and allergy to penicillins.
Possible interaction: loop diuretics.
Side effects: gastrointestinal upset, allergic reactions.
Manufacturer: Lilly.

Kefzol

Description: a cephalosporin antibiotic preparation available as a powder in vials for reconstitution and injection, at 2 strengths, containing 500mg and 1g cephazolin (as salt).
Used for: septicaemia, endocarditis, skin, soft tissue, respiratory, urinary tract infections.
Dosage: adults, 500mg–1g every 6 to 8 hours by intramuscular or intravenous injection. Children, over 1 month in age, 25–50mg/kg body weight each day by intramuscular or intravenous injection in divided doses.
Special care: kidney disease or disorder, hypersensitivity to beta-lactam antibiotics. In beta-haemolytic infections, treatment should be given for a minimum period of 10 days.
Avoid use: children under 1 month.
Possible interaction: aminoglycosides, loop diuretics, probenecid.
Side effects: gastrointestinal upset, blood changes involving white blood cells, candidosis (thrush), pain at injection site, seizures. A rise in levels of blood urea and liver enzymes, positive Coomb's test (a test for rhesus antibodies).
Manufacturer: Lilly.

Kelfizine W

Description: a sulphonamide antibiotic preparation available as white tablets containing 2g sulfametopyrazine, marked weekly dose on 1 side and name on the reverse.
Used for: treatment and prevention of chronic bronchitis, urinary tract infections.
Dosage: adults, 1 tablet each week.
Special care: patients with kidney or liver disease or damage. Persons taking the drug over long period should receive regular blood checks.
Avoid use: children, women in late pregnancy, nursing mothers.
Possible interaction: hypoglycaemics taken orally, folate antagonists.
Side effects: gastrointestinal upset, skin rashes, haemolytic anaemia, inflammation of the tongue, blood changes if taken long-term.
Manufacturer: Pharmacia.

Kelocyanor

Description: a chelating agent (1 which binds to a metal) available as a solution in ampoules for injection containing 1.5% dicobalt edetate in glucose.
Used for: as an antidote in patients with cyanide poisoning.
Dosage: adults and children, 20ml (300mg) by intravenous injection over 1 minute followed straight away by 50ml dextrose intravenous infusion 50%. Both may be repeated once or twice as required.
Side effects: tachycardia, vomiting, short-lived hypotension, toxic effects from cobalt.
Manufacturer: Lipha.

Kemadrin

Description: an anticholinergic preparation available as scored white tablets containing 5mg procyclidine hydrochloride marked WELLCOME S3A. Also, **Kemadrin Injection** available as 2ml ampoules containing 2mg procyclidine hydrchloride.
Used for: Parkinson's disease, especially drug-induced symptoms.
Dosage: adults, 2.5mg 3 times each day after meals, in first instance, then increasing every second or third day by 2.5–5mg. The usual maximum daily dose is 30mg. Injection, 10–20mg each day by intramusucular or intravenous injection.
Special care: heart disease, enlarged prostate gland, obstruction of gastrointestinal tract, narrow angle glaucoma. Drug should be gradually withdrawn.
Avoid use: children, patients with tardive dyskinesia (a movement disorder especially affecting elderly people).
Possible interaction: antihistamines, phenothiazines, antidepressants.
Side effects: anticholinergic side effects, confusion with higher doses.
Manufacturer: Wellcome.

Kemicetine Succinate

Description: a chloramphenicol antibiotic available as a powder in vials for reconstitution and injection containing 1g chloramphenicol (as sodium succinate).
Used for: serious, life-threatening infections including *H. influenzae*, meningitis and typhoid.
Dosage: adults, 1g by intravenous injection every 6 to 8 hours. Children, newborn babies, 25mg/kg body weight each day; others, 50mg/kg body weight daily. All given intravenously every 6 hours in divided doses.
Special care: patients with liver or kidney disease or damage.

Possible interaction: hypoglycaemics, anti-coagulants, phenytoin.

Side effects: gastrointestinal upset, dry mouth, disturbance of vision, rash, Grey syndrome in babies. Drug causes serious blood changes such as aplastic anaemia and is reserved for use in conditions in which no effective alternative is available, and patient's life is at risk. Regular blood tests should be performed.

Manufacturer: Pharmacia.

Kenalog

Description: an anti-inflammatory corticosteroid (glucocorticoid) preparation available in pre-filled syringes and vials for injection, containing 40mg triamcinolone acetonide/ml.

Used for: pain in joints, stiffness and swelling due to rheumatoid arthritis, osteoarthritis. Inflammation of connective tissue (bursa) around joint (bursitis), tendon sheath (tenosynovitis), inflammation of the elbow joint (epicondylitis). Also used for collagen disorders, deficiency of hormones of adrenal cortex, serious dermatitis, allergic disorders.

Dosage: adults by intramuscular injection, 40mg by deep injection into gluteal muscle; further doses according to patient's condition. For allergic states, e.g. hay fever, 40–100mg as single dose. Joint disorders, 5–40mg by intra-articular injection (directly into joint) according to joint size. Maximum dose if more than one joint is being treated is 80mg. Children, age 6 to 12 years, in proportion to adult dose according to age, severity of condition, bodyweight and joint size.

Special care: pregnancy, inflammation of kidneys, osteoporosis, infections, viral or fungal conditions, tuberculosis, diabetes. Also, glaucoma, recent surgical anastomoses, thrombophlebitis, epilepsy, liver cirrhosis, hypertension, hyperthyroidism. Patients with osteoporosis, secondary cancers, disease characterized by skin rash (exanthematous disease) e.g. measles, psychoses, suffering from stress. Patients should avoid contact with *Herpes zoster* virus or chicken pox and should seek medical help if inadvertently exposed. Drug should be gradually withdrawn.

Avoid use: children under 6 years.

Possible interaction: cardiac glycosides, NSAIDs, phenytoin, anticoagulants taken orally, anticholinesterases, phenobarbitone, hypo-glycaemics, rifampicin, ephedrine, diuretics.

Side effects: skin changes as in Cushing's syndrome, peptic ulcer, osteoporosis, hyperglycaemia, euphoria and depression.

Manufacturer: Squibb.

Kerlone

Description: an antihypertensive preparation which is a cardioselective ß-blocker available as scored, white, film-coated tablets containing 20mg betaxolol hydrochloride marked KE 20.

Used for: hypertension.

Dosage: adults, 1 tablet each day, (half for elderly persons in first instance).

Special care: pregnancy, breast-feeding, diabetes, liver or kidney disease, metabolic acidosis, undergoing general anaesthesia. Drug should be gradually withdrawn. Patients with weak hearts may require digitalis and diuretic treatment.

Avoid use: children, patients with history of bronchospasm, obstructive airways disease, heart block, heart failure, heart shock, peripheral disease of the arteries, sick sinus syndrome.

Possible interaction: CNS depressants, indomethacin, clonidine withdrawal, ergotamine, sympathomimetics, class I antiarrhythmics, cimetidine, verapamil, other antihypertensives, reserpine, hypoglycaemics.

Side effects: bradycardia, cold hands and feet, fatigue on exertion, disturbance of sleep, gastrointestinal upset, bronchospasm, heart failure. Withdraw if dry eyes or skin rash occur.

Manufacturer: Lorex.

Ketalar

Description: a general anaesthetic available as a solution in vials for injection at strengths of 10mg, 50mg and 100mg/ml, containing ketamine (as hydrochloride).

Used for: induction and maintenance of general anaesthesia especially in children requiring repeated anaesthesia.

Dosage: by intravenous injection or infusion depending upon period of time for which general anaesthesia is required.

Avoid use: patients prone to hallucination, those with hypertension.

Possible interaction: ACE inhibitors, TCADs, antipsychotics, ß-blockers, anti-hypertensives, anxiolytics and hypnotics.

Side effects: hallucinations (but incidence is reduced if used with diazepam and is less of a problem in children), possible tachycardia and rise in arterial blood pressure. Relatively slow recovery time.

Manufacturer: Parke-Davis.

Ketovite

Description: a multivitamin preparation available as yellow, sugar-free tablets containing 1mg thiamine hydrochloride, 0.5mg acetomenaphthone, 1mg riboflavine, 0.33mg pyridoxine hydrochloride, 3.3mg nicotinamide, 16.6mg ascorbic acid, 50mg inositol, 1.16mg calcium pantothenate, 0.25mg folic acid, 0.17mg biotin, 5mg tocopheryl acetate. Also **Ketovite Liquid**, a pink, sugar-free vitamin supplement, containing 150mg choline chloride, 12.5 micrograms cyanocobalamin, 400 units vitamin D, 2500 units vitamin A, all/5ml.

Used for: dietary supplement for patients on synthetic diets due to disorders of amino acid or carbohydrate metabolism.

Dosage: 1 tablet 3 times each day and 5ml of solution once daily.

Possible interaction: levodopa.

Manufacturer: Paines and Byrne.

Kinidin Durules

Description: a class I antiarrhythmic preparation available as white, sustained-release tablets containing 250mg quinidine bisulphate.

Used for: disorders of heart rhythm including types of tachycardia, atrial fibrillation and extrasystoles.

Dosage: adults, 1 tablet each day at first increasing to 2 to 5 daily.

Special care: patients with tachycardia, hypotension, hypokalaemia, congestive heart failure.

Avoid use: children, pregnancy, heart block, myasthenia gravis, inflammation or damage of heart muscle, uncompensated heart failure, toxic effects of digitalis.

Possible interaction: digitalis, cimetidine, anticoagulants taken orally, vasodilators, non-depolarizing substances, antihypertensives.

Side effects: hepatitis, allergic responses, cinchonism (a condition resulting from overdose of quinine and quinidine characterized by ringing in the ears, deafness, headache, brain congestion).

Manufacturer: Astra.

Klaricid

Description: a macrolide antibiotic preparation, available in a variety of forms: oval, yellow, film-coated tablets containing 250mg clarithromycin marked with logo; **Klaricid Paediatric Suspension** containing 125mg/5ml solution; **Klaricid Intravenous Injection** containing 500mg clarithromycin as powder in vials for reconstitution.

Used for: infections of respiratory tract, middle ear, soft tissue and skin.

Dosage: adults, and children over 12 years, tablets, 1 twice each day for 1 week; serious infections, 2 tablets daily for up to 2 weeks. Injection, 1g by intravenous infusion in 2 divided doses each day for 5 days. Children, use paediatric suspension under 1 year, 7.5mg/kg body weight, 1 to 2 years, 2.5ml; 3 to 6 years, 5ml; 7 to 9 years, 7.5ml; 10 to 12 years, 10ml. All twice each day in divided doses.

Special care: pregnancy, breast-feeding, liver or kidney disease.

Possible interaction: anticoagulants taken by mouth, carbamazepine, theophylline, terfenadine, digoxin.

Side effects: gastrointestinal upset, vomiting, diarrhoea, nausea, pain in abdomen, short-lived central nervous system effects, headache, skin rash, pain and skin reactions at injection site.

Manufacturer: Abbott.

Konakion

Description: a vitamin A derivative available as a solution in ampoules for injection containing 1mg phytomenadione/0.5ml, and as white, sugar-coated tablets containing 10mg phytomenadione.

Used for: hypoprothrombinaemia (an abnormally low level of prothrombin clotting factor II in the blood, characterized by bleeding and loss of blood clotting ability). Also, haemorrhagic disease of the newborn (a bleeding disorder of newborn infants caused by vitamin K deficiency).

Dosage: adults, 10–20mg by intramuscular or slow intravenous injection, or as tablets. The maximum dose is 40mg in 24 hours. Newborn babies, 1mg given intramuscularly; babies over 3 months, 5–10mg each day.

Side effects: sweating, flushing, lack of oxygen in blood (cyanosis) causing bluish tinge to skin and mucous membranes. Symptoms of analphylaxis may occur with injection.

Manufacturer: Roche.

Kytril

Description: an anti-emetic preparation which is a 5HT₃-antagonist that acts to block vomiting and nausea reflexes which occur when 5HT₃ receptors in the gut are stimulated. It is available as triangular, white, film-coated tablets containing 1mg granisetron as hydrochloride. Also, **Kytril Injection** available as a solution in ampoules containing 1mg/ml.

Used for: prevention and treatment of vomiting and nausea caused by cytotoxic drug therapy.

Dosage: 1 tablet 1 hour before chemotherapy begins followed by 1 every 12 hours. Injection, 3mg diluted in 20–50ml infusion fluid given over 5 minutes by intravenous route. Can be repeated if required at 10 minute intervals with a maximum dose of 9mg in 24 hours.

Special care: pregnant women, patients with obstruction of intestine.
Avoid use: children, breast-feeding.

Side effects: constipation, headache, short-lived rise in level of liver enzymes.
Manufacturer: Smith Kline Beecham.

L

Lactilol

Description: an osmotic laxative, lactitol monohydrate (10g) as powder in a sachet.

Used for: constipation, acute or chronic portal systemic encephalopathy, PSE (hepatic coma-toxic waste not neutralized in the liver, reaching the brain or substances required for brain function not synthesized in the liver).

Dosage: 1 sachet mixed with food or drink morning or evening. For constipation, adults, 2 sachets reducing to 1 daily; children 1 to 6 years, quarter to half sachet; 6 to 12 years half to 1 sachet; 12 to 16 years, 1 to 2 sachets; all daily. Not for children under 12 months. For PSE, 0.5–0.7g/kg weight per day in 3 divided doses with meals.

Special care: pregnancy. Maintain fluid intake and monitor electrolyte in long-term treatment of elderly or debilitated.

Avoid use: obstruction of intestine, galactosaemia (accumulation of galactose in the blood in children who cannot utilize this sugar due to inborn lack of the appropriate enzyme). *Possible interaction*: antacids, neomycin for those with PSE.

Side effects: flatulence, bloating, gastrointestinal discomfort, chronic itching around the anus.

Manufacturer: Zyma.

Lamictal

Description: a triazine, lamotrigine, available as yellow tablets of strength 25mg, 50mg and 100mg marked with name and strength.

Used for: anticonvulsant.

Dosage: 50mg daily for 2 weeks, then 50mg twice daily for 2 weeks increasing to maintenance dose of 200–400mg daily in 2 divided doses. If sodium valproate is being taken, 25mg on alternate days for 2 weeks then 25mg daily for 2 weeks up to a maintenance dose of 100–200mg daily in 1 or 2 doses. Not recommended for children or the elderly.

Special care: pregnancy, lactation. Monitor liver, kidney and clotting in patients developing fever, flu, rash, drowsiness or deterioration of seizure control. Withdraw gradually over 2 weeks.

Avoid use: liver or kidney disease.

Possible interaction: sodium valproate, primidone, phenobarbitone, phenytoin, carbamazepine.

Side effects: dizziness, blurred vision, headache, drowsiness, gastrointestinal upsets, rash, Stevens-Johnson syndrome, angioneurotic oedema.

Manufacturer: Wellcome.

Lamisil

Description: an allylamine antifungal, terbinafine hydrochloride, as white 250mg tablets marked LAMISIL.

Used for: fungal infections of skin and nails.

Dosage: 1 daily for 2 to 6 weeks (athlete's foot); groin infection, 2 to 4 weeks; body infection 4 weeks and 6 to 12 weeks for nail infections. Not for children.

Also **Lamisil Cream**, a 1% cream.

Used for: fungal and yeast infections of the skin.

Dosage: apply to infected area 1 or 2 times per day for 1 to 2 weeks. Not for children.

Special care: pregnancy, lactation, chronic liver disorder, impaired kidney function.

Possible interaction: any drug affecting liver enzymes.

Side effects: headache, myalgia, arthralgia, allergic skin reaction, gastrointestinal upset.

Manufacturer: Sandoz.

Lamprene

Description: a phenazine, clofazimine, available as 100mg strength in brown gelatin capsules marked GEIGY AND GM.

Used for: leprosy.

Dosage: as advised, but often as part of a 3-drug treatment when 300mg once a month given by the physician and 50mg daily, self-administered. Treatment may be prolonged (over 2 years).

Special care: pregnancy, lactation, diarrhoea, abdominal pain, liver or kidney disease.

Side effects: dry skin, pruritis, discolouration of hair, skin and secretions, gastrointestinal upsets. Dosage can be reduced accordingly.

Manufacturer: Geigy.

Lanoxin

Description: a cardiac glycoside, digoxin, available as 250μg white tablet marked WELLCOME Y3B. Also **Lanoxin-PF**, 62.5μg blue tablet marked WELLCOME USA, **Lanoxin-PG Elixir**, 50μg/ml and **Lanoxin Injection**, 250μg/ml digoxin in 2ml ampoules.

Used for: digitalis treatment, especially congestive heart failure.

Dosage: maintenance dose: adults, 125–750μg daily; elderly, 62.5–250μg daily; for children, see literature.

Special care: acute myocardial infarction, atrio-ventricular block, thyroid disorder, severe lung disease, kidney impairment.

Avoid use: hypercalcaemia, ventricular tachycardia, hypertrophic obstructive cardiomyopathy.

Possible interaction: calcium tablets or injections, cardiac glycosides, potassium-depleting agents, lithium, quinidine, antacids, antibiotics.

Side effects: changes in heart rhythm, gastro intestinal upsets, visual disturbances.

Manufacturer: Wellcome.

Lanvis

Description: a cytotoxic preparation of thioguanine available as 40mg yellow tablets marked WELLCOME U3B.

Used for: treatment of acute leukaemias.

Dosage: 2–2.5mg/kg daily at the outset.

Special care: interference with production of red blood cells in the bone marrow, causing some loss of immunity to infection. Monitor blood regularly.

Side effects: nausea, vomiting, gastrointestinal upsets, hair loss.

Manufacturer: Wellcome.

Largactil

Description: a group I phenothiazine, chlorpromazine hydrochloride available in 10, 25, 50 and 100mg white tablets marked with LG and strength. Also, **Largactil Syrup** (25mg/5ml), **Largactil Forte Suspension**, chlorpromazine carbonate equivalent to 100mg chlorpromazine hydrochloride per 5ml and **Largactil Injection**, 25mg/ml chlorpromazine hydrochloride in 2ml ampoules.

Used for: disturbances of the CNS that require sedation, schizophrenia, nausea and vomiting (of terminal illness), induction of hypothermia, mood disorders.

Dosage: 25mg 3 times per day, increasing by 25mg per day. Maintenance dose 75–300mg daily. See literature for children. Injection: 25–50mg by deep

intramuscular injection in a single dose. Can be repeated after 6 to 8 hours; to be followed by oral therapy as soon as possible.

Special care: pregnancy, lactation. Children: use in severe cases only.

Avoid use: heart failure, epilepsy, Parkinson's disease, liver or kidney disorder, hypothyroidism, elderly, glaucoma, enlarged prostate, unconscious patients, depression of bone marrow function.

Possible interaction: depressants of the CNS, alcohol, antidepressants, anticonvulsants, anti-diabetics, levodopa, analgesics, antihypertensives.

Side effects: muscle spasms (eye, neck, back, face), restlessness, rigidity and tremor, tardive dyskinesia (repetitious muscular movements), dry mouth, blocked nose, difficulty in passing urine, tachycardia, blurred vision, hypotension, constipation, weight gain, impotence, galactorrhoea, gynaecomastia, amenorrhoea, blood and skin changes, lethargy, fatigue, ECG irregularities.

Manufacturer: Rhône-Poulenc Rorer.

Lariam

Description: a 4-aminoquinolone, mefloquine hydrochloride, as 250mg white tablets.

Used for: treatment and prevention of malaria.

Dosage: prevention: 1 tablet weekly; children, 15–19kg quarter tablet; 20–30kg, half tablet; 31–45kg three-quarters tablet. Not recommended under 15kg. For visits up to 3 weeks, dose to be taken weekly on the same day for a minimum of 6 weeks starting 1 week before departure and continuing for 4 weeks after return. For stays over 3 weeks, weekly dose on the same day during the stay starting 1 week before and continuing for 4 weeks after return. Do not use for more than 3 months. For treatment dosages, see literature.

Special care: patients with heart conduction disorders. Women must use reliable contraception during and for 3 months after the stay.

Avoid use: liver or kidney damage, pregnancy, lactation, history of convulsions or psychiatric disorders.

Possible interaction: sodium valproate; typhoid vaccination, delay use for at least 12 hours after quinine.

Side effects: in treatment: dizziness, nausea, vomiting, appetite loss, gastrointestinal upset.

Manufacturer: Roche.

Larodopa

Description: the dopamine precursor, levodopa, as 500mg white tablets marked ROCHE in a hexagon.

Used for: Parkinson's disease.

Dosage: over 25 years, 125mg twice daily after food increasing after 1 week to 125mg 4 to 5 times per day and further at weekly intervals by 375mg daily, the total in 4 or 5 divided doses. Maintenance dose of 2.5–8g. Not recommended for anyone under 25.

Special care: cardiovascular, liver, kidney, lung or endocrine disease, glaucoma, pregnancy, peptic ulcer. Monitor blood, and liver, kidney and cardiovascular function.

Avoid use: glaucoma, severe psychoses, history of malignant melanoma.

Possible interaction: MAOIs, antihypertensives, sympathomimetics, pyridoxine, ferrous sulphate.

Side effects: anorexia, nausea, vomiting, involuntary movements, heart and CNS disturbances, urine discolouration, low blood pressure when standing up.

Manufacturer: Cambridge.

Lasikil

Description: a loop diuretic and potassium supplement comprising 20mg frusemide and 750mg potassium chloride in a sustained release matrix, forming a white/yellow two-layered tablet marked LK.

Used for: oedema with the need of a potassium supplement.

Dosage: 2 daily as 1 morning dose increasing to 4 if necessary (in 2 divided doses) or reducing to 1 daily.

Special care: diabetes, enlarged prostate or impaired urination, liver or kidney disease, pregnancy, lactation, gout.

Avoid use: Addison's disease, hyperkalaemia, cirrhosis of the liver.

Possible interaction: digitalis, lithium, NSAIDs, aminoglycosides, antihypertensives, cephalosporins, potassium-sparing diuretics.

Side effects: rash, gout, gastrointestinal upset. Discontinue if ulceration or obstruction of small bowel occurs.

Manufacturer: Hoechst.

Lasilactone

Description: a loop and potassium-sparing diuretic consisting of 20mg frusemide and 50mg spironolactone in a blue/white capsule.

Used for: oedema that has not responded to other therapy, hypertension of certain types.

Dosage: 1 to 4 daily, not recommended for children.

Special care: liver or kidney disease, impaired urination, enlarged prostate, diabetes, pregnancy, lactation, gout. Not to be used long-term for young patients.

Avoid use: kidney failure, liver cirrhosis, hyperkalaemia, Addison's disease.

Possible interaction: potassium supplements, potassium-sparing diuretics, antihypertensives, lithium, digitalis, ACE inhibitors, NSAIDs, cephalosporins, aminoglycosides.

Side effects: rash, gout, blood changes, gynaecomastia, gastrointestinal upsets.

Manufacturer: Hoechst.

Lasix

Description: a loop diuretic, frusemide, available as 20mg white tablets marked DLF and 40mg white tablets marked DLI, both also marked with manufacturer's symbol.

Used for: oedema, mild to moderate hypertension.

Dosage: 20–80mg in 1 dose daily or every other day. Children 1–3mg/kg per day.

Also **Lasix 500**, 500mg frusemide in yellow tablet form marked with the manufacturer's symbol and DIX on the reverse.

Used for: acute or chronic kidney insufficiency (used under hospital supervision).

Dosage: see literature.

Also **Lasix Paediatric Liquid**, 1mg/ml frusemide.

Dosage: 1–3mg/kg daily.

Also, **Lasix Injection**, 10mg/ml frusemide in 2, 5 and 25ml ampoules.

Dosage: 20–50mg intramuscularly or slow intravenous injection. Children, 0.5–1.5mg/kg daily.

Special care: gout, diabetes, enlarged prostate, liver or kidney disease, impaired urination, pregnancy, lactation. Potassium supplements may be necessary.

Avoid use: liver cirrhosis.

Possible interaction: NSAIDs, antihypertensives, cephalosporins, aminoglycosides, lithium, digitalis.

Side effects: gout, rash, gastrointestinal upset.

Manufacturer: Hoechst.

Lasix + K

Description: A loop diuretic and potassium supplement, frusemide, available in 40mg white tablets marked with the manufacturer's symbol and DLI on the reverse; and 750mg potassium chloride as pale yellow sustained-release tablets.

Used for: diuretic therapy where potassium is required.

Dosage: 1 frusemide tablet in the morning, and 1 potassium chloride tablet at midday and in the evening. Not for children.

Special care: liver or kidney disease, diabetes, gout, enlarged prostrate (prostatic hypertrophy) or impaired urination, pregnancy, lactation.

Avoid use: liver cirrhosis, Addison's disease,

hyperkalaemia.

Possible interaction: NSAIDs, cephalosporins, antihypertensives, digitalis, lithium, aminoglycosides, potassium-sparing diuretics.

Side effects: rash, gout, gastrointestinal upset. Discontinue if ulceration or obstruction of small bowel occurs.

Manufacturer: Hoechst.

Lasoride

Description: a loop and potassium-sparing diuretic comprising 40mg frusemide and 5mg amiloride hydrochloride in yellow tablets.

Used for: rapid diuretic treatment and conservation of potassium.

Dosage: 1 to 2 tablets in the morning, adjust for elderly. Not for children.

Special care: enlarged prostate, impaired urination, diabetes, gout, pregnancy, lactation, elderly. Electrolyte and fluid levels should be checked regularly.

Avoid use: liver cirrhosis, kidney failure, Addison's disease, hyperkalaemia, electrolyte imbalance.

Possible interaction: NSAIDs, digitalis, antidiabetic drugs, antihypertensives, lithium, ototoxic or nephrotoxic antibiotics, potassium supplements, potassium-sparing diuretics, certain muscle relaxants.

Side effects: gastrointestinal upset, itching, blood changes, malaise, reduced alertness, calcium loss. Occasionally minor mental disturbances, pancreatitis, altered liver function.

Manufacturer: Hoechst.

Ledclair

Description: a chelating agent, sodium calcium edetate as 200mg/ml in 5ml ampoules.

Used for: treatment of poisoning with lead and other heavy metals.

Dosage: up to 40mg/kg twice daily by intravenous drip or intramuscular injection for adults and children. To diagnose poisoning, 25mg/kg intramuscularly 3 times per day. See literature in both cases.

Special care: impaired kidney function.

Side effects: nausea, cramp, kidney damage on overdosage.

Manufacturer: Sinclair.

Ledercort

Description: a glucocorticoid, triamcinolone, in strengths of 2mg (blue, oblong tablet marked LL11) and 4mg (white, oblong tablet marked LL 9352).

Used for: rheumatoid arthritis, allergies.

Dosage: 2–24mg daily but see literature.

Special care: thrombophlebitis, psychoses, recent intestinal anastomoses, chronic nephritis, certain cancers, osteoporosis, peptic ulcer, skin eruption/rash related to a disease, viral, fungal or active infections, tuberculosis. Hypertension, glaucoma, epilepsy, acute glomerulonephritis (inflammation of kidney glomerulus), diabetes, cirrhosis, hypothyroidism, pregnancy, stress. To be withdrawn gradually.

Possible interaction: NSAIDs, oral anticoagulants, phenytoin, ephedrine, phenobarbitone, rifampicin, diuretics, cardiac glycosides, anticholinesterases, hypoglycaemics.

Side effects: osteoporosis, depression, euphoria, hyperglycaemia, peptic ulcers, Cushingoid changes. Also available as triamcinolone acetonide, 0.1% cream.

Used for: inflamed skin disorders.

Dosage: use sparingly 3 or 4 times per day.

Special care: maximum 5 days use on face or for children. Withdraw gradually.

Avoid use: acne, scabies, leg ulcers,peri-oral dermatitis; tuberculous, viral skin or ringworm infections, untreated bacterial or fungal infections. Do not use extensively or for a prolonged period in pregnancy.

Side effects: skin striae and atrophy, Cushingoid changes (see Cushing's syndrome), adrenal gland suppression, telangiectasia (collections of distended blood capillaries).

Manufacturer: Lederle.

Lederfen

Description: propionic acid as fenbufen in light blue tablet marked LEDERFEN (300mg), and light blue oblong tablet marked LEDERFEN 450 (450mg). Also, **Lederfen Capsules**, 300mg fenbufen in dark blue capsules marked LEDERFEN.

Used for: osteoarthritis, rheumatoid arthritis, ankylosing spondylitis and acute muscle/bone disorders.

Dosage: 300mg in the morning with 600mg at night, or 450mg twice daily. Not for children.

Also **Lederfen F**, fenbufen as white effervescent tablets (450mg).

Dosage: 1 dissolved in water, twice per day. Not for children.

Special care: heart failure, kidney or liver disease, pregnancy, lactation, elderly. Monitor those on long-term treatment.

Avoid use: active peptic ulcers or history of gastrointestinal lesions, allergy induced by aspirin or anti-inflammatory drug.

Possible interaction: anticoagulants, salicylates, quinolones.
Side effects: gastrointestinal intolerance, rash.
Manufacturer: Lederle.

Lederfolin

Description: folinic acid (as calcium folinate), 350mg strength, powder in a vial. Also, **Lederfolin Solution** as 10mg/ml in a 35ml ampoule.
Used for: alongside 5-fluorouracil in treatment of advanced colorectal cancer.
Dosage: see literature.
Special care: toxicity of 5-fluorouracil increased.
Manufacturer: Lederle.

Ledermycin

Description: a tetracycline, demeclocycline hydrochloride available as dark red/light red capsules marked LEDERLE 9123 (150mg strength).
Used for: respiratory and soft tissue infections.
Dosage: 300mg twice per day or150mg 4 times. Not for children.
Special care: liver and kidney disease.
Avoid use: pregnancy, lactation.
Possible interaction: milk, mineral supplements, antacids, oral contraceptives.
Side effects: sensitivity to light, gastrointestinal upset, further infections.
Manufacturer: Lederle.

Lederspan 20mg

Description: a glucocorticoid, triamcinolone hexacetonide in vials, 20mg/ml.
Used for: local inflammation of joints and soft tissues in arthritis, tendinitis and bursitis (inflammation of the connective tissue surrounding a joint).
Dosage: 2–30mg depending upon condition and size of joint or synovial space at 3 to 4 weekly intervals.
Also **Lederspan 5mg**
Description: triamcinolone hexacetonide in a vial (5mg/ml).
Used for: skin conditions.
Dosage: 0.5mg (or less) per square inch of affected skin.
Special care: thrombophlebitis, psychoses, recent intestinal anastomoses, chronic nephritis, certain cancers, osteoporosis, peptic ulcer, skin eruption/rash related to a disease, viral, fungal or active infections, tuberculosis. Hypertension, glaucoma, epilepsy, acute glomerulonephritis (inflammation of kidney glomerulus), diabetes, cirrhosis, hypothyroidism, pregnancy, stress. To be withdrawn gradually.

Possible interaction: NSAIDs, oral anticoagulants, phenytoin, ephedrine, phenobarbitone, rifampicin, diuretics, cardiac glycosides, anticholinesterases, hypoglycaemics.
Side effects: osteoporosis, depression, euphoria, hyperglycaemia, peptic ulcers, Cushingoid changes.
Manufacturer: Lederle.

Lentaron

Description: an aromatase inhibitor, formestane, available as a powder (250mg strength) in a vial with 2ml diluent.
Used for: advanced stages of breast cancer occurring after the menopause.
Dosage: 250mg intramuscularly every 2 weeks in gluteal muscle (buttock). Site of injection alternated.
Special care: avoid making injection into vein or sciatic nerve.
Avoid use: pregnancy, lactation, pre-menopausal women.
Side effects: pain and irritation at site of injection, vaginal bleeding or irritation, hot flushes, arthralgia, pelvic or muscular cramps, oedema, thrombophlebitis, sore throat, upset in the CNS or gastrointestinal tract.
Manufacutrer: Ciba.

Lentizol

Description: a tricyclic antidepressant, amitriptyline hydrochloride available as sustained-release pink capsules (25mg) or pink/red capsules (50mg) both with white pellets and marked with LENTIZOL and the capsule strength.
Used for: treatment of depression when sedation is required.
Dosage: 50–100mg at night, up to a maximum of 200mg per day. Elderly, 25–75mg daily. Not for children.
Special care: liver disorders, hyperthyroidism, glaucoma, lactation, epilepsy, diabetes, adrenal tumour, heart disease, urine retention. Psychotic or suicidal patients.
Avoid use: heart block, heart attacks, severe liver disease, pregnancy.
Possible interaction: MAOIs (or within 14 days of their use), alcohol, anti-depressants, barbiturates, anticholinergics, local anaesthetics that contain adrenaline or noradrenaline, oestrogens, cimetidine, antihypertensives.
Side effects: constipation, urine retention, dry mouth, blurred vision, palpitations, tachycardia, nervousness, drowsiness, insomnia. Changes in weight, blood and blood sugar, jaundice, skin

reactions, weakness, ataxia, hypotension, sweating, altered libido, gynaecomastia, galactorrhoea.
Manufacturer: Parke-Davis.

Lescol

Description: a suppressant of cholesterol production and sodium salt of fluvastatin available as red-brown/pale yellow (20mg strength) or red-brown/orange-yellow (40mg strength) capsules, marked with XU, the strength and the company logo.
Used for: hypercholesterolaemia (high blood cholesterol levels) for patients where levels cannot be controlled by diet.
Dosage: over 18 years, 20–40mg once per day in the evening. Adjust to response, monitor lipid levels. Not for children.
Special care: history of liver disease, or high alcohol intake (test liver function), myalgias or muscle weakness particularly with fever or if generally unwell. Any condition predisposing to rhabdomyolysis.
Avoid use: kidney or liver disease, pregnancy, lactation.
Possible interaction: immunosuppressive drugs, rifampicin, erythromycin, nicotinic acid, gemfibrozil.
Side effects: flatulence, abdominal pain, sinusitis, insomnia, nausea, dyspepsia, hypoaesthesia (some loss of sense of touch), infection of the urinary tract, disorders of the teeth.
Manufacturer: Sandoz.

Leucomax

Description: a recombinant human granulocyte macrophage-colony stimulating factor (GM-CSF) available as molgramostim in the form of powder in vials. There are 3 strengths: 150, 300 and 700µg (equivalent to 1.67, 3.33 and 7.77 million-unit).
Used for: reduction in neutropenia and therefore risk of infection associated with cytotoxic chemotherapy, speeding up bone marrow recovery after transplantation of same, neutropenia in patients on ganciclovir in AIDS-related cytomegalovirus retinitis.
Dosage: chemotherapy, 60,000–110,000 units/kg/day (by subcutaneous injection) for 7 to 10 days commencing 24 hours after last chemotherapy; bone marrow transplantation, 110,000 units/kg/day (by intravenous infusion) commencing 24 hours after transplantation and until white cell count is at required level (maximum 30 days treatment); in ganciclovir treatment, 60,000 units/kg/day by subcutaneous injection for 5 days, then adjust to response.
Special care: full blood monitoring necessary,

monitor those with lung disease, pregnancy and lactation, history of autoimmune disease. Not recommended for those under 18 years.
Avoid use: bone marrow cancer.
Side effects: anorexia, nausea, vomiting, diarrhoea, shortness of breath, weakness, rash, rigors, fever, muscle and bone pains, local reaction at site of injection. Anaphylaxis, cardiac failure, convulsions, hypotension, heartbeat abnormalities, pericarditis, pulmonary oedema.
Manufacturer: Sandoz/Schering Plough.

Leukeran

Description: an alkylating agent and cytotoxic drug, chlorambucil, available as yellow tablets (2 and 5mg strengths), marked WELLCOME C2A and H2A respectively.
Used for: ovarian cancer, Hodgkin's disease, chronic lymphocytic leukaemia.
Dosage: 100–200µg/kg daily for 4 to 8 weeks, but see literature.
Special care: kidney disease.
Avoid use: porphyria.
Side effects: bone marrow suppression, rashes.
Manufacturer: Wellcome.

Levophed

Description: a vasoconstrictor and sympatho-mimetic amine, noradrenaline (as the acid tartrate) as 1mg/ml, in ampoules for dilution. Also, **Levophed Special**, 0.1mg/ml.
Used for: cardiac arrest, acute hypotension.
Dosage: intravenous infusion of 8 µg/ml at a rate of 2.3ml/minute initially, adjusted to the response. By intracardiac or rapid intravenous injection, 0.5–0.75ml of a solution with 200 µg/ml .
Special care: extravasation at site of injection (escape of fluid, e.g. blood into tissues) may cause localized necrosis.
Avoid use: pregnancy, myocardial infarction.
Possible interaction: anaesthetics, tricyclics, ß-blockers, dopexamine.
Side effects: headache, uneven heartbeat.
Manufacturer: Sanofi Winthrop.

Lexotan

Description: an anxiolytic benzodiazepine for intermediate-acting use, bromazepam, available as lilac and pink tablets (1.5mg and 3mg strengths respectively) marked with L and the strength.
Used for: short-term treatment of severe or disabling anxiety, with or without insomnia.
Dosage: 3–18mg per day (elderly, 1.5–9mg) in divided doses. Not for children.

Special care: chronic kidney or liver disease or lung insufficiency, pregnancy, labour, lactation, elderly. May impair judgement. Avoid long-term use and withdraw gradually.

Avoid use: acute lung disorders, depression of respiration, phobias, chronic psychosis.

Possible interaction: anticonvulsants, alcohol, depressants of the CNS.

Side effects: gastrointestinal upset, vertigo, ataxia, confusion, drowsiness, light-headedness, hypotension, skin reactions and visual changes, urine retention, changes in libido. Dependence a risk with high doses and long treatment.

Manufacturer: Roche.

Lexpec

Description: a haematinic (haemoglobin-increasing drug), folic acid, available as a syrup containing 2.5mg/5ml.

Used for: megaloblasic anaemia caused by a deficiency of folic acid.

Dosage: 20–40 ml per day for 14 days, then 5–20ml per day. Children, 10–30ml per day.

Also, **Lexpec with Iron**, a combination of folic acid (2.5mg) with ferric ammonium citrate (400mg)/5ml of syrup; and **Lexpec with Iron-M**, 0.5mg folic acid and 400mg of ferric ammonium citrate/5ml of syrup.

Used for: anaemia during pregnancy caused by iron and folic acid deficiency.

Dosage: 5–10ml per day before food for the pregnancy and 1 month after.

Avoid use: megaloblastic anaemia due to vitamin B_{12} deficiency.

Possible interaction: tetracyclines.

Side effects: nausea, constipation, discolouration of teeth (syrup should be drunk through a straw).

Manufacturer: R.P. Drugs.

Li-Liquid

Description: Lithium salt (the citrate) available as a sugar-free liquid in concentrations of 5.4mmol and 10.8mmol/5ml.

Used for: mania, hypomania (excitable, hyperactive and irritable), self-mutilation, extreme mood changes.

Dosage: 10.8–32.4mmol per day initially in 2 divided doses. Lithium levels in serum to be maintained, see literature.

Special care: start treatment in hospital and maintain salt and fluid levels. Record kidney, heart and thyroid functions.

Avoid use: Addison's disease, pregnancy, lactation, hypothyroidism, kidney or heart insufficiency, sodium imbalance.

Possible interaction: NSAIDs, phenytoin, diuretics,

carbamazepine, diazepam, flupenthixol, methyldopa, haloperidol, tetracyclines, metoclopramide.

Side effects: hand tremor, weak muscles, diarrhoea, nausea, oedema, weight gain, disturbances to CNS and in ECG, skin changes, polyuria, polydipsia, hypo- or hyperthyroidism.

Manufacturer: R.P. Drugs.

Librium

Description: a long-acting benzodiazepine, chlordiazepoxide, available in 3 strengths: 5mg (yellow-green tablets), 10mg (light blue-green) and 25mg (dark blue-green), all marked with LIB and the strength. Also, **Librium Capsules**, as green-yellow (5mg) and green/black (10mg) capsules marked with LIB and the strength.

Used for: treatment of severe anxiety over the short-term, with or without insomnia, symptoms of acute alcohol withdrawal.

Dosage: 30mg per day initially to a maximum of 100mg. For insomnia, 10–30mg at bedtime. For alcohol withdrawal, 25–100mg repeated in 2 to 4 hours if necessary. Elderly, 5mg per day to begin with. Not for children.

Special care: chronic kidney or liver disease or lung insufficiency, pregnancy, labour, lactation, the elderly. May impair judgement. Avoid long-term use and withdraw gradually.

Avoid use: acute lung disorders, depression of respiration, phobias, chronic psychosis.

Possible interaction: anticonvulsants, alcohol, depressants of the CNS.

Side effects: gastrointestinal upset, vertigo, ataxia, confusion, drowsiness, light-headedness, hypotension, skin reactions and visual changes, urine retention, changes in libido. Dependence a risk with high doses and long treatment.

Manufacturer: Roche.

Limclair

Description: a chelating agent, trisodium edetate, available in ampoules (strength 200mg/ml).

Used for: parathyroidism, digitalis arrhythmia, hypercalcaemia, corneal opacities.

Dosage: up to 70mg/kg daily by slow intravenous infusion, but see literature. For children, up to 60mg/kg daily by same means.

Special care: tuberculosis.

Avoid use: kidney disease.

Manufacturer: Sinclair.

Lingraine

Description: an ergot-derived alkaloid ergotamine tartrate available as green tablets, strength 2mg.

Used for: migraine and headache.

Dosage: 1 under the tongue at the start of the attack, repeat 30–60 minutes later if required; maximum 3 in 24 hours and 6 in 1 week. Not for children.

Avoid use: liver or kidney disease, severe hypertension, sepsis; coronary, peripheral or occlusive vascular disease; pregnancy, lactation, porphyria, hyperthyroidism.

Possible interaction: ß-blockers, erythromycin.

Side effects: leg cramps, stomach pain, nausea.

Manufacturer: Sanofi Winthrop.

Lioresal

Description: a gamma-amino-butyric acid (GABA) derivative, baclofen, available as a white tablet (strength 10mg), marked CG and KJ. Also **Lioresal Liquid** , a sugar-free liquid containing 5mg/5ml.

Used for: muscle relaxant, for cerebral palsy, meningitis, spasticity of voluntary muscle due to cerebrovascular accidents, multiple sclerosis, spinal lesions.

Dosage: 5mg 3 times per day to begin with, increasing by 5mg 3 times per day at intervals of 3 days. Maximum 100mg per day. For children, see the literature.

Special care: epilepsy, pregnancy, cerebrovascular accidents, the elderly, psychosis, hypertonic (abnormally increased tone or strength) bladder sphincter, liver or kidney disorders, defective respiration. Withdraw gradually.

Avoid use: peptic ulcer.

Possible interactions: lithium, antihypertensives, tricyclic antidepressants, depressants of the CNS, alcohol, fentanyl, levodopa, carbidopa, ibuprofen.

Side effects: sedation and drowsiness, nausea, disturbances of the central nervous system, muscle fatigue, hypotension, disturbance of the heart, lung or circulatory system, frequent and painful urination (dysuria).

Manufacturer: Ciba.

Lipantil

Description: an isobutyric acid derivative, fenofibrate, for lowering of lipids. Available as a white capsule, 100mg strength.

Used for: certain types of hyperlipidaemia (high levels of fat in the blood) resistant to the influence of diet.

Dosage: 3 tablets per day initially, in divided doses with food. 2 to 4 tablets per day for maintenance. For children, 5mg/kg body weight/day.

Special care: in cases of kidney impairment.

Avoid use: severe liver or kidney disorder, pregnancy, lactation, disease of the gall bladder.

Possible interaction: oral hypoglycaemics, anticoagulants, phenylbutazone.

Side effects: headache, tiredness, vertigo, gastrointestinal upsets, rashes.

Manufacturer: Fournier.

Lipostat

Description: a preparation of pravastratin (as the sodium salt) available as pink oblong tablets in 10 and 20mg strengths, marked with the company name and 154 or 178.

Used for: hypercholesterolaemia (high levels of blood cholesterol) which does not respond to other treatments (levels above 7.8mmol/l of cholesterol).

Dosage: 10mg at night to begin with, adjusting to the response at intervals of 4 weeks. Usually 10–40mg as 1 dose, daily, at night. Not for children.

Special care: history of liver disease. Liver function tests to be undertaken during treatment.

Avoid use: pregnancy, lactation, liver disease.

Possible interaction: gemfibrozil and similar derivatives of isobutyric acid, to be taken 1 hour before or 4 hours after colestipolor cholestyramine.

Side effects: muscle pain, headache, rashes, nausea, vomiting, tiredness, diarrhoea, chest pains not related to the heart.

Manufacturer: Squibb.

Liskonum

Description: a sedative, available as white, oblong, controlled-release tablets containing 450mg lithium carbonate (equivalent to 12.2mmol of lithium ions, Li^+).

Used for: acute mania, hypomania, prevention of the recurrence of manic depression.

Dosage: blood lithium levels to be kept in the range 0.8–1.5mmol/l (for mania or hypomania) and 0.5–1.0mmol/l for prevention. Not for children.

Special care: commence treatment in hospital, salt and fluid intake to be kept up. Thyroid and kidney functions to be checked. Any symptoms of intoxication should be reported.

Avoid use: pregnancy, lactation, Addison's disease, kidney or heart disease, hypothyroidism, sodium imbalance.

Possible interaction: NSAIDs, diuretics, flupenthixol, fluoxetine, methyldopa, carbamazepine, fluvoxamine, haloperidol, phenytoin, metoclopramide.

Side effects: muscle weakness, hand tremor, diarrhoea, nausea, disturbances to heart and brain, oedema, weight gain, hypo- or hyperthyroidism, intense thirst, frequent urination, changes in kidney, skin reactions.

Manufacturer: Smith, Kline & French.

Litarex

Description: a white, oval, controlled-release tablet containing 564mg lithium citrate (equivalent to 6mmol of lithium ions, Li^+).

Used for: acute mania, prevention of recurrence of emotional disorders.

Dosage: 1 morning and evening to begin with. Blood lithium level should then be kept in the range 0.8–1.0mmol/l.

Special care: commence treatment in hospital, salt and fluid intake to be kept up. Thyroid and kidney functions should be checked. Any symptoms of intoxication should be reported.

Avoid use: pregnancy, lactation, Addison's disease, kidney or cardiovascular disease, the elderly, hypothyroidism, conditions altering sodium balance.

Possible interaction: NSAIDs, diuretics, flupenthixol, methyldopa, carbamazepine, haloperidol, phenytoin, antidepressants, metoclopramide.

Side effects: muscle weakness, diarrhoea, nausea, hand tremor, heart and brain disturbances, oedema, weight gain, hypo- or hyperthyroidism, intense thirst, frequent urination, skin reactions.

Manufacturer: CP Pharmaceuticals.

Livial

Description: a white tablet containing 2.5mg tibolone (a gonadomimetic), marked MK2, ORGANON and *.

Used for: vasomotor symptoms (affecting blood vessel constriction or dilatation) associated with the menopause.

Dosage: a tablet daily for a minimum of 3 months.

Special care: kidney disorder or history of same, migraine, diabetes, epilepsy, high blood cholesterol levels. Menstrual bleeding may occur irregularly if commenced within 1 year of last period. Treatment to be stopped if liver disorder, cholestatic jaundice or thromboembolic disorders occur.

Avoid use: undiagnosed vaginal bleeding, hormone-dependent tumours, pregnancy, lactation, severe liver disease, cardio- or cerebrovascular disorder.

Possible interaction: carbamazepine, phenytoin, anticoagulants, rifampicin.

Side effects: headache, dizziness, vaginal bleeding, bodyweight changes, seborrhoeic dermatitis (eczema associated with oil-sebum-secreting glands), abnormal liver function, gastrointestinal upset, hair growth, oedema in front of the tibia.

Manufacturer: Organon.

Lobak

Description: a muscle relaxant and analgesic, comprising 100mg chlormezanone and 450mg paracetamol available as white tablets marked LOBAK.

Used for: relief of painful muscle spasms.

Dosage: 1 or 2 three times per day, up to a maximum of 8. Half dose for the elderly not recommended for children.

Special care: pregnancy, lactation, kidney or liver disease.

Avoid use: porphyria.

Possible interaction: MAOIs, depressants of the central nervous system, alcohol.

Side effects: dizziness, drowsiness, reduced alertness, dry mouth, rash, jaundice.

Manufacturer: Sanofi Winthrop.

Locabiotal

Description: an antibiotic and anti-inflammatory, fusafungine available as a metered dose aerosol (125µg per dose).

Used for: inflammation and infection of the upper respiratory tract.

Dosage: 5 oral sprays or 3 sprays in each nostril, 5 times per day. Children: over 12 years, 4 oral sprays 3 times per day or 3 sprays in each nostril 5 times per day; 6 to 12 years, 3 oral sprays 3 times per day or 2 sprays in each nostril 5 times per day; 3 to 5 years, 2 oral sprays 3 times per day or 1 spray in each nostril 5 times per day. Not recommended for children under 3 years.

Manufacturer: Servier.

Loceryl

Description: an antifungal cream, containing 0.25% amorolfine hydrochloride.

Used for: microscopic fungal or ringworm skin infestation.

Dosage: apply daily in the evening, usually for 2 to 3 weeks. Continue for 3 to 5 days after cure. Not for children.

Also, **Loceryl Lacquer**, 5% amorolfine hydrochloride as a lacquer.

Used for: microscopic fungal, yeast and mould nail infestation.

Dosage: apply once or twice per week; review every 3 months. Not for children.

Special care: do not allow to come into contact with eyes, ears or mucous membranes.

Avoid use: pregnancy, lactation.

Side effects: sometimes pruritus (itching), temporary burning sensation.

Manufacturer: Roche.

Locoid

Description: a strong steroid, hydrocortisone 17-

butyrate, available as a 0.1% cream and ointment.

Used for: eczema, psoriasis, skin disorders.

Dosage: apply 2 or 3 times per day.

Also, **Locoid Lipocream**, 0.1% hydrocortisone 17-butyrate in a base containing 70% oil.

Used for: skin disorders.

Dosage: apply 2 or 3 times per day.

Also **Locoid Scalp Lotion**, 0.1% hydrocortisone 17-butyrate in an alcoholic solution.

Used for: seborrhoea of the scalp.

Dosage: apply twice daily.

Also, **Locoid C**, a strong steroid 0.1% hydrocortisone 17-butyrate with an antifungal and antibacterial, 3% chlorquinaldol, available as cream and ointment.

Used for: eczema, psoriasis, and skin disorders when there is also infection.

Dosage: apply 2 to 4 times per day.

Special care: maximum 5 days use on face, withdraw gradually after prolonged use.

Avoid use: acne, dermatitis around the mouth, leg ulcers, scabies, viral skin disease, ringworm or tubercular infection, untreated infections caused by fungi or bacteria. Avoid prolonged or extensive use during pregnancy. Children.

Side effects: suppression of adrenal glands, skin striae and atrophy, telangiectasia (multiple telangiectases—collections of distended blood capillaries), Cushingoid changes.

Manufacturer: Brocades.

Locorten-Vioform

Description: an antibacterial and corticosteroid, comprising 1% clioquinol and 0.02% flumethasone pivalate, as drops.

Used for: inflammation of the outer ear where there may be secondary infection.

Dosage: 2 to 3 drops twice daily for 7 to 10 days for all but children under 2 years of age.

Special care: lactation.

Avoid use: primary infections of the outer ear, perforated eardrum.

Side effects: skin irritation, discolouration of hair.

Manufacturer: Zyma.

Lodine

Description: a NSAID, pyranocarboxylate, available as 200mg etodolac in dark grey/light grey capsules with 2 red bands and marked LODINE 200, and 300mg etodolac in light grey capsules with 2 red bands and marked LODINE 300. Also, **Lodine Tablets**, 200mg etodolac in brown, film-coated tablets marked LODINE 200.

Used for: osteoarthrosis, rheumatoid arthritis.

Dosage: 200 or 300mg twice per day, or 400 or 600mg as 1 dose if response is better. Maximum daily dose of 600mg. Not for children.

Also, **Lodine SR**, 600mg etodolac as grey, sustained-release tablets, marked LODINE and SR 600.

Dosage: 1 daily. Not for children.

Special care: liver, kidney or heart disorder, heart failure, elderly. Monitor those on long-term treatment.

Avoid use: active or history of peptic ulcer, history of gastrointestinal bleeding, aspirin or anti-inflammatory induced allergy, pregnancy, lactation.

Possible interaction: hypoglycaemics, anti-coagulants, quinolones.

Side effects: gastrointestinal upset or bleeding, nausea, epigastric (upper central abdomen) pain, headache, dizziness, nephritis, rash, tinnitus, angioneurotic oedema.

Manufacturer: Wyeth.

Loestrin 20

Description: an oestrogen/progestogen, ethinyl-oestradiol (20mg) with norethisterone acetate (1.5mg) in green tablets. Also **Loestrin 30**, which contains 30mg ethinyloestradiol.

Used for: oral contraception.

Dosage: 1 tablet daily for 21 days, commencing on the fifth day of menstruation, then 7 days without tablets.

Special care: hypertension, Raynaud's disease (reduced blood supply to an organ of the body's extremities), asthma, severe depression, diabetes, varicose veins, multiple sclerosis, chronic kidney disease, kidney dialysis. Blood pressure, breasts and pelvic organs to be checked regularly; smoking not advised.

Avoid use: history of heart disease, infectious hepatitis, sickle cell anaemia, porphyria, liver tumour, undiagnosed vaginal bleeding, pregnancy, hormone-dependent cancer, haemolytic uraemic syndrome (rare kidney disorder), chorea, otosclerosis.

Possible interaction: barbiturates, tetracyclines, griseofulvin, rifampicin, primidone, phenytoin, chloral hydrate, ethosuximide, carbamazepine, glutethimide, dichloralphenazone.

Side effects: fluid retention and bloating, leg cramps/pains, breast enlargement, depression, headaches, nausea, loss of libido, weight gain, vaginal discharge, cervical erosion (alteration of epithelial cells), chloasma (pigmentation of nose, cheeks or forehead), breakthrough bleeding (bleeding between periods).

Manufacturer: Parke-Davis.

Logiparin

Description: an anticoagulant, and low molecular weight heparin (LMWH), tinzaparin sodium available as 11,700 units of anti-Factor Xa (a blood coagulation factor) per ml in syringes.

Used for: prevention of thromboembolism during general or orthopaedic surgery.

Dosage: general surgery—3,500 units injected subcutaneously 2 hours before an operation then 3,500 once daily for 7 to 10 days. Orthopaedic surgery—2,500 units (body weight under 60kg), 3,500 units (60–80kg), 4,500 units (over 80kg), all injected subcutaneously before the operation and repeated once daily for a further 7 to 10 days. Not for children.

Special care: pregnancy, lactation, asthma, severe liver or kidney disorder.

Avoid use: tendency to haemorrhage, peptic ulcer, severe hypertension, endocarditis.

Possible interaction: drugs that affect coagulation or platelet function.

Side effects: increased haemmorhage risk, bruising, skin rashes, thrombocytopenia, temporary increase in liver enzymes.

Manufacturer: Novo Nordisk.

Logynon

Description: a combined oestrogen/progestogen contraceptive comprising ethinyloestradiol and levonorgestrel in the combinations: 30µg/50µg (6 brown tablets), 40µg/75µg (5 white tablets), 30µg/125µg (10 ochre tablets).

Used for: oral contraception.

Dosage: 1 tablet daily for 21 days starting on the first day of menstruation, then 7 days without tablets.

Special care: hypertension, Raynaud's disease (reduced blood supply to an organ of the body's extremities), asthma, severe depression, diabetes, varicose veins, multiple sclerosis, chronic kidney disease, kidney dialysis. Blood pressure, breasts and pelvic organs to be checked regularly; smoking not advised.

Avoid use: history of heart disease, infectious hepatitis, sickle cell anaemia, porphyria, liver tumour, undiagnosed vaginal bleeding, pregnancy, hormone-dependent cancer, haemolytic uraemic syndrome (rare kidney disorder), chorea, otosclerosis.

Possible interaction: barbiturates, tetracyclines, griseofulvin, rifampicin, primidone, phenytoin, chloral hydrate, ethosuximide, carbamazepine, glutethimide, dichloralphenazone.

Side effects: fluid retention and bloating, leg cramps/pains, breast enlargement, depression, headaches, nausea, loss of libido, weight gain, vaginal discharge, cervical erosion (alteration of epithelial cells), chloasma (pigmentation of nose, cheeks or forehead), breakthrough bleeding (bleeding between periods).

Manufacturer: Schering H.C.

Logynon ED

Description: an oestrogen/progestogen contraceptive comprising ethinyloestradiol and levonorgestrel in the combinations: 30µg/50µg (6 brown tablets), 40µg/75µg (5 white tablets), 30µg/125µg (10 ochre tablets) plus 7 white tablets containing inert lactose.

Used for: oral contraception.

Dosage: 1 tablet daily for 28 days starting on the first day of the cycle.

Special care: hypertension, Raynaud's disease (reduced blood supply to an organ of the body's extremities), asthma, severe depression, diabetes, varicose veins, multiple sclerosis, chronic kidney disease, kidney dialysis. Blood pressure, breasts and pelvic organs to be checked regularly; smoking not advised.

Avoid use: history of heart disease, infectious hepatitis, sickle cell anaemia, porphyria, liver tumour, undiagnosed vaginal bleeding, pregnancy, hormone-dependent cancer, haemolytic uraemic syndrome (rare kidney disorder), chorea, otosclerosis.

Possible interaction: barbiturates, tetracyclines, griseofulvin, rifampicin, primidone, phenytoin, chloral hydrate, ethosuximide, carbamazepine, glutethimide, dichloralphenazone.

Side effects: fluid retention and bloating, leg cramps/pains, breast enlargement, depression, headaches, nausea, loss of libido, weight gain, vaginal discharge, cervical erosion (alteration of epithelial cells), chloasma (pigmentation of nose, cheeks or forehead), breakthrough bleeding (bleeding between periods).

Manufacturer: Schering H.C.

Lomotil

Description: an opiate and anticholinergic, diphenoxylate hydrochloride (2.5mg) and atropine sulphate (25µg) in a white tablet marked SEARLE. Also, **Lomotil Liquid** (5ml is equivalent to 1 tablet).

Used for: diarrhoea.

Dosage: 4 tablets or 20ml to begin with then half this dose every 6 hours until control is achieved. Children: 13 to 16 years, 2 tablets or 10ml 3 times per day; 9 to 12 years, 1 tablet or 5ml 4 times per day; 4 to 8 years, 1 tablet or 5ml 3 times daily. Not recommended below 4 years.

Special care: pregnancy, lactation, liver disorder, do not start if there is severe dehydration or imbalance of electrolytes.

Avoid use: acute ulcerative colitis, obstruction in the intestines, jaundice, pseudomembranous colitis (a severe form of colitis).

Possible interaction: depressants of the CNS, MAOIs.

Side effects: allergic reactions, gastrointestinal upset, disturbances of the CNS, anticholinergic effects.

Manufacturer: Gold Cross (Searle).

Loniten

Description: a vasodilator and antihypertensive, minoxidil, available as white tablets (2.5mg, 5mg and 10mg) marked with the tablet strength and on the reverse with U.

Used for: severe hypertension.

Dosage: 5mg per day initially in 1 or 2 divided doses, increasing at intervals of 3 days, to 10mg and thereafter by increases of 10mg daily to a maximum of 50mg. Children: 0.2mg/kg to begin with daily in 1 or 2 divided doses, increasing by 0.1–0.2mg/kg at intervals of 3 days to a maximum of 1mg/kg body weight daily.

Special care: heart attack. Antihypertensives (other than diuretics and ß-blockers) should be withdrawn gradually before starting treatment. Diuretics and sympathetic suppressants to be given at the same time.

Avoid use: phaeochromocytoma.

Side effects: oedema, tachycardia, hair-growth.

Manufacturer: Upjohn.

Lopid

Description: an isobutyric acid derivative, gemfibrozil, available as white/maroon capsules (300mg strength) marked LOPID 300. Also **Lopid Tablets**, 600mg gemfibrozil in white oval tablets marked LOPID.

Used for: prevention of coronary heart disease through lowering high levels of cholesterol or other fats in the blood.

Dosage: 600mg twice per day to a maximum of 1500mg per day.

Special care: blood count, liver function and lipid profile tests before treatment and blood counts over the first year of treatment. Annual check on eyes, period check on serum lipids. To be stopped in cases of persistent abnormal liver function.

Avoid use: gallstones, alcoholism, pregnancy, lactation, liver disorder.

Possible interaction: anticoagulants, simvastatin, pravastatin.

Side effects: headache, dizziness, blurred vision, muscle pain, painful extremities, skin rash, impotence, gastrointestinal upset.

Manufacturer: Parke-Davis.

Loprazolam

Description: an intermediate-acting benzodiazepine hypnotic, loprazolam mesylate, available in 1mg tablets.

Used for: treatment of insomnia or waking at night over the short-term.

Dosage: 1 or 2 at bedtime; up to 1 for the elderly. Not for children.

Special care: chronic kidney or liver disease, lung insufficiency, pregnancy, labour, lactation, elderly. May cause impaired judgement. Avoid prolonged use and withdraw gradually.

Avoid use: acute lung disease, psychotic, phobic or obsessional states, depression of respiration.

Possible interaction: depressants of the CNS, alcohol, anticonvulsants.

Side effects: ataxia, confusion, light-headedness, drowsiness, gastrointestinal upset, changes in vision and libido, skin rash, hypotension, retention of urine. Dependence risk increases with prolonged treatment or higher dosages.

Manufacturer: Roussel.

Lopresor

Description: a ß-blocker, metoprolol tartrate, available as pink tablets (50mg strength) and light blue tablets (100mg strength), marked GEIGY.

Used for: prevention of mortality after myocardial infarction (MI), arrhythmias.

Dosage: see literature for initial dosage after MI, 200mg per day for maintenance. Arrhythmias, 50mg twice or 3 times per day to a daily maximum of 300mg.

Also used for: angina.

Dosage: 50–100mg 2 or 3 times per day.

Also **Lopresor SR**, 200mg metoprolol tartrate in a yellow, sustained-release capsule-shaped tablet marked CG/CG and CDC/CDC on the reverse.

Dosage: 1 per day; up to 2, once per day if necessary.

Also used for: hypertension, additional therapy in thyrotoxicosis.

Dosage: hypertension, 100mg daily to begin with increasing if necessary to 200mg in 1 or 2 divided doses. Thyrotoxicosis, 50mg, 4 times per day. Or 1 tablet of Lopresor SR in the morning.

Also used for: migraine.

Dosage: 100–200mg per day in divided doses.

Special care: history of bronchospasm and certain ß-blockers, diabetes, liver or kidney disease, pregnancy, lactation, general anaesthesia. Withdraw gradually. Not for children.

Avoid use: heart block or failure, slow heart rate (bradycardia), sick sinus syndrome (associated with sinus node disorder), certain ß-blockers, severe peripheral arterial disease.

Possible interaction: verapamil, hypoglycaemics, reserpine, clonidine withdrawal, some anti-arrhythmics and anaesthetics, antihypertensives, depressants of the CNS, cimetidine, indomethacin, sympathomimetics.

Side effects: bradycardia, cold hands and feet, disturbance to sleep, heart failure, gastrointestinal upset, tiredness on exertion, bronchospasm.

Manufacturer: Geigy.

Lopresoretic

Description: a ß-blocker and thiazide diuretic, metoprolol tartrate (100mg) and chlorthalidone (12.5mg), available as an off-white tablet marked GEIGY 56.

Used for: hypertension.

Dosage: 1 daily to begin with in the morning increasing if required to 3 or 4 per day in single or divided doses. Not for children.

Special care: history of bronchospasm and certain ß-blockers, diabetes, liver or kidney disease, pregnancy, lactation, general anaesthesia, gout, check electrolyte levels, K⁺ supplements may be required depending on the case. Withdraw gradually. Not for children.

Avoid use: heart block or failure, slow heart rate (bradycardia), sick sinus syndrome (associated with sinus node disorder), certain ß-blockers, severe peripheral arterial disease, pregnancy, lactation, severe kidney failure, anuria, hepatic cornea.

Possible interaction: verapamil, hypoglycaemics, reserpine, clonidine withdrawal, some antiarrhythmics and anaesthetics, antihypertensives, depressants of the CNS, cimetidine, indomethacin, sympathomimetics, lithium, potassium supplements with potassium-sparing diuretics, digitalis.

Side effects: bradycardia, cold hands and feet, disturbance to sleep, heart failure, gastrointestinal upset, tiredness on exertion, bronchospasm, gout, weakness, blood disorders, sensitivity to light.

Manufacturer: Geigy.

Lorazepam

Description: an intermediate-acting benzo-diazepine, lorazepam, available in tablets strength 1mg.

Used for: moderate to severe anxiety.

Dosage: 1–4mg per day in divided doses, elderly 0.5–2mg. Not for children.

Special care: chronic liver or kidney disease, chronic lung disease, pregnancy, labour, lactation, elderly. May impair judgement. Withdraw gradually and avoid prolonged use.

Avoid use: depression of respiration, acute lung disease; psychotic, phobic or obsessional states.

Possible interaction: anticonvulsants, depressants of the CNS, alcohol.

Side effects: ataxia, confusion, light-headedness, drowsiness, hypotension, gastrointestinal upsets, disturbances in vision and libido, skin rashes, retention of urine, vertigo. Sometimes jaundice or blood disorders.

Manufacturer: available from Wyeth.

Lormetazepam

Description: an intermediate-acting benzodiazepine, lormetazepam, available in 0.5mg and 1mg tablets.

Used for: insomnia.

Dosage: 1mg at bedtime elderly 0.5mg. Not for children.

Special care: chronic liver or kidney disease, chronic lung disease, pregnancy, labour, lactation, elderly. May impair judgement. Withdraw gradually and avoid prolonged use.

Avoid use: depression of respiration, acute lung disease; psychotic, phobic or obsessional states.

Possible interaction: anticonvulsants, depressants of the CNS, alcohol.

Side effects: ataxia, confusion, light-headedness, drowsiness, hypotension, gastrointestinal upsets, disturbances in vision and libido, skin rashes, retention of urine, vertigo. Sometimes jaundice or blood disorders.

Manufacturer: available from APS, Cox, Wyeth.

Loron

Description: a diphosphonate, sodium clodronate, available in ampoules as a solution of 30mg/ml.

Used for: hypercalcaemia induced by tumour.

Dosage: 300mg per day initially, by slow intravenous infusion, for a maximum of 10 days. For maintenance use tablets or capsules. Not for children.

Also **Loron Tablets**, containing 520mg sodium clodronate and in white oblong tablets marked BM E9.

Dosage: 2 to 4 tablets per day in 1, or 2 divided

doses 1 hour before or after food. Maximum usage, 6 months. Not for children.

Also, **Loron Capsules,** 400mg sodium clodronate, in white capsules marked BM B7.

Dosage: 4 to 8 capsules per day in 1, or 2 divided doses 1 hour before or after food for a maximum period of 6 months. Not for children.

Special care: kidney function, serum calcium and phosphate to be monitored.

Avoid use: pregnancy, lactation, kidney failure, inflammation of the intestines.

Possible interaction: antacids, mineral supplements, other diphosphonates.

Side effects: gastrointestinal upset. Sometimes allergic reactions, hypocalcaemia. Temporary proteinuria.

Manufacturer: Boehringer Mannheim Pharmaceuticals.

Losec

Description: a proton pump inhibitor (limits gastric H$^+$), omeprazole, available in pink/brown capsules (20mg) marked A/OM and 20, and brown capsules (40mg) both of which contain enteric-coated granules.

Used for: reflux oesophagitis, duodenal and benign gastic ulcers, Zollinger-Ellison (ZE) syndrome.

Dosage: reflux oesophagitis: 20mg per day for 4 weeks, plus a further 4 to 8 weeks if necessary. In unresponsive (refractory) cases, 40mg once per day. 20mg daily for long-term treatment. Duodenal ulcer: 20mg per day for 8 weeks, and 40mg for severe cases. 20mg daily for long-term treatment. Gastric ulcer: 20mg per day for 8 weeks, increasing to 40mg for severe cases. Z-E syndrome: 60mg per day, modified according to response, maintenance 20–120mg daily (doses over 80mg in 2 divided doses). Not for children.

Special care: for suspected gastric ulcer, malignancy must be excluded prior to treatment.

Avoid use: pregnancy, lactation.

Possible interaction: warfarin, digoxin, phenytoin, diazepam.

Side effects: diarrhoea, headache, nausea, skin rashes, constipation.

Manufacturer: Astra.

Lotriderm

Description: a potent steroid and antifungal agent, betamethasone dipropionate (0.05%) and clotrimazole (1%) available as a cream.

Used for: short-term treatment fungal infections of the skin.

Dosage: apply for 2 weeks, morning and evening (4 weeks for treatment of the feet).

Special care: maximum 5 days use on face or for children, withdraw gradually after prolonged use.

Avoid use: acne, dermatitis around the mouth, leg ulcers, scabies, viral skin disease, ringworm or tubercular infection, untreated infections caused by fungi or bacteria. Avoid prolonged or extensive use during pregnancy. Children.

Side effects: irritation, localized mild burning sensation, hypersensitivity reactions.

Manufacturer: Schering-Plough.

Loxapac

Description: a dibenzoxapine, loxapine succinate, available in yellow/green (10mg), light green/dark green (25mg) and blue/dark green (50mg) capsules marked L2, L3 or L4 respectively.

Used for: chronic and acute psychoses.

Dosage: 20–50mg per day, to begin with, in 2 doses and increasing over 7 to 10 days to 60–100mg daily. Maximum, 250mg daily. Not for children.

Special care: cardiovascular disease, epilepsy, urine retention, glaucoma, pregnancy, lactation.

Avoid use: patients in a coma or depression induced by drugs.

Possible interaction: anticholinergics, depressants of the CNS.

Side effects: faintness, muscle twitches, weakness, dizziness, drowsiness, confusion, tachycardia, hyper- or hypotension, skin reactions, nausea, changes in ECG and eye, headache, vomiting, dyspnoea (shortness of breath), anticholinergic effects.

Manufacturer: Novex.

Ludiomil

Description: a tetracyclic antidepressant, maprotiline hydrochloride, available as peach tablets (10mg, marked Co), greyish-red tablets (25mg, marked DP), light orange tablets (50mg, marked ER) and brown-orange tablets (75mg, marked FS). All are also marked CIBA.

Used for: depression.

Dosage: 25–75mg per day to start with in 1 or 3 divided doses, modifying after 1 or 2 weeks as required; maximum of 150mg daily. Elderly, 30mg once daily or 3 doses of 10mg per day. Not for children.

Special care: pregnancy, lactation, elderly, cardiovascular disease, schizophrenia, hyper-thyroidism.

Avoid use: severe liver or kidney disease, narrow-angle glaucoma, mania, history of epilepsy, urine retention, recent coronary thrombosis.

Possible interaction: sympathomimetics, barbiturates,

MAOIs, antipsychotics, alcohol, antihypertensives, anaesthetics, cimetidine, phenytoin, benzodiazepines.

Side effects: skin rash, convulsions, impaired reactions, anticholinergic effects.

Manufacturer: Ciba.

Lurselle

Description: a butylphenol, probucol, available as white tablets (250mg strength) marked LURSELLE.

Used for: treatment of high blood levels of protein-bound lipids (hyper-lipoproteinaemia).

Dosage: 2 tablets twice daily accompanying the morning and evening meals. Not for children.

Special care: heart disorders. Monitor ECG before starting treatment. Stop treatment 6 months before a planned pregnancy.

Avoid use: pregnancy, lactation.

Side effects: diarrhoea, gastrointestinal upset.

Manufacturer: Merrell Dow.

Lustral

Description: sertraline hydrochloride available as white, capsule-shaped tablets in 50 and 100mg strengths and marked PFIZER with LTL-50 or LTL-100 respectively.

Used for: depression and the prevention of relapse or further bouts of depression.

Dosage: 50mg per day at the start, with food, increasing by 50mg if necessary, every 2 to 4 weeks to a daily maximum of 200mg. Maintenance is usually 50–100mg per day. A dosage of 150mg or more should not be used for more than 8 weeks. Not for children.

Special care: pregnancy, lactation, unstable epilepsy, anyone undergoing ECT.

Avoid use: kidney or liver disorders.

Possible interaction: lithium, tryptophan, MAOIs.

Side effects: nausea, diarrhoea, tremor, increased sweating, dyspepsia, dry mouth, delay in ejaculation.

Manufacturer: Invicta.

M

Macrobid

Description: a preparation which is a nitrofuran antibacterial drug available as yellow/blue modified-release capsules containing 100mg nitrofurantoin, marked Eaton BID.

Used for: infections of urinary tract, prevention of infection during surgical procedures on genital/ urinary tract, pyelitis.

Dosage: adults, treatment, 1 tablet twice each day with food; prevention of infection, 1 tablet twice daily for 4 days starting on day of surgery.

Special care: breast-feeding, patients with diabetes, deficiency of vitamin B, debilitation, anaemia, imbalance in electrolyte (salts) levels. Elderly patients and those on long-term treatment require monitoring of liver, lung and nerve function.

Avoid use: children, pregnant women at end of pregnancy, patients with kidney disease or damage or failure or reduction in ability to produce urine (anuria and oliguria).

Possible interaction: probenecid, quinolones, magnesium trisilicate, sulphinpyrazone.

Side effects: gastrointestinal upset, blood changes, allergic responses, anorexia. Drug should be withdrawn if hepatitis, lung reactions, peripheral nerve damage or haemolysis occur.

Manufacturer: P. & G.P.

Macrodantin

Description: an antibacterial nitrofuran drug available as white/yellow capsules containing 50mg nitrofurantoin, and yellow capsules containing 100mg nitrofurantoin.

Used for: treatment and prevention of urinary tract infections (during surgical procedure), pyelitis.

Dosage: adults and children over 10 years, treatment of acute infection, 50mg 4 times each day for 1 week; serious, recurring infection, 100mg 4 times each day for 1 week. Long-term suppression of infection, 50–100mg each day taken as single dose at bedtime. Prevention, 50mg 4 times each day for 4 days beginning on day of prcedure. Children, 3 months to 10 years, acute infection, 3mg/kg body weight in divided doses each day for 1 week.

Suppression of infection, 1mg/kg body weight once each day.

Special care: breast-feeding, patients who are debilitated, vitamin B deficiency, anaemia, imbalance in electrolyte (salts) levels, diabetes. Elderly patients and those on long-term treatment require regular monitoring of liver and lung function.

Avoid use: pregnant women at end of pregnancy, patients with kidney disease or damage, anuria and oliguria.

Possible interaction: probenecid, quinolones, sulphinpyrazone, magnesium trisilicate.

Side effects: gastrointestinal upset, allergic responses, blood changes, anorexia. Drug should be withdrawn if hepatitis, lung reactions, peripheral nerve damage or haemolysis occur.

Manufacturer: P. & G.P.

Madopar

Description: a combined preparation of dopamine precursor (levodopa) and an enzyme which is a dopa decarboxylase inhibitor, benserazide (as hydrochloride), available as capsules of different strengths. '62.5' blue/grey capsules contain 50mg and 12.5mg respectively. '125' blue/pink capsules contain 100mg and 25mg. '250' blue/caramel capsules contain 200mg and 50mg. All capsules are marked ROCHE. Also, **Madopar Dispersible Tablets**, white scored tablets of 2 different strengths: '62.5' contain 50mg and 12.5mg; '125' contain 100mg and 25mg. Tablets all marked with name and strength. Also, **Madopar CR** green/blue continuous-release capsules containing 100mg levodopa and 25mg benserazide (as hydrochloride), marked ROCHE.

Used for: Parkinson's disease.

Dosage: adults over 25 years of age not already receiving levodopa, 1 '62.5' tablet 3 or 4 times each day at first taken after meals. Dose may be increased by 1 '125' tablet each day once or twice a week. Usual maintenance dose is in the order of 4 to 8 '125' tablets each day in divided doses. Elderly persons, 1 '62.5' once or twice each day with additional '62.5' tablet every third or fourth day if increase is required. Madopar continuous-release capsules: dose individually determined for each patient, usually 50% more than previous levodopa therapy.

Special care: peptic ulcer, wide angle glaucoma, liver, kidney, heart, lung, circulatory diseases or endocrine (hormonal) disorders. Also, psychiatric disorders, soft bones (osteomalacia). Regular blood checks and monitoring of liver, kidney, heart and circulatory function should be carried out.

Avoid use: children and young adults under 25 years of age, pregnancy, breast-feeding. Patients with history of malignant melanoma (tumours of melanocytes which form the skin pigment, melanin), narrow angle glaucoma, severe psychoses.

Possible interaction: sympathomimetics, anti-hypertensives, other similar preparations, ferrous sulphate, MAOIs; antacids (Madopar CR).

Side effects: heart and central nervous system disturbance, involuntary movements, hypotension when rising from lying down, anorexia, nausea, vomiting, discoloured urine. Rarely, haemolytic anaemia.

Manufacturer: Roche.

Magnapen

Description: a compound broad-spectrum penicillin and penicillinase-resistant (i.e. resistant to enzymes produced by some bacteria) preparation. It is available as turquoise/black capsules containing 250mg ampicillin and 250mg flucloxacillin and marked MAGNAPEN. Also, **Magnapen Syrup** containing 125mg ampicillin and 125mg flucloxacillin/5ml. **Magnapen Injection** containing 500mg or 1g powder in vials for reconstitution and injection, both with equal quantities of ampicillin and flucloxacillin.

Used for: severe and mixed infections where some penicillin-resistant (staphylococci) bacteria are present.

Dosage: adults and children over 10, 1 capsule or 10ml syrup 4 times each day taken thirty minutes to 1 hour before meals. Injection, 500mg 4 times each day. Children, under 10 years, 5ml syrup 4 times each day thirty minutes to 1 hour before meals. Injection, under 2 years, quarter of adult dose; 2 to 10 years, half adult dose.

Special care: patients with glandular fever (infectious mononucleosis).

Side effects: gastrointestinal upset, allergic reactions; rarely, cholestatic jaundice.

Manufacturer: Beecham.

Maloprim

Description: a compound antimalarial preparation combining sulphone and diaminopyrimidine drugs, available as scored white tablets containing 100mg dapsone and 12.5mg pyrimethamine, marked WELLCOME H9A.

Used for: prevention of malaria.

Dosage: adults and children over 10 years, 1 tablet each week. Children, 5 to 10 years of age, 1 half tablet weekly.

Special care: patient should continue to take tablets for 4 weeks after leaving area where malaria is present. Special care in breast-feeding mothers, pregnant women should take folate supplements, patients with liver or kidney disease.

Avoid use: children under 5 years, patients with dermatitis herpetiformis (a type of dermatitis).

Possible interaction: folate inhibitors.

Side effects: severe haemolysis, skin sensitivity, blood disorders.

Manufacturer: Wellcome.

Manerix

Description: an antidepressant preparation which is a reversible MAO-A inhibitor (monoamine oxidase A inhibitor) which acts to prevent the breakdown of this neurotransmitter by enzyme, thereby prolonging its activity. It is available as scored, oblong, yellow, film-coated tablets containing 150mg moclobemide, marked ROCHE 150.

Used for: severe depression.

Dosage: adults, 2 tablets each day in divided doses (maximum of 4 daily) taken after meals.

Special care: pregnancy, breast-feeding, serious liver disease, thyrotoxicosis. Also, patients with schizophrenia in which agitation is a predominant symptom. Some foods may need to be avoided.

Avoid use: children, patients with phaeochromocytoma, severe confusional disorders.

Possible interaction: morphine, cimetidine, some sympathomimetic amines, pethidine, fentanyl, some other antidepressants, codeine.

Side effects: headache, giddiness, agitation and restlessness, confusion, nausea, disturbance of sleep.

Manufacturer: Roche.

Marevan

Description: a coumarin anticoagulant preparation available as scored tablets of different strengths all containing warfarin sodium; brown 1mg tablets marked M1, blue 3mg tablets marked M3 and pink 5mg tablets marked M5.

Used for: thromboembolic states.

Dosage: adults, 10mg each day adjusted according to response.

Special care: patients who are seriously ill, have kidney disease or disorder, hypertension, vitamin K deficiency, weight changes and elderly persons and children.

Avoid use: pregnancy, within 24 hours of labour or surgery, reduced liver or kidney function, haemorrhage or bleeding disorders.

Possible interaction: antibiotics, cimetidine, corticosteroids, hypoglycaemics taken orally, phenformin, sulphonamides, NSAIDs, quinidine, drugs have an effect on liver enzymes.

Side effects: skin rash, diarrhoea, baldness.

Manufacturer: Goldshield.

Marplan

Description: an antidepressant MAOI available as scored, pink tablets containing 10mg isocarboxazid, marked ROCHE.

Used for: depression.

Dosage: adults, 30mg each day at first reducing to a usual maintenance dose in the order of 10–20mg daily. Elderly persons, half adult dose.

Special care: elderly persons and patients with epilepsy.

Avoid use: children, patients with congestive heart failure, circulatory disease of arteries of brain (cerebro-vascular disease), liver disease, phaeochromocytoma, blood changes, hyper-thyroidism, heart disease.

Possible interaction: anticholinergics, barbiturates, alcohol, hypoglycaemics, insulin, reserpine, guanethidine, methyldopa. Also sympathomimetic amines, especially ephedrine, amphetamine, levodopa, methylphenidate, phenylpropanolamine, fenfluramine. Also, pethidine, TCADs, narcotic analgesics. Many foods need to be avoided including: meat extracts (Bovril, Oxo), bananas, yeast extracts (Marmite), broad beans, foods made from textured vegetable proteins, alcohol, low alcohol drinks, pickled herrings, all foods that are not completely fresh.All these drugs and foods should be avoided for at least 14 days after treatment stops then tried cautiously.

Side effects: allergic responses with certain foods, tiredness, muscle weakness, low blood pressure on rising, dizziness, swelling of ankles. Dry mouth, blurring of vision, gastrointestinal upset, constipation, difficulty ir urination. Skin rashes, weight gain, blood changes, change in libido, jaundice. Sometimes psychiatric disturbances and confusion.

Manufacturer: Cambridge.

Marvelon

Description: a combined oestrogen/progestogen oral contraceptive preparation available as white tablets containing 30mg ethinyloestradiol and 150 micrograms desogestrel, marked ORGANON, TR over 5 and with *.

Used for: oral contraception.

Dosage: 1 tablet each day for 21 days, starting on first or fifth day of monthly cycle, followed by 7 tablet-free days.

Special care: patients with multiple sclerosis, serious kidney disease or kidney dialysis, asthma, Raynaud's disease, abnormally high levels of prolactin in the blood (hyperprolactinaemia), varicose veins, hypertension. Also, patients suffering from severe depression. Thrombosis risk increases with smoking, age and obesity. During the course of treatment, regular checks on blood pressure, pelvic organs and breasts should be carried out.

Avoid use: pregnancy, those at risk of thrombosis, suffering from heart disease, pulmonary hypertension, angina, sickle cell anaemia. Also, undiagnosed vaginal bleeding, history of cholestatic jaundice during pregnancy, cancers which are hormone-dependent, infectious hepatitis, liver disorders. Also, porphyria, Dublin-Johnson and Rotor syndrome, otosclerosis, chorea, haemolytic uraemic syndrome, recent trophoblastic disease.

Possible interaction: barbiturates, ethosuximide, glutethimide, rifampicin, phenytoin, tetracyclines, carbamazepine, chloral hydrate, griseofulvin, dichloralphenazone, primidone.

Side effects: weight gain, breast enlargement, pains in legs, cramps, loss of sexual desire, headaches, depression, nausea, breakthrough bleeding, cervical erosion, vaginal discharge, brownish patches on skin (chloasma), oedema and bloatedness.

Manufacturer: Organon.

Maxidex

Description: lubricant and corticosteroid eyedrops containing 0.5% hypromellose and 0.1% dexamethasone.

Used for: inflammation of anterior segment of eye.

Dosage: serious disease, 1 to 2 drops each hour, reducing dose as condition improves. For milder conditions, 1 or 2 drops 4, 5 or 6 times each day.

Special care: long-term use by pregnant women and in babies.

Avoid use: patients with glaucoma, suffering from tuberculous, viral or fungal infections or those producing pus; patients with soft contact lenses.

Side effects: cataract, thinning of cornea, rise in pressure within eye, fungal infection.

Manufacturer: Alcon.

Maxitrol

Description: a compound preparation in the form of eyedrops combining a corticosteroid, aminoglycoside, lubricant and peptide. It contains 0.1% dexamethasone, 0.35% neomycin sulphate, 0.5% hypromellose, 6000 units polymyxin B sulphate/ml. Also **Maxitrol Ointment** containing 0.1% dexamethasone, 0.35% neomycin sulphate, 6000 units polymixin B sulphate/gram.

Used for: infected and inflamed conditions of the eye.

Dosage: apply 3 or 4 times each day.

Special care: long-term use by pregnant women or in babies.

Avoid use: patients with glaucoma, suffering from tuberculous, viral or fungal infections or those producing pus; patients with soft contact lenses.

Side effects: cataract, thinning of cornea, rise in pressure within eye, fungal infection.

Manufacturer: Alcon.

Maxolon

Description: an anti-emetic, antidopaminergic preparation, metoclopramide hydrochloride, which acts on the gastrointestinal tract and is available in a number of different forms: white, scored tablets containing 10mg marked MAXOLON. **Maxolon Syrup** containing 5mg/5ml. **Maxolon Paediatric Liquid** containing 1mg/ml. **Maxolon Injection** as a solution in ampoules for injection containing 10mg/2ml. **Maxolon SR** clear capsules containing white, sustained-release granules at a strength of 15mg, marked MAXOLON SR 15. **Maxolon High Dose** available as a solution in ampoules for injection containing 100mg/20ml.

Used for: indigestion, gastrointestinal disturbance, backflow of blood. Also, vomiting and nausea due to cytotoxic drug therapy, cobalt therapy, deep X-ray or postoperative sickness.

Dosage: adults, over 20 years of age, 15mg twice each day with a daily maximum of 0.5mg/kg body weight. Children and young adults under 20 years, for vomiting caused by cancer chemotherapy or radiotherapy from 1 to 5mg, 2 or 3 times per day, depending upon body weight.

Special care: pregnancy, breast-feeding, liver or kidney disease/damage, epilepsy.

Avoid use: patients who have recently had operations on gastrointestinal tract, phaeochromocytoma, breast cancer which is prolactin-dependent.

Possible interaction: phenothiazines, anticholinergics, butyrophenones.

Side effects: diarrhoea, raised levels of prolactin in blood, sleepiness, extrapyramidal reactions (involuntary muscle movements, changes in posture and muscle tone).

Manufacturer: Beecham.

Maxtrex

Description: a folic acid antagonist available as tablets of 2 strengths. Yellow tablets contain 2.5mg methotrexate and are marked M2.5 on 1 side and F on the other. Yellow, scored tablets contain 10mg and are marked M10.

Used for: abnormal growths and serious psoriasis which has not been controlled by other treatments.

Dosage: individually determined according to patient's condition and response.

Special care: patients with gastrointestinal diseases and disorders, liver or kidney disease or damage, low blood cell counts, psychiatric illness, elderly or young persons. Patients should be monitored for liver and kidney function and blood checks.

Avoid use: pregnancy, breast-feeding, patients with serious liver or kidney disorder, abnormally low levels of white blood cells and platelets, severe anaemia.

Possible interaction: alcohol, NSAIDs, live vaccines, drugs that bind to proteins, anticonvulsants, folic acid, etretinate.

Side effects: gastrointestinal upset, skin rashes, liver disorders, depression of bone marrow.

Manufacturer: Pharmacia.

Medihaler-epi

Description: a sympathomimetic preparation available as a metered dose aerosol delivering 0.28mg adrenaline acid tartrate per dose.

Used for: additional treatment in anaphylaxis caused by sensitivity to insect stings or drugs.

Dosage: adults, anaphylaxis only, at least 20 puffs. Children, 10–15 puffs.

Special care: diabetes.

Avoid use: patients with hyperthyroidism, serious heart disease, heart arrhythmias, hypertension.

Possible interaction: sympathomimetics, TCADs, MAOIs.

Side effects: palpitations, agitation, dry mouth, stomach pain.

Manufacturer: 3M Health Care.

Mdeihaler-Ergotamine

Description: an NSAID which is an ergot alkaloid available as a metered dose aerosol delivering 0.36mg ergotamine tartrate/metered dose.

Used for: rapid treatment of migraine.

Dosage: adults and children over 10, 1 dose

repeated after 5 minutes if needed with a maximum of 6 doses in 24 hours and 15 in any 7 day period.

Avoid use: pregnancy, breast-feeding, children under 10 years, patients with liver or kidney disorder, hypertension, heart disease or disease of peripheral arteries, sepsis.

Possible interaction: ß-blockers, erythromycin.

Side effects: muscle pain, nausea.

Manufacturer: 3M Health Care.

Medihaler ISO

Description: a bronchodilator which is a non-selective ß-agonist available as a metered dose aerosol delivering 0.08mg isoprenaline sulphate per dose. Also, **Medihaler Iso Forte** delivering 0.4mg iso-prenaline sulphate per dose by metered dose aerosol.

Used for: severe bronchitis and bronchial asthma.

Dosage: adults, 1–3 puffs which may be repeated after half an hour if required. Maximum dose is 24 puffs in 24 hours.

Special care: pregnancy, diabetes or hypertension.

Avoid use: children, hyperthyroidism or severe coronary disease.

Possible interaction: sympathomimetics, tricyclics, MAOIs.

Side effects: palpitations, agitation, dry mouth.

Manufacturer: 3M Health Care.

Medrone

Description: an anti-inflammatory, glucocorticoid corticosteroid preparation available as tablets of different strengths, all containing methyl-prednisolone. Oval, pink, scored 2mg tablets marked UPJOHN; oval, white, scored 4mg tablets marked UPJOHN; white, scored 16mg tablets, marked UPJOHN 73; light-blue, scored 100mg tablets marked UPJOHN 3379.

Used for: treatment and control of allergic and inflammatory disorders including dermatological, respiratory, neoplastic and collagen diseases and rheumatoid arthritis.

Dosage: 2–40mg each day depending upon patient's condition and response.

Special care: pregnancy, active infections and those of fungal, viral or tuberculous origin, kidney inflammation, diseases characterized by skin rash (exanthematous), hypertension. Also, patients who have recently had surgical anastomoses of intestine, suffering from epilepsy, diabetes, liver cirrhosis, peptic ulcer, hyperthyroidism, secondary cancers. Patients suffering from stress or psychoses, contact with herpes zoster or chicken pox should be avoided and medical help and treatment will be required if this inadvertently occurs.

Possible interaction: cardiac glycosides, phenytoin, rifampicin, NSAIDs, anti-cholinesterases, ephedrine, phenobarbitone, anticoagulants taken orally, diuretics, hypoglycaemics.

Side effects: symptoms as in Cushing's syndrome, osteoporosis, peptic ulcer, hyperglycaemia, depression and euphoria.

Manufacturer: Upjohn.

Mefoxin

Description: a cephalosporin antibiotic preparation available as a powder in vials for reconstitution and injection, in 2 strengths containing 1g or 2g cefoxitin.

Used for: skin, soft tissue, respiratory tract infections, septicaemia and peritonitis. Prevention of infection in gynaecological and obstetric operations, treatment of postoperative infections. Gonorrhoea and urinary tract infections.

Dosage: adults, 1–2g by intravenous or intramuscular injection at 8 hour intervals. Prevention of infection, 2g 30 minutes to 1 hour before surgery 10 every 6 hours postoperatively for 24 hours. Children, newborn babies up to 1 week, 20–40mg/kg body weight at 12 hour intervals. 1 week to 1 month of age, 20–40mg/kg at 8 hour intervals; 1 month and over, 20–40kg/kg at 6 to 8 hour intervals. Prevention of infection, newborn babies, 30–40mg/kg, 30 minutes to 1 hour before operation then every 8 to 12 hours postoperatively for 24 hours. Older babies and children, 30–40mg/kg at same times as in adults.

Special care: pregnancy, breast-feeding, patients with allergy to penicillin, kidney disorder.

Possible interaction: aminoglycosides, loop diuretics.

Side effects: gastrointestinal upset, blood changes, (reduction in levels of white blood cells and platelets), allergic reactions, pain at injection site, rise in levels of blood urea and liver enzymes. Positive Coomb's test (a test for detecting rhesus antibodies).

Manufacturer: M.S.D.

Megace

Description: a hormonal progestogen preparation available as tablets of 2 strengths: scored, white tablets contain 40mg megestrol acetate marked 40; oval, off-white scored tablets contain 160mg marked 160.

Used for: breast and endometrial cancer.

Dosage: breast cancer, 160mg each day as single or divided doses. Endometrial cancer, 40–320mg each day in divided doses. All taken for at least 2 months.

Special care: patients with inflamed veins (thrombophlebitis).

Avoid use: pregnant women.

Side effects: nausea, nettle rash (urticaria), gain in weight.

Manufacturer: Bristol-Myers.

Melleril

Description: a phenothiazine group II antipsychotic drug available as white, film-coated tablets of different strengths containing 10mg, 25mg, 50mg and 100mg thioridazine hydrochloride respectively. All are marked with strength and MEL. Also, **Melleril Syrup** containing 25mg/5ml. **Melleril Suspension** in 2 strengths containing 25mg and 100mg thioridazine base/5ml.

Used for: mania, schizophrenia, hypomania, additional short-term therapy in the treatment of psycho-neuroses. Symptoms of senility, disturbed behaviour and epilepsy in children.

Dosage: depending upon severity and type of condition, in the order of 30–600mg each day. Children, 1 to 5 years, 1mg/kg body weight each day; over 5 years, 75–150mg/kg daily. Maximum dose in this age group is 300mg each day.

Special care: myasthenia gravis, epilepsy, phaeochromocytoma, enlarged prostate gland, Parkinson's disease, heart and circulatory diseases, glaucoma, liver or kidney disorders, respiratory diseases.

Avoid use: pregnancy, breast-feeding, history of blood changes, coma, serious heart or circulatory diseases, severe depression, porphyria.

Possible interaction: alcohol, antiarrhythmics, antacids, tricyclics, antimuscarines, calcium channel blockers, anxiolytics, lithium.

Side effects: hypotension, changes in libido, apathy, depression, insomnia, dry mouth, blocked nose, effects on heart rhythm, disturbance of sleep, constipation, difficulty in passing urine. Blood changes, rashes, jaundice, effects on liver, menstrual changes, breast enlargement, weight gain, abnormal production of breast milk. Rarely, fits, blurring of vision due to deposition of pigment (higher doses).

Manufacturer: Sandoz.

Mengivac (A + C)

Description: a vaccine preparation containing inactivated surface antigen of meningitis A and C. It is produced as a powder in vials, with diluent, containing 50 micrograms of both group A and group C polysaccharide antigens of *Neisseria meningitidis*.

Used for: immunization against meningitis, types A and C.

Dosage: adults and children over eighteen months, 0.5ml by deep subcutaneous or intramuscular injection.

Special care: pregnancy, breast-feeding.

Avoid use: patients with severe infections and feverish illnesses.

Possible interaction: substances which suppress immune system.

Side effects: local skin reactions, slight fever.

Manufacturer: Merieux.

Menophase

Description: a hormonal combined oestrogen/ progestogen preparation available as tablets containing mestranol and norethisterone; 5 pink tablets contain 12.5µg mestranol; 8 orange tablets contain 25µg mestranol; 2 yellow tablets contain 50µg mestranol; 3 green tablets contain 25µg mestranol and 1mg norethisterone; 6 blue tablets contain 30µg mestranol and 1.5mg norethisterone; 4 lavender tablets contain 20µg mestranol and 750µg norethisterone.

Used for: treatment for the relief of menopausal symptoms and prevention of osteoporosis following menopause.

Dosage: 1 tablet each day starting on a Sunday with pink tablets and continuing in order, as indicated. Treatment should be continuous for 6 months to 1 year.

Special care: patients with history of, or considered to be at risk of thrombosis. Women with any of the following should receive careful monitoring: epilepsy, gallstones, porphyria, multiple sclerosis, otosclerosis, diabetes, migraine, hypertension, tetany, fibroids in the uterus. Blood pressure, breasts and pelvic organs should be examined regularly during the course of treatment especially in women who may be at risk of breast cancer.

Avoid use: pregnancy, breast-feeding, women with breast cancer, cancer of reproductive system or other hormonally dependent cancer. Women with inflammation of veins or other thromboembolic conditions, endometriosis, undiagnosed vaginal bleeding, serious liver, kidney or heart disease, Dublin-Johnson or Rotor syndrome.

Possible interaction: drugs which induce liver enzymes.

Side effects: soreness and enlargement of breasts, breakthrough bleeding, weight gain, gastrointestinal upset, dizziness, nausea, headache, vomiting. If frequent, severe, migraine-like headaches, distrubance of vision, rise in blood pressure, jaundice or indications of thrombosis occur, drug should immediately be withdrawn, and also in the

event of pregnancy. Drug should be stopped 6 weeks before planned major surgery.
Manufacturer: Syntex.

Menzol

Description: an hormonal progestogen preparation available in the form of scored, white tablets containing 5mg norethisterone marked NE5, MENZOL 20-day.
Used for: menstrual pain (dysmenorrhoea), menorrhagia, premenstrual syndrome (PMS).
Dosage: 1 tablet 2 or 3 times each day (starting at different times in the monthly cycle depending upon condition being treated). Treatment usually continues for several cycles.
Special care: patients with disturbance of liver function.
Avoid use: pregnancy, severe disturbance of liver function, Dublin-Johnson or Rotor syndrome, history of jaundice during pregnancy, severe pruritus (itching) or herpes gestationus (a raised itchy rash which appears in the last 3 months of pregnancy).
Side effects: weight gain, depression, headache, vomiting, breakthrough bleeding, nausea, oedema, masculinizing (androgenic) effects.
Manufacturer: Schwarz.

Meptid

Description: an analgesic preparation which is an opiate partial agonist available as film-coated orange tablets containing 200mg meptazinol marked MPL-023. Also, **Meptid Injection** containing 100mg meptazinol as hydrochloride/ml.
Used for: short-term relief of pain.
Dosage: adults, 75–100mg by intramuscular injection or 50–100mg intravenously. May be repeated every 2 to 4 hours as required. Obstetric patients, 2mg/kg body weight given intramuscularly.
Special care: patients with liver or kidney disease, serious breathing problems.
Avoid use: children.
Side effects: nausea, dizziness.
Manufacturer: Monmouth.

Merbentyl

Description: an anticholinergic preparation available as white tablets containing 10mg dicyclomine hydrochloride, marked M within 2 circles; white oval tablets containing 20mg, marked MERBENTYL 20. Also **Merbentyl Syrup** containing 10mg/5ml.
Used for: spasm of stomach and gastrointestinal tract.

Dosage: adults, 10–20mg 3 times each day before or after meals. Children, 6 months to 2 years, 5–10mg 3 or 4 times each day fifteen minutes before food with a maximum of 40mg daily. Over 2 years, 10mg 3 times each day.
Special care: enlarged prostate gland, glaucoma, reflux oesophagitis with hiatus hernia.
Avoid use: children under 6 months of age.
Side effects: thirst, dry mouth, dizziness.
Manufacturer: Merrell Dow.

Mercilon

Description: an hormonal combinal oestrogen/progestogen preparation available as white tablets containing 20µg ethinyloestradiol and 150µg desogestrel, marked TR over 4.
Used for: oral contraception.
Dosage: 1 tablet each day for 21 days starting on first or fifth day of monthly cycle, followed by 7 tablet-free days.
Special care: multiple sclerosis, serious kidney disease or kidney dialysis, asthma, Raynaud's disease, abnormally high levels of prolactin in the blood (hyperprolactinaemia), varicose veins, hypertension. Also, patients suffering from severe depression. Thrombosis risk increases with smoking, age and obesity. During the course of treatment, regular checks on blood pressure, pelvic organs and breasts should be carried out.
Avoid use: pregnancy, those at risk of thrombosis, suffering from heart disease, pulmonary hypertension, angina, sickle cell anaemia. Also, undiagnosed vaginal bleeding, history of cholestatic jaundice during pregnancy, cancers which are hormone-dependent, infectious hepatitis, liver disorders. Also, porphyria, Dublin-Johnson and Rotor syndrome, otosclerosis, chorea, haemolytic uraemic syndrome, recent trophoblastic disease.
Possible interaction: barbiturates, ethosuximide, glutethimide, rifampicin, phenytoin, tetracyclines, carbamazepine, chloral hydrate, griseofulvin, dichloralphenazone, primidone.
Side effects: weight gain, breast enlargement, pains in legs and cramps, headaches, loss of sexual desire, depression, nausea, breakthrough bleeding, cervical erosion, brownish patches on skin (chloasma), vaginal discharge, oedema and bloatedness.
Manufacturer: Organon.

Mestinon

Description: an anticholinesterase preparation which acts to inhibit the enzyme that breaks down acetylcholine so that the effects of the neurotransmitter are prolonged. It is produced in the

form of white, quarter-scored tablets containing 60mg pyridostigmine bromide, marked ROCHE.
Used for: myasthenia gravis, paralytic ileus.
Dosage: myasthenia gravis, 5 to 20 tablets each day in divided doses; paralytic ileus, 1 to 4 tablets, as needed. Children, myasthenia gravis, under 6 years, 30mg at first, 6 to 12 years, 60mg at first. Both doses may be gradually increased by 15–30mg each day until condition is controlled.
Special care: patients with epilepsy, Parkinson's disease, asthma, recent heart attack, peptic ulcer, kidney disease, bradycardia, hypotension, abnormal over-activity of vagus nerve.
Avoid use: patients with gastrointestinal or urinary tract obstruction.
Possible interaction: cyclopropane, depolarizing muscle relaxants, halothane.
Side effects: overproduction of saliva, nausea, diarrhoea, colic-type pain.
Manufacturer: Roche.

Meterix

Description: a thiazide-like diuretic preparation available as blue tablets containing 5mg metolazone marked with strength and symbol.
Used for: oedema, toxaemia of pregnancy, hypertension, ascites (collection of fluid in peritoneal cavity of the abdomen).
Dosage: oedema, 5–10mg as a single daily dose with a maximum of 80mg each day; hypertension, 5mg each day at first reducing after 3 to 4 weeks to this dose taken every second day.
Special care: pregnancy, breast-feeding, elderly, liver or kidney disease, cirrhosis of the liver, gout, diabetes, collagen disease. Fluid, electrolytes (salts), and glucose levels require monitoring during the course of therapy.
Avoid use: children, hypercalcaemia, serious liver or kidney failure, allergy to sulphonamide drugs, Addison's disease.
Possible interaction: NSAIDs, carbenoxolone, lithium, barbiturates, tubocurarine, alcohol, cardiac glycosides, alcohol, corticosteroids, opioids.
Side effects: gastrointestinal disturbance, anorexia, sensitivity to light, disturbance of electrolyte balance and metabolism, pancreatitis, rash, impotence, blood changes, dizziness.
Manufacturer: Hoechst.

Meterfolic

Description: a haematinic and folic acid preparation available as grey, film-coated tablets containing ferrous fumerate (equivalent to 100mg iron) and 400µg folic acid, marked METERFOLIC.

Used for: prevention of iron and folic acid deficiency during pregnancy. As a supplement taken when pregnancy is planned to prevent neural tube defects in foetus.
Dosage: pregnant women, 1 tablet once or twice each day; prevention of neural tube defects, 1 tablet each day before conception and continuing for at least the first third of pregnancy.
Special care: patients with history of peptic ulcer or haemolytic anaemia.
Avoid use: patients with vitamin B12 deficiency.
Possible interaction: tetracyclines.
Side effects: constipation and nausea.
Manufacturer: Sinclair.

Metopirone

Description: a diuretic preparation which is an aldosterone inhibitor. Used with glucocorticoids, it acts to eliminate fluid which has accumulated due to increased secretion of the mineralocorticoid hormone, aldosterone. It is produced as creams containing 250mg metyrapone, coded LN and CIBA.
Used for: in addition to glucocorticoids to treat resistant oedema caused by excess secretion of aldosterone. Also, for Cushing's syndrome.
Dosage: adults, resistant oedema, 250mg–6g each day; Cushing's syndrome, 2.5–4.5g each day as divided doses.
Special care: patients with decreased function of the pituitary gland.
Avoid use: pregnancy, breast-feeding, children.
Side effects: allergic responses, nausea, vomiting, hypotension.
Manufacturer: Ciba.

Metosyn

Description: a potent topical steroid preparation available as cream and ointment containing 0.05% fluocinonide. Also, **Metosyn Scalp Lotion** containing 0.05% fluocinonide in an alcholic solution.
Used for: inflamed and allergic skin conditions, those producing pus.
Dosage: apply thinly each morning and night to affected area.
Special care: short-term use only.
Avoid use: children, long-term or extensive use especially in pregnant women, patients with untreated bacterial or fungal infections or skin infections of tuberculous or viral origin or due to ringworm. Also, patients with dermatitis in area of mouth, acne, leg ulcers or scabies.
Side effects: suppression of adrenal glands, skin

thinning, abnormal hair growth, changes as in Cushing's syndrome.
Manufacturer: Stuart.

Metrodin High Purity
Description: an hormonal gonadotrophin preparation available as freeze-dried powder in ampoules, with diluent, for reconstitution and injection, containing 75 units and 150 units urofolitrophin (follicle-stimulating hormone).
Used for: absence or reduced ovulation caused by dysfunction of the hypothalamus, which regulates the hormonal output of the pituitary gland, in turn producing hormones which control the sex organs. Also, for superovulation in women having fertility treatment (IVF).
Dosage: hypothalamic pituitary gland dysfunction, 75–150 units each day at first by subcutaneous or intramuscular injection. Subsequent treatment depends on response. Superovulation, 150–225 units each day.
Special care: monitoring is essential hence treatment is usually under close medical supervision. Any hormonal disorders or brain lesions must be corrected before therapy starts.
Avoid use: pregnant women.
Side effects: allergic reactions, over-stimulation of ovaries which may lead to enlargement or rupture, multiple pregnancy.
Manufacturer: Seronon.

Metrogel
Description: a nitroimidazole antibiotic preparation available in the form of a gel, containing 0.75% metronidazole.
Used for: inflammatory conditions relating to acne rosacea.
Dosage: adults, apply thinly twice each day for 8 to 9 weeks.
Avoid use: children, pregnant women.
Side effects: local skin irritation.
Manufacturer: Sandox.

Metrotop
Description: an antibacterial preparation available in the form of a topical gel containing 0.8% metronidazole.
Used for: to deodorize a tumour producing an unpleasant smell because of fungus infection.
Dosage: apply to clean wound once or twice each day and cover.
Avoid use: pregnancy, breast-feeding.
Side effects: local skin irritation.
Manufacturer: Pharmacia.

Mexitil
Description: a class I antiarrhythmic preparation, mexiletine hydrochloride, available in a variety of different forms. Purple/red capsules contain 50mg and red capsules contain 200mg both marked with strength and symbol. Also, **Mexitil Perlongets**, red/turquoise sustained-release capsules contain 360mg. **Mexitil Injection** contains 25mg/ml in ampoules for injection.
Used for: arrhythmias originating from ventricles of heart.
Dosage: capsules, 400–600mg at first then a further 200–250mg 2 hours later repeated 3 or 4 times each day. Perlongets, 1 capsule twice each day.
Special care: hypotension, Parkinson's disease, liver, kidney or heart failure, conduction defects of the heart, bradycardia.
Avoid use: children.
Side effects: effects on central nervous system, hypotension, gastrointestinal upset.
Manufacturer: Boehringer Ing.

MFV-Ject
Description: a preparation of inactivated material derived from 3 strains of influenza virus available in pre-filled syringes containing 15 micrograms of each type/5ml suspension.
Used for: immunization against influenza.
Dosage: adults, 0.5ml by intramuscular or deep subcutaneous injection. Children, 6 months to 3 years, 0.25ml repeated after 1 month to 6 weeks; 3 to 12 years, 0.5ml repeated after 1 month to 6 weeks. All given by intramuscular or deep subcutaneous injection. (Children who have been vaccinated before or infected with influenza require only 1 dose).
Avoid use: patients with feverish illness, allergic to egg protein (used in culture of viruses).
Side effects: malaise, fever.
Manufacturer: Merieux.

Microgynon 30
Description: an hormonal oestrogen/progestogen combined preparation in the form of beige, sugar-coated tablets containing 30µg ethinyloestradiol and 150µg levonorgestrel.
Used for: oral contraception.
Dosage: 1 tablet each day starting on first day of period followed by 7 tablet-free days.
Special care: patients with multiple sclerosis, serious kidney disease or kidney dialysis, asthma, Raynaud's disease, abnormally high levels of prolactin in the blood (hyperprolactinaemia), varicose veins, hypertension. Also, patients

suffering from severe depression. Thrombosis risk increases with smoking, age and obesity. During the course of treatment, regular checks on blood pressure, pelvic organs and breasts should be carried out.

Avoid use: pregnancy, those at risk of thrombosis, suffering from heart disease, pulmonary hypertension, angina, sickle cell anaemia. Also, undiagnosed vaginal bleeding, history of cholestatic jaundice during pregnancy, cancers which are hormone-dependent, infectious hepatitis, liver disorders. Also, porphyria, Dublin-Johnson and Rotor syndrome, otosclerosis, chorea, haemolytic uraemic syndrome, recent trophoblastic disease.

Possible interaction: barbiturates, ethosuximide, glutethimide, rifampicin, phenytoin, tetracyclines, carbamazepine, chloral hydrate, griseofulvin, dichloralphenazone, primidone.

Side effects: weight gain, breast enlargement, pains in legs and cramps, headaches, loss of sexual desire, depression, nausea, breakthrough bleeding, cervical erosion, vaginal discharge, brownish patches on skin (chloasma), oedema and bloatedness.

Manufacturer: Schering H.C.

Micronor

Description: an hormonal progestogen available as white tablets containing 350µg norethisterone, marked C over 035.

Used for: oral contraception.

Dosage: 1 tablet at same time each day starting on first day of cycle and continuing without a break.

Special care: history of or at risk of thrombosis or embolism, liver disease, cancer which is hormone-dependent, ovarian cysts, hypertension, migraine. Blood pressure, breasts and pelvic organs should be checked regularly during the course of treatment.

Avoid use: pregnancy, patients who have previously had a stroke, poor circulation to heart leading to heart disease, diseased arteries, previous ectopic pregnancy. Also, undiagnosed vaginal bleeding, benign tumour (adenoma) of the liver derived from glandular tissue, recent trophoblastic disease.

Possible interaction: chloral hydrate, barbiturates, meprobamate, phenytoin, rifampicin, carbamazepine, griseofulvin, primidone, glutethimide dichloralphenazone, chlorpromazine, ethosuximide.

Side effects: changes in pattern of menstruation, headache, ovarian cysts, sore breasts, acne.

Manufacturer: Ortho.

Microval

Description: an hormonal progestogen available in the form of white tablets containing 30µg levonorgestrel.

Used for: oral contraception.

Dosage: 1 tablet at same time each day starting of first day of monthly cycle and continuing without any break.

Special care: history of or at risk of thrombosis or embolism, liver disease, cancer which is hormone-dependent, ovarian cysts, hypertension, migraine. Blood pressure, breasts and pelvic organs should be checked regularly during the course of treatment.

Avoid use: pregnancy, patients who have previously had a stroke, poor circulation to heart leading to heart disease, diseased arteries, previous ectopic pregnancy. Also, women with undiagnosed vaginal bleeding, benign tumour (adenoma) of the liver derived from glandular tissue, recent trophoblastic disease.

Possible interaction: chloral hydrate, barbiturates, meprobamate, phenytoin, rifampicin, carbamazepine, griseofulvin, primidone, glutethimide dichloralphenazone, chlorpromazine, ethosuximide.

Side effects: changes in pattern of menstruation, headache, ovarian cysts, sore breasts, acne.

Manufacturer: Wyeth.

Mictral

Description: a compound preparation combining a quinolone and alkalysing agent available as dissolvable granules in sachets, containing 660mg nalidixic acid, anhydrous citric acid, sodium bicarbonate and sodium citrate (equivalent to 4.1g citrate).

Used for: cystitis and infections of lower urinary tract.

Dosage: adults, 1 sachet in water taken 3 times daily in divided doses for a period of 3 days.

Special care: pregnancy, breast-feeding, liver disease. Sunlight should be avoided.

Avoid use: children, patients with kidney disorders, history of fits, porphyria.

Possible interaction: antibacterials and anticoagulants.

Side effects: sensitivity to light, gastrointestinal upset, skin rashes, haemolytic anaemia, disturbance of vision, convulsions, blood changes.

Manufacturer: Sanofi Winthrop.

Midamor

Description: a potassium-sparing diuretic preparation available as diamond-shaped, yellow tablets containing 5mg amiloride hydrochloride marked MSD 92.

Used for: used with other diuretics to save potassium.

Dosage: 1 or 2 tablets each day with a daily maximum of 4.

Special care: pregnancy, breast-feeding, kidney or liver disease, acidosis, gout, a tendency to hyperkalaemia due to diabetes.

Avoid use: children, patients with serious or worsening kidney failure, hyperkalaemia, anuria.

Possible interaction: ACE inhibitors, lithium, potassium-sparing diuretics, potassium supplements.

Side effects: skin rash, gastrointestinal upset.

Manufacturer: Morson.

Mifegyne

Description: a preparation which is a progesterone antagonist available as bi-convex, cylindrical-shaped, yellow tablets containing 200mg mifepristone, marked with logo and 167 B.

Used for: termination of early pregnancy, up to 63 days of gestation.

Dosage: adults, 600mg as a single dose under close medical supervision.

Special care: close observation required and patient may require further treatment to complete termination. Patients with obstructive airways disease or asthma, heart disease, replacement heart valves, kidney or liver disease, history of infected endocarditis. Patients should not take NSAIDs or aspirin for at least 12 days.

Avoid use: women with more advanced pregnancy over 64 days, ectopic or suspected ectopic pregnancy, porphyria, haemorrhage or bleeding disorders, women who smoke aged over 35 years. Also, patients receiving anticoagulant therapy or who have had long-term treatment with corticosteroids.

Possible interaction: aspirin, NSAIDs.

Side effects: vomiting, nausea, vaginal bleeding which may be severe, fainting, malaise, womb and urinary tract infections, skin rashes.

Manufacturer: Roussel.

Migravess Forte

Description: a compound preparation which is an anti-emetic and analgesic available in the form of effervescent, scored white tablets containing 5mg metoclopramide and 450mg aspirin marked F over F. Also, **Migravess Effervescent**, scored, white tablets containing 5mg metoclopramide and 325mg aspirin, marked M over M.

Used for: relief of migraine.

Dosage: adults, 2 tablets in water at start of migraine attack with a maximum daily dose of 6 tablets. Children, 12 to 15 years, half adult dose.

Special care: pregnancy, liver or kidney disease, asthma.

Avoid use: children under 12 years, patients with

allergy to aspirin or NSAIDs, peptic ulcer, bleeding disorders.

Possible interaction: anticoagulants, phenothiazines, uricosurics, anticholinergics, hypoglycaemics, butyrophenones.

Side effects: sleepiness, extrapyramidal symptoms (characterized by involuntary and reflex muscle movements and changes in tone of muscles), diarrhoea, rise in levels of prolactin in blood.

Manufacturer: Bayer.

Migril

Description: a compound preparation combining an ergot alkaloid, antihistamine and xanthine produced as scored, white tablets containing 2mg ergotamine tartrate, 50mg cyclizine hydrochloride, 50mg caffeine hydrate, coded WELLCOME A4A.

Used for: relief of migraine.

Dosage: 1 at start of migraine attack followed by $^1/_2$ to 1 tablet at 30 minute intervals. Maximum dose is 4 tablets for 1 migraine attack and 6 weekly.

Special care: patients with hyperthyroidism, sepsis, anaemia.

Avoid use: pregnancy, breast-feeding, children, patients with heart or circulatory disease, liver or kidney disorders, serious hypertension.

Possible interaction: ß-blockers, central nervous system depressants, erythromycin.

Side effects: sleepiness, rebound headache, pain in abdomen, dry mouth, peripheral ischaemia.

Manufacturer: Wellcome.

Mildison Lipocream

Description: a mildly potent topical steroid preparation available in the form of a cream containing 1% hydrocortisone.

Used for: dermatitis and eczema.

Dosage: apply to affected skin 2 or 3 times each day.

Special care: use on face or in children should be limited to a maximum period of 5 days. Stop using gradually after longer-term use.

Avoid use: long-term use or as a preventative especially by pregnant women, patients with untreated bacterial or fungal infections, skin infections of tuberculous or viral origin, scabies or ringworm. Also, leg ulcers, dermatitis in area of mouth, acne.

Side effects: changes as in Cushing's syndrome, skin thinning, abnormal hair growth, suppression of adrenal glands.

Manufacturer: Yamanouchi.

Minihep

Description: an anticoagulant preparation available

as a solution in pre-filled syringes containing 5000 units sodium heparin/0.2ml. Also, **Minihep Calcium** solution in pre-filled syringes and ampoules containing 5000 units calcium heparin/0.2ml. Both are for subcutaneous injection only.

Used for: pulmonary embolism and deep vein thrombosis.

Dosage: 15,000 units every 12 hours; children 250 units/kg body weight 12 hourly. Both following on from first doses given by intravenous infusion or injection.

Special care: pregnancy, kidney or liver disease. Drug should be withdrawn gradually if taken for more than 5 days. Platelet counts are required if taken for more than 5 days.

Avoid use: bleeding disorders, haemophilia, serious hypertension, recent operation on eye or nervous system, cerebral aneurysm, serious liver disease, peptic ulcer, allergy to heparin, thrombocytopenia.

Possible interaction: aspirin, dipyridamole, glyceryl trinitrate infusion.

Side effects: allergic reactions, skin necrosis, osteoporosis (if taken long-term). Stop drug immediately if thrombocytopenia occurs.

Manufacturer: Leo.

Minims Amethocaine

Description: a topical anaesthetic preparation for the eye, produced in the form of drops in 2 strengths containing 0.5% or 1% amethocaine hydrochloride in single dose units.

Used for: anaesthesia for eye during ophthalmic procedures.

Dosage: adults and children, except newborn babies, 1 drop as required.

Special care: protect eye.

Avoid use: newborn babies.

Possible interaction: sulphonamides.

Side effects: short-lived burning sensation, dermatitis.

Manufacturer: Chauvin.

Minims Atropine

Description: an anticholinergic preparation for the eye produced in the form of single-dose drops containing 1% atropine sulphate.

Used for: to produce mydriasis (dilation of the pupil of the eye by contraction of certain muscles in the iris) and cytoplegia (paralysis of the muscles of accommodation in the eye along with relaxation of the ciliary muscle). This is to allow examination of eye.

Dosage: adults and children, 1 drop as required.

Special care: patients should not drive for 2 hours.

Avoid use: patients with glaucoma.

Side effects: contact dermatitis, occasionally toxic systemic reactions especially in elderly persons and children. Closed angle glaucoma is possible especially in elderly patients.

Manufacturer: Chauvin.

Minims Benoxinate

Description: a topical anaesthetic preparation for the eye produced in the form of single dose drops containing 0.4% oxybuprocaine hydrochloride.

Used for: anaesthesia of eye during ophthalmic procedures.

Dosage: 1 or more drops as needed.

Manufacturer: Chauvin.

Minims Chloramphenicol

Description: a broad-spectrum antibiotic preparation produced in the form of single dose eyedrops containing 0.5% chloramphenicol.

Used for: bacterial eye infections.

Dosage: adults, 1 or more drops, as needed; children, 1 drop as needed.

Special care: remove contact lenses.

Possible interaction: chymotrypsin.

Side effects: rarely, aplastic anaemia. Stop treatment immediately if local allergic reactions occur.

Manufacturer: Chauvin.

Minims Cyclopentolate

Description: an anticholinergic eye preparation produced in the form of single dose eyedrops of 2 strengths containing 0.5% or 1% cyclopentolate hydrochloride.

Used for: mydriasis (dilation of the pupil of the eye by contraction of certain muscles in the iris) and cytoplegia (paralysis of the muscles of accommodation within the eye along with relaxation of the ciliary muscle). This is in order to allow ophthalmic procedures to be carried out.

Dosage: adults and children (except newborn babies), 1 or 2 drops as needed.

Special care: patient with raised pressure within eye.

Avoid use: patients with narrow angle glaucoma.

Side effects: contact dermatitis, rarely toxic systemic effects especially in elderly and children, closed angle glaucoma is possible especially in elderly patients.

Manufacturer: Chauvin.

Minims Gentamicin

Description: an antibiotic aminoglycoside preparation produced in the form of single dosage

eye drops containing 0.3% gentamicin as sulphate.
Used for: bacterial infections of the eye.
Dosage: 1 drop as required.
Manufacturer: Chauvin.

Minims Homatropine

Description: an anticholinergic eye preparation produced in the form of single dose drops containing 2% homatropine hydrobromide.
Used for: to produce mydriasis (dilation of the pupil of the eye by contraction of certain muscles in the iris) and cytoplegia (paralysis of the muscles of accommodation in the eye along with relaxation of the ciliary muscle).
Used for: narrow angle glaucoma.
Dosage: adults and children, 1 or more drops as needed.
Special care: patients should not drive for 2 hours.
Side effects: contact dermatitis, possibly closed angle glaucoma in elderly patients.
Manufacturer: Chauvin.

Minims Lignocaine and Fluorescein

Description: an eye preparation which is a local anaesthetic and stain available in the form of single dose eye drops containing 4% lignocaine hydrochloride and 0.25% fluorescein sodium.
Used for: ophthalmic procedures.
Dosage: adults and children, 1 or more drops as needed.
Manufacturer: Chauvin.

Minims Metipranolol

Description: a non-selective ß-blocker produced in the form of single dose eyedrops of 2 strengths containing 0.1% and 0.3% metipranolol.
Used for: control of raised pressure within eye following surgery. Also, for chronic glaucoma in patients wearing soft contact lenses or who are allergic to preservatives.
Dosage: glaucoma, 1 drop into eye twice each day.
Avoid use: patients with obstructive airways disease, asthma, heart failure, bradycardia, heart block.
Possible interaction: verapamil and possibly other drugs following systemic absorption.
Side effects: dry eyes, allergic blepharo-conjunctivitis (involving lining of eyelids).
Manufacturer: Chauvin.

Minims Neomycin

Description: an aminoglycoside broad-spectrum antibiotic preparation produced in the form of single dose eyedrops containing 0.5% neomycin sulphate.
Used for: bacterial eye infections.

Dosage: adults, 1 or more drops as needed. Children, 1 drop as needed.
Manufacturer: Chauvin.

Minims Pilocarpine

Description: a miotic preparation (one which causes contraction of the pupil) which is a cholinergic agonist and acts to cause constriction of the ciliary eye muscle. This helps to open drainage channels hence reducing pressure within the eye. It is produced as single dose eyedrops in 3 strengths containing 1%, 2% and 4% pilocarpine nitrate.
Used for: emergency treatment of glaucoma. To reverse the effect of weak mydriatic drugs.
Dosage: 1 drop every 5 minutes until the pupil is contracted.
Side effects: headache, blurred vision, bradycardia, colic pains, sweating, overproduction of saliva, bronchospasm may occur if systemic absorption (into body) of eyedrops occur.
Manufacturer: Chauvin.

Minims Prednisolone

Description: a corticosteroid preparation available as single dose eyedrops containing 0.5% prednisolone sodium.
Used for: inflammation of the eye which is not infected.
Dosage: adults and children, 1 or 2 drops every 1 or 2 hours then reduce frequency when condition improves.
Avoid use: pregnancy, glaucoma or tuberculous, viral or fungal infections or those producing pus. Avoid long-term treatment in babies.
Side effects: thinning of cornea, 'steroid cataract' (especially prolonged use and higher doses), rise in pressure within eye, fungal infection.
Manufacturer: Chauvin.

Minims Tropicamide

Description: an anticholinergic preparation available as single dose eyedrops in 2 strengths containing 0.5% and 1% tropicamide.
Used for: as a short-term mydriatic and cycloplegic drug. (A mydriatic produces mydriasis—dilation of the pupil of the eye by contraction of certain muscles in the iris. A cycloplegic produces cycloplegia—paralysis of the muscles of accommodation in the eye along with relaxation of the ciliary muscle). Enables ophthalmic examinations and procedures to be carried out.
Dosage: adults and children, 1 or 2 drops every 5 minutes then repeated after 30 minutes if needed.
Special care: in babies, pressure should be applied

over the tear sac for 1 minute. Patients should not drive for 2 hours.

Avoid use: patients with narrow angle glaucoma.

Side effects: stinging on application which is short-lived.

Manufacturer: Chauvin.

Minocin

Description: a tetracycline antibiotic available as film-coated orange tablets containing 100mg minocycline as hydrochloride, marked M over 100 on one side and LL on the other. Also, **Minocin MR**, yellow/brown modified-release capsules containing 100mg marked 8560 and Lederle. Also **Minocin 50**, beige, film-coated tablets containing 50mg marked M50 on one side and LL on the other.

Used for: Minocin: ear, nose and throat, respiratory, soft tissue, skin and urinary tract infections. Minocin MR: acne.

Dosage: adults, Minocin, 100mg twice each day; Minocin MR 1 each day swallowed whole; Minocin 50 1 tablet twice each day for at least 6 weeks.

Special care: patients with liver disorder.

Avoid use: children, pregnancy, breast-feeding, kidney failure.

Possible interaction: mineral supplements, antacids, penicillins.

Side effects: gastrointestinal upset, superinfections; rarely, disorders of balance, allergic responses.

Manufacturer: Lederle.

Minodiab

Description: a sulphonylurea available as scored, white tablets of 2 strengths containing 2.5mg and 5mg glipizide.

Used for: maturity-onset diabetes.

Dosage: adults, 2.5mg or 5mg each day at first increasing by 2.5–5mg every week. The usual maintenance dose is 2.5–30mg each day, maximum 40mg. Doses higher than 15mg each day should be divided and taken about 15 minutes before meals.

Special care: elderly, kidney failure.

Avoid use: pregnancy, breast-feeding, children, patients with other types of diabetes (juvenile, unstable, growth-onset diabetes), serious liver or kidney diseases, hormonal disorders. Also patients with ketoacidosis, infections, stress, undergoing surgery.

Possible interaction: oral anticoagulants, bezafibrate, aspirin, corticotrophin, corticosteroids, clofibrate, ß-blockers, alcohol, chlorpropamide, acetohexamide, melformin, MAOIs, oral contraceptives, sulphonamides, glucagon, diuretics, phenylbutazone, chloramphenicol, cyclophosphamide, rifampicin.

Side effects: allergic reactions including skin rash.

Manufacturer: Pharmacia.

Mintezol

Description: an antihelmintic preparation used to treat infestation with various kinds of worm; available as scored, orange, chewable tablets containing 500mg thiabendazole.

Used for: guinea worm, threadworm, hookworm, trichinosis, large roundworm, larva migrans, whipworm.

Dosage: adults and children over 60kg body weight, 1.5g twice each day with meals. Less than 60kg, 25mg/kg twice each day with meals.

Special care: patients with liver or kidney disorder.

Avoid use: pregnancy, breast-feeding.

Possible interaction: xanthine derivatives.

Side effects: disturbances of vision and hearing, reduction in alertness, allergic reactions, liver damage, gastrointestinal upset, hypotension, central nervous system disturbance, enuresis (incontinence, especially bed-wetting).

Manufacturer: M.S.D.

Minulet

Description: an hormonal combined oestrogen/progestogen preparation available as sugar-coated white tablets containing 30µg ethinyloestradiol and 75µg gestodene.

Used for: oral contraception.

Dosage: 1 tablet each day for 21 days beginning on first day of period followed by 7 tablet-free days.

Special care: patients with multiple sclerosis, serious kidney disease, kidney dialysis, asthma, Raynaud's disease, abnormally high levels of prolactin in the blood (hyperprolactinaemia), varicose veins, hypertension. Also, patients suffering severe depression. Thrombosis risk increases with smoking, age and obesity. During the course of treatment, regular checks on blood pressure, pelvic organs and breasts should be carried out.

Avoid use: pregnancy, patients considered to be at risk of thrombosis, suffering from heart disease, pulmonary hypertension, angina, sickle cell anaemia. Also, undiagnosed vaginal bleeding, history of cholestatic jaundice during pregnancy, cancers which are hormone-dependent, infectious hepatitis, liver disorders. Also, porphyria, Dublin-Johnson and Rotor syndrome, otosclerosis, chorea, haemolytic uraemic syndrome, recent trophoblastic disease.

Possible interaction: barbiturates, ethosuximide, glutethimide, rifampicin, phenytoin, tetracyclines,

carbamazepine, chloral hydrate, griseofulvin, dichloralphenazone, primidone.
Side effects: weight gain, breast enlargement, pains in legs and cramps, headaches, loss of sexual desire, depression, nausea, breakthrough bleeding, cervical erosion, brownish patches on skin (chloasma), vaginal discharge, oedema and bloatedness.
Manufacturer: Wyeth.

Mithracin

Description: a cytotoxic antibiotic preparation available as a powder in vials for reconstitution and injection containing 2.5mg plicamycin.
Used for: hypercalcaemia due to malignancy.
Dosage: 25µg/kg body 8 each day for 3 to 4 days repeated at minimum intervals of 1 week if necessary. Maintenance dose is 25µg/kg 1 to 3 times each week, all by intravenous infusion.
Special care: patients with liver or kidney disease.
Side effects: irritant to tissues, bone marrow suppression, vomiting, nausea, hair loss.
Manufacturer: Pfizer.

Mitoxana

Description: an alkylating cytotoxic drug, available as powder in vials for reconstitution and injection in 2 strengths containing 1g and 2g ifosfamide.
Used for: lymphomas, solid tumours, chronic lymphocytic leukaemia, usually given with mesna (*see* Uromitexan, a drug which lessens or prevents the toxic effects of ifosfamide on the bladder).
Dosage: given intravenously as directed by physician.
Special care: ensure plenty of fluids are taken—3 to 4 litres each day following injection.
Possible interaction: warfarin.
Side effects: bone marrow suppression, nausea, vomiting, hair loss, haemorrhagic cystitis (risk is reduced with increased fluid intake and mesna).
Manufacturer: ASTA Medica.

Mivacron

Description: a short-acting, non-depolarizing muscle relaxant available in ampoules for injection containing 2mg mivacurium as chloride/ml.
Used for: muscle paralysis during surgical operations.
Dosage: adults, by intravenous injection, 70–150µg/kg body 8 at first then 100 µg/kg every 15 minutes. By intravenous infusion, to maintain paralysis, 8–10 µg/kg/minute, adjusted if needed to usual dose of 6–7 µg/kg/minute. Children, intravenous injection, age 2 to 12 years, 100–200µg/kg at first then 100 µg/kg every 6 to 7 minutes. Intravenous infusion, 10–15µg/kg/minute.

Special care: patients with heart disease or asthma (slower injection rate required).
Avoid use: patients with myasthenia gravis.
Possible interaction: clindamycin, azlocillin, colistin, verapamil, nifedipine, dantrolene, ecothiopate, demacarium, neostigmine, pyridostiamine, magnesium salts.
Manufacturer: Wellcome.

MMR II

Description: a preparation of measles, mumps and rubella vaccine. It contains measles, mumps and rubella vaccine along with 0.25mg neomycin and is available as powder in vials, with diluent.
Used for: immunization of children (and some adults) against measles, mumps and rubella.
Dosage: children over 12 months, 0.5ml by subcutaneous or intramuscular injection.
Special care: history of convulsions and feverishness, altered immunity states in whom fever is undesirable, patients who have had blood or plasma transfusion within last 3 months.
Avoid use: pregnancy, women should avoid pregnancy for 3 months after vaccination. Acute feverish illnesses, thrombocytopenia, history of symptoms of anaphylaxis to eggs or neomycin (egg protein is used in culture of virus for vaccine). Do not give within 1 month of other live vaccines.
Possible interaction: live vaccines.
Side effects: allergic responses, fever, headache, malaise, skin rash.
Manufacturer: M.S.D.

Mobiflex

Description: an NSAID belonging to the Oxicam group available as film-coated, pentagonal brown tablets containing 20mg tenoxicam marked Mobiflex. Also, **Mobiflex Milk** granules in sachets containing 20mg; **Mobiflex Effervescent** tablets containing 20mg. **Mobiflex Injection** available as powder in vials for reconstitution containing 20mg.
Used for: rheumatoid arthritis, osteoarthritis, treatment of soft tissue injuries, (short-term only).
Dosage: 1 tablet or sachet in water each day; injection, 20mg by intravenous or intramuscular injection for first 1 or 2 days, then tablets or granules.
Special care: elderly patients, those with liver or kidney disease or heart failure.
Avoid use: pregnancy, children, inflammation of gastrointestinal tract or bleeding, history of or actual peptic ulcer, allergy to NSAID or aspirin.
Possible interaction: hypoglycaemics taken orally, lithium, anticoagulants, other NSAIDs.

Side effects: headache, blood changes, skin rash, gastrointestinal upset, rise in level of liver enzymes, oedema, distubance of vision.
Manufacturer: Roche.

Modalim

Description: an isobutyric acid derivative used to lower the levels of lipds (fats) in the blood. It is available as capsule-shaped, white, scored tablets containing 100mg ciprofibrate and marked MODALIM.
Used for: hyperlipidaemias (elevated blood lipid levels) of types IIa, IIb, III and IV which cannot be controlled by diet alone.
Dosage: adults, 1 or 2 tablets as a single daily dose.
Special care: liver or kidney disease; live tests should be carried out during the course of treatment.
Avoid use: pregnancy, breast-feeding, children, severe liver or kidney disease.
Possible interaction: hypoglycaemics taken by mouth, oral contraceptives, anticoagulants.
Side effects: vertigo, gastrointestinal upset, loss of hair, impotence, muscle pain; rarely, sleepiness, dizziness.
Manufacturer: Sanofi Winthrop.

Modecate

Description: an antipsychotic preparation which is a depot phenothiazine group III, available in ampoules and disposable syringes containing 25mg fluphenazine decanoate/ml. Also **Modecate Concentrate** in ampoules containing 100mg/ml.
Used for: maintenance of certain psychiatric illnesses especially schizophrenia.
Dosage: adults, 12.5mg by deep intramuscular injection (into gluteal muscle) as first test dose in order to see if patient is liable to experience extrapyramidal (e.g. involuntary, reflex-type muscle movements) symptoms. Then, usual dose in the order of 12.5mg–100mg, according to response, every 2 to 5 weeks. Elderly receive lower initial test dose of 6.25mg.
Special care: elderly, patients who exhibit extrapyramidal symptoms (reduce dose or use alternative drug), pregnancy, breast-feeding, patients wtih myasthenia gravis. Also heart disease, heart arrhythmias, epilepsy, liver or respiratory diseases, enlarged prostate gland, underactive thyroid gland, glaucoma, thyrotoxicosis.
Avoid use: children, patients with phaeochromocytoma, liver or kidney failure, severe heart disease, severe atherosclerosis of cerebral arteries, coma. Also those suffering from severe depression.

Possible interaction: alcohol, antacids, TCADs, antihypertensives, calcium-channel blockers, cimetidine.
Side effects: extrapyramidal symptoms, effects on heart and heart rhythm, effects on central nervous system and EEG, sleepiness, apathy, depression, dry mouth, blocked nose, difficulty passing urine, constipation. Hormonal changes, effects on mestruation, enlargement of breasts, abnormal production of breast milk, impotence. Blood changes, skin rashes, jaundice, effects on liver. Effects on eyes, blurred vision, pigmentation of skin and eyes.
Manufacturer: Sanofi Winthrop.

Moditen

Description: an antipsychotic preparation which is a phenothiazine group III drug available as sugar-coated tablets in 3 strengths all containing fluphenazine hydrochloride; pink 1mg, yellow 2.5mg and white 5mg.
Used for: schizophrenia, paranoia, mania, hypomania, short-term treatment of anxiety, agitation and disordered behaviour.
Dosage: adults, schizophrenia and psychoses, 2.5mg–10mg as 2 or 3 divided doses each day with a maximum of 20mg. Anxiety and agitation, 1–2mg twice each day at first and then according to response. Elderly persons receive lower doses.
Special care: patients who exhibit extrapyramidal reactions (e.g. involuntary reflex-type muscle movements) should receive lower doses or alternative drug; pregnancy, breast-feeding. Myasthenia gravis, enlarged prostate gland, thyrotoxicosis, heart disease, heart arrhythmias, epilepsy, liver or respiratory diseases, underactive thyroid gland, glaucoma.
Avoid use: children, serious heart conditions, phaeochromocytoma, liver or kidney failure, severe atherosclerosis of cerebral arteries, coma. Also, patients who are severely depressed.
Possible interaction: alcohol, antacids, TCADs, antihypertensives, calcium-channel blockers, cimetidine.
Side effects: extrapyramidal symptoms, effects on heart and heart rhythm, effects on central nervous system and EEG, sleepiness, apathy, depression, dry mouth, blocked nose, difficulty passing urine, constipation. Hormonal changes, effects on menstruation, enlargement of breasts, abnormal production of breast milk, impotence. Blood changes, skin rashes, jaundice, effects on liver. Effects on eyes, blurred vision, pigmentation of skin and eyes.
Manufacturer: Sanofi Winthrop.

Modrasone

Description: a moderately potent topical steroid preparation available as cream and ointment containing 0.05% alclometasone diproprionate.

Used for: skin conditions which respond to steroids.

Dosage: apply thinly 2 or 3 times each day.

Special care: do not use on face or in children for more than 5 days. Withdraw treatment gradually if use has been long-term.

Avoid use: extensive or long-term use, especially pregnant women, or as a preventative. Patients with untreated fungal or bacterial infections, skin conditions with tuberculous or viral origin or ringworm. Also, patients with leg ulcers, acne, scabies, dermatitis in area of mouth.

Side effects: changes as in Cushing's syndrome, skin thinning, suppression of adrenal glands, abnormal hair growth.

Manufacturer: Schering-Plough.

Modrenal

Description: a preparation of a drug which inhibits the production of corticosteroid hormones by the adrenal glands. It is available as capsules of 2 strengths; black/pink capsules containing 60mg trilostane and yellow/pink capsules containing 120mg. Both are marked with the strength of the capsules.

Used for: excessive activity of adrenal cortex resulting in excess hormone release as in primary aldosteronism (oversecretion of aldosterone, also called Conn's syndrome) and hypercortisolism. Also for breast cancer in post-menopausal women.

Dosage: adults, 60mg 4 times each day at first then, according to response, adjusted to a usual daily dose in the order of 120mg–480mg as divided doses. The maximum is 960mg each day. Breast cancer, the initial dose is 240mg each day increasing by this amount at 3 day intervals to a maximum 960mg. Glucocorticoid treatment should be given at the same time in these patients.

Special care: eliminate the presence of a tumour producing ACTH (adrenocorticotrophic hormone) before treatment begins, patients with kidney or liver disease, suffering from stress. Non-hormonal methods of contraception should be used.

Avoid use: pregnancy, patients with serious liver or kidney disease.

Possible interaction: aldosterone antagonists, potassium supplements, triamterene, amiloride.

Side effects: nausea, diarrhoea, flushing, runny nose.

Manufacturer: Wanskerne.

Moducren

Description: a compound antihypertensive preparation combining a non-cardioselective ß-blocker, a thiazide and potassium-sparing diuretic available as scored, blue tablets containing 25mg hydrochlorthiazide, 2.5mg amiloride hydrochloride and 10mg timolol maleate, marked MODUCREN.

Used for: hypertension.

Dosage: adults, 1 or 2 tablets as a single dose each day.

Special care: pregnancy, breast-feeding, patients with weak hearts may require diuretics and digitalis, those with diabetes, undergoing general anaesthesia, kidney or liver disorders, gout. Electrolyte (salts) levels may need to be monitored.

Avoid use: history of bronchospasm or obstructive airways disease, heart block, heart shock, uncompensated heart failure, disease of peripheral arteries, bradycardia. Patients with serious or worsening kidney failure or anuria.

Possible interaction: sympathomimetics, class I antiarrhythmics, central nervous system depressants, clonidine withdrawal, ergot alkaloids, cardiac depressant anaesthetics, verapamil, reserpine, indomethacin, hypoglycaemics, cimetidine, other antihypertensives. Digitalis, potassium supplements, potassium-sparing diuretics, lithium.

Side effects: cold hands and feet, disturbance of sleep, fatigue on exercise, bronchospasm, bradycardia, gastrointestinal disturbances, heart failure, blood changes, gout, sensitivity to light, muscle weakness. If skin rash or dry eyes occur, withdraw drug gradually.

Manufacturer: Morson.

Moduret 25

Description: a compound preparation combining a potassium-sparing and thiazide diuretic available as diamond-shaped, off-white tablets containing 2.5mg amiloride hydrochloride and 25mg hydro-chlorothiazide, coded MSD 923.

Used for: hypertension, congestive heart failure, liver cirrhosis (accompanied by an abnormal collection of fluid in the abdomen, ascites).

Dosage: adults, 1 to 4 tablets each day in divided doses.

Special care: patients with liver or kidney disorders, diabetes, acidosis and gout.

Avoid use: children, pregnancy, breast-feeding, serious or worsening kidney failure, hyperkalaemia.

Possible interaction: lithium, ACE inhibitors, potassium supplements and potassium-sparing diuretics, antihypertensives, digitalis.

Manufacturer: DuPont.

Moduretic

Description: a compound preparation combining a

potassium-sparing and thiazide diuretic available in the form of diamond-shaped, scored, peach tablets containing 5mg amiloride hydrochloride and 50mg hydrochlorothiazide, marked NSD 917. Also, **Moduretic Solution** (in 5ml).

Used for: hypertension, congestive heart failure, liver cirrhosis (accompanied by an abnormal collection of fluid in the abdomen, ascites).

Dosage: 1 or 2 tablets or 5–10ml solution each day as single or divided doses. May be increased, if required, to a daily maximum of 4 tablets or 20ml.

Special care: liver or kidney disorders, acidosis, gout, diabetes.

Avoid use: children, pregnancy, breast-feeding, hyperkalaemia.

Possible interaction: lithium, potassium-sparing diuretics, potassium supplements, anti-hypertensives, digitalis.

Side effects: sensitivity to light, gout, rash, blood changes.

Manufacturer: DuPont.

Mogadon

Description: a long-acting benzodiazepine preparation available as scored, white tablets containing 5mg nitrazepam marked with 2 'eyes' and ROCHE.

Used for: insomnia, short-term only.

Dosage: adults, 5–10mg, elderly persons, 2.5–5mg, with doses taken at bedtime.

Special care: kidney or liver disorders, lung insufficiency, pregnancy, labour, breast-feeding. For short-term treatment as drug dependence and tolerance may develop.

Avoid use: history of drug or alcohol abuse, serious lung insufficiency and depressed respiration. Suffering from psychoses, obsessional or phobic states.

Possible interaction: CNS depressants, alcohol, anticonvulsants.

Side effects: headache, drowsiness, loss of coordination (ataxia), confusion, hypotension, gastrointestinal upset. Skin rash, retention of urine, changes in libido, vertigo, disturbance of vision. Rarely, jaundice and blood disorders.

Manufacturer: Roche.

Molipaxin

Description: an antidepressant preparation available in a variety of different forms, all containing trazodone hydrochloride. Pink, film-coated, scored tablets (150mg) are marked MOLIPAXIN 150. **Molipaxin Capsules** are green/purple (50mg) marked with logo and R365B; fawn/purple (100mg)

marked with logo and R365C. **Molipaxin CR**, blue, octagonal-shaped sustained-release tablets (150mg) marked with strength and name. **Molipaxin Liquid** contains 50mg/5ml.

Used for: depression which may be accompanied by anxiety.

Dosage: 150mg each day as divided doses taken after meals or single night-time dose. After 1 week, dose may be increased to 300mg each day with a maximum of 600mg. Elderly persons, 100mg each day in divided doses after meals or as a single night-time dose. Maximum of 300mg each day.

Special care: serious kidney or liver disease or epilepsy.

Avoid use: children.

Possible interaction: CNS depressants, clonidine, muscle relaxants, MAOIs, some anaesthetics.

Side effects: dizziness, headache, drowsines. Discontinue if priapism (abnormal, persistent erection of penis, which is painful and not associated with sexual arousal) occurs.

Manufacturer: Roussel.

Monaspor

Description: a cephalosporin antibiotic preparation available as powder in vials for reconstitution and injection containing 1g cefsulodin sodium.

Used for: urinary tract, soft tissue, respiratory and some bone infections. Infections caused by the organism *Pseudomonas aerugginosa*.

Dosage: adults, 1–4g daily in 2, 3 or 4 divided doses by intravenous or intramuscular injection. Children, 20–50mg/kg body weight each day by intravenous or intramuscular injection.

Special care: pregnancy, patients allergic to penicillin, kidney failure. Tests of kidney function and blood counts should be carried out if taking drug long-term.

Possible interaction: aminoglycosides, loop diuretics.

Side effects: blood changes (abnormal reduction in number of blood platelets and white cells), gastrointestinal upset, candidiasis (thrush), rise in level of blood urea and liver enzymes. Positive Coomb's test (a test for rhesus antibodies).

Manufacturer: Ciba.

Monit

Description: an antianginal nitrate preparation available as scored, white tablets containing 20mg isosorbide mononitrate marked STUART 20. Also, **Monit LS**, white tablets containing 10mg and marked STUART 10; **Monit SR**, white, sugar-coated sustained-release tablets containing 40mg.

Used for: prevention of angina.
Dosage: 1 tablet each day in the morning.
Avoid use: children.
Side effects: flushes, headache, dizziness.
Manufacturer: Lorex.

Monoclate-P

Description: a preparation of freeze-dried coagulation factor VIII with antihaemophiliac activities of 250, 500 and 1000 units in vials for injection.
Used for: treatment of haemophilia A.
Dosage: by intravenous infusion according to body weight and severity of condition.
Special care: in patients with blood groups A, B or AB there is a possibility of haemolysis after large or numerous doses.
Side effects: allergic reactions, nausea, chills, pain at injection site. If more pronounced hypersensitivity reactions occur, discontinue treatment.
Manufacturer: Armour.

Monocur

Description: an antianginal and anti-hypertensive preparation which is a cardioselective ß-blocker available as pink, scored, film-coated tablets containing 5mg bisoprolol fumerate, marked 5 on one side and LL on the other. Also, white film-coated tablets containing 10mg, marked 10 on one side and LL on the other.
Used for: angina and hypertension.
Dosage: usual dose is 10mg once each day with a maximum of 20mg.
Special care: pregnancy, breast-feeding, patients with weak hearts may require diuretics and digitalis. Also, liver or kidney disease, general anaesthesia, metabolic acidosis, diabetes. Drug should be gradually withdrawn.
Avoid use: persons with chronic obstructive airways disease, history of bronchospasm, heart block, heart shock, uncompensated heart failure, sick sinus syndrome, disease of peripheral arteries, bradycardia.
Possible interaction: CNS depressants, verapamil, indomethacin, reserpine, class I antiarrhythmics, hypoglycaemics, clonidine withdrawal, sympatho-mimetics, cardiac depressants anaesthetics, ergot alkaloids, antihypertensives.
Side effects: gastrointestinal upset, fatigue on exercise, cold hands and feet, disturbance of sleep, bronchospasm, bradycardia, heart failure. If skin rash or dry eyes occur, drug should be gradually withdrawn.
Manufacturer: Cyanamid.

Mononine

Description: a preparation of freeze-dried human coagulation factor IX with slight antihaemophiliac activity. Available as 250, 500 and 1000 unit vials.
Used for: haemophilia B.
Dosage: by intravenous infusion depending upon patient's weight and severity of bleeding.
Special care: risk of thrombosis.
Avoid use: widespread coagulation within blood vessels.
Side effects: allergic reactions, flushing, vomiting and nausea, headache, fever, chills, tingling sensation, tiredness. Possible thromboembolism. If hypersensitivity reactions occur, drug should be withdrawn.
Manufacturer: Armour.

Monoparin

Description: an anticoagulant preparation of heparin sodium available as 1000, 5000 and 25,000 units/ml in single dose ampoules. Also, **Monoparin CA** containing 25,000 units heparin calcium/ml.
Used for: treatment of pulmonary embolism and deep vein thrombosis.
Dosage: adults, initial loading dose of 5000 units (10,000 in severe conditions) by intravenous injection followed by continuous infusion at a rate of 1000–2000 units/hour. Or 15,000 units at 12 hour intervals may be given by subcutaneous injection. Small adult or child, lower initial dose then 15–25 units/kg body weight by intravenous infusion/hour or 250 units/kg by subcutaneous injection.
Special care: pregnancy, liver or kidney disorders. If treatment period exceeds 5 days, platelet counts must be carried out.
Avoid use: bleeding disorders or haemophilia, thrombocytopenia, serious liver disease, severe hypertension, peptic ulcer, cerebral aneurysm, recent surgery to central nervous system or eye. Known hypersensitivity to heparin.
Possible interaction: aspirin, antiplatelet drugs, nitrates.
Side effects: hypersensitivity responses, haemorrhage, osteoporosis (after long-term use), skin necrosis. Also, thrombocytopenia, in which case drug should be immediately withdrawn.
Manufacturer: CP Pharmaceuticals.

Monotrim

Description: an antibacterial and folic acid inhibitor available in a variety of forms all containing trimethoprim. **Monotrim Tablets** in 2 strengths, scored, white containing 100mg coded AE over 2; scored, white containing 200mg coded DE over 5, both marked with symbol. **Monotrim Sugar-Free Suspension** containing 50mg/5ml. **Monotrim Injection** containing 20mg as lactate/ml.

Used for: urinary tract infections and others sensitive to trimethoprim.

Dosage: tablets or suspension, 200mg twice each day; injection, 200mg by intravenous injection or infusion every 12 hours. Children, tablets or suspension, age 6 weeks to 5 months, 25mg; 6 months to 5 years, 50mg; 6 to 12 years, 100mg. All doses twice each day. Injection, 8mg/kg body weight each day in 2 or 3 divided doses by intravenous injection or infusion.

Special care: elderly, babies, folate deficiency or kidney disorders. During long-term treatment, regular blood tests should be carried out.

Avoid use: pregnancy, serious kidney disease.

Possible interaction: procainamide, warfarin, nicoumalone, sulphonylureas, phenytoin, maloprim, fansidar, methotrexate.

Side effects: skin rashes, gastrointestinal upset.

Manufacturer: Duphar.

Monozide 10

Description: a compound preparation combining a cardioselective ß-blocker and thiazide diuretic available as film-coated, white tablets containing 10mg bisoprolol fumerate and 6.25mg hydrochlorothiazide.

Used for: hypertension.

Dosage: adults, 1 tablet each day.

Special care: pregnancy, breast-feeding, liver or kidney disease, diabetes, gout, metabolic acidosis. Patients with weak hearts may require digitalis and diuretics. Electrolyte (salts) levels require regular monitoring. Also, special care in patients undergoing general anaesthesia.

Avoid use: children, persons with chronic obstructive airways disease, history of bronchospasm, uncompensated heart failure, heart block, heart shock, bradycardia, disease of peripheral arteries, sick sinus syndrome. Also, serious or worsening kidney failure, anuria.

Possible interaction: CNS depressants, verapamil, indomethacin, class I antiarrhythmics, sympathomimetics, cardiac depressant anaesthetics, clonidine withdrawal, ergot alkaloids, reserpine, ergot alkaloids, hypoglycaemics, antihypertensives. Potassium supplements, potassium-sparing diuretics, lithium, digitalis.

Side effects: cold hands and feet, disturbance of sleep, fatigue on exercise, gastrointestinal upset, bradycardia, heart failure, bronchospasm, gout. Blood changes, muscle weakness, sensitivity to light. Drug should be gradually withdrawn if dry eyes or skin rash occur.

Manufacturer: Lederle.

Monuril

Description: an antibacterial preparation available as granules in sachets containing 3g fosfomycin as trometamol. Also, **Monuril Paediatric** containing 2g fosfomycin as trometamol as granules in sachets.

Used for: lower urinary tract infections and prevention of infection during surgical procedures in this area.

Dosage: adults, treatment, single 3g dose taken 1 to 2 hours after a meal or at night. Prevention, 3g taken 3 hours before procedure, dose is then repeated 24 hours afterwards. Children, treatment, age over 5 years, a single 2g dose taken 1 or 2 hours after a meal or at night.

Special care: pregnancy, breast-feeding, elderly, kidney disease or disorder.

Avoid use: children under 5 years, elderly people over 75 years, patients with serious kidney disease or disorder.

Possible interaction: metoclopramide.

Side effects: rash, gastrointestinal upset.

Manufacturer: Pharmax.

Motens

Description: an antihypertensive preparation which is a class II calcium antagonist available as white, film-coated tablets containing 2mg and 4mg lacidipine, marked 10L and 9L respectively, and with logo.

Used for: hypertension.

Dosage: adults, 2mg once each day as morning dose with breakfast. May be increased after 3 or 4 weeks to 6mg once each day if needed. The maintenance dose is 4mg once each day. Elderly, 2mg once each day increasing if needed to 4mg after 4 weeks.

Special care: weak hearts, liver disease, disturbances of conduction (of electrical nerve impulses).

Avoid use: children, pregnancy, breast-feeding.

Possible interaction: cimetidine.

Side effects: palpitations, flushing, headache, rash, oedema, polyuria, increase in amount of gum tissue. Drug should be withdrawn if chest pain occurs.

Manufacturer: Boehringer Ingelheim.

Motilium

Description: an antidopaminergic preparation available in a number of different forms all containing domperidone. Motilium Tablets are white, film-coated and contain 10mg, marked with the name. **Motilium Suspension** contains 1mg/ml solution; **Motilium Suppositories** contain 30mg.

Used for: nausea and vomiting, indigestion (tablets).

Dosage: tablets for indigestion, 10–20mg 2 or 3 times each day. For nausea and vomiting, 10–20mg as tablets or suspension or 1 or 2 suppositories, both every 4 to 8 hours. Children, for nausea and vomiting following cancer therapy only, 0.2–0.4mg/kg body weight as suspension every 4 to 8 hours, or 1 to 4 suppositories each day, dose determined by body weight.

Avoid use: pregnancy.

Side effects: extrapyramidal reactions (characterized by involuntary reflex muscle movements and spasms), skin rash, raised levels of prolactin in blood.

Manufacturer: Sanofi Winthrop.

Motipress

Description: an anxiolytic and antidepressant combining a phenothiazine group III and TCAD available as triangular, sugar-coated yellow tablets containing 1.5mg fluphenazine hydrochloride and 30mg nortriptyline (as hydrochloride).

Used for: anxiety and depression.

Dosage: 1 tablet each day, preferably taken at bedtime. Maximum treatment period is 3 months.

Special care: breast-feeding, epilepsy, disease of arteries of heart, glaucoma, liver disease, hyperthyroidism, tumours of adrenal glands. Patients with psychoses or at risk of suicide.

Avoid use: pregnancy, damaged liver or kidneys, serious heart disorders, heart attack, heart block, blood changes, history of brain damage or grand mal epilepsy.

Possible interaction: antidepressants, anticonvulsants, alcohol, within 2 weeks of taking MAOIs, barbiturates, adrenaline, noradrenaline, antihypertensives, anticholinergics, oestrogens, cimetidine.

Side effects: sleepiness, vertigo, light-headedness, unsteadiness, disturbance of vision, rash, hypotension, gastrointestinal upset, changes in libido, retention of urine. Allergic reactions, dry mouth, constipation, sweating, tachycardia, nervousness, heart arrhythmias. Impotence, effects on breasts, weight loss or gain.

Manufacturer: Sanofi Winthrop.

Motival

Description: an anxiolytic and antidepressant preparation combining a phenothiazine group III and TCAD available as sugar-coated, pink, triangular-shaped tablets containing 0.5mg fluphenazine hydrochloride and 10mg nortriptyline as hydrochloride.

Used for: anxiety and depression.

Dosage: 1 tablet 3 times each day for a maximum period of 3 months.

Special care: breast-feeding, epilepsy, disease of arteries of heart, glaucoma, liver disease, hyperthyroidism, tumours of adrenal glands. Patients with psychoses or at risk of suicide.

Avoid use: pregnancy, damaged liver or kidneys, serious heart disorders, heart attack, heart block, blood changes, history of brain damage or grand mal epilepsy.

Possible interaction: antidepressants, anticonvulsants, alcohol, within 2 weeks of taking MAOIs, barbiturates, adrenaline, noradrenaline, antihypertensives, anticholinergics, oestrogens, cimetidine.

Side effects: sleepiness, vertigo, lightheadedness, unsteadiness, disturbance of vision, rash, hypotension, gastrointestinal upset, changes in libido, retention of urine. Allergic reactions, dry mouth, constipation, sweating, tachycardia, nervousness, heart arrhythmias. Impotence, effects on breasts, weight loss or gain.

Manufacturer: Sanofi Winthrop.

Motrin

Description: an NSAID and proprionic acid, available in the form of film-coated tablets of 4 strengths. Red tablets contain 200mg ibuprofen; orange tablets contain 400mg; oval-shaped, peach-coloured tablets contain 600mg, all marked with a U. Orange, capsule-shaped tablets contain 800mg, marked with strength and name.

Used for: pain, rheumatism and other bone and muscle disorders including osteoarthritis, rheumatoid arthritis and ankylosing spondylitis.

Dosage: adults, 1200–1800mg each day in divided doses, the maximum being 2400mg daily. Children, 20mg/kg body weight each day with a maximum dose of 500mg for children weighing less than 30kg. For juvenile rheumatoid arthritis, 40mg/kg may be given.

Special care: pregnancy, breast-feeding, elderly, liver or kidney disorders, heart disease, asthma, disease of gastrointestinal tract.

Avoid use: patients with known allergy to NSAID or aspirin, peptic ulcer.

Possible interaction: thiazide diuretics, anticoagulants, quinolones.

Side effects: rash, gastrointestinal disorder or bleeding, thrombocytopenia.

Manufacturer: Upjohn.

MST Continus^{CD}

Description: an opiate preparation which is a controlled drug available as continuous-release film-coated tablets of different strengths, all containing morphine sulphate. White, 5mg; brown, 10mg; light green, 15mg; purple, 30mg; orange, 60mg; grey, 100mg; green, 200mg; tablets are all marked NAPP and with strength. Also, **Continus Suspension**, produced as granules in sachets for dissolving in water, to make raspberry-flavoured continuous-release suspension containing morphine (equivalent to morphine sulphate). Suspension is available in 20mg, 30mg, 60,mg, 100mg and 200mg strengths.

Used for: long-term relief of severe pain when other drugs have proved inadequate.

Dosage: 30mg every 12 hours at first, then adjusted to dose necessary to provide pain relief for 12 hours according to patient's response. Children, 0.2–0.8mg/kg body weight every 12 hours at first, then adjusted to dose necessary to provide pain relief for 12 hours. (Granules may be dissolved in water or mixed with food).

Special care: elderly, liver or kidney disease; hypothyroidism (underactive thyroid gland).

Avoid use: pregnant women, patients with severe liver disease, obstructive airways disease, depressed respiration.

Possible interaction: central nervous system depressants, MAOIs.

Side effects: nausea, constipation, vomiting, drug tolerance and dependence.

Manufacturer: Napp.

Mucaine

Description: a combined antacid and local anaesthetic preparation containing 10mg oxethazine, 4.75ml aluminium hydroxide gel and 100mg magnesium hydroxide/5ml suspension.

Used for: hiatus hernia and oesophagitis.

Dosage: adults, 10–20ml 3 times each day after meals and at night.

Avoid use: children.

Manufacturer: Wyeth.

Mucodyne

Description: a mucolytic preparation available as a syrup containing 250mg carbocisteine/5ml. Also, **Mucodyne CAapsules**, yellow capsules containing 375mg carbocisteine marked MUCODYNE 375. **Mucodyne Paediatric** contains 125mg carbocisteine/5ml as a syrup.

Used for: copious, thick mucus, glue ear in children.

Dosage: adults, 750mg, 3 times each day, reducing to 500mg. Children, syrup, aged 2 to 5 years, 2.5–5ml 4 times each day; 5 to 10 years, 10ml 3 times each day.

Special care: pregnancy, history of peptic ulcer.

Avoid use: children under 2 years, patients with peptic ulcer.

Side effects: nausea, gastrointestinal upset, rash.

Manufacturer: Theraplix.

Multiload

Description: an inter-uterine contraceptive device formed from copper wire on a polyethylene stem. Also, **Multiload Cu 250 Short**, and **Multiload Cu 375**.

Used for: contraception.

Special care: diabetes, anaemia, history of endocarditis or pelvic inflammatory disease, epilepsy, hypermenorrhoea (or menorrhagia, long or heavy menstrual periods). Examine after 3 months, then annually.

Avoid use: pregnancy, past ectopic pregnancy, uterus disorders, infection of vagina or cervix, acute pelvic inflammatory diseases, cervical cancer, abnormal vaginal bleeding, endometrial disease, immuno-suppressive therapy, copper allergy, cancer of the genitalia.

Possible interaction: anticoagulants.

Side effects: pain, pelvic infection, perforation of the uterus, abnormal bleeding. On insertion there may be attack of asthma or epilepsy, bradycardia, Remove if persistent bleeding or cramps, perforation of cervix or uterus, pregnancy, persistent pelvic infection.

Manufacturer: Organon.

Multiparin

Description: an anticoagulant preparation of heparin sodium available as 1000, 5000 and 25,000 units/ml in multidose vials.

Used for: treatment of pulmonary embolism and deep vein thrombosis.

Dosage: adults, initial loading dose of 5000 units (10,000 in severe conditions) by intravenous injection followed by continuous infusion at a rate of 1000–2000 units/hour. Or 15,000 units at 12 hour intervals may be given by subcutaneous injection. Small adult or child, lower initial dose then 15–25 units/kg body weight by intravenous infusion/hour or 250 units/kg by subcutaneous injection.

Special care: pregnancy, liver or kidney disorders. If treatment period exceeds 5 days, platelet counts must be carried out.

Avoid use: bleeding disorders or haemophilia, thrombocytopenia, serious liver disease, severe hypertension, peptic ulcer, cerebral aneurysm, having had recent surgery to central nervous system or eye. Known hypersensitivity to heparin.

Possible interaction: aspirin, antiplatelet drugs, nitrates.

Side effects: hypersensitivity responses, haemorrhage, osteoporosis (after long-term use), skin necrosis. Also, thrombocytopenia, in which case drug should be immediately withdrawn and, rarely, baldness.

Manufacturer: CP Pharmaceuticals.

Mumps Vax

Description: a preparation of mumps vaccine of live attenuated virus of the Jeryl Lynn strain available as powder in single dose vials with diluent, containing the virus and 0.25mg neomycin per dose.

Used for: immunization against mumps for all ages over 1 year.

Dosage: 1 dose of reconstituted vaccine by subcutaneous injection.

Avoid use: children under 1 year, pregnant women, patients with infections, low levels of gammaglobulins in blood, severe egg allergy.

Possible interaction: live vaccines, immunoglobulins, transfusions, cytotoxic drugs, radiation therapy, corticosteroids.

Manufacturer: Morson.

Myambutol

Description: an anti-tuberculous drug available as yellow tablets containing 100mg ethambutol and grey tablets containing 400mg ethambutol.

Used for: treatment of tuberculosis along with other antituberculous drugs and prevention of tuberculosis.

Dosage: prevention and treatment, 15mg/kg body weight each day as a single dose. Children, treatment, 25mg/kg each day for 60 days. Prevention, 15mg/kg each day as a single dose.

Special care: breast-feeding, kidney disorders. Visual tests must be carried out.

Avoid use: patients with inflammation of the optic nerve.

Side effects: visual disturbances, blurred vision, distortion of colour vision—drug should be withdrawn.

Manufacturer: Lederle.

Mycobutin

Description: an antimycobacterial ansamycin drug available as brown/red capsules containing 150mg rifambutin.

Used for: as sole therapy in prevention of monobacterial infections in immunocompromised patients (whose immune system is not working properly). Additional treatment of mycobacterial infections.

Dosage: prevention of mycobacterial infections, 2 tablets each day. As additional therapy in non-tuberculous mycobacterial disease, 3 to 4 tablets each day continuing for 6 months after infection has cleared. Pulmonary tuberculosis, 1 to 3 tablets each day as additional therapy for a minimum period of 6 months.

Special care: severe liver or kidney failure. Blood checks and liver enzyme tests should be carried out.

Avoid use: children, patients wearing soft contact lenses, pregnancy, breast-feeding.

Possible interaction: triazole antifungal drugs, hypoglycaemics taken by mouth, oral contraceptives, cyclosporin, macrolides, anticoagulants, dapsone, zidovudine, digitalis, quinidine, analgesics, phenytoin, corticosteroids.

Side effects: anaemia, leucopenia and thrombocytopenia, pain in muscles and joints, discolouration of urine, skin and bodily secretions.

Manufacterer: Pharmacia.

Mydriacyl

Description: an anticholinergic preparation available as eyedrops containing 0.5% and 1% tropicamide.

Used for: to produce mydriasis (dilation of the pupil of the eye by contraction of certain muscles in the iris) and cytoplegia (paralysis of the muscles of accommodation in the eye along with relaxation of the ciliary muscle).

Dosage: 1 or 2 drops of either strength at intervals between 1 and 5 minutes.

Special care: patients in whom pressure within eye is not known. In infants, pressure should be applied over tear sac for 1 minute.

Avoid use: patients wearing soft contact lenses, those with narrow angle glaucoma.

Side effects: short-lived stinging, sensitivity to light, dry mouth, headache, tachycardia, blurred vision. Also, mental disturbances, behavioural changes, psychoses.

Manufactuer: Alcon.

Mydrilate

Description: an anticholinergic preparation available in the form of eyedrops in 2 strengths containing 0.5% and 1% cyclopentolate hydrochloride.

Used for: refraction and uveitis (inflammation of the uveal tract which includes the choroid, iris and ciliary body, characterized by impaired vision and can cause blindness).

Dosage: adults, refraction, 1 drop of solution of either strength repeated after 15 minutes if needed. Uveitis, 1 or 2 drops of either strength repeated as needed. Children, refraction, under 6 years, 1 or 2 drops of 1% solution; over 6 years, 1 drop of 1% solution. Uveitis, children over 3 months, same dose as adult.

Special care: eye inflammation, raised pressure within eye.

Avoid use: patients with glaucoma.

Side effects: systemic toxic effects due to absorption of drops, especially elderly persons and children, contact dermatitis.

Manufacturer: Boehringer Ingelheim.

Myleran

Description: an alkylating cytotoxic drug available as white tablets in 2 strengths containing 0.5mg and 2mg busulphan, coded F2A and K2A respectively, and WELLCOME.

Used for: chronic myeloid leukaemia.

Dosage: adults, to induce remission, 60µg/kg body weight each day with a maximum daily dose of 4mg. Maintenance dose is 0.5–2mg.

Special care: pregnant women—patients should be treated in hospital. Frequent blood counts are required.

Avoid use: patients with porphyria, children.

Possible interaction: radiotherapy, other cytotoxic drugs.

Side effects: severe bone marrow suppression, nausea, vomiting, hair loss, excessive pigmentation of skin.

Manufacturer: Wellcome.

Myocrisin

Description: a long-acting suppressive drug and gold salt available in ampoules for injection containing 10mg, 20mg and 50mg sodium aurothiomalate/0.5ml.

Used for: rheumatoid arthritis, juvenile arthritis.

Dosage: initial test of 10mg by deep intramuscular injection followed by 50mg each week until condition improves. Children, initial test dose of one tenth to one fifth of ongoing dose which is 1mg/kg bodyweight weekly up to a maximum of 50mg. The interval between doses is gradually increased to 4 weeks depending on response.

Special care: elderly, urine tests and blood counts are essential. Eczema, urticaria, colitis (inflamed bowel). No improvement can be expected in adults until 300mg–500mg has been given, and if

condition has not changed after 1g total dose, drug should be withdrawn.

Avoid use: pregnancy, breast-feeding, patients with history of blood changes, certain skin disorders, liver or kidney disease, porphyria.

Possible interaction: phenylbutazone, penicillamine.

Side effects: rash, eosinophilia (increased number of eosinophils (a type of white blood cells) in blood, an allergic response), albuminuria (presence of albumin in urine). Patients should report if itching (pruritis), bleeding gums, mouth ulcers, sore throat, sore tongue, diarrhoea, bruising, metallic taste in mouth or heavy menstrual bleeding occur. Also toxic effects on liver, cholestatic jaundice, baldness, lung fibrosis may occur.

Manufacturer: Theraplix.

Myotonine

Description: a cholinergic preparation available as scored white tablets containing 10mg bethanechol chloride and white, cross-scored tablets containing 25mg bethanechol chloride.

Used for: total or partial immobility of the bowel or stomach, large, abnormally extended colon, reflux oesophagitis, retention of urine.

Dosage: adults, 10–25mg 3 to 4 times each day; children, reduced dose in proportion to that for 70kg adult.

Avoid use: pregnancy, epilepsy, recent heart attack, serious hypotension, obstruction of urinary or gastro-intestinal tract, Parkinson's disease, severe brady-cardia, asthma, hyperthyroidism, vagotonia (abnormal increase in the activity of the vagus nerve).

Side effects: blurred vision, abdominal pains, nausea, frequency of urination, vomiting, sweating.

Manufacturer: Glenwood.

Mysoline

Description: an anticonvulsant pyrimidinedone preparation available as scored, white tablets containing 250mg primidone, marked with 2 lines and ICI. Also, **Mysoline Suspension** containing 250mg primidone/5ml.

Used for: epilepsy.

Dosage: 125mg taken at night in first instance increasing every 3 days by 125mg to 500mg each day. Then a further increase every third day of 250mg to a maximum dose of 1.5g daily. Children, same initial dose as adults but increasing by 125mg. Usual daily maintenance doses as follows: up to 2 years, 250–500mg; 2 to 5 years, 500–750mg; 6 to 9 years, 750mg–1g; 9 to 12 years, 750mg–1.5g.

Special care: patients with kidney and liver disorders, serious lung insufficiency.

Avoid use: pregnancy, breast-feeding, elderly, patients who are debilitated, porphyria , pain which is not controlled, history of drug or alcohol abuse.

Possible interaction: CNS depressants, griseofulvin, alcohol, phenytoin, systemic steroids, chloramphenicol, rifampicin, metronidazole, anticoagulants of the coumarin type.

Side effects: headache, respiratory depression, dizziness, unsteadiness, sleepiness, confusion, agitation, allergic responses, megaloblastic anaemia. Drug tolerance and dependence may occur. Drug is metabolized to phenobarbitone.

Manufacturer: Zeneca.

Mysteclin

Description: a compound tetracycline and antifungal preparation available as sugar-coated orange tablets containing 250mg tetracycline hydrochloride and 250,000 units nystatin.

Used for: injections and acne susceptible to tetracycline, particularly where candidiasis also occurs.

Dosage: adults 1 or 2 tablets 4 times each day.

Special care: liver or kidney disease.

Avoid use: pregnancy, breast-feeding, children.

Possible interaction: oral contraceptives, antacids, mineral supplements, milk, anticoagulants.

Side effects: allergic responses, gastrointestinal upset, superinfection. If rise in intracranial pressure occurs, drug should be withdrawn.

Manufacturer: Squibb.

N

Nacton Forte

Description: an anticholinergic, poldine methylsulphate, available as orange tablets (4mg strength), marked NACTON 4.

Used for: peptic ulcer, acidity.

Dosage: 4mg 3 times per day and at bedtime. Elderly, half dose. Not for children. Also **Nacton**, 2mg poldine methylsulphate as white tablets marked NACTON 2. *Dosage*: see literature. Not for children.

Special care: glaucoma, tachycardia, difficulty in urinating.

Side effects: anticholinergic effects

Manufacturer: Pharmark.

Nalcrom

Description: an anti-inflammatory non-steroid, sodium cromoglycate as clear capsules containing white powder (100mg) and marked FISONS and 101.

Used for: food allergy.

Dosage: 2 capsules 4 times per day before meals, maximum 40mg/kg per day. Children over 2 years, 1 capsule 4 times per day. Not recommended for children under 2.

Side effects: rashes, joint pain, nausea.

Manufacturer: Fisons.

Nalorex

Description: a narcotic antagonist, naltrexone hydrochloride, available as mottled orange tablets (50mg strength) and marked DuPont and NTR.

Used for: maintenance treatment for patients undergoing detoxification therapy after opioid dependency.

Dosage: 25mg daily to start with and then 50mg per day for at least 3 months. Treatment should be started in a drug addiction centre. Not for children.

Special care: kidney or liver disorder.

Avoid use: a current dependence on opiates, liver failure, acute hepatitis.

Side effects: drowsiness, dizziness, cramps, vomiting, joint and muscle pains.

Manufacturer: DuPont.

Napratec

Description: an NSAID and propionic acid/ prostaglandin analogue, available as naproxen, a yellow oblong tablet (500mg) marked Searle N500, and misoprostol, a white hexagonal tablet (200µg) marked Searle 1461.

Used for: osteoarthritis, rheumatoid arthritis, ankylosing spondylitis where the stomach has to be protected against the medication.

Dosage: 1 tablet of each drug taken twice daily with food.

Special care: asthma, liver or kidney damage, elderly, disease of blood vesssels. Effective contraception must be used by women of child-bearing age.

Avoid use: pregnancy, lactation, duodenal or gastric ulcer, allergy induced by aspirin or anti-inflammatory drugs.

Possible interaction: diuretics, anticoagulants, sulphonylureas, quinolones, sulphonamides, hydantoins, lithium, ß-blockers, probenecid, methotrexate.

Side effects: diarrhoea, abdominal pain, gastrointestinal upset, vaginal bleeding, menorrhagia (long or heavy menstruation), rash, headache, urticaria, dizziness, tinnitus, vertigo, blood changes.

Manufacturer: Searle.

Naprosyn SR

Description: Propionic acid, naproxen (as the sodium salt) available as 500mg in white, capsule-shaped tablets marked 500.

Used for: osteoarthritis, rheumatoid arthritis, ankylosing spondylitis, musculoskeletal disorders, acute gout.

Dosage: 1 to 2 tablets once per day. Not for children. Also, **Naprosyn EC**, naproxen as 250mg, 375mg and 500mg strength white tablets marked with tablet name, the strength and SYNTEX. **Naprosyn Tablets**, naproxen as 250mg (buff tablets), 375mg (pink tablets) and 500mg (buff tablets) marked with tablet name, strength and SYNTEX. **Naprosyn Suspension**, naproxen as 250mg per 10ml and

Naprosyn Granules, 500mg naproxen as peppermint-flavoured granules in a sachet.
Dosage: 500–1000mg per day in 2 divided doses or as 1 dose morning or evening. For gout, 750mg to start with and then 250mg every 8 hours. For musculoskeletal disorders, 500mg to start with, then 250mg every 6 to 8 hours as necessary, no more than 1250mg per day after the first 24 hours. Children: for juvenile rheumatoid arthritis, 5 to 16 years, 10mg/kg body weight per day in 2 divided doses. Not for children under 5.
Also, **Naprosyn Suppositories**, naproxen 500mg.
Dosage: 1 at night with another in the morning (or 500mg by mouth) if necessary.
Special care: liver or kidney damage, elderly, heart failure, asthma, pregnancy, lactation, a history of gastrointestinal lesions.
Avoid use: peptic ulcer, allergy caused by aspirin or anti-inflammatory drugs.
Possible interaction: ACE inhibitors, ß-blockers, lithium, anticoagulants, quinolones, sulphonylureas, hydantoins, frusemide, methotrexate, probenecid.
Side effects: headache, gastrointestinal intolerance, rash, vertigo, blood changes, tinnitus.
Manufacturer: Syntex.

Narcan
Description: a narcotic antagonist, naloxone hydrochloride, available as ampoules or pre-filled syringes (0.4mg/ml, 1mg/ml).
Used for: diagnosis of opioid overdosage, reversal of opioid depression including that due to pentazocine and dextropropoxyphone.
Dosage: 0.4–2mg by injection (intravenous, intramuscular or subcutaneous) every 2 to 3 minutes as necessary, or by intravenous infusion (see literature). Postoperative, 0.1–0.2mg intravenously as required. Children 10µg/kg by same means.
Also, **Narcan Neonatal**, naloxone hydrochloride as 0.02mg/ml in 2ml ampoules.
Used for: depression of neonatal respiration due to obstetric analgesia.
Dosage: 10µg/kg by injection (intravenous, intramuscular or subcutaneous), repeated as required.
Special care: pregnancy, opioid dependence. Patient should be monitored to determine whether repeat doses are needed.
Manufacturer: DuPont.

Nardil
Description: an antidepressant and MAOI, phenelzine sulphate, available as orange tablets (15mg strength).

Used for: depression, phobias.
Dosage: 1 tablet 3 times per day initially, reduced gradually for maintenance. Not for children.
Special care: elderly, epilepsy.
Avoid use: liver disease, blood changes, congestive heart failure, brain vascular disease, hyperthyroidism, phaeochromocytoma.
Possible interaction: sympathomimetic amines (e.g. amphetamine and others), TCADs, pethidine and similar analgesics. The effect of barbiturates and alcohol, insulin, hypnotics may be enhanced and the side effects of anticholinergics may be enhanced or increased, antihypertensives. Avoid foods such as cheese, meat extracts (e.g. Oxo or Bovril), yeast extracts (e.g. Marmite), alcohol, broad beans, bananas, pickled herrings, vegetable proteins. Do not use any of these within 14 days of stopping the drug.
Side effects: severe hypertension with certain foods (see above), dizziness, drowsiness, insomnia, weakness, fatigue, postural hypotension, constipation, dry mouth, gastrointestinal upsets, difficulty in urinating, blurred vision, ankle oedema. Skin rashes, blood disorders, weight gain, jaundice, changes in libido.
Manufacturer: Parke-Davis.

Narphen[CD]
Description: an opiate, phenazocine hydrobromide available as white, scored tablets (strength 5mg) marked SNP/2.
Used for: severe, prolonged pain including pancreatic and biliary pain.
Dosage: 1 tablet every 4 to 6 hours, taken by mouth, or beneath the tongue, as necessary. Maximum single dose, 20mg. Not for children.
Special care: hypothyroidism, chronic kidney or liver disease, elderly. In labour or during pregnancy.
Avoid use: coma, epilepsy, acute alcoholism, breathing difficulty, blocked airways.
Possible interaction: depressants of the central nervous system, MAOIs.
Side effects: constipation, dizziness nausea. Danger of tolerance and dependence.
Manufacturer: Napp.

Naseptin
Description: an antibacterial cream comprising chlorhexidine hydrochloride (0.1%) and neomycin sulphate (0.5%).
Used for: staphylococcal infections of the nose.
Dosage: small amounts to be applied into each nostril 2 to 4 times per day.
Special care: prolonged use should be avoided.

Side effects: sensitive skin.
Manufacturer: Zeneca.

Natrilix
Description: a vasorelaxant, indapamide hemihydrate, available as white, film-coated tablets (strength 2.5mg).
Used for: hypertension.
Dosage: 1 tablet in the morning. Not for children.
Special care: pregnancy, severe kidney disease.
Avoid use: lactation, severe liver disease.
Possible interaction: corticosteroids, laxatives, lithium, cardiac glycosides, diuretics, anti-arrhythmics.
Side effects: nausea, headache, hypokalaemia.
Manufacturer: Servier.

Natulan
Description: a cytostatic agent, procarbazine hydrochloride, available as yellow capsules (strength 50mg).
Used for: Hodgkin's disease, advanced reticoloses (normally malignant overgrowths in the lymphatic or immune system), solid tumours that do not respond to other therapies.
Dosage: see literature but likely to be 50mg per day to begin with, rising to 250–300mg per day in 50mg daily increments. Dose for maintenance (on remission), 50–150mg per day.
Special care: induction therapy should commence in hospital.
Avoid use: pregnancy, severe liver or kidney damage, severe leucopenia, thrombocytopenia.
Possible interaction: alcohol, narcotics, barbiturates, phenothiazines, imipramine-type compounds.
Side effects: nausea, loss of appetite, myelosuppression (reduction in the production of blood cells in the bone marrow).
Manufacturer: Cambridge.

Navidrex
Description: a thiazide diuretic, cyclopenthiazide (0.5mg), available as white scored tablets marked CIBA and AO.
Used for: oedema, heart failure, hypertension.
Dosage: 0.25–1mg per day to a maximum of 1.5mg daily, but see manufacturer's literature. For children, contact the manufacturer.
Special care: liver cirrhosis, liver or kidney disease, SLE, gout, the elderly, pregnancy, lactation. Electrolytes, glucose and fluids should be monitored.
Avoid use: hypercalcaemia, Addison's disease, severe liver or kidney failure, if sensitive to sulphonamides.
Possible interaction: corticosteroids, cardiac glycosides, lithium, carbenozolone, tubocurarine, antidiabetic drugs, NSAIDs, opioids, barbiturates, alcohol.
Side effects: gastrointestinal upset, anorexia, blood changes, rash, sensitivity to light, dizziness, pancreatitis, metabolic and electrolyte upset, impotence.
Manufacturer: Ciba.

Navispare
Description: a thiazide and potassium-sparing diuretic, cyclopenthiazide (0.25mg) with 2.5mg amiloride, available as yellow tablets marked CIBA and RC.
Used for: mild to moderate hypertension.
Dosage: 1 or 2 tablets per day in the morning. Not for children.
Special care: liver or kidney disease, diabetes, hyperlipidaemia, pregnancy, lactation, gout, respiratory or metabolic acidosis.
Avoid use: severe kidney or liver failure, anuria, hyperkalaemia, Addison's disease, hypercalcaemia, hyponatiaemia (low blood sodium levels).
Possible interaction: ACE inhibitors, other antihypertensives, lithium, digitalis, potassium supplements, potassium-sparing diuretics.
Side effects: blood changes, gout, gastrointestinal upset, fatigue, rash, sensitivity to light.
Manufacturer: Ciba.

Navoban
Description: a 5HT₃-antagonist, tropisetron hydrochloride, which blocks vomiting reflexes, available as yellow/white capsules (5mg strength). Also, **Navoban Injection**, containing 5mg/5ml in ampoules.
Used for: chemotherapy-induced nausea and vomiting.
Dosage: 5mg by intravenous injection of infusion before therapy and 1 capsule 1 hour before morning food, for 5 days. Not for children.
Special care: uncontrolled hypertension.
Avoid use: pregnancy, breast-feeding.
Possible interaction: drugs that affect liver enzymes.
Side effects: constipation, dizziness, headache, tiredness, stomach upset.
Manufacturer: Sandoz.

Nebcin
Description: an aminoglycoside, tabramycin

sulphate, available as solution in vials containing 20, 40 or 80mg.

Used for: infections of gastrointestinal and respiratory tract, skin and soft tissue, CNS, urinary tract; septicaemia.

Dosage: 3–5mg/kg per day by intramuscular injection, intravenous injection or infusion in 3 or 4 divided doses. Children: 6–7.5mg/kg daily in divided doses; babies up to 1 month, 4mg/kg per day in 2 doses.

Special care: kidney damage; control dosage and blood levels.

Avoid use: pregnancy, lactation.

Possible interaction: loop diuretics, other aminoglycosides, neuromuscular blocking agents.

Side effects: anaphylaxis, ototoxicity (affecting hearing and balance), nephrotoxicity, raised liver enzymes.

Manufacturer: Lilly.

Negram

Description: a quinolone, nalidixic acid (500mg) available as light brown tablets marked NEGRAM with a symbol on the reverse. Also, **Negram Suspension**, containing 300mg/5ml as a suspension.

Used for: infections of the grastro-intestinal tract by Gram-negative organisms.

Dosage: 500mg–1g 4 times per day. Children up to 12 years, up to 50mg/kg per day. Not for children under 3 months.

Special care: liver or kidney disease, lactation. Avoid sunlight.

Avoid use: history of convulsions.

Possible interaction: probenecid, anticoagulants.

Side effects: rashes, blood changes, convulsions, disturbances in vision and stomach.

Manufacturer: Sanofi Winthrop.

Neo-Cortef

Description: an antibiotic and cortico-steroid comprising 0.5% neomycin in sulphate and 1.5% hydrocortisone acetate, as drops.

Used for: otitis externa and eye inflammation.

Dosage: 2 to 3 drops 4 times per day (otitis), 1 to 2 drops in each eye up to 6 times per day.

Also, **Neo-Cortef Ointment**

Dosage: apply once or twice per day (otitis), apply 2 or 3 times per day or if drops are used during the day, use at night.

Special care: prolonged use on infants or during pregnancy.

Avoid use: perforated ear drum, glaucoma; fungal, viral, tuberculous or acute pus-containing infections.

Side effects: sensitization, superinfection, cataract, rise in pressure within the eye.

Manufacturer: Cusi.

Neo-Cytamen

Description: vitamin B12, hydroxocobalamin, available as 1ml ampoules containing 1000µg per ml.

Used for: megaloblastic anaemia, and other anaemias responsive to B12, Leber's disease (a rare hereditary visual defect), tobacco amblyopia (reduced vision although eye structure appears normal).

Dosage: 250–1000µg intramuscularly on alternate days for 7 to 14 days then 250µg once per week until blood count is normal. 1000µg every 2 to 3 months for maintenance. For ambylopia, see literature.

Possible interaction: oral contraceptives, chloramphenicol.

Side effects: some rare hypersensitivity reactions.

Manufacturer: Evans.

Neo-Medrone Cream

Description: a mild steroid and antibacterial, 0.25% methylprednisolone acetate and 0.5% neomycin sulphate, as a cream.

Used for: allergic and inflammatory skin conditions where there is bacterial infection.

Dosage: use 1 to 3 times per day.

Special care: thrombophlebitis, psychoses, recent intestinal anastomoses, chronic nephritis, certain cancers, osteoporosis, peptic ulcer, skin eruption/ rash related to a disease, viral, fungal or active infections, tuberculosis. Hypertension, glaucoma, epilepsy, acute glomerulonephritis (inflammation of kidney glomerulus), diabetes, cirrhosis, hypothyroidism, pregnancy, stress. To be withdrawn gradually.

Possible interaction: NSAIDs, oral anticoagulants, phenytoin, ephedrine, phenobarbitone, rifampicin, diuretics, cardiac glycosides, anticholinesterases, hypoglycaemics.

Side effects: osteoporosis, depression, euphoria, hyperglycaemia, peptic ulcers, Cushingoid changes.

Manufacturer: Upjohn.

Neo-Mercazole

Description: an antithyroid, carbimazole, available as pink tablets (strengths 5 and 20mg) marked BS with strength on the reverse.

Used for: thyrotoxicosis.

Dosage: 20–60mg per day initially in 2 or 3 divided doses until thyroid functions normally. 5–15mg per day for 6 to 18 months for maintenance, or maintain

20–60mg per day with 50–150µg supplemental thyroxine daily for 6 to 18 months. Children, 5–15mg per day in divided doses.

Special care: pregnancy (but see literature).

Avoid use: lactation, obstruction of the trachea.

Side effects: arthralgia, headache, nausea, rashes. Depression of the bone marrow. Drug should be discontinued if there are mouth ulcers or a sore throat.

Manufacturer: Nicholas.

Neo-Naclex

Description: a thiazide, bendrofluazide (5mg), available as white, scored tablets marked NEO-NACLEX.

Used for: hypertension, oedema.

Dosage: 1 to 2 tablets once per day for oedema, half or 1 tablet for maintenance periodically. For hypertension, half to 2 once per day. For children, 50–100µg/kg body weight.

Special care: cirrhosis of the liver, liver or kidney disease, diabetes, SLE, gout, pregnancy, breast-feeding, elderly. Monitor glucose, electrolytes and fluids.

Avoid use: hypercalcaemia, severe liver or kidney failure, sensitivity to sulphonamides, Addison's disease.

Possible interaction: lithium, cardiac glycosides, potassium-sparing diuretics, potassium supplements, corticosteroids, tubocurarine, NSAIDs, carbenoxolone, alcohol, opiods, barbiturates, antidiabetic drugs.

Side effects: rash, blood changes, anorexia, dizziness, pancreatitis, gastrointestinal upset, sensitivity to light, upset to metabolism and electrolytes.

Manufacturer: Goldshield.

Neo-Naclex-K

Description: a thiazide and potassium supplement, bendrofluazide (2.5mg) with 630mg potassium chloride in a slow-release, two-layer tablet, pink and white, marked NEO-NACLEX-K.

Used for: hypertension and chronic oedema.

Dosage: 1 to 4 per day (hypertension). 2 per day for oedema inreasing to 4 if required, maintenance 1 or 2 periodically. Not for children.

Special care: liver cirrhosis, diabetes, liver or kidney disease, SLE, gout, elderly, pregnancy, lactation. Monitor glucose, fluid and electrolytes.

Avoid use: hypercalcaemia, severe liver or kidney failure, Addison's disease, sensitivity to sulphonamides.

Possible interaction: lithium, corticosteroids,

cardiac glycosides, potassium supplements, potassium-sparing diuretics, NSAIDs, tubocurarine, carbenoxolone, alcohol, opioids, barbiturates, antidiabetic drugs.

Side effects: rash, blood changes, gastrointestinal upsets, sensitivity to light, impotence, dizziness, pancreatitis, anorexia, upset to metabolism and electrolytes. Stop if signs of blockage or ulceration of small bowel occur.

Manufacturer: Goldshield.

Neocon 1/35

Description: an oestrogen/progestogen oral contraceptive containing 35µg ethinyloestradiol and 500µg norethisterone in white tablets marked C over 535.

Used for: oral contraception.

Dosage: 1 per day for 21 days commencing on the fifth day of menstruation, then 7 days without tablets.

Special care: hypertension, Raynaud's disease (reduced blood supply to an organ of the body's extremities), asthma, severe depression, diabetes, varicose veins, multiple sclerosis, chronic kidney disease, kidney dialysis. Blood pressure, breasts and pelvic organs to be checked regularly; smoking not advised.

Avoid use: history of heart disease, infectious hepatitis, sickle cell anaemia, porphyria, liver tumour, undiagnosed vaginal bleeding, pregnancy, hormone-dependent cancer, haemolytic uraemic syndrome (rare kidney disorder), chorea, otosclerosis.

Possible interaction: barbiturates, tetracyclines, griseofulvin, rifampicin, primidone, phenytoin, chloral hydrate, ethosuximide, carbamazepine, glutethimide, dichloralphenazone.

Side effects: fluid retention and bloating, leg cramps/pains, breast enlargement, depression, headaches, nausea, loss of libido, weight gain, vaginal discharge, cervical erosion (alteration of epithelial cells), chloasma (pigmentation of nose, cheeks or forehead), breakthrough bleeding (bleeding between periods).

Manufacturer: Ortho.

Neogest

Description: a progestogen-only contraceptive, norgestrel (75µg) available in brown tablets.

Used for: oral contraception.

Dosage: starting on the first day of the cycle, 1 tablet each day at the same time, without a break.

Special care: hypertension, thromboembolic disorders, liver disease, hormone-dependent cancer, ovarian cysts, migraine. Regular checks on blood pressure, breasts and pelvic organs.

Avoid use: previous severe arterial or heart disease, benign liver tumours, undiagnosed vaginal bleeding, pregnancy, past ectopic pregnancy. Discontinue immediately for pregnancy, jaundice, thrombophlebitis or thromboembolism.

Possible interaction: griseofulvin, rifampicin, meprobamate, chloral hydrate, carbamazepine, primidone, barbiturates, phenytoin, dichloral-phenazone, ethosuximide, glutethimide.

Side effects: acne, breast discomfort, headache, ovarian cysts, irregular menstrual bleeding.

Manufacturer: Schering H.C.

Neosporin

Description: a peptide and aminoglycoside, polymyxin B sulphate (5000 units) and neomycin sulphate (1700 units) with gramicidin (25 units/ml), as drops.

Used for: bacterial infections, prevention of infections in the eye before and after surgery, removal of foreign bodies from the eye.

Dosage: 1 or 2 drops 4 or more times per day.

Special care: existing eye defect.

Manufacturer: Cusi.

Neotigason

Description: a vitamin A derivative, acitretin, used only in hospitals and available as brown/white (10mg) and brown/yellow capsules marked ROCHE.

Used for: severe psoriasis, congenital ichthyosis, Darier's disease (skin disease with brown or black wart-like patches).

Dosage: 25–30mg per day initially, for 2 to 4 weeks up to a maximum of 75mg per day. 25–50mg per day for maintenance. Maximum treatment period, 6 months. Not for children.

Special care: teratogenic, effective contraception necessary during treatment and for 2 years after stopping. Diabetes, monitor liver, serum lipids and bone. Do not donate blood for 1 year afterwards.

Avoid use: kidney or liver disease, pregnancy, lactation.

Possible interaction: alcohol, tetracyclines, methotrexate, high doses or vitamin A.

Side effects: hair loss, itching, erythema, dryness, erosion of mucous membranes, nausea, headache, sweating, drowsiness, myalgia, arthralgia, bone thickening, liver disorder.

Manufacturer: Roche.

Nephril

Description: a thiazide diuretic, polythiazide,

available as white tablets (1mg) with NEP over 1 marked on one side and Pfizer on the reverse.

Used for: oedema, hypertension.

Dosage: 1–4mg per day for oedema, 500µg–4mg per day for hypertension. Not recommended for children.

Special care: liver or kidney disease, liver cirrhosis, gout, SLE, diabetes, elderly, pregnancy, breast-feeding. Check glucose, electrolytes and fluid.

Avoid use: liver or kidney failure, hypercalcaemia, Addison's disease, sensitivity to sulphonamides.

Possible interaction: NSAIDs, cardiac glycosides, lithium corticosteroids, carbenoxolone, tubocurarine, alcohol, barbiturates, opioids, antidiabetic drugs.

Side effects: rash, blood changes, dizziness, impotence, anorexia, pancreatitis, gastrointestinal, electrolyte or metabolism upset, sensitivity to light.

Manufacturer: Pfizer.

Nerisone

Description: a potent steroid, diflucortolone valerate (0.1%) available as a cream, oily cream or ointment.

Used for: skin disorders that respond to steroids.

Dosage: apply 2 or 3 times per day reducing to once per day for maintenance. On children under 4, do not use for more than 3 weeks.

Also, **Nerisone Forte**, a very potent form (0.3%) available as ointment and oily cream.

Used for: initial treatment of resistant, severe skin disorders.

Dosage: apply sparingly 2 or 3 times per day for a maximum of 2 weeks (maximum total use 60g/week). For maintenance use Nerisone. Not recommended for children under 4.

Special care: thrombophlebitis, psychoses, recent intestinal anastomoses, chronic nephritis, certain cancers, osteoporosis, peptic ulcer, skin eruption/rash related to a disease, viral, fungal or active infections, tuberculosis. Hypertension, glaucoma, epilepsy, acute glomerulonephritis (inflammation of kidney glomerulus), diabetes, cirrhosis, hypothyroidism, pregnancy, stress. To be withdrawn gradually.

Possible interaction: NSAIDs, oral anticoagulants, phenytoin, ephedrine, phenobarbitone, rifampicin, diuretics, cardiac glycosides, anticholinesterases, hypoglycaemics.

Side effects: osteoporosis, depression, euphoria, hyperglycaemia, peptic ulcers, Cushingoid changes.

Manufacturer: Schering H.C.

Netillin

Description: an aminoglycoside and anti-bacterial,

netilmicin sulphate, available as ampoules containing 10, 50 or 100mg/ml.

Used for: septicaemia, bacteraemia (bacteria in the blood), serious infections of the kidney, urinary tract, skin and soft tissues, respiratory tract. Gonorrhoea.

Dosage: 4–6mg/kg once per day as 2 or 3 divided doses. For life-threatening infections, up to 7.5mg/kg per day in 3 divided doses, all by intramuscular or slow intravenous injection. Children (by the same means): over 2 years, 2–2.5mg/kg 8-hourly; 1 week to 2 years, 2.5–3mg/kg 8-hourly; under 1 week 3mg/kg 12-hourly.

Special care: myasthenia gravis, Parkinson's disease. Control total dosage in cases of kidney disease.

Avoid use: pregnancy.

Possible interaction: anaesthetics, etha crynic acid, frusemide, neuromuscular blockers.

Side effects: nephrotoxicity and ototoxicity (affects hearing and balance).

Manufacturer: Schering-Plough.

Neulactil

Description: a group II phenothiazine and antipsychotic, pericyazine, available as yellow tablets, marked with name (2.5mg) or marked with name and strength (10mg). Also **Neulactil Forte Syrup**, containing 10mg/5ml.

Used for: schizophrenia, severe anxiety and tension, agitation, behavioural disorders, maintenance of sedation for psychotic states.

Dosage: 15–75mg per day initially (elderly 5–30mg), to a maximum of 300mg daily. See literature for children.

Special care: pregnancy, lactation, elderly during very hot or cold weather.

Avoid use: heart failure, epilepsy, Parkinson's disease, liver or kidney disorder, hypothyroidism, glaucoma, coma, bone marrow depression, enlarged prostate.

Possible interaction: alcohol, CNS depressants, antihypertensives, analgesics, levodopa, anti-depressants, anticonvulsants, antidiabetic drugs.

Side effects: muscle spasms (eye, neck, back, face), restlessness, rigidity and tremor, tardive dyskinesia (repetitious muscular movements), dry mouth, blocked nose, difficulty in passing urine, tachycardia, blurred vision, hypotension, constipation, weight gain, impotence, galactorrhoea, gynaecomastia (abnormal development of breasts in a male), amenorrhoea, blood and skin changes, lethargy, fatigue, ECG irregularities.

Manufacturer: R.P.R.

Neupogen

Description: a recombinant human granulocyte colony stimulating factor (G-CSF), filgrastim, available as 30 million units in a single dose vial, for specialist use.

Used for: reduction of neutropenia during cytotoxic chemotherapy and after bone marrow transplantation.

Dosage: chemotherapy, 500,000 units/kg per day by subcutaneous injection or intravenous infusion starting within 24 hours of chemotherapy and continuing until neutrophil count is normal (about 14 days). Bone marrow transplantation—1 million units/kg per day starting within 24 hours.

Special care: risk of bone marrow tumour growth, pre-malignant bone marrow conditions. Monitor platelets, haemoglobin, osteoporosis, pregnancy, lactation.

Side effects: temporary hypotension, urinary abnormalities, musculoskeletal pain, disturbances in liver enzymes and serum uric acid.

Manufacturer: Amgen, Roche.

Neurontin

Description: a GABA analogue, gabapentin, available as capsules: white (100mg), yellow (300mg); orange (400mg), all marked with name and strength.

Used for: added treatment of seizures not controlled by other anticonvulsants.

Dosage: 300mg once, twice and 3 times per day on days 1, 2 and 3 respectively, increasing to 400mg 3 times per day up to a maximum of 800mg. Not for children.

Special care: haemodialysis, pregnancy, kidney disease, elderly, lactation, avoid sudden withdrawal (minimum 1 week).

Possible interaction: antacids.

Side effects: ataxia, dizziness, fatigue, headache, tremor, diplopia, nausea, vomiting, nystagmus (involuntary eye movements) rhinitis, amblyopia (reduced vision in an eye that appears normal structurally).

Manufacturer: Parke-Davis.

Nifensar XL

Description: a class II calcium antagonist and antihypertensive, nifedipine, available as yellow, sustained-release tablets (20mg) marked N20.

Used for: mild to moderate hypertension.

Dosage: 2 once per day swallowed with food, adjusted according to response. 1 or 2 once per day for maintenance. Maximum 5 per day. Elderly, 1 per day initially. Not for children.

Special care: diabetes, angina pectoris, kidney disease, weak heart.

Avoid use: pregnancy, breast-feeding, liver disease.

Possible interaction: other antihypertensives, digoxin, climetidine, quinidine, fentaryl.

Side effects: nausea, oedema, headache, flushes, dizziness, ischaemic pain, jaundice, rash, lethargy, enlarged gums.

Manufacturer: R.P.R.

Nimotop

Description: a class II calcium antagonist, nimodipine, available as 30mg off-white tablets marked Bayer and SK.

Used for: prevention of ischaemic, neurological defects after a subarachnoid (intracranial) haemorrhage.

Dosage: 2 tablets every 4 hours commencing within 4 days of the haemorrhage and continuing for 21 days. Also, **Nimotop Infusion**, containing 0.2mg/ml in vial and bottle.

Used for: neurological deficits after subarachnoid haemorrhage.

Dosage: 1mg/hour by intravenous infusion for 2 hours, then 2mg/hour for 5 to 14 days. For bodyweights under 70kg, or for unstable blood pressure, start at 0.5mg/hour. Not for children.

Special care: raised intracranial pressure, cerebral oedema, kidney disease, pregnancy. Check blood pressure. PVC apparatus should not be used—use polyethylene or polypropylene.

Possible interaction: ß-blockers, other calcium antagonists.

Side effects: flushes, headache, hypotension, heart rate changes.

Manufacturer: Bayer.

Nipent

Description: an adenosine deaminase inhibitor, and cytotoxic drug pentostatin, available as 10mg powder in vial for reconstitution, used in cancer chemotherapy.

Used for: prolonged remission in the treatment of malignancies.

Dosage: intravenously on alternate weeks. For specialist use only.

Side effects: nausea and vomiting, bone marrow suppression, suppression of the immune system, hair loss, teratogenic.

Manufacturer: Lederle.

Nipride

Description: a vasodilator, sodium nitroprusside available as powder (50mg) in ampoules.

Used for: critical hypertension, heart failure, controlled hypotension in surgery.

Dosage: for hypertension, 0.3µg/kg/minute by intravenous infusion to begin then adjust to response, usually 0.5–6µg/kg/minute (maximum 8µg/kg/minute). Lower doses for patients already taking antihypertensives. Lower doses also in surgery (up to 1.5µg/kg/minute). For heart failure, 10–15µg/minute by intravenous infusion increasing at 5 to 10 minute intervals to a maximum of 280µg/minute. Maximum treatment 72 hours, withdraw over 10 to 30 minutes.

Special care: severe kidney disease, hypothyroidism, ischaemic heart disease, elderly, pregnancy, lactation, impaired circulation in the brain. Check blood pressure and concentration of cyanide in plasma.

Avoid use: vitamin B_{12} deficiency, severe liver disease, optic atrophy (causing blindness).

Possible interaction: ACE inhibitors, NSAIDs, alcohol, antipsychotics, antidepressants, ß-blockers, diuretics, anxiolytics and hypnotics, corticosteroids, sex hormones, baclofen, carbenoxolone, levodopa.

Side effects: headache, nausea, dizziness, stomach pain, palpitations, sweating, reeduced platelet count. Also those due to high cyanide concentrations in plasma which *in addition* are tachycardia, metabolic acidosis.

Manufacturer: Roche.

Nitoman

Description: a dopamine reducing agent, tetrabenazine, available as yellow-buff tablets (25mg) marked ROCHE 120.

Used for: Huntington's chorea, senile chorea, hemiballismus (violent involuntary movement).

Dosage: 25mg 3 times per day initially, increasing by 25mg/day every 3 or 4 days to a daily maximum of 200mg. Not for children.

Special care: pregnancy.

Avoid use: breast-feeding.

Possible interaction: levodopa, MAOIs, reserpine.

Side effects: drowsiness, depression, hypotension on standing, rigidity, tremor.

Manufacturer: Roche.

Nitrazepam

Description: a long-acting benzodiazepine, nitrazepam, available as tablets (5mg). Also, **Nitrazepam Oral Suspension** containing 2.5mg/5ml.

Used for: insomnia over the short-term or when it is severe.

Dosage: 5–10mg at bedtime; elderly, 2.5–5mg. Not for children.

Special care: chronic liver or kidney disease, chronic lung disease, pregnancy, labour, lactation, elderly. May impair judgement. Withdraw gradually and avoid prolonged use.

Avoid use: depression of respiration, acute lung disease; psychotic, phobic or obsessional states.

Possible interaction: anticonvulsants, depressants of the CNS, alcohol.

Side effects: ataxia, confusion, light-headedness, drowsiness, hypotension, gastrointestinal upsets, disturbances in vision and libido, skin rashes, retention of urine, vertigo. Sometimes jaundice or blood disorders.

Manufacturer: non-proprietary—available from several suppliers.

Nitrocine
Description: a solution of glyceryl trinitrate (1mg/ml) in ampoules and bottles.

Used for: prevention and treatment of angina, left ventricular failure.

Dosage: 10–200µg/minute by intravenous infusion.

Special care: hypotension, tolerance.

Avoid use: anaemia, cerebral haemorrhage, head trauma, closed angle glaucoma.

Side effects: flushes, headache, tachycardia, dizziness, hypotension on standing.

Manufacturer: Schwarz.

Nitronal
Description: a solution of glyceryl trinitrate (1mg/ml) in ampoules and vials.

Used for: prevention and treatment of angina, left ventricular failure.

Dosage: 10–200µg/minute by intravenous infusion.

Special care: hypotension, tolerance.

Avoid use: anaemia, cerebral haemorrhage, head trauma, closed angle glaucoma.

Side effects: flushes, headache, tachycardia, dizziness, hypotension on standing.

Manufacturer: Lipha.

Nivaquine
Description: a suppressive drug and 4-aminoquinoline, chloroquine sulphate, available as yellow tablet (150mg) marked NIVAQUINE 200.

Used for: rheumatoid arthritis, malaria.

Dosage: 1 tablet per day (arthritis); for malaria prevention, 2 tablets in 1 dose on the same week day for 2 weeks before being subjected to possible infection and for 4 weeks after. Children should use the syrup.

Also, **Nivaquine Syrup**, 50mg/5ml chloroquine sulphate.

Dosage: 3mg/kg per day for arthritis; prevention of malaria, 5mg/kg at weekly intervals, for 2 weeks before and 4 weeks after being subjected to possible infection. For treatment see literature.

Also, **Nivaquine Injection**, 40mg/ml in ampoules.

Used for: emergency treatment.

Dosage: see literature.

Special care: porphyria, kidney or liver disorders, severe gastrointestinal, blood or neurological disorders, psoriasis, pregnancy, lactation, history of epilepsy. Regular eye tests before and during treatment.

Side effects: gastrointestinal upset, headache, skin eruptions, loss of pigment, hair loss, blurred vision, damage to retina, blood disorders, allergic reactions, opacities in cornea.

Manufacturer: R.P.R.

Nivemycin
Description: an antibiotic and aminoglycoside, neomycin sulphate, available as 500mg tablets. Also, **Nivemycin Elixir** containing 100mg/5ml.

Used for: preparation before bowel surgery and an added treatment for hepatic coma.

Dosage: 2 tablets per hour for 4 hours, then 2 every 4 hours for 2 to 3 days (pre-operation). Children: over 12 years, 2 tablets; 6 to 12 years, half to 1 tablet; 1 to 5 years, 10–20ml; under 1 year, 2.5–10ml. All taken 4 hourly for 2 to 3 days pre-operatively.

Special care: Parkinson's disease, hepatic coma, kidney disease.

Avoid use: bowel obstruction.

Side effects: gastrointestinal upset.

Manufacturer: Boots.

Nizoral
Description: an imidazole and antifungal, ketoconazole, available as white tablets (200mg) marked JANSSEN and K over 200. Also, **Nizoral Suspension** containing 100mg/5ml.

Used for: systemic fungal infections, prevention of infections in patients with reduced immune response, chronic vaginal thrush and infections of the gastrointestinal tract not responding to other teatment, skin and mucous membrane fungal infections.

Dosage: 200–400mg daily with meals continuing 1 week after symptoms have ceased. For vaginal thrush 400mg once per day for 5 days. Children 3mg/kg daily.

Also, **Nizoral Cream**, 2% ketoconazole.

Used for: candidal vulvitis.

Dosage: apply once or twice per day

Avoid use: liver disease or liver abnormalities, pregnancy, hypersensitivity to other imidazoles.

Possible interaction: antacids, anticoagulants, phenytoin, rifampicin, cyclosporin, astemizole, terfenadine, anticholinergics, H$_2$ antagonists.

Side effects: hypersensitivity, rashes, headache, gastrointestinal disturbances, hepatitis, thrombocytopenia (reduction in blood platelets), rarely breast enlargement.

Nizoral Cream *also used for*: ringworm infections, skin infection, seborrhoeic dermatitis.

Dosage: apply once or twice per day.

Side effects: skin irritation.

Also **Nizoral Shampoo**, 20mg ketoconazole per ml of liquid.

Used for: seborrhoeic dermatitis, dandruff, scaly skin rash (pityriasis).

Dosage: dermatitis, use shampoo twice weekly for 2 to 4 weeks, and once every 1 or 2 weeks for prevention. Pityriasis, shampoo once per day for 5 days; prevention once daily for 3 days maximum.

Side effects: skin irritation.

Manufacturer: Janssen.

Nobrium

Description: a long-acting benzodiazepine and anxiolytic medazepam, available as yellow/orange capsules (5mg) marked with strength and ROCHE.

Used for: treatment of severe or disabling anxiety over the short-term whether it occcurs alone or with insomnia.

Dosage: 15–40mg in divided doses; elderly 5–20mg. Not for children.

Special care: chronic liver or kidney disease, chronic lung disease, pregnancy, labour, lactation, elderly. May impair judgement. Withdraw gradually and avoid prolonged use.

Avoid use: depression of respiration, acute lung disease; psychotic, phobic or obsessional states.

Possible interaction: anticonvulsants, depressants of the CNS, alcohol.

Side effects: ataxia, confusion, light-headedness, drowsiness, hypotension, gastrointestinal upsets, disturbances in vision and libido, skin rashes, retention of urine, vertigo. Sometimes jaundice or blood disorders.

Manufacturer: Roche.

Noctec

Description: a sedative and hypnotic chloral hydrate, available as liquid-filled red capsules containing 500mg.

Used for: insomnia.

Dosage: 500mg–1g with water 15 to 30 minutes before bedtime. Daily maximum, 2g. Not for children.

Special care: porphyria, lactation, impaired judgement and dexterity.

Avoid use: gastritis, pregnancy, severe liver, heart or kidney disease.

Possible interaction: anticoagulants, CNS depressants, alcohol.

Side effects: headache, skin allergies, ketonuria, excitement, delirium.

Manufacturer: Squibb.

Nods Tropicamide

Description: an anticholinergic, tropicamide (125µg), available as sterile ophthalmic applicator strips.

Used for: a short-acting dilator of the pupil and paralyser of the ciliary muscle of the eye.

Dosage: 1 unit in lower conjunctival sac, repeating after 30–45 minutes if required.

Special care: if driving or operating machinery.

Avoid use: narrow angle glaucoma.

Manufacturer: Chauvin.

Nolvadex-D

Description: an antioestrogen and infertility drug, tamoxifen citrate, available as white octagonal tablets (20mg) marked NOVADEX-D and ICI. Also, **Nolvadex FORTE**, as white elongated octagonal tablets (40mg) marked NOLVADEX FORTE and ICI. Also, **Nolvadex**, 10mg white tablets marked NOLVADEX and ICI.

Used for: infertility.

Dosage: 20mg per day on 4 consecutive days starting on second day of menstruation, increasing to 40mg and 80mg for later courses, if necessary.

Avoid use: pregnancy.

Possible interaction: warfarin.

Side effects: vaginal bleeding, hot flushes, dizziness, gastrointestinal upset. Stop if there are disturbances to vision.

Manufacturer: Zeneca.

Nootropil

Description: a GABA analogue, piracetam, available as white, oblong tablets (800 and 1200mg strengths) marked N. Also, **Nootropil Solution**, containing 333mg/ml.

Used for: additional treatment for cortical myoclonus (sudden muscular spasms).

Dosage: 7.2g per day initially, increasing by 4.8g daily at 3 or 4 day intervals to a maximum of 20g per day in 2 or 3 divided doses. Not for children under 16 years.

Special care: kidney disease, elderly. Withdraw gradually.

Avoid use: severe kidney dysfunction, liver disease, pregnancy, breast-feeding.

Possible interaction: thyroid hormones.

Side effects: insomnia, nervousness, weight gain, depression, diarrhoea, rash, hyperactivity.

Manufacturer: UCB.

Norcuron

Description: a muscle relaxant, vercuronium bromide (10mg) as powder in vials with water for injections.

Used for: short to medium duration muscle relaxant.

Dosage: 80–100µg/kg by intravenous injection and 20–30µg/kg for maintenance. Infants over 5 months as for adult; up to 4 months 10–20µg/kg then increase gradually to obtain response. 50–80µg/kg/ hour by intravenous infusion after initial injection of 40–100µg/kg.

Special care: respiration should be assisted, reduce dose in kidney disease.

Possible interaction: some cholinergics, nifedipine, verapamil.

Manufacturer: Organon-Teknika.

Norditropin

Description: a growth hormone, somatropin, available as a powder in a vial (12 units) plus diluent.

Used for: failure of growth in children due to growth hormone deficiency, Turner's syndrome.

Dosage: 0.07–0.1 units/kg body weight 6 to 7 times per week by subcutaneous injection (growth failure). For Turner's syndrome, 0.1 units/kg.

Also, **Norditropin Penset**, 12 and 24 units somatropin as powder in vials with 2ml of solvent.

Dosage: as above.

Special care: diabetes, deficiency of ACTH (adrenocorticotrophic hormones), intrancranial lesion. Check thyroid function.

Avoid use: pregnancy, lactation, tumour, closure of epiphyses.

Side effects: oedema, hypothyroidism, pain at injection site.

Special care: chronic liver or kidney disease, chronic lung disease, pregnancy, labour, lactation, elderly. May impair judgement. Withdraw gradually and avoid prolonged use.

Avoid use: depression of respiration, acute lung disease; psychotic, phobic or obsessional states.

Possible interaction: anticonvulsants, depressants of the CNS, alcohol.

Side effects: ataxia, confusion, light-headedness,

drowsiness, hypotension, gastrointestinal upsets, disturbances in vision and libido, skin rashes, retention of urine, vertigo. Sometimes jaundice or blood disorders. (Move site of injection to avoid lipoatrophy).

Manufacturer: Novo Nordisk.

Nordox

Description: a tetracycline, doxycycline, available in green capsules (100mg) marked NORDOX 100.

Used for: infections of the respiratory tract including bronchitis and sinusitis. Acne. Infections of the genito-urinary tract.

Dosage: 200mg on the first day, then 100mg per day with food or drink. Not for children.

Special care: liver disease.

Avoid use: pregnancy, breast-feeding.

Possible interaction: mineral supplements, antacids.

Side effects: allergic reactions, gastrointestinal upset, superinfections. Stop if there is intracranial hypertension.

Manufacturer: Panpharma.

Norflex

Description: an anticholinergic, orphenadrine citrate, available in ampoules (30mg/ml).

Used for: musculoskeletal pain.

Dosage: 60mg by intramuscular or slow intravenous injection, repeated every 12 hours if required. Not for children.

Special care: pregnancy, tachycardia.

Avoid use: glaucoma, lactation, myasthenia gravis, urine retention.

Side effects: nausea, blurred vision, dizziness, dry mouth, confusion, tremor.

Manufacturer: 3M Health Care.

Norgeston

Description: a progestogen-only contraceptive, levonorgestrel, available in white tablets (30µg).

Used for: oral contraception.

Dosage: 1 at the same time each day without a break, starting on the first day of the cycle.

Special care: hypertension, thromboembolic disorders, liver disease, hormone-dependent cancer, ovarian cysts, migraine. Regular checks on blood pressure, breasts and pelvic organs.

Avoid use: previous severe arterial or heart disease, benign liver tumours, undiagnosed vaginal bleeding, pregnancy, past ectopic pregnancy. Discontinue immediately for pregnancy, jaundice, thrombophlebitis or thromboembolism.

Possible interaction: griseofulvin, rifampicin, meprobamate, chloral hydrate, carbamazepine,

primidone, barbiturates, phenytoin, dichloralphenazone, ethosuximide, glutethimide.
Side effects: acne, breast discomfort, headache, ovarian cysts, irregular menstrual bleeding.
Manufacturer: Schering H.C.

Noriday

Description: a progestogen-only contraceptive, norethisterone, available as white tablets (350µg) marked NORIDAY and SYNTEX.
Used for: oral contraception.
Dosage: 1 at the same time each day without a break, starting on the first day of the cycle.
Special care: hypertension, thromboembolic disorders, liver disease, hormone-dependent cancer, ovarian cysts, migraine. Regular checks on blood pressure, breasts and pelvic organs.
Avoid use: previous severe arterial or heart disease, benign liver tumours, undiagnosed vaginal bleeding, pregnancy, past ectopic pregnancy. Discontinue immediately for pregnancy, jaundice, thrombophlebitis or thromboembolism.
Possible interaction: griseofulvin, rifampicin, meprobamate, chloral hydrate, carbamazepine, primidone, barbiturates, phenytoin, dichloralphenazone, ethosuximide, glutethimide.
Side effects: acne, breast discomfort, headache, ovarian cysts, irregular menstrual bleeding.
Manufacturer: Schering H.C.

Norimin

Description: a combined oestrogen/progestogen contraceptive containing 35µg ethinyloestradiol and 1mg norethisterone in a peach tablet marked C over 135.
Used for: oral contraception.
Dosage: 1 per day for 21 days, starting on the fifth day of menstruation, then 7 days without tablets.
Special care: hypertension, Raynaud's disease (reduced blood supply to an organ of the body's extremities), asthma, severe depression, diabetes, varicose veins, multiple sclerosis, chronic kidney disease, kidney dialysis. Blood pressure, breasts and pelvic organs to be checked regularly; smoking not advised.
Avoid use: history of heart disease, infectious hepatitis, sickle cell anaemia, porphyria, liver tumour, undiagnosed vaginal bleeding, pregnancy, hormone-dependent cancer, haemolytic uraemic syndrome (rare kidney disorder), chorea, otosclerosis.
Possible interaction: barbiturates, tetracyclines, griseofulvin, rifampicin, primidone, phenytoin, chloral hydrate, ethosuximide, carbamazepine,

glutethimide, dichloralphenazone.
Side effects: fluid retention and bloating, leg cramps/pains, breast enlargement, depression, headaches, nausea, loss of libido, weight gain, vaginal discharge, cervical erosion (alteration of epithelial cells), chloasma (pigmentation of nose, cheeks or forehead), breakthrough bleeding (bleeding between periods).
Manufacturer: Syntex.

Norinyl-1

Description: a combined oestrogen/progestogen contraceptive containing 50µg mestranol and 1mg norethisterone in a white tablet marked NORINYL and SYNTEX.
Used for: oral contraception.
Special care: hypertension, Raynaud's disease (reduced blood supply to an organ of the body's extremities), asthma, severe depression, diabetes, varicose veins, multiple sclerosis, chronic kidney disease, kidney dialysis. Blood pressure, breasts and pelvic organs to be checked regularly; smoking not advised.
Avoid use: history of heart disease, infectious hepatitis, sickle cell anaemia, porphyria, liver tumour, undiagnosed vaginal bleeding, pregnancy, hormone-dependent cancer, haemolytic uraemic syndrome (rare kidney disorder), chorea, otosclerosis.
Possible interaction: barbiturates, tetracyclines, griseofulvin, rifampicin, primidone, phenytoin, chloral hydrate, ethosuximide, carbamazepine, glutethimide, dichloralphenazone.
Side effects: fluid retention and bloating, leg cramps/pains, breast enlargement, depression, headaches, nausea, loss of libido, weight gain, vaginal discharge, cervical erosion (alteration of epithelial cells), chloasma (pigmentation of nose, cheeks or forehead), breakthrough bleeding (bleeding between periods).
Manufacturer: Syntex.

Noristerat

Description: a depot progestogen contraceptive, norethisterone oenanthate, available as an oily solution in ampoules containing 200mg/ml.
Used for: short-term highly effective contraception irrespective of errors by patient.
Dosage: 200mg by deep intramuscular injection (in gluteal muscle) administered within the first 5 days of the cycle. May be repeated once after 8 weeks.
Special care: liver disorder or diseases that are likely to worsen in pregnancy, severe depression.
Avoid use: acute and severe chronic liver disease,

pregnancy, history of thrombo-embolism, history during pregnancy of itching, idiopathic jaundice or pemphigoid gestationis (skin disorder with large blisters).

Side effects: weight changes, breast discomfort, headache, dizziness, nausea, menstrual changes.

Manufacturer: Schering H.C.

Normax

Description: a laxative and faecal softener containing danthron (50mg) and docusate sodium (60mg) in brown capsules marked NORMAX.

Used for: constipation in the elderly, for those with heart failure, coronary thrombosis and constipation induced by analgesics.

Dosage: 1 to 3 tablets at night. Children over 6 years, 1 at night. Not for children under 6 years.

Special care: lactation.

Avoid use: obstruction of the bowel.

Manufacturer: Evans.

Normegon

Description: Human menopausal gonadotrophin.

Used for: female or male infertility due to understimulation of the gonads by gonadotrophin. Superovulation for in-vitro fertilization.

Dosage: by intramuscular injection, but see literature.

Special care: exclude other possible causes including gonad abnormalities. Check oestrogen levels and size of ovaries regularly.

Avoid use: ovarian, pituitary or testicular tumours.

Side effects: risk of multiple pregnancy, miscarriage, rash.

Manufacturer: Organon.

Normison

Description: an intermediate-acting benzo-diazepine, temazepam, available as yellow capsules marked N10 (10mg) and N20 (20mg).

Used for: premedication, short-term treatment of insomnia when sedation during the day is not required.

Dosage: 20–40mg half to 1 hour before surgery (premedication), 10–30mg at bedtime (elderly 10mg), maximum 60mg for severe cases. Not for children.

Special care: chronic liver or kidney disease, chronic lung disease, pregnancy, labour, lactation, elderly. May impair judgement. Withdraw gradually and avoid prolonged use.

Avoid use: depression of respiration, acute lung disease; psychotic, phobic or obsessional states.

Possible interaction: anticonvulsants, depressants of the CNS, alcohol.

Side effects: ataxia, confusion, light-headedness, drowsiness, hypotension, gastrointestinal upsets, disturbances in vision and libido, skin rashes, retention of urine, vertigo. Sometimes jaundice or blood disorders.

Manufacturer: Wyeth.

Noroxin

Description: an anti-infective for the eye and a 4-quinolone, norfloxacin, available as 0.3% drops.

Used for: bacterial infections.

Dosage: 1 or 2 drops 4 times per day.

Special care: pregnancy.

Side effects: localized irritation, bitter taste.

Manufacturer: M.S.D.

Norplant

Description: a progestogen depot contraceptive, levonorgestrel, available as an implant (228mg) beneath the skin.

Used for: long-term contraception that is reversible.

Dosage: subdermal implant, for those aged 18–40, to be removed within 5 years.

Special care: risk of arterial disease, hypertension, benign intracranial hypertension, migraine. Check blood pressure, breasts and pelvic organs before and during treatment.

Avoid use: thromboembolic disorders, heart disease, liver disease, history of severe arterial disease, pregnancy, undiagnosed vaginal bleeding, hormone-dependent cancer, recent cancer of the uterus.

Possible interaction: phenytoin, primidone, rifampicin, griseofulvin, barbiturates, carbamazepine, phenylbutazone, chronic use of tetracyclines.

Side effects: amenorrhoea, ovarian cysts, irregular or extended menstrual bleeding, headache, nausea, weight gain, hirsutism, hair loss, enlargement of related organs.

Manufacturer: Roussel.

Norval

Description: a TCAD, mianserin hydrochloride, available as orange tablets in 10, 20 and 30mg strengths, marked with NORVAL and tablet strength.

Used for: depression.

Dosage: 30–40mg per day as 1 dose at night or in divided doses. Increase after a few days to maintenance levels of 30–90mg per day. Elderly, start no higher than 30mg per day, increase gradually. Not for children.

Special care: elderly, pregnancy, heart block, myocardial infarction, epilepsy, glaucoma, enlarged prostate.

Avoid use: lactation, severe liver disease, mania.

Possible interaction: alcohol, anticoagulants, MAOIs.

Side effects: drowsiness, blood changes. Blood tests advisable monthly for first 3 months. Withdraw if there develops infection, jaundice, convulsions or hypomania.

Manufacturer: Bencard.

Nova-T

Description: an IUD comprising copper wire with a silver core on a plastic T-shaped carrier.

Used for: contraception.

Special care: diabetes, anaemia, history of endocarditis or pelvic inflammatory disease, epilepsy, hypermenorrhoea (or menorrhagia). Examine after 3 months, then annually.

Avoid use: pregnancy, past ectopic pregnancy, uterus disorders, infection of vagina or cervix, acute pelvic inflammatory diseases, cervical cancer, abnormal vaginal bleeding, endometrial disease, immuno-suppressive therapy, copper allergy, cancer of the genitalia.

Possible interaction: anticoagulants.

Side effects: pain, pelvic infection, perforation of the uterus, abnormal bleeding. On insertion there may be attack of asthma or epilepsy, bradycardia. Remove if persistent bleeding or cramps, perforation of cervix or uterus, pregnancy, persistent pelvic infection.

Manufacturer: Schering H.C.

Novagard

Description: an IUD comprising copper wire with a silver core on a plastic T-shaped carrier.

Used for: contraception.

Special care: diabetes, anaemia, history of endocarditis or pelvic inflammatory disease, epilepsy, hypermenorrhoea (or menorrhagia, long or heavy menstrual periods). Examine after 3 months, then annually.

Avoid use: pregnancy, past ectopic pregnancy, uterus disorders, infection of vagina or cervix, acute pelvic inflammatory diseases, cervical cancer, abnormal vaginal bleeding, endometrial disease, immuno-suppressive therapy, copper allergy, cancer of the genitalia.

Possible interaction: anticoagulants.

Side effects: pain, pelvic infection, perforation of the uterus, abnormal bleeding. *On insertion* there may be attack of asthma or epilepsy, bradycardia. Remove if persistent bleeding or cramps, perforation of cervix or uterus, pregnancy, persistent pelvic infection.

Manufacturer: Kabi Pharmacia

Novantrone

Description: a cytotoxic antibiotic, mitozantrone hydrochloride, available as a solution in vials (2mg/ml).

Used for: treatment of tumours (leukaemia, lymphoma, breast cancer, and solid tumours).

Dosage: by intravenous infusion, see literature.

Special care: check heart after total dose of 160mg/m^2 to avoid dose-related cardiotoxicity.

Side effects: suppression of bone marrow, see literature.

Manufacturer: Lederle.

Noxyflex

Description: a combined antibacterial and antifungal compound, noxythiolin, available as powder (2.5g) in vials.

Used for: solution to be instilled into bladder or other body cavities.

Dosage: see literature.

Special care: the solution must be freshly prepared and used within 7 days.

Manufacturer: Geistlich.

Nozinan

Description: a group I phenothiazine and antipsychotic, methotrimeprazine, available as white tablets (25mg) marked NOZINAN 25.

Used for: schizophrenia, mental disorders where sedation is needed, control of terminal pain and accompanying vomiting or distress.

Dosage: mental disorders, 25–50mg per day for patients who can walk about, 100–200mg for those who cannot. For pain, 12.5–50mg every 4 to 8 hours. Not for children.

Also, **Nozinan Injection**, 2.5% isotonic solution in ampoules.

Dosage: for pain, 12.5–25mg by intramuscular injection or, after dilution, by intravenous injection, every 6 to 8 hours, up to 50mg for severe cases. Or 25–200mg per day diluted with saline, by continuous subcutaneous infusion. Not for children.

Special care: liver disease, Parkinson's disease, epilepsy, cardiovascular disease, pregnancy, lactation.

Avoid use: bone marrow depression (unless terminal), coma.

Possible interaction: alcohol, depressants of the CNS, antihypertensives, antidepressants, analgesics, antidiabetics, levodopa, anticonvulsants.

Side effects: rigidity, tremor, dry mouth, muscle spasms in eye, neck, face and back, tardive dyskinesia (involuntary, repetitive muscle movements in the limbs, face and trunk),

tachycardia, constipation, blocked nose, difficulty in urinating, hypotension, weight gain, impotence, galactorrhoea, gynaecomastia, blood changes, jaundice, dermatitis, ECG changes, fatigue, drowsiness, seizures.
Manufacturer: R.P.R.

Nubain
Description: an analgesic and opiate, nalbuphine hydrochloride, available as 10mg/ml in ampoules.
Used for: moderate to severe pain. Pain associated with suspected myocardial infarction, pre and postoperative pain.
Dosage: pain, 10–20mg by intravenous, intramuscular or subcutaneous injection. Myocardial infarction, 10–30mg by slow intravenous injection, followed within 30 minutes by 20mg if necessary. Children, starting with up to 0.3mg/kg by intravenous, intramuscular or subcutaneous injection, repeated up to twice if required.
Special care: liver or kidney disease, head injury, pregnancy, labour, respiratory depression, history of opioid abuse.
Possible interaction: depressants of the CNS.
Side effects: sweating, dizziness, dry mouth, nausea, sedation.
Manufacturer: DuPont.

Nuelin SA
Description: a xanthine and bronchodilator, theophylline, available as white sustained-release tablets (175mg) marked NLS175 and 3M.
Used for: bronchitis, emphysema, narrowing of airways in asthma.
Dosage: 1 to 2 tablets twice per day after food. Children over 6 years, 1 tablet twice per day. Not for children under 6.
Also, **Nuelin SA-250**, containing 250mg and marked NLS 250 and 3M.
Dosage: 1 to 2 tablets twice per day after food. Children over 6 years, half the adult dose. Not recommended for children under 6.
Also, **Nuelin** containing 125mg, marked NL over 125 and 3M.
Dosage: 1 to 2 tablets, 3 or 4 times per day, after food. Children aged 7 to 12, half the adult dose. Not for children under 7 years.
Also, **Nuelin Liquid**, containing 60mg theophylline hydrate (as sodium glycinate) per 5ml.
Dosage: 10–20ml 3 or 4 times per day after food. Children aged 7 to 12, 10ml; aged 2 to 6, 5ml 3 or 4 times per day after food. Not for children under 2 years.

Special care: pregnancy, breast-feeding, heart or liver disease, peptic ulcer.
Possible interaction: B$_2$-agonists, steroids, interferon, erythromycin, diuretics, ciprafloxacin, cimetidine.
Side effects: nausea, gastrointestinal upset, headache, tachycardia, arrhythmias, insomnia.
Manufacturer: 3M Health Care.

Nuvelle
Description: an oestrogen/progestogen compound available as 16 white tablets containing 2mg oestradiol valerate and 12 pink tablets containing in addition 75µg levonorgestrel.
Used for: post-menopausal osteoporosis, hormone replacement therapy for climacteric syndrome (symptoms associated with the menopause).
Dosage: 1 white tablet per day for 16 days then 12 days of taking 1 pink tablet. Start on fifth day of menses (discharge).
Special care: those at risk of thrombosis or with liver disease. Women with any of the following disorders should be monitored: fibroids in the womb, multiple sclerosis, diabetes, tetany, porphyria, epilepsy, liver disease, hypertension, migraine, otosclerosis, gallstones. Breasts, pelvic organs and blood pressure should be checked at regular intervals during course of treatment.
Avoid use: pregnant women, breast-feeding mothers, women with conditions which might lead to thrombosis, thrombophlebitis, serious heart, kidney or liver disease, breast cancer, oestrogen-dependent cancers including those of reproductive system, endometriosis, vaginal bleeding which is undiagnosed.
Possible interaction: drugs which induce liver enzymes.
Side effects: tenderness and enlargement of breasts, weight gain, breakthrough bleeding, giddiness, vomiting and nausea, gastrointestinal upset. Treatment should be halted immediately if severe headaches occur, disturbance of vision, hypertension or any indications of thrombosis, jaundice. Also, in the event of pregnancy and 6 weeks before planned surgery.
Manufacturer: Schering H.C.

Nycopren
Description: a propionic acid and NSAID, naproxen, available as white, oblong tablets (250 or 500mg strength).
Used for: osteoarthrosis, rheumatoid arthritis, acute gout, ankylosing spondylitis, inflammatory musculoskeletal disorders, juvenile rheumatoid arthritis (JRA).

Dosage: 250–500mg twice per day. Gout, start with 750mg followed by 250mg 8-hourly. Musculoskeletal, 500mg then 250mg 8-hourly. For JRA, over 50kg, 250–500mg twice per day, not recommended for under 50kg.

Special care: elderly, kidney or liver disease, heart failure, history of gastrointestinal lesions, pregnancy, asthma. Check kidney and liver for long-term treatment.

Avoid use: lactation, allergy to aspirin or anti-inflammatory drugs, active peptic ulcer.

Possible interaction: sulphonamides, sulphonylureas, anticoagulants, quinolones, ß-blockers, lithium, hydantoins, frusemide, methotrexate, probenecid.

Side effects: headache, vertigo, blood changes, tinnitus, rash, gastrointestinal intolerance.

Manufacturer: Nycomed.

Nystadermal

Description: an antibacterial and potent steroid, nystatin (100,000 units/g) and triamcinolone acetonide (0.1%) available as a cream.

Used for: pruritus and eczema, skin infection and inflammation.

Dosage: apply 2 to 4 times per day.

Special care: thrombophlebitis, psychoses, recent intestinal anastomoses, chronic nephritis, certain cancers, osteoporosis, peptic ulcer, skin eruption/rash related to a disease, viral, fungal or active infections, tuberculosis. Hypertension, glaucoma, epilepsy, acute glomerulonephritis (inflammation of kidney glomerulus), diabetes, cirrhosis, hypothyroidism, pregnancy, stress. To be withdrawn gradually.

Possible interaction: NSAIDs, oral anticoagulants, phenytoin, ephedrine, phenobarbitone, rifampicin, diuretics, cardiac glycosides, anticholinesterases, hypoglycaemics.

Side effects: osteoporosis, depression, euphoria, hyperglycaemia, peptic ulcers, Cushingoid changes.

Manufacturer: Squibb.

Nystaform

Description: an antifungal and antibacterial cream containing 100,000 units of nystatin per gram and 1% chlorhexidine.

Used for: skin infections.

Dosage: apply liberally 2 to 3 times per day until 1 week after healing.

Manufacturer: Bayer.

Nystaform-HC

Description: an antifungal and mildly potent steroid containing 100,000 units of nystatin per gram, 1% chlorhexidine, and 0.5% hydrocortisone available as a cream. Also, **Nystaform-HC Ointment** containing 100,000 units of nystatin, 1% chlorhexidine and 1% hydrocortisone.

Used for: skin disorders where there is infection.

Dosage: apply 2 or 3 times per day until 1 week after healing.

Special care: thrombophlebitis, psychoses, recent intestinal anastomoses, chronic nephritis, certain cancers, osteoporosis, peptic ulcer, skin eruption/rash related to a disease, viral, fungal or active infections, tuberculosis. Hypertension, glaucoma, epilepsy, acute glomerulonephritis (inflammation of kidney glomerulus), diabetes, cirrhosis, hypothyroidism, pregnancy, stress. To be withdrawn gradually.

Possible interaction: NSAIDs, oral anticoagulants, phenytoin, ephedrine, phenobarbitone, rifampicin, diuretics, anticholinesterases, cardiac glycosides, hypoglycaemics.

Side effects: osteoporosis, depression, euphoria, hyperglycaemia, peptic ulcers, Cushingoid changes.

Manufacturer: Bayer.

Nystan

Description: an antibiotic containing 500,000 units of nystatin, available as brown tablets.

Used for: intestinal infection with *Candida*.

Dosage: 1 to 2 tablets 4 times per day. Children should take the suspension.

Also, **Nystan Oral Suspension** containing 100,000 units nystatin/ml in a ready-mixed suspension. Also, **Nystan Forte Suspension** which in addition is free of lactose, sugar and corn starch.

Used for: infections (candidiasis) of the mouth, oesophagus and intestines.

Dosage: 1ml 4 times per day for oral infections, 5ml 4 times per day for infection of the intestines. Children, 1ml 4 times per day. Prevention in infants under 1 month, 1ml per day. For oral infections the suspension should be retained in the mouth. Continue for 2 days after cure. Also, **Nystan Pastilles** containing 100,000 units nystatin per pastille.

Used for: oral infections.

Dosage: 1 pastille sucked slowly 4 times per day for 7 to 14 days.

Side effects: nausea, vomiting and diarrhoea with high doses.

Also, **Nystan** as 100,000 units of nystatin in yellow, diamond-shaped pessaries, marked SQUIBB 457; **Nystan Vaginal Cream** (100,000 units/4g); **Nystan Gel** (100,000 units/g); and **Nystan Oral Tablets** (500,000 units in brown tablets).

Used for: candidal vaginitis (vaginal infection caused by *Candida*, thrush).

Dosage: 1 to 2 pessaries or 1 to 2 applications of cream for 14 or more consecutive nights; irrespective of menstruation. Gel; applied topically to anogenital region 2 to 4 times per day for 14 days. Oral treatment, 1 tablet 4 times per day during vaginal treatment. Children use vaginal cream with oral treatment.

Side effects: temporary burning and irritation.

Also **Nystan** as cream, ointment and gel (100,000 units nystatin per gram).

Used for: thrush of the skin and mucous membranes.

Dosage: apply 2 to 4 times per day.

Manufacturer: Squibb.

O

Ocufen

Description: an NSAID which is a proprionic acid available in the form of eyedrops containing 0.03% flubiprofen sodium.

Used for: to inhibit inflammation and constriction of the pupil (miosis) during operations of the eye.

Dosage: as directed by physician.

Manufacturer: Allergan.

Ocusert Pilo

Description: a cholinergic eye preparation containing pilocarpine hydrochloride and available as elliptical-shaped, sustained-release plastic inserts, each delivering 40 micrograms/hour for a 1 week period.

Used for: glaucoma.

Dosage: place 1 insert under eyelid and replace each week.

Avoid use: patients with severe inflammation or infecion. Not for children.

Side effects: eye irritation, loss of sharpness of vision.

Manufacturer: Cusi.

Odrik

Description: an ACE inhibitor available as capsules of 3 strengths all containing trandolapril. Yellow/red capsules contain 0.5mg; orange/red contain 1mg; red/red contain 2mg.

Used for: hypertension.

Dosage: 0.5mg once each day at first increasing every 2 to 4 weeks to a maximum 4mg as a single daily dose. Maintenance dose is in the order of 1–2mg once each day. Any diuretics being taken should be discontinued 2 or 3 days before treatment starts.

Special care: liver or kidney disease, receiving kidney dialysis, undergoing anaesthesia or surgery, congestive heart failure. Also, patients with low fluid and salt levels.

Avoid use: pregnancy, breast-feeding, obstruction of blood outflow from heart or aortic stenosis (narrowing of aorta). Also, angioneurotic oedema due to previous treatment with an ACE inhibitor.

Possible interaction: NSAIDs, potassium-sparing diuretics.

Side effects: rash, cough, muscular weakness, headache, dizziness, palpitations, hypotension. Rarely, agranulocytosis (a blood disorder characterized by abnormal reduction in number of white blood cells (granulocytes), angioneurotic oedema, depression of bone marrow.

Manufacturer: Roussel.

Olbetam

Description: a lipid-lowering nicotinic acid derivative available as pink/red-brown capsules containing 250mg acipimox marked with name.

Used for: raised protein-bound lipid levels in blood (hyperlipoproteinaemia) of type IIa, IIb and IV.

Dosage: adults, 2 or 3 tablets each day taken as divided doses with meals. Maximum dosage is 1200mg each day.

Avoid use: pregnancy, breast-feeding, children, patients with peptic ulcer.

Side effects: gastrointestinal upset, flushing, headache, inflammation of skin and mucous membranes (erythema), malaise, skin rash.

Manufacturer: Pharmacia.

Omnopon^{CD}

Description: an analgesic, opiate available as a solution in ampoules for injection containing 15.4mg papaveretum/ml.

Used for: severe pain.

Dosage: adults, 0.5–1ml given by subcutaneous, intravenous or intramuscular injection. Dose may be repeated after 4 hours. Children, under 1 year, 0.0075–0.01ml/kg body weight each day. Over 1 year, 0.01–0.015ml/kg. All given by subcutaneous, intravenous or intramuscular injection as a maximum single dose. Elderly, 0.5ml at first by same route.

Special care: pregnancy, breast-feeding, elderly persons, newborn babies, patients with enlarged prostate gland, underactive thyroid gland, serious liver or kidney disease, having head injury.

Possible interaction: alcohol, phenothiazines, MAOIs, CNS depressants.

Side effects: drug dependence and tolerance, constipation, nausea, constipation.
Manufacturer: Roche.

Oncovin

Description: a cytotoxic vinca alkaloid drug produced as a solution in vials for injection containing 1mg vincristine sulphate/ml.
Used for: lymphomas, leukaemia, some solid tumours (e.g. lung and breast cancer).
Dosage: by intravenous injection as directed by physician skilled in cancer chemotherapy.
Special care: care in handling, contact with eyes must be avoided, tissue irritant.
Avoid use: must not be given by intraethecal injection (i.e. into meninges (membrane linings) of the spinal cord).
Side effects: damage to peripheral and autonomic nervous system characterized by muscle weakness and abdominal bloating. Hair loss, vomiting, nausea.
Manufacturer: Lilly.

One-Alpha

Description: a vitamin D analogue, alfacalcidol, available as capsules in 2 strengths; white capsules contain 0.25µg and brown capsules contain 1µg. **Alpha Solution** containing 0.2µg/ml and also **One-Alpha Injection** in ampoules containing 2µg/ml.
Used for: bone disorders due to kidney disease or loss of function, bone disease associated with under or overactivity of parathyroid glands, low calcium levels in newborn babies. Also, rickets and osteomalacia (bone softening).
Dosage: 1µg at first adjusted according to response; children, under 20kg, 0.05µg/kg body weight each day at first; over 20kg, 1µg daily. Injection is given intravenously.
Special care: pregnancy, breast-feeding, kidney failure. Levels of blood calcium must be checked at regular intervals during the course of treatment.
Possible interaction: thiazide diuretics, colestipol, digitalis, barbiturates, antacids, cholestyramine, anticonvulsants, sucralfate, danazol, mineral oils, antacids.
Manufacturer: Leo.

Operidine[CD]

Description: a narcotic analgesic which is a controlled drug available as a solution in ampoules for injection containing 1mg phenoperidine hydrochloride/ml.
Used for: enhancement of anaesthetics and analgesia during surgery; as a depressant of respiration (especially doses above 1mg) in patients receiving long-term assisted ventilation.
Dosage: up to 1mg by intravenous injection then 500 µg every 40 to 60 minutes as needed. With assisted ventilation, 2–5mg then 1mg as needed. Children, 30–50µg/kg body weight. With assisted ventilation, 100–150µg/kg. Elderly persons receive lower doses.
Special care: myasthenia gravis, serious respiratory or liver disease, underactive thyroid. If used in obstetrics, may cause depression of respiration in baby.
Avoid use: obstructive airways disease or depression of respiration (unless being mechanically ventilated).
Possible interaction: MAOIs, cimetidine.
Side effects: convulsions with high doses, respiratory depression, nausea, vomiting, bradycardia, hypotension which is short-lived.
Manufacturer: Janssen.

Opthaine

Description: local anaesthetic eyedrops containing 0.5% proxymetacaine hydrochloride.
Used for: as local anaesthetic during ophthalmic procedures.
Dosage: usual dose, 1 or 2 drops before procedure begins. Protect eye.
Side effects: irritation of eye and, rarely, hypersensitive allergic reactions.
Manufacturer: Squibb.

Opilon

Description: a selective alpha₁-blocker available as film-coated, pale yellow tablets containing 40mg thymoxamine as hydrochloride.
Used for: short-term treatment of Raynaud's disease (a disease affecting the arteries of the fingers which makes them liable to spasm when the hands are cold).
Dosage: 1 tablet 4 times each day increasing to 2 tablets 4 times each day if condition does not respond. If no significant improvement after 2 weeks, drug should be withdrawn.
Special care: angina, recent heart attack, diabetes.
Avoid use: pregnancy, breast-feeding, known hypersensitivity to thymoxamine.
Possible interaction: diarrhoea, nausea, headache, vertigo. Drug should be withdrawn if liver function is affected.
Manufacturer: Parke-Davis.

Opticrom

Description: an NSAID preparation available in the form of eyedrops containing 2% sodium cromoglycate. Also, **Opticrom Eye Ointment** containing 4% sodium cromoglycate.

Used for: allergic conjunctivitis.

Dosage: 1 or 2 drops in both eyes 4 times each day, or ointment 3 times daily.

Avoid use: drops, patients wearing soft contact lenses; ointment, all types of contact lenses.

Side effects: burning, stinging sensation in eye which is of short-lived duration.

Manufacturer: Fisons.

Oramorph

Description: an analgesic opiate preparation available in a variety of different forms, all containing morphine sulphate. **Oramorph SR** are sustained-release, film-coated tablets of different strengths: 10mg buff tablets; 30mg purple tablets; 60mg orange tablets; 100mg grey tablets. All are marked with strength. **Oramorph Solution** contains 10mg morphine sulphate/5ml in a sugar-containing solution. **Oramorph Unit Dose** is a sugar-free solution in single dose vials containing 10mg, 30mg or 100mg morphine sulphate/5ml. **Oramorph Concentrate** is a sugar-free solution containing 100mg morphine sulphate/5ml.

Used for: severe pain.

Dosage: Oramorph SR, 10–20mg every 12 hours at first, increasing as needed. Other preparations, 10–20mg at 4 hourly intervals. Children, all preparations except Oramorph SR, age 1 to 5 years, up to 5mg; 6 to 12 years, 5–10mg, both every 4 hours.

Special care: elderly, breast-feeding, underactivity of thyroid gland, reduced function of adrenal glands, enlarged prostate gland, liver or kidney disease, shock, after surgery.

Avoid use: pregnancy, children under 1 year, obstructive airways disease, disorders characterized by convulsions, depressed respiration, head injuries, coma, severe liver disease, severe alcoholism, raised intracranial pressure.

Possible interaction: central nervous system depressants, MAOIs.

Side effects: vomiting and nausea, constipation, sedation, drug dependence and tolerance.

Manufacturer: Boehringer Ingelheim.

Orap

Description: an antipsychotic drug, pimozide, which is a diphenylbutylpiperidine available as tablets in 3 strengths: scored, white tablets contain 2mg, marked on 1 side with O/2; scored green tablets contain 4mg, marked on 1 side with O/4. Scored, white tablets contain 10mg, marked 1 side with O/10. On the other side all are marked

JANSSEN.

Used for: schizophrenia.

Dosage: adults, 10mg each day at first increasing by 2–4mg daily at weekly intervals. Maximum daily dose is 20mg. To prevent a relapse, 2mg each day. Usual daily dose is in the order of 2–20mg.

Special care: pregnancy, imbalance in electrolyte (salts) levels, liver or kidney disorder, epilepsy, Parkinson's disease, endogenous depression (resulting from factors within the body). ECG should be carried out before and during the course of treatment. Patients require careful monitoring.

Avoid use: children, breast-feeding, patients with a very long QT interval (part of the ECG) which can result in a potentially fatal type of tachycardia, history of heart arrhythmias.

Possible interaction: analgesics, levodopa, CNS depressants, antidiabetic drugs, alcohol, antidepressants, antihypertensives, anticonvulsants, some heart drugs and antipsychotics.

Side effects: extrapyramidal effects (characterized by involuntary and reflex muscle movements), apathy, sleepiness, disturbance of sleep, depression. Blocked nose, dry mouth, constipation, blurring of vision, tachycardia, heart arrhythmias, hypotension, changes in EEG and ECG. Changes in breasts and menstrual cycle, weight gain, impotence. Blood and liver changes, jaundice, rash, pigmentation of skin and eyes, sensitivity to light, haemolytic anaemia, difficulty in urination.

Manufacturer: Janssen.

Orbenin

Description: an antibiotic penicillin which is penicillinase-resistant (i.e. resistant to the penicillinase enzymes produced by certain bacteria). Available as orange/black capsules containing 250mg or 500mg cloxacillin (as sodium salt) and marked with strength and name. Also **Orbenin Injection**, available in vials containing 250mg and 500mg cloxacillin.

Used for: infections caused by Gram-positive bacteria including resistant staphylococci.

Dosage: tablets, 500mg every 6 hours taken half an hour to an hour before meals; injection, 250mg intramuscularly or 500mg intravenously every 4 to 6 hours. Children, over 2 years, half adult dose.

Avoid use: children under 2 years.

Side effects: gastrointestinal upset, allergic responses, rash.

Manufacturer: Forley.

Orelox

Description: a cephalosporin antibiotic available as

505

film-coated white tablets containing 100mg cefpodoxime (as proxetil) marked 208A.
Used for: bronchitis, tonsilitis, pharyngitis, pneumonia, sinusitis.
Dosage: adults, 1 or 2 tablets (depending upon infection) twice each day taken with a meal in the morning and evening.
Special care: pregnancy, sensitivity to beta-lactam antibiotics, kidney disorders.
Avoid use: children.
Possible interaction: H$_2$ antagonists, antacids.
Side effects: headache, gastrointestinal upset, allergic responses, raised liver enzymes, colitis.
Manufacturer: Roussel.

Orgaran

Description: an antithrombotic heparinoid preparation produced as a solution in ampoules for injection, containing 1250 units danaparoid sodium antifactor Xa activity/ml.
Used for: prevention of deep vein thrombosis in patients undergoing surgery.
Dosage: adults, 0.6ml by subcutaneous injection twice each day for 7 to 10 days before operation. The last dose should be given not less than 1 hour before surgery.
Special care: patients with ulcer, liver or kidney disorder, asthma, history of heparin-induced thrombocytopenia who test positive to danaparoid.
Avoid use: pregnancy, breast-feeding, children, bleeding disorders, stroke with haemorrhage, peptic ulcer, serious liver or kidney disease, bacterial endocarditis, serious hypertension, retinopathy (disorder of the blood vessels of the retina of the eye) associated with diabetes.
Side effects: risk of haemorrhage, skin rash, haematoma, bruising. Also, changes in liver enzymes, thrombocytopenia.
Manufacturer: Organon Teknika.

Orimeten

Description: an anti-cancer drug which inhibits steroid synthesis produced in the form of scored, off-white tablets containing 250mg aminoglutethimide marked GG and CG.
Used for: advanced breast cancer in post-menopausal women or those whose ovaries have been removed. Also, advanced prostate cancer and Cushing's syndrome resulting from malignancy.
Dosage: cancer, 1 tablet each day increasing by 1 tablet daily each week. Maximum daily dose is 4 tablets for breast cancer and 3 for prostate cancer. Cushing's syndrome, 1 each day slowly increasing if required to 4 daily in divided doses. Maximum

dose is 8 tablets daily.
Special care: regular monitoring of electrolytes and blood counts is required. Patients with breast or prostate cancer require glucocorticoids (adrenal gland hormones) and these may also be needed by those with Cushing's syndrome. Also, mineralo-corticoids (adrenal gland hormones) may be needed.
Avoid use: pregnancy, breast-feeding.
Possible interaction: synthetic glucocorticoids, anticoagulants, hypoglycaemics taken orally.
Side effects: gastrointestinal upset, blood changes, effects on CNS, rash, thyroid disorders. If allergic alveolitis (inflammation of the air sacs, alveoli, of the lungs) occurs, the drug should be withdrawn.
Manufacturer: Ciba.

Ortho Dionestrol

Description: an hormonal oestrogen preparation available in the form of a vaginal cream with applicator containing 0.01% dienoestrol.
Used for: inflammaion and irritation of the vagina and vulva, atrophic vaginitis.
Dosage: 1 or 2 applicator doses into the vagina each day for 1 to 2 weeks, then reducing to half the initial dose for a further 1 or 2 weeks. Maintenance is 1 applicator dose 1, 2 or 3 times each week.
Special care: patients considered at risk of thromboembolism, porphyria, multiple sclerosis, epilepsy, fibroids in the womb, migraine, tetany. Also, patients with otosclerosis, gallstones, liver disease. Pelvic organs, breasts and blood pressure should be checked regularly during treatment.
Avoid use: pregnancy, breast-feeding, breast or other cancer of reproductive tract or one which is hormone-dependent. Also, thromboembolism-type disorders, undiagnosed vaginal bleeding or endometriosis, thrombophlebitis, heart, liver or kidney disease. Rotor or Dublin-Johnson syndrome.
Possible interaction: drugs which induce liver enzymes.
Side effects: enlargement and soreness of breasts, gastrointestinal upset, dizziness, breakthrough bleeding, headache, vomiting and nausea, weight gain.
Manufacturer: Ortho.

Ortho-Gynest

Description: an hormonal oestrogen preparation available as vaginal pessaries containing 0.5mg oestriol. Also, **Ortho-Gynest Cream** containing 0.01% oestriol, with applicator.
Used for: vaginal, vulval and cervical inflammation and disorders in post-menopausal women; atrophic vaginitis.

Dosage: 1 pessary or applicator dose inserted high up into the vagina at night. Maintenance is 1 pessary or applicator dose each week.

Special care: patients considered at risk of thromboembolism, porphyria, multiple sclerosis, epilepsy, fibroids in the womb, migraine, tetany. Also, otosclerosis, gallstones, liver disease. Pelvic organs, breasts and blood pressure should be checked regularly during course of treatment.

Avoid use: pregnancy, breast-feeding, breast or other cancer of reproductive tract or one which is hormone-dependent. Also, patients with thromboembolism-type disorders, undiagnosed vaginal bleeding or endometriosis, thrombophlebitis, heart, liver or kidney disease. Rotor or Dublin-Johnson syndrome.

Possible interaction: drugs which induce liver enzymes.

Side effects: enlargement and soreness of breasts, gastrointestinal upset, dizziness, breakthrough bleeding, headache, vomiting and nausea, weight gain.

Manufacturer: Ortho.

Otho-Navin 1/50

Description: an hormonal combined oestrogen/progestogen preparation available as white tablets containing 50µg mestranol and 1mg norethisterone marked C over 50.

Used for: oral contraception.

Dosage: 1 tablet each day for 21 days starting on the fifth day of period followed by 7 tablet-free days.

Special care: patients with multiple sclerosis, serious kidney disease or kidney dialysis, asthma, Raynaud's disease, abnormally high levels of prolactin in the blood (hyperprolactinaemia), varicose veins, hypertension. Also, patients suffering from severe depression. Thrombosis risk increases with smoking, age and obesity. During the course of treatment, regular checks on blood pressure, pelvic organs and breasts should be carried out.

Avoid use: pregnancy, patients considered to be at risk of thrombosis, suffering from heart disease, pulmonary hypertension, angina, sickle cell anaemia. Also, undiagnosed vaginal bleeding, history of cholestatic jaundice during pregnancy, cancers which are hormone-dependent, infectious hepatitis, liver disorders. Also, porphyria, Dublin-Johnson and Rotor syndrome, otosclerosis, chorea, haemolytic uraemic syndrome, recent trophoblastic disease.

Possible interaction: barbiturates, ethosuximide, glutethimide, rifampicin, phenytoin, tetracyclines, carbamazepine, chloral hydrate, griseofulvin, dichloralphenazone, primidone.

Side effects: weight gain, breast enlargement, pains in legs and cramps, headaches, loss of sexual desire, depression, nausea, breakthrough bleeding, cervical erosion, brownish patches on skin (chloasma), vaginal discharge, oedema and bloatedness.

Manufacturer: Ortho.

Orudis

Description: an NSAID which is a propionic acid available as capsules in 2 strengths both containing ketoprofen. Purple/green capsules and pink capsules contain 50mg and 100mg respectively, both marked with strength and name. Also, **Orudia Suppositories** containing 100mg.

Used for: musculoskeletal disorders, including osteoarthritis, rheumatoid arthritis, joint disorders, ankylosing spondylitis, gout, pain following orthopaedic surgery, dysmenorrhoea (period pain).

Dosage: adults, capsules, 50–100mg twice daily with meals; suppositories, 1 at night with capsules taken during the day, if needed.

Special care: pregnancy, elderly, heart failure, liver or kidney disorders. Patients taking the drug long-term should receive careful monitoring.

Avoid use: children, patients with known allergy to aspirin or NSAID, history of or active stomach ulcer, asthma, serious kidney disease, recent proctitis (inflammation of rectum and anus).

Possible interaction: hydantoins, anticoagulants, sulphonamides, high doses of methotrexate, quinolones.

Side effects: rash, gastrointestinal upset.

Manufacturer: R.P.R.

Oruvail

Description: an NSAID which is a propionic acid available as capsules in 3 strengths all containing ketoprofen. Purple/pink, pink/pink and pink/white capsules contain 100mg, 150mg and 200mg respectively. All are continuous-release and marked with strength and name. Also, **Oruvail Injection** available as a solution in ampoules containing 50mg/ml.

Used for: musculoskeletal disorders including osteoarthritis, rheumatoid arthritis, joint disorders, ankylosing spondylitis, gout, pain following orthopaedic surgery, dysmenorrhoea (period pain).

Dosage: capsules, 100–200mg once each day with meal; injection, 50–100mg every 4 hours by deep intramuscular injection. Maximum dose is 200mg each day for 3 days.

Special care: pregnancy, elderly, liver or kidney disease, heart failure.

Avoid use: children, known allergy to NSAID or aspirin, history of or active stomach ulcer, asthma, serious kidney disease.
Possible interaction: hydantoins, anticoagulants, quinolones, high doses methotrexate, sulphonamides.
Side effects: rash, gastrointestinal upset.
Manufacturer: R.P.R.

Oruvail Gel

Description: an NSAID which is a propionic acid available in the form of a gel containing 2.5% ketoprofen.
Used for: sports injuries, strains, sprains, bruises, etc.
Dosage: adults, 15g each day in 2 to 4 divided doses for up to 1 week; massage affected area after applying gel.
Special care: pregnancy, avoid mucous membranes, eyes and broken skin.
Avoid use: breast-feeding, patients with known allergy to NSAID or aspirin, history of asthma.
Side effects: slight local irritation of skin.
Manufacturer: R.P.R.

Otomize

Description: a combined antibiotic and corticosteroid preparation available in the form of a suspension for use with a pump action spray. The solution contains 0.1% dexamethasone, 2% acetic acid and 3250 units neomycin/ml.
Used for: inflammation of external ear.
Dosage: 1 metered dose 3 times each day continuing for 2 days after condition has cleared.
Special care: pregnant women, patients with perforated ear drum.
Side effects: stinging or burning which is short-lived.
Manufacturer: Stafford-Miller.

Otosporin

Description: a combined antibiotic and corticosteroid preparation available in the form of ear drops containing 10,000 units polymixin B sulphate, 3400 units neomycin sulphate and 1% hydrocortisone.
Used for: inflammation and bacterial infections of outer ear.
Dosage: 3 drops 3 or 4 times each day or insert wick soaked in solution which is kept wet.
Special care: avoid long-term use in infants.
Avoid use: perforated eardrum.
Side effects: superinfection.
Manufacturer: Wellcome.

Ovestin

Description: an hormonal oestrogen preparation available as white tablets containing 1.0mg oestriol coded DG7, ORGANON and with *. Also, **Ovestin Cream** with applicator containing 0.1% oestriol.
Used for: tablets, disorders of genital and urinary tract arising from infections when oestrogen is deficient. Cream, atrophic vaginitis, itching, dryness and atrophy of vulva in elderly women. Treatment of this area before vaginal operations.
Dosage: tablets, 0.5–3mg each day for 4 weeks then 0.5–1mg daily. Cream, 1 applicator dose into vagina each day for 3 weeks with a maintenance dose of 1 applicatorful twice weekly.
Special care: patients considered at risk of thromboembolism, porphyria, multiple sclerosis, epilepsy, fibroids in the womb, migraine, tetany. Also, patients with otosclerosis, gallstones, liver disease. Pelvic organs, breasts and blood pressure should be checked regularly during the course of treatment.
Avoid use: pregnancy, breast-feeding, patients with breast or other cancer of reproductive tract or one which is hormone-dependent. Also, patients with thromboembolism-type disorders, undiagnosed vaginal bleeding or endometriosis, thrombophlebitis, heart, liver or kidney disease. Rotor or Dublin-Johnson syndrome.
Possible interaction: drugs which induce liver enzymes.
Side effects: enlargement and soreness of breasts, gastrointestinal upset, dizziness, breakthrough bleeding, headache, vomiting and nausea, weight gain.
Manufacturer: Organon.

Ovran

Description: an hormonal combined oestrogen/progestogen preparation available as white tablets containing 50µg ethinyloestradiol and 250µg levonorgestrel. Also, **Ovran 30**, white tablets containing 30µg ethinyloestradiol and 250µg levonorgestrel. Both are marked WYETH.
Used for: oral contraception.
Dosage: 1 tablet each day for 21 days starting on first day of period followed by 7 tablet-free days.
Special care: patients with multiple sclerosis, serious kidney disease or kidney dialysis, asthma, Raynaud's disease, abnormally high levels of prolactin in the blood (hyperprolactinaemia), varicose veins, hypertension. Also, patients suffering from severe depression. Thrombosis risk increases with smoking, age and obesity. During the course of treatment, regular checks on blood

pressure, pelvic organs and breasts should be carried out.

Avoid use: pregnancy, patients considered to be at risk of thrombosis, suffering from heart disease, pulmonary hypertension, angina, sickle cell anaemia. Also, undiagnosed vaginal bleeding, history of cholestatic jaundice during pregnancy, cancers which are hormone-dependent, infectious hepatitis, liver disorders. Also, porphyria, Dublin-Johnson and Rotor syndrome, otosclerosis, chorea, haemolytic uraemic syndrome, recent trophoblastic disease.

Possible interaction: barbiturates, ethosuximide, glutethimide, rifampicin, phenytoin, tetracyclines, carbamazepine, chloral hydrate, griseofulvin, dichloralphenazone, primidone.

Side effects: weight gain, breast enlargement, pains in legs and cramps, headaches, loss of sexual desire, depression, nausea, breakthrough bleeding, cervical erosion, brownish patches on skin (chloasma), vaginal discharge, oedema and bloatedness.

Manufacturer: Wyeth.

Ovranette

Description: an hormonal combined oestrogen/progestogen preparation, available as white tablets containing 30µg ethinyloestradiol and 150µg levonorgestrel, marked WYETH and 30.

Used for: oral contraception.

Dosage: 1 tablet each day for 21 days starting on first day of period followed by 7 tablet-free days.

Special care: patients with multiple sclerosis, serious kidney disease or kidney dialysis, asthma, Raynaud's disease, abnormally high levels of prolactin in the blood (hyperprolactinaemia), varicose veins, hypertension. Also, patients suffering from severe depression. Thrombosis risk increases with smoking, age and obesity. During the course of treatment, regular checks on blood pressure, pelvic organs and breasts should be carried out.

Avoid use: pregnancy, patients considered to be at risk of thrombosis, suffering from heart disease, pulmonary hypertension, angina, sickle cell anaemia. Also, undiagnosed vaginal bleeding, history of cholestatic jaundice during pregnancy, cancers which are hormone-dependent, infectious hepatitis, liver disorders. Also, porphyria, Dublin-Johnson and Rotor syndrome, otosclerosis, chorea, haemolytic uraemic syndrome, recent trophoblastic disease.

Possible interaction: barbiturates, ethosuximide, glutethimide, rifampicin, phenytoin, tetracyclines, carbamazepine, chloral hydrate, griseofulvin, dichloralphenazone, primidone.

Side effects: weight gain, breast enlargement, pains in legs and cramps, headaches, loss of sexual desire, depression, nausea, breakthrough bleeding, cervical erosion, brownish patches on skin (chloasma), vaginal discharge, oedema and bloatedness.

Manufacturer: Wyeth.

Ovysmen

Description: an hormonal combined oestrogen/progestogen preparation available as white tablets containing 35µg ethinyloestradiol and 500µg norethisterone marked C over 535.

Used for: oral contraception.

Dosage: 1 tablet each day for 21 days starting on fifth day of period followed by 7 tablet-free days.

Special care: patients with multiple sclerosis, serious kidney disease or kidney dialysis, asthma, Raynaud's disease, abnormally high levels of prolactin in the blood (hyperprolactinaemia), varicose veins, hypertension. Also, patients suffering from severe depression. Thrombosis risk increases with smoking, age and obesity. During the course of treatment, regular checks on blood pressure, pelvic organs and breasts should be carried out.

Avoid use: pregnancy, patients considered to be at risk of thrombosis, suffering from heart disease, pulmonary hypertension, angina, sickle cell anaemia. Also, undiagnosed vaginal bleeding, history of cholestatic jaundice during pregnancy, cancers which are hormone-dependent, infectious hepatitis, liver disorders. Also, porphyria, Dublin-Johnson and Rotor syndrome, otosclerosis, chorea, haemolytic uraemic syndrome, recent trophoblastic disease.

Possible interaction: barbiturates, ethosuximide, glutethimide, rifampicin, phenytoin, tetracyclines, carbamazepine, chloral hydrate, griseofulvin, dichloralphenazone, primidone.

Side effects: weight gain, breast enlargement, pains in legs and cramps, headaches, loss of sexual desire, depression, nausea, breakthrough bleeding, cervical erosion, brownish patches on skin (chloasma), vaginal discharge, oedema and bloatedness.

Manufacturer: Ortho.

Oxazepam

Description: an anxiolytic drug and intermediate-acting benzodiazepine available as tablets in 3 strengths containing 10mg, 15mg and 30mg oxazepam.

Used for: anxiety.

Dosage: 15–30mg 3 or 4 times each day increasing to 60mg 3 times daily if exceptionally severe.

Elderly persons take reduced dose of 10–20mg 3 to 4 times each day.

Special care: chronic liver or kidney disease, chronic lung disease, pregnancy, labour, lactation, elderly. May impair judgement. Withdraw gradually and avoid prolonged use.

Avoid use: depression of respiration, acute lung disease; psychotic, phobic or obsessional states.

Possible interaction: anticonvulsants, depressants of the CNS, alcohol.

Side effects: ataxia, confusion, light-headedness, drowsiness, hypotension, gastrointestinal upsets, disturbances in vision and libido, skin rashes, retention of urine, vertigo. Sometimes jaundice or blood disorders.

Manufacturer: non-proprietary but available from APS, Berk, Cox, Kerfoot, Norton, Wyeth.

Oxivent

Description: an anticholinergic bronchodilator delivering 100µg oxitropium bromide per dose by metered dose inhaler. Also, **Oxivent Autohaler** delivering 100µg oxitropium bromide per dose by breath-actuated metered dose aerosol.

Used for: obstructive lung disease, asthma.

Dosage: adults, 2 puffs 2 or 3 times each day.

Special care: avoid eyes, patients with enlarged prostate gland, glaucoma.

Avoid use: pregnancy, breast-feeding, children, allergy to ipratropium bromide or atropine.

Side effects: dry mouth, nausea, irritation of throat, anticholinergic effects. If cough or wheezing develops, drug should be withdrawn.

Manufacturer: Boehringer Ingelheim.

P

Pabrinex

Description: a combined preparation of vitamins B and C in paired ampoules for both intravenous and intramuscular injection. Pairs of intravenous ampoules contain 250mg thiamine hydrochloride, 4mg riboflavine, 50mg pyridoxine hydrochloride, 160mg nicotinamide, 500mg ascorbic acid and 1g anhydrous dextrose. Pairs of intramuscular ampoules contain the same but without anhydrous dextrose.

Used for: severe deficiencies in vitamin B and C when oral doses cannot be taken or are not adequate.

Dosage: by intravenous injection (over 10 minutes) or infusion, 2 to 4 pairs of ampoules every 4 to 8 hours for up to 2 days. Then 1 pair of intramuscular ampoules by intramuscular injection or 1 pair of intravenous ampoules by intravenous injection or infusion once each day for 5 to 7 days.

Special care: anaphylaxis may occur hence treatment should only be given when it is essential and facilities for resuscitation must be available.

Possible interaction: levodopa.

Side effects: anaphylaxis.

Manufacturer: Link.

Palfium^{CD}

Description: an analgesic opiate preparation which is a controlled drug available as scored, white tablets containing 5mg dextromoramide and scored peach tablets containing 10mg dextromoramide. Also, **Palfium Suppositories** containinng 10mg dextromoramide astartrate.

Used for: severe, intractable pain.

Dosage: tablets, up to 5mg at first then adjusted according to response. Suppositories, 1 as required. Children, 80 µg/kg body weight.

Special care: pregnancy, elderly, underactive thyroid gland, liver disorders.

Avoid use: women in labour, patients with obstructed airways and depression of respiration.

Possible interaction: CNS depressants, MAOIs.

Side effects: sweating, nausea dependence and tolerance.

Manufacturer: B.M. Pharm.

Pamergan P100^{CD}

Description: a narcotic analgesic and sedative available in ampoules for injection containing 100mg pethidine hydrochloride and 50mg promethazine hydrochloride/2ml.

Used for: relief of pain in labour, pain during and after operations, pre-medication enhancement of anaesthesia.

Dosage: labour and severe pain, 1–2ml every 4 hours by intramuscular injection if necessary; pre-medication, 25–200mg by intramuscular injection 1 hour before surgery; enhancement of anaesthesia (with nitrous oxide), 10–25mg by slow intravenous injection. Children, pre-medication, age 8 to 12 years, 0.75ml; 13 to 16 years, 1ml all by intramuscular injection.

Special care: pregnancy, breast-feeding. Elderly and debilitated persons should receive reduced doses. Also, liver disorders, asthma, respiratory depression, hypotension, underactivity of thyroid gland. If patient is terminally ill, the benefits may be considered to outweigh any risk.

Avoid use: patients with serious kidney disorders, head injury or raised intracranial pressure.

Possible interaction: MAOIs, cimetidine, anxiolytics and hypnotics.

Side effects: convulsions with high doses, vomiting, nausea, constipation, drowsiness, difficulty passing urine, depression of respiration, hypotension, sweating, dry mouth, flushing palpitations, bradycardia, urticaria, rash, itching, miosis (constriction of pupil of the eye), vertigo. Hallucinations and mood swings.

Manufacturer: Martindale.

Paramax

Description: an NSAID combining an analgesic and anti-emetic preparation available as scored, white tablets containing 500mg paracetamol and 5mg metaclopramide hydrochloride, marked PARAMAX. Also **Paramax Sachets**, effervescent powder.

Used for: migraine.

Dosage: adults over 20 years, 2 tablets when attack

starts followed by 2 every 4 hours up to maximum dose of 6 in 24 hours. Age 16 to 19 years and over 60kg body weight, 2 tablets at start of attack and maximum dose of 5 in 24 hours. 30–50kg body weight, 1 tablet at start of attack with a maximum of 3 in 24 hours. Age 12 to 14 years, over 30kg body weight, 1 tablet at start of attack with maximum of 3 in 24 hours.

Special care: pregnancy, breast-feeding, liver or kidney disorder.

Avoid use: children under 12 years, patients with phaeochromocytoma, breast cancer which is prolactin-dependent, recent surgery on gastrointestinal tract.

Possible interaction: phenothiazines, anticholinergics, butyrophenones.

Side effects: drowsiness, raised blood levels of prolactin, diarrhoea, extrapyramidal reactions (characterized by reflex-type muscle movements and spasms).

Manufacturer: Lorex.

Paraplatin

Description: an alkylating cytotoxic drug produced as a solution in vials for injection containing 10mg carboplatin/ml.

Used for: ovarian cancer, small cell lung cancer.

Dosage: as directed by physician skilled in cancer chemotherapy.

Special care: patients with kidney disorders.

Possible interaction: aminoglycosides, capreomycin, anticoagulants taken orally.

Side effects: bone marrow suppression, nausea, vomiting, toxic effects on nerves, kidneys, hearing, hair loss.

Manufacturer: Bristol-Myers.

Parlodel

Description: a dopamine agonist available as scored white tablets in 2 strengths containing 1mg and 2.5mg bromocriptine (as mesylate) respectively, all marked with strength and name. Also, **Parlodel Capsules** in 2 strengths, white/blue containing 5mg bromocriptine, coded PARLODEL 5 and white containing 10mg, coded PARLODEL 10.

Used for: Parkinson's disease, additional therapy in acromegaly (enlarged face, feet and hands due to a pituitary gland tumour producing an excess of growth hormone), tumours which are prolactin-dependent, abnormally high prolactin levels in blood, prevention and suppression of milk production after childbirth. Also, benign breast disorders connected with monthly cycle, breast pain, hormone-based infertility.

Dosage: adults, for Parkinson's disease, initial dose, 1–1.25mg taken at night for 1 week increasing gradually to 2.5mg 3 times each day in fourth week. Dose is then gradually increased to 10–40mg 3 times each day in divided doses. Drug should be taken with meals. Acromegaly and tumours dependent upon prolactin, initial dose, 1–1.25mg taken at night gradually increasing to 5mg every 6 hours (with daily meals). Prevention and suppression of lactation; 2.5mg on day of birth then 2.5mg twice each day with meals for 2 weeks. Excess prolactin levels in blood, 1–1.25mg taken at night increasing to 7.5mg each day in divided doses with meals with a maximum of 30mg daily. Benign breast disease and pain, 1–1.25mg taken at night increasing gradually to 2.5mg twice each day with meals. Infertility, 1–1.25mg taken at bedtime at first gradually increasing to 7.5mg each day in divided doses with meals, the maximum being 30mg daily.

Special care: history of heart and circulatory disorders or psychoses. Regular gynaecological monitoring necessary for women and non-hormonal methods of contraception should be used for those not wishing to conceive as may cause ovulation.

Avoid use: high blood pressure at time of childbirth, hypersensitivity to ergot alkaloids, toxaemia of pregnancy. Withdraw if conception occurs.

Possible interaction: drugs affecting blood pressure, alcohol, metoclopramide, erythromycin.

Side effects: vomiting, nausea, leg pains, slight constipation, dry mouth, vasospasm. Rarely, heart attack, stroke, headache, hypertension, convulsions, dizziness, confusion. Drug should be withdrawn if peritoneal fibrosis occurs.

Manufacturer: Sandoz.

Parnate

Description: an MAOI available as sugar-coated red tablets containing 100mg tran-ylcypromine (as sulphate), marked SKF.

Used for: depression.

Dosage: 1 tablet twice daily increasing to 1 tablet 3 times daily after 1 week. Maintenance dose is 1 tablet daily.

Special care: elderly, epilepsy.

Avoid use: children, patients with phaeochromocytoma, congestive heart failure, heart and circulatory diseases, blood changes, hyperthyroidism, liver disease, disease of cerebral arteries.

Possible interaction: ephedrine, TCADs, narcotic analgesics and pethidine, amphetamine, levodopa, methylphenidate, phenylpropanolamine, fenfluramine. Alcohol, barbiturates, hypnotics, hypoglycaemics, insulin, reserpine, anti-cholinergics, methyldopa, guanethidine. Many foods should be avoided including yeast extracts, Marmite, meat extracts, Oxo and Bovril, alcoholic drinks, broad bean pods, banana skins, flavoured textured soya protein, pickled herrings. Also any foods that are not completely fresh.

Side effects: severe hypertensive responses with certain foods, constipation, blurred vision, difficulty passing urine, gastrointestinal upset. Low blood pressure on rising, skin rash, swelling of ankles, fatigue, weariness, dizziness, jaundice, blood disorders, weight gain, changes in libido. Occasionally, confusion and mania.

Manufacturer: S.K. & F.

Parstelin

Description: an MAOI available as sugar-coated green tablets containing 10mg tranylcypromine as sulphate and 1mg trifluoperazine as hydrochloride, marked SKF.

Used for: depression.

Dosage: 1 tablet twice each day at first increasing to 1 tablet 3 times each day after 1 week. Maintenance dose is normally 1 daily tablet.

Special care: elderly, epilepsy.

Avoid use: children, phaeochromocytoma, congestive heart failure, heart and circulatory diseases, blood changes, hyperthyroidism, liver disease, disease of cerebral arteries.

Possible interaction: ephedrine, TCADs, narcotic analgesics and pethidine, amphetamine, levodopa, methylphenidate, phenylpropanolamine, fenfluramine. Alcohol, barbiturates, hypnotics, hypoglycaemics, insulin, reserpine, anticholinergics, methyldopa, guanethidine. Many foods should be avoided including yeast extracts, Marmite, meat extracts, Oxo and Bovril, alcoholic drinks, broad bean pods, banana skins, flavoured textured soya protein, pickled herrings. Also any foods that are not completely fresh.

Side effects: severe hypertensive responses with certain foods, constipation, blurred vision, difficulty passing urine, gastrointestinal upset. Low blood pressure on rising, skin rash, swelling of ankles, fatigue, weariness, dizziness, jaundice, blood disorders, weight gain, changes in libido. Occasionally, confusion and mania.

Manufacturer: S.K. & F.

Partobulin

Description: a preparation of human anti-D immunoglobulin available as a solution in ampoules for injection containing 1250 units/ml.

Used for: rhesus (D) incompatibility.

Dosage: antenatal prevention, 1250 units by intramuscular injection in weeks 28 and 34 of pregnancy and a further dose within 72 hours of birth. Following abortion or miscarriage or possible sensitising procedure, e.g. amniocentesis, 1250 units within 72 hours by intramuscular injection. Following transplacental bleeding where more than 25ml of foetal blood has been transferred (1% of foetal red blood cells), 5000 units or 50 units/ml of foetal blood, by intramuscular injection.

Special care: patients who have IGA antibodies or with known history of unusual reactions to transfused blood or blood products.

Possible interaction: live vaccines.

Manufacturer: Immuno.

Parvolex

Description: an amino acid preparation used to treat drug overdose and available as a solution in ampoules for injection containing 200mg acetylcysteine/ml. Acetylcysteine acts to protect the liver from damage.

Used for: paracetamol overdose.

Dosage: by intravenous infusion in glucose intravenous infusion; 150mg/kg body weight in 200ml over 15 minutes at first. Then 50mg/kg body weight in 500ml over 4 hours followed by 100mg/kg body weight in 1000ml over 16 hours.

Special care: history of asthma. Vomiting should be induced if patient is treated within 4 hours of overdose. Plasma concentrations of paracetamol require monitoring. Patients who have taken alcohol, phenobarbitone, rifampicin, carbamazepine or phenytoin may be at risk of live toxicity at lower plasma-paracetamol concentrations.

Possible interaction: metals and rubber.

Side effects: rash, anaphylaxis.

Manufacturer: Evans.

Pavulon

Description: a non-depolarizing muscle relaxant available as a solution in ampoules for injection containing 4mg pancuronium bromide/2ml.

Used for: muscle relaxation for intubation of patients undergoing anaesthesia and mechanical ventilation in intensive care.

Dosage: adults, 50–100 µg/kg body weight at first (for intubation) then 10–20 µg/kg body weight as needed to maintain relaxation. Children, 60–100 µg/kg body weight at first then 10–20 µg/kg. Newborn baby, 30–40 µg/kg body weight at first followed by 10–20 µg/kg. Intensive care patients, 60 µg/kg body weight every hour to hour and a half.

Special care: patients with liver and kidney disorders (reduced dose).

Possible interaction: procainamide, quinidine, aminoglycosides, clindamycin, azloallin, colistin, propanolol, verapamil, nifedipine, ecothiopate, demacarium, pyridostigmine, neostigmine, magnesium salts.

Manufacturer: Organon Teknika.

Penbritin

Description: an antibiotic broad-spectrum penicillin preparation available as black/red capsules in 2 strengths containing 250mg and 500mg ampicillin, marked with strength and name. Also, **Penbritin Syrup** available as powder for reconstitution with water, then containing 125mg/5ml. **Penbritin Syrup Forte** contains 250mg/5ml (available as powder for reconstitution). **Penbritin Paediatric Suspension** contains 125mg/1.25ml when reconstituted (available as powder). **Penbritin Injection** available as powder in vials containing 250mg and 500mg ampicillin sodium.

Used for: ear, nose, throat and respiratory infections, soft tissue infections. Infections of urinary tract and gonorrhoea.

Dosage: adults, oral preparations, 250mg–1g every 6 hours; injection, 250–500mg by intravenous or intramuscular injection, 4, 5 or 6 times each day. Children, oral preparations, 125–250mg every 6 hours; injection, half adult dose.

Special care: patients with glandular fever.

Side effects: gastrointestinal upset, hypersensitivity reactions.

Manufacturer: Beecham.

Pendramine

Description: a penicillin derivative available as film-coated, scored, oblong white tablets containing 125mg and 250mg penicillamine respectively; the 250mg tablets are marked HB.

Used for: severe rheumatoid arthritis.

Dosage: 125–250mg each day for first 4 to 8 weeks, then increase every 4 weeks by 125–250mg to a maximum dose of 2g each day, if needed. Children, usual dose, 15–20mg/kg body weight each day. Start with lower dose then gradually increase every 4 weeks over period of 3 to 6 months.

Special care: patients sensitive to penicillin checks on blood, urine and kidney function are required regularly during the course of treatment.

Avoid use: pregnancy, breast-feeding, patients with kidney disorders, thrombocytopenia, SLE, agranulocytosis (serious reduction in number of white blood cells [granulocytes]).

Possible interaction: phenylbutazone, zinc or iron salts, cytotoxic drugs, antimalarial drugs, gold salts, antacids.

Side effects: blood changes, myasthenia gravis, anorexia, rash, fever, nausea, protein in urine, blood in urine, SLE, nephrotic syndrome (a kidney abnormality resulting from a number of diseases and conditions).

Manufacturer: ASTA Medica.

Pentacarinat

Description: an antiprotazal preparation available as a powder in vials for reconstitution and injection containing 300mg pentamidine isethionate. Also, **Pentacarinat Solution** containing 300mg pentamidine isethionate/5ml for nebulization.

Used for: pneumocystis carinii pneumonia, kala-azar, cutaneous leishmaniasis.

Dosage: adults and children, pneumocystis carinii pneumonia, 4mg/kg body weight each day for 14 days; nebulized solution, 600mg each day for 3 weeks; prevention of secondary infection, 300mg every 4 weeks or 150mg every 2 weeks. Kala-azar, 3–4mg/kg body weight each day on alternate days up to a maximum of 10 deep intramuscular injections. May be repeated, if needed. Cutaneous leishmaniasis, 3–4mg/kg body weight by deep intramuscular injection once or twice each week until condition improves. Trypanosomiasis, 4mg/kg body weight by deep intramuscular injection or intravenous infusion each day on alternate days to a maximum of 7 to 10 injections.

Special care: must only be given by specialist physician under close medical supervision. Risk of serious hypotension once dose has been given; patient must be lying down and blood pressure monitored. Patients with liver or kidney disorder (reduced dose), hyper or hypotension, anaemia, leucopenia, thrombocytopenia, hypo or hyperglycaemia.

Side effects: severe and occasionally fatal reactions due to hypotension, pancreatitis, hypoglycaemia, cardiac arrhythmias. Also, leucopenia, thrombocytopenia, hypocalcaemia, serious kidney failure. Vomiting, dizziness, nausea, fainting, rash, flushing, constriction of airways on inhalation, pain, disturbance of sense of taste. Tissue and muscle damage, abscess and pain at injection site.

Manufacturer: Theraplix.

Pentasa

Description: a colorectal salicylate preparation available as an enema containing 1g mesalazine. Also, **Pentasa Suppository**, suppositories containing 1g mesalazine; **Pentasa SR** sustained-release scored tablets which are light grey and contain 250mg and 500mg mesalazine respectively, marked with strength and PENTASA.

Used for: ulcerative colitis (inflammation and ulceration of the colon and rectum).

Dosage: adults, 1 enema or suppository at night; tablets, 2 500mg tablets 3 times each day increasing to 8 500mg tablets (maximum dose), if needed. Maintenance dose is 500mg 3 times each day.

Special care: pregnancy, breast-feeding, elderly, protein in urine or raised levels of blood urea.

Avoid use: children.

Side effects: headache, abdominal pain, nausea.

Manufacturer: Yamanouchi.

Pepcid

Description: an H2 blocker available as square, beige tablets and square, brown tablets containing 20mg and 40mg famotidine respectively, both marked with strength and name.

Used for: treatment of stomach and duodenal ulcers, prevention of relapse of duodenal ulcers. Prevention and treatment of reflux disease of stomach and oesophagus, treatment of Zollinger-Ellison syndrome.

Dosage: treatment of ulcers, 40mg taken at night for 4 to 8 weeks; prevention of relapse of duodenal ucer, 20mg taken at night. Gastro-oesophageal reflux disease, 20mg twice each day for 6 weeks to 3 months (or 40mg, if damage or ulceration is present). Prevention, 20mg twice each day. Zollinger-Ellison syndrome, 20mg 6 hours at first adjusted according to response to a maximum dose of 800mg each day.

Special care: pregnancy, breast-feeding, stomach cancer or kidney disease.

Avoid use: children.

Side effects: nausea, diarrhoea, constipation, rash, gastrointestinal upset, dry mouth, headache, anorexia, dizziness, weariness. Rarely there may be enlargement of breasts in males (reversible).

Manufacturer: Morson.

Perfan

Description: a phosphodiesterase inhibitor available in ampoules for injection containing 5mg enoximone/ml.

Used for: congestive heart failure where filling pressures are increased and cardiac output reduced.

Dosage: adults, by slow intravenous injection, 0.5–1mg/kg body weight at first then 500 µg/kg every half hour until condition improves or 3mg/kg may be given every 3 to 6 hours, as needed. By

intravenous infusion, 90 µg/kg body weight/ minute at first over 10 to 30 minutes. Then intermittent or continuous infusion of 20 µg/kg body weight. Total maximum dose should not be greater than 24mg/kg body weight in 24 hours. Plastic apparatus must be used as crystals form in glass.

Side effects: tachycardia, heart arrhythmias, unusual heartbeats, nausea, vomiting, headache, diarrhoea, hypotension, insomnia, fever, chills, urine retention, reduced ability to produce and pass urine, pains in limbs.

Manufacturer: Merrell Dow.

Pergonal

Description: an hormonal gonadotrophin preparation available as a powder in ampoules for reconstitution and injection containing menotrophin (equivalent to 75 units of both follicle-stimulating hormone and luteinizing hormone, with solvent).

Used for: underactivity (infertility) of testes due to lack of gonadotrophin. Female infertility due to lack of ovulation. Superovulation for in vitro fertilization.

Dosage: male adults, 1 ampoule 3 times each week along with 2000 units chorionic gonadotrophin twice each week for at least 4 months. Female infertility, by intramuscular injection according to levels of oestrogen. Superovulation, 2 or 3 ampoules each day.

Special care: patients with hormonal disorders or intracranial lesions must have these corrected before therapy begins.

Avoid use: pregnancy.

Side effects: overstimulation of ovaries may lead to enlargement and rupture, allergic responses, multiple pregnancy.

Manufacturer: Serono.

Perinal

Description: a colorectal preparation combining a steroid and local anaesthetic available in the form of a metered dose spray containing 0.2% hydrocortisone and 1% lignocaine hydrochloride.

Used for: pain in anal area.

Dosage: 2 sprays up to 3 times each day.

Special care: short-term use only, pregnancy.

Avoid use: patients with infections of fungal, viral and bacterial origin.

Side effects: systemic corticosteroid effects, e.g. changes as in Cushing's syndrome.

Manufacturer: Dermal.

Persantin

Description: an anti-platelet drug available as sugar-

coated orange and white tablets containing 25mg and 100mg dipyridamole, marked with strength and name.
Used for: additional therapy along with oral anticoagulants to prevent thrombosis of artificial heart valves.
Dosage: 300–600mg each day in 3 or 4 doses taken before meals. Children, 5mg/kg body weight as divided dose each day.
Special care: recent heart attack, worsening angina, narrowing of aorta below valves.
Possible interaction: antacids.
Side effects: gastrointestinal upset, giddiness, headache.
Manufacturer: Boehringer Ingelheim.

Pertofran
Description: a TCAD available as sugar-coated pink tablets containing 25mg desipramine hydrochloride, marked EW and CG.
Used for: depression.
Dosage: 1 tablet 3 times each day at first increasing to 2, 3 or 4 times daily if needed. Elderly, start with 1 tablet daily.
Special care: elderly, epilepsy.
Avoid use: children, phaeochromocytoma, congestive heart failure, heart and circulatory diseases, blood changes, hyperthyroidism, liver disease, disease of cerebral arteries.
Possible interaction: ephedrine, TCADs, narcotic analgesics and pethidine, amphetamine, levodopa, methylphenidate, phenylpropanolamine, fenfluramine. Alcohol, barbiturates, hypnotics, hypoglycaemics, insulin, reserpine, anticholinergics, methyldopa, guanethidine. Many foods should be avoided including yeast extracts, Marmite, meat extracts, Oxo and Bovril, alcoholic drinks, broad bean pods, banana skins, flavoured textured soya protein, pickled herrings. Also any foods that are not completely fresh.
Side effects: severe hypertensive responses with certain foods, constipation, blurred vision, difficulty passing urine, gastrointestinal upset. Low blood pressure on rising, skin rash, swelling of ankles, fatigue, weariness, dizziness, jaundice, blood disorders, weight gain, changes in libido. Occasionally, confusion and mania.
Manufacturer: Geigy.

Pevaryl TC
Description: a preparation in the form of a cream which combines an antifungal and potent steroid, containing 1% econazole nitrate and 0.1% triamcinolone acetonide.

Used for: inflammatory skin conditions where fungal infection is present.
Dosage: rub into affected area twice each day for 14 days.
Special care: short-term use only.
Avoid use: children, long-term or extensive use especially in pregnancy, patients with untreated bacterial or fungal infections or skin infections of tuberculous or viral origin or due to ringworm. Also, dermatitis in area of mouth, acne, leg ulcers or scabies.
Side effects: suppression of adrenal glands, skin thinning, abnormal hair growth, changes as in Cushing's syndrome.
Manufacturer: Cilag.

Pharmorubicin
Description: a cytotoxic antibiotic preparation available as a powder in vials for reconstitution and injection containing 10mg, 20mg or 50mg epirubicin hydrochloride. Also, **Pharmorubicin Solution** containing 2mg/ml.
Used for: breast cancer, papillary tumours of bladder.
Dosage: adults, breast cancer, by intravenous injection as directed by physician. Papillary tumours, solution of 50mg in 50ml sterile water is instilled each week for 8 weeks. Prevention, once each week for 4 weeks then once each month for 11 months.
Special care: care in handling, irritant to tissues. Patients with liver disease (reduced doses).
Side effects: bone marrow suppression, nausea, vomiting, hair loss, effects on fertility.
Manufacturer: Pharmacia.

Physeptone^{CD}
Description: an opiate analgesic preparation which is a controlled drug available as scored, white tablets containing 5mg methadone hydrochloride marked WELLCOME L4A. Also, **Physeptone Injection**, containing 10mg/ml in ampoules for injection.
Used for: severe pain.
Dosage: tablets, 5–10mg every 6 to 8 hours or same dose by subcutaneous or intramuscular injection.
Special care: pregnancy, underactive thyroid gland or serious liver disease.
Avoid use: children, depression of respiration, obstructive airways disease, obstetric patients, those who are not confined to bed.
Possible interaction: central nervous system depressants, MAOIs.
Side effects: dizziness, nausea, sedation, euphoria, drug tolerance and dependence.
Manufacturer: Wellcome.

Piptoril Depot

Description: a phenothiazine group II available as a depot oily injection in ampoules containing 50mg pipothiazine palmitate/ml.

Used for: ongoing treatment of certain psychiatric disorders particularly schizophrenia.

Dosage: a test dose at first of 25mg by deep intramuscular injection into the gluteal muscle (buttock), then adjusted by 25mg or 50mg increments until best response is achieved. The usual maintenance dose is in the order of 50–100mg every 4 weeks with a maximum of 200mg.

Special care: pregnancy, breast-feeding, history of convulsions, severe extrapyramidal responses to phenothiazines taken orally.

Avoid use: children, severe heart disorder, liver or kidney failure, phaeochromocytoma, depression of bone marrow function, severe hardening of cerebral arteries.

Possible interaction: alcohol, anaesthetics, antacids, antimuscarines, anxiolytics, hypnotics, calcium channel blockers, lithium.

Side effects: extrapyramidal symptoms, changes in ECG and EEG, tachycardia and heart arrhythmias, apathy, drowsiness, insomnia, depression. Dry mouth, blocked nose, difficulty passing urine, constipation, hypotension, blurred vision. Changes in breasts and menstrual cycle, weight gain, impotence, blood changes, effects on liver, jaundice, rash, pigmentation of skin and eyes (especially higher doses).

Manufacturer: Theraplix.

Pipril

Description: an antibiotic broad-spectrum penicillin available as powder in vials in strengths of 1g, 2g and 4g piperacillin (as sodium salt), with diluent, for injection (1g and 2g) and infusion (4g).

Used for: local and systemic infections; prevention of infection during operations.

Dosage: adults, by intramuscular or slow intravenous injection or by intravenous infusion. 100–150mg/kg body weight in divided doses each day at first. Severe infections may require up to 200–300mg/kg with 16g or more daily if life is threatened. Single doses over 2g must be given by intravenous injection or infusion. Children may require lesser doses.

Special care: pregnancy, kidney disorder.

Side effects: gastrointestinal upset, hypersensitive allergic reactions.

Manufacturer: Lederle.

Piptalin

Description: an anti-spasmodic used for digestive disorders, combining an anticholinergic and deflatulent drug, available as a sugar-free elixir containing 4mg pipenzolate bromide and 40mg activated dimethicone/5ml.

Used for: flatulence, pain due to spasm and overactivity of gastrointestinal tract, abdominal extension due to gas build-up.

Dosage: 10ml 3 or 4 times each day taken 15 minutes before meal. Children, up to 10kg body weight, 2.5ml; 10–20kg, 2.5–5ml; 20–40kg, 5ml. All taken 15 minutes before meals 3 or 4 times each day.

Special care: urine retention, enlarged prostate gland, glaucoma.

Avoid use: pregnancy, breast-feeding, myasthenia gravis, various disorders of gastrointestinal tract including obstruction, paralytic ileus, pyloric stenosis, ulcerative colitis. Also, liver or kidney disorders, tachycardia, unstable angina.

Possible interaction: benzodiazepines, TCADs, antihistamines.

Side effects: constipation, urine retention, vomiting and nausea, dry mouth, visual disorder, weakness, tachycardia, blushing, palpitations, insomnia.

Manufacturer: B.M. Pharmaceuticals.

Pitressin

Description: A preparation of antidiuretic hormone available as a solution in ampoules for injection containing 20 units agipressin (synthetic vasopressin)/ml.

Used for: pituitary diabetes insipidus.

Dosage: by intramuscular or subcutaneous injection, 5–20 units every 4 hours. By intravenous infusion, 20 units over 15 minutes.

Special care: pregnancy, conditions which might be made worse by water retention, asthma, heart failure, migraine, epilepsy, kidney disorders. Careful checks on amount of water retention required.

Avoid use: disease of arteries especially coronary arteries, severe nephritis.

Side effects: constriction of coronary arteries possibly leading to angina and reduction in blood flow to heart, hypersensitive allergic reactions, feeling of needing to defecate, belching, abdominal pains, nausea, pallor.

Manufacturer: Parke-Davis.

Plaquenil

Description: an NSAID which is a 4-aminoquinolone available as sugar-coated orange tablets containing 200mg hydroxychloroquine sulphate.

Used for: rheumatoid arthritis and juvenile rheumatoid arthritis, lupus erythematosus (a severe inflammatory disease affecting internal organs and skin).

Dosage: 2 tablets each day with meals at first, with a maintenance dose of 1 or 2 tablets daily. The maximum dose is 6.5mg/kg body weight each day. If no improvement is seen after 6 months, drug should be withdrawn. Children, 6.5mg/kg body weight each day.

Special care: breast-feeding, porphyria, liver or kidney disease, a history of blood, gastrointestinal or neurological disorders. Patients on long-term therapy should receive regular eye tests.

Avoid use: pregnancy, patients with maculopathy (a disorder of the eye spot of the retina).

Possible interaction: antacids, drugs which may damage the eyes, aminoglycosides.

Side effects: opacity of the cornea and changes in the retina of the eye, reduced eye accommodation (discontinue if this occurs). Also, gastrointestinal intolerance, baldness, skin responses, bleaching of hair.

Manufacturer: Sanofi Winthrop.

Plendil

Description: an antihypertensive class II calcium antagonist available as film-coated sustained-release tablets containing 5mg and 10mg felodipine.

Used for: hypertension.

Dosage: 5mg once each day increasing if necessary to a usual maintenance dose of 5–10mg. The maximum daily dose is 20mg.

Special care: recent problems of poor blood circulation to the heart or serious liver disease.

Avoid use: pregnancy, breast-feeding.

Possible interaction: phenytoin, phenobarbitone, cimetidine, carbamazepine.

Side effects: flushing, swelling of ankles, weariness, giddiness, headache, slight swelling of gums, palpitations.

Manufacturer: Schwarz.

Pneumovax II

Description: a preparation of pneumococcal vaccine, available as a solution for injection, containing 25 µg of 23 types of pneumococcus/0.5ml as a purified mixture of capsular polysaccharides.

Used for: immunization against pneumococcal disease.

Dosage: adults and children age 2 years and over, 0.5ml by intramuscular or subcutaneous injection.

Special care: patients with weak hearts or lungs,

respiratory diseases or feverish illnesses, revaccination of high risk children.

Avoid use: pregnancy, breast-feeding, children under 2 years, patients with Hodgkin's disease who have had chemotherapy or radiation treatment. Patients who have recently received immuno-suppressive treatment, revaccination of adults.

Side effects: fever, local skin reactions, relapse of patients with stabilized thrombocytopenic purpura (a bleeding disorder characterized by haemorrhage beneath the skin and mucous membranes).

Manufacturer: Morson.

Polyfax

Description: a preparation of peptide antibiotics available as an ointment containing 10,000 units polymyxin B sulphate and 500 units bacitracin zinc per gram.

Used for: eye infections including conjunctivitis, keratitis, styes, blepharitis. Prevent infection after removal of foreign objects from the eye or surgery. Also, impetigo, infected burns and skin infections.

Dosage: apply thinly at least twice per day.

Special care: patients with extensive, open wounds.

Side effects: skin sensitization, toxic effects on kidneys.

Manufacturer: Cusi.

Polytrim

Description: A combined antibacterial preparation available in the form of eyedrops containing 1mg trimethoprim and 10,000 units polymyxin B sulphate/ml. Also, **Polytrim Ointment** containing 5mg trimethoprim and 10,000 units polymyxin B sulphate/gram.

Used for: bacterial eye infections.

Dosage: apply 3 or 4 times each day continuing for 2 days after symptoms have cleared.

Manufacturer: Cusi.

Ponderax Pacaps

Description: an anti-obesity serotoninergic drug available as blue/clear sustained-release capsules, with white pellets containing 60mg fenfluramine hydrochloride marked P and PA60.

Used for: severe obesity.

Dosage: adults 1 tablet daily half an hour before a meal for a maximum period of 3 months.

Special care: therapy should last for up to 3 months and drug gradually withdrawn over last 1 or 2 weeks.

Avoid use: patients suffering from depression, epilepsy, psychiatric disorder or drug or alcohol abuse.

Possible interaction: antidiabetics, MAOIs, alcohol, antihypertensives, sedatives, anti-anoretics.
Side effects: dry mouth, nervousness, sedation, hallucinations, frequency of urination, depression (especially if drug abruptly stopped), diarrhoea.
Manufacturer: Pacaps Servier.

Pondocillin

Description: an antibiotic preparation which is a broad-spectrum penicillin available as film-coated, oval, white tablets containing 500mg pivampicillin coded with symbol and 128. Also, **Pondocillin Suspension** containing 175mg pivampicillin/5ml available as granules for reconstitution.
Used for: skin, soft tissue infections, bronchitis, pneumonia, gonorrhoea and urinary tract infections.
Dosage: adults, 1 tablet or 15ml suspension twice each day with drink or food. Children, under 1 year, 40–60mg/kg; 1 to 5 years, 10–15ml; 6 to 10 years, 15–20ml. All as daily divided doses with food or drink.
Special care: kidney disease.
Avoid use: patients with glandular fever.
Side effects: gastrointestinal upset, hypersensitive allergic reactions.
Manufacturer: Leo.

Ponstan Forte

Description: an NSAID available as blue/ivory capsules containing 250mg mefenamic acid marked PONSTAN 250. Also, **Ponstan Forte** film-coated, yellow tablets containing 500mg marked with name. **Ponstan Paediatric Suspension** containing 50mg/5ml.
Used for: pain, period pain, headache, rheumatoid pain (Stills disease), osteoarthritis, heavy menstrual bleeding.
Dosage: adults, 500mg 3 times each day (on first day of period in patients with heavy menstrual bleeding). Children, use paediatric suspension, aged 6 months to 1 year, 5ml; 2 to 4 years, 10ml; 5 to 8 years, 15ml; 9 to 12 years, 20ml. All doses at 8 hour intervals for no more than 1 week.
Special care: pregnancy, breast-feeding, elderly, allergies, asthma, heart failure, epilepsy.
Avoid use: known allergy to NSAID or aspirin, ulcer, liver or kidney disorder, inflammatory bowel disease.
Possible interaction: sulphonylureas, anti-coagulants, hydantoins, quinolones.
Side effects: kidney disorder, gastrointestinal intolerance, raised level of liver enzymes. Rarely, blood changes. Withdraw drug if skin rash occurs.
Manufacturer: Parke-Davis.

Potaba

Description: an antifibrotic preparation which dissolves fibrous tissue, available as powder in sachets containing 3g potassium p-aminobenzoate. Also, **Potaba Tablets** white, containing 500mg. **Potaba Capsules**, red/white, containing 500mg.
Used for: scleroderma (thickened skin), Peyronie's disease (fibrous hardening of the penis).
Dosage: adults, 12g each day in 4 divided doses with meals.
Special care: kidney disease.
Possible interaction: sulphonamides.
Side effects: anorexia, nausea (discontinue if these occur).
Manufacturer: Glenwood.

Praxilene

Description: a preparation that is a peripheral and cerebral activator which improves the use of glucose and oxygen by the tissues, increasing the level of ATP (the energy molecules of cells) and decreasing lactic acid levels. It is available as pink capsules containing 100mg naftidrofuryl oxalate. Also, **Praxilene Forte** available in ampoules for injection containing 20mg naftidrofuryl oxalate/ml.
Used for: disorders of cerebral and peripheral arteries.
Dosage: 1 or 2 tablets 3 times each day.
Special care: use of Praxilene Forte in patients with very weak heart or conduction disorders.
Avoid use: children. Use of Forte in patients with heart block.
Side effects: nausea, stomach ache.
Manufacturer: Lipha.

Precortisyl

Description: a glucocorticoid corticosteroid preparation available as white tablets containing 1mg prednisolone and scored, white tablets containing 5mg prednisolone. Also, **Precortisyl Forte** scored, white tablets containing 25mg prednisolone.
Used for: Precortisyl, allergic and rheumatic disorders; Forte, rheumatic fever, systemic lupus erythematosus (severe inflammatory disorder affecting many parts of the body), blood disorders.
Dosage: Precortisyl, 20–40mg each day in divided doses at first, then reducing by 2.5–5mg every third or fourth day until a maintenance dose, in the order of 5–20mg daily, is achieved. Forte, 75mg in 3 divided doses. Children, Precortisyl, age 1 to 7 years, quarter to half adult dose; 7 to 12 years, half to three-quarters adult dose.
Special care: pregnancy, diabetes, kidney

inflammation, hypertension, thrombophlebitis, epilepsy, secondary cancer, underactive thyroid, peptic ulcer, glaucoma, recent surgical anastomoses of intestine. Also, patients suffering from stress, psychoses, liver cirrhosis, infections of fungal or viral origin, tuberculosis, other infections. Also avoid contact with chicken pox or *Herpes zoster* and seek medical advice if this occurs or if infected.

Avoid use: children under 1 year.

Possible interaction: diuretics, hypoglycaemics, phenytoin, NSAIDs, rifampicin, anticholinesterases, ephedrine, anticoagulants taken orally, phenobarbitone, cardiac glycosides, diuretics.

Side effects: mood changes, depression and euphoria, changes as in Cushing's syndrome, osteoporosis, peptic ulcer, hyperglycaemia.

Manufacturer: Roussel.

Pred Forte

Description: a corticosteroid preparation available as eyedrops containing 1% prednisolone acetate.

Used for: inflammation of eyes where no infection is present.

Dosage: 1 or 2 drops 2, 3 or 4 times each day. 2 drops every hour may be needed during the first 48 hours.

Special care: pregnancy, babies.

Avoid use: fungal, viral or tuberculous eye infections or those producing pus. Also, glaucoma, dendritic ulcer, those wearing soft contact lenses.

Side effects: formation of cataracts, thinning of cornea, rise in pressure within eye, secondary fungal or viral infections.

Manufacturer: Allergan.

Predenema

Description: a steroid colorectal agent available as an enema containing 20mg prednisolone (as metasulphobenzoate sodium).

Used for: ulcerative colitis.

Dosage: adults, 1 enema at night for 2, 3 or 4 weeks.

Special care: pregnancy, avoid long-term use.

Avoid use: children. Patients with perforated bowel, infections, fistulae, obstruction of the bowel, peritonitis.

Manufacturer: Pharmax.

Predfoam

Description: a steroid colorectal agent available as a white aerosol foam containing 20mg prednisolone (as metasulphobenzoate sodium) per metered dose.

Used for: ulcerative colitis, proctitis (inflammation of the rectum).

Dosage: adults, 1 metered dose into rectum twice each day for 2 weeks continuing for another 2 weeks if condition improves.

Special care: pregnancy, short-term use only.

Avoid use: children, patients with perforated bowel, infections, fistulae, obstruction of the bowel, peritonitis.

Manufacturer: Pharmax.

Prednesol

Description: a glucocorticoid corticosteroid preparation available as scored, pink tablets containing 5mg prednisolone (as disodium phosphate) marked with name and GLAXO.

Used for: rheumatic, allergic and inflammatory disorders responsive to steroids.

Dosage: adults, 10–100mg in water each day at first, in divided doses, then reducing to lowest dose which is effective. Children, age 1 to 7, quarter to half adult dose; 7 to 12, half to three-quarters adult dose.

Special care: thrombophlebitis, psychoses, recent intestinal anastomoses, chronic nephritis, certain cancers, osteoporosis, peptic ulcer, skin eruption/rash related to a disease, viral, fungal or active infections, tuberculosis. Hypertension, glaucoma, epilepsy, acute glomerulonephritis (inflammation of kidney glomerulus), diabetes, cirrhosis, hypothyroidism, pregnancy, stress. To be withdrawn gradually.

Possible interaction: NSAIDs, oral anticoagulants, phenytoin, ephedrine, phenobarbitone, rifampicin, diuretics, cardiac glycosides, anticholinesterases, hypoglycaemics.

Side effects: osteoporosis, depression, euphoria, hyperglycaemia, peptic ulcers, Cushingoid changes.

Manufacturer: Glaxo.

Predsol

Description: a steroid colorectal agent available as an enema containing 20mg prednisolone as disodium phosphate. Also, **Predsol Suppositories** containing 5mg prednisolone (as disodium phosphate).

Used for: enema, ulcerative colitis; suppositories, proctitis (inflammation of rectum) and anal disorders resulting from Crohn's disease (a disorder of the intestine or part of digestive tract in which there is inflammation and ulceration).

Dosage: adults, enema, 1 at night for 2, 3 or 4 weeks; suppositories, 1 every night and morning after passing stool.

Special care: pregnancy, short-term use only.

Avoid use: children, bacterial, fungal, tuberculous or viral infections.

Side effects: systemic glucocorticoid effects, e.g. mood swings, euphoria and depression, changes as in Cushing's syndrome, peptic ulcer, hyperglycaemia, osteoporosis.
Manufacturer: Evans.

Preferid

Description: a potent topical steroid preparation available as cream and ointment containing 0.025% budesonide.
Used for: psoriasis, all types of dermatitis, eczema.
Dosage: apply thinly 2 or 3 times each day.
Special care: thrombophlebitis, psychoses, recent intestinal anastomoses, chronic nephritis, certain cancers, osteoporosis, peptic ulcer, skin eruption/ rash related to a disease, viral, fungal or active infections, tuberculosis. Hypertension, glaucoma, epilepsy, acute glomerulonephritis (inflammation of kidney glomerulus), diabetes, cirrhosis, hypothyroidism, pregnancy, stress. To be withdrawn gradually.
Possible interaction: NSAIDs, oral anticoagulants, phenytoin, ephedrine, phenobarbitone, rifampicin, diuretics, cardiac glycosides, anticholinesterases, hypoglycaemics.
Side effects: osteoporosis, depression, euphoria, hyperglycaemia, peptic ulcers, Cushingoid changes.
Manufacturer: Yamanouchi.

Pregnyl

Description: a preparation of human chorionic gonadotrophin available as powder in ampoules, with solvent for reconstitution and injection, at strengths of 500, 1500 and 5000 units.
Used for: underdevelopment of male sexual organs, deficient production of sperm, delayed puberty in males; infertility due to lack of maturing of follicles and ovulation in females. Along with human menopausal gonadotrophin to produce superovulation for in vitro fertilization treatment.
Dosage: male adults, hypogonadism, 500–1000 units 2 or 3 times each week by intramuscular injection. Delayed puberty, 1500 units twice each week by intramuscular injection for at least 6 months. Females, infertility, following treatment with human menopausal gonadotrophin, 5000– 10000 units by intramuscular injection. Then 3 further injections of 5000 units during the next 9 days. Superovulation, 30 to 40 hours after injection with human menopausal gonadotrophin, 5000– 10000 units by intramuscular injection.
Special care: patients with heart or kidney disorders, epilepsy, hypertension, migraine, hormone levels should be monitored in female patients.

Avoid use: children, patients with androgen-dependent cancers.
Side effects: skin rashes, salt and water retention.
Manufacturer: Organon.

Premarin

Description: an oestrogen preparation available as sugar-coated, oval, maroon tablets and sugar-coated, oval, yellow tablets containing 0.625mg and 1.25mg conjugated oestrogens. Also, **Premarin Vaginal Cream** containing 0.625mg/g conjugated oestrogens.
Used for: tablets, hormone replacement therapy for menopausal women who have had a hysterectomy. Prevention of osteoporosis following menopause. Relief of symptoms of some breast cancers in post-menopausal women. Cream, atrophic vaginitis and urethritis (inflammation due to atrophy of the tissues of the vagina and urethra), Kraurosis vulvae (a disease of the external genital area, characterized by degeneration of tissues and itching, affecting elderly women).
Dosage: tablets, for hormone replacement therapy, 0.625mg–1.25mg each day for 12 to 18 months. Prevention of osteoporosis, same dose for 5 to 10 years. Breast cancer, up to 10mg 3 times each day for at least 9 months. Cream, 1–2g applied daily to affected area or intra-vaginally (using applicator) for 3 weeks followed by 1 week without treatment.
Special care: those at risk of thromboembolism or with history of disorders relating to this, those with porphyria, gallstones, diabetes, otosclerosis, fibroids in the uterus, tetany, epilepsy, mild liver disease. Blood pressure, breasts and pelvic organs should be checked regularly during the course of treatment.
Avoid use: thromboembolism, thrombophlebitis, vaginal bleeding which is not diagnosed, or endometriosis, genital tract cancer or other oestrogen-dependent cancers. Serious kidney, liver, heart disease, Dublin-Johnson or Rotor syndrome.
Possible interaction: drugs which induce liver enzymes.
Manufacturer: Wyeth.

Prempak-C

Description: an oestrogen and progestogen preparation available in the form of sugar-coated oval tablets in 2 strengths, 28 maroon or 28 yellow containing 0.625mg or 1.25mg conjugated oestrogens respectively. Also, 12 sugar-coated brown tablets containing 0.15mg norgestrel in same pack.
Used for: hormone replacement therapy in women

who have not had a hysterectomy, for menopausal symptoms, prevention of osteoporosis following menopause.

Dosage: 1 maroon or yellow tablet for 16 days then 1 maroon or yellow tablet and 1 brown tablet for 12 days, starting on first day of period if present.

Special care: patients with history of, or considered to be at risk of thrombosis. Women with any of the following should receive careful monitoring: epilepsy, gallstones, porphyria, multiple sclerosis, otosclerosis, diabetes, migraine, hypertension, tetany, fibroids in the uterus. Blood pressure, breasts and pelvic organs should be examined regularly during the treatment especially in women who may be at risk of breast cancer.

Avoid use: pregnancy, breast-feeding, with breast cancer, cancer of reproductive system or other hormonally dependent cancer, inflammation of veins or other thromboembolic conditions, endometriosis, undiagnosed vaginal bleeding, serious liver, kidney or heart disease, Dublin-Johnson or Rotor syndrome.

Possible interaction: drugs which induce liver enzymes.

Side effects: soreness and enlargement of breasts, breakthrough bleeding, weight gain, gastrointestinal upset, dizziness, nausea, headache, vomiting. If frequent, severe, migraine-like headaches, disturbance of vision, rise in blood pressure, jaundice or indications of thrombosis occur, drug should immediately be withdrawn, and also in the event of pregnancy. Drug should be stopped 6 weeks before planned major surgery.

Manufacturer: Wyeth.

Prepidil

Description: a prostaglandin preparation available as a sterile cervical gel in single use syringes containing 500µg dinoprostone/3g gel.

Used for: induction of labour, softening and dilation of cervix.

Dosage: 1 dose into cervical canal, repeated as directed by physician.

Special care: glaucoma, asthma, raised pressure within eye; high doses may cause rupture of uterus. Should not be given continuously for more than 2 days.

Avoid use: patients at risk of rupture of uterus, those in whom delivery is complicated, e.g. placenta praevia, those with serious toxaemia, untreated pelvic infection, multiple pregnancy, previous history of difficult delivery, inflammation of vagina or cervix.

Side effects: chills, shivering, flushing, headache,

nausea, vomiting, diarrhoea, raised level of white blood cells, short-lived fever, abnormal increase in muscle tone of uterus, severe contractions.

Manufacturer: Upjohn.

Prepulsid

Description: a prokinetic drug acting on the gastrointestinal tract, which promotes the movement of food through the oesophagus and stomach. It is available as scored, white tablets containing 10mg cisapride (as monohydrate). Also, **Prepulsid Suspension**, cherry-flavoured solution containing 5mg cisapride/5ml.

Used for: gastro-oesophageal reflux, maintenance treatment of reflux oesophagitis, dyspepsia, relief of symptoms when gastric emptying is delayed as in systemic sclerosis, diabetes, autonomic neuropathy.

Dosage: gastro-oesophageal reflux, 20mg before breakfast and at night time or 10mg 3 times each day for 12 weeks. Then a maintenance dose of 20mg once each day at bedtime or 10mg twice each day before breakfast and at night. Dyspepsia, 10mg 3 times each day for 4 weeks. Delayed gastric emptying, 10mg 3 or 4 times each day, for 6 weeks.

Special care: breast-feeding, elderly, kidney or liver disorders.

Avoid use: pregnancy, children, patients with gastrointestinal obstruction, haemorrhage or perforation.

Possible interaction: anticholinergics, anti-coagulants taken orally, central nervous system depressants.

Side effects: abdominal rumbling and pain, diarrhoea; rarely, extrapyramidal effects, headache, convulsions.

Manufacturer: Janssen.

Prescal

Description: an antihypertensive preparation which is a class II calcium antagonist, available as scored yellow tablets containing 2.5mg isradipine marked NM and CIBA.

Used for: hypertension.

Dosage: 1 tablet in the morning and at night, increasing after 3 or 4 weeks to 2 twice each day if needed. Maximum dose is 4 twice daily. Elderly, half a tablet twice each day at first.

Special care: pregnancy, breast-feeding, narrowing of aorta (aortic stenosis), sick sinus syndrome.

Avoid use: children.

Possible interaction: anticonvulsants.

Side effects: tachycardia, palpitations, headache, giddiness, flushing, fluid retention in hands and feet, pain in abdomen, gain in weight, tiredness, skin rashes. Rise in level of transaminase enzymes in blood.

Manufacturer: Ciba.

Prestim

Description: an antihypertensive preparation which combines a non-cardioselective ß-blocker and thiazide diuretic available as white, scored tablets containing 10mg timolol maleate and 2.5mg bendrofluazide, marked with a lion and 132.

Also, **Prestim Forte** scored, white tablets containing 20mg timolol maleate and 5mg bendrofluazide, marked with a lion and 146.

Used for: hypertension.

Dosage: Prestim, 1 to 4 tablets each day. Prestim Forte, half dose.

Special care: pregnancy, breast-feeding, patients with weak hearts may require diuretics and digitalis, those with diabetes, undergoing general anaesthesia, kidney or liver disorders, gout. Electrolyte (salts) levels may need to be monitored.

Avoid use: history of bronchospasm or obstructive airways disease, heart block, heart shock, uncompensated heart failure, disease of peripheral arteries, bradycardia. Serious or worsening kidney failure or anuria.

Possible interaction: sympathomimetics, class I antiarrhythmics, central nervous system depressants, clonidine withdrawal, ergot alkaloids, cardiac depressant anaesthetics, verapamil, reserpine, indomethacin, hypoglycaemics, cimetidine, other antihypertensives. Digitalis, potassium supplements, potassium-sparing diuretics, lithium.

Side effects: cold hands and feet, disturbance of sleep, fatigue on exercise, bronchospasm, bradycardia, gastrointestinal disturbances, heart failure, blood changes, gout, sensitivity to light, muscle weakness. If skin rash or dry eyes occur, withdraw drug gradually.

Manufacturer: Leo.

Priadel

Description: an antidepressant preparation which is a lithium salt available as scored, white, continuous-release tablets in 2 strengths. Capsule-shaped tablets contain 200mg lithium carbonate marked P200. Tablets, marked PRIADEL, contain 400mg lithium carbonate. Also, **Priadel Liquid**, a sugar-free solution containing 520mg lithium citrate/5ml.

Used for: tablets, manic depression, mania, aggressive and self-harming behaviour, recurrent bouts of depression.

Dosage: tablets, 400–1200mg as a single dose each day at first; liquid 400–1200mg in 2 divided daily doses at first. Dosage then adjusted to maintain a certain blood level.

Special care: levels in blood must be monitored along with heart, kidney and thyroid function.

Avoid use: children, pregnancy, breast-feeding, hypothyroidism, Addison's disease, heart or kidney disorders, disturbance of salt balance.

Possible interaction: diazepam, metoclopramide, diuretics, flupenthixol, methyldopa, tetracyclines, phenytopin, haloperidol, NSAIDs, carbamazepine.

Side effects: trembling hands, diarrhoea, nausea, disturbance of ECG and central nervous system, gain in weight, hypo and hyperthyroidism, skin rashes, oedema, passing of large quantities of urine, thirstiness, oedema.

Manufacturer: Delandale.

Primacor

Description: a heart drug and phosphodiesterase inhibitors, which have a mode of action resembling stimulation by the sympathetic nervous system. Primacor is available in ampoules for injection containing 10mg milrinone/ml.

Used for: acute, postoperative heart failure after cardiac surgery; short-term treatment of congestive heart failure which has not responded to other drugs.

Dose: 50µg/kg body weight by slow intravenous injection over 10 minutes. Then by intravenous infusion at a rate of 375–750 nanograms/kg/minute. This is for up to 12 hours in postoperative patients and for 48–72 hours in those with congestive heart failure. The maximum daily dose is 1.13mg/kg.

Special care: certain types of heart failure associated with disease of heart valves and outflow obstruction. Patients with kidney disorder should receive reduced dose. Monitoring of fluid, electrolyte levels, blood pressure, central venous blood pressure, heart rate, ECG, liver enzymes, platelet counts must be carried out.

Side effects: unusual heart beats, hypotension, arrhythmias, vomiting, nausea, insomnia, headache, diarrhoea. Less commonly, chills, pains in limbs, reduced production of urine, urine retention, fever.

Manufacturer: Sanofi Winthrop.

Primalan

Description: an anti-allergic antihistamine preparation which is a phenothiazine type drug, available as white tablets containing 5mg mequitazine marked PRIMALAN.

Used for: hay fever, itching, urticaria, inflammation of the nose.

Dosage: 1 tablet twice each day.

Avoid use: pregnancy, liver disease, enlarged prostate gland, epilepsy.

Possible interaction: central nervous system depressants, some sympathomimetics (indirect acting), alcohol, MAOIs.

Side effects: sleepiness, impaired reactions, extrapyramidal responses, anticholinergic side effects.

Manufacturer: Theraplix.

Primaxin IV

Description: an antibiotic compound preparation, combining a carbapenem and enzyme inhibitor. It is available as 250mg or 500mg of powder in vials for reconstitution and injection, containing equal parts of imipenem (as monohydrate) and cilastin (as sodium salt). Also, **Primaxin IM**, a preparation containing 500mg cilastin and 500mg imipenem as powder in vials for reconstitution and intramuscular injection.

Used for: septicaemia, bone, skin, joint, soft tissue infections, infections of urinary, genital and lower respiratory tracts, abdominal and gynaecological infections. Also, prevention of infection after surgery.

Dosage: adults, Primaxin IV, 250 mg–1g by intravenous infusion every 6 to 8 hours, depending upon nature and severity of infection. Prevention of infection, 1g when patient is anaesthetized followed by a further 1g dose 3 hours later. Primaxin, depending upon nature and severity of infection, in the order of 500–750mg by deep intramuscular injection. Maximum dose is 1.5g each day. Patients with gonococcal inflammation and infection of urethra or cervix receive 500mg as a single dose. Children, Primaxin IV only, age over 3 months, 15mg/kg body weight every 6 hours, the maximum daily dose being 2g.

Special care: pregnancy, breast-feeding, patients with kidney disorders, gastrointestinal diseases (especially inflammation of bowel), those with known allergy to penicillin.

Avoid use: children under 3 months.

Possible interaction: ganciclovir, probenecid.

Side effects: diarrhoea, colitis (inflammation of the large intestine or bowel), nausea, vomiting, blood changes. Disturbance of central nervous system, convulsions, rise in level of liver enzymes, creatinine and urea in blood.

Manufacturer: M.S.D.

Primolut N

Description: an hormonal progestogen preparation available as white tablets containing 5mg norethisterone marked AN inside a hexagon shape.

Used for: abnormal menstrual bleeding, other menstrual disorders, postponement of menstruation, endometriosis.

Dosage: adults, heavy menstrual bleeding, 1 tablet twice or 3 times each day from day 19 to day 26 of cycle. Postponement of menstruation, 1 tablet 3 times each day, beginning 3 days before expected start of period. Endometriosis, 2 tablets each day beginning on fifth day of cycle, increasing to 4 or 5 daily if spotting takes place. 2 tablets each day should be taken for at least 4 to 6 months.

Special care: migraine or epilepsy.

Avoid use: pregnancy, history of itching or idiopathic jaundice during pregnancy, serious liver disorders, Dublin-Johnson and Rotor syndromes..

Side effects: disturbance of liver function, masculinization.

Manufacturer: Schering H.C.

Primoteston Depot

Description: an hormonal preparation of a depot androgen available as a solution in ampoules for injection containing 250mg testosterone oenanthate/ml.

Used for: underactivity of testes, breast cancer.

Dosage: underactivity of testes, 250mg by intramuscular injection every 2 or 3 weeks. Same for maintenance once every 2 or 3 weeks. Female breast cancer, 200mg by intramuscular injection every 2 weeks.

Special care: epilepsy, migraine, hypertension heart, kidney or liver disease.

Avoid use: liver or prostate cancer, untreated heart failure, heart disease due to insufficient blood supply.

Possible interaction: drugs that induce liver enzymnes.

Side effects: weight gain, oedema, liver tumours. Males, decrease in fertility, premature closure of epiphyses, priapism (abnormal, prolonged and painful erection of penis, not associated with sexual arousal but with underlying disorder or caused by a drug). Females, masculinization, withdraw drug if hypercalcaemia occurs.

Manufacturer: Schering H.C.

Pro-Banthine

Description: an anticholinergic preparation available as sugar-coated, peach-coloured tablets containing 15mg propantheline bromide.

Used for: peptic ulcer, irritable bowel syndrome, enuresis (incontinence of urine).

Dosage: ulcer, 1 tablet 3 times each day taken before

meals, and 2 at bedtime; irritable bowel syndrome, up to 8 tablets each day in divided doses. Enuresis, 1 to 2 tablets 3 times each day, with a daily maximum of 8 in divided doses.

Special care: elderly, liver or kidney disease, ulcerative colitis, serious heart disease, degenerative disease of autonomic nervous system.

Avoid use: children, patients with glaucoma, obstruction of gastrointestinal or urinary tracts.

Possible interaction: digoxin.

Side effects: anticholinergic side effects.

Manufacturer: Baker Norton.

Pro-Viron

Description: an hormonal androgen preparation available as white, scored tablets containing 25mg mesterolone.

Used for: androgen deficiency, male infertility.

Dosage: 25mg 3 or 4 times each day redcued to 50–70mg in divided doses as a daily maintenance dose.

Special care: elderly patients with kidney or liver disorders, epilepsy, secondary bone cancers (risk of hypercalcaemia, hypertension, ischaemic heart diesease). Boys before age of puberty.

Avoid use: kidney disorder, hypercalcaemia, breast cancer in men, prostate cancer.

Possible interaction: liver-inducing enzymes.

Side effects: premature closure of epiphyses in boys before puberty, precocious sexual development in boys, suppression of sperm production in men, hypercalcaemia. Increase in bone growth, priapism (prolonged, painful erection of penis not associated with sexual arousal but symptom of underlying disorder or drug), oedema with salt retention.

Manufacturer: Schering Health.

Procainamide Durules

Description: a class I antiarrhythmic drug available as pale yellow, sustained-release tablets containing 500mg procainamide hydrochloride.

Used for: heart arrhythmias, some disorders of muscles.

Dosage: usually 2 to thee tablets 3 times each day.

Special care: heart, liver or kidney failure. Regular blood tests required.

Avoid use: patients with myasthenia gravis, SLE, heart block, asthma.

Side effects: effects on CNS, blood changes, SLE, gastrointestinal upset.

Manufacturer: Astra.

Proctofoam H.C.

Description: a colorectal preparation combining a steroid and local anaesthetic available as an aerosol foam containing 1% hydrocortisone acetate and 1% pramoxine hydrochloride with applicator.

Used for: haemorrhoids, anal fissures, proctitis (inflammation of rectum and anus), cryptitis (inflammation of a crypt—a blind pit or small sac in the anal region).

Dosage: 1 applicator dose into the rectum 2 or 3 times each day and after passing stool. Apply to external anal area as needed.

Special care: pregnancy, short-term use only.

Avoid use: children, patients with fungal, viral or tuberculous infections.

Side effects: systemic corticosteroid side effects.

Manufacturer: Stafford-Miller.

Proctosedyl

Description: a colorectal preparation combining a steroid and local anaesthetic available as suppositories containing hydrochloride. Also, **Proctosedyl Ointment** containing 0.5% hydrocortisone and 0.5% cinchocaine hydrochloride.

Used for: haemorrhoids, anal itching and inflammation.

Dosage: 1 suppository and/or 1 application of ointment in the morning and at night, and after passing motion.

Special care: pregnancy, short-term use only.

Avoid use: patients with fungal, viral or tuberculous infections.

Side effects: systemic corticosteroid side effects.

Manufacturer: Schering H.C.

Profasi

Description: a gonadotrophin preparation available as powder in ampoules along with solvent for reconstitution and injection in different strengths containing 500 units, 1000 units, 2000 units, 5000 units and 10,000 units chorionic gonadotrophin.

Used for: underactivity of testes (infertility), undescended testicles, female infertility due to lack of ovulation, superovulation for in vitro fertilization treatment.

Dosage: underactive testes, 2000 units twice each week; undescended testicles, 500–1000 units every other day. Females, lack of ovulation, up to 10,000 units in middle of monthly cycle; superovulation, up to 10,000 units. All doses in males given intramuscularly, in females by intramuscular or subcutaneous injection.

Special care: any other hormonal disorders should be corrected before treatment starts. Hormone levels in females require monitoring.

Side effects: oedema, allergic reactions, over-stimulation of ovaries.
Manufacturer: Serono.

Progesic
Description: an NSAID available as yellow tablets containing 200mg fenoprofen (as calcium salt) marked LILLY 4015.
Used for: pain, rheumatic and arthritic disorders including osteoarthritis, rheumatoid arthritis, ankylosing spondylitis.
Dosage: 200–600mg 3 or 4 times each day with a maximum of 3g daily.
Special care: pregnancy, breast-feeding, elderly, history of gastrointestinal bleeding or peptic ulcer, liver or kidney disease, heart failure.
Avoid use: children, allergy to aspirin or anti-inflammatory drug, severe kidney disease, asthma, persons taking anticoagulant medication.
Possible interaction: aspirin, loop diuretics, anticoagulants, sulphonylureas, hydantoins, phenobarbitone, quinolones.
Side effects: liver and kidney disorders, allergic reactions, gastrointestinal bleeding and intolerance.
Manufacturer: Lilly.

Progynova
Description: an hormonal oestrogen preparation available in the form of beige, sugar-coated tablets, containing 1mg and blue, containing 2mg oestradiol valerate respectively.
Used for: short-term treatment of menopausal symptoms.
Dosage: 1mg each day for 21 days then 7 tablet-free days. 2mg tablets should only be used when needed.
Special care:those at risk of thromboembolism, porphyria, multiple sclerosis, epilepsy, fibroids in the womb, migraine, tetany. Also, otosclerosis, gallstones, liver disease. Pelvic organs, breasts and blood pressure should be checked regularly during course of treatment.
Avoid use: pregnancy, breast-feeding, breast or other cancer of reproductive tract or 1 which is hormone-dependent. Also, thromboembolism-type disorders, undiagnosed vaginal bleeding or endometriosis, thrombophlebitis, heart, liver or kidney disease, Rotor or Dublin-Johnson syndrome.
Possible interaction: drugs which induce liver enzymes.
Side effects: enlargement and soreness of breasts, gastrointestinal upset, dizziness, breakthrough bleeding, headache, vomiting and nausea, weight gain.
Manufacturer: Schering H.C.

Proleukin
Description: a highly toxic drug which is a recombinant interleukin-2 available as a powder in vials for reconstitution and injection containing 18 million units aldesleukin.
Used for: secondary cancer of kidney cells in some patients.
Dosage: as individually directed by physician; by intravenous infusion.
Special care: for use in specialist cancer units only.
Possible interaction: antihypertensives.
Side effects: pulmonary oedema, hypotension, serious toxic effects on liver, kidneys, bone marrow, thyroid and central nervous system.
Manufacturer: EuroCetus.

Proluton Depot
Description: a depot hormonal preparation of a progestogen containing 250mg hydroxy-progesterone hexanoate/ml in ampoules for oily injection.
Used for: habitual abortion.
Dosage: 250–500mg by intramuscular injection each week during the first 5 months of pregnancy.
Special care: hypertension, kidney or heart disease.
Avoid use: pregnancy, liver disease, cancer of breast or reproductive tract, undiagnosed vaginal bleeding, porphyria, serious disease of the arteries.
Side effects: weight changes, oedema, disturbance of menstrual cycle and premenstrual symptoms, depression, discomfort in breasts, change in libido, urticaria, acne, baldness, unusual hair growth, anaphylactoid-type reactions. Sleepiness, insomnia; rarely, jaundice.
Manufacturer: Schering H.C.

Prominal^{CD}
Description: an anticonvulsant preparation and barbiturate available as white tablets containing 30mg, 60mg and 200mg methylphenobarbitone, marked P30, P60 and P200 respectively.
Used for: focal and grand mal epilepsy.
Dosage: 100–600mg each day, children 5–15mg/kg body weight each day.
Special care: kidney and liver disorders, serious lung insufficiency.
Avoid use: pregnancy, breast-feeding, elderly, patients who are debilitated, suffering from porphyria, pain which is not controlled, history of drug or alcohol abuse.
Possible interaction: CNS depressants, griseofulvin, alcohol, phenytoin, systemic steroids, chloramphenicol, rifampicin, metronidazole, anticoagulants of the coumarin type.

Side effects: headache, respiratory depression, dizziness, unsteadiness, sleepiness, confusion, agitation, allergic responses. Drug tolerance and dependence may occur. Drug is metabolized to phenobarbitone.
Manufacturer: Sanofi Winthrop.

Prondol

Description: a TCAD available as yellow tablets containing 15mg iprindole (as hydrochloride) marked WYETH.
Used for: depression.
Dosage: 15–30mg 3 times daily at first with a maximum of 60mg 3 times daily. Elderly start with 15mg 3 times daily.
Special care: liver disorders, hyperthyroidism, glaucoma, lactation, epilepsy, diabetes, adrenal tumour, heart disease, urine retention. Psychotic or suicidal patients.
Avoid use: children, heart block, heart attacks, severe liver disease, pregnancy.
Possible interaction: MAOIs (or within 14 days of their use), alcohol, anti-depressants, barbiturates, anticholinergics, local anaesthetics that contain adrenaline or noradrenaline, oestrogens, cimetidine, antihypertensives.
Side effects: constipation, urine retention, dry mouth, blurred vision, palpitations, tachycardia, nervousness, drowsiness, insomnia. Changes in weight, blood and blood sugar, jaundice, skin reactions, weakness, ataxia, hypotension, sweating, altered libido, gynaecomastia, galactorrhoea.
Manufacturer: Wyeth.

Pronestyl

Description: a class I antiarrhythmic preparation available as scored, white tablets containing 250mg procainamide hydrochloride marked SQUIBB 754. Also, **Pronestyl Injection,** a solution in vials containing 100mg procainamide hydrochloride/ml.
Used for: heart arrhythmias.
Dosage: tablets, up to 50mg/kg body weight each day as divided doses every 3 to 6 hours. Injection, for acute condition, rate not greater than 50mg/minute by slow intravenous injection (or 100mg with monitoring of ECG). This is repeated every 5 minutes until arrhythmia is controlled. Maximum dose 1g. By intravenous infusion, 500–600mg over 25 to 30 minutes while ECG is monitored. Then a maintenance dose of 2–6mg/minute followed by tablets, if needed, 3 to 4 hours after infusion has been given.
Special care: elderly persons, pregnant women, patients with heart or liver failure, myasthenia

gravis, regular blood tests should be carried out during the course of treatment.
Avoid use: children, SLE or heart block.
Possible interaction: other antiarrhythmics, terfenadine, astemizole, phenothiazines, cimetidine, neostigmine, pyridostigmine.
Side effects: SLE, blood changes (leucopenia and agranulocytosis—severe reduction in some white blood cells due to chemicals or drugs), gastrointestinal upset.
Manufacturer: Squibb.

Propaderm

Description: a potent topical steroid prepartion available as cream or ointment containing 0.025% beclomethasone dipropionate.
Used for: inflammatory skin conditions responsive to steroids.
Dosage: apply thinly to affected area twice each day.
Special care: thrombophlebitis, psychoses, recent intestinal anastomoses, chronic nephritis, certain cancers, osteoporosis, peptic ulcer, skin eruption/rash related to a disease, viral, fungal or active infections, tuberculosis. Hypertension, glaucoma, epilepsy, acute glomerulonephritis (inflammation of kidney glomerulus), diabetes, cirrhosis, hypothyroidism, pregnancy, stress. To be withdrawn gradually.
Possible interaction: NSAIDs, oral anticoagulants, phenytoin, ephedrine, phenobarbitone, rifampicin, diuretics, cardiac glycosides, anticholinesterases, hypoglycaemics.
Side effects: osteoporosis, depression, euphoria, hyperglycaemia, peptic ulcers, Cushingoid changes.
Manufacturer: Yamanouchi.

Propine

Description: a sympathomimetic preparation available as eyedrops containing 0.1% dipivefrin hydrochloride.
Used for: hypotension in eye, open angle glaucoma.
Dosage: adults, 1 drop into eye every 12 hours.
Special care: patients without whole or part of lens (aphakia) e.g. as in surgical removal of cataracts, narrow angle between iris and cornea of eye.
Avoid use: children, patients with closed angle glaucoma, wearing soft contact lenses.
Side effects: short-lived stinging, allergic responses, increased blood flow; rarely, raised blood pressure.
Manufacturer: Allergan.

Proscar

Description: a preparation which is a selective 5-

alpha reductase inhibitor available as film-coated, apple-shaped blue tablets containing 5mg finasteride marked with name and MSD.

Used for: benign enlargement of the prostate gland.

Dosage: 1 tablet each day for at least 6 months, then continuing long-term if condition is responding.

Special care: obstruction or disease of genital tract. Women may absorb drug via semen through sexual intercourse or by handling tablets—risk in pregnancy.

Avoid use: patients with prostate cancer.

Side effects: decreased libido, impotence, reduced volume of ejaculation possibly affecting fertility.

Manufacturer: M.S.D.

Prostap SR

Description: a gonadotrophin-releasing hormone analogue available as powder in microcapsule in vial with diluent for depot injection containing 3.75mg leuprorelin acetate.

Used for: advanced cancer of the prostate gland.

Dosage: 3.75mg as a single dose by subcutaneous or intramuscular injection each month.

Special care: patients may require additional treatment with an anti-androgen starting 2 or 3 days before Prostap is given and continuing for 2 to 3 weeks.

Special care: in patients at risk of compression of spinal cord or obstruction of ureter.

Side effects: short-lived bone pain and obstruction of urine, decreased libido, impotence; rarely, swelling of hand and feet due to oedema, decreased libido, nausea, fatigue.

Manufacturer: Lederle.

Prostigmin

Description: an anticholinesterase preparation available as scored, white tablets containing 15mg neostigmine bromide marked PROSTIGMIN. Also, **Prostigmin Injection** available in ampoules containing 2.5mg neostigmin methylsulphate.

Used for: myasthenia gravis, urine retention following surgery, paralytic ileus (decrease or absence of movement—peristalsis—along the intestine due to injury or surgery).

Dosage: urine retention, paralytic ileus, 1 to 2 tablets as needed; myasthenia gravis, 5 to 20 tablets in divided doses each day. Injection, urine retention, paralytic ileus 0.5–2.5mg by subcutaneous or intramuscular injection; myasthenia gravis, 1.0–2.5mg by subcutaneous or intramuscular injection. Children, urine retention, paralytic ileus, 2.5–15mg as required; myasthenia gravis, newborn babies, 1–5mg every 4 hours, other ages 15–90mg in divided doses each day. Injection, urine retention, paralytic ileus, 0.125–1mg by intramuscular or subcutaneous injection; myasthenia gravis, newborn babies, 50–250µg every 4 hours, 30 minutes before feeds. Other ages, 200–500µg as needed.

Special care: Parkinson's disease, asthma, heart disease, epilepsy, vagotonia (increased activity of and effects resulting from stimulation of vagus nerve).

Avoid use: patients with obstruction of intestine or urinary tract.

Possible interaction: cyclopropane, halothane, depolarizing muscle relaxants.

Side effects: vomiting, nausea, diarrhoea, pains in abdomen, overproduction of saliva.

Manufacturer: Roche.

Prostin E₂ Oral

Description: a prostaglandin preparation available as rectangular, white tablets containing 500µg dinoprostone marked 76 on one side and U on the other. Also, **Prostin E₂ Vaginal Tablets**, white tablets containing 3mg, marked 715 and UPJOHN. **Prostin E₂ Solutions**, alcoholic solution in ampoules in 2 strengths containing 1mg and 10mg/ml. **Prostin E₂ Vaginal Gel**, in 2 strengths containing 1mg and 2mg/3g gel.

Used for: induction of labour.

Dosage: tablets, 500µg then 0.5–1mg hourly, the maximum dose being 1.5mg. Vaginal tablets, 3mg inserted high into vagina followed by further 3mg 6 to 8 hours later if labour has not begun. Maximum dose is 6mg. Vaginal gel, 1mg intravaginally at first followed by further 1–2mg after 6 hours if labour has not begun. Maximum dose is 3mg; (exceptionally, 4mg maximum dose may be needed).

Special care: higher doses may cause rupture of uterus, should not be given for more than 2 days. Glaucoma, raised pressure within eye, asthma.

Avoid use: previous history of difficult or traumatic birth, multiple pregnancy, risk of uterine rupture, obstruction or failure of uterine contractions, untreated pelvic infections, foetal distress, serious toxaemia.

Side effects: vomiting, diarrhoea, nausea, dizziness, headache, shivering, flushing, temporary fever, raised white blood cell count, exceptionally high muscle tone of uterus, very severe contractions.

Manufacturer: Upjohn.

Prostin F₂

Description: a prostaglandin available as a solution in ampoules for injection into amniotic fluid containing 5mg dinoprost (as tromethamine salt)/ml.

Used for: induction of labour—rarely used.

Special care: higher doses may cause rupture of uterus, should not be given for more than 2 days. Patients with vaginitis or cervicitis (inflammation of vagina or cervix), glaucoma, raised pressure within eye, asthma.

Avoid use: previous history of difficult or traumatic birth, multiple pregnancy, risk of uterine rupture, obstruction or failure of uterine contractions, untreated pelvic infections, foetal distress, serious toxaemia.

Side effects: vomiting, diarrhoea, nausea, dizziness, headache, shivering, flushing, temporary fever, raised white blood cell count, exceptionally high muscle tone of uterus, very severe contractions.

Manufacturer: Upjohn.

Prostin VR

Description: a prostaglandin preparation available as an alcoholic solution in ampoules for infusion containing 0.5mg alprostadil/ml.

Used for: newborn babies with congenital heart defects, before corrective surgery.

Dosage: 50–100 nanograms/kg body weight/minute at first then lowest effective dose.

Special care: risk of haemorrhage, arterial blood pressure must be monitored.

Avoid use: newborn babies with hyaline membrane disease (respiratory distress syndrome) in which lungs are not properly expanded, (usually premature infants between 32 and 37 weeks of gestation).

Side effects: apnoea (especially babies less than 2kg body weight), hypotension, oedema, fever, diarrhoea, tachycardia and bradycardia, flushing, convulsions, cardiac arrest. Effects on blood, weakening of walls of pulmonary artery and ductus arteriosus.

Manufacturer: Upjohn.

Prothiaden

Description: a TCAD preparation available as brown/red capsules containing 25mg dothiepin hydrochloride marked P25. Also, **Prothiaden Tablets**, sugar-coated red tablets containing 75mg dothiepin hydrochloride marked P75.

Used for: depression and anxiety.

Dosage: adults, 75–150mg each day either as divided doses or taken as single dose at night.

Special care: liver disorders, hyperthyroidism, glaucoma, lactation, epilepsy, diabetes, adrenal tumour, heart disease, urine retention. Psychotic or suicidal patients.

Avoid use: children, heart block, heart attacks, severe liver disease, pregnancy.

Possible interaction: MAOIs (or within 14 days of their use), alcohol, antidepressants, barbiturates, anticholinergics, local anaesthetics that contain adrenaline or noradrenaline, oestrogens, cimetidine, antihypertensives.

Side effects: constipation, urine retention, dry mouth, blurred vision, palpitations, tachycardia, nervousness, drowsiness, insomnia. Changes in weight, blood and blood sugar, jaundice, skin reactions, weakness, ataxia, hypotension, sweating, altered libido, gynaecomastia, galactorrhoea.

Manufacturer: Boots.

Provera

Description: an hormonal progestogen preparation available as scored tablets in 3 strengths all containing medroxyprogesterone acetate. Orange, 2.5mg, marked U64; blue, 5mg, marked 286; white, 10mg, marked Upjohn 50.

Used for: abnormal uterine bleeding, endometriosis, secondary ammenorrhoea (situation where menstrual periods stop due to underlying physical, psychiatric or environmental factors). Breast cancer in women after menopause, renal cell and endometrial cancer.

Dosage: abnormal uterine bleeding 2.5–10mg each day for 5 to 10 days, repeated for 2 or 3 monthly cycles. Endometriosis, 10mg 3 times each day starting on first day of cycle and and continuing for 90 days without a break. Ammenorrhoea, 2.5–10mg each day for 5 to 10 days beginning on what is thought to be 16th continuing to 21st day of cycle. Repeat for 3 monthly cycles without break. Breast cancer, 400–800mg each day, renal cell and endometrial cancer, 200–400 mg daily.

Special care: diabetes, asthma, heart or kidney disorders, migraine, history of depression.

Avoid use: pregnancy, cancer of genital tract, liver disease, history of or present thromboembolic conditions.

Side effects: gain in weight, abnormal production of breast milk, slight oedema, breast pain. Gastrointestinal upset, central nervous system effects, skin and mucous membrane reactions.

Manufacturer: Upjohn.

Prozac

Description: an antidepressant preparation which is a 5HT reuptake inhibitor, promoting the availability of this neurotransmitter. It is available as white/green capsules containing 20mg fluoxetine hydrochloride marked DISTA 3105. Also, **Prozac Liquid**, a syrup containing 20mg/5ml.

Used for: depression especially when sedation is not needed. Obsessive-compulsive disorders, bulimia nervosa (over-eating phase of anorexia nervosa).

Dosage: depression, usual dose in the order of 20mg each day; obsessive compulsive disorder, 20–60mg each day; bulimia nervosa, 60mg each day.

Special care: pregnancy, heart disease, epilepsy, diabetes, kidney disorder, liver failure, heart disease.

Avoid use: children, breast-feeding, severe kidney failure, unstable epilepsy.

Possible interaction: vinblastine, MAOIs, lithium, carbamazepine, TCADs, flecainide, encainide, tryptophan.

Side effects: diarrhoea, vomiting, nausea, insomnia, headache, dizziness, drowsiness, anxiety, weakness, fever, hypomania, convulsions, mania. Withdraw drug if allergic reactions or rash occur.

Manufacturer: Dista.

Pulmadil

Description: a bronchodilator which is a selective beta$_2$-agonist available as a metered dose aerosol delivering 0.2mg rimiterol hydrobromide per dose.

Used for: bronchospasm resulting from chronic bronchitis and bronchial asthma.

Dosage: 1 to 3 doses which can be repeated after half an hour, if needed. Maximum of 24 doses in 24 hours.

Special care: pregnancy, weak heart, arrhythmias, angina, hyperthyroidism, hypertension.

Possible interaction: sympathomimetics.

Side effects: dilation of peripheral blood vessels, headache.

Manufacturer: 3M Health Care.

Pulmicort

Description: a bronchodilator corticosteroid preparation delivering 200µg budesonide per metered dose aerosol, suitable for use with a standard inhaler, nebuhaler or collapsible space delivery unit. Also, **Pulmicort LS** delivering 50µg per dose. **Pulmicort Turbohaler** for use with a powder inhaler delivering 100, 200 or 400µg budesonide per metered dose. **Pulmicort Respules** available at strengths of 0.25mg and 0.5mg per ml available in ampoules for nebulization.

Used for: bronchial asthma.

Dosage: Pulmicort, 1 puff twice daily up to 8 puffs daily in severe attack. Pulmicort turbohaler 200–1600µg in divided doses daily. Pulmicort respules, in the order of 1–2mg twice each day with a maintenance dose of 0.5–1mg twice daily. Children, Pulmicort, 1 to 2 puffs twice each day. Pulmicort LS (children only), 1 to 8 puffs each day. **Pulmicort** turbohaler, 200–800µg in divided doses daily. Pulmicort respules, age 3 months to 12 years, 0.5–1mg twice each day with a maintenance dose of 0.25–0.5mg twice daily.

Special care: pregnancy, pulmonary tuberculosis either active or statis, those transferring from other (systemic) steroids.

Side effects: candidiasis of throat and mouth, dryness and hoarseness.

Manufacturer: Astra.

Pump-Hep

Description: an anticoagulant preparation of sodium heparin available in single dose ampoules for continuous infusion, at a strength of 1000 units/ml.

Used for: pulmonary embolism and deep vein thrombosis.

Dosage: 15,000 units; children 250 units/kg body weight, both 12 hourly. Both following on from first doses given by intravenous infusion or injection.

Special care: pregnancy, kidney or liver disease. Drug should be withdrawn gradually if taken for more than 5 days. Platelet counts are required if taken for more than 5 days.

Avoid use: patients with bleeding disorders, haemophilia, serious hypertension, recent operation on eye or nervous system, cerebral aneurysm, serious liver disease, peptic ulcer, allergy to heparin, thrombocytopenia.

Possible interaction: aspirin, dipyridamole, glyceryl trinitrate infusion.

Side effects: allergic reactions, skin necrosis, osteoporosis (if taken long-term). Stop drug immediately if thrombocytopenia occurs.

Manufacturer: Leo.

Puri-Nethol

Description: a cytotoxic drug available as scored, fawn-coloured tablets containing 50mg mercaptopurine coded WELLCOME 04A.

Used for: leukaemia, especially in children.

Dosage: adults and children, 2.5mg/kg bod yweight each day at first, used for maintenance treatment.

Special care: pregnancy, kidney disorder. Dosage should be reduced if allopurinol is also being received.

Possible interaction: allopurinol, warfarin.

Side effects: vomiting, nausea, bone marrow suppression, anorexia, toxic effects on liver.

Manufacturer: Wellcome.

Pyopen

Description: an antibiotic preparation of penicillin

available as powder in vials for reconstitution and injection containing 1g and 5g carbenicillin sodium.

Used for: endocarditis, meningitis, septicaemia, infected burns and wounds, urinary and respiratory tract infections, sepsis within abdomen, infections following operations.

Dosage: by rapid infusion, 5g every 4 to 6 hours; children, 250–400mg/kg body weight in divided doses each day.

Special care: kidney disorders.

Side effects: gastrointestinal upset, allergic hypersensitivity reactions, hypokalaemia, change in function of blood platelets.

Manufacturer: Link.

Pyrogastrone

Description: a compound preparation combining an antacid and cytoprotectant available as off-white tablets containing 20mg carbenoxolone sodium, 60mg magnesium trisilicate, 600mg alginic acid, 240mg dried aluminium hydroxide, 210mg sodium bicarbonate marked PG and with symbol. Also, **Pyrogastrone Liquid** containing 10mg carbenoxolone sodium, 150mg dried aluminium hydroxide/5ml.

Used for: gastro-oesophageal reflux, oesophagitis.

Dosage: 1 tablet or 10ml suspension 3 times each day after meals plus 2 tablets or 20ml suspension at bedtime.

Special care: patients with fluid and salt retention.

Avoid use: pregnancy, children, elderly, hypokalaemia, liver or kidney failure.

Possible interaction: diuretics, digoxin.

Side effects: hypertension, heart failure, hypokalaemia, retention of water and salt.

Manufacturer: Sanofi Winthrop.

Q

Questran A

Description: a bile acid sequestrant available as a low sugar powder in sachets containing 4g cholestyramine. Also, **Questran**, powder in sachets containing 4g cholestyramine.

Used for: diarrhoea resulting from surgery, radiation, Crohn's disease, damage or disease of vagus nerve, itching resulting from liver disease. Also, prevention of coronary heart disease in men with very high lipid/cholesterol levels in the blood who are aged between 35 and 59. Treatment of type II hyperlipoproteinaemias (high levels of lipid-bound proteins).

Dosage: diarrhoea and elevated lipid and lipid/protein levels, 1 sachet each day at first gradually increasing to 3 to 6 each day after 3 or 4 weeks, taken as single or divided doses; daily maximum is 9 sachets. Itching, 1 or 2 sachets daily; children over 6 years of age, dose in proportion to that of adult weighing 70kg.

Special care: pregnancy, breast-feeding, dietary supplements of vitamins A, D amd K may be needed with high doses taken long term, patients with phenylketonuria (abnormal presence of phenylketones in urine) taking Questran A. Any other drugs should be taken 1 hour before Questran A or 4 hours afterwards.

Avoid use: children under 6 years of age, total obstruction of bile duct.

Possible interaction: antibiotics, digitalis, diuretics.

Side effects: increased tendency for bleeding in patients taking drug long-term due to deficiency in vitamin K, constipation.

Manufacturer: Bristol-Myers.

Quinocort

Description: a topical preparation combining a mildly potent steroid and antifungal, antibacterial agent available as a cream containing 0.5% potassium hydroxyquinolone sulphate and 1% hydrocortisone.

Used for: inflammatory, infected skin conditions responsive to steroids.

Dosage: apply thinly 2 or 3 times each day.

Special care: thrombophlebitis, psychoses, recent intestinal anastomoses, chronic nephritis, certain cancers, osteoporosis, peptic ulcer, skin eruption/rash related to a disease, viral, fungal or active infections, tuberculosis. Hypertension, glaucoma, epilepsy, acute glomerulonephritis (inflammation of kidney glomerulus), diabetes, cirrhosis, hypothyroidism, pregnancy, stress. To be withdrawn gradually.

Possible interaction: NSAIDs, oral anticoagulants, phenytoin, ephedrine, phenobarbitone, rifampicin, diuretics, cardiac glycosides, anticholinesterases, hypoglycaemics.

Side effects: osteoporosis, depression, euphoria, hyperglycaemia, peptic ulcers, Cushingoid changes.

Manufacturer: Quinoderm.

R

Rapifen^{CD}

Description: a narcotic analgesic and controlled drug, alfentanil hydrochloride, available in ampoules containing 500µg/ml. Also **Rapifen Intensive Care** (5mg/ml).

Used for: analgesia during short operations, enhancement of anaesthesia, suppression of respiration for patients in intensive care receiving assistance with ventilation.

Dosage: 500µg over 30 seconds to start then 250µg; with assisted ventilation (for adult and child) 30–50µg/kg then 15µg/kg, all by intravenous injection. 50–100µg/kg over 10 minutes by intravenous infusion for adult or child with assisted ventilation. For analgesia and respiratory suppression, 2mg/hour adjusted according to response.

Special care: myasthenia gravis, elderly, liver disease, pregnancy, respiratory disease.

Avoid use: respiratory depression, diseases causing obstruction of the airways.

Possible interaction: erythromycin, anxiolytics and hypnotics, cimetidine, cisapride, antidepressants.

Side effects: respiratory depression, temporary hypotension, nausea, vomiting, bradycardia.

Manufacturer: Janssen.

Rastinon

Description: a sulphonylurea, tolbutamide, available as white tablets (500mg) marked with symbol and RASTINON 0.5.

Used for: maturity-onset diabetes.

Dosage: 2 per day at the start, adjusted depending upon response. Maintenance dose of 1 to 3 per day as a single or divided dose. Not for children.

Special care: the elderly or patients with kidney failure.

Avoid use: during pregnancy or lactation; juvenile, growth-onset or unstable brittle diabetes (insulin-dependent diabetes mellitus); ketoacidosis; severe kidney or liver disorders; stress, infections or surgery; endocrine disorders.

Possible interaction: MAOIs, corticosteroids, ß-blockers, diuretics, corticotrophin (ACTH), oral contraceptives, alcohol. Also aspirin, oral anticoagulants, and the generic drugs bezafibrate, clofibrate, phenylbutazone, cyclophosphamide, rifampicin, sulphonamides and chloramphenicol. Also glucagon.

Side effects: skin rash and other sensitivity reactions. Other conditions tend to be rare, e.g. hyponatraemia (low blood sodium concentration) or aplastic anaemia.

Manufacturer: Hoechst.

Razoxin

Description: a cytotoxic and antineoplastic drug, razoxone, available as white tablets (125mg), marked ICI.

Used for: leukaemias.

Dosage: 150–500mg/m² per day for 3 to 5 days.

Side effects: nausea, vomiting, bone marrow suppression, hair loss, suppression of the immune system, teratogenic.

Manufacturer: Zeneca.

Recormon

Description: recombinant human erythropoietin (hormone-regulating red blood cell production) available as powder in vials (1000, 2000, 5000 units epoetin beta).

Used for: anaemia in patients with chronic kidney failure and on dialysis.

Dosage: 20 units/kg 3 times per week for 4 weeks, by subcutaneous injection, or 40 units/kg by intravenous injection with the same frequency. Dose may be doubled depending upon haemoglobin response. May be increased by 20 units/kg at monthly intervals to a maximum of 720 units/kg per week. For maintenance, reduce the dosage to half and adjust weekly. Children over 2 as per adults; not recommended for children under 2.

Special care: history of epilepsy, thrombocytosis (increase in blood platelet count giving an increased tendency to blood clots), hypertension, chronic liver failure, pregnancy, lactation. May need iron supplements, check haemoglobin, blood pressure, platelet count and serum electrolytes.

Side effects: symptoms resembling flu,

hypertension, clotting in atrio-ventricular fistula.
Manufacturer: B.M. Pharm.

Redeptin
Description: an antipsychotic and diphenylbutylpiperidine, fluspirilene, available as 2mg/ml in ampoules and 6ml vials.
Used for: schizophrenia.
Dosage: starting with 2mg per week by intramuscular injection increasing as necessary by 2mg per week to a maximum of 20mg. Dose for maintenance, 2–8mg per week. Elderly, start with 0.5mg per week and adjust depending upon response. Not for children.
Special care: lactation, epilepsy, liver or kidney disease, Parkinson's disease.
Avoid use: pregnancy.
Possible interaction: alcohol, depressants of the CNS, antihypertensives, antidepressants, analgesics, antidiabetics, levodopa, anticonvulsants.
Side effects: rigidity, tremor, dry mouth, muscle spasms in eye, neck, face and back, tardive dyskinesia (involuntary, repetitive muscle movements in the limbs, face and trunk), tachycardia, constipation, blocked nose, difficulty in urinating, hypotension, weight gain, impotence, galactorrhoea, gynaecomastia, blood changes, jaundice, dermatitis, ECG changes, fatigue, drowsiness, seizures.
Manufacturer: S.H. & F.

Refolinon
Description: Folinic acid (as a calcium salt) available as pale yellow tablets (15mg) marked F and CF.
Used for: megaloblastic anaemia, antidote or rescue after treatment with methotrexate.
Dosage: 1 tablet daily for anaemia, see literature for antidote use.
Also, **Refolinon Injection**, containing 3mg/ml.
Avoid use: vitamin B12 deficiency anaemia.
Manufacturer: Farmitalia.

Regaine
Description: a hair restorer, minoxidil, available as a liquid containing 20mg/ml.
Used for: alopecia.
Dosage: 1ml applied to the scalp 2 times per day for at least 4 months. Hair loss will recur if treatment ceases.
Special care: hypotension, broken skin, check blood pressure in susceptible patients.
Side effects: dermatitis.
Manufacturer: Upjohn.

Relifex
Description: an NSAID and naphthylalkanone, nabumetone, available as red tablets (500mg) marked RELIFEX 500. Also, **Relifex Suspension** (500mg/5ml).
Used for: rheumatoid arthritis and osteoarthritis.
Dosage: 2 tablets or 10ml as 1 dose at bedtime. An extra 1 to 2 tablets or 5–10ml may be taken in the morning for severe cases. Elderly, 1 to 2 tablets or 5–10ml per day. Not for children.
Special care: elderly, allergy-induced by aspirin or anti-inflammatory drugs, liver or kidney disease, history of peptic ulcer.
Avoid use: active peptic ulcer, pregnancy, breast-feeding, severe liver disease.
Possible interaction: sulphonylurea, hypo-glycaemics, hydantoin, oral anticoagulants, anticonvulsants.
Side effects: nausea, diarrhoea, abdominal pain, dyspepsia, constipation, headache, dizziness, rashes, sedation.
Manufacturer: Bencard.

Remedeine
Description: an analgesic containing 500mg paracetamol, 20mg dihydrocodeine tartrate in white tablets marked PD/20. Also, **Remedeine Forte** containing 500mg paracetamol and 30mg dihydrocodeine tartrate in white tablets marked PD/30.
Used for: severe pain.
Dosage: 1 to 2 tablets 4 to 6 hourly up to a daily maximum of 8 tablets. Not for children.
Special care: chronic liver disease, hypothyroidism, allergies, kidney disease.
Avoid use: raised intracranial pressure, depression of respiration, diseases causing obstruction of the respiratory tract.
Possible interaction: alcohol, MAOIs.
Side effects: nausea, vomiting, drowsiness, headache, vertigo, constipation, retention of urine.
Manufacturer: Napp.

Respacal
Description: a ß2-agonist and bronchodilator, tulobuterol hydrochloride, available as white tablets (2mg) marked ucb.
Used for: prevention and control of bronchospasm in asthma.
Dosage: 1 tablet twice per day increasing to 3 times per day if required. Children over 10 years, 1/2 to 1 tablet twice per day. Not for children under 10.
Also, **Respacal Syrup**, 1mg per 5ml.
Dosage: 10ml 2 or 3 times perday. Children over 10

years, 5–10ml; 6 to 10 years, 2.5–5ml both twice per day. Not for children under 6.

Special care: epilepsy, hypertension, hyperthyroidism, diabetes, disease of the heart and blood vessels.

Avoid use: acute liver failure or chronic liver disease, kidney failure.

Side effects: tremor, palpitations, tachycardia, possible serious hypokalaemia.

Manufacturer: UCB.

Restandol

Description: an androgen, testosterone undecanoate, available as brown, oval gelatin capsules (40mg strength), marked ORG and DV3.

Used for: osteoporosis caused by androgen deficiency, deficiency in the male of the secretory activity of the testis whether due to castration or other disorder.

Dosage: starting with 3 to 4 capsules per day for 2 to 3 weeks, adjusting to 1 to 3 depending upon response.

Special care: epilepsy, hypertension, heart, liver or kidney disease, migraine.

Avoid use: untreated heart failure, cancer of the liver or prostate, abnormal condition of the kidney (nephrosis/nephrotic syndrome), ischaemic heart disease.

Possible interaction: drugs that induce liver enzymes.

Side effects: oedema, weight increase, tumours of the liver, lower fertility, premature epiphyseal closure, extended erection of the penis not associated with sexual arousal.

Manufacturer: Organon.

Retin-A

Description: a vitamin A derivative, tretinoin available as a 0.025% lotion. Also, **Retin-A Gel** (0.01% and 0.025%), **Retin-A Cream** (0.025% and 0.05%).

Used for: acne vulgaris (common in adolescents) where there are pustules, papules (solid, raised lesion less than 1cm across) and comedones (blackheads).

Dosage: apply once or twice per day for at least 8 weeks. Not for children.

Special care: pregnancy, avoid UV light.

Avoid use: eczema, abrasions, cuts. Do not get on eyes or mucous membranes.

Possible interaction: keratolytics.

Side effects: irritation, erythema, alteration to skin pigmentation.

Manufacturer: Cilag.

Retrovir

Description: an antiviral compound, zidovudine, available as white capsules (100mg) marked 100 and Y9C and white/blue capsules (250mg) marked 250 and H2F. Both bear the company logo and a blue securiband. Also, **Retovir Syrup**, 50mg/5ml, a pale-yellow strawberry-flavoured solution.

Used for: treatment of HIV virus infections.

Dosage: adults (asymptomatic) 500–1500mg per day in 4 or 5 divided doses; 6 200mg per day if tolerable for symptomatic HIV. Children over 3 months, 180mg/m^2 4 times per day. Not for children under 3 months.

Special care: blood tests every 2 weeks for the first 3 months, then monthly. Alter dose should there be anaemia or bone marrow suppression. Kidney or liver disease, elderly, pregnancy.

Avoid use: low neutrophil (white blood cell) counts or low levels of haemoglobin, lactation.

Possible interaction: analgesics (paracetamol particularly), potentially nephroptoxics or bone marrow suppressives, probenecid, methadone, drugs affecting liver activity. Warn patients about accompanying use of self-administered drugs.

Side effects: neutropenia, leucopenia, nausea, anaemia, abdominal pain and gastrointestinal disturbances, fever, rash, headache, muscle pain, insomnia, numbness or tingling sensations.

Manufacturer: Wellcome.

Revanil

Description: a dopamine agonist, lysuride maleate, available as white tablets (200µg) marked CM in a hexagon.

Used for: Parkinson's disease.

Dosage: start with 1 tablet at bedtime with food increasing weekly by 1 tablet daily to a maximum of 25 daily. Not for children.

Special care: pregnancy, tumour of the pituitary.

Avoid use: weak heart, disturbance of peripheral circulation.

Possible interaction: dopamine antagonists, psychotropics (affecting behaviour and psychic functions).

Side effects: nausea, vomiting, hypotension, headache, dizziness, lethargy, drowsiness, abdominal pain, constipation, psychiatric reactions.

Manufacturer: Roche.

Rheumox

Description: a benzotriazine and NSAID, azapropazone dihydrate, available as orange capsules (300mg) marked RHEUMOX and AHR. Also, **Rheumox Tablets** containing 600mg in orange, oblong tablets marked RHEUMOX 600.

Used for: gout, hyperuricaemia (high blood uric acid), rheumatoid arthritis, osteoarthritis, ankylosing spondylitis.

Dosage: acute gout, 2.4g in divided doses over 24 hours then 1.8g per day and 1.2g per day; 600mg morning and night for chronic gout. For other conditions, 1.2g per day in 2 or 4 divided doses. Elderly, 300mg morning and night up to a maximum of 900mg per day if kidneys function normally. Not for children.

Special care: pregnancy, heart failure, elderly, liver or kidney disease (monitor if on long-term treatment), past peptic ulcer.

Avoid use: kidney disorder, past blood changes, peptic ulcer.

Possible interaction: sulphonamides, hypoglycaemics, anticoagulants, methotrexate, phenytoin.

Side effects: oedema, gastrointestinal bleeding, sensitivity to light, alveolitis (allergic lung reaction to substances inhaled). Discontinue upon a positive Coomb's test (antiglobulin test—an antibody against globulin).

Manufacturer: Wyeth.

Rhinocort

Description: a corticosteroid, budesonide, available as a metered dose (50µg) nasal aerosol.

Used for: rhinitis.

Dosage: apply twice to each nostril twice per day, reducing to 1 application twice daily. Not recommended for long-term continuous treatment for children.

Also, **Rhinocort Aqua**, a 100µg metered pump nasal spray.

Dosage: start with 2 applications in each nostril every morning; 1 application for maintenance. Not for children.

Special care: pregnancy, infections of a fungal, viral or tuberculous nature.

Side effects: sneezing.

Manufacturer: Astra.

Rhinolast

Description: an antihistamine, azelastine hydrochloride, available as a 0.1% metered dose nasal spray.

Used for: rhinitis.

Dosage: 1 application per nostril twice per day. Not for children.

Special care: pregnancy, breast-feeding.

Side effects: nasal irritation, effect on taste.

Manufacturer: ASTA Medica.

Ridaura

Description: a gold salt, auranofin, available as pale yellow square tablets (3mg).

Used for: progressive rheumatoid arthritis no controlled by NSAIDs.

Dosage: start with 6mg per day and continue for 3 to 6 months minimum. Dosage can be increased to 3mg 3 times per day if response is inadequate. Cease after a further 3 months if response still inadequate. Not for children.

Special care: kidney and liver disorders, rash, past bone marrow depression, bowel inflammation. Blood and urinary protein should be monitored before and during treatment. Women should use effective contraception during and 6 months after treatment.

Avoid use: past necrotising enterocolitis (an acute inflammatory bowel disorder affecting large and small intestines), exfoliative dermatitis, severe blood disorders, kidney disease, severe liver disease, SLE, pregnancy, breast-feeding, pulmonary fibrosis.

Side effects: nausea, abdominal pain, diarrhoea, rashes, itching, hair loss, ulcerative enterocolitis, inflammation of the mouth (stomatitis), conjunctivitis, nephrotic syndrome (oedema, low protein in the urine and low blood albumin levels), upset to taste.

Manufacturer: Bencard.

Rifadin

Description: an antibiotic and antimalarial, rifampicin, available as blue/red capsules (150mg) and red capsules (300mg), marked LEPETIT. Also, **Rifadin Syrup** (100mg/5ml) and **Rifadin Infusion** as 600mg powder in a vial with 10ml solvent in an ampoule.

Used for: prevention of meningococcal meningitis, treatment of carriers of *Haemophilus influenzae*, additional therapy for brucellosis, Legionnaire's disease and serious staphylococcal infections, tuberculosis and mycobacterial infections, leprosy.

Dosage: meningitis—600g twice per day for 2 days; influenza—20mg/kg per day for 4 days; brucellosis—600–1200mg per day as 2 to 4 doses; tuberculosis—8–12mg/kg per day thirty minutes before or 2 hours after a meal; leprosy—600mg once per month or 10mg/kg per day. Children: meningitis—1 to 12 years, 10mg/kg twice per day for 2 days; 3 months to 1 year, 5mg/kg, not for children under 3 months; influenza—20mg/kg daily for 4 days, infants up to 1 month 10mg/kg daily for 4 days; tuberculosis—10–30mg/kg per day to a daily maximum of 600mg; leprosy—as adult dose.

Special care: pregnancy, breast-feeding, liver disease, elderly, poorly nourished or the very young.
Avoid use: jaundice.
Possible interaction: digitalis, hypoglycaemics, cyclosporin, corticosteroids, anticoagulants, oral contraceptives, dapsone, quinidine, phenytoin, narcotics.
Side effects: rashes, gastrointestinal upset, flu-like symptoms, upset liver function, orange discolouration of urine and secretions.
Manufacturer: Merrell Dow.

Rifater

Description: a compound drug containing 50mg isoniazid, 300mg pyrazinamide and 120mg rifampicin in pink-beige tablets.
Used for: pulmonary tuberculosis in the initial intensive phase.
Dosage: a single dose thirty minutes before or 2 hours after a meal—over 65kg, 6 tablets per day; 50–64kg, 5 tablets; 40–49kg, 4 tablets; under 40 kg, 3 tablets per day, to continue for 2 months followed by rifampicin/isoniazid compound. For the initial period, the additional use of ethambutol or streptomycin is advised. For children contact the manufacturer.
Special care: history of epilepsy, gout, liver disease, haemoptysis (coughing up blood).
Avoid use: jaundice.
Possible interaction: digitalis, hypoglycaemics, cyclosporin, corticosteroids, anticoagulants, oral contraceptives, dapsone, quinidine, phenytoin, narcotics.
Side effects: rashes, gastrointestinal upset, flu-like symptoms, upset liver function, orange discolouration of urine and secretions.
Manufacturer: Merrell Dow.

Rifinah

Description: a combination of rifampicin (150mg) and isoniazid (100mg) in pink tablets marked RH150 and also orange tablets, coded RH300 containing 300mg rifampicin and 150mg isoniazid.
Used for: tuberculosis.
Dosage: 2 Rifinah 300 daily if over 50kg; 3 Rifinah 150 daily if under 50kg, as a single dose thirty minutes before or 2 hours after a meal. Not for children.
Special care: pregnancy, lactation, undernourished, elderly, liver disease (monitor).
Avoid use: jaundice.
Possible interaction: digitalis, hypoglycaemics, cyclosporin, corticosteroids, anticoagulants, oral contraceptives, dapsone, quinidine, phenytoin, narcotics.

Side effects: rashes, gastrointestinal upset, flu-like symptoms, upset liver function, orange discolouration of urine and secretions.
Manufacturer: Merrell Dow.

Rimactane

Description: a rifamycin, rifampicin, available in red capsules coded JZ 150 (150mg) and red/brown capsules coded CS 300 (300mg), both also marked CG. Also, **Rimactane Syrup** (100mg/5ml).
Used for: prevention of meningococcal meningitis, additional treatment in tuberculosis and certain mycobacterial infections.
Dosage: (meningitis) 600mg twice per day for 2 days; children 1 to 12 years 10mg/kg; up to 1 year, 5mg/kg both twice per day for 2 days. For tuberculosis etc., 450–600mg thirty minutes before breakfast; children up to 20mg/kg per day to a maximum single dose of 600mg.
Also, **Rimactane Infusion** as 300mg rifampicin powder in a vial.
Special care: porphyria, pregnancy, breast-feeding, liver disease (monitor), elderly, poorly-nourished or the very young.
Avoid use: jaundice.
Possible interaction: corticosteroids, digitalis, anticoagulants, hypoglycaemics, cyclosporin, oral contraceptives, phenytoin, quinidine, antacids, dapsone, anticholinergics, opiates.
Side effects: rashes, gastrointestinal upset, flu-like symptoms, upset liver function, discolouration of urine and secretions.
Manufacturer: Ciba.

Rimactazid

Description: a combination of rifampicin and isoniazid in pink tablets '150' marked EI and CG (150mg/100mg respectively) and orange oblong tablets '300' marked DH and CG (300mg/150mg respectively).
Used for: tuberculosis.
Dosage: 2 300 tablets per day before breakfast (for over 50kg) or 3 150 tablets per day (for under 50kg). Not for children.
Special care: porphyria, elderly, epilepsy, pregnancy, lactation, liver disease (monitor).
Avoid use: acute liver disease, neuritis (peripheral), past drug-induced hepatitis.
Possible interaction: anticoagulants, anticholinergics, corticosteroids, antacids, digitalis, hypoglycaemics, cyclosporin, oral contraceptives, phenytoin, dapsone, narcotics, quinidine, disulfiram.
Side effects: rashes, gastrointestinal upset, flu-like

symptoms, upset liver function, discolouration of urine and secretions.

Manufacturer: Ciba.

Rimso-50

Description: a bladder irrigator, dimethyl sulphoxide (50%, sterile solution).

Used for: relief of interstitial cystitis.

Dosage: see literature.

Special care: malignancy of the urinary tract. Check liver and kidney function and eyes regularly.

Side effects: hypersensitivity reactions because of histamine release.

Manufacturer: Britannia.

Rinatec

Description: an anticholinergic nasal spray, ipratropium bromide, in 20µg metered dose spray.

Used for: rhinorrhoea (runny nose) associated with perennial rhinitis.

Dosage: 1 or 2 sprays in the nostrils up to 4 times per day. Not for children.

Special care: enlarged prostate, glaucoma.

Side effects: irritation, nasal dryness.

Manufacturer: Boehringer Ingelheim.

Risperdal

Description: an antipsychotic and benzisoxazole derivative, risperidone available as 1mg white (Ris/1), 2mg orange (Ris/2), 3mg yellow (Ris/3) and 4mg green oblong tablets (Ris/4), all marked Janssen.

Used for: schizophrenia and other psychoses.

Dosage: (over 15 years) 1mg on first day, 2mg on second day, 3mg on third day , all twice per day. Maximum 8mg twice per day. Elderly, start with 0.5mg, increasing by 0.5mg to 1-2mg twice daily. Not for children.

Special care: epilepsy, elderly, disease of kidney, liver or heart and blood vessels, Parkinson's disease, pregnancy, breast-feeding. If driving or operating machine. Cease if signs of tardive dyskinesia.

Possible interaction: levodopa, dopamine agonists, drugs acting centrally.

Side effects: hypotension when standing, tachycardia, galactorrhoea, sexual disorders, extrapyramidal symptoms, anxiety, insomnia, headache, fatigue, dizziness, weight gain, gastrointestinal upset, rash, rhinitis, blurred vision, poor concentration.

Manufacturer: Janssen/Organon.

Rivotril

Description: an anticonvulsant and benzodiazepine, clonazepam, available as beige tablets (0.5mg) and white tablets (2mg) marked RIV and with tablet strength.

Used for: epilepsy.

Dosage: start with maximum daily dose of 1mg increasing to maintenance of 4–8mg per day. Elderly, 0.5mg daily maximum initially. Children: 5 to 12 years, 0.5mg maximum per day initially rising to maintenance of 3–6mg per day; 1 to 5 years, 0.25mg, and 1–3mg (same criteria); up to 1 year, 0.25mg and 0.5–1mg (same criteria). Gradually increase all to maintenance dose.

Also, **Rivotril Injection**, 1mg in solvent in ampoules (with diluent).

Used for: status epilepticus (continual seizures producing brain damage unless halted).

Dosage: 1mg by slow intravenous injection Children, 0.5mg by same means, but see literature.

Special care: chronic lung insufficiency, chronic liver or kidney disease, the elderly, pregnant, during labour or lactation. Judgement and dexterity may be affected, long-term use is to be avoided. To be withdrawn gradually.

Avoid use: acute lung insufficiency, depression of respiration (except in cases of acute muscle spasms). Also when treating anxiety, obsessional states or chronic psychosis.

Possible interaction: alcohol and other depressant of the central nervous system, anticonvulsants.

Side effects: vertigo, gastrointestinal upsets confusion, ataxia, drowsiness, light-headedness hypotension, disturbance of vision, skin rashes. Also urine retention, changes in libido. Dependence potential problem.

Manufacturer: Roche.

Ro-A-Vit

Description: Vitamin A as 50,000 units per ml in a aqueous solution (in ampoules).

Used for: vitamin A deficiency.

Dosage: ½ to 1 ampoule by deep intramuscular injection, weekly or monthly.

Special care: do not mix with other vitamin injections, liver disease. Monitor.

Side effects: possible hypervitaminosis (toxic effect of excessive doses) in children and infants.

Manufacturer: Cambridge.

Roaccutane

Description: a vitamin A derivative, isotretinoin available in red/white gelatin capsules (5 and 20mg marked with R and strength.

Used for: acne, especially severe form unresponsive to previous treatment with antibiotic drugs.

Dosage: start with 0.5mg/kg with food for 4 weeks adjusting depending upon response within the range 0.1–1.0mg/kg for an additional 8 to 12 weeks. Not normally repeated. Not for children.

Special care: (hospital use only) exclude pregnancy, effective contraception necessary 1 month before and up to 4 weeks after treatment. Check liver function and blood lipids regularly.

Avoid use: pregnancy, breast-feeding, liver or kidney disease.

Possible interaction: high doses of vitamin A.

Side effects: hair loss, dryness, mucosal erosion, nausea, headache, drowsiness, sweating, seizures, menstrual disorders, mood changes, rise in liver enzymes; sometimes hearing loss, thrombocytopenia.

Manufacturer: Roche.

Robaxin

Description: a carbamate and muscle relaxant, methocarbamol, available as white, oblong tablets marked AHR (750mg strength).

Used for: skeletal muscle spasm.

Dosage: 2 tablets 4 times per day. Elderly—1 tablet 4 times per day. Not for children.

Also, **Robaxin Injectable** (100mg/ml in ampoules).

Special care: liver or kidney disease, pregnancy, breast-feeding.

Avoid use: coma, brain damage, myasthenia gravis, epilepsy.

Possible interaction: depressants and stimulants of the CNS, alcohol, anticholinergics.

Side effects: allergies, drowsiness.

Manufacturer: Shire.

Robaxisal Forte

Description: a carbamate and salicylate and muscle relaxant comprising 400mg methocarbamol and 325g aspirin in pink/white, two-layered tablets marked AHR.

Used for: skeletal muscle spasms.

Dosage: 2 tablets (elderly 1) 4 times daily. Not for children.

Special care: pregnancy, breast-feeding, liver or kidney disease, past bronchospasm, allergy to anti-inflammatory drugs.

Avoid use: brain damage, coma, myasthenia gravis, peptic ulcer, epilepsy, haemophilia.

Possible interaction: anticholinergics, alcohol, stimulants and depressants of the CNS, hypoglycaemics, hydantoins, anticoagulants.

Side effects: gastrointestinal bleeding, allergies, drowsiness.

Manufacturer: Shire.

Robinul

Description: an anticholinergic, glycopyrronium bromide, available as ampoules containing 0.2mg/ml. Also, **Robinul Neostigmine** which contains 0.5mg glycopyrronium bromide and 2.5mg/ml neostigmine methysulphate in ampoules.

Used for: reduction of secretions during anaesthesia.

Dosage: for premedication 200–400µg Robinul by intramuscular or intravenous injection (child: 4–8µg/kg to a maximum of 200µg). Robinul neostigmine: 1–2ml (child 0.02ml) by intravenous injection over 10 to thirty seconds.

Special care: cardiovascular disease, atropine should be given, asthma, epilepsy, peptic ulcer, pregnancy, breast-feeding, hypotension, Parkinson's disease, bradycardia, recent myocardial infarction.

Possible interaction: cisapride, antihistamines, nefopam, disopyramide, TCADs, MAOIs, phenothiazines, amantadine.

Side effects: nausea, vomiting, diarrhoea, abdominal cramps, tachycardia.

Manufacturer: Wyeth.

Rocaltrol

Description: a vitamin D analogue, calcitriol, available as capsules containing 0.25µg (red/white) and 0.5µg (red).

Used for: in cases of renal osteodystrophy (bone development defect due to kidney disorder affecting calcium and phosphorus metabolism).

Dosage: 1–2µg per day increasing if required to 2–3µg by 0.25–0.5µg increments. Not for children.

Special care: pregnancy, do not use other vitamin D preparations. Check serum calcium levels.

Avoid use: hypercalcaemia metastatic calcification (due to spread of malignancy).

Side effects: hypercalciuria (calcium in urine), hypercalcaemia.

Manufacturer: Roche.

Rocephin

Description: a cephalosporin, ceftriaxone, available as a powder in vials (250mg, 1g and 2g).

Used for: meningitis, pneumonia, septicaemia. Infections of bone, skin and soft tissue. Gonorrhoea, preventitive for operations, infections in patients with neutropenia.

Dosage: 1g per day by deep intramuscular injection, slow intravenous injection or infusion. 2–4g as 1 dose, per day, for severe infections. Gonorrhoea—250mg intramuscularly; preventative—1g intramuscularly or slow intravenous injection; also colorectal surgery—2g intramuscularly or by slow intravenous injection or infusion. Children (over 6 weeks only): 20–50mg/kg daily by the same means, up to 80mg/kg for severe infections.

Special care: severe liver or kidney disease, hypersensitivity to ß-lactam.

Avoid use: pregnancy.

Side effects: primarily skin infections, blood changes, gastrointestinal upset.

Manufacturer: Roche.

Roferon-A

Description: an interferon, interferon alfa-2a, available in vials of 3, 4.5 and 18 million units, with syringe, needles and water for injection.

Used for: AIDS-related Kaposi's sarcoma, some leukaemias, T-cell lymphoma, hepatitis B, renal cell carcinoma.

Dosage: by subcutaneous and intramuscular injection. See literature.

Avoid use: pregnancy.

Possible interaction: theophylline.

Side effects: (dose-related) depression, flu-like symptoms, bone marrow suppression, hypo-and hypertension, arrhythmia, rash, seizures; rarely, coma.

Manufacturer: Roche.

Rogitine

Description: an alpha-blocker and antihypertensive, phentolamine mesylate, in ampoules of 10mg/ml.

Used for: hypertension associated with phaeochromocytoma.

Dosage: 2–5mg by intravenous injection, repeated if required. Children: 1mg.

Special care: asthma, gastritis, kidney disorder, peptic ulcer. Elderly, pregnancy, lactation. Monitor blood.

Avoid use: hypotension, weak heart, myocardial infarction, hypersensitivity to sulphites, disease of coronary arteries.

Possible interaction: antihypertensives, anti-psychotics.

Side effects: weakness, dizziness, tachycardia, hypotension, flushes, blocked nose, gastrointestinal upset.

Manufacturer: Ciba.

Rohypnol

Description: an hypnotic and intermediate-acting benzodiazepine, flunitrazepam, in diamond-shaped purple tablets (1mg) marked ROHYPNOL.

Used for: short-term treatment of severe or disabling insomnia, to induce sleep at unusual times.

Dosage: $\frac{1}{2}$ to 1 tablet at bedtime (elderly, $\frac{1}{2}$ tablet). Not for children.

Special care: chronic liver or kidney disease, chronic lung disease, pregnancy, labour, lactation, elderly. May impair judgement. Withdraw gradually and avoid prolonged use.

Avoid use: depression of respiration, acute lung disease; psychotic, phobic or obsessional states.

Possible interaction: anticonvulsants, depressants of the CNS, alcohol.

Side effects: ataxia, confusion, light-headedness, drowsiness, hypotension, gastrointestinal upsets, disturbances in vision and libido, skin rashes, retention of urine, vertigo. Sometimes jaundice or blood disorders.

Manufacturer: Wyeth.

Rowachol

Description: Essential oils comprising 32mg menthol, 17mg a and ß-pinenes, 6mg menthone, 5mg camphene, 5mg borneol and 2mg cineole in green, spherical, soft, gelatin capsules.

Used for: additional treatment for disposal of stones in the common bile duct (with chenodeoxycholic acid).

Dosage: start with 1 capsule 3 times per day, increasing to 1 to 2 capsules 3 times per day, before meals. Not for children.

Possible interaction: oral contraceptives, oral anticoagulants.

Manufacturer: Monmouth.

Rowatinex

Description: Essential oils comprising 31mg a and ß pinenes, 15mg camphene, 10mg borneol, 4mg anethol, 4mg fenchone, 3mg cineole in yellow, spherical, soft, gelatin capsules.

Used for: stones in the urinary tract or kidney, mild urinary tract infections.

Dosage: 1 capsule 3 or 4 times per day before meals. Not for children.

Possible interaction: oral contraceptives, oral anticoagulants.

Manufacturer: Monmouth.

Rubavax

Description: a live attenuated virus, Rubella vaccine, with 25µg neomycin per dose, as powder in vial with syringe of diluent (0.5ml).

Used for: immunization of girls aged 10 to 14 and women (not pregnant) who are seronegative.

Dosage: 0.5ml by deep subcutaneous or intramuscular injection. Not for children under 10.

Avoid use: pregnancy, or pregnancy within 3 months of injection, acute infections.

Possible interaction: live vaccines,

immunoglobulin, transfusions of blood or plasma.
Side effects: rash, joint pain, sore throat, fever, malaise, disorder of the lymph system.
Manufacturer: Merieux.

Rythmodan

Description: a class I antiarrhythmic, disopyramide, available as green/beige capsules (100mg) marked RY RL.
Used for: disturbance in heart beat.
Dosage: 300–800mg per day in divided doses. Not for children. Also, **Rythmodan Retard**, 250mg disopyramide phosphate in white, sustained-release tablets marked RY and R with symbol.
Dosage: 1–1½ tablets twice per day. Not for children. Also, **Rythmodan Injection**, 10mg/ml in ampoules.
Special care: 1st degree atrioventricular block (slowed conduction or stopped heart impulse), heart, liver or kidney failure, enlarged prostate, urine retention, hyperkalaemia, glaucoma.
Avoid use: 2nd or 3rd degree atrioventricular block, severe heart failure.
Possible interaction: ß-blockers, anticholinergics, diuretics, other class I antiarrhythmics, erythromycin.
Side effects: anticholinergic effects, sometimes jaundice, hypoglycaemia, psychosis.
Manufacturer: Roussel.

S

Sabril

Description: an anticonvulsant preparation which is an analogue of a gamma-aminobutyric acid available as oval, white, scored tablets containing 500mg vigabatrin. Also, **Sabril Sachet** containing 500mg vigabatrin as powder.

Used for: control of epilepsy which has not responded to other drugs.

Dosage: 2g each day as single or divided doses, at first along with any other drug being taken. Then dose altered according to response with a maximum of 4g daily. Children, 40mg/kg body weight each day at first increasing, if needed, to a maximum of 80–100mg/kg.

Special care: elderly, kidney disorders, history of psychiatric illness or behavioural problems. Neurological function should be monitored during the course of treatment. Withdraw drug gradually.

Avoid use: pregnancy, breast-feeding.

Possible interaction: other anti-epileptic drugs.

Side effects: behavioural disturbances, irritability, aggression, dizziness, sleepiness, fatigue, disturbance of vision and memory, nervousness. Children may show agitated behaviour. Patients with a certain type of convulsion (myoclonic) may experience an increase in frequency.

Manufacturer: Merrell Dow.

Saizen

Description: a preparation of growth hormone as powder in vials containing 4 units and 10 units somatropin for reconstitution and injection.

Used for: failure of growth in children due to deficiency in growth hormone. Turner's syndrome.

Dosage: children, deficiency of growth hormone, 0.07–0.08 units/kg body weight each day by intra-muscular or subcutaneous injection. Or, 0.2 units/kg 3 times each week. Turner's syndrome, 0.09–0.1 units/kg each day at first then 0.11–0.14 units/kg if needed.

Special care: diabetes, lesion on the brain, deficiency in ACTH (adrenocorticotrophic hormone). Thyroid function should be monitored.

Avoid use: Girls who are pregnant or breast-feeding, children with fusion of epiphyses or tumour.

Side effects: pain at site of injection, breakdown of fat beneath skin at injection site, oedema, hypothyroidism.

Manufacturer: Serono.

Salamol

Description: a preparation which is a bronchodilator and selective ß₂-agonist available as a metered dose aerosol delivering 100µg salbutamol per dose. Also, **Salamol Steri-Neb** available as a preservative-free solution for nebulization containing 2.5mg and 5mg salbutamol as sulphate/2.5ml, as single dose units.

Used for: Salamol, bronchospasm as in bronchitis, emphysema and asthma. Salamol Steri-Neb, severe bronchospasm and acute severe asthma which has failed to respond to other drugs.

Dosage: Salamol, adults, for attack, 1 or 2 puffs; prevention, 2 puffs 3 to 4 times each day. Salamol Steri-Neb, 2.5mg nebulized 3 or 4 times each day increasing to 5mg if needed. Children, Salamol, half adult dose.

Special care: pregnancy, weak heart, heart arrhythmias, angina, hypertension, hyperthyroidism.

Possible interaction: ß-blockers, sympatho-mimetics.

Side effects: headache, dilation of peripheral blood vessels, tremor, hypokalaemia.

Manufacturer: Baker Norton.

Salazopyrin

Description: a colorectal NSAID which is a salicylate and sulphonamide, available as scored, yellow tablets containing 500mg sulphasalazine marked with logo. Also, **Salazopyrin En-Tabs**, enteric-coated yellow tablets (500mg) marked with logo. **Salazopyrin Suspension**, fruit-flavoured containing 250mg/5ml. **Salazopyrin Enema** containing 3g; **Salazopyrin Suppositories** containing 500mg.

Used for: ulcerative colitis (inflammation of colon), Crohn's disease. Salazopyrin En-Tabs, rheumatoid arthritis which has not responded to other NSAIDs.

Dosage: oral preparations, for ulcerative colitis and Crohn's disease, 2 to 4 tablets or 20–40ml 4 times each day with a maintenance dose of 4 tablets or 40ml in divided doses daily. Enema, 1 at night; suppositories, 2 in the morning and after passing stool in addition to oral dose. Rheumatoid arthritis, 1 En-Tab daily for 1 week increasing over 6 weeks to 6 each day in divided doses. Children, over 2 years of age, oral preparations, 40–60mg/kg body weight each day with a maintenance dose of 20–30mg/kg daily. Suppositories, a reduced dose in proportion to that for 70kg adult.

Special care: patients with allergies, liver or kidney disorders. Any ill effects should be reported and patients should receive regular checks of liver function and blood.

Avoid use: children under 2 years.

Possible interaction: rash, nausea, fever, headache, appetite loss, gastrointestinal disturbance. Effects on CNS and kidneys, blood changes, allergic hypersensitivity reactions. Reduced production of, and presence of abnormal spermatozoa in males.

Manufacturer: Pharmacia.

Salbulin

Description: a bronchodilator which is a selective ß2-agonist available as a metered dose aerosol delivering 100µg salbutamol/dose.

Used for: bronchospasm in bronchitis, emphysema, asthma.

Dosage: adults, attack, 1 or 2 puffs; prevention, 2 puffs 3 or 4 times each day. Children, half adult dose.

Special care: pregnancy, hyperthyroidism.

Possible interaction: ß-blockers, sympathomimetics.

Side effects: headache, dilation of peripheral blood vessels, nervousness, tremor.

Manufacturer: 3M Health Care.

Salofalk

Description: a colorectal preparation and salicylate available as oval, yellow, enteric-coated tablets containing 250mg mesalazine.

Used for: ulcerative colitis, maintenance treatment.

Dosage: adults, for active condition, 6 tablets each day in 3 divided doses. Maintenance treatment, 3 to 6 tablets each day in divided doses.

Special care: pregnancy, kidney disorder.

Avoid use: children, blood clotting disorders, serious liver or kidney disease, allergy to salicylates, peptic ulcer.

Possible interaction: preparations that make the stools more acid, lactulose.

Side effects: allergic hypersensitivity responses, increased haemoglobin levels.

Manufacturer: Thames.

Saluric

Description: a thiazide diuretic available as scored, white tablets containing 500mg chlorothiazide marked MSD 432.

Used for: hypertension, oedema.

Dosage: hypertension, half to 1 tablet in single or divided doses each day with a maximum of 2 tablets. Oedema, $1/2$ to 2 tablets once or twice each day or on days when required, with a maximum of 4 daily. Children, age under 6 months, 35mg/kg body weight each day; 6 months to 2 years, 125–375mg each day. 2 to 12 years, 375mg–1g each day. All in 2 divided doses.

Special care: elderly, pregnancy, breast-feeding, gout, liver or kidney disorders, SLE, liver cirrhosis, diabetes. Glucose, electrolyte and fluid levels should be monitored during the course of treatment.

Avoid use: hypercalcaemia, allergy to sulphonamides, serious liver or kidney failure. Addison's disease.

Possible interaction: NSAIDs, lithium opioids, corticosteroids, alcohol cardiac glycosides, barbiturates, tubocurarine, carbenoxolone, anti-diabetic drugs.

Side effects: gastrointestinal upset, dizziness, disturbance of metabolism and electrolyte balance, blood changes, pancreatitis, impotence, anorexia.

Manufacturer: M.S.D.

Sandimmun

Description: a fungal metabolite immuno-suppressant available as a yellow, sugar-free, oily solution containing 100mg cyclosporin/ml. Also, **Sandimmun Capsules** available in 3 strengths, oval, light pink 25mg; oblong, yellow, 50mg; and oblong, deep pink, 100mg all containing cyclosporin. **Sandimmun Intravenous Infusion** available in ampoules containing 50mg/ml.

Used for: serious rheumatoid arthritis which has not responded to other drugs, suppression of immune system in patients undergoing bone marrow or organ transplants, prevention and treatment of graft-versus-host disease. Serious atopic dermatitis and psoriasis which has not responded to other drugs or where these are not considered to be suitable.

Dosage: 1.25–5mg/kg body weight per day depending upon condition. See literature.

Special care: pregnancy, breast-feeding, hyperkalaemia, herpes, hyperuricaemia (raised levels of uric acid in blood). Treatment must be given in specialist unit and close monitoring of blood potassium levels, blood pressure, liver and kidney function is required before and during treatment. Avoid sunbathing.

Avoid use: malignant diseases (except of skin), kidney disorders, uncontrolled infections or hypertension.

Possible interaction: barbiturates, systemic antibiotics, rifampicin, live vaccines, ketoconazole, erythromycin, phenytoin, carbamazepine, itraconazole, fluconazole, ACE inhibitors, oral contraceptives, calcium antagonists, certain enzyme inhibitors, colchicine, drugs with toxic effects on kidneys. Potassium supplements and potassium-sparing diuretics, prednisolone, lipid solutions, methyl prednisolone, NSAIDs, propafenone.

Side effects: weakness, tiredness, muscle cramps, burning sensation in feet and hands, tremor, gastrointestinal upset. Rarely, other blood changes, headache, weight gain, oedema, rash, fits, colitis, pancreatitis. Also, hyperkalaemia, rise in uric acid levels in blood, damage to nerves, effects on menstruation, enlargement of breasts. If uncontrolled hypertension or liver and kidney disorders occur, drug should be withdrawn.

Manufacturer: Sandoz.

Sandoglobulin

Description: a freeze-dried preparation of human normal immunoglobulin available with diluent for intravenous infusion.

Used for: globulin deficiencies in newborn babies, thrombocytopenic purpura (a bleeding disorder).

Dosage: deficiency, 0.1–0.3g/kg body weight every 2 to 4 weeks. Thrombocytopenic purpura, 0.4g/kg each day for 5 days. Then maintenance dose of same order when needed.

Special care: during infusion, patients must be monitored for signs of anaphylaxis.

Avoid use: patients with selective immunoglobulin A deficiency who have antibodies to Ig A and who are sensitized.

Possible interaction: live viral vaccines.

Side effects: allergic anaphylactoid-type reactions, inflammatory responses which may be delayed.

Manufacturer: Sandoz.

Sandostatin

Description: a somatostatin analogue available as a solution in ampoules for subcutaneous injection at strengths of 0.05mg, 0.1mg and 0.5mg/ml and 1mg/5ml multidose vial, all containing octreotide (as acetate).

Used for: short-term treatment of acromegaly (abnormal enlargement of face, hands and feet due to excess secretion of growth hormone by a pituitary gland tumour), before surgery or X-ray therapy. Relief of symptoms of certain tumours of the gastrointestinal tract and pancreas, and carcinoid tumours which release hormones.

Dosage: acromegaly, 0.1–0.2mg 3 times each day. Tumours, 0.05mg once or twice each day increasing to 0.2mg 3 times daily if needed. Carcinoid tumours, stop drug if no improvement after 1 week.

Special care: diabetes. Those taking drug long-term require monitoring of thyroid function and for development of gallstones.

Avoid use: pregnancy, breast-feeding.

Possible interaction: cimetidine, cyclosporin.

Side effects: pain, swelling and soreness at injection site, pain in abdomen, vomiting, diarrhoea, steatorrhoea (increased amount of fat in faeces which are pale, frothy and foul-smelling), anorexia, gallstones.

Manufacturer: Sandoz.

Sanomigran

Description: a serotonin antagonist available as sugar-coated, ivory-coloured tablets containing 0.5mg and 1.5mg pizotifen (as hydrogen maleate), marked SMG and SMG 1.5 respectively. Also, **Sanomigran Elixir** containing 0.25mg/5ml as a sugar-free solution.

Used for: prevention of migraine.

Dosage: 1.5mg each day in 3 divided doses or 1 dose at night. Dosage may be increased to a maximum of 4.5mg each day if needed with up to 3mg as a maximum single dose. Children, up to 1.5mg each day in divided doses or 1mg as a single night time dose.

Special care: urine retention, glaucoma.

Side effects: gain in weight, sleepiness.

Manufacturer: Sandoz.

Saventrine

Description: a heart stimulant and ß-agonist available as mottled white tablets containing 30mg isoprenaline hydrochloride marked with a P inside a hexagon shape. Also, **Saventrine I.V.** available as a solution in ampoules for injection containing 1mg/ml.

Used for: heart block, severe bradycardia, Stokes Adams attacks.

Dosage: tablets (rarely used) 30mg every 6 hours with usual dose in the order of 90–840mg each day. Infusion, 0.5–10µg/minute.

Special care: diabetes or hypertension.

Avoid use: hyperthyroidism, serious heart disease, tachycardia, ventricular fibrillation, cardiac asthma.

Side effects: headache, tremor, sweating, diarrhoea, palpitations.

Manufacturer: Pharmax.

Schering PC4

Description: an oestrogen/progestogen preparation available as sugar-coated white tablets containing 50μg ethinyloestradiol and 0.5mg norgestrel.

Used for: emergency and contraception (the 'morning-after' pill) to be taken within 72 hours of unprotected sexual intercourse.

Dosage: 2 tablets taken as soon as possible after intercourse followed, 12 hours later, by another 2 tablets.

Special care: porphyria, gallstones, liver disorders, heart, kidney, circulatory diseases, diabetes, epilepsy, hypertension, history of severe depression. If patient still becomes pregnant, monitoring required to ensure pregnancy is not ectopic. Intercourse should be avoided for the remainder of the cycle.

Avoid use: patients with overdue menstrual period, those not within 72 hours of unprotected intercourse.

Possible interaction: barbiturates, chlorpromazine, rifampicin, chloral hydrate, glutethimide, tetracyclines, dichloralphenazone, griseofulvin, ethosuximide, phenytoin, carbamazepine, primidone.

Side effects: vomiting (reduces drug's effect) and nausea. Period normally starts later than expected, following treatment.

Manufacturer: Schering H.C.

Scheriproct

Description: a combined steroid and local anaesthetic preparation available as an ointment containing 0.19% prednisolone hexanoate and 0.5% cinchocaine hydrochloride. Also, **Scheriproct Suppositories** containing 1.3mg prednisolone hexanoate and 1mg cinchocaine hydrochloride.

Used for: anal fissure, haemorrhoids, proctitis (inflammation of rectum), anal itching.

Dosage: apply ointment 2, 3 or 4 times each day; insert 1 suppository 1, 2 or 3 times each day after passing stool.

Special care: pregnant women, short-term use only.

Avoid use: patients with tuberculous, viral or fungal infections.

Side effects: systemic corticosteroid side effects.

Manufacturer: Schering H.C.

Scoline

Description: a depolarizing muscle relaxant of short-lived duration available as a solution in ampoules for injection containing 50mg suxamethonium chloride/ml.

Used for: paralysis following induction of anaesthesia usually to allow tracheal tube to be inserted. Has duration of action lasting 5 minutes and repeated doses may be given to allow longer-lasting procedures to be carried out.

Special care: with unusual or low concentration of pseudocholinesterase enzymes in whom more prolonged paralysis may occur. Dual block involving longer-lasting paralysis may develop after repeated doses of suxamethonium.

Avoid use: liver disease or burns.

Possible interaction: digoxin, ecothiopate, demacarium, eyedrops, neostigmine, pyndostigmine, thiotepa, cyclophoshamide, bambuterol.

Side effects: short-lived rise in creatine, phosphokinase (enzyme) and potassium levels in blood plasma, postoperative muscle pains.

Manufacturer: Evans.

Scopoderm

Description: an anti-emetic, anticholinergic preparation available as a self-adhesive pink patch containing 1.5mg hyoscine.

Used for: motion sickness.

Dosage: adults and children over 10 years, apply patch to clean, dry skin behind ear 5 to 6 hours before travelling. Replace after 72 hours if needed and remove when travelling is finished.

Special care: pregnancy, breast-feeding, liver or kidney disorders, obstruction of intestine, bladder or pyloric stenosis.

Avoid use: children under 10 years, glaucoma. Consumption of alcohol.

Possible interaction: drugs affecting CNS, anticholinergics, alcohol.

Side effects: skin rashes and irritation, urine retention, dry mouth, disturbance of vision, sleepiness, dizziness. Rarely, withdrawal symptoms.

Manufacturer: Ciba.

Secadrex

Description: an antihypertensive preparation combining a cardioselective ß-blocker and thiazide diuretic available as film-coated white tablets containing 200mg acebutolol (as hydrochloride) and 12.5mg hydrochlorothiazide, marked SECADREX.

Used for: hypertension.

Dosage: 1 to 2 tablets as a single dose each day.

Special care: pregnancy, breast-feeding, patients with weak hearts may require diuretics and digitalis, diabetes, undergoing general anaesthesia, kidney or liver disorders, gout. Electrolyte (salts) levels may need to be monitored.

Avoid use: history of bronchospasm or obstructive airways disease, heart block, heart shock, uncompensated heart failure, disease of peripheral arteries, bradycardia. Serious or worsening kidney failure or anuria.

Possible interaction: sympathomimetics, class I antiarrhythmics, CNS depressants, clonidine withdrawal, ergot alkaloids, cardiac depressant anaesthetics, verapamil, reserpine, indomethacin, hypoglycaemics, cimetidine, other anti-hypertensives. Digitalis, potassium supplements, potassium-sparing diuretics, lithium.

Side effects: cold hands and feet, disturbance of sleep, fatigue on exercise, bronchospasm, bradycardia, gastrointestinal disturbances, heart failure, blood changes, gout, sensitivity to light, muscle weakness. If skin rash or dry eyes occur, withdraw drug gradually.

Manufacturer: Theraplix.

Seconal Sodium^{CD}

Description: a barbiturate preparation available as 50mg and 100mg orange capsules, coded F42 and F40 respectively, both containing quinalbarbitone sodium.

Used for: short-term treatment of serious insomnia.

Dosage: 50–100mg taken at night.

Special care: extremely dangerous, addictive drug with narrow margin of safety. Liable to abuse by overdose leading to coma and death or if combined with alcohol. Easily produces dependence and severe withdrawal symptoms. Drowsiness may persist next day affecting driving and performance of skilled tasks.

Avoid use: should be avoided if possible in all patients. Not to be used for children, young adults, pregnant and nursing mothers, elderly, those with drug or alcohol related problems, patients with liver, kidney or heart disease or porphyria. Insomnia where the cause is pain.

Possible interaction: alcohol, CNS depressant drugs, Griseofulvin, metronidazone, rifampicin, phenytoin, chloramphenicol. Anticoagulant drugs of the coumarin type, steroid drugs including contraceptive pill.

Side effects: hangover with drowsiness, shakiness, dizziness, headache, anxiety, confusion, excitement, rash and allergic responses, gastro intestinal upsets, urine retention, loss of sexual desire.

Manufacturer: Kite.

Sectral

Description: an anti-arrhythmic, anti-anginal preparation which is a cardioselective ß-blocker available as capsules in 2 strengths, both containing acebutolol (as hydrochloride). White/buff, 100mg and pink/buff 200mg both marked with strength and SECTRAL. Also, **Sectral Tablets**, white, film-coated, containing 400mg marked SECTRAL 400.

Used for: heart arrhythmias, angina.

Dosage: adults, arrhythmias, maintenance dose of 400–1200mg in 2 or 3 divided doses each day. Angina, 400mg once each day taken with breakfast or 200mg twice daily. The maximum is 1.2g each day.

Special care: history of bronchospasm and certain ß-blockers, diabetes, liver or kidney disease, pregnancy, lactation, general anaesthesia. Withdraw gradually. Not for children.

Avoid use: heart block or failure, bradycardia, sick sinus syndrome (associated with sinus node disorder), certain ß-blockers, severe peripheral arterial disease.

Possible interaction: verapamil, hypoglycaemics, reserpine, clonidine withdrawal, some antiarrhythmics and anaesthetics, antihypertensives, depressants of the CNS, cimetidine, indomethacin, sympathomimetics.

Side effects: bradycardia, cold hands and feet, disturbance to sleep, heart failure, gastrointestinal upset, tiredness on exertion, bronchospasm.

Manufacturer: Theraplix.

Securon SR

Description: a class I calcium antagonist available as film-coated, oblong, scored, green, sustained-release tablets containing 240mg verapamil hydrochloride and marked with logo. Also, **Half Securon SR**, white, film-coated, sustained-release tablets containing 120mg marked 120 SR and company name. Also, **Securon Tablets** white, film-coated and available in strengths of 40mg, 80mg and 120mg, all marked with strength, name and KNOLL. Also, **Securon I.V.** available as a solution in pre-filled syringes containing 2.5mg/ml.

Used for: supraventricular tachycardia, angina, hypertension.

Dosage: tachycardias, Securon Tablets, 40–120mg 3 times each day. Angina, Securon SR, Half Securon SR or Securon Tablets, 120mg 3 times each day. Hypertension, Securon SR or Half Securon SR, 240mg once each day with a maximum of 480mg in divided doses daily. Patients who have not taken verapamil before start with lower dose of 120mg once daily. Securon Tablets, 120mg twice each day at first increasing to 160mg twice daily if needed. Maximum dose is 480mg in divided doses daily. Children, for tachycardias, Securon Tablets only, age under 2 years, 20mg; age over 2 years, 20–40mg, both 2 or 3 times each day.

Special care: pregnancy, breast-feeding, patients with liver or kidney disorders, heart conduction disturbances, bradycardia, 1st degree heart block. Patients with weak hearts require digitalis and/or diuretics.

Avoid use: some kinds of heart block, heart shock, sick sinus syndrome, serious bradycardia, heart attack, severe hypotension, uncompensated heart failure, certain types of heart flutter or fibrillation. Patients should not receive intravenous ß-blockers at same time.

Possible interaction: digoxin, ß-blockers, cimetidine, muscle relaxant drugs, inhaled anaesthetics, cyclosporin, rifampicin, antihypertensives, lithium, carbamazepine, theophylline, phenobarbitone, phenytoin.

Side effects: constipation; rarely, nausea, headache, dizziness, allergic reactions, hypotension, enlargement of breasts, increased growth of gum tissues, flushes. (Effects on heart rate, heart muscle and hypotension when given intravenously).

Manufacturer: Knoll.

Securopen

Description: an antibiotic preparation which is an antipseudomonal penicillin available as powder in vials for reconstitution and injection at strengths of 500mg, 1g, 2g and 5g all containing azlocillin (as monosodium).

Used for: local and systemic infections especially those caused by pseudomonas bacteria.

Dosage: adults, 2g every 8 hours by intravenous injection; serious infections, 5g every 8 hours by intravenous infusion. Children, premature baby, 50mg/kg body weight every 12 hours; newborn baby, 100mg/kg every 12 hours; aged 1 week to 1 year, 100mg/kg every 8 hours; 1 to 14 years, 75mg/kg every 8 hours.

Special care: pregnancy, kidney disorders.

Possible interaction: tubocurarine and other non-depolarizing muscle relaxants, methotrexate.

Side effects: gastrointestinal upset, allergic hypersensitive responses.

Manufacturer: Bayer.

Semprex

Description: an antihistamine preparation of the arylalkylamine type available as white capsules containing 8mg acrivastine marked with symbol, 09C and company name.

Used for: allergic rhinitis, urticaria.

Dosage: adults, 1 tablet 3 times each day.

Special care: pregnancy, breast-feeding.

Avoid use: children, elderly, kidney failure.

Possible interaction: CNS depressants, alcohol.

Side effects: rarely, drowsiness.

Manufacturer: Wellcome.

Septrin

Description: an antibiotic preparation combining a folic acid inhibitor and sulphonamide available as white tablets and orange dissolvable tablets, both containing 80mg trimethoprim and 400mg sulphamethoxazole. Tablets are both marked with maker's name, tablet name and coded Y2B. **Septrin Adult Suspension** same components/5ml. **Septrin Paediatric Suspension**, sugar-free, containing 40mg trimethoprim and 200mg sulphamethoxazole/5ml. Also, **Septrin for Infusion** available in ampoules containing 80mg trimethoprim and 400mg sulphamethoxazole/5ml.

Used for: infections of skin, gastrointestinal, respiratory and urinary tracts.

Dosage: tablets, 1 to 3 twice each day; suspension, 5–15ml twice daily; Septrin Forte, 1 to 1 ½ tablets twice each day. Infusion, 960mg every 12 hours increasing to 1.44g if infection is extremely severe, given intravenously. Children, Paediatric Suspension, 6 weeks to 6 months, 2.5ml; 6 months to 6 years, 5ml; over 6 years, 10ml, all twice each day. Tablets, children over 6 years, 1 tablet or 5ml adult suspension. Infusion, 36mg/kg body weight each day in 2 divided doses increasing to 54mg/kg in the case of severe infections.

Special care: breast-feeding, elderly, patients with kidney disorders (require reduced or less frequent doses). Regular blood tests should be carried out in patients taking the drug long-term.

Avoid use: pregnancy, newborn babies, severe liver or kidney disorders, blood changes.

Possible interaction: anticonvulsants, folate inhibitors, hypoglycaemics, anticoagulants.

Side effects: vomiting, nausea, inflammation of tongue, blood changes, skin rashes, folate deficiency; rarely erythema multiformae (allergic disorder affecting skin and mucous membranes), Lyell syndrome.

Manufacturer: Wellcome.

Serc

Description: an anti-emetic preparation which is a histamine analogue available as white tablets in 2 strengths containing 8mg and 16mg betahistine, dihydrochloride, marked Duphar 256 or 267 respectively.

Used for: symptoms associated with Ménière's syndrome including hearing loss, tinnitus and vertigo.

Dosage: 16mg 3 times each day at first with a maintenance dose of 24–48mg daily.

Special care: patients with peptic ulcer, bronchial asthma.

Avoid use: phaeochromocytoma.

Side effects: gastrointestinal upset.

Manufacturer: Duphar.

Serenace

Description: an anti-depressant preparation which is a butyrophenone available as green/light green capsules containing 0.5mg haloperidol marked Norton 500 and SERENACE. Also, **Serenace Tablets** in 4 strengths all containing haloperidol; white, 1.5mg; pink, 5mg; 10mg and 20mg all marked with strength on one side and SERENACE on other, and coded NORTON. **Serenace Liquid**, containing 2mg/ml; **Serenace Injection** available as a solution in ampoules for injection in strengths of 5mg and 10mg/ml.

Used for: capsules, additional treatment for anxiety; tablets and liquid, manic states, psychoses, schizophrenia, behaviour disorders in children.

Dosage: capsules, 1 twice each day; tablets or liquid, 1.5–20mg each day at first increasing as needed to control disorder. Then decreasing to a maintenance dose in the order of 3–10mg each day. The maximum daily dose is 200mg. Injection, for emergency treatment, 5–30mg by intravenous or intramuscular injection every 6 hours, then preparations taken by mouth. Children, tablets or liquid only, 0.025–0.05mg/kg body weight each day at first. Usual daily maximum is 10mg.

Special care: pregnancy, tardive dyskinesia (disorder characterized by repeated involuntary muscle movements), hyperthyroidism, kidney or liver failure, serious heart or circulatory disorders, epilepsy.

Avoid use: breast-feeding, parkinsonism, coma.

Possible interaction: rifampicin, fluoxetine, carbamazepine, anxiolytics, hypnotics.

Side effects: extrapyramidal side effects, drowsiness, hypothermia, insomnia, pallor, nightmares, depression, constipation, dry mouth, blocked nose, difficulty in urination. Changes in ECG and EEG, effects on heart, e.g. tachycardia, arrhythmias, blood changes, changes in endocrine system, e.g. effects on menstruation, breasts, impotence, weight gain. Effects on liver, jaundice, sensitivity to light, purple pigmentation of skin and eyes.

Manufacturer: Baker Norton.

Serevent

Description: a bronchodilator and selective ß2-agonist available as a metered dose aerosol delivering 25µg salmeterol (as xinafoate) per dose. Also, **Serevent Diskhaler**, using disks containing 4 x 50µg blisters salmeterol (as xinafoate) with breath-actuated delivery system.

Used for: various types of asthma along with anti-inflammatory therapy.

Dosage: adults, Serevent, 2 puffs twice each day, 4 puffs if exceptionally severe. Serevent Diskhaler, 1 blister twice each day or 2 if very severe. Children, Serevent, age over 4 years, 2 puffs twice each day. Serevent Diskhaler, 1 blister twice each day.

Special care: pregnancy, breast-feeding, thyrotoxicosis, acute symptoms of asthma or if unstable and severe. Steroid therapy should be continued.

Avoid use: children under 4 years.

Possible interaction: ß-blockers.

Side effects: paradoxical bronchospasm, hypokalaemia; rarely, skin eruptions, pain in chest, joints and muscles, headache, palpitations, tremor, irritation of throat.

Manufacturer: A. & H.

Serophene

Description: an antioestrogen preparation available as scored, white tablets containing 50mg clomiphene citrate.

Used for: female infertility caused by disorder of hypothalamus-pituitary gland function. Also, with gonadotrophins in invitro fertilization treatment.

Dosage: infertility, 1 tablet each day for 5 days, ideally starting within 5 days of menstruation. Superovulation, 2 tablets each day starting on day 2 continuing to day 6 of monthly cycle.

Special care: ensure patient is not pregnant before and during course of treatment.

Avoid use: patients with undiagnosed bleeding from uterus, large cyst on ovary, cancer of endometrium, liver disorder.

Side effects: pain or discomfort in abdomen, enlargement of ovaries, flushes. Withdraw drug if blurring of vision occurs.

Manufacturer: Serono.

Serotax

Description: an antidepressant available as film-coated, oval, scored tablets in 2 strengths; containing 20mg (white) and 30mg (blue) paroxetine (as hydrochloride). Both marked with strength and name.

Used for: depression and depressive illness with anxiety.

Dosage: 20mg once each day at first, taken in the morning with breakfast. Then increasing gradually every 2 or 3 weeks by 10mg to a maximum daily dose of 50mg. Elderly persons start with lower dose of 20mg once each day increasing gradually to 40mg daily, if needed.

Special care: pregnancy, breast-feeding, serious liver or kidney disorders, heart disease or disease of arteries of heart, epilepsy, history of mania.

Avoid use: children.

Possible interaction: anticonvulsants, tryptophan, drugs affecting liver enzymes, phenytoin, MAOIs, anticonvulsants.

Side effects: dry mouth, sweating, sleepiness, tremor, nausea, weakness, effects on sexual habits.

Manufacturer: S.K. & F.

Sevredol^{CD}

Description: an analgesic opiate available as film-coated, capsule-shaped, scored tablets in 2 strengths, blue containing 10mg, and pink containing 20mg morphine sulphate. Both are marked with strength and IR.

Used for: severe pain.

Dosage: 10mg every 4 hours at first increasing dose if necessary. Children, age 3 to 5 years, 5mg every 4 hours; 6 to 12 years, 5–10mg every 4 hours.

Special care: elderly, enlarged prostate gland, underactive thyroid, liver or kidney disease, paralytic ileus, respiratory problems, reduced function of adrenal glands, following surgery.

Avoid use: pregnancy, breast-feeding, children under 3 years, obstructive airways disease, serious liver disease, head injuries, raised pressure within brain, coma, depression of respiration, alcoholism.

Possible interaction: CNS depressants, MAOIs.

Side effects: nausea, vomiting, constipation, sedation, drug tolerance and addiction.

Manufacturer: Napp.

Simplene

Description: a sympathomimetic preparation available in the form of eyedrops in 2 strengths containing 0.5% and 1% adrenaline.

Used for: primary open angle and secondary glaucoma.

Dosage: 1 drop twice each day.

Avoid use: patients with narrow angle glaucoma or diabetes.

Possible interaction: MAOIs, ß-blockers, tricyclics.

Side effects: pain or discomfort in eye, headache, skin reactions, pigmentation with melanin. Rarely, systemic side effects.

Manufacturer: Chauvin.

Sinemet

Description: an anti-Parkinson's disease preparation combining a dopamine precursor and dopa decarboxylase inhibitor available in the form of tablets. 'LS' scored, oval, yellow tablets contain 50mg levodopa and 12.5mg carbidopa (as monohydrate), marked with name. 'Plus' scored, oval, yellow tablets contain 100mg and 25mg marked with name. '110' scored, oval, blue tablets contain 100mg and 10mg, marked MSD 647. '275' scored, oval, blue tablets contain 250mg and 25mg marked MSD 654. Also, **Sinemet CR**, oval, mottled, peach-coloured, continuous-release tablets containing 200mg and 50mg marked 521 and DPP. Also, **Half Sinemet CR**, oval, pink, continuous-release tablets containing 100mg and 25mg marked 601 and DPP.

Used for: Parkinson's disease.

Dosage: adults over 18 years, not receiving levodopa, 1 'LS' or 1 'Plus' tablet 3 times each day at first increasing by 1 tablet every other day to the equivalent of 8 'Plus' tablets each day. Patients who have been taking levodopa should stop this 8 hours before taking Sinemet. Sinemet CR, 1 tablet twice each day in first instance, if not receiving levodopa, then adjusted according to response.

Special care: liver or kidney disease, disease of heart or heart blood vessels, endocrine disorders, peptic ulcer, wide angle glaucoma. Liver, kidney and heart function should be monitored and blood values checked regularly if patients are taking drug long-term.

Avoid use: children, pregnancy, breast-feeding, narrow angle glaucoma, history of malignant melanoma, severe psychoses.

Possible interaction: MAOIs, sympathomimetics, antihypertensives, drug acting on central amines.

Side effects: CNS effects, low blood pressure on rising, discolouration of urine, vomiting, nausea, involuntary muscle movements, anorexia.

Manufacturer: DuPont.

Sinequan

Description: a TCAD preparation available as tablets in different strengths, all containing doxepin (as hydrochloride). Red, 10mg capsules, coded SQN; red/blue 25mg capsules, coded SQN 25; blue, 50mg capsules, coded SQN 50; blue/yellow 75mg capsules coded SQN 75. All are marked PFIZER.

Used for: depression.

Dosage: 10–100mg 3 times each day or a maximum of 100mg as a single night-time dose.

Special care: liver disorders, hyperthyroidism, glaucoma, lactation, epilepsy, diabetes, adrenal tumour, heart disease, urine retention. Psychotic or suicidal patients.

Avoid use: heart block, heart attacks, severe liver disease, pregnancy.

Possible interaction: MAOIs (or within 14 days of their use), alcohol, antidepressants, barbiturates, anticholinergics, local anaesthetics that contain adrenaline or noradrenaline, oestrogens, cimetidine, antihypertensives.

Side effects: constipation, urine retention, dry mouth, blurred vision, palpitations, tachycardia, nervousness, drowsiness, insomnia. Changes in weight, blood and blood sugar, jaundice, skin reactions, weakness, ataxia, hypotension, sweating, altered libido, gynaecomastia, galactorrhoea.

Manufacturer: Pfizer.

Sinthrome

Description: a coumarin anticoagulant preparation available as white tablets containing 1mg nicoumalone, marked CG and AA.

Used for: thromboembolic disorders.

Dosage: 8–12mg on first day, 4–8mg on following day, then according to response.

Special care: breast-feeding, elderly, serious heart failure, liver disorders, hypertension, disorders of absorption from gastrointestinal tract, reduced protein binding. If intramuscular injections are given there is a risk of haematoma (accumulation of leaked blood which forms a solid mass within tissues).

Avoid use: pregnancy, children, patients who have had surgery or undergone labour in last 24 hours, those with liver or kidney disorders, serious hypertension, blood changes, inflammation of or leakage of fluid from pericardium, bacterial endocarditis. Patients who are unco-operative.

Possible interaction: quinidine, corticosteroids, NSAIDs, antibiotics, hypoglycaemics taken by mouth, cimetidine, sulphonamides, phenformin. Drugs affecting the halting of bleeding, liver enzymes, vitamin K, absorption.

Side effects: allergic responses, damage to liver, reversible hair loss, haemorrhage. Rarely, headache, nausea, skin necrosis, anorexia.

Manufacturer: Geigy.

Skinoren

Description: an antibacterial preparation available as a cream containing 20% azelaic acid.

Used for: acne.

Dosage: apply in the morning and evening to affected skin and rub in, maximum dose is 10g daily. Treatment should be continued according to response but for no more than 6 months.

Special care: pregnancy, breast-feeding, avoid eyes.

Side effects: sensitivity to light, local skin irritation.

Manufacturer: Schering H.C.

Slo-Phyllin

Description: a xanthine bronchidilator available as sustained-release capsules enclosing white pellets, in 3 strengths, all containing theophylline. White/clear 60mg, brown/clear 125mg and blue/clear 250mg capsules are all marked with strength, SLO-PHYLLIN and LIPHA.

Used for: bronchospasm in asthma, emphysema, bronchitis.

Dosage: 250–500mg twice each day; children, age 2 to 6 years, 60–120mg; 6 to 12 years, 125–250mg; all twice each day.

Special care: pregnancy, breast-feeding, peptic ulcer, liver or heart disease.

Avoid use: children under 2 years.

Possible interaction: interferon, erythromycin, diuretics, ß2-agonists, cimetidine, steroids, ciprofloxacin.

Side effects: gastrointestinal upset, nausea, heart arrhythmias, tachycardia, headache, insomnia.

Manufacturer: Lipha.

Slow-Fe Folic

Description: a haematinic preparation available as film-coated, cream-coloured tablets containing 160mg dried ferrous sulphate and 400µg folic acid, marked TP and CIBA.

Used for: prevention of iron and folic acid deficiencies in pregnant women.

Dosage: 1 to 2 tablets each day.

Possible interaction: anticonvulsants, penicillamine, tetracyclines, antacids, zinc salts.

Side effects: constipation nausea.

Manufacturer: Ciba.

Slo-Trasicor

Description: an antianginal, antihypertensive preparation available as film-coated, white, sustained-release tablets containing 160mg oxprenolol hydrochloride, marked with name and manufacturer's name.

Used for: angina, hypertension.

Dosage: angina, 1 each morning at first increasing to 2 or 3 if needed. If nocturnal angina is present, an evening dose may be taken. Hypertension, 1 tablet each morning.

Special care: history of bronchospasm and certain ß-blockers, diabetes, liver or kidney disease, pregnancy, lactation, general anaesthesia. Withdraw gradually. Not for children.

Avoid use: heart block or failure, bradycardia, sick

sinus syndrome (associated with sinus node disorder), certain ß-blockers, severe peripheral arterial disease.

Possible interaction: verapamil, hypoglycaemics, reserpine, clonidine withdrawal, some antiarrhythmics and anaesthetics, antihypertensives, depressants of the CNS, cimetidine, indomethacin, sympathomimetics.

Side effects: bradycardia, cold hands and feet, disturbance to sleep, heart failure, gastrointestinal upset, tiredness on exertion, bronchospasm.

Manufacturer: Ciba.

Sno-Phenicol

Description: a broad-spectrum antibiotic preparation available as eyedrops containing 0.5% chloramphenicol.

Used for: bacterial infections of the eye.

Dosage: 1 or more drops into eye, as needed. Children, 1 drop as needed.

Side effects: local allergic hypersensitive responses (stop immediately). Rarely, aplastic anaemia.

Manufacturer: Chauvin.

Sno-Pilo

Description: a cholinergic eye preparation available in the form of drops in different strengths containing 1%, 2% and 4% pilocarpine.

Used for: glaucoma.

Dosage: 1 or 2 drops 4 times each day.

Avoid use: severe inflammation of iris, wearing soft contact lenses.

Side effects: short-lived loss of visual sharpness.

Manufacturer: Chauvin.

Sodium Amytal^{CD}

Description: an hypnotic barbiturate preparation, available as blue capsules in 2 strengths containing 60mg and 200mg amylobarbitone sodium, coded LILLY F23 or F33 respectively.

Used for: insomnia, which has not responded to other drugs.

Dosage: tablets, 60–200mg taken at night.

Special care: extremely dangerous, addictive drug with narrow margin of safety. Liable to abuse by overdose leading to coma and death or if combined with alcohol. Easily produces dependence and severe withdrawal symptoms. Drowsiness may persist next day affecting driving and performance of skilled tasks.

Avoid use: should be avoided if possible in all patients. Not to be used for children, young adults, pregnant and nursing mothers, elderly pesons, those with drug or alcohol related problems, patients with

liver, kidney or heart disease, porphyria. Insomnia where the cause is pain.

Possible interaction: alcohol, CNS depressant drugs, Griseofulvin, metronidazone, rifampicin, phenytoin, chloramphenicol. Anticoagulant drugs of the coumarin type, steroid drugs including contraceptive pill.

Side effects: hangover with drowsiness, shakiness, dizziness, headache, anxiety, confusion, excitement, rash and allergic responses, gastro intestinal upsets, urine retention, loss of sexual desire.

Manufacturer: Kite.

Sodium Amytal Injection^{CD}

Description: a barbiturate preparation, available as a powder in vials for reconstitution and injection containing 500mg amylobarbitone sodium.

Used for: status epilepticus (but not grand mal epilepsy).

Dosage: 250 mg–1g by slow intravenous or intramuscular injection. Children, age over 6 years, 65–500mg by slow intravenous or intramuscular injection.

Special care: kidney and liver disorders, serious lung insufficiency.

Avoid use: pregnancy, breast-feeding, elderly, patients who are debilitated, porphyria, pain which is not controlled, history of drug or alcohol abuse.

Possible interaction: CNS depressants, griseofulvin, alcohol, phenytoin, systemic steroids, chloramphenicol, rifampicin, metronidazole, anticoagulants of the coumarin type.

Side effects: headache, respiratory depression, dizziness, unsteadiness, sleepiness, confusion, agitation, allergic responses. Drug tolerance and dependence may occur.

Manufacturer: Kite.

Sofra-Tulle

Description: a gauze dressing for wounds impregnated with 1% framycetin sulphate available in individual foil sachets.

Used for: burns, wounds, ulcers, infected areas.

Dosage: apply to affected area.

Avoid use: large open wounds—danger of ototoxicity (damage to organs of balance and hearing), especially in children, elderly and patients with kidney disorders.

Manufacturer: Roussel.

Sofradex

Description: a compound preparation combining a corticosteroid, aminoglycoside and antibiotic available in the form of drops containing 0.05%

dexamethasone, 0.5% framycetin sulphate and 0.005% gramicidin. Also, **Sofradex Ointment** containing 0.05% dexamethasone, 0.5% framycetin sulphate and 0.005% gramicidin.

Used for: inflammation and infection of outer ear. Inflammation of eye and prevention of infection, short term only, blepharitis (inflammation of hair follicles of eye lashes which may be caused by infection.

Dosage: drops, ear, apply 2 to 3 drops 3 or 4 times each day; ointment, ear, apply once or twice daily. Drops, eye, 1 or 2 drops up to 6 times each day or more frequently if necessary. Ointment, eye, apply 2 or 3 times each day or at night if drops are being used.

Special care: pregnant women.

Avoid use: long-term use in babies or by pregnant women, perforated eardrum (if for ear infections), eye infections producing pus or those with tuberculous, fungal or viral origin.

Side effects: superinfection, use in eyes may lead to thinning of cornea, fungal infection, cataract, rise in pressure within eye.

Manufacturer: Roussel.

Soframycin

Description: an antibiotic aminoglycoside preparation available in the form of drops containing 0.5% framycetin sulphate. Also, **Soframycin Ointment** containing 0.5% framycetin sulphate.

Used for: eye infections, styes, blepharitis (inflammation and infection of hair follicles of eye lashes), conjunctivitis. Ointment also used for bacterial infections of skin.

Dosage: eyes, apply 1 or 2 drops 3 or 4 times each day; apply ointment 2 or 3 times each day or at night if drops are being used. Skin, apply to affected area up to 3 times each day.

Special care: use on more extensive areas of skin.

Side effects: sensitization, ototoxicity (damage to organs of balance and hearing).

Manufacturer: Roussel.

Solpadol

Description: a compound analgesic preparation available as scored, white, effervescent tablets containing 500mg paracetamol and 30mg codeine phosphate. Also, **Solpadol Caplets**, capsule-shaped, white tablets containing the same.

Used for: severe pain.

Dosage: 2 tablets every 4 hours with a maximum of 8 in any 24 hour period.

Special care: labour, pregnancy, breast-feeding, elderly, liver or kidney disorders, underactive thyroid gland, obstruction or inflammation of the bowel.

Avoid use: children, depression of respiration, obstruction of airways, head injury, raised pressure within brain, alcoholism, surgery to the biliary tract (bile duct, gall bladder).

Possible interaction: CNS depressants, MAOIs.

Side effects: constipation, blurred vision, dizziness, dry mouth, nausea, sedation, drug dependence and tolerance.

Manufacturer: Sanofi Winthrop.

Solu-Cortef

Description: a glucocorticoid-mineralocorticoid (corticosteroid) preparation available in vials with diluent for reconstitution and injection, containing 100mg hydrocortisone (as sodium succinate).

Used for: medical emergencies requiring rapid corticosteroid dose, e.g. anaphylaxis, asthma.

Dosage: 100–500mg by slow intravenous injection. Children, may require reduced doses but not less than 25mg each day.

Special care: thrombophlebitis, psychoses, recent intestinal anastomoses, chronic nephritis, certain cancers, osteoporosis, peptic ulcer, skin eruption/rash related to a disease, viral, fungal or active infections, tuberculosis. Hypertension, glaucoma, epilepsy, acute glomerulonephritis (inflammation of kidney glomerulus), diabetes, cirrhosis, hypothyroidism, pregnancy, stress. To be withdrawn gradually.

Possible interaction: NSAIDs, oral anticoagulants, phenytoin, ephedrine, phenobarbitone, rifampicin, diuretics, cardiac glycosides, anticholinesterases, hypoglycaemics.

Side effects: osteoporosis, depression, euphoria, hyperglycaemia, peptic ulcers, Cushingoid changes.

Manufacturer: Upjohn.

Solu-Medrone

Description: a glucocorticoid corticosteroid preparation available as powder in vials for reconstitution and injection, in 4 strengths of 40mg, 125mg, 500mg and 1g all containing methylprednisolone (as sodium succinate). Also, **Solu-Medrone 2g** available in vials with diluent, containing 2g methylprednisolone (as sodium succinate).

Used for: Solu-Medrone, allergic conditions, ulcerative colitis, Crohn's disease, Stevens-Johnson syndrome, removal of stomach contents by aspiration, cerebral oedema resulting from tumour, transplant operations. Solu-Medrone 2G, serious spinal cord injuries.

Dosage: Solu-Medrone, transplants, up to 1g each day; other conditions, 10–500mg by slow intravenous or intramuscular injection over 30 minutes or longer. Solu-Medrone 2G, 30mg/kg body weight by intravenous injection over 15 minutes starting within 8 hours of injury. Then, further dose after 45 minutes at rate of 5.4mg/kg/hour for 23 hours, by intravenous infusion. Children, Solu-Medrone only, up to 30mg/kg each day depending upon condition; status asthmaticus (severe, prolonged asthma attack), 1–4mg/kg each day for 1 to 3 days.

Special care: thrombophlebitis, psychoses, recent intestinal anastomoses, chronic nephritis, certain cancers, osteoporosis, peptic ulcer, skin eruption/rash related to a disease, viral, fungal or active infections, tuberculosis. Hypertension, glaucoma, epilepsy, acute glomerulonephritis (inflammation of kidney glomerulus), diabetes, cirrhosis, hypothyroidism, pregnancy, stress. To be withdrawn gradually.

Possible interaction: NSAIDs, oral anticoagulants, phenytoin, ephedrine, phenobarbitone, rifampicin, diuretics, cardiac glycosides, anticholinesterases, hypoglycaemics.

Side effects: osteoporosis, depression, euphoria, hyperglycaemia, peptic ulcers, Cushingoid changes.

Manufacturer: Upjohn.

Soneryl^{CD}

Description: an hypnotic barbiturate available as pink, scored tablets containing 100mg butobarbitone marked SONERYL.

Used for: insomnia which has not responded to other drugs.

Dosage: 1–2 tablets taken at bedtime.

Special care: extremely dangerous, addictive drug with narrow margin of safety. Liable to abuse by overdose leading to coma and death or if combined with alcohol. Easily produces dependence and severe withdrawal symptoms. Drowsiness may persist next day affecting driving and performance of skilled tasks.

Avoid use: should be avoided if possible in all patients. Not to be used for children, young adults, pregnant and nursing mothers, elderly pesons, those with drug or alcohol related problems, patients with liver, kidney or heart disease, porphyria. Insomnia where the cause is pain.

Possible interaction: alcohol, CNS depressants, griseofulvin, metronidazone, rifampicin, phenytoin, chloramphenicol. Anticoagulant drugs of the coumarin type, steroid drugs including contraceptive pill.

Side effects: hangover with drowsiness, shakiness, dizziness, headache, anxiety, confusion, excitement, rash and allergic responses, gastro intestinal upsets, urine retention, loss of sexual desire.

Manufacturer: Theraplix.

Sotacor

Description: a non-cardioselective ß-blocker available as white tablets in 2 strengths of 80mg and 160mg containing solatol hydrochloride, both marked with strength and name. Also, **Sotacor Injection** available as a solution in ampoules for injection containing 10mg/ml.

Used for: prevention of second heart attack, arrhythmias, angina, hypertension.

Dosage: prevention of heart attack, 320mg once each day starting 5 to 14 days after first attack. Arrhythmias, 160–240mg each day in divided or single doses. Angina, 160mg each day in single or divided doses; hypertension, 160mg each day at first increasing to 320mg daily if needed.

Special care: history of bronchospasm and certain ß-blockers, diabetes, liver or kidney disease, pregnancy, lactation, general anaesthesia. Withdraw gradually. Not for children.

Avoid use: heart block or failure, bradycardia, sick sinus syndrome (associated with sinus node disorder), certain ß-blockers, severe peripheral arterial disease.

Possible interaction: verapamil, hypoglycaemics, reserpine, clonidine withdrawal, some anti-arrhythmics and anaesthetics, antihypertensives, depressants of the CNS, cimetidine, indomethacin, sympathomimetics.

Side effects: bradycardia, cold hands and feet, disturbance to sleep, heart failure, gastrointestinal upset, tiredness on exertion, bronchospasm.

Manufacturer: Bristol-Myers.

Sotazide

Description: an antihypertensive compound which combines a non-cardioselective ß-blocker and thiazide diuretic, available as oblong, scored, blue tablets containing 160mg solatol hydrochloride and 25mg hydrochlorothiazide.

Used for: hypertension.

Dosage: 1 tablet each day increasing to 2 if needed.

Special care: pregnancy, breast-feeding, patients with weak hearts may require diuretics and digitalis, those with diabetes, undergoing general anaesthesia, kidney or liver disorders, gout. Electrolyte (salts) levels may need to be monitored.

Avoid use: history of bronchospasm or obstructive airways disease, heart block, heart shock, uncompensated heart failure, disease of peripheral arteries, bradycardia. Serious or worsening kidney failure or anuria.

Possible interaction: sympathomimetics, class I antiarrhythmics, CNS depressants, clonidine withdrawal, ergot alkaloids, cardiac depressant anaesthetics, verapamil, reserpine, indomethacin, hypoglycaemics, cimetidine, other antihypertensives. Digitalis, potassium supplements, potassium-sparing diuretics, lithium.

Side effects: cold hands and feet, disturbance of sleep, fatigue on exercise, bronchospasm, bradycardia, gastrointestinal disturbances, heart failure, blood changes, gout, sensitivity to light, muscle weakness. If skin rash or dry eyes occur, withdraw drug gradually.

Manufacturer: Bristol-Myers.

Sparine

Description: an antipsychotic and group I phenothiazine available as a yellow suspension containing promazine embonate equivalent to 50mg hydrochloride/5ml. Also, **Sparine Injection** containing 50mg promazine hydrochloride/ml as a solution in ampoules.

Used for: additional therapy in treatment of agitation, restlessness and agitation in elderly people, prolonged hiccough. Injection additionally used for vomiting and nausea, EEG and cardiac investigative proceudres in children.

Dosage: 100–200mg 4 times each day; elderly, half adult dose or 25–50mg for agitation and restlessness. Injection, 50mg every 6 to 8 hours by intramuscular injection; elderly, half adult dose. Children, injection only, 0.7mg/kg body weight given intramuscularly.

Special care: pregnancy, breast-feeding, Parkinson's disease, liver disorders, disease of heart or arteries of heart.

Avoid use: depresssed bone marrow function or in coma.

Possible interaction: alcohol, anaesthetics, anti-convulsants, levodopa, analgesics, antidiabetic drugs, antihypertensives, antidepressants, tranquillizers.

Side effects: extrapyramidal side effects, drowsiness, hypothermia, insomnia, pallor, nightmares, depression, constipation, dry mouth, blocked nose, difficulty in urination. Changes in ECG and EEG, effects on heart, e.g. tachycardia, arrhythmias, blood changes, changes in endocrine system, e.g. effects on menstruation, breasts, impotence, weight gain. Effects on liver, jaundice, sensitivity to light, purple pigmentation of skin and eyes.

Manufacturer: Wyeth.

Spiroctan

Description: a potassium-sparing diuretic, available in the form of blue tablets containing 25mg and green tablets containing 50mg spironolacetone, coded BM B2 and BM A8 respectively. Also, **Spiroctan Capsules**, green, containing 100mg, coded BM A7. Also, **Spiroctan-M**, available as a solution in ampoules containing 20mg canrenoate potassium/ml.

Used for: congestive heart failure, cirrhosis of the liver, nephrotic syndrome (a kidney abnormality), primary aldosteronism (a disease of the adrenal glands in which an excess of aldosterone, the hormone which regulates blood levels of sodium and potassium, is produced). Also, ascites (a collection of fluid in the peritoneal cavity of the abdomen, resulting from various diseases or disorders).

Dosage: tablets and capsules, 50–200mg each day which may be increased, if needed, to a maximum of 400mg. The maximum single dose is 100mg. Spiroctan-M, 200–400mg, maximum 800mg, each day. Children, tablets or capsules, 1.5–3mg/kg body weight each day.

Special care: liver or kidney disorders, long-term use in young people. Fluid, electrolyte and levels of blood urea nitrogen should be monitored.

Avoid use: pregnancy, breast-feeding, Addison's disease, serious kidney disorders, hyperkalaemia.

Possible interaction: potassium-sparing diuretics, potassium supplements, carbenoxolone, ACE inhibitors, NSAIDs, cardiac glycosides.

Side effects: disturbance of metabolism and electrolyte levels, menstrual changes, gastro-intestinal upset, enlargement of breasts, deepening of voice, rash, loss of coordination, confusion.

Manufacturer: B.M. Pharm.

Sporanox

Description: a triazole antifungal drug available as pink/blue capsules enclosing coated pellets containing 100mg itraconazole.

Used for: candidiasis (fungal infections) of vagina, oropharynx (the part of the pharynx containing the tonsils), skin disorders.

Dosage: vulvo-vaginal infections, 2 tablets twice for 1 day; infections of oropharynx, 1 tablet each day for 15 days (2 tablets daily in patients with AIDS or who are neutropenic). Skin disorders, 1 tablet each day for 15 days or 30 days or 2 for 7 days, depending upon condition.

Special care: liver disease or those who have suffered toxic effects to the liver from taking other drugs.

Avoid use: elderly, children, pregnancy, breast-feeding. Contraception must be used during treatment and for 1 month following taking Sporanox.

Possible interaction: antacids, astemizole, rifampicin, terfenadine, cyclosporin, H_2 antagonists.

Side effects: pain in abdomen, indigestion, nausea, headache.

Manufacturer: Janssen.

Stafoxil

Description: a penicillinase-resistant penicillin (i.e. resistant to the enzymes produced by some bacteria), available as brown/cream capsules in 2 strengths, containing 250mg and 500mg flucloxacillin (as sodium salt).

Used for: soft tissue, skin, ear, nose and throat infections caused by Gram-positive bacteria.

Dosage: 250mg 4 times each day taken 1 hour before meals. Children, over 2 years, half adult dose.

Avoid use: children under 2 years.

Side effects: gastrointestinal upset, allergic hypersensitive reactions; rarely, cholestatic jaundice.

Manufacturer: Yamanouchi.

Staril

Description: an antihypertensive and ACE inhibitor available as diamond-shaped, white tablets containing 10mg fosinopril sodium marked with star, 158 and SQUIBB. Also, white 20mg tablets, marked with star, 609 and SQUIBB.

Used for: hypertension which has not responded to other drugs or where these are not appropriate.

Dosage: 10mg once each day at first with a maintenance dose in the order of 10–20mg daily. The maximum daily dose is 40mg. Any diuretic being taken should be stopped a few days before treatment starts but can be resumed after 4 weeks, if needed.

Special care: congestive heart failure, kidney or liver disorders, receiving dialysis, depletion of fluid or salts.

Avoid use: pregnancy, breast-feeding, children.

Possible interaction: antacids, potassium-sparing diuretics, potassium supplements, lithium, NSAIDs, antihypertensives.

Side effects: chest and muscle pains, rash, gastrointestinal upset, fatigue, dizziness, palpitations, cough, disturbance of sense of taste; rarely, pancreatitis. If angioneurotic oedema occurs, withdraw drug.

Manufacturer: Squibb.

STD Injection

Description: a sclerosant drug available as a solution in ampoules for injection at strengths of 0.5%, 1% and 3% all containing sodium tetradecyl sulphate.

Used for: varicose veins in the leg by compression sclerotherapy.

Dosage: for large veins, 0.25–1ml of 3% solution into section of vein by intravenous injection followed immediately by compression applied continuously. Maximum treatment of 4 sites in any 1 session of treatment. Small veins, 0.25–1ml of 1% solution in same way as for large veins. Maximum treatment of 10 sites in any 1 session. Very small veins or venules, 0.1–1ml of 0.5% solution as above. Maximum treatment of 10 sites in any 1 session.

Special care: pregnancy, breast-feeding, disease of the arteries, history of allergy. Treatment must be carried out by specialist with emergency equipment available in the event of anaphylaxis.

Avoid use: thrombophlebitis, infections, varicose veins caused by tumours, diabetes which is not controlled. Patients who are obese or immobile, taking oral contraceptives.

Manufacturer: STD.

Stelazine

Description: an anxiolytic, antidepressant and anticonvulsant preparation which is a phenothiazine group II drug. It is available as sugar-coated, blue tablets in 2 strengths containing 1mg and 5mg trifluoperazine (as hydrochloride), and marked SKF. Also, **Stelazine Syrup** containing 1mg/5ml; **Stelazine Spansules**, yellow/clear, sustained-release capsules containing 2mg, 10mg and 15mg as white and blue pellets, marked 2. **Stelazine Concentrate**, containing 10mg/ml; **Stelazine Injection** available as a solution in ampoules containing 1mg/ml.

Used for: anxiety and agitation which may be accompanied by depression, psychosis, schizophrenia, disturbed behaviour; vomiting and nausea.

Dosage: anxiety, Stelazine tablets, syrup, spansules, 2–4mg each day with a maximum of 6mg. Schizophrenia, psychosis, disturbed behaviour, tablets or syrup, 5mg twice each day at first increasing to 15mg after 7 days. If needed, dosage may be further increased every 3 days by 5mg until condition is controlled and then reduced again for maintenance. Spansules, 1 10mg strength each day at first, increasing to 1 15mg spansule daily after 7 days. Injection, 1–3mg each day in divided doses, by intramuscular injection. Nausea and vomiting, tablets, syrup, spansules, 2–6mg each day. Elderly persons, tablets or syrup, all disorders, 1mg each day at first which may require gradual increase according to response. Children, usually use syrup, all disorders, age 3 to 5 years, up to 1mg; 6 to 12 years, up to 4mg, all as daily divided doses.

Special care: pregnancy, breast-feeding, elderly, heart disease or disease of heart blood vessels, epilepsy, Parkinson's disease, vomiting which is undiagnosed.

Avoid use: children under 3 years, depressed bone marrow function, liver damage, coma.

Possible interaction: analgesics, alcohol, CNS depressants, antihypertensives.

Side effects: dry mouth, blurring of vision, disturbance of CNS, changes to ECG, hormonal changes. Rarely, extrapyramidal side effects and allergic responses with low doses. Judgement and performance of skilled tasks may be impaired.

Manufacturer: S.K. & F.

Stemetil

Description: an antipsychotic and anticonvulsant and phenothiazine group III drug, available as cream tablets 5mg and 25mg (scored) both containing prochlorperazine maleate and marked with strength and name. Also, **Stemetil Syrup** containing 5mg prochlorperazine mesylate/5ml. **Stemetil EFF**, effervescent granules in sachets for reconstitution in water containing 5mg prochlorperazine mesylate. Also, **Stemetil Suppositories**, available in strengths of 5mg and 25mg containing prochlorperazine. **Stemetil Injection** available as a solution in ampoules for injection containing 1.25% prochlorperazine mesylate.

Used for: psychoses, schizophrenia, minor psychiatric and emotional disorders, severe vomiting and nausea, migraine, vertigo resulting from Ménière's disease (an inner ear disorder accompanied by ringing in the ears and progressive deafness).

Dosage: psychiatric disorders, oral preparations, 15–25mg each day, maximum 40mg for minor illnesses; 75–100mg daily for schizophrenia, all in divided doses. Suppositories, 25mg 2 or 3 times each day, then oral preparations. Injection, 12.5–25mg 2 or 3 times each day by deep intramuscular injection then oral preparations. Vertigo, oral preparations, 5mg 3 times each day with a maximum of 30mg. Nausea, vomiting, 20mg as single dose then 10mg after 2 hours if needed. Prevention, 5–10mg 2 or 3 times each day.

Suppositories, for vertigo, nausea and vomiting, 25mg as single dose then oral preparations after 6 hours, if needed. Injection, 12.5mg by deep intramuscular injection, then oral preparations if needed. Children, use syrup for nausea, vomiting only, over 10kg in weight, 0.25mg/kg body weight 2 or 3 times each day.

Special care: breast-feeding, heart disease or disease of heart blood vessels, Parkinson's disease, prolonged vomiting which is not diagnosed.

Avoid use: pregnancy, children under 10kg body weight, epilepsy, depressed bone marrow function, liver or kidney disorders, coma.

Possible interaction: alcohol, antidiabetics, CNS depressants, antihypertensives, anti-cholinergics, analgesics, anticonvulsants.

Side effects: anticholinergic side effects and disturbance of CNS, hypotension on rising (following injection), blood disorders, jaundice. At low doses there may rarely be endocrine changes, extrapyramidal side effects and allergic responses. Judgement and performance of skilled tasks may be impaired.

Manufacturer: Theraplix.

Ster-Zac DC

Description: a disinfectant preparation available as a cream containing 3% hexachlophane.

Used for: disinfection of hands prior to surgery.

Dosage: wash hands with 3–5ml used as soap.

Special care: children under 2 years.

Manufacturer: Hough, Hoseason.

Stesolid

Description: a preparation for use rectally, with applicator, which is a long-acting benzodiazepine, available as a solution in single doses containing 5mg or 10mg diazepam.

Used for: agitation, acute anxiety, convulsions, status epilepticus in which rapid treatment is necessary but injection intravenously is not desirable. Also, muscle spasm and premedication.

Dosage: for all conditions, 10mg via rectum, elderly persons, 5mg. Children, age 1 to 3 years, 5mg; over 3 years, 10mg.

Special care: chronic liver or kidney disease, chronic lung disease, pregnancy, labour, lactation, elderly. May impair judgement. Withdraw gradually and avoid prolonged use.

Avoid use: children under 1 year, depression of respiration, acute lung disease; psychotic, phobic or obsessional states.

Possible interaction: anticonvulsants, depressants of the CNS, alcohol.

Side effects: ataxia, confusion, light-headedness, drowsiness, hypotension, gastrointestinal upsets, disturbances in vision and libido, skin rashes, retention of urine, vertigo. Sometimes jaundice or blood disorders.
Manufacturer: Durmex.

Stiedex

Description: a topical potent steroid preparation available as an oily cream containing 0.25% desoxymethasone. **Stiedex LP**, a moderately potent steroid preparation available as an oily cream containing 0.05%. Also, **Stiedex Lotion**, combining a potent steroid and keratolytic agent in a lotion containing 0.25% desoxymethasone and 1% salicylic acid.
Used for: Stiedex cream and LP cream, skin inflammations responsive to steroids. Lotion, psoriasis, especially of scalp and various other skin conditions.
Dosage: creams, apply thinly 2 or 3 times each day and rub in. Lotion, apply once or twice each day in morning and/or evening and rub in. When condition improves, use once each day.
Special care: thrombophlebitis, psychoses, recent intestinal anastomoses, chronic nephritis, certain cancers, osteoporosis, peptic ulcer, skin eruption/rash related to a disease, viral, fungal or active infections, tuberculosis. Hypertension, glaucoma, epilepsy, acute glomerulonephritis (inflammation of kidney glomerulus), diabetes, cirrhosis, hypothyroidism, pregnancy, stress. To be withdrawn gradually.
Avoid use: children (Stiedex).
Possible interaction: NSAIDs, oral anticoagulants, phenytoin, ephedrine, phenobarbitone, rifampicin, diuretics, cardiac glycosides, anticholinesterases, hypoglycaemics.
Side effects: osteoporosis, depression, euphoria, hyperglycaemia, peptic ulcers, Cushingoid changes.
Manufacturer: Stiefel.

Stiemycin

Description: an antibiotic solution containing 2% erythromycin.
Used for: acne.
Dosage: adults, apply twice each day in the morning and evening after washing.
Side effects: possible slight irritation and dryness of skin at site of application.
Manufacturer: Stiefel.

Streptase

Description: a fibrinolytic preparation available as powder in vials for reconstitution and injection containing 250,000 units or 750,000 units streptokinase. Also, **Streptase 1.5 Mega Units**, as powder in vials for reconstitution and injection containing 1,500,000 units streptokinase.
Used for: Streptase, pulmonary embolism, deep vein thrombosis, blockage of peripheral arteries, thrombosis of retinal blood vessels. Streptase 1.5 Mega Units, acute heart attack.
Dosage: Streptase, initial dose of 250,000 units by intravenous infusion, then 100,000 units by infusion/hour for 24–72 hours depending upon response. Streptase 1.5 Mega Units, single dose over 1 hour by intravenous infusion of 1.5 million units, accompanied by oral doses of 150mg aspirin each day for at least 4 weeks. Children, Streptase only, initial dose adjusted according to condition, body weight then 20 units/ml of blood volume.
Special care: heart disorders; blood tests and anticoagulant therapy are also required.
Avoid use: pregnancy, patients who have received streptokinase treatment in last 5 days to 12 months, those with known allergy to streptokinase. Patients with recent bleeding disorders, clotting disorders, liver or kidney damage, brain growth, lung disease, inflammation and bacterial infection of endocardium, serious bronchitis, pancreatitis, diabetes. Having recently had surgery or with history of bleeding.
Possible interaction: drugs affecting blood platelets, anticoagulants.
Side effects: feverish reactions, heart arrhythmias, hypotension, pulmonary oedema, haemorrhage, embolism caused by cholesterol. Rarely, anaphylaxis.
Manufacturer: Hoechst.

Stromba

Description: an anabolic steroid available as white, scored tablets containing 5mg stanozolol marked STROMBA.
Used for: Behcet's disease, (a rare disease affecting the blood vessels of the eye), prevention of angio-oedema which is hereditary.
Dosage: Behcet's disease, 10mg each day; angio-oedema, 2.5–10mg each day at first then reduce dose as condition responds. Children, angio-oedema, aged 1 to 6 years, 2.5mg each day at first; 6 to 12 years, 2.5–5mg daily in first instance. Dose is then adjusted according to response.
Special care: use for long periods in children, women past menopause, patients with kidney or heart disorders. Monitoring of liver function is required if patient has history of jaundice.

Avoid use: pregnancy, porphyria, cancer of prostate gland, liver disease, type 1 diabetes.

Possible interaction: oral anticoagulants.

Side effects: indigestion, headache, skin rash, pains and cramps; toxic effects on liver, masculinizing effects on women and children before puberty.

Manufacturer: Sanofi Winthrop.

Sublimaze^{CD}

Description: a narocotic analgesic available as a solution in ampoules containing 50µg fentanyl/ml.

Used for: analgesia during operations, enhancement of analgesic, respiratory depression in patients receiving artificial ventilation.

Dosage: adults breathing unaided, 50–200µg at first then 50µg as needed. Adults being ventilated, 0.3–3.5mg at first then 100–200µg as needed. Children, 3 to 5 µg/kg body weight then 1µg/kg as needed. Child being ventilated, 15µg/kg then 1–3 µg/kg as needed.

Special care: liver disease, underactive thyroid, respiratory disorders, myasthenia gravis. If used in obstetric patients, may cause depression of respiration in baby.

Avoid use: obstructive airways disease or depression of respiration unless being artificially ventilated.

Possible interaction: MAOIs, anxiolytics, hypnotics, cimetidine.

Side effects: depression of respiration, bradycardia, vomiting, nausea, short-lived hypotension.

Manufacturer: Janssen.

Sulpitil

Description: an antipsychotic preparation and substituted benzamide available as scored, white tablets containing 200mg sulpiride marked L113.

Used for: schizophrenia.

Dosage: adults and young persons over 14 years, 200–400mg twice each day with a maximum of 1800mg daily. Elderly, 50–100mg twice each day at first increasing slowly to normal adult dose.

Special care: pregnancy, epilepsy, kidney disorders, hypertension, hypomania.

Avoid use: breast-feeding, phaeochromocytoma, porphyria.

Possible interaction: alcohol, anxiolytics, hypnotics, tetrabenazine, calcium channel blockers, cimetidine.

Side effects: extrapyramidal side effects, ECG and EEG changes. Effects on heart rhythm, blocked nose, dry mouth, constipation, blurring of vision, difficulty passing urine, drowsiness, apathy, depression, insomnia. Blood changes involving white blood cells, hormonal changes, e.g.

enlargement of breasts, change in libido, impotence, sensitivity to light, effects on liver, changes in weight.

Manufacturer: Pharmacia.

Sultrin

Description: a compound sulphonamide antibacterial preparation available as lozenge-shaped, white, vaginal tablets (with applicator) containing 172.5mg sulphathiazole, 143.75mg sulphacetamide and 184mg sulphabenzamide marked with C and symbol. Also, **Sultrin Cream** containing 3.42% sulphathiazole, 2.86% sulphacetamide, 3.7% sulphabenzamide, with applicator.

Used for: inflammation and infection of vagina and cervix caused by bacteria, post-cervical cautery, postoperative treatment.

Dosage: tablets, 1 intravaginally twice each day for 10 days. Cream, 1 applicator dose intravaginally twice each day for 10 days which may need to be reduced to 1 dose daily, depending upon response.

Avoid use: children, kidney disorders.

Side effects: allergic reactions.

Manufacturer: Cilag.

Suprax

Description: an antibiotic cephalosporin available as film-coated, scored white tablets containing 200mg cefixime marked LL200 and SUPRAX. Also, **Suprax Paediatric Suspension** containing 100mg/5ml solution.

Used for: infections of urinary and respiratory tract.

Dosage: 200–400mg as single or 2 divided doses for 7 to 14 days. Children, age 6 to 12 months, 3.75ml; 1 to 4 years, 5ml; 5 to 10 years, 10ml; 11 to 12 years, 15ml. All as daily doses of paediatric suspension.

Special care: pregnancy, breast-feeding, allergy to ß-lactams, serious kidney disorders.

Avoid use: children under 6 months.

Side effects: rashes, gastrointestinal upset, headache, dizziness. Rarely, pseudomembranous colitis.

Manufacturer: Lederle.

Suprecur

Description: a preparation which is a GnRH (gonadotrophin-releasing hormone) analogue that acts on the pituitary gland inhibiting the release of gonadotrophin, resulting in a lowering of the levels of oestrogen produced by the ovaries. It is available in the form of a nasal spray, with pump, delivering a metered dose of 150µg buserelin (as acetate) per application.

Used for: endometriosis, pituitary desensitization prior to controlled stimulation of the ovaries (with gonadotrophins) as a part of infertility treatment.

Dosage: for endometriosis, 1 spray into each nostril in the morning, middle of the day and evening for a maximum period of 6 months. Treatment should begin on first or second day of monthly cycle. Infertility, 1 spray in 1 nostril 4 times each day, as directed by specialist, usually for 2 to 3 weeks.

Special care: patients subject to depression or at risk of osteoporosis. Barrier methods of contraception must be used.

Avoid use: pregnancy, breast-feeding, hormone-dependent tumours, undiagnosed vaginal bleeding.

Possible interaction: nasal decongestants.

Side effects: local irritation of nose, menopausal symptoms, e.g. hot flushes, change in libido, vaginal dryness, sweating, nausea, headache, changes in breasts and tenderness, cysts on ovaries, backache, dry skin, acne, rash, palpitations, changes in density of bones.

Manufacturer: Hoechst.

Suprefact

Description: a gonadotrophin-releasing hormone analogue, acting on pituitary gland receptors resulting in the inhibition of the release of luteinizing hormone and lower levels of testosterone in the blood. Suprefact is available in vials for injection containing 1mg buserelin (as acetate)/ml. Also, **Suprefact Nasal Spray** containing 100 µg per dose.

Used for: Stage C or D cancer of the prostate gland in which it is desirable for levels of testosterone to be reduced.

Dosage: 0.5ml every 8 hours by subcutaneous injection for 1 week. Then 1 spray in each nostril 6 times each day as maintenance dose.

Special care: anti-androgens may be needed.

Avoid use: patients with tumours that are not responsive to hormones; those who have had 1 or both testes surgically removed (orchidectomy).

Side effects: short-lived irritation of nostrils, loss of libido, hot flushes.

Manufacturer: Hoechst.

Surgam SA

Description: an NSAID which is a propionic acid available as sustained-release maroon/pink capsules enclosing white pellets containing 300mg tiaprofenic acid, marked SURGAM SA. Also, **Surgam Tablets**, white, in strengths of 200mg and 300mg, marked with symbol on one side and name and strength on the reverse.

Used for: disorders of joints, skeleton and muscles including osteoarthritis, rheumatoid arthritis, lumbago, ankylosing spondylitis, injuries.

Dosage: capsules, 2 as a single daily dose; tablets, 600mg as divided doses each day.

Special care: pregnancy, breast-feeding, elderly, heart failure, liver or kidney disorders, known allergy to aspirin or NSAID.

Avoid use: children, history of or active peptic ulcer.

Possible interaction: sulphonamides, hypo-glycaemics, diuretics, anticoagulants, hydantoins.

Side effects: headache, gastrointestinal upset, sleepiness, rash. Withdraw if cystitis and haematuria (blood in urine) occur (rare).

Manufacturer: Roussel.

Surmontil

Description: a TCAD preparation available as white tablets in strengths of 10mg and 25mg containing trimipramine (as maleate), both marked with strength and SURMONTIL. Also, **Surmontil Capsules**, white/green containing 50mg marked SU50.

Used for: depression and/or anxiety, agitation, disturbance of sleep.

Dosage: mild or moderate symptoms, 50–75mg as single dose, 2 hours before going to bed. Continue for a minimum of 3 weeks. Moderate to severe symptoms, 75mg each day under specialist supervision gradually increasing according to condition. Usual dose is in the order of 150–300mg each day then reducing for maintenance once condition improves. Elderly, 10–25mg 3 times each day.

Special care: liver disorders, hyperthyroidism, glaucoma, lactation, epilepsy, diabetes, adrenal tumour, heart disease, urine retention. Psychotic or suicidal patients.

Avoid use: heart block, heart attacks, severe liver disease, pregnancy.

Possible interaction: MAOIs (or within 14 days of their use), alcohol, antidepressants, barbiturates, anticholinergics, local anaesthetics that contain adrenaline or noradrenaline, oestrogens, cimetidine, antihypertensives.

Side effects: constipation, urine retention, dry mouth, blurred vision, palpitations, tachycardia, nervousness, drowsiness, insomnia. Changes in weight, blood and blood sugar, jaundice, skin reactions, weakness, ataxia, hypotension, sweating, altered libido, gynaecomastia, galactorrhoea.

Manufacturer: Theraplix.

Survanta

Description: a lung surfactant available as a solution

in single dose vials containing 25mg beractant (a natural lung extract)/ml.

Used for: newborn babies with respiratory distress undergoing mechanical ventilation whose birthweight exceeds 700g and who are receiving continuous monitoring.

Dosage: 100mg/kg body weight in volume not greater than 4ml/kg by endotracheal tube. Best given within 8 hours of birth and a maximum of 4 further doses at a minimum of 6 hourly intervals, may be given within 48 hours.

Special care: continuous monitoring of oxygen level in arterial blood required.

Side effects: endotracheal tube may become blocked by mucous, possible haemorrhage in lung.

Manufacturer: Abbott.

Sustamycin

Description: a tetracycline antibiotic preparation available as sustained-release capsules in light and darker blue containing 250mg tetracycline hydrochloride.

Used for: infections responsive to tetracyclines, severe acne.

Dosage: infections, 2 capsules twice each day at first reducing to 1 as condition improves. Acne, 4 tablets each day for first 2 to 3 weeks then 1 for 3 to 4 months.

Special care: liver or kidney disorders.

Avoid use: pregnancy, breast-feeding, children.

Possible interaction: mineral supplements, milk, antacids, oral contraceptives.

Side effects: allergic responses, superinfections, gastrointestinal upset.

Manufacturer: B.M. Pharmaceuticals.

Sustanon 100

Description: an hormonal depot androgen preparation available in ampoules for injection containing 20mg testosterone propionate, 40mg testosterone phenylpropionate, 40mg testosterone isocaproate/ml. Also, **Sustanon 250** available in ampoules for injection containing 30mg testosterone propionate, 60mg testosterone phenylpropionate, 60mg testosterone isocaproate and 100mg testosterone decanoate/ml.

Used for: androgen deficiency in males, osteoporosis resulting from androgen deficiency.

Dosage: 1ml by deep intramuscular injection every 2 weeks; Sustanon 250, 1ml by deep intramuscular injection every 3 weeks.

Special care: heart, liver or kidney disorders, migraine, hypertension, epilepsy.

Avoid use: heart disease, heart failure which is untreated, cancer of prostate gland or liver, nephrotic syndrome (a kidney abnormality resulting from various diseases and disorders).

Possible interaction: drugs which induce liver enzymes.

Side effects: weight gain, liver tumours, oedema, reduced fertility, premature closure of epiphyses, priapism (painful and prolonged erection of penis not connected with sexual arousal but caused by drug treatment or sickle-cell trait. Causes tissue damage if not relieved by decompression).

Manufacturer: Organon.

Symmetral

Description: a dopaminergic, tricyclic amine preparation available as reddish-brown capsules containing 100mg amantadine hydrochloride marked GEIGY. Also, **Symmetral Syrup** containing 50mg amantadine hydrochloride/ml.

Used for: Parkinson's disease, prevention and treatment of patients with certain strains of influenza (A_2, A/New Jersey) who are at risk from complications. *Herpes zoster* infections.

Dosage: Parkinson's disease, 100mg capsules of syrup each day for 7 days at first then same dose twice daily. Influenza, treatment, 1 capsule twice each day for 5 to 7 days; prevention, 1 capsule twice each day for 7 to 10 days. *Herpes zoster*, 1 capsule or 10ml syrup twice each day for 14 to 28 days. Children, for influenza age over 10 years, treatment and prevention, 1 capsule in morning for 7 to 10 days.

Special care: pregnancy, congestive heart failure, liver or kidney disorders, suffering from confusion.

Avoid use: children under 10 years, serious kidney disease, history of or active stomach ulcer, history of convulsions.

Possible interaction: anticholinergics, levodopa, CNS stimulants.

Side effects: livedo reticularis (a disorder of the veins resulting in a mottled 'fish-net' appearance of legs and occasionally arms), oedema in hands and feet, skin rash, gastrointestinal upset, disturbance of vision, effects on central nervous system.

Manufacturer: Geigy.

Synacthen Depot

Description: a depot preparation of adrenal stimulating hormone available in ampoules for injection containing 1mg tetracosactrin acetate and zinc complex/ml.

Used for: collagen and rheumatic disorders, Crohn's disease, ulcerative colitis.

Dosage: acute treatment, 1–2g by intramuscular

injection each day with reduced doses for maintenance. Children, age 1 month to 2 years, 0.25mg by intramuscular injection each day at first; 2 to 5 years, 0.25–0.5mg by intramuscular injection each day at first; 5 to 12 years, 0.25–1mg by intramuscular injection each day at first. For maintenance, these doses are repeated every 2 to 8 days.

Special care: thrombophlebitis, psychoses, recent intestinal anastomoses, chronic nephritis, certain cancers, osteoporosis, peptic ulcer, skin eruption/rash related to a disease, viral, fungal or active infections, tuberculosis. Hypertension, glaucoma, epilepsy, acute glomerulonephritis (inflammation of kidney glomerulus), diabetes, cirrhosis, hypothyroidism, pregnancy, stress. To be withdrawn gradually.

Avoid use: allergic conditions, asthma.

Possible interaction: NSAIDs, oral anticoagulants, phenytoin, ephedrine, phenobarbitone, rifampicin, diuretics, cardiac glycosides, anticholinesterases, hypoglycaemics.

Side effects: osteoporosis, depression, euphoria, hyperglycaemia, peptic ulcers, Cushingoid changes.
Manufacturer: Ciba.

Synalar

Description: a potent topical steroid preparation available as cream and ointment containing 0.025% fluocinolone acetonide. **Synalar 1:4**, a moderately potent steroid cream and ointment containing 0.00625%. **Synalar Cream 1:10**, a mildly potent steroid cream containing 0.0025%. **Synalar C** a combined potent steroid, antibacterial, antifungal cream and ointment containing 0.025% fluocinolone acetonide and 3% clioquinol. **Synalar N**, a potent steroid and antibacterial cream and ointment containing 0.025% fluocinolone acetonide and 0.5% neomycin sulphate. Also, **Synalar Gel** containing 0.025% fluocinolone acetate.

Used for: Synalar steroid preparations, skin conditions responsive to steroid treatment; Synalar combined preparations, infected skin conditions responsive to steroid treatment. Synalar Gel, skin conditions of the scalp responsive to steroid treatment.

Dosage: apply thinly 2 or 3 times each day and rub in. Synalar Gel, rub into scalp in the morning and at night at first and then once or twice each week for maintenance.

Special care: thrombophlebitis, psychoses, recent intestinal anastomoses, chronic nephritis, certain cancers, osteoporosis, peptic ulcer, skin eruption/rash related to a disease, viral, fungal or active

infections, tuberculosis. Hypertension, glaucoma, epilepsy, acute glomerulonephritis (inflammation of kidney glomerulus), diabetes, cirrhosis, hypothyroidism, pregnancy, stress. To be withdrawn gradually.

Avoid use: use only mild steroid preparations in children.

Possible interaction: NSAIDs, oral anticoagulants, phenytoin, ephedrine, phenobarbitone, rifampicin, diuretics, cardiac glycosides, anticholinesterases, hypoglycaemics.

Side effects: osteoporosis, depression, euphoria, hyperglycaemia, peptic ulcers, Cushingoid changes.
Manufacturer: Zeneca.

Synard

Description: a gonadotrophin-releasing hormone analogue available as a nasal spray delivering 200µg nafarelin (as acetate) per metered dose. It acts on the pituitary gland to lower the levels of oestrogen produced by the ovaries and endometrial growth.

Used for: endometriosis.

Dosage: 1 spray into 1 nostril in the morning and then a second spray into the other nostril in the evening. Treatment should continue for a maximum period of 6 months and start between day 2 and 4 of monthly cycle.

Special care: patients at risk of osteoporosis. Barrier methods of contraception should be used.

Avoid use: pregnancy, breast-feeding, undiagnosed vaginal bleeding. Treatment should not be repeated.

Possible interaction: nasal decongestants.

Side effects: changes in libido and bone density, changes in breast size and tenderness. Menopausal symptoms, e.g. hot flushes, sweating, vaginal dryness, mood changes, depression, aches and cramps. Migraine, palpitations, cysts on ovaries, allergic hypersensitive responses, hair loss, blurring of vision.

Manufacturer: Syntex.

Synflex

Description: an NSAID available as film-coated orange tablets containing 275mg napoxen sodium marked SYNTEX.

Used for: period pain, pain following operations, migraine, muscle and bone pains, strains and sprains.

Dosage: age over 16 years, usual dose, 2 tablets as 1 dose then 1 tablet 6 to 8-hourly as required. Maximum dose is 4 tablets daily. Migraine, 3 tablets as first dose then 1 or 2 tablets 6 to 8-hourly with a daily maximum of 5.

Special care: pregnancy, breast-feeding, elderly, liver or kidney disorders, history of lesions in the gastrointestinal tract, heart failure, asthma. Patients taking drug long-term require careful monitoring.

Avoid use: children under 16 years, known allergy to NSAID or aspirin, peptic ulcer.

Possible interaction: sulphonylureas, anti-coagulants, frusemide, ß-blockers, quinolones, ACE inhibitors, hydantoins, lithium probenecid, methotrexate.

Side effects: blood changes, gastrointestinal dibances and nausea, vertigo, rash, tinnitus, some sensitivity and oedema but these are uncommon.

Manufacturer: Syntex.

Synphase

Description: a combined oestrogen/progestogen oral contraceptive preparation available as: 7 white tablets containing 35µg ethinyloestradiol, 0.5mg norethisterone; 9 yellow tablets containing 35µg and 1mg norethisterone; 5 white tablets containing 35µg and 0.5mg respectively. All are marked SYNTEX and the white tablets also with a B.

Used for: oral contraception.

Dosage: 1 tablet each day starting on fifth day of period then 7 tablet-free days.

Special care: multiple sclerosis, serious kidney disease or kidney dialysis, asthma, Raynaud's disease, abnormally high levels of prolactin in the blood (hyperprolactinaemia), varicose veins, hypertension, severe depression. Thrombosis risk increases with smoking, age and obesity. During the course of treatment, regular checks on blood pressure, pelvic organs and breasts should be carried out.

Avoid use: pregnancy, patients at risk of thrombosis, suffering from heart disease, pulmonary hypertension, angina, sickle cell anaemia. Also, undiagnosed vaginal bleeding, history of cholestatic jaundice during pregnancy, cancers which are hormone-dependent, infectious hepatitis, liver disorders. Also, porphyria, Dublin-Johnson and Rotor syndrome, otosclerosis, chorea, haemolytic uraemic syndrome, recent trophoblastic disease.

Possible interaction: barbiturates, ethosuximide, glutethimide, rifampicin, phenytoin, tetracyclines, carbamazepine, chloral hydrate, griseofulvin, dichloralphenazone, primidone.

Side effects: weight gain, breast enlargement, pains in legs and cramps, headaches, loss of sexual desire, depression, nausea, breakthrough bleeding, cervical erosion, brownish patches on skin (chloasma), vaginal discharge, oedema and bloatedness.

Manufacturer: Syntex.

Syntaris

Description: a corticosteroid preparation available as a nasal spray delivering 25µg flunisolide per metered dose.

Used for: allergic and inflammatory conditions affecting the nose, e.g. hay fever.

Dosage: 2 sprays into each nostril 2, or maximum of 3, times each day reducing to a minimum effective dose for control. Treatment should continue long-term. Children, age 5 to 12 years, 1 spray in each nostril 3 times each day.

Special care: pregnancy, patients who have had recent trauma or surgery, ulcers of the nose. Also, special care in patients changing from other steroid drugs.

Avoid use: children under 5, untreated infections of nose or eyes.

Side effects: short-lived irritation of nose.

Manufacturer: Syntex.

Syntocinon

Description: a uterotropic hormonal preparation containing synthetic oxytocin used in obstetrics, and available as a solution in ampoules for injection at strengths of 2 units/2ml, 5 units/ml, 10 units/ml, 50 units/5ml.

Used for: to induce and augment labour, missed abortion.

Dosage: by slow intravenous infusion as a solution containing 1 unit per litre, adjusted as needed.

Special care: disorders of heart and heart circulation, hypertension, previous Caesarian section, abnormal presentation of baby, multiple birth.

Avoid use: placental praevia, serious toxaemia, obstruction of delivery, distress in baby, hypertonic (very active) activity of uterus, tendency to amniotic fluid embolism.

Side effects: danger of severe uterine contractions leading to rupture (with higher doses), hypertension and subarachnoid haemorrhage in mother, heart arrhythmias, water intoxication and lung oedema (infusion volume must remain low).

Manufacturer: Sandoz.

Syntometrine

Description: a uterotropic hormonal preparation used in obstetrics available as a solution in ampoules for injection containing 0.5mg ergometrine maleate and 5 units synthetic oxytocin/ml.

Used for: bleeding due to incomplete abortion (before surgery to remove contents of uterus), during delivery (third stage of labour) after or when baby's shoulders have emerged.

Dosage: 1ml by intramuscular injection.
Special care: porphyria, multiple birth, hypertension, heart disease, liver or kidney disease.
Avoid use: serious heart, liver, kidney or lung disease, severe hypertension, sepsis, circulatory disease, toxaemia, in first or second stage of labour.
Side effects: vomiting and nausea, short-lived hypertension, constriction of blood vessels, heart attack, stroke, lung oedema.
Manufacturer: Sandoz.

Syntopressin
Description: a vasopressin analogue available as a solution for use with a nasal spray delivering 50 units lypressin/ml.

Used for: diabetes insipidus.
Dosage: 1 or 2 sprays into one or both nostrils 3 to 7 times a day.
Special care: pregnancy, patients with epilepsy, hypertension, disease of peripheral blood vessels, hypertension, advanced arteriosclerosis, heart failure.
Avoid use: coronary heart disease, undergoing anaesthesia with cyclopropane or halothane.
Possible interaction: chlorpropamide, lithium, carbamazepine, clofibrate.
Side effects: blocked nose and ulceration of lining of nose, nausea, pain in abdomen, feeling of needing to defecate.
Manufacturer: Sandoz.

T

Tagamet

Description: an H_2 blocker cimetidine for treatment of ulcers, available in green tablets (200mg) and green oblong tablets (400mg) marked TAGAMET, SK & F and strength, and green oval tablets (800mg) marked SK & F and T 800. Also, **Tagamet Effervescent**, 400mg white effervescent tablet and **Tagamet Syrup** (200mg/5ml).

Used for: ulcers—duodenal, benign gastric, recurrent and stomach. Dyspepsia, oesophageal reflux and where gastric acid has to be reduced.

Dosage: for duodenal ulcer, 800mg at bedtime or 400mg twice daily for 4 weeks, then half dose for maintenance. See literature for other conditions. Children over 1 year, 25–30mmg/kg per day in divided doses. Also, **Tagamet Injection** (200mg/ 2ml) and **Tagamet Infusion** (400mg in 100ml).

Special care: eliminate malignancy first; kidney disorder, pregnancy, breast-feeding.

Possible interaction: theophylline, oral anti-coagulants, phenytoin.

Side effects: rash, dizziness, tiredness, diarrhoea, confusion (in the elderly), gynaecomastia; rarely pancreatitis, thrombocytopenia, muscle and joint pain.

Manufacturer: S.K. & F.

Tambocor

Description: a class I antiarrhythmic, flecainide acetate, available as white tablets marked 3M TR 50 (50mg) or 3M TR 100 (100mg).

Used for: tachycardia, arrhythmias.

Dosage: 50–100mg twice per day to a maximum of 400mg daily, depending upon condition, reduced after 3 to 5 days to the lowest possible maintenance dose. Not for children.

Also, **Tambocor Injection**, 10mg/ml in ampoules.

Dosage: see literature. Not for children.

Special care: start therapy in hospital. Pacemakers, weak liver or kidneys, heart disease, pregnancy. Monitor plasma levels.

Avoid use: heart failure, past myocardial infarction, 2nd or 3rd degree atrioventricular block, sinus node disease, atrial fibrillation.

Possible interaction: digoxin, other class I antiarrhythmics, cardiac depressants.

Side effects: nausea, dizziness, vomiting, sight disturbances, sensitivity to light, jaundice, upset to liver enzymes, ataxia, tingling sensations.

Manufacturer: 3m Health Care.

Tamofen

Description: an antioestrogen, tamoxifen citrate, available as white tablets with 10mg (marked T10), 20mg (T20) and 40mg (T40).

Used for: infertility (only under strict medical supervision and monitoring), breast cancer.

Dosage: 20mg per day for 4 days starting on second day on menstruation increasing to 40g and then 80mg for later treatments if required. For breast cancer 20mg per day increasing to 40mg if required.

Avoid use: pregnancy.

Possible interaction: warfarin.

Side effects: gastrointestinal upset, hot flushes, vaginal bleeding, dizziness, disturbance to sight.

Manufacturer: Tillotts.

Tampovagan

Description: an oestrogen, stilboestrol, available as a pessary with 5% lactic acid.

Used for: vaginitis after the menopause.

Dosage: 2, high in the vagina at night for 2 to 3 weeks. Not for children.

Special care: patients considered to be at risk of thrombosis or with liver disease. Women with any of the following disorders should be carefully monitored: fibroids in the womb, multiple sclerosis, diabetes, tetany, porphyria, epilepsy, liver disease, hypertension, migraine, otosclerosis, gallstones. Breasts, pelvic organs and blood pressure should be checked at regular intervals during the course of treatment.

Avoid use: pregnancy, breast-feeding, conditions which might lead to thrombosis, thrombophlebitis, serious heart, kidney or liver disease, breast cancer, oestrogen-dependent cancers including those of reproductive system, endometriosis, vaginal bleeding which is undiagnosed.

Possible interaction: drugs which induce liver enzymes.

Side effects: tenderness and enlargement of breasts, weight gain, breakthrough bleeding, giddiness, vomiting and nausea, gastrointestinal upset. Treatment should be halted immediately if severe headaches occur, disturbance of vision, hypertension or any indications of thrombosis, jaundice. Also, in the event of pregnancy and 6 weeks before planned surgery.

Manufacturer: Norgine.

Tarcortin

Description: a mild steroid and anti-psoriatic, comprising 0.5% hydrocortisone and 5% coal tar extract in a cream.

Used for: eczema, psoriasis and other skin disorders.

Dosage: apply twice or more per day.

Special care: thrombophlebitis, psychoses, recent intestinal anastomoses, chronic nephritis, certain cancers, osteoporosis, peptic ulcer, skin eruption/rash related to a disease, viral, fungal or active infections, tuberculosis. Hypertension, glaucoma, epilepsy, acute glomerulonephritis (inflammation of kidney glomerulus), diabetes, cirrhosis, hypothyroidism, pregnancy, stress. To be withdrawn gradually.

Possible interaction: NSAIDs, oral anticoagulants, phenytoin, ephedrine, phenobarbitone, rifampicin, diuretics, cardiac glycosides, anticholinesterases, hypoglycaemics.

Side effects: osteoporosis, depression, euphoria, hyperglycaemia, peptic ulcers, Cushingoid changes.

Manufacturer: Stafford-Miller.

Targocid

Description: a glycopeptide and antibiotic, teicoplanin, available as powder in vials (200 and 400mg).

Used for: serious Gram-positive infections or staphylococcal infections where there is no response or a sensitivity to penicillins or cephalosporins.

Dosage: 400mg intravenously on first day, then 200mg per day. For severe infections, 400mg intravenously every 12 hours for 3 doses then 400mg daily. Over 85kg, 3–6mg/kg but see literature. If kidney disease, reduce dose from day 4. Children, up to 2 months, 16mg/kg on first day, then 8mg/kg per day; over 2 months, 10mg/kg every 12 hours for 3 doses then 6mg/kg per day. For severe infections 10mg/kg every 12 hours for 3 doses then same dose daily.

Special care: check blood, liver and kidneys regularly.

Avoid use: pregnancy, lactation.

Side effects: thrombophlebitis, rash, fever, reaction at site of injection, bronchospasm, nausea, vomiting, dizziness, diarrhoea, blood changes.

Manufacturer: Merrell Dow.

Tarivid

Description: a 4-quinolone antibiotic, ofloxacin, available as white, oblong tablets (200mg) and yellow, oblong tablets (400mg).

Used for: infections of the urinary tract, respiratory tract. Sexually transmitted diseases.

Dosage: 200–400mg per day depending upon the infection and its severity. Doses over 400mg to be given as 2 divided doses. Not for children.

Also, **Tarivid Infusion**, 2mg/ml ofloxacin hydrochloride.

Used for: infections of the respiratory tract, upper and lower urinary tract, septicaemia.

Dosage: 200–800mg per day for 7 to 10 days, varying according to infection and its severity. Not for children.

Special care: kidney damage, psychiatric disorders, exposure to UV light or strong sunlight, when driving or operating machinery.

Avoid use: pregnancy, breast-feeding, history of epilepsy, growing adolescents.

Possible interaction: NSAIDs, anticoagulants, iron, antacids with aluminium or magnesium. Hypotensives, barbiturate anaesthetics (for injection).

Side effects: skin reactions, convulsions, disturbances to CNS, gastrointestinal upset, hypersensitivity reactions, colitis. For injection—thrombophlebitis, pain at the site of injection, hypotension.

Manufacturer: Hoechst.

Taxol

Description: a taxane, paclitaxel, available as a solution (6mg/ml) in vials.

Used for: ovarian cancer (metastatic) resistant to treatment with platinum.

Dosage: 175mg/m^2 by intravenous infusion over 3 hours, repeated 3-weekly. Additional, preliminary treatment necessary with antihistamines, H$_2$-antagonists and corticosteroids.

Special care: abnormalities in heart conduction, disease of peripheral nerves, liver or kidney failure. Check blood. Have resuscitation equipment available.

Avoid use: if neutrophils are low, pregnancy, lactation, severe liver damage.

Side effects: peripheral nerve disease, suppression of

bone marrow, joint and muscle pain, hair loss, hypotension, gastrointestinal upset, bradycardia, oedema.
Manufacturer: BMS.

Tazocin

Description: a ß-lactamase inhibitor (active against ß-lactamase-producing bacteria) and broad spectrum penicillin comprising piperacillin (2g) with tazobactam (250mg) both as sodium salts also as 4g/500mg both as powder in vials.
Used for: infections of the lower respiratory tract, urinary tract, of the skin, abdominal. Septicaemia and infections caused by more than 1 organism.
Dosage: 4.5g every 8 hours by slow intravenous infusion or injection. Not for children.
Special care: pregnancy, breast-feeding, kidney failure, low potassium levels.
Possible interaction: drugs that affect blood coagulation or platelet function, probenecid.
Side effects: allergic reactions, superinfection, gastrointestinal upset, skin reactions.
Manufacturer: Lederle.

Tegretol

Description: an iminostilbene and dibenzazepine, carbamazepine, available as white tablets (100 and 200mg) marked with name and strength, and white oblong tablets (400mg) marked with name and strength. Also, **Tegretol Chewtabs**, 100 and 200mg as square, pale orange chewable tablets marked T, tablet strength and name. **Tegretol Retard**, 200mg in continuous-release, orange, oblong tablets marked CG and HC and 400mg tablets coloured brown and marked CG and ENE. Also, **Tegretol Liquid**, a sugar-free liquid containing 100mg/5ml.
Used for: prevention of manic depressive psychosis which does not respond to therapy with lithium, epilepsy, trigeminal neuralgia.
Dosage: manic depression—start with 400mg per day in divided doses and increase until the symptoms are controlled (to a maximum of 1.6g per day), usually 400–600mg. Epilepsy, start with 100–200mg once or twice per day increasing to 800mg–1.2g and a maximum of 1.6g. Children, 10 to 15 years, 600mg–1g; 5 to 10 years, 400–600mg; 1 to 5 years, 200–400mg; up to 1 year, 100–200mg. All per day, in divided doses. Neuralgia, start with 100mg once or twice per day increasing to gain control, usually 600–800mg per day in divided doses (daily maximum 1.6g).
Special care: pregnancy, breast-feeding, liver and kidney disease, elderly, severe cardiovascular disease. Check blood and liver function.

Avoid use: abnormalities in atrioventricular conduction (heart conduction block).
Possible interaction: MAOIs, combined oral contraceptives, oral anticoagulants, steroids, lithium, phenytoin, cimetidine, dextropropoxyphene, doxycycline, isoniazid, erythromycin, diltiazem, verapamil, viloxazine.
Side effects: double vision, dry mouth, dizziness, drowsiness, gastric upset, oedema, rashes, blood changes, hair loss, toxic epidermal necrolysis (a rare skin disease producing exfoliation), kidney failure, hepatitis, enlargement of lymph nodes, changes in heart conduction, jaundice.
Manufacturer: Geigy.

Temazepam

Description: an intermediate benzodiazepine and hypnotic, temazepam, available as a solution (10mg/5ml). Also, **Temazepam Tablets** (10 and 20mg) and **Temazepam Gel Filled**, 10, 15, 20 and 30mg gel-filled capsules.
Used for: insomnia.
Dosage: 10–30mg at bedtime (elderly, 5–15mg). For severe cases, up to 60mg maximum. Not for children.
Special care: chronic liver or kidney disease, chronic lung disease, pregnancy, labour, lactation, elderly. May impair judgement. Withdraw gradually and avoid prolonged use.
Avoid use: depression of respiration, acute lung disease; psychotic, phobic or obsessional states.
Possible interaction: anticonvulsants, depressants of the CNS, alcohol.
Side effects: ataxia, confusion, light-headedness, drowsiness, hypotension, gastrointestinal upsets, disturbances in vision and libido, skin rashes, retention of urine, vertigo. Sometimes jaundice or blood disorders.
Manufacturer: non-proprietary.

Temgesic^{CD}

Description: an opiate and analgesic, buprenorphine hydrochloride, available as white, sublingual tablets (200 and 400µg) marked with 2 or 4 and symbol.
Used for: moderate to severe pain.
Dosage: 200–400µg sublingually every 6 to 8 hours or as required. Children, not for under 16kg; 16–25kg, 100µg; 25–37.5kg, 100–200µg; 37.5–50kg, 200–300µg, taken sublingually every 6 to 8 hours. Also, **Temgesic Injection** (300µg/ml in ampoules).
Dosage: 300–600µg every 6 to 8 hours, by intramuscular or slow, intravenous injection. Children, not for under 6 months; over 6 months, 3–6µg/kg every 6 to 8 hours to a maximum of 9µg/kg.

Special care: pregnancy, labour, reduced breathing or liver functions, dependence on narcotics or large doses previously.

Possible interaction: depressants of the CNS, MAOIs.

Side effects: nausea, dizziness, drowsiness, sweating.

Manufacturer: Reckitt & Colman.

Temopen

Description: a penicillin, temocillin (as sodium) that is resistant to penicillinase, available as powder (1g) in vials.

Used for: septicaemia, infections of the urinary and lower respiratory tracts caused by Gram-negative bacilli which are susceptible to temocillin.

Dosage: 1–2g every 12 hours intramuscularly or intravenously. For urinary tract infection, 1g per day. Contact manufacturer re dosage for children.

Special care: pregnancy, breast-feeding, kidney disease.

Side effects: pain at the point of injection, diarrhoea. Discontinue if rash occurs.

Manufacturer: Bencard.

Tenif

Description: a cardioselective ß-blocker and class II calcium antagonist, atenolol (50mg) with nifedipine (20mg) available in red-brown capsules marked with TENIF and logo.

Used for: angina, hypotension.

Dosage: 1 capsule twice per day (angina); 1 per day increasing to 2 per day if necesssary (elderly, 1) for hypertension. Not for children.

Special care: anaesthesia, diabetes, liver or kidney disease, weak heart or heart conduction defect.

Avoid use: heart failure, heart block, cardiagenic shock, pregnancy, breast-feeding.

Possible interaction: heart depressants, quinidine, cimetidine.

Side effects: oedema, headache, dizziness, flushes, rash, dry eyes, jaundice, hyperplasia of the gums.

Manufacturer: Stuart.

Tenoret 50

Description: a cardioselective ß-blocker and thiazide diuretic comprising 50mg atenolol and 12.5mg chlorthalidone in brown tablets marked TENORET 50 and logo.

Used for: hypertension, especially in the elderly.

Dosage: 1 tablet per day. Not for children.

Special care: history of bronchospasm and certain ß-blockers, diabetes, liver or kidney disease, pregnancy, lactation, general anaesthesia, gout, check electrolyte levels, K+ supplements may be required depending on the case. Withdraw gradually. Not for children.

Avoid use: heart block or failure, slow heart rate (bradycardia), sick sinus syndrome (associated with sinus node disorder), certain ß-blockers, severe peripheral arterial disease, pregnancy, lactation, severe kidney failure, anuria, hepatic cornea.

Possible interaction: verapamil, hypoglycaemics, reserpine, clonidine withdrawal, some antiarrhythmics and anaesthetics, antihypertensives, depressants of the CNS, cimetidine, indomethacin, sympathomimetics, lithium, potassium supplements with potassium-sparing diuretics, digitalis.

Side effects: bradycardia, cold hands and feet, disturbance to sleep, heart failure, gastrointestinal upset, tiredness on exertion, bronchospasm, gout, weakness, blood disorders, sensitivity to light.

Manufacturer: Stuart.

Tenoretic

Description: a cardioselective ß-blocker and thiazide diuretic containing 100mg atenolol, 25mg chlorthalidone in brown tablets marked with logo and TENORETIC.

Used for: hypertension.

Dosage: 1 tablet per day. Not for children.

Special care: history of bronchospasm and certain ß-blockers, diabetes, liver or kidney disease, pregnancy, lactation, general anaesthesia, gout, check electrolyte levels, K+ supplements may be required depending on the case. Withdraw gradually. Not for children.

Avoid use: heart block or failure, slow heart rate (bradycardia), sick sinus syndrome (associated with sinus node disorder), certain ß-blockers, severe peripheral arterial disease, pregnancy, lactation, severe kidney failure, anuria, hepatic cornea.

Possible interaction: verapamil, hypoglycaemics, reserpine, clonidine withdrawal, some anti-arrhythmics and anaesthetics, antihypertensives, depressants of the CNS, cimetidine, indomethacin, sympathomimetics, lithium, potassium supplements with potassium-sparing diuretics, digitalis.

Side effects: bradycardia, cold hands and feet, disturbance to sleep, heart failure, gastrointestinal upset, tiredness on exertion, bronchospasm, gout, weakness, blood disorders, sensitivity to light.

Manufacturer: Stuart.

Tenormin

Description: a cardioselective ß-blocker, atenolol, available in white tablets (25mg, marked with TENORMIN, 25 and logo) and orange tablets

(100mg, marked with TENORMIN and logo). Also, **Tenormin LS**, 50mg orange tablets marked 9 with name and **Tenormin Syrup**, a lemon-lime sugar-free syrup containing 25mg/ml. Also available as **Tenormin Injection** (0.5mg/ml in 10ml ampoule).

Used for: cardiac arrhythmias, early treatment of acute myocardial infarction, angina, hypertension.

Dosage: 50–100mg per day, reduced for the elderly or where there is kidney disorder. Not for children.

Special care: history of bronchospasm and certain ß-blockers, diabetes, liver or kidney disease, pregnancy, lactation, general anaesthesia. Withdraw gradually. Not for children.

Avoid use: heart block or failure, slow heart rate (bradycardia), sick sinus syndrome (associated with sinus node disorder), certain ß-blockers, severe peripheral arterial disease.

Possible interaction: verapamil, hypoglycaemics, reserpine, clonidine withdrawal, some anti-arrhythmics and anaesthetics, antihypertensives, depressants of the CNS, cimetidine, indomethacin, sympathomimetics.

Side effects: bradycardia, cold hands and feet, disturbance to sleep, heart failure, gastrointestinal upset, tiredness on exertion, bronchospasm.

Manufacturer: Stuart.

Tenuate Dospan^{CD}

Description: a CNS stimulant, diethylpropion hydrochloride, available as sustained-release, white, oblong tablets marked MERRELL.

Used for: obesity.

Dosage: 1 tablet mid-morning. Not for children.

Special care: angina, peptic ulcer, hypertension, arrhythmias.

Avoid use: severe hypertension, arteriosclerosis, hyperthyroidism, glaucoma, pregnancy, breast-feeding, past drug or alcohol abuse or psychiatric illness.

Possible interaction: other anoretic drugs, anti-hypertensives, antidiabetics, guanethidine, MAOIs, sympathomimetics, psychotropics, methyldopas.

Side effects: dependence, tolerance, psychoses, agitation, sleeplessness. Do not use over long period.

Manufacturer: Merrell Dow.

Teoptic

Description: a ß-blocker, carteolol hydrochloride, available as 1% and 2% drops.

Used for: hypertension in the eye, certain glaucomas.

Dosage: start with 1 drop of 1% solution in affected eye twice per day. Use 2% solution if 1% is ineffective. Not for children.

Special care: heart block, cardiogenic shock, diabetes.

Avoid use: heart failure, asthma, serious lung disease, pregnancy, soft or gas-permeable contact lenses.

Possible interaction: other ß-blockers.

Side effects: blurred vision, burning sensation, pain, irritation of the eye, hyperaemia (greater than normal amount of blood in the vessels).

Manufacturer: Ciba Vision.

Terra-Cortril

Description: an antibiotic 0.5% oxytetracycline hydrochloride, with a mild steroid, 0.17% hydrocortisone, in a spray.

Used for: infected eczema, infected intertrigo (dermatitis of skin surfaces in contact), insect bites.

Dosage: spray 2 to 4 times per day. Not for children.

Also **Terra-Cortril Ointment**, 3% oxytetracycline hydrochloride with 1% hydrocortisone.

Dosage: use 2 to 4 times per day. Not for children.

Also, **Terra-Cortril Nystatin**, as for the ointment but with 100,000 units nystatin (an antifungal).

Used for: infected skin conditions.

Dosage: apply 2 to 4 times per day. Not for children.

Special care: thrombophlebitis, psychoses, recent intestinal anastomoses, chronic nephritis, certain cancers, osteoporosis, peptic ulcer, skin eruption/rash related to a disease, viral, fungal or active infections, tuberculosis. Hypertension, glaucoma, epilepsy, acute glomerulonephritis (inflammation of kidney glomerulus), diabetes, cirrhosis, hypo-thyroidism, pregnancy, stress. To be withdrawn gradually.

Possible interaction: NSAIDs, oral anticoagulants, phenytoin, ephedrine, phenobarbitone, rifampicin, diuretics, cardiac glycosides, anticholinesterases, hypoglycaemics.

Side effects: osteoporosis, depression, euphoria, hyperglycaemia, peptic ulcers, Cushingoid changes.

Also, an antibiotic/corticosteroid combination with 5mg oxytetracycline hydrochloride, 15mg hydrocortisone acetate and 10,000 units/ml polymyxin in B sulphate, in drop form.

Used for: external ear infections.

Dosage: 2 to 4 drops 3 times per day for up to 7 days. Not for children.

Avoid use: pregnancy, perforated ear drum, infections of a viral, fungal or tuberculous nature or those containing pus.

Side effects: superinfection, allergy.

Manufacturer: Pfizer.

Terramycin

Description: a tetracycline, oxytetracycline,

available as yellow tablets (250mg) marked Pfizer. Also, **Terramycin Capsules**, 250mg in yellow capsules marked TER 250 and Pfizer.
Used for: infections sensitive to Terramycin; severe acne.
Dosage: 250–500mg 4 times per day. Not for children.
Special care: liver or kidney disease.
Avoid use: pregnancy, breast-feeding.
Possible interaction: antacids, mineral supplements, milk, oral contraceptives.
Side effects: superinfections, allergic reactions, gastrointestinal upsets.
Manufacturer: Pfizer.

Tertroxin

Description: a thyroid hormone, liothyronine sodium (20µg), in white tablets marked with EVANS and name.
Used for: severe thyroid deficiency, myxoedema coma.
Dosage: start with 10–20µg 8-hourly increasing after 7 days if required to 60µg per day in divided doses. For elderly and children, start with 5µg per day in divided doses.
Special care: diabetes, breast-feeding.
Avoid use: angina caused by effort, cardiovascular problems.
Possible interaction: phenytoin, anticoagulants, tricyclics, cholestyramine.
Side effects: tachycardia, arrhythmias, muscle cramps or weakness, anginal pain, flushes, headache, sweating, diarrhoea, weight loss, excitability.
Manufacturer: Link.

Tetavex

Description: a purified tetanus toxoid vaccine containing 40 units/0.5ml on aluminium hydroxide in syringes, ampoules and vials.
Used for: immunization and booster doses.
Dosage: first immunization: 0.5ml, then 0.5ml after 1 month and 0.5ml after 1 more month. Reinforcing (booster) doses: 0.5ml 10 years after first immunization. When required after injuries, 0.5ml single dose unless a booster has been administered in previous 12 months. All given by deep subcutaneous or intramuscular injection.
Special care: hypersensitivity may occur if a dose is given within 12 months of a booster.
Avoid use: acute infectious disease unless in a wound susceptible to tetanus.
Side effects: malaise, fever.
Manufacturer: Merieux.

Tetrabid

Description: 250mg tetracycline hydrochloride in purple/yellow sustained-release capsules.
Used for: acne, infections sensitive to this drug such as bronchitis.
Dosage: 1 capsule per day for at least 3 months (acne). For infections, start with 2 capsules then 1 every 12 hours. Not for children.
Special care: liver or kidney disorder.
Avoid use: pregnancy, breast-feeding.
Possible interaction: antacids, mineral supplements, milk, digoxin, oral anticoagulants, oral contraceptives.
Side effects: superinfections, allergic reactions, gastrointestinal upset. Cease use if there is intracranial hypertension.
Manufacturer: Organon.

Tetralysal

Description: a tetracycline, lymecycline (408mg), in white capsules marked Farmitalia.
Used for: acne; infections of the skin and soft tissue; ear, nose and throat or the respiratory tract.
Dosage: 1 twice per day (for at least 8 weeks in the case of acne). Not for children.
Special care: liver and kidney disorders.
Avoid use: pregnancy, breast-feeding.
Possible interaction: mineral supplements, antacids, oral contraceptives.
Side effects: superinfections, allergic reactions, gastrointestinal upset.
Manufacturer: Farmitalia.

Tical

Description: a penicillin, ticarcillin sodium, available as a 5g infusion bottle and powder in vials.
Used for: septicaemia, peritonitis, infections of the urinary or respiratory tract, infected wounds, endocarditis and postoperative infections especially those caused by *Pseudomonas aeruginosa*.
Dosage: up to 20g by slow intravenous injection or rapid infusion (children 300mg/kg) or up to 4g per day intramuscularly and in divided doses (children 100mg/kg).
Special care: kidney disease.
Side effects: gastrointestinal upset, hypersensitivity reactions.
Manufacturer: Link.

Tilade Mint Syncroner

Description: an anti-inflammatory and non-steroid, nedocromil sodium, available as a mint-flavoured suspension delivered by aerosol with spacer device (2mg). Also, **Tilade Mint**, utilizing a metered dose aerosol

Used for: bronchial asthma where anti-inflammatory control is required.

Dosage: start with 2 puffs 4 times per day (2 puffs twice per day for maintenance). Not for children.

Special care: pregnancy.

Side effects: cough, passing headache, gastrointestinal upset.

Manufacturer: Fisons.

Tildiem

Description: a class III calcium antagonist, diltiazem hydrochloride, available as off-white tablets (60mg) marked TILDIEM 60.

Used for: angina.

Dosage: 60mg 3 times per day to a maximum of 480mg per day in divided doses. Not for children.

Also, **Tildiem Retard**, white, sustained-release tablets (90 and 120mg).

Dosage: start with 90mg or 120mg twice per day increasing if required to a maximum of 2 120mg tablets twice per day. Elderly; 60mg twice per day, increasing to 90 or 120mg. Not for children.

Also, **Tildiem LA**, white/yellow, sustained-release capsules containing 300mg.

Used for: hypertension.

Dosage: 1 at the same time every day. For the elderly, start with Retard 120mg each day. Using Retard–120mg twice per day increasing if required to 180mg twice daily. Elderly, 120mg daily to a maximum of 120mg twice per day. Not for children.

Special care: check heart rate in elderly or cases of liver and kidney disorder. Monitor patients with mild bradycardia.

Avoid use: pregnancy, bradycadia, heart block, sick sinus syndrome.

Possible interaction: other antihypertensives, ß-blockers, heart depressants, digoxin, dantrolene infusion, cyclosporin, diazepam, lithium cimetidine, theophylline, carbamazepine.

Manufacturer: Lorex.

Timecef

Description: a cephalosporin antibiotic, cefodizime (as sodium salt) available in vials (1g).

Used for: infections of the urinary and lower respiratory tracts.

Dosage: 1g twice per day (respiratory tract), 2g per day as 1 or divided doses (urinary tract) by intravenous injection, infusion or intramuscular injection. Not for children.

Special care: sensitivity to penicillin, severe kidney disorder, pregnancy, breast-feeding, colitis.

Possible interaction: aminoglycosides, loop

diuretics.

Side effects: gastrointestinal upset, passing rise in liver enzymes, hypersensitivity reactions, eosinophilia (increase of eosinophils, a type of white blood cell, in the blood).

Manufacturer: Roussel.

Timentin

Description: a ß-lactamase inhibitor with penicillin, comprising clavulanic acid (as potassium salt) with ticarcillin (as sodium salt) available as powder in vials (1.6 or 3.2g containing 100mg/1.5g and 200mg/3g).

Used for: severe infections in patients in hospital with poor host defence to infection.

Dosage: 3.2g every 6 to 8 hours by intermittent intravenous infusion to a maximum frequency of 4-hourly. Children up to 1 month, 80mg/kg every 12 hours, increasing to 8-hourly; others 80mg/kg every 6 to 8 hours.

Special care: kidney disorder, severe liver disorder.

Side effects: gastrointestinal upset, hypersensitivity reactions, hepatitis.

Manufacturer: Beecham.

Timodine

Description: a combined antifungal, mild steroid and disinfectant comprising 100,000 units/g nystatin, 0.5% hydrocortisone, 0.2% benzalkonium chloride solution with 10% dimethicone.

Used for: skin disorders, severe nappy rash infected with *Candida*.

Dosage: apply sparingly 3 times per day or at nappy change.

Special care: thrombophlebitis, psychoses, recent intestinal anastomoses, chronic nephritis, certain cancers, osteoporosis, peptic ulcer, skin eruption/rash related to a disease, viral, fungal or active infections, tuberculosis. Hypertension, glaucoma, epilepsy, acute glomerulonephritis (inflammation of kidney glomerulus), diabetes, cirrhosis, hypothyroidism, pregnancy, stress. To be withdrawn gradually.

Possible interaction: NSAIDs, oral anticoagulants, phenytoin, ephedrine, phenobarbitone, rifampicin, diuretics, cardiac glycosides, anticholinesterases, hypoglycaemics.

Side effects: osteoporosis, depression, euphoria, hyperglycaemia, peptic ulcers, Cushingoid changes.

Manufacturer: Reckitt & Colman.

Timoptil

Description: a ß-blocker, timolol maleate, available as metered dose drops (0.25% and 0.5%).

Used for: ocular hypertension, certain glaucomas.

Dosage: 1 drop of 0.25% solution twice per day increasing to 0.5% solution if required. Not for children.

Special care: pregnancy, breast-feeding, withdraw gradually.

Avoid use: heart failure, heart block, asthma, sinus bradycardia, past obstructive lung disease, soft lenses.

Possible interaction: adrenaline, antihypertensives, verapamil.

Side effects: irritation, systemic ß-blocker effects (e.g. cold hands and feet, tiredness, stomach upset, rash).

Manufacturer: M.S.D.

Tinset

Description: an antihistamine and mast cell stabiliser, oxatomide, available as white tablets (30mg) marked JANSSEN and Ox over 30.

Used for: allergic rhinitis, urticaria, other allergic conditions.

Dosage: adults 1 to 2 tablets twice per day; children over 5 up to 1 tablet twice per day. Not for children under 5.

Possible interaction: depressants of the CNS, alcohol.

Side effects: drowsiness, slowed reactions.

Manufacturer: Janssen.

Tobralex

Description: an aminoglycoside, tobramycin, available as 0.3% drops.

Used for: bacterial infections of the eye.

Dosage: 1 or 2 drops every 4 hours, up to 2 drops every hour for severe cases. Reduce dose before ceasing treatment.

Side effects: passing irritation.

Manufacturer: Alcon.

Tofranil

Description: a TCAD, imipramine hydrochloride, available as red-brown triangular (10mg) and round (25mg) tablets, both marked GEIGY. Also, **Tofranil Syrup** (25mg/5ml).

Used for: depression; bed-wetting in children.

Dosage: 25mg 3 times per day, up to 150–200mg per day after 7 days. Maintenance dose, 50–100mg per day. Elderly, 10mg per day increasing to 30–50mg. Children: over 11 years, 10–15ml; 8 to 11 years, 5–10ml; 6 to 7 years, 5ml; at bedtime for 3 months maximum (withdraw gradually). Not for children under 6 years.

Special care: liver disorders, hyperthyroidism, glaucoma, lactation, epilepsy, diabetes, adrenal

tumour, heart disease, urine retention. Psychotic or suicidal patients.

Avoid use: heart block, heart attacks, severe liver disease, pregnancy.

Possible interaction: MAOIs (or within 14 days of their use), alcohol, antidepressants, barbiturates, anticholinergics, local anaesthetics that contain adrenaline or noradrenaline, oestrogens, cimetidine, antihypertensives.

Side effects: constipation, urine retention, dry mouth, blurred vision, palpitations, tachycardia, nervousness, drowsiness, insomnia. Changes in weight, blood and blood sugar, jaundice, skin reactions, weakness, ataxia, hypotension, sweating, altered libido, gynaecomastia, galactorrhoea.

Manufacturer: Geigy.

Tolanase

Description: a sulphonylurea, tolazamide, available as white tablets marked UPJOHN 70 (100mg) or UPJOHN 114 (250mg).

Used for: maturity-onset diabetes.

Dosage: 100–250mg per day to a maximum of 1g if necessary (in divided doses). Not for children.

Special care: elderly, kidney failure.

Avoid use: during pregnancy or lactation; juvenile, growth-onset or unstable brittle diabetes (insulin-dependent diabetes mellitus); ketoacidosis; severe kidney or liver disorders; stress, infections or surgery; endocrine disorders.

Possible interaction: MAOIs, corticosteroids, ß-blockers, diuretics, corticotrophin (ACTH), oral contraceptives, alcohol. Also aspirin, oral anti-coagulants, and the generic drugs bezafibrate, clofibrate, phenylbutazone, cyclophosphamide, rifampicin, sulphonamides and chloramphenicol. Also glucagon.

Side effects: skin rash and other sensitivity reactions. Other conditions tend to be rare, e.g. hyponatraemia (low blood sodium concentration) or aplastic anaemia.

Manufacturer: Upjohn.

Tolectin

Description: a derivative of acetic acid, tolmetin (as sodium salt), available as orange/ivory capsules marked T200 (200mg) or orange capsules marked T400 (400mg).

Used for: osteoarthritis, rheumatoid arthritis, ankylosing spondylitis, juvenile rheumatoid arthritis, joint disorders.

Dosage: 600–1800mg per day in 2 to 4 divided doses. Children, 20–25mg/kg per day in 3 or 4 divided doses.

Special care: liver or kidney disease (check on long-term treatment), heart failure, past gastrointestinal disease, pregnancy, breast-feeding, elderly.
Avoid use: allergy to aspirin or anti-inflammatory drugs, active peptic ulcer.
Side effects: oedema, rash, epigastric pain.
Manufacturer: Cilag.

Tolerzide
Description: a non-cardioselective ß-blocker and thiazide diuretic comprising 80mg sotalol hydrochloride and 12.5mg hydrochlorothiazide in a lilac tablet marked TOLERZIDE.
Used for: hypertension.
Dosage: 1 tablet per day. Not for children.
Special care: history of bronchospasm and certain ß-blockers, diabetes, liver or kidney disease, pregnancy, lactation, general anaesthesia, gout, check electrolyte levels, K⁺ supplements may be required depending on the case. Withdraw gradually.
Avoid use: heart block or failure, slow heart rate (bradycardia), sick sinus syndrome (associated with sinus node disorder), certain ß-blockers, severe peripheral arterial disease, pregnancy, lactation, severe kidney failure, anuria, hepatic cornea, urinary retention.
Possible interaction: verapamil, hypoglycaemics, reserpine, clonidine withdrawal, some anti-arrhythmics and anaesthetics, antihypertensives, depressants of the CNS, cimetidine, indomethacin, sympathomimetics, lithium, potassium supplements with potassium-sparing diuretics, digitalis.
Side effects: bradycardia, cold hands and feet, disturbance to sleep, heart failure, gastrointestinal upset, tiredness on exertion, bronchospasm, gout, weakness, blood disorders, sensitivity to light.
Manufacturer: Bristol-Myers.

Tonocard
Description: a class I antiarrhythmic, tocainide hydrochloride, available as yellow tablets marked A/TT (400mg).
Used for: life-threatening ventricular arrhythmias.
Dosage: 1.2g per day in 2 or 3 divided doses, to a maximum of 1.8–2.4g. Not for children.
Special care: severe liver or kidney disease, elderly, heart failure, pregnancy.
Avoid use: heart block in the absence of a pacemaker.
Possible interaction: other anti-arrhythmics.
Side effects: leucopenia, agranulocytosis, tremor, SLE, dizziness, gastrointestinal upset.
Manufacturer: Astra.

Topicycline
Description: an antibiotic, tetracycline hydrochloride, available as a 0.22% solution.
Used for: acne.
Dosage: apply liberally twice per day until the skin is wet. Not for children.
Special care: kidney disease, pregnancy, breast-feeding. Avoid mouth, eyes and mucous membranes.
Side effects: stinging.
Manufacturer: P. & G.P.

Topilar
Description: a potent steroid, fluclorolone acetonide, available as a cream (0.025%). Also **Topilar Ointment** (0.025%).
Used for: skin disorders that respond to steroids, plaque psoriasis of soles and palms.
Dosage: apply 2 times per day.
Special care: thrombophlebitis, psychoses, recent intestinal anastomoses, chronic nephritis, certain cancers, osteoporosis, peptic ulcer, skin eruption/rash related to a disease, viral, fungal or active infections, tuberculosis. Hypertension, glaucoma, epilepsy, acute glomerulonephritis (inflammation of kidney glomerulus), diabetes, cirrhosis, hypothyroidism, pregnancy, stress. To be withdrawn gradually.
Possible interaction: NSAIDs, oral anticoagulants, phenytoin, ephedrine, phenobarbitone, rifampicin, diuretics, cardiac glycosides, anticholinesterases, hypoglycaemics.
Side effects: osteoporosis, depression, euphoria, hyperglycaemia, peptic ulcers, Cushingoid changes.
Manufacturer: Bioglan.

Toradol
Description: an NSAID, ketorolac trometamol, available as solutions (10mg/ml and 30mg/ml) in ampoules.
Used for: short-term control of moderate or severe postoperative pain.
Dosage: start with 10mg intravenously or intramuscularly then 10–30mg 4 to 6 hourly. Maximum 90mg daily for 2 days. Elderly, maximum 60mg daily for 2 days. Not for children under 16. Also, **Toradol Tablets**, 10mg in white tablets marked TORADOL 10 and SYNTEX.
Dosage: 1 tablet 4 to 6 hourly, maximum 4 per day, for up to 7 days. If following injections, 90mg maximum dose on day 1 and 40mg thereafter. Elderly, 1 tablet 6 to 8-hourly for up to 7 days. Maximum dose after injections 60mg on day 1 and then 40mg. Not for children under 16.

Special care: elderly; heart, liver kidney or allergic disease, gastrointestinal disease.

Avoid use: allergy to aspirin or anti-inflammatory drugs, pregnancy, breast-feeding, peptic ulcer, angioneurotic oedema, asthma, blood coagulation disorders, kidney disease, gastrointestinal or cerebrovascular bleeding, low volume of circulating blood, dehydration, high risk of haemorrhage induced by surgery.

Possible interaction: NSAIDs, anticoagulants, lithium, methotrexate, probenecid, frusemide, oxypentifylline.

Side effects: ulcers, wound haemorrhage, gastrointestinal upsets, drowsiness, oedema, kidney failure, bronchospasm, anaphylaxis, pain at site of injection, abnormal liver functions.

Manufacturer: Syntex.

Totamol

Description: a cardioselective ß-blocker, atenolol, available as orange tablets (25, 50 and 100mg) each marked ATL, CP and with tablet strength.

Used for: cardiac arrhythmias, early treatment of acute myocardial infarction; angina; hypertension.

Dosage: 50–100mg per day, less for the elderly or where there is impaired kidney function. Not for children.

Special care: history of bronchospasm and certain ß-blockers, diabetes, liver or kidney disease, pregnancy, lactation, general anaesthesia. Withdraw gradually. Not for children.

Avoid use: heart block or failure, bradycardia, sick sinus syndrome (associated with sinus node disorder), certain ß-blockers, severe peripheral arterial disease.

Possible interaction: verapamil, hypoglycaemics, reserpine, clonidine withdrawal, some anti-arrhythmics and anaesthetics, antihypertensives, depressants of the CNS, cimetidine, indomethacin, sympathomimetics.

Side effects: bradycardia, cold hands and feet, disturbance to sleep, heart failure, gastrointestinal upset, tiredness on exertion, bronchospasm.

Manufacturer: C.P. Pharm.

Tracrium

Description: a muscle relaxant, atracurium besylate, available in ampoules (10mg/ml).

Used for: surgery, long-term ventilation.

Dosage: start with 300–600µg/kg, then 100–200µg/kg as required, by intravenous injection; 5–10µg/kg/minute by intravenous infusion.

Special care: respiration should be assisted until drug is inactivated or antagonised.

Avoid use: myasthenia gravis.

Possible interaction: lithium, nifedipine, verapamil.

Manufacturer: Wellcome.

Trancopal

Description: a muscle relaxant and tranquilliser, chlormezanone, available in yellow tablets (200mg) marked TR.

Used for: short-term treatment of insomnia, and anxiety where there is muscle tension; painful muscle spasms.

Dosage: 200mg up to 4 times per day or 1 400mg dose at night. Half doses for the elderly. Not for children.

Special care: liver or kidney disease, pregnancy. Judgement and dexterity may be impaired.

Avoid use: porphyria.

Possible interaction: alcohol, MAOIs, CNS depressants.

Side effects: headache, dry mouth, nausea, lethargy, dizziness, rashes, jaundice.

Manufacturer: Sanofi Winthrop.

Trandate

Description: an a/ß-blocker, labetolol hydrochloride, available as orange tablets (50, 100, 200 and 400mg) marked with name and strength.

Used for: angina, hypertension.

Dosage: start with 100mg twice per day with food, increasing at intervals of 14 days to a maximum of 2.4g per day in divided doses. Elderly start with 50mg twice per day. Not for children.

Also, **Trandate Injection**, ampoules containing 5mg/ml.

Special care: history of bronchospasm and certain ß-blockers, diabetes, liver or kidney disease, pregnancy, lactation, general anaesthesia. Withdraw gradually. Not for children.

Avoid use: heart block or failure, slow heart rate, sick sinus syndrome (associated with sinus node disorder), certain ß-blockers, severe peripheral arterial disease.

Possible interaction: verapamil, hypoglycaemics, reserpine, clonidine withdrawal, some anti-arrhythmics and anaesthetics, antihypertensives, depressants of the CNS, cimetidine, indomethacin, sympathomimetics.

Side effects: bradycardia, cold hands and feet, disturbance to sleep, heart failure, gastrointestinal upset, tiredness on exertion, bronchospasm. Withdraw if liver reaction (rare).

Manufacturer: D.F.

Tranxene

Description: a long-acting benzodiazepine,

clorazepate potassium available in capsules containing 15mg (pink/grey) and 7.5mg (maroon/ grey), marked with TRANXENE, capsule strength and symbol.

Used for: anxiety whether or not depression is present.

Dosage: 7.5–22.5mg per day, elderly 7.5mg. Not for children under 16.

Special care: chronic liver or kidney disease, chronic lung disease, pregnancy, labour, lactation, elderly. May impair judgement. Withdraw gradually and avoid prolonged use.

Avoid use: depression of respiration, acute lung disease; psychotic, phobic or obsessional states.

Possible interaction: anticonvulsants, depressants of the CNS, alcohol.

Side effects: ataxia, confusion, light-headedness, drowsiness, hypotension, gastrointestinal upsets, disturbances in vision and libido, skin rashes, retention of urine, vertigo. Sometimes jaundice or blood disorders.

Manufacturer: Boehringer Ingelheim.

Trasicor

Description: a non-cardioselective ß-blocker, oxprenolol hydrochloride, available as tablets containing 20 or 40mg (white), 80mg (beige) and 160mg (orange) all marked with strength, CIBA and TRASICOR.

Used for: cardiac arrhythmias, angina, hypertension, anxiety.

Dosage: from 20–160mg 2 or 3 times per day, depending upon condition being treated. Maximum daily dose 480mg. Not for children.

Special care: history of bronchospasm and certain ß-blockers, diabetes, liver or kidney disease, pregnancy, lactation, general anaesthesia. Withdraw gradually. Not for children.

Avoid use: heart block or failure, bradycardia, sick sinus syndrome (associated with sinus node disorder), certain ß-blockers, severe peripheral arterial disease.

Possible interaction: verapamil, hypoglycaemics, reserpine, clonidine withdrawal, some antiarrhythmics and anaesthetics, antihypertensives, depressants of the CNS, cimetidine, indomethacin, sympathomimetics.

Side effects: bradycardia, cold hands and feet, disturbance to sleep, heart failure, gastrointestinal upset, tiredness on exertion, bronchospasm.

Manufacturer: Ciba.

Trasidrex

Description: a non-cardioselective ß-blocker and thiazide, comprising 160mg oxprenolol hydrochloride in a sustained-release core and 0.25mg cyclopenthiazide in a red outer coat. The tablet is marked with Ciba and TRASIDREX.

Used for: hypertension.

Dosage: start with 1 tablet each morning increasing to 3 per day if required. Not for children.

Special care: history of bronchospasm and certain ß-blockers, diabetes, liver or kidney disease, pregnancy, lactation, general anaesthesia, gout, check electrolyte levels, K$^+$ supplements may be required depending on the case. Withdraw gradually. Not for children.

Avoid use: heart block or failure, bradycardia, sick sinus syndrome (associated with sinus node disorder), certain ß-blockers, severe peripheral arterial disease, pregnancy, lactation, severe kidney failure, anuria, hepatic cornea.

Possible interaction: verapamil, hypoglycaemics, reserpine, clonidine withdrawal, some antiarrhythmics and anaesthetics, antihypertensives, depressants of the CNS, cimetidine, indomethacin, sympathomimetics, lithium, potassium supplements with potassium-sparing diuretics, digitalis.

Side effects: bradycardia, cold hands and feet, disturbance to sleep, heart failure, gastrointestinal upset, tiredness on exertion, bronchospasm, gout, weakness, blood disorders, sensitivity to light.

Manufacturer: Ciba.

Trasylol

Description: a haemostatic and antifibrinolytic, aprotinin, available as vials containing 500,000 units per 50ml.

Used for: where there is risk of major blood loss during open heart surgery, or where blood conservation is vital, haemorrhage.

Dosage: by slow intravenous injection or infusion, up to 2 or 3 million units.

Side effects: localized thrombophlebitis, sometimes hypersensitivity reactions.

Manufacturer: Bayer.

Travogyn

Description: an antifungal drug, isoconazole nitrate, available as white, almond-shaped vaginal tablets (300mg) marked with CT in a hexagon.

Used for: vaginal infections from *Candida* or mixed fungal and Gram-positive bacteria.

Dosage: 2 tablets inserted in 1 dose. Not for children.

Side effects: passing irritation and burning sensation.

Manufacturer: Schering H.C.

Traxam

Description: an NSAID, felbinac, available as a 3% gel. Also, **Traxam Foam** (3.17%).

Used for: strains, sprains and injury to soft tissue.

Dosage: 1g rubbed into the area 2 to 4 times per day initially for 14 days. Maximum daily usage 25g. Not for children.

Special care: pregnancy, breast-feeding.

Avoid use: allergy to aspirin or anti-inflammatory drugs.

Side effects: dermatitis, itching, erythema.

Manufacturer: Lederle.

Trental

Description: a peripheral vasodilator and xanthine, oxpentifylline, available in pink, oblong, sustained-release tablets (400mg).

Used for: disorders of the peripheral vascular system.

Dosage: 400mg 2 or 3 times per day. Not for children.

Special care: coronary artery disease, hypotension, kidney disease.

Avoid use: porphyria.

Possible interaction: antihypertensives.

Side effects: flushes, vertigo, gastrointestinal upsets.

Manufacturer: Hoechst.

Tri-Adcortyl

Description: a potent steroid with antifungal and antibacterial comprising 0.1% triamcinolone acetate, 100,000 units/g nystatin, 0.25% neomycin sulphate and 0.025% gramicidin, as cream and ointment.

Used for: inflamed skin disorders with infection.

Dosage: use 2 to 4 times per day.

Special care: thrombophlebitis, psychoses, recent intestinal anastomoses, chronic nephritis, certain cancers, osteoporosis, peptic ulcer, skin eruption/rash related to a disease, viral, fungal or active infections, tuberculosis. Hypertension, glaucoma, epilepsy, acute glomerulonephritis (inflammation of kidney glomerulus), diabetes, cirrhosis, hypothyroidism, pregnancy, stress. To be withdrawn gradually.

Possible interaction: NSAIDs, oral anticoagulants, phenytoin, ephedrine, phenobarbitone, rifampicin, diuretics, cardiac glycosides, anticholinesterases, hypoglycaemics.

Side effects: osteoporosis, depression, euphoria, hyperglycaemia, peptic ulcers, Cushingoid changes.

Manufacturer: Squibb.

Tri-Adcortyl Otic

Description: a combined preparation of corticosteroid, antibiotic and antifungal containing 0.1% triamcinolone acetonide, 0.25% neomycin sulphate, 0.025% gramicidin and 100,000 units/g nystatin.

Used for: inflammation of the outer ear.

Dosage: use 2 to 4 times per day.

Special care: pregnancy, perforated ear drum, do not use long-term in infants.

Avoid use: viral and tuberculous lesions.

Manufacturer: Squibb.

Tri-Cicatrin

Description: a topical corticosteroid containing 1% hydrocortisone, 250 units/g bacitracin zinc, 3400 units/g neomycin sulphate and 100,000 units/g nystatin, as an ointment.

Used for: mild inflammatory skin disorders.

Dosage: use 2 to 3 times per day, less frequently upon improvement.

Special care: thrombophlebitis, psychoses, recent intestinal anastomoses, chronic nephritis, certain cancers, osteoporosis, peptic ulcer, skin eruption/rash related to a disease, viral, fungal or active infections, tuberculosis. Hypertension, glaucoma, epilepsy, acute glomerulonephritis (inflammation of kidney glomerulus), diabetes, cirrhosis, hypothyroidism, pregnancy, stress. To be withdrawn gradually.

Possible interaction: NSAIDs, oral anticoagulants, phenytoin, ephedrine, phenobarbitone, rifampicin, diuretics, cardiac glycosides, anticholinesterases, hypoglycaemics.

Side effects: osteoporosis, depression, euphoria, hyperglycaemia, peptic ulcers, Cushingoid changes

Manufacturer: Wellcome.

Tri-Minulet

Description: an oestrogen/progestogen compound containing ethinyloestradiol and gestodene in 6 beige tablets (30/50μg) 5 dark brown tablets (40/70μg) and 10 white tablets (30/100μg respectively).

Used for: oral contraception.

Dosage: 1 tablet daily for 21 days starting on first day of menstruation, then 7 days without tablets.

Special care: hypertension, Raynaud's disease (reduced blood supply to an organ of the body's extremities), asthma, severe depression, diabetes, varicose veins, multiple sclerosis, chronic kidney disease, kidney dialysis. Blood pressure, breasts and pelvic organs to be checked regularly; smoking not advised.

Avoid use: history of heart disease, infectious hepatitis, sickle cell anaemia, porphyria, liver tumour, undiagnosed vaginal bleeding, pregnancy, hormone-dependent cancer, haemolytic uraemic syndrome (rare kidney disorder), chorea, otosclerosis.

Possible interaction: barbiturates, tetracyclines, griseofulvin, rifampicin, primidone, phenytoin, chloral hydrate, ethosuximide, carbamazepine, glutethimide, dichloralphenazone.

Side effects: fluid retention and bloating, leg cramps/pains, breast enlargement, depression, headaches, nausea, loss of libido, weight gain, vaginal discharge, cervical erosion (alteration of epithelial cells), chloasma (pigmentation of nose, cheeks or forehead), breakthrough bleeding (bleeding between periods).

Manufacturer: Wyeth.

Triadene

Description: an oestrogen/progestogen compound containing ethinyloestradiol and gestodene in 6 beige tablets (30/50µg) 5 dark brown tablets (40/70µg) and 10 white tablets (30/100µg respectively).

Used for: oral contraception.

Dosage: 1 tablet daily for 21 days starting on first day of menstruation, then 7 days without tablets.

Special care: hypertension, Raynaud's disease (reduced blood supply to an organ of the body's extremities), asthma, severe depression, diabetes, varicose veins, multiple sclerosis, chronic kidney disease, kidney dialysis. Blood pressure, breasts and pelvic organs to be checked regularly; smoking not advised.

Avoid use: history of heart disease, infectious hepatitis, sickle cell anaemia, porphyria, liver tumour, undiagnosed vaginal bleeding, pregnancy, hormone-dependent cancer, haemolytic uraemic syndrome (rare kidney disorder), chorea, otosclerosis.

Possible interaction: barbiturates, tetracyclines, griseofulvin, rifampicin, primidone, phenytoin, chloral hydrate, ethosuximide, carbamazepine, glutethimide, dichloralphenazone.

Side effects: fluid retention and bloating, leg cramps/pains, breast enlargement, depression, headaches, nausea, loss of libido, weight gain, vaginal discharge, cervical erosion (alteration of epithelial cells), chloasma (pigmentation of nose, cheeks or forehead), breakthrough bleeding (bleeding between periods).

Manufacturer: Schering H.C.

Triam-Co

Description: a potassium-sparing diuretic and thiazide, triamterene (50mg) and hydro-chlorothiazide (25mg) in peach tablets marked with logo and TTRIAM-CO.

Used for: oedema, hypertension.

Dosage: start with 1 per day for hypertension; 1 twice per day after meals for oedema, reducing to 1 daily or 2 on alternate days. Maximum 4 per day. Not for children.

Special care: diabetes, gout, pancreatitis, acidosis, liver or kidney disease, pregnancy, breast-feeding.

Avoid use: severe kidney failure, hyperkalaemia, hypercalcaemia, Addison's disease, diabetic ketoacidosis, liver disorder.

Possible interaction: potassium supplements, potassium-sparing diuretics, digitalis, lithium, NSAIDs, ACE inhibitors, antihypertensives.

Side effects: headache, cramps, weakness, diarrhoea, nausea, vomiting, dry mouth, rash, hypotension, hypercalcaemia, hyperglycaemia, SLE, reversible kidney failure.

Manufacturer: Baker Norton.

Tribiotic

Description: an aminoglycoside and antibiotic in aerosol form containing 500,000 units neomycin sulphate, 10,000 units bacitracin zinc and 150,000 units/110g polymyxin B sulphate.

Used for: prevention and control of infection during surgery.

Dosage: apply 1 aerosol sparingly for a maximum of 7 days; (children 1 second/kg/day).

Special care: pregnancy, breast-feeding, loss of hearing, large areas of damaged skin.

Avoid use: burns.

Possible interaction: other aminoglycoside antibiotics.

Side effects: sensitization, toxicity of the kidney or organs of hearing and balance.

Manufacturer: 3M Health Care.

Tridil

Description: an antiarrhythmic and anti-anginal, glyceryl nitrate available in ampoules containing 0.5mg/ml.

Used for: angina, arrhythmias.

Dosage: see literature.

Special care: hypotension, tolerance.

Avoid use: anaemia, cerebral haemorrhage, certain glaucomas, head trauma.

Possible interaction: anticoagulants.

Side effects: flushes, headache, dizziness, tachycardia, hypotension on standing.

Manufacturer: DuPont.

Trimopan

Description: a folic acid inhibitor, trimethoprim, available in white tablets marked 2H7 (100mg) and 3H7 (200mg).

Used for: infections sensitive to trimethoprim, urinary tract infections.

Dosage: 200mg twice per day. Children should use the suspension.

Also, **Trimopan Suspension** containing 50mg/5ml.

Dosage: children, 6 to 12 years, 10ml; 2 to 6 years, 5ml; 4 months to 2 years, 2.5ml; all twice per day. Not for infants under 4 months.

Special care: kidney disorder, folate deficiency, elderly, breast-feeding. Check blood during long-term treatment.

Avoid use: pregnancy, infants up to 1 month, severe kidney disease where blood levels cannot be monitored.

Side effects: folate deficiency, gastrointestinal and skin reactions.

Manufacturer: Berk.

Trimovate

Description: a moderately potent steroid with antifungal and antibiotic comprising 0.05% clobetasone butyrate, 100,000 units/g nystatin, 3% oxytetracycline, as a cream.

Used for: skin disorders that respond to steroids, especially in moist or covered areas where there may be infection.

Dosage: use up to 4 times per day.

Special care: thrombophlebitis, psychoses, recent intestinal anastomoses, chronic nephritis, certain cancers, osteoporosis, peptic ulcer, skin eruption/rash related to a disease, viral, fungal or active infections, tuberculosis. Hypertension, glaucoma, epilepsy, acute glomerulonephritis (inflammation of kidney glomerulus), diabetes, cirrhosis, hypothyroidism, pregnancy, stress. To be withdrawn gradually.

Possible interaction: NSAIDs, oral anticoagulants, phenytoin, ephedrine, phenobarbitone, rifampicin, diuretics, cardiac glycosides, anticholinesterases, hypoglycaemics.

Side effects: osteoporosis, depression, euphoria, hyperglycaemia, peptic ulcers, Cushingoid changes.

Manufacturer: Glaxo.

Trinordiol

Description: an oestrogen/progestogen combined contraceptive containing ethinyloestradiol and levonorgestrel as 6 brown tablets (30/50μg respectively), 5 white tablets (40/75μg) and 10 ochre tablets (30/125μg).

Used for: oral contraception.

Dosage: 1 tablet for 21 days starting on the first day of menstruation, then 7 days without tablets.

Special care: hypertension, Raynaud's disease

(reduced blood supply to an organ of the body's extremities), asthma, severe depression, diabetes, varicose veins, multiple sclerosis, chronic kidney disease, kidney dialysis. Blood pressure, breasts and pelvic organs to be checked regularly; smoking not advised.

Avoid use: history of heart disease, infectious hepatitis, sickle cell anaemia, porphyria, liver tumour, undiagnosed vaginal bleeding, pregnancy, hormone-dependent cancer, haemolytic uraemic syndrome (rare kidney disorder), chorea, otosclerosis.

Possible interaction: barbiturates, tetracyclines, griseofulvin, rifampicin, primidone, phenytoin, chloral hydrate, ethosuximide, carbamazepine, glutethimide, dichloralphenazone.

Side effects: fluid retention and bloating, leg cramps/pains, breast enlargement, depression, headaches, nausea, loss of libido, weight gain, vaginal discharge, cervical erosion (alteration of epithelial cells), chloasma (pigmentation of nose, cheeks or forehead), breakthrough bleeding (bleeding between periods).

Manufacturer: Wyeth.

Trinovum

Description: a combined oestrogen/progestogen contraceptive containing ethinyloestradiol and norethisterone as 7 white tablets marked C535 (35μg/0.5mg respectively), 7 light peach tablets marked C735 (35μg/0.75mg) and 7 peach tablets marked C135 (35μg/1mg).

Used for: oral contraception.

Dosage: 1 tablet per day for 21 days commencing on first day of menstruation then 7 days without tablets. Also, **Trinovum ED**, as for Trinovum but with 7 light-green inert lactose tablets marked CC.

Dosage: starting on first day of menstruation, 1 tablet per day for 28 days with no break.

Special care: hypertension, Raynaud's disease (reduced blood supply to an organ of the body's extremities), asthma, severe depression, diabetes, varicose veins, multiple sclerosis, chronic kidney disease, kidney dialysis. Blood pressure, breasts and pelvic organs to be checked regularly; smoking not advised.

Avoid use: history of heart disease, infectious hepatitis, sickle cell anaemia, porphyria, liver tumour, undiagnosed vaginal bleeding, pregnancy, hormone-dependent cancer, haemolytic uraemic syndrome (rare kidney disorder), chorea, otosclerosis.

Possible interaction: barbiturates, tetracyclines, griseofulvin, rifampicin, primidone, phenytoin,

chloral hydrate, ethosuximide, carbamazepine, glutethimide, dichloralphenazone.
Side effects: fluid retention and bloating, leg cramps/pains, breast enlargement, depression, headaches, nausea, loss of libido, weight gain, vaginal discharge, cervical erosion (alteration of epithelial cells), chloasma (pigmentation of nose, cheeks or forehead), breakthrough bleeding (bleeding between periods).
Manufacturer: Ortho.

Triptafen

Description: an anti-depressant combining a TCAD and group III phenothiazine, as 25mg amitryptiline hydrochloride with 2mg perphenazine in pink tablets marked 1D. Also, **Triptafen-M**, containing 10mg amitriptyline hydrochloride and 2mg perphenazine in pink tablets marked 2D.
Used for: depression with anxiety.
Dosage: 1 tablet 3 times per day plus 1 at bedtime if needed. Assess after 3 months. Not for children.
Special care: pregnancy, breast-feeding, Parkinson's disease, liver disorders, hyperthyroidism, epilepsy, diabetes, glaucoma, retention of urine, cardiovascular disease, psychotic patients.
Avoid use: cardiovascular disease, bone marrow depression, heart block, acute myocardial infarction, severe liver disease.
Possible interaction: antidepressants, anticonvulsants, alcohol, within 2 weeks of taking MAOIs, barbiturates, adrenaline, noradrenaline, antihypertensives, anticholinergics, oestrogens, cimetidine.
Side effects: sleepiness, vertigo, light-headedness, unsteadiness, disturbance of vision, rash, hypotension, gastrointestinal upset, changes in libido, retention of urine. Allergic reactions, dry mouth, constipation, sweating, tachycardia, nervousness, heart arrhythmias. Impotence, effects on breasts, weight loss or gain.
Manufacturer: Forley.

Trisequens

Description: an oestrogen/progestogen combination available as 12 blue tablets (marked 270) containing 2mg oestradiol and 1mg oestriol, 10 white tablets (marked 271) containing 2mg oestradiol, 1mg oestriol and 1mg norethisterone acetate and 6 red tablets (marked 272) containing 1mg oestradiol and 0.5mg oestriol.
Also, **Trisequens Forte**, with the same components as 12 yellow tablets marked 273 (4mg/2mg), 10 white tablets marked 274 (4mg/2mg/1mg) and 6 red tablets marked 272 (1mg/0.5mg).

Used for: symptoms of the menopause, prevention of post-menopausal osteoporosis.
Dosage: 1 tablet per day without a break, starting on fifth day of discharge with a blue tablet (or yellow if Forte).
Special care: patients considered to be at risk of thrombosis or with liver disease. Women with any of the following disorders should be carefully monitored: uterine fibroids, multiple sclerosis, diabetes, tetany, porphyria, epilepsy, liver disease, hypertension, migraine, otosclerosis, gallstones. Breasts, pelvic organs and blood pressure should be checked at regular intervals during treatment.
Avoid use: pregnancy, breast-feeding, conditions which might lead to thrombosis, thrombophlebitis, serious heart, kidney or liver disease, breast cancer, oestrogen-dependent cancers including those of reproductive system, endometriosis, vaginal bleeding which is undiagnosed.
Possible interaction: drugs which induce liver enzymes.
Side effects: tenderness and enlargement of breasts, weight gain, breakthrough bleeding, giddiness, vomiting and nausea, gastrointestinal upset. Treatment should be halted immediately if severe headaches occur, disturbance of vision, hypertension or any indications of thrombosis, jaundice. Also, in the event of pregnancy and 6 weeks before planned surgery.
Manufacturer: Novo Nordisk.

Tricate

Description: an ACE inhibitor, ramipril, available as yellow/white (1.25mg), orange/white (2.5mg) and crimson/white (5mg) capsules.
Used for: hypertension.
Dosage: start with 1.25mg per day moving to maintenance dose of 2.5–5mg per day; maximum of 10mg per day. Any diuretic should be stopped 2 to 3 days before taking Tritace. Not for children.
Special care: start treatment in hospital for congestive heart failure or liver disease; haemodialysis, kidney disease (reduce dose and monitor during treatment).
Avoid use: pregnancy, breast-feeding, narrowing of the aorta, past angioneurotic oedema, outflow obstruction.
Possible interaction: lithium, potassium supplements, antihypertensives potassium-sparing diuretics.
Side effects: headache, fatigue, nausea, vomiting, dizziness, abdominal pain, cough, diarrhoea, hypersensitivity reactions.
Manufacturer: Hoechst.

Trivax

Description: a vaccine containing the triple antigen for diphtheria, tetanus and whooping cough, available in ampoules. Also **Trivax-AD** which is adsorbed on aluminium hydroxide.

Used for: active immunization against these diseases.

Dosage: for children under 5, 3 doses of 0.5ml at 4 weekly intervals. Not for children over 5 or adults.

Avoid use: acute fever, past convulsions, cerebral irritation, neurological diseases. Reaction to a preceding dose. Epilepsy in the family or history of severe allergies.

Side effects: fever, loss of appetite, irritability, crying.

Manufacturer: Evans.

Trobicin

Description: an antibacterial compound similar to an aminoglycoside, spectinomycin, as powder (as dihydrochloride pentahydrate) in a vial (400mg/ml) with diluent.

Used for: gonorrhoea.

Dosage: 2g by deep intramuscular injection or 4g for severe cases. Children over 2, 40mg/kg.

Special care: pregnancy, liver or kidney disease.

Possible interaction: lithium.

Side effects: fever, urticaria, nausea, dizziness, lower urine output.

Manufacturer: Upjohn.

Trosyl

Description: an imidazole antifungal, tioconazole, available as a solution containing 280mg/ml.

Used for: nail infections caused by *Candida* and fungi.

Dosage: apply 12 hourly for 6 to 12 months.

Avoid use: pregnancy.

Side effects: nail irritation.

Manufacturer: Novex.

Tryptizol

Description: a TCAD, amitriptyline hydrochloride, available as blue tablets marked MSD 23 (10mg), yellow tablets marked MSD 45 (25mg) and brown tablets marked MSD 102 (50mg). Also, **Tryptizol Capsules**, 75mg orange, sustained-release capsules (marked MSD 649) and **Tryptizol Syrup** 10mg amitryptiline embonate/5ml.

Used for: depression (adults), bed-wetting (children).

Dosage: 75mg up to 150mg per day, in divided doses and 50–100mg for maintenance usually as 1 bedtime dose. Elderly, 50mg per day in divided doses or as 1 bedtime dose. Children; 11 to 16 years, 25–50mg per day; 6 to 10 years, 10–20mg per day. Not for children under 6.

Also, **Tryptizol Injection** as 10mg/ml.

Dosage: 10–20mg 4 times per day, intravenously or intramuscularly. Not for children.

Special care: liver disorders, hyperthyroidism, glaucoma, lactation, epilepsy, diabetes, adrenal tumour, heart disease, urine retention. Psychotic or suicidal patients.

Avoid use: children, heart block, heart attacks, severe liver disease, pregnancy.

Possible interaction: MAOIs (or within 14 days of their use), alcohol, antidepressants, barbiturates, anticholinergics, local anaesthetics that contain adrenaline or noradrenaline, oestrogens, cimetidine, antihypertensives.

Side effects: constipation, urine retention, dry mouth, blurred vision, palpitations, tachycardia, nervousness, drowsiness, insomnia. Changes in weight, blood and blood sugar, jaundice, skin reactions, weakness, ataxia, hypotension, sweating, altered libido, gynaecomastia, galactorrhoea.

Manufacturer: Morson.

Tuinal^{CD}

Description: a barbiturate, quinal barbitone sodium and amylobarbitone sodium in equal amounts, available as orange/blue capsules (100mg) marked LILLY F65.

Used for: short-term treatment of severe insomnia for those tolerant to barbiturates.

Dosage: 100–200mg at bedtime. Not for children.

Special care: extremely dangerous, addictive drug with narrow margin of safety. Liable to abuse by overdose leading to coma and death or if combined with alcohol. Easily produces dependence and severe withdrawal symptoms. Drowsiness may persist next day affecting driving and performance of skilled tasks.

Avoid use: should be avoided if possible in all patients. Not to be used for children, young adults, pregnancy, nursing mothers, elderly, those with drug or alcohol related problems, patients with liver, kidney or heart disease, porphyria. Insomnia where the cause is pain.

Possible interaction: alcohol, central nervous system depressant drugs, Griseofulvin, metronidazone, rifampicin, phenytoin, chloramphenicol. Anticoagulant drugs of the coumarin type, steroid drugs including contraceptive pill.

Side effects: hangover with drowsiness, shakiness, dizziness, headache, anxiety, confusion, excitement,

rash and allergic responses, gastro intestinal upsets, urine retention, loss of sexual desire.
Manufacturer: Lilly.

Tylex

Description: an analgesic comprising 500mg paracetamol and 30mg codeine phosphate in red and white capsules marked C30.
Used for: severe pain.
Dosage: 1 or 2 capsules 4-hourly to a maximum of 8 per day. Not for children.
Special care: head injury, raised intracranial pressure, bowel disorders, Addison's disease, hypothyroidism, liver or kidney disease, elderly.
Avoid use: pregnancy, breast-feeding, chronic alcoholism, depression of respiration, diseases causing obstruction of airways.
Possible interaction: CNS depressants, MAOIs.
Side effects: nausea, dry mouth, blurred vision, dizziness, sedation, constipation, tolerance, dependence.
Manufacturer: Cilag.

Typhim VI

Description: an inactivated surface antigen of *Salmonella typhi* as 25µg/0.5ml in pre-filled syringe.
Used for: active immunization against typhoid.
Dosage: 0.5ml by intramuscular or deep subcutaneous injection. Children over 18 months, as adult dosage; under 18 months, assess risk of exposure.
Special care: pregnancy, breast-feeding.
Avoid use: acute infections.
Side effects: headache, fever, malaise, localized reactions.
Manufacturer: Merieux

U

Ubretid
Description: an anticholinesterase, distigmine bromide, available as white tablets (5mg) marked UBRETID, and **Ubretid Injection** as 1ml ampoules (0.5mg/ml).
Used for: intestinal and ileal weakness after operations, myasthenia gravis, postoperative urine retention, neurogenic bladder (bladder disorder caused by a lesion of the nervous system).
Dosage: 1 tablet daily, 30 minutes before breakfast up to 4 for myasthenia gravis (2 for children). Postoperative conditions, 0.5mg 12 hours intramuscularly after surgery then 24-hourly until normal function restored. Not for children.
Special care: asthma, heart disease, epilepsy, Parkinson's disease, peptic ulcer.
Avoid use: pregnancy, postoperative shock, obstruction in intestines or urinary tract, weak circulation.
Possible interaction: depolarizing muscle relaxants.
Side effects: nausea, vomiting, colic, diarrhoea, increased salivation.
Manufacturer: R.P.R.

Ucerax
Description: an antihistamine, hydroxyzine hydrochloride, available as white, oblong tablets (25mg). Also, **Ucerax Syrup** (10mg/5ml).
Used for: anxiety, skin disorders, pruritus (itching) due to urticaria.
Dosage: 50–100mg 4 times per day for anxiety; otherwise 25mg at night up to 25mg 3 or 4 times per day if required. Children; over 6 years start with 15–25mg at night increasing to 50–100mg per day in divided doses; 6 months to 6 years, 5–15mg increasing to 50mg daily maximum in divided doses.
Special care: kidney disease. Judgement and dexterity may be affected.
Avoid use: pregnancy, breast-feeding.
Possible interaction: depressants of the CNS, alcohol.
Side effects: anticholinergic effects, drowsiness.
Manufacturer: U.C.B.

Ukidan
Description: a fibrinolytic, urokinase, available as powder in vials containing 5000, 25,000 and 100,000 units.
Used for: pulmonary embolism, deep vein thrombosis, bleeding into the eye in front of the lens, clot in haemodialysis shunt, blockage in peripheral vessel.
Dosage: see the literature.
Special care: peptic ulcer.
Avoid use: severe liver or kidney disease, pregnancy, severe hypertension, recent surgery.
Possible interaction: glucose.
Side effects: fever, haemorrhage.
Manufacturer: Serono.

Ultradil
Description: a moderately potent steroid containing 0.1% fluocortolone pivalate and 0.1% fluocortolone hexanoate as cream and ointment.
Used for: eczema, skin disorders and skin conditions that respond to steroids.
Dosage: start by applying 3 times per day, reducing to once per day.
Special care: thrombophlebitis, psychoses, recent intestinal anastomoses, chronic nephritis, certain cancers, osteoporosis, peptic ulcer, skin eruption/rash related to a disease, viral, fungal or active infections, tuberculosis. Hypertension, glaucoma, epilepsy, acute glomerulonephritis (inflammation of kidney glomerulus), diabetes, cirrhosis, hypothyroidism, pregnancy, stress. To be withdrawn gradually.
Possible interaction: NSAIDs, oral anticoagulants, phenytoin, ephedrine, phenobarbitone, rifampicin, diuretics, cardiac glycosides, anticholinesterases, hypoglycaemics.
Side effects: osteoporosis, depression, euphoria, hyperglycaemia, peptic ulcers, Cushingoid changes.
Manufacturer: Schering H.C.

Ultralanum
Description: a moderately potent steroid containing 0.25% fluocortolone pivalate and 0.25%

fluocortolone hexanoate as a cream. Also, **Ultralanum Ointment** containing 0.25% fluocortolone and 0.25% fluocortolone hexanoate.
Used for: skin conditions responding to steroids.
Dosage: apply 2 or 3 times per day and reduce to once per day.
Special care: thrombophlebitis, psychoses, recent intestinal anastomoses, chronic nephritis, certain cancers, osteoporosis, peptic ulcer, skin eruption/ rash related to a disease, viral, fungal or active infections, tuberculosis. Hypertension, glaucoma, epilepsy, acute glomerulonephritis (inflammation of kidney glomerulus), pregnancy, diabetes, cirrhosis, hypothyroidism, stress. To be withdrawn gradually.
Possible interaction: NSAIDs, oral anticoagulants, phenytoin, ephedrine, phenobarbitone, rifampicin, diuretics, cardiac glycosides, anticholinesterases, hypoglycaemics.
Side effects: osteoporosis, depression, euphoria, hyperglycaemia, peptic ulcers, Cushingoid changes.
Manufacturer: Schering H.C.

Ultraproct
Description: a steroid and local anaesthetic containing fluocortolone pivalate (0.61mg), fluocortolone hexanoate (0.63mg) and cinchocaine hydrochloride (1mg) as suppositories.
Used for: haemorrhoids, anal fissure, itching, proctitis (inflammation of the rectum).
Dosage: 1 to 3 per day, after defaecation. Not for children.
Also, **Ultraproct Ointment**, containing 0.092% fluocortolone pivalate, 0.095% fluocortolone hexanoate and 0.5% cinchocaine hydrochloride.
Dosage: use 2 to 4 times per day. Not for children.
Special care: pregnancy. Do not use for a long period.
Avoid use: infections of a viral, fungal or tuberculous nature.
Side effects: corticosteroid effects.
Manufacturer: Schering H.C.

Unihep
Description: an anticoagulant, heparin sodium, available as 1000, 5000, 10,000 and 25,000 units in ampoules.
Used for: treatment and prophylaxis of deep vein thrombosis and pulmonary embolism, angina, acute occlusion of peripheral arteries.
Dosage: varies with condition, see literature.
Special care: pregnancy, liver and kidney disease. Monitor platelet count if treatment exceeds 5 days and cease treatment should thrombocytopenia occur.
Avoid use: thrombocytopenia, cerebral aneurysm,

severe hypertension, haemophilia, haemorrhagic disorders, severe liver disease, recent eye or nervous system surgery, hypersensitivity to heparin.
Possible interaction: aspirin, glyceryl trinitrate ketorolac, dipyridamole.
Side effects: thrombocytopenia, skin necrosis, haemorrhage, osteoporosis with prolonged use hypersensitivity reactions.
Manufacturer: Leo.

Uniparin
Description: an anticoagulant, heparin sodium, available as 5000 units/0.2ml in pre-filled syringe. Also, **Uniparin Forte** (10,000 units/0.4ml) and **Uniparin Ca**, heparin calcium as 25,000 units per ml in pre-filled syringes.
Used for: treatment and prophylaxis of deep vein thrombosis and pulmonary embolism, angina, acute occlusion of peripheral arteries.
Dosage: by subcutaneous injection. See literature for dosage.
Special care: pregnancy, liver and kidney disease. Monitor platelet count if treatment exceeds a period of 5 days and cease treatment should thrombocytopenia occur.
Avoid use: thrombocytopenia, cerebral aneurysm, severe hypertension, haemophilia, haemorrhagic disorders, severe liver disease, recent eye or nervous system surgery, hypersensitivity to heparin.
Possible interaction: aspirin, glyceryl trinitrate ketorolac, dipyridamole.
Side effects: thrombocytopenia, skin necrosis, haemorrhage, osteoporosis with prolonged use hypersensitivity reactions.
Manufacturer: C.P. Pharm.

Uniroid-HC
Description: a steroid (5mg hydrocortisone) and local anaesthetic (5mg cinchocaine hydrochloride) available as suppositories.
Used for: haemorrhoids, itching around the anus.
Dosage: insert 1 dose 3 times per day, and after defaecation for up to 7 days. Not for children.
Also, **Uniroid-HC Ointment** containing 5mg hydrocortisone and 5mg/g cinchocaine hydrochloride.
Dosage: use 3 times per day and after defaecation, for up to 7 days. Not for children.
Special care: pregnancy. Do not use over a prolonged period.
Avoid use: infections of a viral, fungal or tuberculous nature.
Side effects: corticosteroid effects.
Manufacturer: Unigreg.

Univer

Description: a class I calcium antagonist, verapamil hydrochloride, available as sustained-release capsules coloured yellow/dark blue (120mg and 240mg, marked V120 and V240) and yellow (180mg, marked V180).

Used for: angina, hypertension.

Dosage: 360mg once per day to a maximum of 480mg (angina). For hypertension, 240mg once per day, unless new to verapamil in which case start with 120mg per day.

Special care: 1st degree heart block, weak heart, liver or kidney disease, bradycardia, hypotension, disturbance in heart conduction, pregnancy.

Avoid use: 2nd or 3rd degree heart block, heart failure, sick sinus syndrome.

Possible interaction: quinidine, digoxin, ß-blockers.

Side effects: flushes, constipation, occasionally nausea, vomiting, headache, allergy or liver disorder.

Manufacturer: Rorer.

Uriben

Description: a quinolone, nalidixic acid, available as a suspension (300mg/5ml).

Used for: infections of the gastrointestinal tract caused by Gram-negative organisms, urinary tract infections.

Dosage: gastrointestinal tract infections: 10–15ml 4 times per day, children over 3 months 1ml/kg per day. Contact manufacturer regarding children under 3 months. For urinary tract infections: acute cases, 15ml 4 times per day for at least 7 days; chronic cases 10ml. Children's doses as above.

Special care: severe kidney disease, liver disease, avoid excessive sunlight.

Avoid use: past convulsions, porphyria. Children under 3 months.

Possible interaction: probenecid, anticoagulants.

Side effects: rashes, blood disorders, seizures, disturbances in sight, gastrointestinal upset.

Manufacturer: R.P. Drugs.

Urispas

Description: an antispasmodic drug, flavoxate hydrochloride, available as white tablets containing 100mg and marked URISPAS, and 200mg (marked URISPAS 200).

Used for: incontinence, frequent or urgent urination, painful urination, bed-wetting.

Dosage: 200mg 3 times per day. Not for children.

Special care: pregnancy, glaucoma.

Avoid use: conditions causing obstruction in the urinary or gastrointestinal tracts.

Side effects: diarrhoea, dry mouth, blurred vision, nausea, fatigue, headache.

Manufacturer: Syntex.

Uromitaxen

Description: a protectant for the urinary tract, mesna, available as solution in ampoules (100mg/ml).

Used for: prevention of toxicity in the urinary tract caused by the metabolite acrolein.

Dosage: orally or intravenously. See literature for details.

Side effects: fatigue, headache, gastrointestinal upset, depression, irritability, rash, malaise, pain in the limbs.

Manufacturer: ASTA Medica.

Ursofalk

Description: a bile acid, ursodeoxycholic acid, available as white capsules containing 250mg.

Used for: dissolving cholesterol gallstones.

Dosage: 8–12mg/kg/day in 2 divided doses after meals of which one must be the evening meal. Use for 3 to 4 months after the stones have been dissolved. Not for children.

Avoid use: if gall bladder does not function. Women who are not using contraception.

Possible interaction: drugs to lower cholesterol levels, oral contraceptives, oestrogens.

Manufacturer: Thames.

Utinor

Description: a 4-quinolone compound, norfloxacin, available as white, oval tablets (400mg) marked UTINOR.

Used for: acute and chronic infections of the urinary tract.

Dosage: 1 tablet twice per day. Duration depends upon the condition. Not for children.

Special care: past epilepsy, kidney disorder.

Avoid use: pregnancy, breast-feeding, growing adolescents and children before puberty.

Possible interaction: NSAIDs, antacids, oral anticoagulants, cyclosporin, theophylline, nitrofurantoin, probenecid, sucralfate.

Side effects: diarrhoea, nausea, headache, dizziness, heartburn, rash, abdominal cramp, irritability, convulsions, anorexia, disturbance to sleep.

Manufacturer: M.S.D.

Utovlan

Description: a progestogen, norethisterone, available as white tablets (5mg) marked SYNTEX.

Used for: dysmenorrhoea (painful menstruation),

menorrhagia (long or heavy menstrual periods), uterine bleeding, metropathia haemorrhagica (endometrial hyperplasia—irregular bleeding due to excess activity of oestrogen).

Dosage: 1 tablet 3 times per day for 10 days then twice per day for days 19–26 of the next 2 cycles.

Used for: postponement of menses (discharge).

Dosage: 1 tablet 3 times per day commencing 3 days before anticipated start.

Used for: endometriosis.

Dosage: 1 tablet 3 times per day for at least 6 months, increasing to 4 or 5 per day if necessary.

Used for: premenstrual syndrome.

Dosage: 1 per day from days 16–25 of the cycle.

Used for: breast cancer.

Dosage: start with 8 per day increasing to 12 if required.

Special care: epilepsy, migraine, diabetes.

Avoid use: not for children. Carcinoma of the breast dependent upon progestogen, past thromboembolic disorders, undiagnosed abnormal vaginal bleeding, liver disease, severe itching, pregnancy, jaundice, past herpes.

Side effects: liver or gastrointestinal upset.

Manufacturer: Syntex.

V

Vagifem

Description: an hormonal oestrogen preparation available as vaginal pessaries with applicator containing 25µg oestradiol.

Used for: atrophic vaginitis.

Dosage: adults, 1 pessary inserted into vagina each day for 2 weeks, then 1 twice each week for 3 months.

Special care: those at risk of thrombosis or with liver disease. Women with any of the following disorders should be carefully monitored: fibroids in the womb, multiple sclerosis, diabetes, tetany, porphyria, epilepsy, liver disease, hypertension, migraine, otosclerosis, gallstones. Breasts, pelvic organs and blood pressure should be checked at regular intervals during the course of treatment.

Avoid use: pregnancy, breast-feeding, women with conditions which might lead to thrombosis, thrombophlebitis, serious heart, kidney or liver disease, breast cancer, oestrogen-dependent cancers including those of reproductive system, endometriosis, vaginal bleeding which is undiagnosed.

Possible interaction: drugs which induce liver enzymes.

Side effects: tenderness and enlargement of breasts, weight gain, breakthrough bleeding, giddiness, vomiting and nausea, gastrointestinal upset. Treatment should be halted immediately if severe headaches occur, disturbance of vision, hypertension or any indications of thrombosis, jaundice. Also, in the event of pregnancy and 6 weeks before planned surgery.

Manufacturer: Novo Nordisk.

Valium

Description: a long-acting benzodiazepine drug available as white 2mg tablets, yellow 5mg tablets and blue 10mg tablets all containing diazepam. Tablets are scored and marked with ROCHE and strength. Also, **Valium Syrup** containing 2mg diazepam/5ml; **Valium Injection** available as a solution in ampoules containing 5mg diazepam/ml.

Used for: severe and disabling anxiety, insomnia, severe alcohol withdrawal symptoms, sleep disorders in children. Feverish convulsions, status epilepticus (injection only), spasm of muscles and cerebral spasticity, as a sedative during medical or surgical procedures.

Dosage: oral preparations, 2–60mg in divided doses each day depending upon condition being treated. Injection, 10–20mg, or 0.2mg/kg body weight depending upon condition being treated, by intravenous or intramuscular injection every 4 hours. Status epilepticus, this dose may be repeated after half an hour to an hour with a maximum of 3mg/kg by intravenous infusion over 24 hours. Elderly, oral preparations, 1–30mg each day in divided doses; injection 5mg by intravenous or intramuscular injection every 4 hours. Children, oral preparations, 1–40mg each day in divided doses depending upon condition being treated; 1–5mg at bedtime for sleep disorders. Injection, status epilepticus and convulsions, 0.2–0.3mg/kg by intravenous or intramuscular injection.

Special care: elderly, pregnancy, breast-feeding, liver or kidney disorders, lung disease. Drug should be gradually withdrawn.

Avoid use: patients with serious lung disease, depression of respiration, obsessional and phobic disorders, severe psychosis. Avoid long-term use.

Possible interaction: CNS depressants, anticonvulsants, alcohol. Drugs which induce or inhibit liver enzymes.

Side effects: impaired judgement and performance of skilled tasks, confusion, shakiness, sleepiness, vertigo. Gastro-intestinal upset, retention of urine, disturbance of vision, changes in libido, skin rashes, hypotension. Thrombophlebitis at site of injection; rarely, jaundice and blood changes. The longer treatment lasts and the higher the dose the greater the risk of drug dependence.

Manufacturer: Roche.

Vallergan

Description: an anti-allergic preparation, which is an antihistamine of the phenothiazine type, available as film-coated, blue tablets containing

10mg trimeprazine tartrate marked V10. Also, **Vallergan Syrup** containing 7.5mg/5ml; **Vallergan Forte Syrup**, containing 30mg/5ml.

Used for: itching, urticaria, premedication before surgery in children.

Dosage: 10mg 2 or 3 times each day with a maximum of 100mg daily. Elderly persons, 10mg once or twice daily. Children, for itching and allergic conditions age over 2 years, 2.5–5mg 3 or 4 times each day. Premedication, age 2 to 7 years, up to 2mg/kg body weight 1 or 2 hours before surgery.

Avoid use: pregnancy, breast-feeding, liver or kidney disorders, Parkinson's disease, epilepsy, phaeochromocytoma, underactive thyroid gland, myasthenia gravis, glaucoma.

Possible interaction: alcohol, antihypertensives, hypoglycaemics, MAOIs, sympathomimetics, anticholinergics, central nervous system depressants.

Side effects: sleepiness, rash, drowsiness, impaired performance and reactions, heart disturbances, hypotension, depression of respiration. Anticholinergic and extrapyramidal effects, convulsions, raised levels of prolactin in blood, abnormally low level of white blood cells, jaundice, sensitivity to light (with high doses).

Manufacturer: Theraplix.

Vancocin CP

Description: an antibiotic glycopeptide preparation available as powder in vials for reconstitution and injection containing 250mg, 500mg and 1g vancomycin (as hydrochloride). Also, **Vancocin Matrigel** available as peach/blue capsules containing 125mg (coded Lilly 3125); grey/blue capsules containing 250mg (coded Lilly 3126).

Used for: potentially fatal infections caused by staphylococci which are resistant to other antibiotics. Vancocin Matrigel, staphylococcal enterocolitis and pseudo-membraneous colitis.

Dosage: 500mg every 6 hours or 1g every 12 hours given by slow intravenous infusion over 1 hour. Children, 10mg/kg body weight by slow intravenous infusion over 1 hour at 6 hourly intervals. Vancocin Matrigel, 500mg each day for 7 to 10 days in divided doses with a daily maximum of 2g. Children, 40mg/kg for 7 to 10 days in 3 or 4 divided doses with a daily maximum of 2g.

Special care: elderly, pregnancy, patients with existing loss of hearing, kidney disorders. Blood, kidney function and hearing shoudl be carefully monitored during the course of treatment.

Possible interaction: drugs with toxic effects on central nervous system or kidneys, anaesthetics.

Side effects: chills, fever, nausea, phlebitis, reduction in number of some white blood cells and rise in number of eosinophils, toxic effects on kidneys and organs of hearing and balance. Anaphylactoid allergic reactions.

Manufacturer: Lilly.

Varidase

Description: a preparation of fibrinolytic and proteolytic enzymes available as powder in vials containing 100,000 units streptokinase and 25,000 units streptodomase.

Used for: cleansing and removal of debris from wounds and ulcers.

Dosage: apply as wet dressing once or twice each day.

Avoid use: patients with active haemorrhage.

Manufacturer: Lederle.

Vascace

Description: an antihypertensive preparation which is an ACE inhibitor, available in the form of oval, film-coated, scored tablets in various strengths, all containing cilazapril and marked with strength and CIL. Pink, 0.25mg strength; white, 0.5mg strength; yellow, 1mg strength; red, 2.5mg streength and brown 5mg strength.

Used for: hypertension and renovascular hypertension.

Dosage: hypertension, 1mg once each day at first with a maintenance dose in the order of 1–2.5mg daily. Any diuretic being taken should be withdrawn 2 or 3 days before treatment starts. Renovascular hypertension, 0.25–0.5mg once each day then adjusted according to response of condition. Elderly, hypertension, 0.5mg each day at first; renovascular hypertension, 0.25mg once each day at first.

Special care: liver or kidney disease, congestive heart failure, undergoing renal dialysis, anaesthesia or surgery, suffering from lack of fluid or salt.

Avoid use: children, pregnancy, breast-feeding, patients wth outflow obstruction of the heart, aortic stenosis, ascites (abnormal collection of fluid in the peritoneal cavity which is a complication of various diseases).

Possible interaction: NSAIDs, potassium-sparing diuretics.

Side effects: nausea, headache, fatigue, rash, indigestion, giddiness. Rarely, pancreatitis, changes in blood count, angioneurotic oedema.

Manufacturer: Roche.

Vasocon-A

Description: an anti-inflammatory compound

preparation combining an antihistamine and sympathomimetic, available as eyedrops containing 0.5% antazoline phosphate and 0.05% naphazoline hydrochloride.

Used for: inflammatory eye conditions including allergic conjunctivitis.

Dosage: adults, 1 or 2 drops up to 4 times each day.

Special care: diabetes, hypertension, hyperthyroidism, disease of coronary arteries.

Avoid use: narrow angle glaucoma, wearing soft contact lenses.

Possible interaction: MAOIs.

Side effects: sleepiness, tachycardia, headache, insomnia, short-lived stinging in eye.

Manufacturer: Lolab.

Vasoxine

Description: an antiarrhythmic and a-agonist, available as a solution in ampoules for injection containing 20mg methoxamine hydrochloride.

Used for: hypotension during anaesthesia.

Dosage: adults, 5–10mg by slow intravenous injection or 5–20mg by intramuscular injection.

Special care: patients with hyperthyroidism, pregnancy.

Avoid use: serious disease of the coronary arteries or heart blood vessels.

Possible interaction: anoretic drugs, cough and cold remedies.

Side effects: hypertension, bradycardia, headache.

Manufacturer: Wellcome.

Velbe

Description: a drug which is a vinca alkaloid available as powder in vials with diluent containing 10mg vinblastine sulphate.

Used for: leukaemias, lymphomas, some solid tumours, e.g. of lung and breast.

Dosage: by intravenous injection as directed by specialist physician.

Special care: caution in handling (trained personnel, protective clothing), irritant to tissues.

Avoid use: intrathecal route.

Side effects: bone marrow suppression, toxic effects on peripheral and autonomic nervous system, reversible hair loss, nausea, vomiting, effects on fertility.

Manufacturer: Lilly.

Velosef

Description: an antibiotic preparation which is a cephalosporin available as capsules in 2 strengths both containing cephradine. Blue/orange 250mg capsules, coded SQUIBB 113 and blue 500mg capsules coded SQUIBB 114. Also, **Velosef Syrup** containing 250mg/5ml. **Velosef Injection** as powder in vials for reconstitution and injection containing 500mg and 1g cephradine.

Used for: infections of skin, soft tissues, respiratory, gastrointestinal and urinary tracts, joints and bones. Also, endocarditis and septicaemia and for prevention of infection during surgery.

Dosage: oral preparations, 1–2g each day in 2, 3 or 4 divided doses with a maximum daily dose of 4g. Injection, 2–4g by intramuscular or intravenous injection or intravenous infusion in divided daily doses. Children, oral preparations, 25–50mg/kg body weight in 2, 3 or 4 daily divided doses. For inflammation of middle ear, 75–100mg/kg each day in divided doses. Injection, 50–100mg/kg each day in divided doses. All treatment should continue for 48–72 hours after symptoms have disappeared.

Special care: known hypersensitivity to penicillins, kidney disorders.

Possible interaction: aminoglycosides.

Side effects: gastrointestinal upset, allergic hypersensitive responses. Rarely, blood changes involving white blood cells, rise in levels of urea and liver enzymes in blood, positive Coomb's test (a test to detect Rhesus antibodies), candidiasis.

Manufacturer: Squibb.

Ventide

Description: a bronchodilator, anti-inflammatory preparation which combines a selective ß-agonist and corticosteroid. It is available as an aerosol delivering 100µg salbutamol and 50µg beclomethasone dipropionate per metered dose. Also, **Ventide Rotacaps** available as clear/grey capsules containing 400µg salbutamol as sulphate and 200µg beclomethasone dipropionate, marked VENTIDE, for use with Rotahaler. Also, **Ventide Paediatric Rotacaps**, clear/light grey capsules containing 200µg salbutamol as sulphate and 100µg beclomethasone dipropionate, for use with Rotahaler.

Used for: long-term treatment of asthma which requires inhaled bronchodilator and corticosteroid therapy.

Dosage: Ventide, 2 puffs 3 to 4 times each day; Ventide Rotacaps, 1 puff 3 to 4 times each day. Children, Ventide, 1 or 2 puffs 2, 3 or 4 times each day. Ventide Paediatric Rotacaps, 1 puff 2, 3 or 4 times each day. *Special care*: pregnancy, weak heart, angina, heart arrhythmias, hyperthyroidism, hypertension, tuberculosis. Special care in patients changing from systemic steroids.

Possible interaction: sympathomimetics.

Side effects: dilation of peripheral blood vessels, headache, nervous tension, tremor, fungal infections of throat and mouth and hoarseness.
Manufacturer: A. & H.

Ventodisks

Description: a bronchodilator, anti-inflammatory preparation, which is a selective ß2-agonist, available as light blue disks of 200µg strength and dark blue disks of 400µg strength, containing salbutamol as sulphate. Both are marked with strength and name.
Used for: bronchospasm occurring in bronchitis, emphysema and bronchial asthma.
Dosage: acute attack, 200 or 400µg 3 to 4 times each day. Children, acute attack, 200µg as single dose; prevention, half the dose of adult.
Special care: pregnancy, weak heart, angina, heart arrhythmias, hyperthyroidism, hypertension.
Possible interaction: sympathomimetics.
Side effects: headache, dilation of peripheral blood vessels, nervous tension, tremor.
Manufacturer: A. & H.

Ventolin

Description: a bronchodilator/anti-inflammatory preparation which is a selective ß2-agonist, available as pink tablets containing 2mg and 4mg salbutamol as sulphate, marked AH and IK and AH and 2K respectively. Also, **Ventolin Syrup**, sugar and colour-free, containing 2mg/5ml. Also, **Ventolin Inhaler**, a metered dose aerosol delivering 100µg salbutamol per puff. **Ventolin Rotacaps** available as clear/light blue capsules containing 200µg and clear/dark blue capsules containing 400 µg, both marked with strength and name for use with Rotahaler. **Ventolin Injection** available as a solution in ampoules containing 50 and 500µg/ml. **Ventolin Infusion**, available as a solution in ampoules containing 1mg/ml. **Ventolin Respirator Solution**, for hospital use only containing 5mg/ml in bottles. **Ventolin Nebules** for use with nebulizer available as single dose units containing 2.5mg and 5mg/2.5ml.
Used for: bronchospasm occurring in bronchitis, emphysema and bronchial asthma. Injection, status asthmaticus and severe bronchospasm.
Dosage: oral preparations, 2–8mg 3 or 4 times each day. Ventolin Inhaler, attack, 1 or 2 puffs; prevention, 2 puffs 3 or 4 times each day. Ventolin Rotacaps, acute attack, 200 or 400µg as 1 dose; prevention, 400µg 3 or 4 times each day. Injection, 8µg/kg body weight by intramuscular or subcutaneous injection. Or, 4 µg/kg by slow intravenous injection. Nebules, 2.5–5mg nebulised up to 4 times each day. Other preparations, see literature. Children, oral preparations, aged 2 to 6 years, 1–2mg; 6 to 12 years, 2mg, all 3 or 4 times each day. Ventolin Inhaler, half adult dose; Rotacaps, acute attack, 200µg as 1 dose; prevention, half adult dose. Nebules, same as adult dose.
Special care: pregnancy, patients with hyperthyroidism, hypertension, weak heart, angina, heart arrhythmias.
Avoid use: children under 2 years (oral preparations).
Possible interaction: sympathomimetics.
Side effects: headache, dilation of peripheral blood vessels, nervous tension, tremor.
Manufacturer: A. & H.

Vepesid

Description: an anti-cancer drug which is a podophyllotoxin available as pink gelatin capsules containing 50mg and 100mg etoposide. Also, **Vepesid Injection** available as a solution in vials containing 20mg etoposide/ml.
Used for: lymphomas, cancer of the bronchus, teratoma of the testes.
Dosage: as directed by specialist but in divided doses over 3 to 5 days. Oral doses are double those of inection which is given intravenously.
Special care: care in handling (trained staff, protective clothing), irritant to tissues.
Side effects: hair loss, bone marrow suppression, vomiting, nausea, effects on fertility.
Manufacturer: Bristol-Myers.

Vermox

Description: an antihelmintic preparation available as a sugar-free suspension containing 100mg mebendazole/5ml. Also, **Vermox Tablets**, scored, pink, containing 100mg mebendazole marked Me/100 and JANSSEN.
Used for: infestations of large roundworm, threadworm, common and American hookworm, whipworm.
Dosage: adults and children aged over 2 years; threadworm, 100mg with dose repeated after 2 or 3 weeks if necessary. Other types of worm, 100mg morning and night for 3 days.
Avoid use: pregnancy.
Side effects: gastrointestinal upset.
Manufacturer: Janssen.

Vibramycin

Description: a tetracycline antibiotic preparation available as green capsules containing 100mg doxycycline (as hydrochloride), marked VBM 100 and Pfizer. Also, **Vibramycin-D**, off-white, dissolvable tablets containing 100mg vibramycin marked Pfizer and D-9.

Used for: gastrointestinal and respiratory tract infections, pneumonia, soft tissue, urinary tract infections, sexually transmitted diseases, eye infections, acne vulgaris.

Dosage: all infections except sexually transmitted diseases, 200mg with food or drink on first day then 100–200mg daily. Acne, 50mg each day with food or drink for 6 to 12 weeks. (Sexually transmitted diseases, as advised in literature).

Special care: patients with liver disease.

Avoid use: pregnancy, breast-feeding, children.

Possible interaction: carbamazepine, antacids, phenytoin, mineral supplements, barbiturates, methoxyflurane.

Side effects: superinfections, gastrointestinal upset, allergic responses. Withdraw if intracranial hypertension occurs.

Manufacturer: Invicta.

Villescon

Description: a combined sympathomimetic and vitamin preparation available as a tonic containing 2.5mg prolintane hydrochloride, 1.67mg thiamine-hydrochloride, 1.36mg riboflavine sodium phosphate, 0.5mg pyridoxine hydrochloride, 5mg nicotinamide/5ml.

Used for: a general tonic.

Dosage: 10ml after breakfast with second dose in afternoon for 1 to 2 weeks. Children, age 5 to 12 years, 2.5–10ml twice each day.

Avoid use: children under 5 years, patients with epilepsy or thyrotoxicosis.

Possible interaction: levodopa, MAOIs.

Side effects: nausea, insomnia, tachycardia, colic.

Manufacturer: Boehringer Ingelheim.

Virazid

Description: an antiviral preparation available as a powder in vials for nebulization containing 20mg tribavirin/ml.

Used for: serious respiratory syncitial virus bronchiolitis (inflammation and infection of bronchioles).

Dosage: children only, delivery via an oxygen hood, tent or mask for 12 to 18 hours each day for at least 3 days and for a maximum of 7 days.

Special care: patient and equipment require careful monitoring.

Avoid use: pregnancy, females of child-bearing age.

Side effects: worsening of respiratory condition, reticulocytosis (increase in number of reticulocytes—immature erythrocyte red blood cells), pneumothorax, bacterial pneumonia.

Manufacturer: Britannia.

Virormune

Description: a sex hormone (androgen) preparation available as a solution in ampoules containing 50mg testosterone propionate/ml.

Used for: cryptorchidism (undescended testicle), male hypogonadism (deficiency in secretion of hormones by testes), delayed puberty in males. Breast cancer after menopause in women.

Dosage: for hypogonadism, 50mg 2 or 3 times each week; cryptorchidism or delayed puberty, 50mg each week. Breast cancer in women, 100mg 2 or 3 times each week, all by intramuscular injection.

Special care: liver, kidney, or heart disorders, migraine, epilepsy, hypertension.

Avoid use: cancer of liver or prostate gland, heart disease or heart failure which is untreated, kidney nephrosis (an abnormality resulting from various diseases or conditions). Hypercalcaemia, high levels of calcium in urine.

Possible interaction: drugs that induce liver enzymes.

Side effects: weight gain, reduced fertility, oedema, tumours of liver, priapism (painful and prolonged erection of penis not connected with sexual arousal but resulting from drug treatment or underlying disorder). Also, premature closure of epiphyses, increased bone growth, masculinization (women).

Manufacturer: Paines and Byrne.

Virudox

Description: an antiviral preparation available as a solution with applicator brush containing 5% idoxuridine, dimethyl sulphoxide to 100%.

Used for: skin infections caused by *Herpes simplex* and *Herpes zoster*.

Dosage: adults, apply to affected skin 4 times each day for 4 days.

Special care: avoid mucous membranes and eyes. May damage clothing.

Avoid use: pregnancy, breast-feeding, children.

Side effects: stinging when applied, unusual, distinctive taste during treatment. Over-use may cause skin to soften and break down.

Manufacturer: Bioglan.

Viskaldix

Description: a non-cardioselective ß-blocker and thiazide, pindolol (10mg) with clopamide (5mg) in white tablets marked with name.

Used for: hypertension.

Dosage: start with 1 tablet in the morning increasing if required, after 2 or 3 weeks, to 2 or a maximum of 3 per day. Not for children.

Special care: history of bronchospasm and certain ß-blockers, diabetes, liver or kidney disease, pregnancy, lactation, general anaesthesia, gout, check electrolyte levels, K⁺ supplements may be required depending on the case. Withdraw gradually. Not for children.

Avoid use: heart block or failure, bradycardia, sick sinus syndrome (associated with sinus node disorder), certain ß-blockers, severe peripheral arterial disease, pregnancy, lactation, severe kidney failure, anuria, hepatic cornea.

Possible interaction: verapamil, hypoglycaemics, reserpine, clonidine withdrawal, some anti-arrhythmics and anaesthetics, antihypertensives, depressants of the CNS, cimetidine, indomethacin, sympathomimetics, lithium, potassium supplements with potassium-sparing diuretics, digitalis.

Side effects: bradycardia, cold hands and feet, disturbance to sleep, heart failure, gastrointestinal upset, tiredness on exertion, bronchospasm, gout, weakness, blood disorders, sensitivity to light.

Manufacturer: Stuart.

Visken

Description: a non-cardioselective ß-blocker, pindolol, available as white tablets (5 and 15mg) marked with name and strength.

Used for: angina, hypertension.

Dosage: half to 1 tablet 3 times per day (angina); 10–15mg per day increasing weekly to a maximum of 45mg if necessary. Not for children.

Special care: history of bronchospasm and certain ß-blockers, diabetes, liver or kidney disease, pregnancy, lactation, general anaesthesia. Withdraw gradually. Not for children.

Avoid use: heart block or failure, bradycardia, sick sinus syndrome (associated with sinus node disorder), certain ß-blockers, severe peripheral arterial disease.

Possible interaction: verapamil, hypoglycaemics, reserpine, clonidine withdrawal, some antiarrhythmics and anaesthetics, antihypertensives, depressants of the CNS, cimetidine, indomethacin, sympathomimetics.

Side effects: bradycardia, cold hands and feet, disturbance to sleep, heart failure, gastrointestinal upset, tiredness on exertion, bronchospasm.

Manufacturer: Sandoz.

Vista-Methasone

Description: a corticosteroid, betamethasone sodium phosphate, available as 0.1% drops.

Used for: non-infected inflammatory conditions of the nose, ear and eye. Also, **Vista-Methasone N** (also includes 0.5% neomycin sulphate).

Used for: infected inflammation of the nose, ear and eye.

Dosage: 1 to 3 drops from 2 hourly to twice daily, depending upon condition.

Special care: pregnancy; avoid prolonged use during pregnancy, or with infants.

Avoid use: infections of a viral, fungal or tuberculous nature, perforated eardrum (for ear conditions), glaucoma or soft contact lenses (for eye conditions).

Side effects: superinfection. For eyes—corneal thinning, cataract, fungal infection, rise in pressure within the eye.

Manufacturer: Daniels.

Vivalan

Description: an antidepressant and oxazine, viloxazine hydrochloride, in white tablets (50mg) marked V and ICI.

Used for: depression, particularly where sedation is not required.

Dosage: 300mg per day in divided doses (maximum 400mg/day). Elderly, start with 100mg per day. Not for children.

Special care: heart block, heart failure, ischaemic heart disease, pregnancy, epilepsy, suicidal tendency.

Avoid use: past peptic ulcer, liver disease, mania, recent myocardial infarction, breast-feeding.

Possible interaction: phenytoin, clonidine, MAOIs levodopa, theophylline, CNS depressants, carbamazepine.

Side effects: anticholinergic effects, jaundice, convulsions, vomiting, headache, affected reactions.

Manufacturer: Zeneca.

Vivotif

Description: a live attenuated vaccine, *Salmonella typhi*, Ty 21a strain in white/pink capsules.

Used for: immunization against typhoid fever.

Dosage: 1 capsule with cold drink 1 hour before a meal on days 1, 3 and 5. Annual boost of 3 capsules for those regularly at risk. Children over 6 years, adult dose. Not for children under 6.

Special care: pregnancy, breast-feeding.

Avoid use: acute fever or gastrointestinal illness, immunosuppressed patients.

Possible interaction: antibiotics, cytotoxics, immunosuppressants, sulphonamides, mefloquine.

Side effects: mild gastrointestinal upset.

Manufacturer: Evans.

Volital

Description: a stimulant of the CNS, pemoline, available as white tablets (20mg) marked P9.

Used for: hyperkinesia (overactive restlessness) in children.

Dosage: aged 6 to 12 years, start with 20mg in the morning increasing weekly by 20mg to 60mg/day, or possible 120mg if no improvement on lower doses. Not for children under 6.

Special care: reduce dose if side effects occur (improvement usually happens within 6 weeks).

Possible interaction: MAOIs.

Side effects: weight loss, anorexia, headache, sweating, palpitations, dizziness, irritability.

Manufacturer: L.A.B.

Volmax

Description: a selective ß2-agonist, salbutamol sulphate, in white hexagonal continuous-release tablets (4 and 9mg) marked with strength.

Used for: chronic bronchitis, emphysema, bronchospasm.

Dosage: 8mg twice per day. Children, aged 3 to 12 years, 4mg twice per day. Not for those under 3 years.

Special care: angina, hypertension, cardiac arrhythmias, pregnancy, hyperthyroidism, weak heart.

Possible interaction: sympathomimetics.

Side effects: headache, dilatation of peripheral vessels, nervousness.

Manufacturer: A. & H.

Volmaran

Description: a phenylacetic acid, diclofenac sodium, in 25 and 50mg orange tablets.

Used for: pain or inflammation associated with rheumatic disease, gout, musculoskeletal disorders.

Dosage: 75–150mg per day in divided doses after food.

Special care: elderly, kidney, liver or heart disease.

Avoid use: porphyria, hypersensitivity to aspirin or other NSAIDs, pregnancy, peptic ulcer.

Possible interaction: ACE inhibitors, other NSAIDs, quinolones, anticoagulants, antidiabetics, antihypertensives, diuretics, lithium.

Side effects: gastrointestinal upset, nausea, diarrhoea, hypersensitivity reactions, dizziness, blood disorders, headache.

Manufacturer: Eastern.

Voltarol

Description: a phenylacetic acid, diclofenac sodium, available as yellow (25mg) and brown (50mg) tablets marked with name, strength and GEIGY.

Used for: rheumatoid arthritis, osteoarthrosis, ankylosing spondylitis, chronic juvenile arthritis, acute gout.

Dosage: 75–150mg per day in divided doses. Children over 1 year, 1–3mg/kg/day.

Also, **Voltarol Dispersible** as pink, triangular tablets (50mg) marked V and GEIGY.

Dosage: 1 taken 3 times daily in water for a maximum of 3 months. Not for children.

Also, **Voltarol Sustained-Release SR**, as pink, triangular tablets (75mg) marked V 75 SR and GEIGY, and **Voltarol Retard** as 100mg red tablets marked VOLTAROL R and GEIGY.

Dosage: 1 SR once or twice per day, 1 Retard per day.

Also, **Voltarol Suppositories** (100mg).

Dosage: 1 at night and **Voltarol Paediatric Suppositories** (12.5mg).

Dosage: children, 1–3mg/kg/day in divided doses.

Also, **Voltarol Injection** (25mg/ml).

Used for: back pain, postoperative pain, pain in trauma or from fractures.

Dosage: 75mg intramuscularly once or twice per day for 2 days maximum. Continue with tablets or suppositories if required.

Special care: monitor long-term treatment. Liver, kidney or heart disease, porphyria, past gastro-intestinal lesions, pregnancy, breast-feeding, elderly, blood disorders.

Avoid use: allergy to aspirin or anti-inflammatory drugs, proctitis (inflammation of anus and rectum), peptic ulcer.

Possible interaction: lithium, diuretics, digoxin, methotrexate, salicylates, cyclosporin, NSAIDs, steroids, oral hypoglycaemics, quinolones.

Side effects: headache, oedema, gastrointestinal upset.

Manufacturer: Geigy.

Voltarol Emulgel

Description: an NSAID, diclofenac diethyl-ammonium salt as 1.16g in an aqueous gel (equivalent to 1g diclofenac sodium).

Used for: soft tissue rheumatism, strains, sprains, bruises.

Dosage: 2–4g rubbed into area 3 to 4 times per day. Not for children.

Special care: pregnancy, breast-feeding, avoid eyes, mucous membrane, broken skin.

Avoid use: allergy to aspirin or anti-inflammatory drugs.

Side effects: itching, dermatitis, localized erythema,

sensitivity to light.
Manufacturer: Geigy.

Voltarol Ophtha

Description: an NSAID, diclofenac sodium, available as 0.1% single dose eyedrops.
Used for: reduction of miosis (excessive constriction of the sphincter muscle of the iris) in cataract surgery, postoperative inflammation.
Dosage: see literature.
Possible interaction: ACE inhibitors, other NSAIDs, quinolones, anticoagulants, antidiabetics, antihypertensives, diuretics, lithium.
Manufacturer: Ciba Vision.

W

Warticon

Description: a cytotoxic drug, 0.5% podophyllotoxin, available as a solution with applicator. Also, **Warticon Fem** including mirror.

Used for: external genital warts.

Dosage: use twice per day over 3 days, repeated weekly for up to 4 weeks if necessary. Not for children.

Avoid use: pregnancy, breast-feeding.

Side effects: localized irritation.

Manufacturer: Perstop.

Welldorm

Description: a sedative and hypnotic, chloral betaine, available in purple oval tablets (strength 707mg, equivalent to 414mg of chloral hydrate).

Used for: insomnia over the short-term.

Dosage: 1 or 2 tablets at bedtime to a maximum of 2g chloral hydrate equivalent per day.

Also, **Welldorm Elixir**, 143mg chloral hydrate/5ml.

Dosage: 15–45ml at bedtime to a daily maximum of 2g. Children: 30–50mg/kg to a daily maximum of 1g.

Avoid use: severe heart, kidney or liver disease, porphyria, gastritis, pregnancy, breast-feeding.

Possible interaction: anticoagulants, alcohol, CNS depressants, anticholinergics.

Side effects: headache, nausea, vomiting, flatulence, bloating, rashes, blood disorders, excitability.

Manufacturer: S.N.P.

Wellferon

Description: an interferon (affects immunity and cell function) interferon alfa-N1, available as vials containing 3 million units/ml.

Used for: chronic hepatitis B, hairy-cell leukaemia.

Dosage: by subcutaneous and intramuscular injection. See literature for dose.

Special care: see literature.

Avoid use: see literature.

Possible interaction: theophylline.

Side effects: lethargy, flu-like symptoms, depression, bone marrow depression, hypo- and hypertension, arrhythmias, rashes, seizures.

Manufacturer: Wellcome.

X

Xanax

Description: a long-acting benzodiazepine, alprazolam, available as white, oval tablets (250µg) marked UPJOHN 29 and pink, oval tablets (500µg) marked UPJOHN 55.

Used for: short-term treatment of anxiety and anxiety with depression.

Dosage: 250–500µg 2 or 3 times per day, elderly, 250µg, to a daily maximum of 3mg. Not for children.

Special care: chronic liver or kidney disease, chronic lung disease, pregnancy, labour, lactation, elderly. May impair judgement. Withdraw gradually and avoid prolonged use.

Avoid use: depression of respiration, acute lung disease; psychotic, phobic or obsessional states.

Possible interaction: anticonvulsants, depressants of the CNS, alcohol.

Side effects: ataxia, confusion, light-headedness, drowsiness, hypotension, gastrointestinal upsets, disturbances in vision and libido, skin rashes, retention of urine, vertigo. Sometimes jaundice or blood disorders.

Manufacturer: Upjohn.

Xatral

Description: a selective a_1-blocker, alfuzosin hydrochloride, available as white tablets (2.5mg) marked XATRAL 2.5.

Used for: benign prostatic hypertrophy (enlargement of prostate gland).

Dosage: 1 tablet 3 times per day to a maximum of 4. Elderly, 1 at morning and evening to start, to a maximum of 4.

Special care: weak heart, hypertension. Monitor blood pressure especially when starting treatment. Stop 24 hours before anaesthesia, or if angina worsens.

Avoid use: severe liver disease, past orthostatic hypotension (low blood pressure on standing).

Possible interaction: antihypertensives, calcium antagonists, other a-blockers.

Side effects: gastrointestinal upset, headache, dizziness, vertigo, tachycardia, orthostatic hypotension, chest pain, fatigue, rash, flushing, oedema, itching, palpitations, fainting.

Manufacturer: Lorex.

Xuret

Description: a thiazide-like diuretic, metolazone, available as white tablets (0.5mg) marked X and GALEN.

Used for: hypertension.

Dosage: 1 per day each morning (maximum 2 per day). Not for children.

Special care: diabetes, gout, SLE, elderly, cirrhosis of the liver, liver or kidney disease, pregnancy, breast-feeding. Check, fluid, glucose and electrolyte levels.

Avoid use: Addison's disease, hypercalcaemia, severe kidney or liver failure, sensitivity to sulphonamides.

Possible interaction: NSAIDs, corticosteroids, alcohol, antidiabetics, opioids, barbiturates, cardiac glycosides, lithium, tubocurarine.

Side effects: gastrointestinal upset, blood disorders, rash, sensitivity to light, impotence, anorexia, dizziness, pancreatitis, disturbance to metabolism and electrolyte levels.

Manufacturer: Galen.

Xylocaine

Description: a local anaesthetic, lignocaine hydrochloride, available as vials of strength 0.5%, 1% and 2% with or without adrenaline.

Used for: local anaesthetics.

Dosage: 200mg maximum (without adrenaline) or 500mg (with). Children: given in proportion to adult dose. See literature.

Also, **Xylocaine Ointment** (5% lignocaine) in tube or accordion syringe. Also, **Xylocaine Gel**, 2% lignocaine hydrochloride in tube or accordion syringe, and **Xylocaine Antiseptic Gel** containing, in addition, 0.25% chlorhexidine gluconate solution.

Used for: anaesthesia of urethra or vagina, surface anaesthesia.

Dosage: women, 3–5ml; men 10ml to start, then 3–5ml. Not for children.

Also, **Xylocaine 4% Topical** (4% lignocaine hydrochloride).

Used for: bronchoscopy, dental treatment, reduced sensitivity to pain in oropharyngeal region, surface anaesthesia.

Dosage: up to 5ml but see literature. Children: up to 3mg/kg.

Also, **Xylocaine Pump Spray** 10mg lignocaine per dose.

Used for: dental treatment, ear, nose and throat surgery, surface anaesthesia in obstetrics.

Dosage: a maximum of 20 doses. Children: in proportion.

Special care: epilepsy, persons with liver or heart failure.

Avoid use: cardiovascular disease if adrenaline is used, any surgery of the extremities, thyrotoxicosis, myaesthenia gravis.

Possible interaction: phenothiazines, tricyclics, MAOIs (if adrenaline version).

Manufacturer: Astra.

Xylocard

Description: a class I antiarrhythmic, lignocaine hydrochloride, available in preloaded syringes (100mg).

Used for: arrhythmia of the ventricle associated with myocardial infarction.

Dosage: 50–100mg over 2 minutes, by intravenous injection. Repeat once or twice after 5 to 10 minutes, if required. Not for children.

Special care: liver or kidney disease.

Avoid use: heart block, heart conduction disorders, heart failure.

Possible interaction: loop diuretics, thiazides, cimetidine, propanolol.

Side effects: nausea, blurred vision, hypotension, agitation, drowsiness, depression of respiration.

Manufacturer: Astra.

Xyloproct

Description: a combined local anaesthetic and steroid containing 60mg lignocaine, 50mg aluminium acetate, 400mg zinc oxide, and 5mg hydrocortisone acetate in suppository form.

Used for: haemorrhoids, itching, anal fissure, anal fistula.

Dosage: 1 at night and after defecation.

Also, **Xyloproct Ointment** containing 5% lignocaine, 18% zinc oxide, 3.5% aluminium acetate and 0.275% hydrocortisone.

Dosage: use several times per day.

Special care: pregnancy. Do not use over a long period.

Avoid use: infections of a viral, fungal or tuberculous nature.

Side effects: corticosteroid effects.

Manufacturer: Astra.

Y

Yutopar

Description: a ß-agonist for relaxation of uterine smooth muscle, ritodrine hydrochloride, available in yellow tablets (10mg) marked Yutopar.

Used for: premature labour (with no complications), foetal asphyxiation in labour.

Dosage: one, half an hour before the end of intravenous therapy. For maintenance, one every two hours for twenty-four hours, then one or two every four to six hours. Also, **Yutopar Injection** (10mg/ml in ampoules).

Special care: diabetes, thyrotoxicosis or cardiovascular disease of the mother, monitor heart rate of both mother and foetus.

Avoid use: if a prolonged pregnancy would be hazardous, toxaemia of pregnancy, cord compression, antepartum haemorrhage (bleeding before the birth and after 28th week), threatened abortion.

Possible interaction: ß-agonists, ß-agonists, MAOIs.

Side effects: anxiety, tachycardia, tremor, higher blood sugar levels.

Manufacturer: Duphar.

Z

Zaditen

Description: an anti-allergic agent and anti-histamine, ketotifen, as hydrogen fumarate, available as white, scored tablets (1mg) marked ZADITEN 1. Also **Zaditen Capsules** (1mg white capsules marked CS) and **Zaditen Elixir** (1mg/5ml, sugar-free).

Used for: prevention of bronchial asthma, allergic rhinitis and conjunctivitis.

Dosage: 1–2mg twice per day with food. Children over 2 years, 1mg twice per day with food. Not for children under 2 years.

Avoid use: pregnancy, breast-feeding.

Possible interaction: antihistamines, alcohol, oral hypoglycaemics, depressants of the CNS.

Side effects: dry mouth, dizziness, drowsiness, affected reactions.

Manufacturer: Sandoz.

Zadstat

Description: a nitro imidazole and antibacterial/amoeboride/antiprotozoal, metronidazole, available as white tablets (200mg) marked LL and M200.

Used for: infections caused by anaerobic bacteria, amoebiasis, trichomonal infections, ulcerative gingivitis.

Dosage: average 600–800mg per day in divided doses, reduced doses for children. See literature for amoebiasis. Partner should also be treated for trichomonal infections when the dose may be up to 2g as a single dose.

Also **Zadstat Suppositories** (500mg and 1g).

Dosage: see literature.

Special care: pregnancy, breast-feeding (a high dose treatment is not recommended).

Possible interaction: oral anticoagulants, alcohol, phenobarbitone.

Side effects: leucopenia, urticaria, angioneurotic oedema, furred tongue, unpleasant taste, gastrointestinal upset, dark urine, disturbance to CNS, seizures on prolonged or intensive treatment.

Manufacturer: Lederle.

Zantac

Description: an H_2 blocker, ranitidine hydrochloride, available as white, pentagonal tablets (150mg) and white tablets (300mg) both marked with GLAXO, strength and ZANTAC. Also, **Zantac Effervescent**, 150 and 300mg white effervescent tablets, and **Zantac Syrup**, 150mg/10ml with 7.5% ethanol in a sugar-free syrup.

Used for: duodenal, benign gastric and post-operative ulcers; ulcers due to NSAIDs. Oesophageal reflux, prevention of ulcers induced by NSAIDs, dyspepsia, oesophagitis.

Dosage: 150mg 2 times per day or 300mg at bedtime. 150mg 4 times per day for oesophagitis. Also see literature. Not for children under 8 years. Over 8 years, for peptic ulcer, 2–4mg/kg twice per day.

Also, **Zantac Injection**, 50mg/2ml as a solution in ampoules.

Special care: exclude malignancy first, kidney disease, pregnancy, lactation.

Side effects: dizziness, headache, sometimes hepatitis, leucopenia, confusion, thrombocytopenia, hypersensitivity .

Manufacturer: Glaxo.

Zarontin

Description: a succinimide and anticonvulsant, ethosuximide, in amber oblong capsules (250mg), marked P-D. Also, **Zarontin Syrup** (250mg/5ml).

Used for: petit mal.

Dosage: 500mg per day increasing as required by 250mg at 4 to 7 day intervals to a maximum of 2g per day. Children, 6 to 12 years, adult dose; under 6, 250mg per day adjusted according to response.

Special care: pregnancy, breast-feeding, liver or kidney disease. Withdrawal should be gradual.

Side effects: gastric upset, disturbance to CNS, rashes, blood disorders, SLE.

Manufacturer: Parke-Davis.

Zavedos

Description: a cytotoxic antibiotic, idarubicin hydrochloride, as powder in vials (5 and 10mg). Also, **Zavedos Capsules**, 5, 10 and 25mg strengths in capsules coloured orange, red/white and orange/

white respectively. Also as powder for reconstitution and injection.

Used for: acute leukaemia.

Special care: teratogenic, liver and kidney disease, irritant to skin and tissues (when handling), heart disease, elderly, monitor heart.

Avoid use: of simultaneous radiotherapy, pregnancy.

Side effects: nausea, vomiting, hair loss, bone marrow suppression (inhibiting blood cell formation), tissue necrosis upon extravasation, inflammation of mucous membranes.

Manufacturer: Farmitalia.

Zestoretic

Description: an ACE inhibitor and thiazide diuretic containing 20mg lisinopril and 12.5mg hydrochlorothiazide, in white tablets.

Used for: hypertension.

Dosage: 1 tablet per day (maximum of 2). Not for children.

Special care: liver or kidney disease, gout, diabetes, anaesthesia, ischaemic heart or cerebrovascular disease, haemodialysis, imbalance in fluid or electrolyte levels.

Avoid use: pregnancy, breast-feeding, anuria, angioneurotic oedema in conjunction with previous treatment using ACE inhibitor.

Possible interaction: lithium, NSAIDs, hypoglycaemics, potassium supplements, potassium-sparing diuretics, tubocurarine.

Side effects: headache, fatigue, hypotension, cough, dizziness, nausea, impotence, angioneurotic oedema, diarrhoea.

Manufacturer: Zeneca.

Zestril

Description: an ACE inhibitor, lisinopril, available as tablets, marked with heart shape and strength: 2.5mg (white), 5 and 10mg (pink), and 20mg (red). 2.5, 10 and 20mg have company symbol;10 and 20mg have a trade mark.

Used for: additional therapy (to digitalis and diuretics) in congestive heart failure, hypertension.

Dosage: start with 2.5mg per day, increasing gradually to a maintenance dose of 5–20mg once per day. Cease using diuretic 2 to 3 days before treatment for hypertension. Reduce dose of diuretic in treating heart failure and start treatment in hospital. Not for children.

Special care: renovascular hypertension (increased pressure in hepatic portal vein), kidney disease, haemodialysis, congestive heart failure, anaesthesia, breast-feeding.

Avoid use: pregnancy, angioneurotic oedema from past treatment with ACE inhibitor, narrowing of aorta, enlargement of right ventricle.

Possible interaction: potassium supplement, potassium-sparing diuretics, antihypertensives, indomethacin, lithium.

Side effects: kidney failure, angioneurotic oedema, hypotension, dizziness, headache, diarrhoea, fatigue, cough, nausea, palpitations, rash, weakness.

Manufacturer: Zeneca.

Zimovane

Description: a cyclopyrrolone and hypnotic, zopiclone, available as white tablets (7.5mg) marked ZM.

Used for: insomnia.

Dosage: 1 tablet at bedtime (2 if required). Elderly , ¹/₂ tablet. Not for children.

Special care: liver disorder, check for withdrawal symptoms on completing treatment.

Avoid use: pregnancy, breast-feeding.

Possible interaction: trimipramine, alcohol, other depressants of the CNS.

Side effects: gastrointestinal upset, metallic aftertaste, allergic reactions, drowsiness, minor behavioural changes, judgement and dexterity may be impaired.

Manufacturer: R.P.R.

Zinacef

Description: a cephalosporin and antibacterial, cefuroxime (as sodium salt) available in 250mg, 750mg and 1.5g vials.

Used for: infections of soft tissue, the respiratory and urinary tracts, meningitis, gonorrhoea, prevention of infection during surgery.

Dosage: see literature.

Possible interaction: aminoglycosides, loop diuretics.

Side effects: gastrointestinal upset, hypersensitivity reactions. Occasionally leucopenia, neutropenia, candidosis.

Manufacturer: Glaxo.

Zinamide

Description: a derivative of nicotinic acid, pyrazinamide, in white tablets (500mg) marked MSD 504.

Used for: tuberculosis when used with other antituberculous drugs.

Dosage: 20–35mg/kg/day in divided doses, to a maximum of 3g. Not for children.

Special care: past gout or diabetes, check liver function and blood uric acid.

Avoid use: liver disease. Withdraw if there is liver

damage or high blood uric acid with gouty arthritis.
Side effects: hepatitis.
Manufacturer: M.S.D.

Zineryt
Description: an antiobiotic containing erythromycin (4%), zinc acetate (1.2%) in an alcoholic solution.
Used for: acne.
Dosage: use twice daily.
Special care: avoid mucous membranes and eyes.
Side effects: passing irritation.
Manufacturer: Brocades.

Zinnat
Description: a cephalosporin and antibacterial, cefuroxime axetil, in white tables containing 125 or 250mg, marked GLAXO and 125 or 250. Also, **Zinnat Suspension** (125mg/5ml).
Used for: infections of the ear, nose and thorat, respiratory or urinary tracts, skin and soft tissues.
Dosage: usually 250mg twice per day after food, 500mg for severe infections and a 1g single dose per day for gonorrhoea. Children over 2 years 250mg twice per day; 3 months–2 years, 125mg twice per day. Not for infants under 3 months.
Special care: pregnancy, hypersensitivity to penicillin, breast-feeding.
Side effects: colitis, hypersensitivity reactions, headache, gastrointestinal upset, candidosis, increase in liver enzymes.
Manufacturer: Glaxo.

Zirtek
Description: an antihistamine, cetirizine hydrochloride, in white oblong tablets (10mg) marked Y/Y.
Used for: urticaria, seasonal rhinitis.
Dosage: 1 tablet per day. Not for children under 6 years; over 6 years, adult dose.
Also, **Zirtek Solution** (1mg/ml) in banana-flavoured, sugar-free solution.
Dosage: 10ml per day for adults and children over 6 years. Not for children under 6 years.
Special care: pregnancy, kidney disease.
Avoid use: breast-feeding.
Side effects: agitation, gastrointestinal upset, dizziness, headache, dry mouth, drowsiness.
Manufacturer: UCB.

Zita
Description: an H_2-blocker, cimetidine, in 200, 400 and 800mg tablets.
Used for: ulcer (stomach, benign gastric and duodenal), reflux oesophagitis, Zollinger-Ellison syndrome.

Dosage: usually 400mg twice per day or 800mg at night for 4 to 8 weeks, depending upon condition. Children, 20–30mg/kg per day in divided doses.
Special care: liver or kidney disease, pregnancy, breast-feeding.
Possible interaction: warfarin, phenytoin, theophylline, pethidine, antiarrhythmics, anticoagulants, rifampicin, antidepressants, antidiabetics, ß-blockers, benzodiazepines, some antipsychotics, chloroquine, carbamazepine.
Side effects: rash, dizziness, fatigue. Occasionally liver disorder, muscle or joint pain, bradycardia and heart block, gynaecomastia (with high dosages).
Manufacturer: Eastern.

Zithromax
Description: a macrolide and antibacterial, azithromycin dihydrate, in white capsules (250mg) marked ZTM250 and Pfizer.
Used for: infections of skin, soft tissue, and respiratory tract, otitis media and certain genital infections.
Dosage: 2 per day for 3 days taken 1 hour before or 2 hours after food.
Also, **Zithromax Suspension**, 200mg/5ml.
Dosage: children: 12 to 14 years, 10ml; 8 to 11 years, 7.5ml; 3 to 7 years, 5ml; under 3 years, 10mg/kg.
Special care: pregnancy, breast-feeding, liver or kidney disorder.
Avoid use: liver disease.
Possible interaction: antacids, cyclosporin, warfarin, digoxin, ergot derivatives.
Side effects: allergic reaction, rash, anaphylaxis, gastrointestinal upset, angioneurotic oedema.
Manufacturer: Richborough.

Zocor
Description: an HMG CoA reductase inhibitor, simvastatin, in oval tablets (10mg, peach; 20mg, tan) marked with strength and ZOCOR.
Used for: primary high blood cholesterol levels.
Dosage: start with 10mg at night, altered to match response, within the range 10–40mg. Not for children.
Special care: past liver disease, check liver function.
Avoid use: pregnancy, women should use non-hormonal contraception, breast-feeding, liver disease.
Possible interaction: cyclosporin, digoxin, coumarin anticoagulants, gemfibrozil, nicotinic acid.
Side effects: headache, nausea, dyspepsia, diarrhoea, abdominal pain, constipation, flatulence, weakness, myopathy.
Manufacturer: M.S.D.

Zofran

Description: a 5HT₃-antagonist (blocks nausea and vomiting reflexes), ondansetron hydrochloride in yellow, oval tablets (4 and 8mg) marked with GLAXO and strength.

Also, **Zofran Injection** (2mg/ml).

Used for: postoperative nausea and vomiting or that due to chemo- and radiotherapy.

Dosage: see literature.

Special care: pregnancy.

Avoid use: breast-feeding.

Side effects: flushes, headache, constipation.

Manufacturer: Glaxo.

Zoladex

Description: a gonadotrophin release hormone analogue, goserelin acetate, as a biodegradable depot (3.6mg).

Used for: endometriosis, advanced breast cancer, prostate cancer.

Dosage: 1 depot subcutaneously in abdominal wall every 28 days for up to 6 months.

Special care: those at risk of osteoporosis, or males at risk of obstruction of the ureter or compression of the spinal cord.

Avoid use: pregnancy, breast-feeding. Non-hormonal contraception should be used.

Side effects: headaches, hot flushes, breast swelling or tenderness, rashes, vaginal dryness, hyper-calcaemia.

Manufacturer: Zeneca.

Zovirax

Description: a nucleoside analogue and antiviral, acyclovir, available in shield-shaped tablets; 200mg, blue and marked ZOVIRAX with a triangle; 400mg, pink and marked ZOVIRAX 400 with a triangle. Also 800mg in white, elongated tablet marked ZOVIRAX 800. Also **Zovirax Suspension** (200mg/5ml) and **Zovirax Chickenpox Treatment** (400mg/5ml).

Used for: *Herpes simplex* and *Herpes zoster* particularly in immunocompromised patients.

Dosage: from 800mg–4g per day depending upon condition. Children from 200mg 4 times per day. See literature.

Also, **Zovirax Infusion** (250 and 500mg as powder in vials) and **Zovirax Cream** (5%).

Dosage: use 5 times per day at 4-hour intervals, for 5 days. Also ointment, (3%).

Used for: herpetic keratitis (inflammation of the cornea).

Dosage: insert 1cm into lower conjuctival sac 5 times per day continuing 3 days after healing.

Special care: kidney disease, do not use cream in eyes.

Possible interaction: probenecid.

Side effects: erythema, flaking skin with topical use, passing irritation, kidney disorder, stinging (with ointment).,

Manufacturer: Wellcome.

Zumenon

Description: an oestrogen, oestradiol, available as blue tablets (2mg) marked 381 and DUPHAR.

Used for: symptoms of the menopause.

Dosage: start with 1 per day, increased to 2 if necessary, reducing to 1 as soon as possible. Commence on fifth day of menstruation (any time if absent).

Special care: patients at risk of thrombosis or with liver disease. Women with any of the following disorders should be carefully monitored: fibroids in the womb, multiple sclerosis, diabetes, tetany, porphyria, epilepsy, liver disease, hypertension, migraine, otosclerosis, gallstones. Breasts, pelvic organs and blood pressure should be checked at regular intervals during the course of treatment.

Avoid use: pregnancy, breast-feeding, women with conditions which might lead to thrombosis, thrombophlebitis, serious heart, kidney or liver disease, breast cancer, oestrogen-dependent cancers including those of reproductive system, endometriosis, undiagnosed vaginal bleeding.

Possible interaction: drugs which induce liver enzymes.

Side effects: tenderness and enlargement of breasts, weight gain, breakthrough bleeding, giddiness, vomiting and nausea, gastrointestinal upset. Treatment should be halted immediately if severe headaches occur, disturbance of vision, hypertension or any indications of thrombosis, jaundice. Also, in the event of pregnancy and 6 weeks before planned surgery.

Manufacturer: Duphar.

Zyloric

Description: an inhibitor of xanthine oxidase which forms uric acid. Allopurinol is available as white tablets coded U4A (100mg) and ZYLORIC 300 with C9B (300mg).

Used for: gout, prevention of stones of uric acid and calcium oxalate.

Dosage: start with 100–300mg per day. Maintenance dose of 200–600mg per day. Not for children.

Special care: pregnancy, liver or kidney disease, elderly. Anti-inflammatory drug to be given for 1

month at start of treatment. Maintain fluid intake.
Avoid use: acute gout.
Possible interaction: anticoagulants, azathioprine, mercaptopurine, chlorpropamide.

Side effects: nausea, acute gout, withdraw if there are skin reactions.
Manufacturer: Wellcome.

The Human Body

The Musculoskeletal System

The Skeleton

The skeleton gives the body its support and shape, provides the anchor and the mechanical basis for movements of the muscles and provides protection for the internal organs. It is formed by 206 bones which are connected by joints of fibrous or cartilaginous material.

Bone

Bones are formed from hard tissue with a matrix of collagen fibres and cells. There are two types of bone—compact, and spongy or cancellous. The dense compact bone consists of bone cells which are formed in rings around minute channels, known as the Haversian canals, through which run blood and lymphatic vessels and nerves. The appearance of spongy bone resembles that of a honeycomb, with the hard material surrounding Haversian spaces, which, in some bones, contain bone marrow cells which form red blood cells.

There are four basic types of bone in the body:

Long bones—consisting of a long shaft known as the diaphysis and two ends called the epiphyses. Examples of these bones include the femur (thigh bone), the leg bones (tibia and fibula) and the fingers (the phalanges).

Short bones—cube-shaped, generally spongy bones. The wrist (carpal) is a short bone.

Flat bones—consisting of compact bone around spongy bone. These bones, although generally

The human skeleton

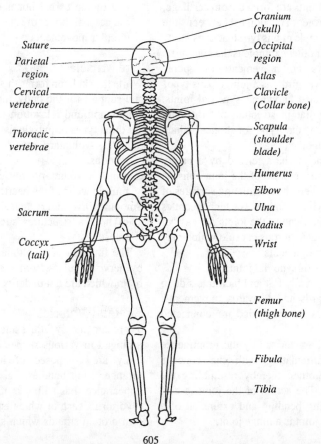

Suture
Parietal region
Cervical vertebrae
Thoracic vertebrae
Sacrum
Coccyx (tail)

Cranium (skull)
Occipital region
Atlas
Clavicle (Collar bone)
Scapula (shoulder blade)
Humerus
Elbow
Ulna
Radius
Wrist
Femur (thigh bone)
Fibula
Tibia

thin, provide protection and are areas for the attachment of muscles. Examples of flat bones include the bones of the skull, the sternum and the shoulder blades (scapulae).

Irregular bones—these vary in shape and composition. Examples include the bones of the spinal column and the face.

The skeleton has two basic divisions: the axial skeleton comprises the bones of the skull, the vertebral column, the ribs and the sternum. The appendicular skeleton comprises the bones of the upper and lower limbs, the pelvis and the shoulder blade and collar-bone.

The Joints

Joints are formed wherever one bone connects, or articulates, with another, facilitating movement and providing protection. There are three basic structure types of joints: fibrous, cartilaginous and synovial joints. Additionally joints are classified in terms of their function as immovable, slightly movable and movable.

Fibrous joints are immovable as they have no cavity and the bones are connected by dense connective tissue. A typical example of a fibrous joint is the suture which joins the bones of the skull.

Slightly movable joints are formed from cartilage, a firm, pliable tissue. The joints between the vertebrae are one example of this type that does allow a little movement. Another example is the symphisis joint, which allows no movement; the pubic symphisis of the pelvic girdle is a joint of this type.

Moveable joints, also known as synovial joints, are all basically similar in structure but differ in shape depending on the type of bones which articulate with one another.

The synovial joint is characterized by a cavity within a capsule. The structure of the joint consists of cartilage which covers the articulating surfaces of the bones, a synovial membrane which secretes fluid in the cavity, lubricating the joints for ease of movement, and an outer fibrous capsule which may be thickened to form ligaments.

There are six types of synovial joint:

Gliding—these are usually flat and facilitate side to side and backwards and forwards movements. The carpal bones of the wrist are connected gliding joints.

Hinge—these are characterized by the prominence of one bone articulating with the concave depression of another, thereby resembling the hinge of a door. The action of the joint is also similar, facilitating bending and extension of a limb. The elbow joint is a hinge joint.

Pivot—the primary movement facilitated by the pivot joint is rotation. The rounded or pointed surface of one bone articulates with a ring formed by bone and ligament. The vertebrae in the region of the neck articulate at hinge joints, enabling rotation of the head as in 'shaking' the head to indicate a negative response.

Condyloid—characterized by a rounded end of one bone articulating with a shallow depression in another bone. This facilitates flexion and extension, and movement towards and away from the midline of the body (abduction and adduction). The joint between the skull and the lower jaw is typical of a condyloid joint.

Ball and socket joint—this type allows free and easy movement in all directions. The surface of one bone forms a ball shape, articulating with the deep depression in another bone. A good example of this type of joint is the hip joint where the head of the femur articulates with the deep hollow in the pelvic girdle.

Saddle joint—this type of joints facilitates flexion extension, adduction and abduction. The surface of one bone is convex, shaped like a saddle, and the surface of the other is concave. This is exemplified in the joint between the trapezium, one of the carpal bones of the thumb, and the metacarpal bone of the thumb, which allows circular movements.

The Muscles

While the skeleton forms the mechanical framework and support for the body, motion is enabled by the contraction and relaxation of muscle tissue. There are three types of muscle tissue:

Skeletal—voluntary muscle attached to bone by tendons.

Cardiac—involuntary muscle which forms the muscle walls of the heart.

Smooth—involuntary muscle situated in the walls of hollow structures such as the stomach and intestines.

The function of involuntary muscle is facilitated by nerve impulses from specialized centres in the brain which are not under conscious control.

Skeletal Muscles

There are nearly 700 skeletal muscles which are arranged in various shapes and are usually paired. They are composed of long fibres which are arranged in bundles, giving them a striped appearance. Each fibre is made up of a bundle of myofibrils, each of which is composed of thick and thin protein strands which slide across one another when they contract, thereby shortening the length of the muscle.

The skeletal muscles are connected to bones by tendons, dense fibrous tissue which forms a type of cord. When muscles exert a pulling force, the tendon will exert a similar force on the bone, inducing movement. The pairs arrangement of most muscles enables one muscle to act in contrast to the other to produce the required movement. For example in bending the arm at the elbow joint, the biceps contract to exert the pull and the triceps muscles relax, becoming longer and flatter. Once the arm is straightened the process is reversed, with the triceps contracting to become shorter and the biceps relaxing.

Each movement involves the coordination of several different muscle groups; walking, for example, involves the muscles of six different groups. Muscular movement is controlled by the central nervous system where stimulation of nerve impulses occurs in response to conscious thought. The nerve cells in the brain will send messages to the muscles via the spinal cord and the motor nerves. Each motor nerve is composed of nerve cell structures, known as motor neurones, which transmit the electrical impulses in a pathway to the muscle tissue. Each fibre of the muscle is connected to one of these neurones which enables the muscles to respond so quickly to the impulses sent from the brain.

The skeletal muscles

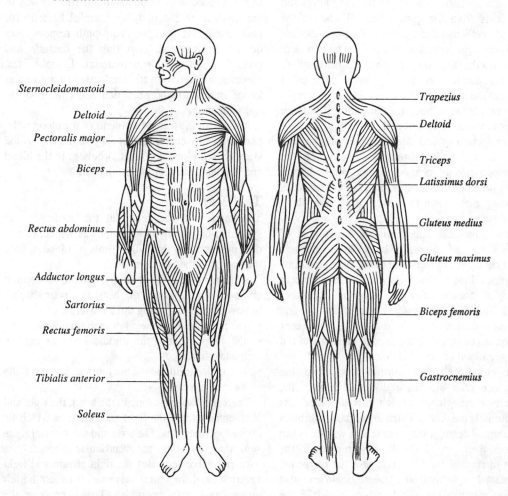

Sternocleidomastoid

Deltoid

Pectoralis major

Biceps

Rectus abdominus

Adductor longus

Sartorius

Rectus femoris

Tibialis anterior

Soleus

Trapezius

Deltoid

Triceps

Latissimus dorsi

Gluteus medius

Gluteus maximus

Biceps femoris

Gastrocnemius

The Cardiovascular System

The cardiovascular system consists of the heart, the blood and the blood vessels (arteries, veins, capillaries, arterioles and venules), which facilitate the supply of oxygen and nutrients to tissues and cells, while also picking up waste products for eventual elimination from the body.

Blood

Blood performs three basic functions:

- The transportation of oxygen from the lungs and nutrients from the gastrointestinal tract to the body's cells and the carrying of carbon dioxide and waste products from the cells to be expelled. It is also the method by which hormones released by the ductless endocrine glands are carried around the body.
- The regulation of body temperature, pH balance and the water content of cells.
- As protection against disease. Blood plays a vital role in the body's immune system and the transportation of phagocytes and antibodies to fight infectious organisms. The blood also has a clotting mechanism to prevent excessive blood loss.

Blood constitutes approximately 8 per cent of body weight; the volume of blood in the average male is between 5–6 litres and in the average female 4–5 litres. Blood is made up of around 55 per cent plasma, a mixture of water, proteins and other solutes including nutrients, waste products, and enzymes and hormones. The remaining 45 per cent of blood is composed of the formed elements of red and white blood cells and platelets.

Red blood cells, or erythrocytes, have the appearance of a biconcave disc and contain the pigment haemoglobin which gives blood its characteristic red colour. Once blood passes through the lungs, haemoglobin combines with oxygen which is then carried via the erythrocytes to the body's interstitial fluid and released, the oxygen is then passed on to the cells. Haemoglobin can also transport a proportion of the carbon dioxide in the body back to the lungs to be exhaled and thus removed from the body. The average adult has between 4.8 and 5.4 million red blood cells.

White blood cells, or leucocytes, are far fewer in number than red blood cells but are larger and have an entirely different function, which is primarily the defence against infection. Leucocytes can be divided into two distinct types, granulocytes and agranulocytes, and again subdivided into neutrophils, eosinophils and basophils (the former) and lymphocytes and monocytes (the latter). Each of these blood cells responds in a particular way to the invasion of the body by harmful bacteria (or pathogens). For example, neutrophils respond very quickly to invasion, engulfing the bacteria and getting rid of the dead material. Lymphocytes, however, are active in the production of antibodies in the immune response which helps the body to fight infection.

Another of the formed elements of the blood is the platelet, a tiny cell fragment (approximately $1/3$ the size of a red blood cell) that circulates in the blood and is vital in the clotting mechanism.

The Heart

The heart is at the centre of the cardiovascular system, a bag of involuntary muscle which, in one day, pumps more than 7000 litres of blood around the body, via the blood vessels.

Situated in the thoracic cavity, behind the sternum and between the lungs, the heart is a pear shaped, hollow organ comprising three muscle layers:

- the pericardium—the outer membranous sac
- the myocardium—the middle layer of cardiac muscle fibres
- the endocardium—the membrane covering the internal cavities

There are four chambers in the heart, the right and left ventricles and the right and left atria which lie above the ventricles. The atria and the ventricles are separated by the atrioventricular valves; the tricuspid valve separates the right atrium and right ventricle, and the mitral valve lies between the left atrium and left ventricle. These prevent the backflow of blood that is being pumped through the heart.

Blood from the body (except the lungs) is delivered to the right atrium via two large veins, the inferior and the superior vena cava. The blood is then passed into the right ventricle and out through the pulmonary artery to the lungs. Once oxygenated it is then carried back to the heart by the four pulmonary veins (two per lung), entering the left atrium where it is then passed into the left ventricle and out to the body via the aorta. The flow of blood between the ventricles and the arteries is regulated by the semi-lunar valves. If the blood pressure is greater in the artery than it is in the ventricle then the semi-lunar valves will close to prevent the backflow of blood.

The heart

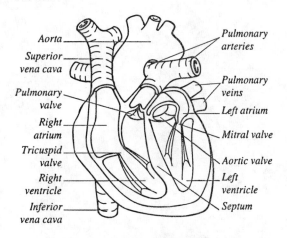

Aorta
Superior vena cava
Pulmonary valve
Right atrium
Tricuspid valve
Right ventricle
Inferior vena cava

Pulmonary arteries
Pulmonary veins
Left atrium
Mitral valve
Aortic valve
Left ventricle
Septum

The flow of blood through the heart is facilitated by the contraction and relaxation of the heart muscle which is itself governed by an electrical impulse. This cycle of contraction and relaxation (or heartbeat) lasts in total for approximately 0.8 second.

The muscle fibres of the heart are able to repeatedly generate the impulses that control the cardiac cycle without stimulus from the autonomic nervous system, thus operating as a pacemaker and system of conduction, carrying the initial impulse throughout the heart muscle. The impulse is initiated by the sinoatrial node which lies in the wall of the right atrium, just below where it opens to the superior vena cava. Nerve impulses from the sinoatrial node spread out through the atria causing them to contract and then spread to the atrioventricular node which is located in the septum, the wall that separates the atria. The blood is then emptied from the atria into the ventricles while the impulse is passed on to a group of fibres known as

the bundle of His, which provide the only electrical connection point between the atria and ventricles. From here the impulse will then pass down the septum and through the right and left bundle branches which extend from the bundle of His. The ventricles contract once the impulse has stimulated the Purkinje fibres which will conduct the impulse to the ventricular myocardial cells in the walls of each of these chambers.

The Blood Vessels

The blood vessels form the route by which blood is carried away from the heart to the tissues of the body and then back to the heart. The structure, and size of the vessels vary greatly and comprise a complex network of circulation and regulation.

The arteries carry blood away from the heart to the body tissues. The blood found in the arteries is freshly oxygenated and has a characteristic orange-red colour.

The structure of the walls of the arteries makes them both elastic and contractile, enabling them to stretch when the ventricles contract and blood is released from the heart, and contract when the ventricles relax, thereby forcing the blood onwards.

The large arteries, known as the elastic arteries, include the aorta, the carotid and iliac arteries; their function is to conduct blood from the heart to the muscular or medium-sized arteries, which distribute blood around the body. The walls of these arteries are slightly different enabling them to adjust the flow of blood in accordance with the need of the part of the body which they supply. This is by two processes known as vasoconstriction and vasodilation. In vasoconstriction the smooth muscle of the walls contracts and the hollow centre of the artery (known as the lumen) becomes narrower, resulting in a lower volume of blood flow. In vasodilation the smooth muscle relaxes, increasing the size of the lumen and increasing the volume of blood flow.

The arterioles are tiny arteries that deliver blood to the capillaries and again the structure of the walls enables the arterioles to regulate the flow of blood to the capillaries. The capillaries are microscopic and are distributed near to all the body cells.

The function of capillaries is in the actual cellular exchange of oxygen and nutrients and waste products between the blood and the body tissue; this function is facilitated by the thin walls of the vessels.

The flow of blood then continues to the venules in some areas of the body, where in others they form extensive networks which enables the fast diffusion of large amounts of nutrients and the uptake of waste products for filtration. Where there is no direct flow between an arteriole, a capillary and a venule a structure known as the metarteriole emerges from the capillary network to continue the flow of blood into the venule. The function of venules is to collect blood from the capillary network and drain it into the veins for return to the heart.

Generally, the blood pressure in veins is much lower than that in the arteries; whereas blood is lost in rapid spurts from a severed artery, blood from a severed vein will ooze out more slowly. Many veins contain valves which are vital in promoting the flow of blood to the heart, particularly from the lower limbs where the blood has to flow against the pull of gravity.

The veins deliver blood to the superior and inferior vena cava which then return the venous blood to the heart.

The Respiratory System

Respiration is the process by which oxygen is provided for the body cells, stimulating metabolic reactions for the release of nutrients. Once oxygen has been used by the cells, carbon dioxide is released and then eliminated from the body when breathed out (or expired). The gaseous exchange—essential for life—is the primary function of the respiratory system, though the structures of the system also serve as a sensory organ.

The six basic structures of the respiratory system are the nose, pharynx, larynx, trachea, bronchi and lungs.

The nose has a basic framework of bone and cartilage attached to muscle and the outer skin. Lined with mucous membrane the internal structure of the nose is connected to the pharynx by two openings called the internal nares. Air breathed in through the nose is warmed, moistened and filtered as it passes through the conchae, three bony projections which are lined with mucous membrane composed of cells which can trap particles of dust and germs.

The filtered air flows through the internal nare into the pharynx, or throat, which lies just behind the internal nasal cavity. Shaped rather like a funnel, it has three functions; the passage of air and of food, and as a kind of chamber for the vocal sounds produced by the larynx (the voice box). The first portion of the pharynx is the nasopharynx which transports both air and mucus downwards. It also has openings into the Eustachian tubes of the ear and is involved in equalizing the air pressure between the ears, nose and throat. The middle section, the oropharynx, receives air, food and drink from the mouth and it is here that the tonsils are found.

The lowest portion of the pharynx, the laryngopharynx, also acts as a passageway for food, fluids and air and is connected to the larynx which produces vocal sounds when air is expelled over the vocal cords, two membranes which vibrate to produce sound. The structure of ligaments, muscles and cartilage in the larynx control the tension in the cords, thereby changing the sound patterns.

The epiglottis is a piece of elastic cartilage which is situated at the base of the tongue and is joined by a 'stem' to the Adam's apple, while a flap of cartilage can freely move up or down. When food is swallowed the larynx rises and this triggers the free flap of the epiglottis to move downwards, thereby creating a lid over the larynx and channelling the food into the oesophagus and not into the respiratory tract. The larynx extends into the trachea or windpipe which is approximately 10cm long and its walls are supported by incomplete cartilage rings which provide support but also flexibility, enabling the trachea to give a little when food is passing down the oesophagus, which lies directly behind it. Again the inner walls are covered with mucosal lining which traps particles of dust and microorganisms which are moved upwards and expelled form the respiratory tract. The trachea then divides into the left and right bronchus (pleural bronchi) which are similar in structure to the trachea, and lead into the left and right lung respectively. The bronchi then branch out into secondary bronchi, then tertiary bronchi and the process of branching continues until the terminal bronchioles are reached.

The lungs are cone-shaped and extend from just above the collar-bone to the surface of the diaphragm. The surface of each lung is rounded to match the curved shape of the ribs and covered in the pleural membrane, one layer of which adheres to the wall of the thoracic cavity and the other to the lungs themselves. The pleural cavity which lies between these layers secretes a fluid which prevents any friction from developing between the two membranes. The midline of the each lung contains a region known as the hilus, the area through which blood and lymphatic vessels, nerves and the primary bronchi enter and leave. Each lung is divided into lobes, three in the right lung and two in the left, within which there are smaller divisions known as lobules (ten in each lung), each of which is supplied with an arteriole, a venule, a lymphatic vessel and the branch of terminal bronchiole. The bronchioles then branch into respiratory bronchioles then into alveolar ducts and finally into the alveolar sacs and the alveoli, where gaseous exchange takes place. As the respiratory branches extend deeper into the lungs the structures become less muscular and cartilaginous giving way to thin connective tissue supported by elastic membrane.

The Physiology of Respiration

Natural respiration occurs automatically in response to nerve impulses sent from the respiratory centre in the brain stem to the muscles involved in the process of inspiration (breathing in) and expiration (breathing out). The diaphragm, the large muscle that provides the floor to the thoracic cavity, contracts and flattens in response to the impulses, thereby increasing the volume of the thoracic space. As the diaphragm contracts the external intercostal muscles which run between the ribs also contract to expand the rib cage upwards and outwards. The walls of the lungs are then pulled outwards creating an increase in lung volume and a decrease in the internal pressure. This then causes air to be inhaled into the respiratory tract.

Once the air reaches the alveoli, exchange of the respiratory gases can occur. The linings of the alveoli contain minute capillaries. Diffusion of the gases takes place by diffusion across the thin capillary and alveolar walls. Thus oxygen is passed into the capillaries for supply to body tissues and carbon dioxide is passed from the capillaries to the alveoli to be expelled from the body during exhalation. It is estimated that each lung contains around 300,000,000 alveoli which provide an huge surface area for the rapid and effective exchange of gases to take place.

During expiration of air the process is reversed. Initially the intercostal muscles relax and the ribs move downwards, then the diaphragm also relaxes reducing the volume of the thoracic cavity. The elastic fibres around the alveoli and those in the alveolar ducts and the bronchioles then spring back reducing the lung volume and air is drawn outside the body.

The respiratory system

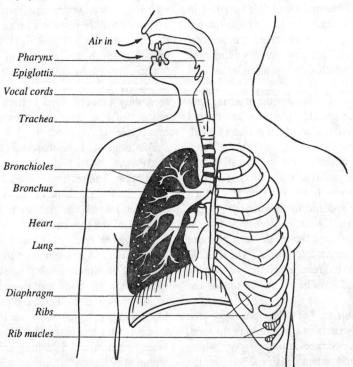

Air in
Pharynx
Epiglottis
Vocal cords
Trachea
Bronchioles
Bronchus
Heart
Lung
Diaphragm
Ribs
Rib mucles

The Digestive System

Before the nutrition in food can be used by the body it has to be broken down into molecules small enough to be transported by the blood and passed into the interstitial tissues and cells. This breakdown of food is achieved by digestion which involves both mechanical and chemical actions and takes place in a long canal which stretches from the mouth to the anus.

The mouth is involved with the mechanical and chemical breakdown of food. The teeth are bony structures embedded in the jawbone which break food down into smaller pieces through chewing, or mastication. Each tooth has three basic portions: the crown, the neck and the root. The crown is the visible part of the tooth and is covered in enamel which is the hardest substance in the body. Beneath the enamel is the dentine, a bony connective tissue which lends shape to the tooth. The pulp cavity which lies beneath the dentine contains blood vessels, nerves and lymphatic vessels which run downwards through the root of the tooth. The neck of the tooth forms the division between the crown and the root and is bordered by the gum. The root also consists of dentine covered by a bony substance called cementum which attaches to a ligament which is the anchor of the tooth.

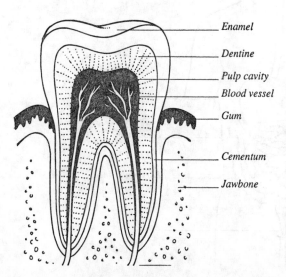

Enamel

Dentine

Pulp cavity

Blood vessel

Gum

Cementum

Jawbone

The first set of human teeth, the milk teeth, begin to break through the gum at around 6 months after birth and are gradually lost and replaced by the permanent set up to the age of 12. The permanent dental set consists of 32 teeth which consist of the following:

- eight incisors—for cutting food
- four canines—for tearing food
- eight premolars—for grinding food
- twelve molars—for grinding food (the third molars are also known as the wisdom teeth.

The tongue is a muscular organ anchored to the floor of the mouth which assists in the breakdown of food and which contains the taste buds.

While food is being chewed and broken into smaller pieces, it is also mixed with saliva which is continuously secreted into the mouth from the salivary glands. The amount of saliva secreted increases when food is in the mouth moistening and dissolving the food to facilitate swallowing and beginning the process of chemical breakdown. Water is the main constituent of saliva but it also contains a number of other substances including two digestive enzymes which begin the breakdown of starches.

Saliva is secreted via ducts from three main pairs of glands: the parotid glands, the submandibular glands and the sublingual glands. These glands continue to heavily secrete saliva for a while after food has been swallowed to wash out the mouth and dilute substances that may remain.

The Oesophagus

Once food leaves the mouth it is a soft substance which can be easily swallowed and passed into the pharynx and then into the oesophagus, the long, hollow, muscular tube that leads to the stomach.

The oesophagus measures approximately 25cm in length and descends through the thoracic cavity in to the abdomen. It functions only as pathway for food, pushing it onwards through persistent, involuntary muscular movements known as peristalsis. These wave-like movements involve the contraction and relaxation of circular muscles and are assisted by the secretion of mucous from the inner wall of the oesophagus which lubricates the food. Food takes a few seconds to pass through the oesophagus while fluids and soft foods take approximately one second.

Between the main portion of the oesophagus and the stomach there is a slight narrowing where a sphincter muscle is situated. The relaxation of this muscle enables food to be passed into the stomach.

The Stomach

The stomach is a large, curved sac-like organ, situated immediately below the diaphragm which consist of four main areas: the cardia, the fundus, the body and the pylorus. The layers of the stomach consist of an outer membrane, three different kinds of muscle fibre, a layer of tissue containing blood vessels and an inner mucosal layer that lies in folds when the stomach is empty but stretches to become smooth when full.

When the food enters the stomach it is stimulated into peristaltic movement and into the release of gastric juice from the gastric glands that lie in the mucous membrane. The gastric juice contains hydrochloric acid and digestive enzymes, which along with gentle peristaltic movements, further break up the food and turn it into a semi-liquid

mixture known as chyme. This process can take up to six hours depending on the amount and type of food eaten, for example carbohydrates will be broken up more quickly than proteins. Once the process is complete the chyme is emptied into the duodenum which forms the first portion of the small intestine.

The Intestines

Chemical digestion in the small intestine also involves secretions from three organs that actually lie outside the digestive tract: the pancreas, the liver and the gallbladder.

Once the chyme reaches the duodenum, it stimulates the mucous membrane to secrete the hormone secretin which is then transported via the circulation to the pancreas. The pancreas lies behind the outer curved section of the stomach and is joined to the duodenum by two ducts, the pancreatic duct (which joins the common bile duct from the liver and gallbladder) and the accessory duct. The pancreas is composed of small groups of glandular cells some of which are the islets of Langerhans which are involved in the endocrine function of insulin release. The majority of the cell groups produce a fluid which is a mixture of water, salts, sodium bicarbonate and enzymes which digest

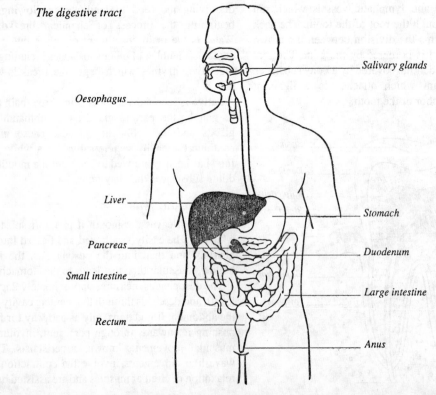

The digestive tract

Salivary glands

Oesophagus

Liver

Stomach

Pancreas

Duodenum

Small intestine

Large intestine

Rectum

Anus

triglyceride fats, proteins and carbohydrates. The pancreatic juice is conveyed to the small intestine by the two ducts.

The liver contributes to the digestive process with the production and secretion of bile which is a yellow-green fluid consisting of water, bile salts and bile pigments but no enzymes. Bile salts are active in the breakdown and absorption of the fat substance triglyceride. The liver secretes bile into the gallbladder which stores and concentrates the substance prior to releasing it into the small intestine through the common bile duct. The gallbladder secretes bile in response to stimulation from the hormone cholecystokinin which is secreted by the mucous membrane of the small intestine.

Intestinal juice secreted by the glands in the walls of the small intestine and the submucosal layer of the duodenum also contain digestive enzymes and mucous which helps to neutralize the gastric acid in chyme. Most digestion and absorption of nutrients is completed in the small intestine and the anatomy of the organ is entirely appropriate to this. This muscular tube comprises three portions: the duodenum which measures approximately 25 cm in length, the jejunum, measuring approximately 1 metre and the ileum which is approximately 2 metres in length and extends into the large intestine. The small intestine consists of the same four layers as the stomach but contain, small hair-like projections, known as villi, on the mucosal layers that increase the surface area available for digestion and absorption of nutrients. The villi has a central core which is served by an arteriole, a venule and a capillary network, through which nutrients are passed from the small intestine and into the blood or lymphatic fluid.

Chyme is passed through the small intestine in peristaltic movements but these are far more gentle that those of the upper part of the digestive tract and food tends to remain in the small intestine for a longer period. Chyme is passed on to the large intestine via the ileocaecal valve which is the junction between the ileum and the first portion of the large intestine, the caecum. At this stage the chyme is still a liquid substance but as it travels on from the caecum and through the long portion known as the colon, water and some vitamins are absorbed into the blood and the chyme becomes a more solid mass, faeces. The mucosal layer of the colon also secretes mucous to lubricate the faeces as it is pushed through in gentle peristaltic movements. Although no enzymes are secreted, bacteria that live in the colon convert proteins into amino acids and will produce flatus (wind) from the fermentation of carbohydrates.

The faeces is then passed into the rectum through the mass peristaltic movement which begins in the transverse portion of the colon in response to involuntary nerve impulses which are stimulated by arrival of food in the stomach. This reflex, known as the gastrocolic response, initiates the contraction of muscles along the intestinal tract which along with voluntary muscular contractions propel the faeces along. The final portion of the intestinal tract, the anus consists of an internal and external sphincter. The internal sphincter relaxes in response to involuntary muscular contraction and the external sphincter, the portion which opens on to the body surface, in response to voluntary muscular control. Once the external sphincter is relaxed the faeces is then expelled from the body.

The Urinary System

The organs of the urinary system are, like the liver and the lungs, concerned with the elimination of waste products that have been produced by the cells of the body during metabolic function.

The main function of the urinary system is in the control of the pressure, the composition and the volume of blood and is achieved by regulating the amount and the water/solute balance in the body. The structures that comprise the urinary system are the kidney, the ureters, the bladder and the urethra.

The Kidneys

The kidneys are the organs in which urine is produced from the waste products removed from the blood. Situated in the posterior abdominal wall, just above the waist and positioned either side of the vertebral column, the adult kidney measures approximately 10–12cm in length. It is kept in position by a mass of connective and adipose tissue. Near the centre of the each kidney is an area called the hilus via which the renal artery and nerve supply enter and the renal vein and ureter exit.

The kidney is encased within a capsule of transparent, fibrous membrane which acts as a protective coat against injury and infection. Beneath the renal capsule is the cortex and then the renal medulla within which there are a number of cone-shaped structures known as the medullary pyramids. These narrow at the apex where they meet the calyces. The region of the kidney that comprises the cortex and the medullary pyramids is called the parenchyma within which there are the microscopic, functional structures known as the nephrons. There are approximately 1,000,000 nephrons in each kidney.

The calyces are part of the renal pelvis through which urine is collected from the ducts of the pyramids and drained into the ureter.

Blood enters the kidney via the renal artery which then branches into smaller arterioles from which the afferent arteriole enters the glomerulus, a microscopic capillary bundle which sits within a cup like structure known as the Bowman's capsule. The glomerular walls are very thin and as blood flows

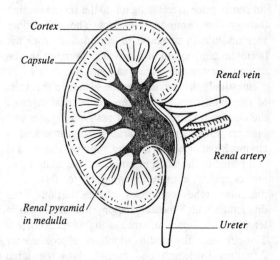

through them water and solutes pass into the capsular space. The blood then flows out through the efferent arteriole. The fluid in the capsular space then passes into the renal tubule which is divided into several areas and on through a series of collecting ducts. This enables the waste products to be removed from the blood and eventually secreted into the ureter and other blood constituents, for example plasma proteins, to be reabsorbed.

The bladder

Once the urine has been drained into the ureters it is carried into the bladder. The ureters are approximately 2530 cm in length and enter the bladder via two openings. When the bladder fills with urine the pressure within the bladder constricts these openings and so prevents the backflow of urine into the ureters and back to the kidneys.

The walls of the ureters are composed of three layers, the outer layer connects with connective tissue to maintain the position of the structures and is supplied with lymphatic and blood vessels and nerves. The middle layer is muscular and its function is to contract to conduct the urine to the bladder, a movement known as peristalsis. The inner layer is a mucous membrane composed of three different types of cells. Mucous secreted by this layer prevents the urine from coming into contact with the cells of the walls.

The bladder is a hollow, muscular, sac-like organ which, when empty, sits in the pelvic cavity, rising into the abdominal cavity when full. The layers of the bladder walls are composed of muscular tissue and an inner layer of mucosal membrane composed of cells that are able to stretch in response to the continuous need to accommodate for volumes of fluid. The bladder opens out into the urethra via the internal and external sphincters which are muscular.

The bladder empties (a process known as micturition) in response to nerve impulses that are stimulated by receptors in the wall of the bladder. Once the bladder is 25–50 per cent full these receptors send an impulse to the brain via sensory pathways which results in the conscious desire to pass urine. A nerve centre situated in the spinal column then transmit impulses to the internal and external sphincters and the and the bladder wall into muscular action which then expels urine from the bladder.

The urine is expelled from the bladder into the urethra, a tube which leads from the floor of the bladder to the orifice on the surface of the body.

The anatomy of the urethra differs greatly between men and women. In women it is very short (approximately 4cm in length) and leads to an opening in the vulva which lies in front of the vaginal opening. The male urethra is approximately 18–20cm in length and passes through the penis. The urethra is also the pathway for sperm and is, therefore a structure of the both the urinary and reproductive systems. Various ducts deliver sperm into the urethra from the male reproductive organs and glands for ejaculation during sexual intercourse.

The urinary system

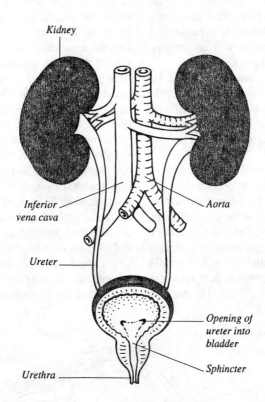

Kidney

Inferior vena cava

Aorta

Ureter

Opening of ureter into bladder

Sphincter

Urethra

The Senses

Vision

The organ of visual sense is the eye, a highly complex organ situated in the skull, in a socket known as the orbit.

The accessory structures to the eye include the eyelids, eyelashes and eyebrows, the extrinsic eye muscles and the lacrimal apparatus. The eyelids protect the eyeball from excessive light, foreign bodies and during sleep, and also lubricate the eyeballs by spreading the secretions over the surface. The lacrimal apparatus is the collective term used for a number of structures that are involved in the production of the fluid commonly known as tears. The fluid itself is a mixture of mucous, a watery-salty solution and an enzyme which cleans and lubricates the eyeball.

The extrinsic eye muscles comprise six muscles that are responsible for the movement of the eyeball, each muscle controlling movement for a different direction. These movements are coordinated by three cranial nerves which originate in the brainstem and the cerebellum.

The eyeball is mostly contained within the orbit of the skull, with only the front portion actually exposed. It is covered by the strong protective sclera, which forms the white of the eye and gives the eye shape and protection. The front portion of the eye is covered by the transparent cornea through which the iris and the pupil can be seen. The middle layer of the eye is the uvea, which comprises the choroid, the ciliary body and the iris. The choroid has a dense supply of blood vessels and lines the sclera and the back of the eye, supplying nutrients to the retina. The ciliary body, which lie at the front of the eye, consist of the ciliary processes, which secrete aqueous humour, and the ciliary muscle which alters the shape of the lens to focus on near or far objects. The iris is the third portion of the uvea which gives the eyeball its colour and is composed of muscle fibres. It is attached to the ciliary processes and lies between the cornea and the lens. The main function of the iris is in controlling the amount of light which enters the eye through the pupil, the hole in its centre. For example, when a bright light is shined directly onto an eye, the circular muscles of the iris constrict to reduce the size of the pupil, thereby reducing the amount of light passing through it. In poor light, however, the radial muscles contract and enlarge the dilate the pupil, increasing the amount of light passing through.

The inner coat of the eye is the retina, the light-sensitive structure which consists of nervous tissue and pigment cells. The function of the pigment cells is to absorb stray light which ensures that the image transmitted by light remains sharp and clear, instead of scattered and indistinct. The nervous tissue contains the neurons which process the visual image and transmit the image to the brain. There are three layers of these neurons, including the photoreceptor layer which contains the rods and cones. Rods are specialized for processing black and white vision

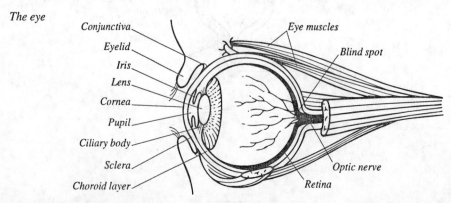

The eye

Conjunctiva
Eyelid
Iris
Lens
Cornea
Pupil
Ciliary body
Sclera
Choroid layer

Eye muscles
Blind spot
Optic nerve
Retina

data in dim light, and cones for processing colour data in bright light.

The optic disc lies on the front surface of the retina and it is through this that the optic nerve, and the retinal blood vessels enter and exit. The optic disc interrupts the layer of nervous tissue and so becomes a blind spot which cannot process any visual data.

The structure of the eye concerned with focusing is the lens which lies just behind the iris and the pupil. The lens can change shape, under the influence of the ciliary muscle, to focus on near or far objects by bending the rays of light that pass through it.

The lens is also the structure which divides the interior of the eyeball into two cavities; the anterior chamber and the posterior chamber. The anterior chamber contains the aqueous humour which helps to maintain the shape of the eye and to nourish the cornea and the lens. The posterior chamber is filled with the jelly-like vitreous humour which also helps to maintain the shape of the eyeball and hold the retina in place against the choroid layer.

Hearing and Balance

The organ which is the receptor for auditory stimuli and the maintenance of equilibrium is the ear.

The ear has three main regions: the external ear, the middle ear and the internal ear. The external ear comprises three structures: pinna, the external auditory canal and the tympanic membrane. The pinna is the part which lies on the outside of the head and is composed of elastic cartilage and covered with skin. The external auditory canal, which is a tube about 2.5 cm in length, leads to the tympanic membrane, which separates the external ear from the middle ear. The canal also contains a few hairs and sebaceous glands near the opening to the pinna. These glands produce a substance called cerumen (more commonly known as earwax) which along with the hairs prevents dust and other particles from entering the ear.

The tympanic membrane (or eardrum) is semi-transparent and composed of several types of connective tissue. When sound waves collected by the pinna and the external auditory canal reach the tympanic membrane it vibrates and these vibrations are passed on to the middle ear.

The middle ear, also known as the tympanic cavity, lies in the temporal bone and is lined by mucous membrane. The structures contained within the middle ear are the Eustachian tube, the ossicles, the oval window and the round window. The Eustachian tube lies on the floor of the middle ear and opens into the pharynx when swallowing and yawning occur. This enables air in the Eustachian tube to be renewed so that the air pressure is kept constant with atmospheric pressure. This equalizes the pressure either side of the tympanic membrane so that it can vibrate effectively when hit by sound waves. The ossicles extend across the middle ear and are attached to the walls by ligaments. The ossicles are three tiny bones called the malleus, incus and stapes (or more commonly known as the hammer, anvil and stirrup because of their distinctive shapes). The ossicles are connected to one another by joints and the malleus is connected to the tympanic membrane. When the tympanic membrane vibrates the vibrations are passed on to the ossicles, first the malleus, then the incus and finally the stapes, which is attached to the membrane of the oval window. The round window lies directly below the oval window and is covered by the secondary tympanic membrane; both windows open into the inner ear.

Also known as the labyrinth, the inner ear consists of the cochlea and semi-circular canals. The cochlea

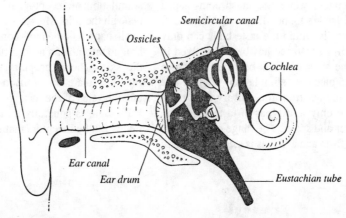

The ear

Ossicles

Semicircular canal

Cochlea

Ear canal

Ear drum

Eustachian tube

is a bony, spiral-shaped tube which contains three channels separated by two types of membrane. The organ of hearing, known as the organ of Corti, rests on one of these membranes and consists of the cells and neurones of the auditory nerve. Once the sound vibrations have reached the oval window they are transferred to the cochlea as pressure waves. A series of complex responses take place within the structures of the cochlea resulting in the stimulation of the cells in the organ of Corti, which in turn generate nerve impulses which then transmit the sound to the brain.

The semicircular canals contain the receptors for equilibrium. The canals sit at right angles to one another and bulge at one end to form three ampulla which contain sensory cells, some of which are connected to nerve fibres. Fluid within the semicircular canals moves in response to movements of the head stimulating the sensory cells to send impulses to the brain. Balance is maintained by the position of the semicircular canals and the differing speeds at which the fluid moves in response to particular movements.

Taste

The sense of taste is referred to as gustatory, relying on the chemical breakdown of a substance. The taste buds contain the receptors for taste and are situated mainly in the tongue and to a much lesser extent in the soft palate of the mouth, the pharynx and the larynx.

On the tongue a collection of sensory and supporting cells are formed into oval bodies, the taste buds, which are situated in the walls of papillae (small projections) on the mucous membrane that covers the tongue. There are three types of papillae— fungiform and circumvallate, which contain most of the taste buds, and filiform which is primarily concerned with tactile responses. Circumvallate papillae are the largest type and are situated at the back of the tongue, while the mushroom-shaped fungiform papillae are found all over the surface.

The sensory cells within the taste buds can only perceive taste if a substance has been dissolved in saliva. Once the substance has been broken down into smaller molecules stimulation of hair-like structures that project from the sensory cells takes place. There are only four types of taste sensation: sour, salty, bitter and sweet. The range of tastes that we experience from actual foods is a combination of these primary sensations working in conjunction with olfactory stimuli.

The tongue can be divided into 'taste zones' areas which react particularly strongly to the primary taste sensations. The tip of the tongue is sensitive to sweet and salty substances, the back to bitter substances, and the sides to sour. Taste impulses are conducted from the nerve fibres in the buds along three of the cranial nerves to various parts of the brain to interpret conscious discernment of taste.

Smell

The sense of smell, or olfactory sense, is also a chemical sense, relying on the interaction of molecules with receptor cells which are situated in the upper part of the nasal cavity. Olfactory receptors are neurones that are replaced approximately every 30 days. The olfactory hairs project from the end of the neurones and act as conductors. The Bowman's gland, situated in the connective tissue, secretes mucus through ducts to the surface of the olfactory epithelium, dissolving the odour molecules. The olfactory receptors run into the olfactory nerves to the olfactory bulbs which are situated in the brain.

Although the sense of smell in a human is relatively weak in comparison to that of other animals, the olfactory impulses are passed on to the area of the forebrain which deals with emotion. This explains why certain smells can elicit memories or specific reactions, such as nausea in the case of smelling a substance with which you associate having been ill.

Cutaneous

The receptors of the skin are concerned with the two types of cutaneous sensation: tactile sensations concerned with touch, pressure and vibration and thermal sensation concerned with temperature.

Touch sensations are generated from the stimulation of receptors in the skin or the tissues beneath the skin. Meissner's corpuscles are found as oval-shaped bodies of connective tissue situated around the end of a nerve fibre in the dermal layer of the skin. These receptors transmit impulses very rapidly and are numerous in the fingertips, the palns and the soles of the feet.

Pressure is generally a more sustained sensation that is felt by receptors that lie in deeper tissue.

The Reproductive System

The reproductive system consists of organs and supporting structure which produce, release and transport reproductive cells (gametes) and hormones by which the creation of new life and the passing on of genetic material is made possible.

The Male Reproductive System

The male reproductive system consists of the testes, the accessory ducts, the accessory sex glands and the supporting structures, such as the penis.

The two testicles lie within the scrotum, a sac of loose skin, divided internally into two cavities by a septum; each of these sacs contains a testicle. The testes are oval-shaped glands, each measuring approximately 5cm in length. During embryo development the testes are formed in the abdominal wall and descend to their position in the scrotum (via the inguinal canals) during the seventh month of foetal development. The testes are composed of minute tubules known as the seminal tubules which are supported by connective tissue. The seminal tubules are divided into compartments which unite into tubules and ducts before joining up with the convoluted epididymis, which runs into the vas deferens. It is in the seminal tubules that the formation and development of sperm occurs, by a process known as spermatogenesis. Sperm have several stages of development with the more mature sperm situated near the lumen of the tubules. Once the sperm leave the seminal tubules they move into the straight tubules and from there into the vasa efferentia which open into the epididymis. During the passage through the convoluted epididymis the sperm undergo a further stage of maturation which lasts for 10–14 days. The sperm are also propelled towards the vas deferens through the contractions of the smooth muscle layer of the epididymis.

The vas deferens is one of the accessory organs of the male reproductive system. It is a muscular tube, measuring approximately 45cm in length, which leads from the epididymis into the urethra. The vas deferens stores sperm and conveys it from the epididymis to the ejaculatory duct through peristaltic movements of the muscular walls. The ejaculatory duct is formed by the vas deferens and the ducts of the seminal vesicles, which secrete substances that promote the viability and motility of the semen.

The ejaculatory ducts eject sperm into the urethra, a tube which measures 20cm in length and serves as the terminal duct of the male reproductive and urinary systems. The urethra consists of three

The male reproductive system

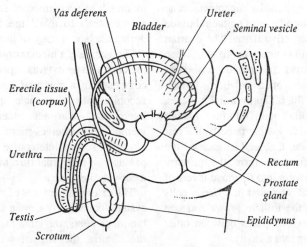

621

portions: the prostatic urethra, the membranous urethra and the penile urethra. The prostatic urethra passes through the prostate gland, a walnut-sized gland which, through ducts, secretes fluid which increases the viability of the sperm. Below the prostate gland lie the Cowper's glands, two pea-sized glands whic secrete alkaline and lubricating substances that protect the sperm in the environment of the urethra.

The prostatic urethra opens into the short membranous section and then into the penile urethra, which extends through the penis for approximately 15–20cm opening into the external urethral orifice at the base of the penis.

The ejaculation of semen (the composition of sperm and the substances secreted by the accessory glands) occurs in response to stimulation from sensory nerves. During sexual arousal, which occurs most commonly as the result of tactile or visual stimulation, the spongy tissue which makes up the penis becomes engorged with blood, which produces the stiffening of the tissue known as erection. The rhythmic movement of the penis then results in the response known as orgasm which results in the ejaculation of semen from the urethra to the exterior of the body. Part of this reflex also involves the constriction of the sphincter at the base of the bladder which prevents urine from passing into the urethra during the propulsion of semen.

The Female Reproductive System

The organs of the female reproductive system consist of the ovaries, the Fallopian tubes, the uterus, the vagina and the external structures of the vulva. The mammary glands are also regarded as specialized organs of the female reproductive system.

The ovaries are the two glands, the size and shape of almonds, situated in the upper part of the pelvic cavity and held in position by ligaments. The ovaries are surrounded by a layer of epithelial tissue which gives way to connective tissue. The ovarian follicles lie within the connective tissue, these consist of immature ova in various states of development. The ovary of a newborn female contains approximately 70, 000 primordial follicles, of which around 500 will develop into fully mature ova and will be released following puberty, the rest will gradually degenerate. One cell in each of the primordial follicles grows to form the primary oocyte while the others form into flattened layers of specialized cells which surround it. These cells change in structure as the follicle grows and one layer secretes fluid into the spaces between other cells, eventually forming into a cavity.

With the onset of puberty, hormones secreted by the pituitary gland further mature the ovum. At this stage the primary oocyte divides twice to produce a ripe ovum and two polar bodies which disintegrate. The follicle has, by this stage, developed into a large, fluid-filled body (known as the Graafian follicle) which moves toward the surface of the ovary. The follicle then ruptures through the surface of the ovary in a process known as ovulation.

The mature ova are swept into the Fallopian tubes which extend laterally from the uterus (one tube lying on either side). The tubes measure approximately 10cm in length, opening out into funnel-shaped portions (the infundibulum) which lie near the ovaries. The infundibulum extend into small projections, called the fimbriae, which move to create currents, sweeping the ovum into the tubes. The ovum then moves through the portion known as the ampulla (the area in which, if it occurs, fertilization of the ovum by the male sperm usually takes place) and then further into the Fallopian tube.

The Fallopian tubes extend into the uterus, a pear-shaped, muscular organ, situated between the bladder and the rectum. The lower portion of the uterus connects with the cervix which opens into the vagina. The uterus is the organ in which implantation of a fertilized ovum and foetal development take place. The mucous membrane lining of the uterus, the endometrium, changes in structure throughout the menstrual cycle in response to hormones and chemicals released by the hypothalamus, the pituitary gland and the ovaries. Prior to ovulation the endometrium becomes thicker, with an increased blood supply, in preparation for receiving a fertilized ovum. If there is no fertilized egg then the endometrium breaks down and is shed during menstruation.

The muscular walls of the endometrium are able to stretch to accommodate foetal development and also contract to expel the foetus from the body during the labour stage of pregnancy.

The vagina is a tubular organ which extends from the cervix to an external opening in the vulva. It is composed of a muscular layer, that can stretch to accommodate the male penis during sexual intercourse, and an inner layer of mucous membrane. It receives sperm during the ejaculatory phase of sexual intercourse and also serves as a passage for menstrual flow and for the expulsion of a baby during labour.

The external structures of the female reproductive system, collectively known as the vulva, consist of the mons pubis, the labia majora and labia minora, the clitoris, the vaginal orifice and the external urethral orifice. The mons pubis consists of a pad of fatty tissue lying under the skin which protects the pubic symphisis of the pelvic girdle. The labia majora are two long folds of skin which extend along the length of the vulva; these guard the vaginal and urethral openings along with the labia minora, two smaller folds of skin which lie beside the labia majora.

The clitoris, a small body of erectile tissue which enlarges and hardens during sexual stimulation, is situated at the head of the labia minora, just above the urethral opening. Lying below the urethral opening is the vaginal orifice, the external opening of the vagina. Either side of this lie the Bartholin's glands which produce a mucous secretion which aids lubrication during sexual intercourse.

The female reproductive system

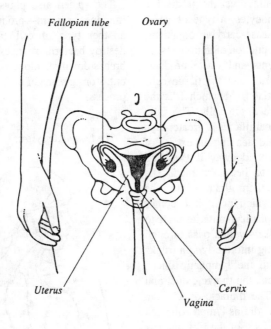

Fallopian tube   Ovary

Uterus   Cervix   Vagina

The Lymphatic System

The lymphatic system describes the vessels, organs and structures involved in carrying out the immune responses of the body. This involves the production and conveyance of lymphocytes, a type of white blood cell, which fight disease-carrying organisms in the body through the production of antibodies.

The exchange of nutrients and waste products between the blood capillaries and the tissue cells takes place in the interstitial fluid which fills the minute spaces between the tissue cells. The fluid which permeates from the capillaries is greater than the volume that is absorbed, leaving an excess of fluid which has to be drained away if the fluid balance in the tissues is to be maintained. The excess interstitial fluid then drains into the lymphatic capillaries (at which point it becomes known as lymph). The lymphatic capillaries unite to form the larger lymph vessels which pass through lymph glands before running into the lymph trunks which pass the lymph into the lymphatic ducts. There are two of these ducts, the thoracic duct and the right lymphatic duct. The thoracic duct is the larger of these channels and drains lymph collected from the tissues below the base of the ribs, the left upper extremities and the left side of the chest, neck and head. The right lymphatic duct drains lymph from the right upper extremities and the right side of the chest, neck and head.

Movement of lymph along the capillaries, vessels and trunks is facilitated by the contractions of the skeletal muscles and by respiratory movement.

The lymph glands are small oval structures found along the network of lymph vessels. They vary in size and number depending upon their position in the body; the lymph glands at the armpits and groin, for example, are grouped. The lymph glands have two basic functions: the production of lymphocytes and the removal of bacteria from the lymph. In this way pathogens which are present in the body are destroyed by lymphocytes and macrophages, which are also found in lymph glands.

The spleen also plays an important role in the immune system—producing lymphocytes and another type of cell called a phagocyte, which destroy bacteria by ingesting them. The spleen also breaks down red blood cells that have become worn out, storing some of the iron and haemoglobin in the process.

The lymphatic system

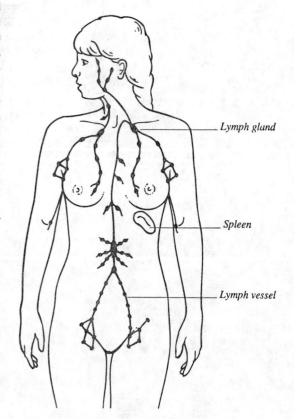

Lymph gland

Spleen

Lymph vessel

The Endocrine System

The endocrine glands are those that secrete hormones into the space outside the body cells (extracellular space) to be passed into the blood capillaries and carried around the body by the bloodstream. They are, therefore, also known as the ductless glands because the other glands of the body secrete their products via ducts onto a free surface, for example the sweat glands and the digestive glands.

The Pituitary Gland

Often referred to as the master gland because it produces hormones which influence other endocrine glands, the pituitary gland is found at the base of the brain. The hormones produced by the pituitary gland include the growth hormone, which regulates growth, and the thyroid stimulating hormone, which controls the secretion of hormones by the thyroid gland. Other hormones are involved with the maintenance of the fluid balance in the body by the regulation of the amount of urine produced by the kidneys, and the stimulation of the production of hormones in both male and female sex glands.

The Thyroid Gland

The thyroid gland is situated in the neck, in front of the trachea (windpipe). This gland produces thyroxin which regulates the metabolism, the chemical processes by which growth, healing, repair and replacement of body tissues occur. A deficiency in the production of this hormone can, in childhood, result in a retardation of both mental and physical development. In adults it can cause myxoedema, a condition in which the individual becomes overweight and experiences extreme fatigue and weakness and mental sluggishness. If the thyroid gland produces too much thyroxin this can cause hyperactivity and profound weight loss.

The Parathyroid Glands

The four parathyroid glands lie on either side of the thyroid gland (one pair on each side). These glands produce a hormone which regulates the amount of calcium which circulates in the bloodstream and is laid down in bone. Calcium is a vital mineral component of bone tissue and an imbalance in the amount of calcium in the bone and the blood can lead to tetany or to a weakening of the bones.

The Adrenal Glands

Also known as the suprarenal glands, each adrenal gland lies just at the top of each kidney and consists of two portions, the cortex and the medulla. The cortex produces mineralocorticoid hormones, which regulates the amount of minerals circulating in the bloodstream, particularly potassium and sodium which are essential in maintaining the correct fluid balance in the body. It also produces glucocorticoid hormones which influence the metabolism of glucose.

The medulla produces adrenaline which stimulates the so-called 'fight or flight' response in the autonomic nervous system. At times of stress or when an individual experiences fear or emotional anger, this hormone is released through the nervous system, causing a quickening in the rate of heartbeat and breathing, thereby increasing the amount of oxygen and glucose supplied to the tissues of the body. This, in effect, prepares the body for the potential physical demands of a situation, for example, running away from danger.

The Pancreas

The pancreas has two basic functions: the secretion of pancreatic juice which assists in the chemical digestion of food and the production of the hormone insulin which controls the level of glucose in the blood and converts glucose into glycogen. When carbohydrates are broken down by the digestive process, glucose is formed, providing energy for the body cells. Any excess glucose is then converted by insulin into glycogen which can be stored in the liver and the muscles for future use. If an insufficient amount of insulin is produced then the excess glucose cannot be converted in this way, giving rise to the condition known as diabetes mellitus.

The Testes

The testes are part of the male reproductive system which, under the influence of a hormone produced by the pituitary gland, produce testosterone. This hormone controls the development of the male sex organs and the development of the secondary sexual characteristics at puberty, for example, the growth and distribution of body hair, the deepening of the voice and the enlargement of the penis and testes. Testosterone also influences sexual behaviour and the maturation of sperm, which are formed in the testes.

The Ovaries

The ovaries are part of the female reproductive system, the organs which produce the female egg cells, or ova. The ovaries also secrete the hormones oestrogen and progesterone, under the influence from the gonadotrophic hormones secreted by the pituitary gland. Oestrogen controls the development of the female reproductive system and the secondary sexual characteristics, for example, the development of the breasts, the distribution of body hair and change in body shape. Along with progesterone, oestrogen also controls the reproductive cycle, each month preparing the endometrial lining of the uterus for the implantation of a fertilized ovum—a process known as the menstrual cycle.

The female endocrine system

The male endocrine system

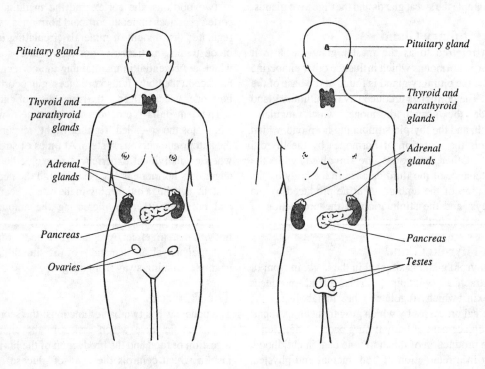

Pituitary gland

Thyroid and parathyroid glands

Adrenal glands

Pancreas

Ovaries

Pituitary gland

Thyroid and parathyroid glands

Adrenal glands

Pancreas

Testes

The Nervous System

The highly complex system which coordinates and controls the functions is the nervous system. It is divided into two parts: the central nervous and the peripheral nervous system. Some of the functions of the nervous system are under conscious control, others, such as digestion, are involuntary.

The Central Nervous System

The central nervous system consists of the brain and the spinal cord. The brain is the control centre of the body, regulating the functions of the organs as well as being the centre of conscious thought, feeling and memory.

The largest area of the brain is the cortex, which consists of nerve cell bodies known as white and grey matter. It is the cortex which receives messages from the sense organs and which directs voluntary movement, for example, it will send impulses to the muscles of the arm and hand to reach out and pick up an object. It is also responsible for speech, learning and intelligence, emotion and personality.

The cerebellum is the centre for the controlling the coordination of the movements of muscles and the balance of the body. Initially impulses controlling the coordination of a particular movement will be initiated in the cortex of the brain, which is connected to the cerebellum by connecting fibres. However, if the movement is learned and repeated frequently, the cerebellum and muscles will work independently of the cortex.

The brain stem lies at the base of the brain, just above the first portion of the spinal cord; it consists of three areas, the medulla oblongata, the pons and the midbrain. The medulla oblongata, part of the autonomic nervous system, is the site of the respiratory and cardiovascular centres, controlling the basic rhythm of breathing and the rate and the force at which the heart beats. The reflexes of swallowing, coughing and sneezing are also controlled from centres in this part of the brain. The pons which lies above the medulla oblongata forms a kind of junction between the brain and the spinal column, relaying impulses to the motor and sensory centres of the brain. The midbrain, which forms the latter-most portion of the brainstem, responds to certain visual stimuli by conveying impulses which control appropriate responsive movements in the eyes, the head and the neck.

The spinal cord is a mass of nervous tissue, which runs through the vertebrae of the spinal column

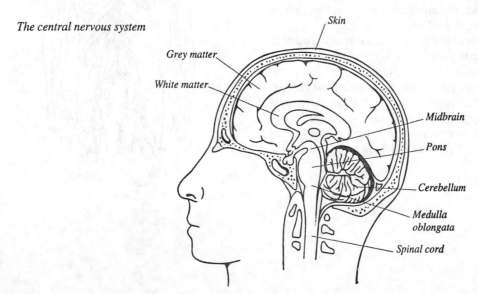

The central nervous system

Skin

Grey matter

White matter

Midbrain

Pons

Cerebellum

Medulla oblongata

Spinal cord

(backbone). There are 31 pairs of spinal nerves which extend laterally from the spinal cord which divide into branches, extending to the muscles and skin, and to the organs of the body.

To a greater extent the spinal cord controls most of the reflex actions of the body. These are automatic responses to particular stimuli, for example, removing the fingers from an object of extreme heat. In this type of response the message, which begins at the sensory receptor nerve cells in the skin, will travel to the spinal cord. The message is then relayed back from the spinal cord along motor nerve cells to the appropriate muscles to respond in a particular way. In the case of fingers on a hot plate the muscles of arm and fingers will contract to produce a jerking movement away from the object. Reflex action is usually involuntary because the whole response occurs without the involvement of the nerve cells in the cortex of the brain.

Other movements are coordinated in the brain under voluntary control, with the impulse travelling down the spinal cord and transmitted to the relevant muscles.

The spinal cord also serves as the pathway for the autonomic nervous system—controlling the functions of the body which are not under conscious control. Impulses originating in the autonomic centres of the brain, travel down the spinal cord and along the spinal nerves.

The Peripheral Nervous System

The peripheral nervous sytem describes the nerves which link the central nervous system to other parts of the body. It comprises the autonomic nervous system and the somatic nervous sytem, which supplies the skeletal muscles and skin.

A nerve is a bundle of fibres composed of neurons and supporting connective nervous tissue, covered by a fibrous sheath. Neurons are the vital transmission components of the peripheral nervous system, able to carry impulses from the central nervous system to the muscles and organs, and capable of converting sensory and motor stimuli into electrical impulses to be sent to the brain.

Each neuron has a nucleus cell body surrounded by short fibres, called dendrites, which receive electrical impulses. A longer fibre, known as an axon, then conducts the message onwards to its terminal portion. Many axons are insulated by a coating called the myelin sheath, which ensures that conduction occurs as quickly as possible. Once the impulse reaches the axon endings, conduction of the impulse to the next neuron is made across a gap, known as a synapse. The axon endings contain a chemical known as a neurotransmitter which is released when the impulse reaches them; this enables the impulse to pass across the synapse and on to the next neurone until the terminal neuron is reached.

There a millions of neurons in the body which enable the impulses to be passed very rapidly and across many different routes, so that the initial message from the brain is activated almost immediately.

Parts of the nervous system

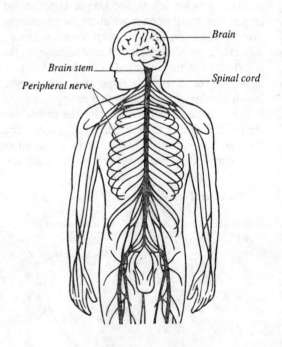

Brain

Brain stem

Spinal cord

Peripheral nerve

Guide to First Aid

At the Scene of the Emergency

Before dealing with any patient in need of first aid, it is important to check that you will not actually exacerbate the situation or put yourself at risk. It is vital that you send for specialist help as soon as possible—for this you may be able to use bystanders after instructing them clearly which emergency services you require. You may need to be aware of the safety implications of dealing with a patient in conditions such as heavy traffic or fire, circumstances which will always require increased levels of calm and concentration. You must never be afraid to admit your limitations as a first-aider, and should always be prepared to make way for professionals.

Identifying the Problem: Diagnosis

It can be exceedingly difficult even for doctors to make a diagnosis at times of emergency, without the support of hospital testing facilities. Often it will be impossible for the first-aider to obtain a reliable history from the patient if he or she is unconscious or severely shocked. However, if the first-aider is confident that he can identify life-threatening conditions in the first instance then detailed history-taking is of secondary importance. However, where a patient is unable to give details of events leading up to an accident or emergency, then this information should be sought from any relations or bystanders who might be able to provide useful information. Wherever possible, the first-aider should try to ascertain the patient's name and age and whether or not he has any significant medical problems or is currently taking any medication for a specific condition.

Bites and Stings

When an insect, such as a bee, a wasp or a hornet, stings it injects a tiny amount of venom beneath the skin, causing localized swelling and redness. Although painful, insect stings are rarely serious and the symptoms will begin to subside after 3–4 hours. However, stings can be dangerous, even fatal, if the individual is allergic to the venom or if he has suffered multiple stings. In this case it is essential that the victim receives medical attention immediately.

Insect stings

1 Only honey bees will actually leave their sting embedded in the skin. If the sting is visible, then carefully remove it with the edge of a knife or fingernail. Do not squeeze the sting as this will release more venom.

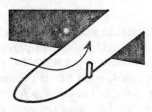

2 Wash the sting site with soap and water and apply ice wrapped in cloth or a cold compress to the area for up to 30 minutes to reduce the swelling.

Allergic reaction to an insect sting

1 Swelling around the face or on other parts of the body.
2 Difficulty with breathing and swallowing.
3 Weakness and dizziness.
4 Nausea and stomach cramps.
5 Unconsciousness.

To treat an allergic reaction

1 Lie the casualty still and ensure that the stung limb is lower than the level of his heart.
2 Seek emergency medical help immediately.

Animal bites

Bites which have been caused by an animal or a human should always be referred for medical examination because there is a risk that bacteria on teeth and in saliva will lead to infection.

Bleeding can be quite severe depending upon the type and number of bites, and the first-aider's initial aim should be to control the bleeding.

Treatment for a superficial wound

1 If bleeding is not severe then wash the wound thoroughly with soap and water to try to remove some of the possible contamination.
2 Control bleeding by applying a sterile dressing or a clean pad and pressing it firmly against the wound.
3 When bleeding has ceased, cover the wound with a fresh dressing held in place with adhesive tape or bandaging.
4 Seek medical examination of the wound.

Do not apply any medicated ointment to the wound.

Treatment for a severe wound

1 Arrange for the prompt removal of the casualty to hospital.
2 Control serious bleeding by applying direct pressure to the wound(s).
3 Cover the wound with a sterile dressing or a pad of clean cloth.
4 Observe the casualty for signs of shock.

Bleeding

Blood is the medium in which oxygen is carried to all the living tissues of the body, therefore the loss of any great quantity of blood represents a threat to life itself and should always be treated as a medical emergency. The body has a very sophisticated clotting mechanism which can seal up small lesions quickly and efficiently. Furthermore, a healthy adult may suffer no ill effects after a loss of 850 ml or 1 $\frac{1}{2}$ pints. The difficulty in an emergency situation is that it is often impossible to assess the volume of blood loss accurately. It is therefore advisable for the first-aider to take prompt action to stop bleeding wherever possible.

The type of bleeding suffered by a patient will be dependent upon the type of wound sustained. An open wound is one in which there is a visible break in the skin, whereas a closed wound causes the escape of blood from the circulation in to the tissues. The first kind of bleeding is known as **external** bleeding, and the second is known as **internal** bleeding.

Emergency action for bleeding

Wherever possible, try to be aware of your own safety. If you have any open wounds, try to ensure that there is a barrier between yourself and the casualty's wound prior to dealing with bleeding.

1 Locate and examine the wound for foreign bodies such as glass. Remove any clothing obstructing your access to the wound. If the wound appears to be free of glass etc., apply pressure directly onto the wound. If the wound is long, or there is a foreign body protruding from it, press down firmly on either side of the wound whilst trying to keep the edges as close together as possible. Applying pressure will be easier if you can use a clean pad of material or sterile dressing, but this is not essential and it is important not to waste time searching for one.
2 Elevate the affected part above the level of the patient's heart—you may find it easier to lie the patient down. **Do not** handle a limb you suspect may be fractured other than attempting to stop bleeding.

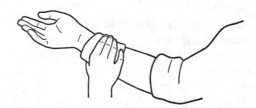

3 Continue to apply pressure for at least 10 minutes. If your original pad or dressing has become saturated, do not attempt to remove it. If possible wrap more bandages round it firmly, but not so tightly as to obstruct circulation. Scarves, clean sheets and handkerchiefs etc., will make suitable substitutes for bandages.

If the wound contains a foreign body:

1 Make no attempt to pull out the foreign body as this could exacerbate bleeding and shock—it may be acting as a partial 'plug'. However, if it appears loose, it may be possible to flush it out under running water, but do not waste too much time attempting this.
2 Elevate the limb and apply pressure on the edges of the wound. If you have access to sterile gauze pads or any other suitable material, try to build up a platform or ring around the base of the protruding object until it is higher than the object itself. (Leave the object exposed until this is achieved.)

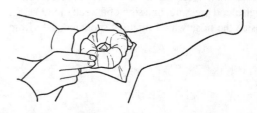

3 Bandage firmly on either side of the wound, but avoiding the wound and embedded object.
4 Cover the wound loosely with sterile dressings or clean material, elevate the limb and **seek medical help immediately**.

Remember—your priorities are:

1 To control bleeding and prevent shock (*see* p.659).
2 To prevent or minimize infection.
3 To secure medical help for your patient as quickly as possible.

If despite your best efforts the patient begins to display symptoms of shock, then treat as follows:

1 Identify and treat the cause of shock if possible.
2 Lay the patient flat on the floor as comfortably as possible.
3 Elevate his legs above head height (unless you suspect a fracture).
4 Loosen or remove any restrictive articles of clothing.
5 Keep the patient warm by covering with blankets, rugs or coats, but do not apply a direct heat source such as a hot water bottle.
6 Keep a check on the patient's vital signs—pulse and respira-tion, and his level of consciousness. Be ready to resus-citate if necessary (*see* ABC of Resuscitation on p.649).

Internal bleeding

Internal bleeding may result from injury such as bone fracture or severe bruising, but it can also occur spontaneously as a result of stomach ulcer or vaginal bleeding or several other medical emergencies. In the absence of any visible blood, the diagnosis is often a hard one to make, but signs and symptoms of shock (*see* p.659) will emerge if internal bleeding is significant. Sometimes there will be blood present at body orifices, and there may be bruising. Always treat for shock and summon medical help immediately.

Nosebleeds

Nosebleeds are rarely serious and most commonly occur either after a blow to the nose, during an infection such as the common cold, or as a consequence of picking or blowing the nose. Occasionally, frequent nosebleeds may be a result of high blood pressure, or a sign of a weak blood vessel inside the nose which ruptures spontaneously from time to time. Normally, nosebleeds are simply inconvenient and unpleasant, but occasionally they can be dangerous if bleeding is prolonged as the casualty can suffer considerable blood loss perhaps resulting in shock. If the blood coming from the nose appears thin and watery, summon medical help immediately as this may indicate leakage of fluid from around the brain as a result of head or facial injury.

To treat a nosebleed:

1 Seat the patient comfortably with his head forward. Do not tip the head back in an attempt to stop bleeding, as the patient will be forced to swallow the blood as it trickles down the back of his throat which may cause vomiting.
2 Pinch the patient's nose just beneath the bridge and ask her to breathe through the mouth.

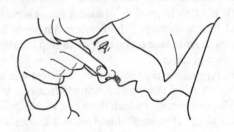

3 Ask her not to speak, sniff or swallow if possible as this may hinder clots from forming.
4 Apply pressure for a full 10 minutes in the first instance. If bleeding persists, apply a further 10 minutes' pressure. If bleeding has not ceased completely within 30 minutes, consult a doctor immediately or take the patient to the nearest accident and emergency unit. The patient should remain in the treatment position while travelling.
5 If bleeding stops, clean gently around the nose with cotton wool or a swab soaked in warm water. Ask the patient not to blow her nose for at least 4 hours and to rest quietly to avoid dislodging the clot.

Breathing Difficulties

Asthma

Asthma is an increasingly common respiratory disorder which can be triggered by allergy, exertion, cigarette smoke, respiratory infection, or by emotional factors. The patient will experience increasing tightness in the chest and difficulty in breathing as the air passages constrict. Breathing is characterized by wheezing, which may be audible as a whistling sound particularly when the patient breathes out. Most asthma sufferers cope well with the problem, and will usually be aware of the onset of an attack and take appropriate medication, usually in the form of inhalers. However, if it is the patient's first attack and he does not have medication, or if medication has been taken but without any response, it is essential that medical help is summoned immediately as asthma can be fatal.

Symptoms of an asthmatic attack

1 Difficulty in breathing, anxiety and difficulty in speaking.
2 Blueish appearance to the face, especially around the lips.

To treat an attack of asthma

1 Sit the patient at a table and encourage him to lean forward with his arms resting on the top of a table.
2 Ensure the room has an adequate supply of fresh air. Open a window, but not if the weather is cold.
3 Reassure the patient and encourage him to take his medication.
4 If there has been no response to the inhaler within 10-15 minutes, or if the patient becomes drowsy or begins to go blue around the lips, telephone for an ambulance immediately.

Croup

Croup is a breathing disorder of very young children caused by inflammation and partial obstruction of the trachea (windpipe) and the larynx. It is characterized by a barking cough, perhaps accompanied by a wheezing or whistling sound (known as **stridor**) and in severe cases the child's skin may have a blue appearance. It frequently occurs at night and can be very alarming, but an attack almost always resolves itself without further problems. Recovery can be quickened by:

1 Taking the child into a steam-filled room, such as a bathroom with the hot tap running in the bath.
2 Keeping the atmosphere in the child's bedroom humid.

It is advisable to call your doctor as the condition can recur after the initial attack has subsided.

If the child is sitting bolt upright or has a high temperature, this may indicate a more serious condition known as **epiglottitis** in which the swelling may completely obstruct the airway. This is a condition which requires immediate medical attention.

Hyperventilation

Hyperventilation occurs when an individual experiences an emotional fright, upset or stress. It is characterized by a shallow, rapid breathing pattern, whereby too much carbon dioxide is removed from the body. This will cause feelings of dizziness and tingling, and may cause the individual to panic. Adequate carbon dioxide levels can be restored and the symptoms controlled by encouraging the individual to breath into a paper bag held over his nose and mouth for up to 4 minutes.

Burns and Scalds

Burns are sustained in a number of ways—most commonly from dry heat, friction or corrosive chemicals, whilst scalds are caused by liquids and vapours. Although heat accounts for most burns and scalds, it is important to remember that contact with extreme cold can also burn, as can radiation.

At the scene of the burns incident:

1 Make sure you do not put yourself in danger from the presence of fire, electrical hazards, etc.
2 Where possible, stop the burning of affected tissues by rapid cooling. The most effective way of doing this is to place the affected limb or part under cold running water **for at least 10 minutes**. This will have the effect of minimizing tissue damage, swelling, shock and pain.

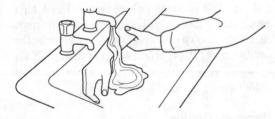

3 If removing the patient to hospital, turn off the water and cover the wound. A **non-stick** sterile dressing is preferable, but if not available, a clean handkerchief, pillowcase or sheet will do. Burns are highly vulnerable to infection, so it is important not to leave a wound exposed to the atmosphere for any length of time.
4 Keep the patient as calm as possible and observe for signs of shock. Always obtain medical help quickly for all but the most minor of burns (*see* p.659).

Never use an adhesive dressing on a burn.

Never apply creams, ointments, sprays, butter or indeed anything else to a burn—these will have to be removed and will cause additional pain and distress to the sufferer.

Never prick or burst any blister which appears on a burn—these are nature's defence against infection.

Never try to remove anything sticking to a burn—in

fact try not to touch or interfere with the affected area at all.

Burns to the mouth and throat

Burns on the face and mouth are extremely serious as they can cause rapid swelling of the airways. Summon medical help immediately and be prepared to resuscitate. Inform the ambulance service that you suspect burns of the airway.

Electrical burns

Burns may be caused by an electrical current passing into the body. Although most damage is done at the points of entry and exit, occasionally tracks of damage are caused internally. Severe electric shock may cause cardiac arrest—if the victim is unconscious, disregard any burns initially and give priority to the ABC of Resuscitation (*see* p.649).

If the source of electricity is Low Voltage, such as domestic supply it is essential to isolate the casualty from the current either by disconnecting the power or using wood or plastic to separate the victim from the appliance. Alternatively wrench the cable from the plug or grab the victims clothing and pull her free. **Do not come into contact with the victim's skin.**

Thereafter

1 Treat the site of injury as for any other burn.
2 Observe and treat the victim for shock and summon an ambulance.

Chemical burns

Chemicals which cause severe burns are normally found in industry, but some paint strippers and other domestic chemicals can also inflict similar burns. Try to find out what the substance was in order to inform the doctor, and summon medical help immediately. In the meantime:

1 Flood the burnt area with copious amounts of running water. Protect yourself with rubber gloves.
2 Remove any clothing which is likely to be contaminated with the chemical.
3 Get the casualty to hospital as quickly as possible.

Chemical burns to the eyes

If the eyes are affected, it is essential to pour as much water into them as possible. This will obviously need to be done as gently as possible, and as the eyes will probably be tightly shut in pain, it may be necessary to prise them open firmly. Chemical burns to the eyes can cause lasting damage and even blindness, therefore it is essential to seek hospital treatment without delay.

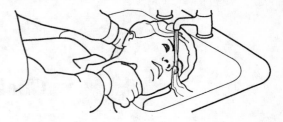

Choking

Normally when we swallow, a flap of cartilage known as the epiglottis moves downwards to stop food being taken into the trachea or windpipe. Where this fails to happen, food becomes stuck in the airway and choking is said to have occurred. Sometimes, the victim may appear to vomit or cough up the foreign body, but occasionally this fails to happen and the patient may be unable to breathe either partially or completely. Where a choking victim is unable to breathe, action must be taken immediately, as brain damage will occur within three or four minutes of its being starved of oxygen. Choking is a common cause of accidental death amongst children.

How to recognize a choking attack

1 The victim will probably clutch at his or her throat and be unable to speak.
2 The victim will probably become acutely distressed and panicky.
3 Inability to breathe will probably result in fairly rapid loss of consciousness.

Emergency action for a choking attack in an adult

1 Lean the victim forwards and give her 5 hard slaps on the back between the shoulder blades.
2 If this is unsuccessful, then abdominal thrusts can be performed from behind a patient who is either standing or sitting. For this, pass your hands around the patient and interlock your hands together just above the navel in the region of the diaphragm and pull sharply inwards and upwards.

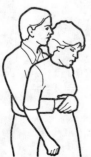

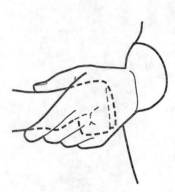

3 If the casualty is unconscious, kneel astride her on the floor and perform similar abdominal thrusts with the heel of the hand (one hand positioned on top of the other) just below the rib-cage
4 If you have tried abdominal thrusts six times without response, telephone 999 for an ambulance and begin resuscitation immediately.

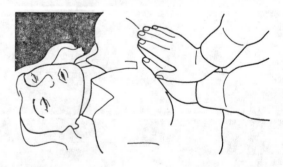

Emergency action for a choking child

1 Lay the child across your lap with its head down. Slap firmly between the shoulder blades five times.
2 Should this be unsuccessful, turn him over so he faces you on your lap and give him five firm upward thrusts with one hand above his navel.
3 Should this fail to dislodge the foreign body, then try steps 1 and 2 again. If the child becomes unconscious, then call an ambulance immediately and begin resuscitation.

Emergency action for a choking baby

Abdominal thrusts should **never** be used on a child younger than 1 year.

1 Straddle the baby face down along your arm and give her five firm slaps between the shoulders.
2 If choking continues, turn the baby over and place two fingertips between the navel and the breastbone. Press forward and downward in quick movements and repeat the movement up to four times if necessary.
3 If the infant loses consciousness, summon medical help immediately and begin resuscitation.

Remember

Never poke your fingers down a choking victim's throat in an attempt to find the obstructing object—you will only push it in further and make it more difficult to dislodge. If the object appears in or at the victim's mouth, then you may remove it gently.

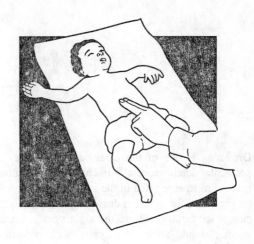

Drowning

Drowning is one of the most common causes of accidental death, especially in children, but is often quite hard to recognize in the initial stages. It may be very hard for a person drowning to summon the energy to shout, therefore the sight of a swimmer waving should always be treated with suspicion. The victim will attempt to hold his breath for as long as possible, but will eventually be forced to take a breath, permitting water to enter the airway. The muscles in the throat will respond by going into spasm which will then restrict breathing. Unconsciousness will follow shortly after this as the oxygen supply to the brain is cut off.

The brain will sustain permanent damage after it has been deprived of oxygen for just 3–4 minutes, unless the water is very cold. Under these circumstances, the brain may require less oxygen, and may survive unharmed for up to 30 minutes or more, particularly in the case of children. Therefore, it is always worth attempting to resuscitate a victim who has been pulled from cold water, even if you suspect he has been submerged for longer than 4 minutes.

Rescue and treatment of a drowning victim

1 **Do not risk your own safety**. Try to reach the victim from land by extending a pole or a rope. **Do not** attempt to swim or wade to him through a strong current or deep, cold water as you may find yourself quickly overcome.

2 If you are carrying the victim to safety try to ensure that you have a floating object, such as a board or a lifebelt, that he can grab hold of; in his panic he may grab you and thus make it more difficult for you to keep afloat. Keep his head tilted below the level of his body to allow as much water to drain naturally as possible. Similarly, when laying the victim down, try do so on a slope with his head down-most.

3 Check the airway for signs of obstruction with weeds or other debris, and clear by using finger sweeps, except in very small children. **Do not** use abdominal thrusts as this may cause stomach contents to be inhaled.

4 If the victim still has a carotid pulse but is failing to breathe, then begin mouth-to-mouth ventilation straight away (*see* p.650).

5 If there is no carotid pulse or breathing, then send someone for an ambulance and give full cardio-pulmonary resuscitation (*see* p.650).

6 Even though your patient appears to have made a full recovery, always send him to hospital for observation as serious breathing difficulties may recur some hours after the accident. Whilst awaiting the arrival of the emergency services, keep the patient as warm as possible, as he may be suffering from hypothermia.

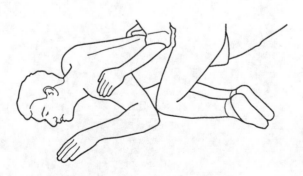

Fainting and Fits

Epilepsy

Epilepsy is a common condition in which the sufferer experiences a fit or seizure in response to sudden disruption of normal electrical activity in the brain. In an attack, the casualty may suddenly fall to the ground unconscious. For a few seconds, his muscles may stiffen and breathing will stop. This is known as the **tonic** phase, and is succeeded by the **clonic** phase, in which the whole body jerks violently, and breathing recommences noisily through clenched teeth. Normally, the jerking will cease and the muscles relax within about a minute. Breathing will become normal again, but the patient may remain unconscious for a few more minutes.

Although an epileptic fit can be frightening to witness, they rarely cause the sufferer any lasting harm, unless they have injured themselves during the fall or the clonic phase.

How to help during an epileptic fit

1 Try to clear a space around the patient, and if possible position him on his back before the jerking begins.
2 Loosen tight clothing, but do not attempt to restrain the patient or put anything in his mouth during the attack.
3 When the convulsion has subsided, place the patient in the recovery position (*see* p.653) and remain with him until he has made a complete recovery.
4 When he is fit to move, ensure that he gets home safely and informs his doctor, especially if this is the first attack.
5 If the patient does not regain consciousness within 15 minutes, or has repeated convulsions then call an ambulance.

Fainting

Fainting is a temporary loss of consciousness occasioned by a reduced blood supply to the brain. This may be caused by an emotional shock, fear, pain or inadequate food intake over a period of time.

More usually, however, people faint after long spells of inactivity, particularly in warm, airless conditions, during which blood will tend to pool in the lower part of the body, thereby reducing the amount available to the brain.

Treatment of fainting:

1 Lie the casualty down on the floor and raise his legs above the level of his head.
2 Open the windows and wait for the casualty to regain consciousness—usually within a few minutes.
3 If the patient recovers, but continues to feel faint, ask him to sit with his head down between his knees.
4 If the casualty does not regain consciousness quickly, place him in the recovery position (*see* p.653), check pulse and respiration and call for an ambulance. Be prepared to resuscitate if necessary.

Febrile convulsion

Febrile convulsions are caused by overheating and are most common in the under 2's. There is usually a history of fever and illness such as throat infection, which is often exacerbated by wrapping the child too warmly in bed. Typically, the child's skin will be flushed and hot, and the convulsion is characterized by arching of the back and violent muscle-twitching. The fists may be clenched and the eyes rolled upwards, and the breath is often held.

Treatment of a febrile convulsion is aimed at reducing the child's body temperature.

1 Remove the child's blankets and clothing.
2 Sponge the child with a sponge or flannel soaked in tepid water starting from the head and working downwards.
3 Keep the airway open by placing the child in the recovery position (*see* p.653).
4 Pad around the child with soft pillows to prevent him from hurting himself during a convulsion.
5 Call the doctor.

Fractures

A fracture is a crack or break in a bone. It takes a considerable degree of force to break bones as they are not simply brittle sticks but living tissues supporting the body. However, the bones of the elderly or those affected by disease may become more brittle and vulnerable, whilst those of children may be more likely to split under force as they are more supple. Bones are supplied with a rich network of nerves and blood vessels, which accounts for the amount of pain and swelling experienced when a fracture is sustained.

Types of fracture

1 Simple fracture: A clean break in a bone.
2 Compound fracture: A break in which the broken bone pierces the skin or is accompanied by a wound. In a compound fracture, the bone is exposed to contamination by infection from the air.
3 Comminuted fracture: The bone is shattered into several fragments at the site of the break.
4 Greenstick fracture: Most commonly experienced by children. This type of fracture will show up on an X-ray as an incomplete break or split in a bone.
5 Pathological fracture: The bone may break spontaneously where affected by disease or some other weakening factor such as a cyst.

Signs and symptoms of fracture

1 The patient may report having heard or felt a snap, although this can be caused by injuries other than fracture.
2 The patient will often experience severe pain which is worsened by attempts to move the limb.
3 The patient will be unable to move the limb normally as a result of the pain and the instability of the broken bone.
4 Bleeding from the damaged bone and surrounding tissues will quickly result in swelling. Some time later, bruising will probably occur, again as a result of haemorrhage within the tissues.
5 The limb may be misshapen or deformed as a

result of the break, or thrown into an unnatural position.

How to help a fracture victim

1 With the exception of suspected fractures to small bones in the upper limbs, it is best not to move the casualty, especially if you suspect his spine may be fractured.
2 Steady the broken limb by holding it gently but firmly above and below the fracture site, but do not attempt to straighten it.
3 Dial 999 for an ambulance at your earliest possible opportunity.
4 It may be possible to immobilize the injured part without moving it unnecessarily. For example, it may be possible to support a broken leg between two cushions or folded clothing, but do not attempt this if it involves moving the limb or altering its position. It is always a good idea to immobilize a broken arm against the body using a sling.
5 If it looks as if help may be some time in arriving, a broken leg may be gently secured to the sound leg with bandages. However, do not persist with this if it seems to be causing additional pain or distress.
6 Reassure the patient and observe for shock (*see* p.659)
7 Keep the patient warm, but do not give him anything to eat or drink, as he may require a general anaesthetic on admission to hospital.

Open fractures

Open fractures (i.e. those in which the broken bone is exposed to the air through a wound in the skin) should be treated in much the same way as closed fractures. The main problem is that as the wound is open, it is more prone to infection and there may be considerable blood loss. As with any fracture, it is essential to arrange for early removal of the casualty to hospital. Whilst waiting for the ambulance to arrive, proceed as follows:
1 Support the wound in the same way as you would with a closed fracture.

2 Gently cover the wound with a sterile dressing or clean pad of material.

3 Place more padding such as cotton wool around the pad and build it high enough to prevent pressure on any protruding bone (*see* illustration on p.633).

4 Bandage the padding gently but firmly in place. Take care not to bandage it so tightly that it impedes circulation or causes the patient further pain.

5 If possible elevate and immobilize the limb.

6 Reassure the patient and observe for shock (*see* p.659).

Facial fractures

Broken noses, cheekbones and jaws are among the most common injuries to the face. The main problems with injuries of this type is that the airway may become blocked by swelling or bleeding, or perhaps by teeth which have been dislodged. Bear in mind that the blow which caused the most obvious injury may also have caused some damage to the skull, the neck or even the brain.

Fracture of the Lower Jaw

This injury is usually caused by direct force to the jaw, either by a blow or a heavy fall. The pain can be excruciating, and is often exacerbated by movement of the jaw which is often hard to avoid. Fast removal of the patient to hospital is vital, but in the meantime you can make her more comfortable.

1 Encourage her to sit upright with her head tilted forward. This will encourage blood and saliva to drain from the mouth rather than necessitating swallowing.

2 Give the patient a soft pad and allow her to hold it in place against the painful jaw to support it. Encourage her to keep the jaw supported or tie a narrow bandage around the head until she reaches the hospital.

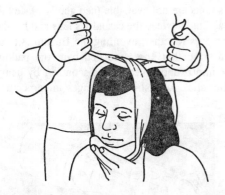

Injuries/Fractures of the Nose and Cheekbones

These injuries frequently occur as a result of fighting and can cause considerable discomfort as swelling progresses. The aim of the first-aider is to reduce the swelling and to have the patient examined in hospital as soon as possible. Treat swelling as follows:

1 Apply a cold compress. (A flannel or large handkerchief soaked in cold water then frequently refreshed will suit this purpose.)

2 Take or send the patient to hospital.

If the Facial Injury Victim is Unconscious

1 Check frequently that the airway is clear.

2 Place her in the recovery position (*see* p.653).

3 Call an ambulance immediately.

4 If a fractured jaw is suspected, slip a pad of soft material under the head in order to prevent its weight resting on and further damaging the jaw.

Remember that an injury above chest level should be treated as a suspected Spinal Injury.

Fractures of the Upper Limb

The term 'upper limb' includes not only the arm but also the shoulder and the collar bone. If the patient can walk without too much distress, then it may be unnecessary to call an ambulance, although hospital treatment is essential.

Fracture of the Collar-bone

The collar-bone is situated at the base of the neck and supplies the arm's support between the breastbone and the shoulder-blade. Fractures are usually a result of indirect force, such as an outstretched hand during a fall transmitting the force up to the collar-bone. The patient will undoubtedly experience pain at the injury site, and will frequently attempt to relieve this by tilting the head to one side. If a fractured collar-bone is suspected:

1 Immobilize the arm on the injured side by sitting the patient down and placing the arm on the affected side across her chest with her fingertips resting lightly on the opposite shoulder.

2 Place some padding between the injured limb and the casualty's chest. Support the arm in this position in an elevation sling across the shoulder (*see* p.648).

3 Give the arm further support if possible by adding a broadfold bandage around the chest.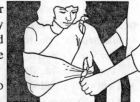

4 Take the patient to hospital.

643

Dislocation of the shoulder

Dislocation of the shoulder is most commonly caused by a fall. In dislocation, the ball-type shoulder joint is wrenched out of its socket causing extreme pain, especially upon movement. The first-aider's main aim is to reduce the pain by immobilizing the joint until the casualty can be taken to hospital—**do not** attempt to relocate the joint. Seat the patient then:

1 Gently position the affected arm across the chest and apply an arm sling.
2 Slip some padding behind the sling to give further support on the affected side.
3 Arrange for the patient to be taken to hospital.

Fracture of the upper arm

Fractures of the long bone (humerus) in the upper arm occur most commonly as a result of a fall, although can occasionally result from a direct blow. There will commonly be extreme pain accompanied by bruising and/or swelling at the site of the fracture. As with other arm injuries, hospital treatment is called for but first

1 Seat the patient.
2 Apply a sling and broad fold bandage (*see* p.648).

Fractures around the elbow

These are fairly common and are characterized by pain and swelling, which will be worsened by movement. With this type of fracture, there is increased danger of damage to surrounding nerves and blood vessels, therefore it is best to call an ambulance rather than attempting to take the patient to hospital on your own. If the elbow can still be bent, then use a sling as previously described for other arm injuries. If the arm cannot be bent:

1 Immobilize the arm by placing some padding between the arm and the trunk, then securing the arm against the body with large, broad bandages.
2 Check the patient's wrist pulse every 10 minutes. If pulse is absent loosen the bandaging ask the patient to reposition his arm if possible until pulse returns. Call an ambulance.

Fractures of the hip and leg

When attending a casualty with a fracture of the leg or hip it is important that an ambulance is summoned as soon as possible. The casualty should not be moved unless medical assistance cannot be summoned or you have to remove him from a situation of potential danger. Fractures of the hip and thigh bone are often characterized by shortening and outward rotation of the injured limb. Should you need to move the patient:

1 Gently lay the casualty on his back, supporting the injured limb with your hand, and make him as comfortable as possible.
2 Place plenty of soft padding between the legs, from the groin to the ankle. If long, straight boards or branches are available then prepare to use these as splints. One splint should be long enough to reach from the groin to the ankle and the other from the armpit to the ankle. Pad the shorter splint, lay it gently between the legs and gently bring the sound limb alongside the fractured leg.

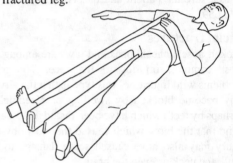

3 Place padding from the casualty's armpit to the ankle of the injured leg and then bandage as illustrated, avoiding the fracture site and ensuring that the knots are tied over the splint. Apply more padding between his arm and the outer surface of the long splint.

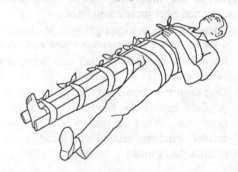

4 If splints are not available then gently place thick padding between the casualty's legs and bandage the legs together, avoiding the fracture site and ensuring that knots are tied over the padding. Minimize movement and discomfort by using a thin stick to push the bandages underneath the legs.

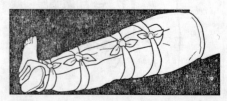

5 Once the limbs are immobilized, if possible raise them a little to reduce the swelling. Check the ankles for signs of a pulse and the toes for numbness; loosen the bandages a little if necessary.

7 Observe the casualty for shock (*see* p.659) and ensure that he is kept warm and as comfortable as possible.

Fractures of the lower leg

Fractures to the lower leg are frequently characterized by an open wound. It is, therefore, important to gently cover the wound with a clean dressing or material and summon medical assistance as soon as possible. Never attempt to straighten the fractured bone or to move the injured limb unnecessarily. To immobilize the leg you should:

1 Gently lie the casualty on his back and ensure that he is as comfortable as possible.

2 Use two splints which both extend from well above the knee to the ankle. Place the splints along the inner and outer side of the fractured leg, applying padding in between the splints and the leg on both sides.

3 Tie the splints to the leg with bandages or material in up to four places, always avoiding the site of the fracture. Ensure that the knots are tied over the splint.

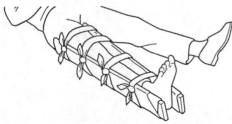

4 If splints are not available gently try to straighten the knee of the injured leg if it is bent. Place padding between the legs and move the sound leg alongside the injured limb.

5 Tie the feet using a figure of 8 bandage, then tie a bandage around the knee. Apply 2–3 more bandages, avoiding the fracture site and ensuring that the knots are tied on the uninjured side.

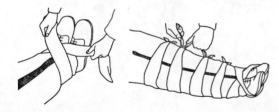

Fracture of the spine

Suspected fracture of the spine should always be treated as a serious injury and medical help should be sought urgently. Fracture to the vertebrae, the small bones which make up the spine, may be complicated by the risk of damage to the spinal cord which is enclosed within the spinal column. The spinal cord is composed of nerve tissue which transmits impulses from the brain which control many of the functions of the body. Any damage to the spinal cord could, thus, result in temporary or permanent paralysis in parts of the body, depending on where the injury occurs. It is therefore essential that the casualty is immobilized as far as possible to minimize the risk of damage.

Symptoms of spinal injury

1 The victim may complain of severe pain in the back.

2 Lack of control over movement in the limbs.

3 Loss of sensation in the limbs, even when touched gently.

Treatment of spinal injury

When attending a casualty with a back injury, where the precise nature of the injury is unclear, **always** treat it as a fracture.

1 Arrange for the casualty to be removed to hospital, by ambulance, as soon as possible.

2 Support the casualty by gently steadying him head with your hand and placing rolled up clothing, blankets and towels around the trunk of his body. Secure these in place with bricks, stones or heavy bags. Cover the casualty with a blanket and keep as comfortable as possible.

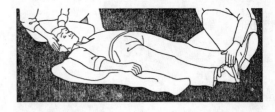

3 If the victim is in imminent danger and has to be moved immediately, then he must be supported at the head and neck, the shoulders, the waist and the legs to ensure that the head, neck and torso are in alignment.

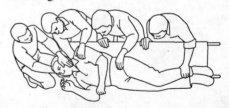

4 The casualty should always be carried any distance on a rigid stretcher or board with the limbs gently supported.

Dislocated bones

Articulating joints, such as the shoulder or hip, are held together by strong strips of tissue called ligaments. The ligaments generally hold the joint in the correct position and ensure its correct movement, but occasionally violent movement or injury can tear the ligament thus permitting dislocation or displacement of the bone. Contrary to popular belief, **no attempt** should be made to replace the joint, as this can result in further injury. The best course of action is to treat the dislocation as a fracture and ensure the swift removal of the patient to hospital for treatment.

Bandages and Slings

A basic triangular bandage can be adapted for use as a sling or for using as a broad or narrow bandage or a ring pad. These can be made by cutting a piece of material (approximately 1 metre by 1 metre) in half diagonally.

Broad bandage

Broad bandages can be used for immobilizing limbs before transporting a casualty.

Using the triangular bandage, fold in the point towards the base of the bandage and then fold in half again.

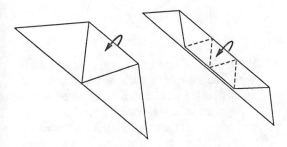

Narrow bandage

A narrow bandage can be used for securing a dressing in place, making a ring pad and for fixing a figure of eight bandage.

Using a triangular bandage make a broad bandage as shown above and then simply fold in half again.

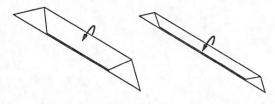

Ring pad

When used on a complicated fracture where the bone is protruding through the skin or on a wound where a foreign body is present, a ring pad can be used to provide protection around the wound and prevent dressings from creating too much pressure.

1 Make a narrow bandage and wrap it once around the fingers of one hand to make a loop.
2 Take hold of the other end of the bandage and wind it around the loop, pulling it tight.
3 Continue to firmly wind the bandage around the loop until the bandage has been used and tuck in the end.

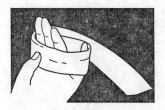

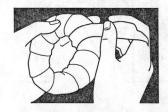

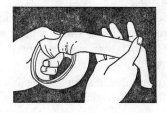

Slings

Arm sling

An arm sling should provide support for the forearm, elbow and wrist. It should be applied so that the hand is slightly higher than the elbow and the fingertips are exposed. Always apply a sling with the casualty standing or sitting down and work from the injured side to provide more support.

1 Support the arm across the chest, ensuring that the hand is slightly higher than the elbow. Take a triangular bandage and slide one end underneath the forearm until the point of the bandage reaches well below the elbow.
2 Take the upper end of the sling, place it around the

shoul-der on the uninjured side, then take it around the back of the neck and then to the front on the injured side.

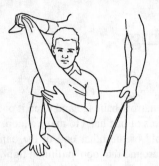

3 Take the lower end of the sling and fold it over the forearm and then tie it off in the hollow above the collar-bone.
4 Take the point of the bandage and fold it forward onto the front, fixing it with a safety pin.

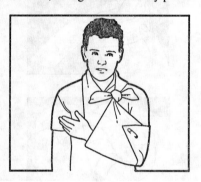

Elevation sling

An elevation sling should be used to support an injury to the shoulder or where a hand wound is bleeding. The aim is to raise and support the forearm and the hand.

1 Gently place the forearm on the injured side across the chest so that the fingertips are level with the opposite shoulder. Ask the casualty to support the limb if possible.

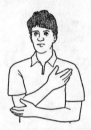

2 Place the base of a triangular bandage over the raised forearm and hand so that the upper end sits on the shoulder on the uninjured side and the point reaches beyond the tip of the elbow.
3 Gently slide the base of the bandage underneath the elbow, forearm and hand.

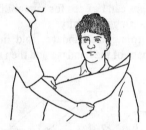

4 Take the lower end of the sling and place it around the casualty's back and across to the shoulder on the uninjured side. Tie it off in the hollow of the collar-bone and adjust if necessary.
5 Take the point of the sling and tuck it between the forearm and the front of the sling. This will leave a fold of material which can be pinned back against the arm.

Remember—when applying bandages and slings ensure that the casualty's circulation is not affected. If so then adjust the bandage or reposition the sling until circulation has improved.

Heart Attack and Cardiac Arrest

A heart attack is said to have occurred when a clot of blood suddenly blocks a coronary artery, one of the main blood vessels to the heart muscle, the **myocardium.** When this happens, the affected part of muscle will die due to the resulting lack of oxygen causing the patient severe, gripping chest pain. Sometimes, the patient may have a history of **angina pectoris,** a condition in which the coronary arteries are narrowed due to the build-up of fatty deposits on the inside walls. This restricts the blood flow to the myocardium and causes severe crushing pain in the chest, not unlike that of a heart attack. Therefore, it is sometimes very difficult to distinguish between an attack of angina and a heart attack. Unlike a heart attack, angina is usually relieved by rest or by placing a tablet of glyceryl trinitrate (GTN) under the patient's tongue.

Signs and symptoms of heart attack

1 Severe crushing chest pain, possibly radiating down one or both arms, or up into the jaw. The pain will not be relieved by rest or GTN.
2 Facial pallor or 'ashen' appearance, sometimes with blueish colouring of the lips.
3 The skin may be cold and clammy to the touch.
4 The patient may suffer from breathlessness, weakness and dizziness.
5 Nausea and vomiting may be present.
6 The pulse may be irregular and either slow or fast.
7 The patient may collapse suddenly, possibly without warning.

Treatment of a heart attack

1 Keep the casualty as calm and as comfortable as possible. Loosen any tight clothing and place pillows behind his head and knees to support him in a half-sitting position.
2 Phone 999 for an ambulance and be prepared to resuscitate.
3 If ordinary aspirin is available, give the casualty one and ask him to chew and swallow it. Recent research has shown that aspirin given immediately after the onset of heart attack can improve the victim's chances of recovery, perhaps by inhibiting further clotting in the coronary arteries.

Cardiac arrest

Cardiac arrest is the term used to describe any sudden cessation of the heart, characterized by absence of pulse and breathing. Cardiac arrest may be the result of severe heart attack, anaphylactic shock, electric shock, poisoning (including drug overdose), hypothermia or suffocation.

During cardiac arrest, the brain and heart muscle are completely starved of oxygen, a state which can be tolerated only for a few minutes before permanent damage results. **It is vital that resuscitation procedures are instigated immediately**.

The ABC of resuscitation

Resuscitation is the emergency action required when there is sustained interruption of the oxygen supply to the brain. In order that this vital oxygen supply may be restored, three vital conditions must be met:

A The **Airway** must be clear in order to permit oxygen-rich air to enter the lungs.
B There must be adequate **Breathing** taking place in order that the oxygen can enter the bloodstream.
C The blood must be pumped around the body providing effective **Circulation** to the brain and all body tissues.

When presented with an unconscious casualty, it is important to assess his condition **quickly** before attempting resuscitation. Therefore it is important to ask the following questions:

1 Is the patient unconscious with no evidence of pulse or breathing? If so: Dial 999 for an ambulance and carry out artificial ventilation and chest compression until the ambulance arrives.
2 Is the patient unconscious and not breathing but pulse is still present? If so: Administer 10 breaths of artificial respiration and dial 999 for an ambulance. Continue artificial respiration until the ambulance arrives or spontaneous breathing is resumed. Check the pulse frequently.

3 Is the patient unconscious, but breathing, with pulse present? If so: Treat any obvious injuries, dial 999 for an ambulance and place the patient in the recovery position (*see* p.653).

Always proceed by following the ABC of Resuscitation.

A: Open the airway

1 Remove any visible obstructions from the mouth.
2 Placing two fingers under the casualty's chin, gently raise the jaw. Simultaneously, tilt the casualty's head well back by applying pressure to the forehead with your other hand.

Sometimes the airway may be blocked by the tongue as a result of loss of muscular control during unconsciousness, and this manoeuvre will lift the tongue clear.

B: Check for breathing

Place your face close to the casualty's mouth and listen and feel for breathing for a full 5 seconds. At the same time look along the chest and abdomen for signs of movement.

C: Check the circulation

If the heart is beating adequately, it will be possible to feel a **pulse** in the neck where the main carotid arteries pass on either side of the larynx on the way to the head. With the patient's head tilted back, slide your fingers between the Adam's Apple and the strap muscle and feel for the carotid pulse for five seconds.

If pulse and breathing are absent, you will need to commence artificial ventilation and chest compression immediately.

Mouth to mouth or artificial ventilation

If the casualty is not breathing, but still has a pulse, then by breathing the exhaled air from your lungs into his you may be able to keep them adequately ventilated until help arrives.

1 Place the casualty flat on his back, and tilt the head back to open the airway unless you suspect Spinal Injury in which case lift the chin. Remove any obvious obstructions from the mouth. (Broken or loose dentures should be removed, but well-fitting dentures should remain in place).

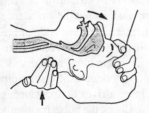

2 Pinch the nose between the index finger and thumb. Take a deep breath, then form a seal around the casualty's mouth with your own.

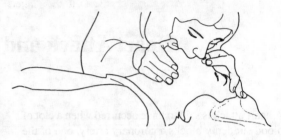

3 Blow steadily into the mouth until the chest rises. Each full inflation should take about two seconds.
4 Remove your lips from the casualty's and allow the chest to 'exhale' fully before giving a subsequent breath.

If the chest fails to rise:

1 Check that the head is tilted back correctly.
2 Ensure that your lips are forming a proper seal around the patient's mouth.
3 Check that air is not escaping from the nostrils.
4 Check that the airway is not blocked by vomit or blood.

If an airway obstruction is suspected, then finger sweeps may be performed **on an adult:**

Grasp the tongue and lower jaw and pull gently upwards to open the mouth. Sweep the finger round the mouth and hook out any obstruction. (**This manoeuvre is not suitable for children.**)

The first-aider should administer 10 breaths of artificial ventilation before phoning for an ambulance, then continue at a rate of approximately 10 breaths per minute until the casualty breathes spontaneously or medical help arrives.

Chest compression

If the patient has no palpable carotid pulse and no breathing is present, then it is vital that you perform artificial ventilation and external chest compression to prevent brain damage which is likely to occur in just a few minutes. Artificial respiration and external chest compression are together known as **cardio-pulmonary resuscitation** or **CPR.**

1 Lie the patient flat on his back and feel for the point at which his lower ribs meet in the centre (the *xiphisternum).*

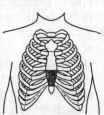

2 Place your left hand index and middle fingers over this point and the heel of your

right hand on the breastbone or sternum above your fingers.

3 Place your left hand directly on top of your right hand interlocking the fingers. Pull the fingers away so that the heel of your right hand is the only part in direct contact with the breastbone.

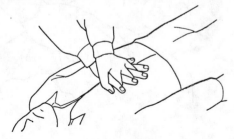

4 Keeping your arms straight, lean over the casualty and apply pressure to the breastbone. The intention is to depress and release the breastbone about 4–5cm or $1\frac{1}{2}$–2 inches approximately 80 times per minute. Keep your hands in contact with the patient between compressions so that a smooth rhythm can be achieved. It may help to count aloud '1 and 2 and 3 and 4,' etc.

Compressing the chest in this way expels some of the blood from within the heart and forces it out into the tissues and around the body. As the pressure is released, more blood will be 'sucked' into the heart to replace that expelled.

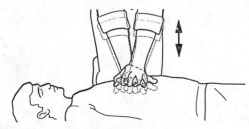

The Sequence of CPR

The most effective sequence of CPR which can be performed by one person is 15 chest compressions followed by 2 breaths of artificial respiration. If two first-aiders are present the ratio should be 5 to 1.

Do not cease CPR unless:

1 The ambulance has arrived and paramedics take over.

2 The casualty moves or begins to groan, or his colour improves. If this occurs, then check immediately for a carotid pulse. If the pulse has returned, and the casualty is also breathing, place him in the recovery position (*see* p.653) until help arrives. If the pulse has restarted but breathing has not, then continue with artificial ventilation alone at a rate of 10 breaths per minute. Check

the pulse at the end of every 10 ventilations, as you will need to restart full CPR again if it stops.

3 You are exhausted and cannot continue.

CPR for children

Although it is rare for a child to suffer a cardiac arrest, it does occasionally happen and the first-aider should be aware that the main difference between treating a child and an adult is that the child will need to be given artificial ventilation for a full minute before dialling 999 for an ambulance. CPR can be performed on older children in much the same way as for adults, using a lighter and slightly faster technique, but must be modified as follows for use on children and babies.

1 **Airway:** Gently lift the chin and tilt the head to open the airway. **Do not perform finger sweeps or touch the back of the child's throat**. Any obvious food particles or other obstruction should be gently removed from the mouth.

2 **Breathing:** Look, feel and listen carefully for breathing. If it is absent, then begin artificial ventilation. This should be done as for adults, with the following exceptions.

a It is more effective to form a seal with your mouth round the child's mouth and nose than mouth alone.

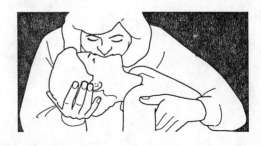

b The rate of artificial ventilation will need to be twice that for an adult—about 20 breaths per minute.

c Depending on the size of the child, you will need to vary the amount of air you breathe into the lungs to make the chest rise. A baby will only require tiny puffs, whereas an older child will need more.

3 **Circulation:** The carotid pulse is often hard to find in an infant—if so try the *brachial* pulse. You will find this half way between the shoulder and the elbow on the inner side of the arm. Press lightly with your index and middle fingers (perhaps using your thumb as a brace behind the arm) for a full 5 seconds. If no pulse is detected, then you will need to commence chest compression. You can use the adult technique if

the child is large, but for babies and very young children it will need to be modified as follows:

a For a **toddler** or small child, identify the correct position on the chest as per the adult technique, but use the heel of one hand only. Press to a depth of 3–4 cm or $1\frac{1}{2}$ inches. In both cases, apply chest compressions at a rate of approximately 100 per minute, alternating 5 compressions with one breath.

b For a **baby**, imagine a line between his nipples and apply chest compression with two fingertips just below the line. Aim to depress the chest slightly less than 1 inch or two centimetres.

Remember: If pulse and breathing are absent, artificial ventilation must be combined with chest compression. Call an ambulance as soon as possible.

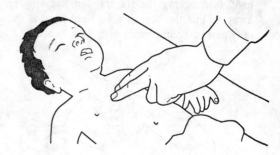

The Recovery Position

An unconscious patient should always be placed in the recovery position, as the position of the head will prevent the tongue blocking the airway whilst allowing fluids to drain freely from the mouth. You should not leave an unconscious patient to call for help unless you have first placed him in the recovery position as follows:

1 Kneel beside the patient and open his airway by lifting the chin up and tilting the head. The arm nearest you should be placed at right angles to the body, with the elbow bent and the palm uppermost.

2 Bring the other arm across the patient's body and place his hand against his cheek. Hold the arm in this position.

3 With your other hand, firmly grasp the far thigh and pull the knee up and towards you. Continue pulling on the thigh until the patient is on his side with his hand still under her cheek.

4 Adjust the hand position and tilt the head back again if necessary to ensure that the airway remains open. The hand should keep the head in the correct position.

5 The upper leg should be bent so that the hip and the knee are both at right angles.

6 Call an ambulance immediately, and make frequent checks on the patient's pulse and breathing whilst you wait.

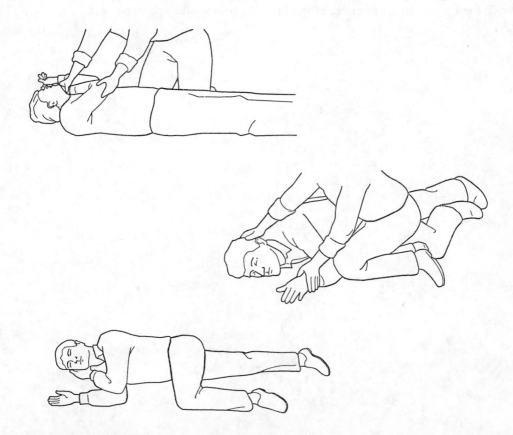

Poisoning

By poison we mean a substance which, if it enters the body can exert harmful effects, permanent or temporary. The routes by which a poison may enter the body are as follows:

1 **Swallowing**: May be accidental or deliberate (overdose) and includes a wide variety of substances from alcohol and illicit drugs to household cleaners or plants.
2 **Inhalation**: This can be of gases such as carbon monoxide, as well as solvents and vapours.
3 **Skin absorption**: Pesticides and insecticides may be absorbed in this way, and particularly strong chemicals may also cause burns.
4 **Injection into the skin**: This includes venom such as that injected by snakes and insects and also illicit drugs injected by abusers.

Detailed instruction on the treatment of specific types of poisoning is outwith the scope of this book, but in general the following steps should be taken:

1 Try to obtain an accurate history of the poisoning incident. If possible find out exactly what the substance was, how much has been ingested and how much time has elapsed since.
2 Obtain medical assistance immediately. **Never** attempt to make the patient vomit as this may cause further damage to the gastro-intestinal tract and may even cause the patient to inhale the vomit.
3 Place an unconscious patient in the recovery position.
4 Send specimens of the toxin to the hospital with the patient, if possible, as well as vomit specimens. This will help in identification of the toxin and the amount ingested.

Temperature Extremes

The body is designed to function at a temperature of between 36°C and 37.5°C (96.8°F and 99.5°F). Generally, the core temperature is kept constantly within these limits by a heat-regulating mechanism in the brain. Occasionally, the body temperature can rise or fall to a level whereby this mechanism can no longer effectively regulate the temperature resulting in the following conditions:

Hypothermia

Hypothermia occurs when the core temperature of the body falls to below 35° C (95°F). Once below 35°, shivering stops and the patient no longer feels cold but appears lethargic and apathetic. If the body temperature continues to drop, hypothermia sufferers may become increasingly confused and may even begin to experience sensations of heat and attempt to remove their clothing. At a temperature of below 30°C (86°F), the muscles become rigid and unconsciousness will eventually ensue. A body temperature of less than 27°C (80.6°F) will eventually cause cardiac arrest. Elderly people and babies are particularly susceptible to hypothermia, but young, healthy people can also be at risk if exposed to extremely low temperatures for lengthy periods of time.

Treatment of hypothermia

1 Bring the patient indoors and remove any wet clothing.
2 If indoors, and the casualty is capable of moving unaided, fill a bath with hot water (40°C/104°F) and completely immerse him in it. If the casualty is frail or elderly, allow him to warm up gradually in bed, well covered. Avoid using electric blankets and hot water bottles.
3 Give the patient something hot and sweet to drink. Avoid alcohol as it exacerbates hypothermia.
4 Call a doctor. If the casualty becomes unconscious, call an ambulance and be prepared to resuscitate.

Heat Exhaustion

Heat exhaustion usually occurs gradually and is particularly common in those who have been working or exercising vigorously in unaccustomed heat. The symptoms are often similar to those of shock (*see* p.659), due to the excessive loss of fluids through perspiration. The sufferer's temperature may be normal or only slightly raised, the skin cold and clammy and the pulse fast and weak. In addition, the loss of salt due to excessive perspiration may cause painful muscle cramps. The patient may also be hyperventilating.

Treatment of heat exhaustion

1 Remove the patient out of direct sunlight and heat to a shaded, cool place.
2 Ask the casualty to lie down and support her legs in a raised position.
3 Encourage her to drink plenty of weak salty water (about one teaspoon of salt per litre of water is sufficient).
4 If the patient recovers quickly, she should still be encouraged to see her doctor.
5 Should the patient become unconscious, place her in the recovery position (*see* p.653) and call an ambulance. While you are waiting for help to arrive, keep a check on the patient's pulse and breathing.

Heatstroke

Heatstroke often occurs rapidly resulting in unconsciousness within a few minutes, although there is sometimes a warning period when the patient may complain of feeling unwell or strange. It occurs when the brain's 'thermostat' fails as a result of prolonged exposure to high temperature in the surroundings or illness with high fever.

Symptoms of heatstroke

1 Dizziness, headache, discomfort and unease and confusion.
2 The skin will feel hot and dry and appear flushed.
3 The pulse will be fast and strong.
4 The patient may collapse and become unconscious.

Treatment of heatstroke

1 Remove the casualty quickly to a cool place and

remove his outer clothing. Summon medical help immediately.

2 If possible wrap the casualty in a sheet and keep it wet until his oral temperature falls to 38°C (100.4°F).

3 When the temperature has returned to a safe level, remove the wet sheet and substitute it for a dry one. Keep a close watch on the patient, and be prepared to repeat step 2 if the temperature rises again.

4. If the casualty becomes unconscious, place him in the recovery position (*see* p.653) and be prepared to resuscitate. Call an ambulance immediately.

Unconsciousness

Common causes of unconsciousness

1 Impairment of the blood supply to the brain. This may be a result of either
   a   Fainting
   b   Shock
   c   Cardiac arrest
2 Impairment of oxygen supply to the brain. This may result from either
   a   Choking
   b   Suffocation
   c   Carbon monoxide poisoning
3 Direct damage to the brain i.e. head injury.
4 Compression of the brain. This may be a result of either
   a   Skull fracture
   b   Infections
   c   Tumour
   d   Stroke
5 Alteration of the chemical balance of the brain's blood supply. This may be caused by either
   a   Poisoning (including drugs and alcohol)
   b   Low blood sugar (hypoglycaemia)
6 Other causes such as
   a   Epilepsy
   b   Abnormally high body temperature
   c   Electrocution

First aid for the unconscious

Unconsciousness is caused by a variety of conditions which interrupt normal brain function. Unlike sleep, the casualty cannot be easily or completely roused in response to stimuli such as sound, or pain. The first-aider should always bear in mind that there is a danger that the airway will become blocked during unconsciousness either by vomit or by the tongue falling backwards causing an obstruction of the airway. Therefore always follow the following steps:

1 Lift the chin and gently tilt the head to open the airway. (If the patient begins to vomit, place in the recovery position.) If you suspect that there may be Spinal Injury open the airway by lifting the chin. Do not tilt the head.

2 Check the pulse and respiration. Be prepared to resuscitate if necessary.
3 Check the casualty for any heavy external bleeding or fractures and treat accordingly.
4 Place the patient in the recovery position (*see* p.653) if you are satisfied that there is no serious neck or spinal injury.
5 If full consciousness has not be regained within 3 minutes, telephone 999 for an ambulance.

Do not attempt to give the unconscious patient anything by mouth.

Do not attempt to move the patient unnecessarily, or to make him or her sit up.

Head injuries and loss of consciousness

The brain is encased within the hard bony skull and cushioned by cerebro-spinal fluid to protect it from injury. It transmits impulses via the spinal chord which runs down the neck and spine to all the nerves of the body. The brain and spinal chord are extremely fragile and incapable of repairing themselves, hence the protection of the skull and spine.

Fracture of the skull

Although skull fracture is frequently indicative of a potentially serious and life-threatening condition, be aware that the real danger is damage to the brain itself. There may be fragments of bony skull causing pressure or compression on the brain (depressed fracture) and the resulting indentation of the skull may be missed as a result of swelling in the scalp. Therefore all injuries to the head should be treated with the utmost caution and suspicion especially if any of the following signs of cerebral compression are present:

1 Vomiting, persistent headache or yawning.
2 Brief or partial loss of consciousness, or full unconsciousness.
3 Pupils of unequal sizes, which may enlarge and fail to constrict in response to light if compression increases.
4 One-sided paralysis or weakness of the face or body.

5 Irregular or noisy breathing, becoming increasingly slower.

6 Slow, strong pulse.

7 High temperature and flushed face.

8 Leakage of watery blood or straw-coloured fluid from the nose or ear.

Remember that an injury above chest level should be treated as a suspected Spinal Injury. In all cases, call 999 for an ambulance and treat as for unconsciousness whilst awaiting its arrival.

Diabetic coma

Diabetes mellitus

Normally, an organ called the pancreas produces a hormone called insulin which regulates the level of sugar in which circulates in the bloodstream. In diabetes mellitus, the pancreas fails to perform this role adequately. Sufferers may display symptoms such as tiredness, loss of weight, severe thirst, and passing large quantities of urine. Once diagnosed, patients can lead a relatively normal life by making a few minor adjustments. Mild diabetes may be controlled simply be restricting the intake of carbohydrate foods in the diet and/or by taking oral medication. More severe forms, however, will need to be controlled by regular injections of insulin and careful monitoring of energy intake.

Diabetic emergencies—hyperglycaemia and hypoglycaemia

If the blood sugar level falls below normal, then a condition known as hypoglycaemia is said to exist. Without adequate levels of sugar in the blood, the brain can no longer function normally. Most diabetics are aware of the steps they must take to prevent this occurring, and can usually identify the first symptoms of an attack and take the appropriate action—normally the ingestion of sugar or glucose tablets. However, if an attack becomes advanced, unconsciousness will eventually occur and failure to act quickly can result in permanent brain damage to the sufferer.

How to recognize an attack of Hypoglycaemia

1 The attack will usually be rapid in onset. The patient may complain of weakness, tiredness, hunger or feeling faint. Ask if he is diabetic, or look for a medic-alert bracelet or warning card.

2 The patient may experience palpitations and muscle tremors.

3 If no sugar is taken, the patient may become confused or aggressive.

4 Skin will become cold, clammy and sweaty.

5 Breathing may become shallow.

6 Patient may eventually become unconscious.

Treatment of hypoglycaemia

1 Aim to raise the blood sugar levels as quickly as possible by giving the victim sugary food or drink. Find out if the patient carries a supply of Glucagon Injection for such emergencies, in which case follow the instructions enclosed. If there is no improvement within five minutes or....

2 If the victim is unconscious, place him in the recovery position and be prepared to resuscitate.

3 Call for an ambulance.

Hyperglycaemia

In hyperglycaemia, the pancreas fails to produce enough insulin to prevent excessive levels of sugar in the blood. Once diagnosed, diabetics will be able to prevent hyperglycaemia by balancing their dietary intake of sugar and by regular insulin injections.

Occasionally, hyperglycaemia can cause unconsciousness, but the condition generally develops gradually over a period of days or weeks. The symptoms of hyperglycaemic coma are as follows:

1 Dry skin

2 Faint smell of acetone (similar to nail varnish remover or mown grass) on the breath

3 Rapid pulse

4 Deep, laboured breathing.

Dial 999 for an ambulance or transport the patient to hospital immediately for treatment.

Shock and Allergic Reactions

An allergy is an abnormal response by the body to a specific stimulus or allergen. These can be familiar, everyday substances such as house dust, pollen or animal fur causing mild symptoms such as sneezing, itchiness or a rash. Hay fever, for instance is an allergic response to pollens in the air and is most commonly experienced in the summer months. Similarly, many people may suffer unpleasant allergic reactions after ingesting particular foods. Shellfish, nuts and eggs are often the culprits, and most sufferers quickly manage to identify those foods which cause the reaction and thereafter avoid them. Sometimes, patients can also experience an allergic response to some drugs such as penicillin, and medical practitioners will always bear this in mind when prescribing medication.

Although allergies can be extremely unpleasant and distressing for the sufferer, they will rarely necessitate first aid or emergency treatment. However, a patient may occasionally experience a severe and life-threatening reaction to an allergen. This is known as anaphylactic shock and requires urgent medical attention. This reaction can occur in response to bee or wasp stings or the ingestion of nuts or any food which causes allergy in the sufferer and can therefore be extremely difficult to diagnose.

Anaphylactic shock

1 Does the patient's skin have a rash or red blotches (hives)?
2 Is there any swelling on any part of the patient's body, but particularly on the face, the lips or the tongue?
3 Is he having difficulty in breathing? This may indicate swelling in the airway.
4 Is he experiencing tightness in his chest?
5 Is his skin colour normal or does it appear greyish or even blue?
6 Is the patient unconscious or suffering from seizures?
7 Can his pulse be felt? Is it weak or rapid?

Any of the above symptoms can develop within a few moments of the initial exposure to the allergen. The treatment for severe anaphylactic shock is the administration of the drug adrenaline and oxygen. Increasingly, allergy suffer-ers identified as being at risk of anaphylactic shock will be issued with pre-packed injections of adrenaline which are quick and simple to use, so it is sensible to check whether or not your patient is thus equipped. Otherwise, there is no specific treatment other than remaining with your patient until medical help arrives. He should be kept in a comfortable upright position to assist breathing, unless he loses consciousness, in which case the recovery position is preferred.

Shock

When referred to in medical emergency, shock is taken to signify a life-threatening condition caused by the failure of the circulatory system to pump blood around the body. Internal and external bleeding can cause this, as can heart attack, anaphylactic shock and excessive loss of body fluids such as that which occurs in diarrhoea or severe burns. The body tries to maximize the use of remaining body fluids by withdrawing them from the surface and extremities of the body to the centre. This can progressively produce the following symptoms:

1 The patient's skin becomes cold, grey and clammy as the body attempts to divert blood supplies to the vital organs.
2 The pulse becomes rapid as the heart works harder to circulate the reduced volume of blood.
3 The pulse becomes weaker and may become irregular as the blood volume and pressure fall.
4 The patient becomes weak and giddy as oxygen fails to reach the muscles and brain.
5 The patient's breathing becomes rapid and shallow, and he may appear to be attempting to yawn or gulp in air ('air hunger').
6 The patient may complain of nausea and actually vomit.
7 The patient may experience thirst as the brain senses that the body needs to make up a shortfall in fluid.
8 The patient may become restless and agitated as the oxygen supply to the brain deteriorates.

9 The patient will lose consciousness, and the pulse at the wrist may become unpalpable.

10 The heart will stop.

It is vital to identify and treat the causes of shock immediately.

Always summon medical help at the earliest possible opportunity, but it may be possible to slow the progression of shock by taking prompt action to stop bleeding from an open wound.

Guide to Popular Complementary Therapies

Acupressure

This is an ancient form of healing combining massage and acupuncture, practised over 3,000 years ago in Japan and China. It was developed into its current form using a system of special massage points and is today still practised widely in the Japanese home environment.

Certain 'pressure points' are located in various parts of the body and these are used by the practitioner by massaging firmly with the thumb or fingertip. These points are the same as those utilized in acupuncture. There are various ways of working and the pressure can be applied by the practitioner's fingers, thumbs, knees, palms of the hand, etc. Relief from pain can be quite rapid at times, depending upon its cause, while other more persistent problems can take longer to improve.

Acupressure is said to enhance the body's own method of healing, thereby preventing illness and improving the energy level. The pressure exerted is believed to regulate a matter called 'Qi', which is energy that flows along 'meridians'. These are invisible channels that run along the length of the body. These meridians are mainly named after the organs of the body such as the liver and stomach, but there are four exceptions, which are called the 'pericardium', 'triple heater', 'conception' and 'governor'. Specifically named meridian lines may also be used to treat ailments other than those relating to it.

Ailments claimed to have been treated successfully are back pain, asthma, digestive problems, insomnia, migraine and circulatory problems, amongst others. Changes in diet, regular exercise and certain self-checking methods may be recommended by your practitioner. It must be borne in mind that some painful symptoms are the onset of serious illness so you should always first consult your G.P.

Before any treatment commences, a patient will be asked details of lifestyle and diet, the pulse rate will be taken along with any relevant past history relating to the current problem. The person will be requested to lie on a mattress on the floor or on a firm table, and comfortable but loose-fitting clothing is best so that the practitioner can work most effectively on the energy channels. No oils are used on the body and there is no equipment. Each session lasts from approximately 30 minutes to 1 hour. Once the pressure is applied, and this can be done in a variety of ways particular to each practitioner, varying sensations may be felt. Some points may feel sore or tender and there may be some discomfort such as a deep pain or coolness. However, it is believed that this form of massage works quickly so that any tenderness soon passes.

The number of treatments will vary from patient to patient, according to how the person responds and what problem or ailment is being treated. Weekly visits may be needed if a specific disorder is being treated while other people may go whenever they feel in need. It is advisable for women who are pregnant to check with their practitioner first since some of the acupressure methods are not recommended during pregnancy. Acupressure can be practised safely at home although it is usually better for one person to perform the massage on another. Common problems such as headache, constipation and toothache can be treated quite simply although there is the possibility of any problem worsening first before an improvement occurs if the pressure points are over stimulated. You should, however, see your doctor if any ailment persists. To treat headache, facial soreness, toothache and menstrual pain, locate the fleshy piece of skin between the thumb and forefinger and squeeze firmly, pressing towards the forefinger. The pressure should be applied for about five minutes and either hand can be used. This point is known as 'Large Intestine 4'.

To aid digestive problems in both adults and babies, for example to settle infantile colic, the point known as 'Stomach 36' is utilized, which is located on the outer side of the leg about 75mm (3ins) down from the knee. This point should be quite simple to find as it can often feel slightly tender. It should be pressed quite firmly and strongly for about five to ten minutes with the thumb.

When practising acupressure massage on

someone else and before treatment begins, ensure that the person is warm, relaxed, comfortable and wearing loose-fitting clothing and that he or she is lying on a firm mattress or rug on the floor. To discover the areas that need to be worked on, press firmly over the body and see which areas are tender. These tender areas on the body correspond to an organ that is not working correctly. To commence massage using fingertips or thumbs, a pressure of about 4.5 kg (10 lbs) should be exerted. The massage movements should be performed very quickly, about 50 to 100 times every minute, and some discomfort is likely (which will soon pass) but there should be no pain. Particular care should be taken to avoid causing pain on the face, stomach or over any joints. If a baby or young child is being massaged then considerably less pressure should be used. If there is any doubt as to the correct amount, exert a downwards pressure on bathroom scales to ascertain the weight being used. There is no need to hurry from one point to another since approximately 5 to 15 minutes is needed at each point for adults, but only about 30 seconds for babies or young children.

Using the 'self-help' acupressure, massage can be repeated as often as is felt to be necessary with several sessions per hour usually being sufficient for painful conditions that have arisen suddenly. It is possible that as many as 20 sessions may be necessary for persistent conditions causing pain, with greater intervals of time between treatments as matters improve. It is not advisable to try anything that is at all complicated (or to treat an illness such as arthritis) and a trained practitioner will obviously be able to provide the best level of treatment and help. To contact a reputable practitioner who has completed the relevant training it is advisable to contact the appropriate professional body.

Acupuncture

This is an ancient Chinese therapy that involves inserting needles into the skin at specific points of the body. The word 'acupuncture' originated from a Dutch physician, William Ten Rhyne, who had been living in Japan during the latter part of the 17th century and it was he who introduced it to Europe. The term means literally 'prick with a needle'. The earliest textbook on acupuncture, dating from approximately 400 BC, was called *Nei Ching Su Wen*, which means 'Yellow Emperor's Classic of Internal Medicine'. Also recorded at about the same time was the successful saving of a patient's life by acupuncture, the person having been expected to die whilst in a coma. Legend has it that acupuncture was developed when it was realized that soldiers who recovered from arrow wounds were sometimes also healed of other diseases from which they were suffering. Acupuncture was very popular with British doctors in the early 1800s for pain relief and to treat fever. There was also a specific article on the successful treatment of rheumatism that appeared in *The Lancet*. Until the end of the Ching dynasty in China in 1911, acupuncture was slowly developed and improved, but then medicine from the West increased in popularity. However, more recently there has been a revival of interest and it is again widely practised throughout China. Also, nowadays the use of laser beams and electrical currents are found to give an increased stimulative effect when using acupuncture needles.

The specific points of the body into which acupuncture needles are inserted are located along 'meridians'. These are the pathways or energy channels and are believed to be related to the internal organs of the body. This energy is known as *qi* and the needles are used to decrease or increase the flow of energy, or to unblock it if it is impeded. Traditional Chinese medicine sees the body as being comprised of two natural forces known as the *yin* and *yang*. These two forces are complementary to each other but also opposing, the yin being the female force and calm and passive and also representing the dark, cold, swelling and moisture. The yang force is the male and is stimulating and aggressive, representing the heat and light, contraction and dryness. It is believed that the cause of ailments and diseases is due to an imbalance of these forces in the body, e.g. if a person is suffering from a headache or high blood pressure then this is because of an excess of yang. If, however, there is an excess of yin, this might result in tiredness, feeling cold and fluid retention .

The aim of acupuncture is to establish that there is an imbalance of yin and yang and to rectify it by using the needles at certain points on the body. Traditionally there were 365 points but more have been found in the intervening period and nowadays there can be as many as 2,000. There are 14 meridians, called after the organs they represent, e.g. the lung, kidney, heart and stomach as well as two organs unknown in orthodox medicine—the triple heater or warmer, which relates to the activity of the endocrine glands and the control of temperature. In addition, the pericardium is concerned with seasonal activity and also regulates the circulation of the blood. Of the 14 meridians, there are two, known as the *du,* or governor, and the *ren*, or conception, which both run straight up the body's midline, although the du is much shorter, extending from the head down to the mouth, while the ren starts at the chin and extends to the base of the trunk.

There are several factors that can change the flow of qi (also known as shi or ch'i), and they can be of an emotional, physical or environmental nature. The flow may be changed to become too slow or fast, or it can be diverted or blocked so that the incorrect organ is involved and the acupuncturist has to ensure that the flow returns to normal. There are many painful afflictions for which acupuncture can be used. In the West, it has been used primarily for rheumatism, back pain and arthritis, but it has also been used to alleviate other disorders such as stress, allergy, colitis, digestive troubles, insomnia, asthma, etc. It has been claimed that withdrawal symptoms (experienced by people stopping smoking and ceasing other forms of addiction) have been helped as well.

Acupuncture

Qualified acupuncturists complete a training course of three years duration and also need qualifications in the related disciplines of anatomy, pathology, physiology and diagnosis before they can belong to a professional association. It is very important that a fully qualified acupuncturist, who is a member of the relevant professional body, is consulted because at the present time, any unqualified person can use the title 'acupuncturist'.

At a consultation, the traditional acupuncturist uses a set method of ancient rules to determine the acupuncture points. The texture and colouring of the skin, type of skin, posture and movement and the tongue will all be examined and noted, as will the patient's voice. These different factors are all needed for the Chinese diagnosis. A number of questions will be asked concerning the diet, amount of exercise taken, lifestyle, fears and phobias, sleeping patterns and reactions to stress. Each wrist has six pulses, and each of these stand for a main organ and its function. The pulses are felt (known as palpating), and by this means acupuncturists are able to diagnose any problems relating to the flow of qi and if there is any disease present in the internal organs. The first consultation may last an hour, especially if detailed questioning is necessary along with the palpation.

The needles used in acupuncture are disposable and made of a fine stainless steel and come already sealed in a sterile pack. They can be sterilized by the acupuncturist in a machine known as an autoclave but using boiling water is not adequate for this purpose. (Diseases such as HIV and hepatitis can be passed on by using unsterilized needles.) Once the needle is inserted into the skin it is twisted between the acupuncturist's thumb and forefinger to spread or draw the energy from a point. The depth to which the needle is inserted can vary from just below the skin to up to 12mm (half an inch) and different sensations may be felt, such as a tingling around the area of insertion or a loss of sensation at that point. Up to 15 needles can be used but around five is generally sufficient. The length of time that they are left in varies from a few minutes to half an hour and this is dependent on a number of factors such as how the patient has reacted to previous treatment and the ailment from which he or she is suffering.

Patients can generally expect to feel an improvement after four to six sessions of therapy, the beneficial effects occurring gradually, particularly if the ailment has obvious and long-standing symptoms. Other diseases such as asthma will probably take longer before any definite improvement is felt. It is possible that some patients may not feel any improvement at all, or even feel worse after the first session and this is probably due to the energies in the body being over-stimulated. To correct this, the acupuncturist will gradually use fewer needles and for a shorter period of time. If no improvement is felt after about six to eight treatments, then it is doubtful whether acupuncture will be of any help. For general body maintenance and health, most traditional acupuncturists suggest that sessions be arranged at the time of seasonal changes.

There has been a great deal of research, particularly by the Chinese, who have produced many books detailing a high success rate for acupuncture in treating a variety of disorders. These results are, however, viewed cautiously in the West as methods of conducting clinical trials vary from East to West. Nevertheless trials have been carried out in the West and it has been discovered that a pain message can be stopped from reaching the brain using acupuncture. The signal would normally travel along a nerve but it is possible to 'close a gate' on the nerve, thereby preventing the message from reaching the brain, hence preventing the perception of pain. Acupuncture is believed to work by blocking the pain signal. However, doctors stress that pain can be a warning that something is wrong or of the occurrence of a particular disease, such as cancer, that requires an orthodox remedy or method of treatment.

It has also been discovered that there are substances, called endorphins and encephalins, produced by the body that are connected with pain relief. Studies from all over the world show that acupuncture stimulates the release of these opiates into the central nervous system, thereby giving pain relief. The amount of opiates released has a direct bearing on the degree of pain relief. Acupuncture is a widely used form of anaesthesia in China where, for suitable patients, it is said to be extremely effective (90 per cent). It is used successfully during childbirth, dentistry and for operations. Orthodox doctors in the West now accept that heat treatment, massage and needles used on a sensitive part of the skin afford relief from pain caused by disease elsewhere. These areas are known as trigger points, and they are not always situated close to the organ that is affected by disease. It has been found that approximately three-quarters of these trigger points are the same as the points used in Chinese acupuncture. Recent research has also shown that it is possible to find the acupuncture points by the use of electronic instruments as they register less electrical resistance than other areas of skin. As yet, no evidence has been found to substantiate the existence of meridians.

The Alexander Technique

This technique, which is based on correct posture so that the body is able to function naturally and with the minimum amount of muscular effort, was devised by Frederick Mathias Alexander (1869–1955). He was an Australian actor who found that he was losing his voice when performing but after rest his condition improved. Although he received medical help, the condition did not improve and it occurred to him that whilst acting he might be doing something that caused the problem. To see what this might be he performed his act in front of a mirror and saw what happened when he was about to speak. He experienced difficulty in breathing and lowered his head, thus making himself shorter. He realized that the strain of remembering his lines and having to project his voice, so that people furthest away in the audience would be able to hear, was causing him a great deal of stress and the way he reacted was a quite natural reflex action. In fact, even thinking about having to project his voice made the symptoms recur and from this he concluded that there must be a close connection between body and mind. He was determined to try and improve the situation and gradually, by watching and altering his stance and posture and his mental attitude to his performance on stage, matters improved. He was able to act and speak on stage and use his body in a more relaxed and natural fashion.

In 1904 Alexander travelled to London where he had decided to let others know about his method of retraining the body. He soon became very popular with other actors who appreciated the benefits of using his technique. Other public figures, such as the author Aldous Huxley, also benefited. Later he went to America, achieving considerable success and international recognition for his technique. At the age of 78 he suffered a stroke but by using his method he managed to regain the use of all his faculties—an achievement that amazed his doctors.

The Alexander technique is said to be completely harmless, encouraging an agreeable state between mind and body and is also helpful for a number of disorders such as headaches and back pain. Today, Alexander training schools can be found all over the world. A simple test to determine if people can benefit is to observe their posture. People frequently do not even stand correctly and this can encourage aches and pains if the body is unbalanced. It is incorrect to stand with round shoulders or to slouch. This often looks uncomfortable and discomfort may be felt. Sometimes people will hold themselves too erect and unbending, which again can have a bad effect. The correct posture and balance for the body needs the least muscular effort but the body will be aligned correctly. When walking one should not slouch, hold the head down or have the shoulders stooped. The head should be balanced correctly above the spine with the shoulders relaxed. It is suggested that the weight of the body should be felt being transferred from one foot to the other whilst walking.

Once a teacher has been consulted, all movements and how the body is used will be observed. Many muscles are used in everyday activities, and over the years bad habits can develop unconsciously, with stress also affecting the use of muscles. This can be demonstrated in people gripping a pen with too much force or holding the steering wheel of a car too tightly whilst driving. Muscular tension can be a serious problem affecting some people and the head, neck and back are forced out of line, which in turn leads to rounded shoulders with the head held forward and the back curved. If this situation is not altered and the body is not re-aligned correctly, the spine will become curved with a hump possibly developing. This leads to back pain and puts a strain on internal organs such as the chest and lungs.

No force is used by the teacher other than some gentle manipulation to start pupils off correctly. Some teachers use light pushing methods on the back and hips, etc, while others might first ensure that the pupil is relaxed and then pull gently on the neck, which stretches the body. Any bad postures will be corrected by the teacher and the pupil will be shown how best to alter this so that muscles will be used most effectively and with the least effort. Any manipulation that is used will be to ease the body into a more relaxed and natural position. It is helpful to be completely aware of using the technique not only on the body but also with the mind. With frequent use of the Alexander technique for posture and the release of tension, the muscles and the body should be used correctly with a consequent improvement in, for example, the manner of walking and sitting.

The length of time for each lesson can vary from about half an hour to three quarters of an hour and the number of lessons is usually between 10 and 30, by which time pupils should have gained sufficient knowledge to continue practising the technique by themselves. Once a person has learned how to improve posture, it will be found that he or she is taller and carrying the body in a more upright manner. The technique has been found to be of benefit to dancers, athletes and those having to speak in public. Other disorders claimed to have been treated successfully are depressive states, headaches caused by tension, anxiety, asthma, hypertension, respiratory problems, colitis, osteoarthritis and rheumatoid arthritis, sciatica and peptic ulcer.

The Alexander technique is recommended for all ages and types of people as their overall quality of life, both mental and physical, can be improved. People can learn how to resist stress and one eminent professor experienced a great improvement in a variety of ways: in quality of sleep; lessening of high blood pressure and improved mental awareness. He even found that his ability to play a musical instrument had improved.

The Alexander technique can be applied to two positions adopted every day, namely sitting in a chair and sitting at a desk. To be seated in the correct manner the head should be comfortably balanced, with no tension in the shoulders, and a small gap between the knees (if legs are crossed the spine and pelvis become out of line or twisted) and the soles of the feet should be flat on the floor. It is incorrect to sit with the head lowered and the shoulders slumped forward because the stomach becomes restricted and breathing may also be affected. On the other hand, it is also incorrect to hold the body in a stiff and erect position.

To sit correctly while working at a table, the body should be held upright but in a relaxed manner with any bending movement coming from the hips and with the seat flat on the chair. If writing, the pen should be held lightly and if using a computer one should ensure that the arms are relaxed and feel comfortable. The chair should be set at a comfortable height with regard to the level of the desk. It is incorrect to lean forward over a desk because this hampers breathing, or to hold the arms in a tense, tight manner.

There has been some scientific research carried out that concurs with the beliefs that Alexander formed, such as the relationship between mind and body (the thought of doing an action actually triggering a physical reaction or tension). Today, doctors do not have any opposition to the Alexander technique and may recommend it on occasions.

Aromatherapy

Aromatherapy is a method of healing using very concentrated essential oils that are often highly aromatic and are extracted from plants. Constituents of the oils confer the characteristic perfume or odour given off by a particular plant. Essential oils help the plant in some way to complete its cycle of growth and reproduction. For example, some oils may attract insects for the purpose of pollination; others may render it distasteful as a source of food. Any part of a plant—the stems, leaves, flowers, fruits, seeds, roots or bark—may produce essential oils or essences but often only in minute amounts. Different parts of the same plant may produce their own form of oil. An example of this is the orange, which produces oils with different properties in the flowers, fruits and leaves.

The therapeutic and medicinal properties of plant extracts have long been recognized and their use dates back to earliest times. Art and writings from the ancient civilizations of Egypt, China and Persia show that plant essences were used and valued by priests, physicians and healers. Plant essences have been used throughout the ages for healing—in incense for religious rituals, in perfumes and embalming ointments and for culinary purposes. There are many Biblical references that give an insight into the uses of plant oils and the high value that was attached to them. Throughout the course of human history the healing properties of plants and their essential oils has been recognized and most people probably had some knowledge about their use. It was only in more recent times, with the great developments in science and orthodox medicine, particularly the manufacture of antibiotics and synthetic drugs, that knowledge and interest in the older methods of healing declined. However, in the last few years there has been a great rekindling of interest in the practice of aromatherapy with many people turning to this form of treatment.

Extraction of essential oils

Since any part of a plant may produce essential oils, the method of extraction depends upon the site and accessibility of the essence in each particular case. The oils are produced by special minute cells or glands and are released naturally by the plant in small amounts over a prolonged period of time when needed. In order to harvest the oils in appreciable amounts, it is usually necessary to collect a large quantity of the part of the plant needed and to subject the material to a process that causes the oil glands to burst. One of the most common methods is *steam distillation*. The plant material is paced tightly into a press or still and steamed at a high temperature. This causes the oil glands to burst and the essential oil vaporises into the steam. This is then cooled to separate the oil from the water. Sometimes water is used for distillation rather than steam. Another method involved dissolving the plant material in a solvent or alcohol and is called *solvent extraction*. This involves placing the material in a centrifuge, which rotates at high speed, and then extracting the essential oils by means of a low temperature distillation process. Substances obtained in this way may be called *resins* or *absolutes*. A further method is called *maceration* in which the plant is soaked in hot oil. The plant cells collapse and release their essential oils, and the whole mixture is then separated and purified by a process called *defleurage*. If fat is used instead of oil, the process is called *enfleurage*. These methods produce a purer oil that is usually more expensive than one obtained by distillation. The essential oils used in aromatherapy tend to be costly as vast quantities of plant material are required to produce them and the methods used are complex and costly.

Storage and use of essential oils

Essential oils are highly concentrated, volatile and aromatic. They readily evaporate and change and deteriorate if exposed to light, heat and air. Hence pure oils need to be stored carefully in brown glass bottles at a moderate temperature away from direct light. They can be stored for one or two years in this way. For most purposes in aromatherapy, essential oils are used in a dilute form, being added either to water or to another oil, called the *base* or *carrier*.

The base is often a vegetable oil such as olive or safflower, which iboth have nutrient and beneficial properties. An essential/carrier oil mixture has a short useful life of two or three months and so they are usually mixed at the time of use and in small amounts.

Techniques used in aromatherapy

There are four techniques used in aromatherapy and these are *massage*, *bathing*, *inhalation* and *compresses*.

Massage is the most familiar method of treatment associated with aromatherapy. Essential oils are able to penetrate through the skin and are taken into the body, exerting healing and beneficial influences on internal tissues and organs. The oils used for massage are first diluted by being mixed with a base and should never be applied directly to the skin in their pure form in case of an adverse allergic reaction.

Bathing most people have experienced the benefits of relaxing in a hot bath to which a proprietary perfumed preparation has been added. Most of these preparations contain essential oils used in aromatherapy. The addition of a number of drops of an essential oil to the bath water can have great beneficial effects. It is soothing and relaxing, easing aches and pains, and can also have a stimulating effect, banishing tiredness and restoring energy, depending upon the type of oil that is used. In addition, there is the added benefit of inhaling the vapours of the oil as they evaporate from the hot water.

Inhalation isthought to be the most direct and rapid means of treatment. This is because the molecules of the volatile essential oil act directly on the olfactory organs and are immediately perceived by the brain. A popular method is the time-honoured one of *steam inhalation,* in which a few drops of essential oil are added to hot water in a bowl. The person sits with his or her face above the mixture and covers the head, face and bowl with a towel so that the vapours do not escape. This can be repeated up to three times a day but should not be undertaken by people suffering from asthma. Some essential oils can be applied directly to a handkerchief or onto a pillow and the vapours inhaled in this way.

Compresses to prepare a compress in aromatherapy, a few drops of essential oil are added to a proportion of hot or cold water and then a cloth is soaked in the mixture. The cloth is wrung out, (although kept fairly wet) and applied to the painful part, and is tied in place with clingfilm and a bandage. The compress

needs to be left in place for two hours before being changed. Usually, hot compresses are applied to chronic persistent pain. For conditions in which there is heat, inflammation, swelling and fever, a cold compress is generally indicated.

Essential oils may also be diluted with water and used in hand and foot baths if only a small area of the body needs to be treated. Some are appropriate for use as gargles and mouth washes, and are helpful in clearing up infections such as mouth ulcers. However, they should never be swallowed. Essential oils can be used effectively in the home by adding a few drops into a bowl of water or potpourri and leaving to stand in a room.

Mode of action of essential oils

Although the subject of a great deal of research, there is a lack of knowledge about how essential oils work in the body to produce their therapeutic effects. It is known that individual essential oils possess antiseptic, antibiotic, sedative, tonic and stimulating properties, and it is believed that they act in harmony with the natural defences of the body such as the immune system. Some oils, such as eucalyptus and rosemary, act as natural decongestants whereas others, such as sage, have a beneficial effect upon the circulation.

Conditions that may benefit from aromatherapy

A wide range of conditions and disorders may benefit from aromatherapy and it is considered to be a gentle treatment suitable for all age groups. It is especially beneficial for long-term chronic conditions, and the use of essential oils is believed by therapists to prevent the development of some illnesses. Conditions that may be relieved by aromatherapy include painful limbs, muscles and joints due to arthritic or rheumatic disorders, respiratory complaints, digestive disorders, skin conditions, throat and mouth infections, urinary tract infections and problems affecting the hair and scalp. Also, period pains, burns, insect bites and stings, headaches, high blood pressure, feverishness, menopausal symptoms, poor circulation and gout can benefit from aromatherapy. Aromatherapy is of great benefit in relieving stress and stress-related symptoms such as anxiety, insomnia and depression.

Many of the essential oils can be safely used at home and the basic techniques of use can soon be mastered. However, some should only be used by a trained aromatherapist and others must be avoided in certain conditions such as pregnancy. In some circumstances, massage is not considered to be advisable. It is wise to seek medical advice in the event of doubt or if the ailment is more than a minor one.

Consulting a professional aromatherapist

Aromatherapy is a holistic approach to healing hence the practitioner endeavours to build up a complete picture of the patient and his or her lifestyle, nature and family circumstances, as well as noting the symptoms which need to be to be treated. Depending upon the picture that is obtained, the aromatherapist decides upon the essential oil or oils that are most suitable and likely to prove most helpful in the circumstances that prevail. The aromatherapist has a wide ranging knowledge and experience upon which to draw. Many oils can be blended together for an enhanced effect and this is called a 'synergistic blend'. Many aromatherapists offer a massage and/or instruction on the use of the selected oils at home.

Examples of some essential oils

Basil is now grown in many countries of the world although it originates from Africa.The herb has a long history of medicinal and culinary use, and was familiar to the Ancient Egyptian and Greek civilizations. Basil is sacred in the Hindu religion and has many medicinal uses in India and other Eastern countries. The whole plant is subjected to a process of steam distillation to obtain the essential oil used in aromatherapy. Basil has a refreshing, invigorating effect and also has antiseptic properties. It is used in massage, inhalation and baths, and can help to relieve the symptoms of tiredness, colds and respiratory disorders, indigestion and digestive problems, and minor skin wounds and rashes. It can help to alleviate the symptoms of depression although it has a depressive effect if used to excess.

Bergamot oil of bergamot is obtained from a plant that is a native species of some Asian and Eastern countries. The oil was first used and traded in Italy and derives its name from the northern city of Bergamo. In Italian medicine, it was popular as a remedy for feverish illnesses and to expel intestinal worms. It has also been used in cosmetics and perfumes, as the flavouring of Earl Grey tea, and in other foods. The oil is squeezed from the peel of the fruits for use in aromatherapy. It has refreshing, soothing and antiseptic properties, and may be combined with eucalyptus to enhance its effects. It can be used in massage, inhalation and baths, and helps to relieve painful or itchy skin conditions such

as psoriasis. It is also used to treat cold sores, mouth and throat infections, shingles, ulcers and symptoms of depression and tiredness.

Eucalyptus is a native species of Australia and Tasmania but is now grown in many countries throughout the world. The plant has a characteristic pungent odour, and the oil obtained from it has disinfectant and antiseptic properties, clears the nasal passages and acts as a painkiller. The leaves and twigs are subjected to a process of steam distillation in order to obtain the essential oil used in aromatherapy. The diluted oil is used for muscular and rheumatic aches and pains, skin disorders such as ringworm, insect bites, headaches and neuralgia, shingles, respiratory and bronchitic infections and fevers. Eucalyptus is used in many household products and in remedies for coughs and colds.

Juniper is a native species of many northern countries and has a long history of medicinal use. It has stimulant, tonic and antiseptic properties with beneficial effects on the skin and the digestive and reproductive organs. It is used to relieve the symptoms of dermatitis, eczema, spots, and dry, sore and chafed skin. Also, it is helpful in the relief of gout and painful rheumatoid arthritis. It is beneficial in the treatment of stress and sleeplessness. In cases of debility, it helps by acting as a tonic for the digestion and boosting the appetite. It can be used in massage, baths and inhalation, and is a useful treatment for cystitis, haemorrhoids (piles) and menstrual problems. Juniper is also used in veterinary medicine and as an ingredient in some toiletries.

Lavender the highly perfumed lavender is a native species of the Mediterranean but has long been popular as a garden plant in Britain and many other countries. It has antiseptic, tonic and relaxing properties, and the essential oil used in aromatherapy is obtained by subjecting the flowers to a process of steam distillation. It is considered to be one of the safest preparations and is used in the treatment of a wide range of disorders. These include minor skin wounds and burns, insect bites, indigestion and digestive problems, muscle pains and strains, cystitis, period pains and premenstrual symptoms, headaches, depression and stress. Lavender is also widely used in perfumes, toiletries and household preparations.

Peppermint is a native plant of Europe with a long history of medicinal use dating back to the ancient civilizations of Egypt, Greece and Rome. Oil of peppermint is obtained by subjecting the flowering parts of the plant to a process of steam distillation. The essential oil of peppermint has a calming effect on the digestive tract and is excellent for the relief of indigestion, colic-type pains, nausea, travel and morning sickness. It is cooling and refreshing, and useful in the treatment of colds, respiratory symptoms and headaches. Peppermint is widely used in remedies for colds and indigestion, as a food flavouring, especially in confectionery, and in toothpaste.

Sage is a native plant of the northern coastal regions of the Mediterranean and has a long history of medicinal and culinary use dating back to the ancient civilizations of Greece and Rome. The essential oil used in aromatherapy is obtained by subjecting the dried leaves to a process of steam distillation. Sage has a stimulating effect upon the circulation and also has tonic, antiseptic, expectorant (when inhaled) and cooling properties. It is used to improve poor circulation, for sore throats, colds and viral infections, bronchitic and

catarrhal complaints, rheumatism, arthritic pains, joint sprains and strains, mouth infections and headaches. Sage is widely used as a flavouring in foods and in some household preparations and toiletries.

Ylang ylang is a native species of the Far Eastern islands of Indonesia, the Philippines, Java and Madagascar. To obtain the essential oil used in aromatherapy, the flowers are subjected to a process of steam distillation. The oil has antiseptic and relaxing properties and is also believed to be an aphrodisiac. It has a calming effect on the heart-beat rate and can be used to relieve palpitations, tachycardia, hypertension (raised blood pressure), depression and shock. It has a tonic effect upon the skin and is beneficial in the treatment of nervous complaints. Ylang ylang is used in perfumes and toiletries and as a flavouring in the food industry.

Chiropractic

The word chiropractic originates from two Greek words *kheir*, which means 'hand', and *praktikos*, which means 'practical'. A school of chiropractic was established in about 1895 by a healer called Daniel Palmer (1845–1913). He was able to cure a man's deafness that had occurred when he bent down and felt a bone click. Upon examination Palmer discovered that some bones of the man's spine had become displaced. After successful manipulation the man regained his hearing. Palmer formed the opinion that if there was any displacement in the skeleton this could affect the function of nerves, either increasing or decreasing their action and thereby resulting in a malfunction i.e. a disease.

Chiropractic is used to relieve pain by manipulation and to correct any problems that are present in joints and muscles but especially the spine. Like osteopathy, no use is made of surgery or drugs. If there are any spinal disorders they can cause widespread problems elsewhere in the body such as the hip, leg or arm and can also initiate lumbago, sciatica, a slipped disc or other back problems. It is even possible that spinal problems can result in seemingly unrelated problems such as catarrh, migraine, asthma, constipation, stress, etc. However, the majority of a chiropractor's patients suffer mainly from neck and back pain. People suffering from whiplash injuries sustained in car accidents commonly seek the help of a chiropractor. The whiplash effect is caused when the head is violently wrenched either forwards or backwards at the time of impact .

Another common problem that chiropractors treat is headaches, and it is often the case that tension is the underlying cause as it makes the neck muscles contract. Athletes can also obtain relief from injuries such as tennis elbow, pulled muscles, injured ligaments and sprains, etc. As well as the normal methods of manipulating joints, the chiropractor may decide it is necessary to use applications of ice or heat to relieve the injury.

Children can also benefit from treatment by a chiropractor, as there may be some slight accident that occurs in their early years that can reappear in adult life in the form of back pain. It can easily happen, for example, when a child learns to walk and bumps into furniture, or when a baby falls out of a cot. This could result in some damage to the spine that will show only in adult life when a person experiences back pain. At birth, a baby's neck may be injured or the spine may be strained if the use of forceps is necessary, and this can result in headaches and neck problems as he or she grows to maturity. This early type of injury could also account for what is known as 'growing pains', when the real problem is actually damage that has been done to the bones or muscles. If a parent has any worries it is best to consult a doctor and it is possible that the child will be recommended to see a qualified chiropractor. To avoid any problems in adult life, chiropractors recommend that children have occasional examinations to detect any damage or displacement in bones and muscles.

As well as babies and children, adults of all ages can benefit from chiropractic. There are some people who regularly take painkillers for painful joints or back pain, but this does not deal with the root cause of the pain, only the symptoms that are produced. It is claimed that chiropractic could be of considerable help in giving treatment to these people. Many pregnant women experience backache at some stage during their pregnancy because of the extra weight that is placed on the spine, and they also may find it difficult keeping their balance. At the time of giving birth, changes take place in the pelvis and joints at the bottom of the spine and this can be a cause of back pain. Lifting and carrying babies, if not done correctly, can also damage the spine and thereby make the back painful.

It is essential that any chiropractor is fully qualified and registered with the relevant professional association. At the initial visit, a patient will be for asked details of his or her case history, including the present problem, and during the examination painful and tender areas will be noted and joints will be checked to see whether they are functioning correctly or not. X-rays are frequently used by chiropractors as these help them to make a detailed diagnosis since they can show signs of bone disease, fractures or arthritis as well as the spine's condition. After the initial visit, any treatment will normally begin as soon as the patient has been informed of the chiropractor's diagnosis. If it has been decided that chiropractic therapy will not be of any benefit, the patient will be advised accordingly.

For treatment, underwear and/or a robe will be worn, and the patient will either lie, sit or stand on a specially designed couch. Chiropractors use their hands in a skilful way to effect the different manipulative techniques. If it is decided that manipulation is necessary to treat a painful lumbar joint, the patient will need to lie on his or her side. The upper and lower spine will then be rotated manually but in opposite ways. This manipulation will have the effect of partially locking the joint that is being treated, and the upper leg is usually flexed to aid the procedure. The vertebra that is immediately below or above the joint will then be felt by the chiropractor, and the combination of how the patient is lying, coupled with gentle pressure applied by the chiropractor's hand, will move the joint to its furthest extent of normal movement. There will then be a very quick push applied on the vertebra, which results in its movement being extended further than normal, ensuring that full use of the joint is regained. This is due to the muscles that surround the joint being suddenly stretched, which has the effect of relaxing the muscles of the spine that work upon the joint. This alteration should cause the joint to be able to be used more naturally and should not be a painful procedure.

There can be a variety of effects felt after treatment—some patients may feel sore or stiff, or may ache some time after the treatment, while others will experience the lifting of pain at once. In some cases there may be a need for multiple treatments, perhaps four or more, before improvement is felt. On the whole, problems that have been troubling a patient for a considerable time (chronic) will need more therapy than anything that occurs quickly and is very painful (acute).

Although there is only quite a small number of chiropractors in the UK—yet this numbers is increasing—there is a degree of contact and liaison between them and doctors. It is generally accepted that chiropractic is an effective remedy for bone and muscular problems, and the majority of doctors would be happy to accept a chiropractor's diagnosis and treatment, although the treatment of any general diseases, such as diabetes or asthma, would not be viewed in the same manner.

Herbal Medicine

History of the use of herbal remedies

The medicinal use of herbs is said to be as old as mankind itself. In early civilizations, food and medicine were linked and many plants were eaten for their health-giving properties. In ancient Egypt, the slave workers were given a daily ration of garlic to help fight off the many fevers and infections that were common at that time. The first written records of herbs and their beneficial properties were compiled by the ancient Egyptians. Most of our knowledge and use of herbs can be traced back to the Egyptian priests who also practised herbal medicine. Records dating back to 1500 BC listed medicinal herbs, including caraway and cinnamon.

The ancient Greeks and Romans also carried out herbal medicine, and as they invaded new lands their doctors encountered new herbs and introduced herbs such as rosemary or lavender into new areas. Other cultures with a history of herbal medicine are the Chinese and the Indians. In Britain, the use of herbs developed along with the establishment of monasteries around the country, each of which had its own herb garden for use in treating both the monks and the local people. In some areas, particularly Wales and Scotland, Druids and other Celtic healers are thought to have had an oral tradition of herbalism, where medicine was mixed with religion and ritual.

Over time, these healers and their knowledge led to the writing of the first 'herbals', which rapidly rose in importance and distribution upon the advent of the printing press in the 15th century. John Parkinson of London wrote a herbal around 1630, listing useful plants. Many herbalists set up their own apothecary shops, including the famous Nicholas Culpepper (1616–1654) whose most famous work is *The Complete Herbal and English Physician, Enlarged,* published in 1649. Then in 1812, Henry Potter started a business supplying herbs and dealing in leeches. By this time a huge amount of traditional knowledge and folklore on medicinal herbs was available from Britain, Europe, the Middle East, Asia and the Americas. This promoted Potter to write *Potter's Encyclopaedia of Botanical Drugs and Preparations*, which is still published today.

It was in this period that scientifically inspired conventional medicine rose in popularity, sending herbal medicine into a decline. In rural areas, herbal medicine continued to thrive in local folklore, traditions and practices. In 1864 the National Association (later Institute) of Medical Herbalists was established, to organize training of herbal medicine practitioners and to maintain standards of practice. From 1864 until the early part of this century, the Institute fought attempts to ban herbal medicine and over time public interest in herbal medicine has increased, particularly over the last 20 years. This move away from synthetic drugs is partly due to possible side effects, bad publicity, and, in some instances, a mistrust of the medical and pharmacological industries. The more natural appearance of herbal remedies has led to its growing support and popularity. Herbs from America have been incorporated with common remedies and scientific research into herbs and their active ingredients has confirmed their healing power and enlarged the range of medicinal herbs used today.

Herbal medicine can be viewed as the precursor of modern pharmacology, but today it continues as an effective and more natural method of treating and preventing illness. Globally, herbal medicine is three to four times more commonly practised than conventional medicine.

Forms of herbal preparations

capsule this is a gelatine container for swallowing and holding oils or balsams that would otherwise be difficult to administer due to their unpleasant taste or smell. It is used for cod liver oil and castor oil.

decoction this is prepared using cut, bruised or ground bark and roots placed into a stainless steel or enamel pan (not aluminium) with cold water poured on. The mixture is boiled for 20–30 minutes, cooled and strained. It is best drunk when warm.

herbal dressing this may be a compress or poultice A compress is made of cloth or cotton wool soaked in cold or warm herbal decoctions or infusions while a poultice can be made with fresh or dried herbs. Bruised fresh herbs are applied directly to the affected area and dried herbs are made into a paste with water and placed on gauze on the required area. Both dressings are very effective in easing pain, swelling and inflammation of the skin and tissues.

infusion this liquid is made from ground or bruised roots, bark, herbs or seeds, by pouring boiling water onto the herb and leaving it to stand for 10–30 minutes, possibly stirring the mixture occasionally. The resultant liquid is strained and used. Cold infusions may be made if the active principles are yielded from the herb without heat. Today, infusions may be packaged into teabags for convenience.

liquid extract this preparation, if correctly made, is the most concentrated fluid form in which herbal drugs may be obtained and, as such, is very popular and convenient. Each herb is treated by various means dependent upon the individual properties of the herb, e.g. cold percolation, high pressure, evaporation by heat in a vacuum. These extracts are commonly held in a household stock of domestic remedies.

pessary similar to suppositories, but it is used in female complaints to apply a preparation to the walls of the vagina and cervix.

pill probably the best known and most widely used herbal preparation. It is normally composed of concentrated extracts and alkaloids, in combination with active crude drugs. The pill may be coated with sugar or another pleasant-tasting substance that is readily soluble in the stomach.

solid extract this type of preparation is prepared by evaporating the fresh juices or strong infusions of herbal drugs to the consistency of honey. It may also be prepared from an alcoholic tincture base. It is used mainly to produce pills, plasters, ointments and compressed tablets.

suppository this preparation is a small cone of a convenient and easily soluble base with herbal extracts added, which is used to apply medicines to the rectum. It is very effective in the treatment of piles, cancers, etc.

tablet this is made by compressing drugs into a small compass. It is more easily administered and has a quicker action as it dissolves more rapidly in the stomach.

tincture this is the most prescribed form of herbal medicine. It is based on alcohol and, as such, removes certain active principles from herbs that will not dissolve in water, or in the presence of heat. The tincture produced is long-lasting, highly concentrated and only needs to be taken in small doses for beneficial effects. The ground or chopped dried herb is placed in a container with 40 per cent alcohol such as gin or vodka and left for two weeks. The tincture is then decanted into a dark bottle and sealed before use.

Medical terms

In homoeopathy and herbal treatments there are numerous terms used. Listed below are some of the more common terms likely to be encountered in the example herbs provided in this section.

alterative a term given to a substance that speeds up the renewal of the tissues, so that they can carry out their functions more effectively.

anodyne a drug that eases and soothes pain.

anthelmintic a substance that causes the death or expulsion of parasitic worms.

antiperiodic a drug that prevents the return of recurring diseases, e.g. malaria.

antiscorbutic a substance that prevents scurvy and contains necessary vitamins, e.g. vitamin C.

antiseptic a substance that prevents the growth of disease-causing microorganisms, e.g. bacteria, without causing damage to living tissue. It is applied to wounds to cleanse them and prevent infection.

antispasmodic a drug that diminishes muscle spasms.

aperient a medicine that produces a natural movement of the bowel.

aphrodisiac a compound that excites the sexual organs.

aromatic a substance that has an aroma.

astringent a substance that causes cells to contract by losing proteins from their surface. This causes localized contraction of blood vessels and tissues.

balsamic a substance that contains resins and benzoic acid and that is used to alleviate colds and abrasions.

bitter a drug that is bitter-tasting and is used to stimulate the appetite.

cardiac compounds that have some effect on the heart.

carminative a preparation to relieve flatulence and griping.

cathartic a compound that produces an evacuation of the bowels.

cooling a substance that reduces the temperature and cools the skin.

demulcent a substance that soothes and protects the alimentary canal.

deobstruent a compound that is said to clear obstructions, and open the natural passages of the body.

detergent a substance that has a cleansing action, either internally or on the skin.

diaphoretic a term given to drugs that promote perspiration.

diuretics applied to substances that stimulate the kidneys and increase urine and solute production.

emetic a drug that induces vomiting.

emmenagogue a compound that is able to excite the menstrual discharge.

emollient a substance that softens or soothes the skin.

expectorant a group of drugs that are taken to help in the removal of secretions from the lungs, bronchi and trachea.

febrifuge a substance that reduces fever.

galactogogue an agent that stimulates the production of breast milk or increases milk flow.

hydrogogue applied to substances that have the property of removing accumulations of water or serum.

hypnotic drugs or substances that induce sleep.

irritant a general term encompassing any agent that causes irritation of a tissue.

laxative a substance that is taken to evacuate the bowel or soften stools.

mydriatic a compound that cause dilation of the pupil.

nervine a name given to drugs that are used to restore the nerves to their natural state.

narcotic a drug that leads to a stupor and complete loss of awareness.

nutritive compounds that are nourishing to the body.

pectoral applied to drugs that are a remedy in treating chest and lung complaints.

purgative the name given to drugs or other measures that produce evacuation of the bowels. This has normally a more severe effect than aperients or laxatives.

refrigerant a substance that relieves thirst and produces a feeling of coolness.

resolvent a substance that is applied to swellings to reduce them in size.

rubefacient a compound that causes the skin to redden and peel off. Causes blisters and inflammation.

sedative a drug that lessens tension, anxiety and soothes over-excitement of the nervous system.

stimulant a drug or other agent that increases the activity of an organ or system within the body.

stomachic name given to drugs that treat stomach disorders.

styptic applications that check bleeding by blood vessel contraction or by causing rapid blood clotting.

sudorific a drug or agent that produces copious perspiration.

taenicide drugs that are used to expel tapeworms from the body.

tonic substances that are traditionally thought to give strength and vigour to the body and that are said to produce a feeling of wellbeing.

vermifuge a substance that kills, or expels, worms from the intestines.

vulnerary a drug that is said to be good at healing wounds.

Examples of herbs

Aconite *Aconitum napellus. Common name*: Monkshood, blue rocket, friar's cap, wolfsbane.
Occurrence: indigenous to mountain slopes in the Alps and Pyrenees. Introduced into England very early, before 900 AD.
Parts used: the leaves used fresh and the root when dried. It contains alkaloidal material—aconitine, benzaconine and aconine amongst other compounds.
Medicinal uses: the plant is poisonous and should not be used except under medical advice. It is an anodyne, diaphoretic, febrifuge and sedative. Used for reducing fever and inflammation in the treatment of catarrh, tonsillitis and croup. It may be used in controlling heart spasm.
Administered as: tincture, liniment and occasionally as hypodermic injection.

Anemone wood *Anemone nemorosa. Common name*: Crowfoot, windflower, smell fox.
Occurrence: found in woods and thickets across Great Britain.
Parts used: the root, leaves and juice.
Medicinal uses: this species of plant is much less widely used than it has been previously. It used to be good for leprosy, lethargy, eye inflammation and headaches. An ointment made of the leaves is said to be effective in cleansing malignant ulcers.
Administered as: decoction, fresh leaves and root, ointment.

Anemone pulsatilla *Anemone pulsatilla. Common name*: Pasque flower, meadow anemone, wind flower
Occurrence: found locally in chalk downs and limestone areas of England.
Parts used: the whole herb. It produces oil of anemone upon distillation with water.
Medicinal uses: nervine, antispasmodic, alterative and diaphoretic. It is beneficial in disorders of mucous membranes and of the respiratory and digestive passages. Can be used to treat asthma, whooping cough and bronchitis.
Administered as: fluid extract.

Balm *Melissa officinalis. Common name*: Sweet balm, lemon balm, honey plant, cure-all.

Occurrence: a common garden plant in Great Britain that was naturalized into southern England at a very early period.

Parts used: the herb.

Medicinal uses: as a carminative, diaphoretic, or febrifuge. It can be made into a cooling tea for fever patients and balm is often used in combination with other herbs to treat colds and fever.

Administered as: an infusion.

Belladonna *Atropa belladonna. Common name*: Deadly nightshade, devil's cherries, dwale, black cherry, devil's herb, great morel.

Occurrence: native to central and southern Europe but commonly grows in England.

Parts used: the roots and leaves. The root contains several alkaloid compounds including hyoscyamine, atropine and belladonnine. The same alkaloids are present in the leaves but the amount of each compound varies according to plant type and methods of storing and drying leaves.

Medicinal uses: as a narcotic, diuretic, sedative, mydriatic, antispasmodic. The drug is used as an anodyne in febrile conditions, night sweats and coughs. It is valuable in treating eye diseases and is used as a pain-relieving lotion to treat neuralgia, gout, rheumatism and sciatica. Belladonna is an extremely poisonous plant and should always be used under medical supervision. Cases of accidental poisoning and death are well known. Despite this, it is a valuable drug used to treat a wide range of disease.

Administered as: a liquid extract that is used to produce alcoholic extracts, plasters, liniment, suppositories, tincture and ointment.

Broom *Cytisus scoparius. Common name*: Broom tops, Irish tops, basam, bizzom, browne, brum, bream, green broom.

Occurrence: indigenous to England and commonly found on heathland throughout Great Britain, Europe and northern Asia.

Parts used: the young herbaceous tops that contain sparteine and scoparin as the active components.

Medicinal uses: diuretic and cathartic. The broom tops may be used as a decoction or infusion to aid dropsy, while if the tops are pressed and treated broom juice is obtained. This fluid extract is generally used in combination with other diuretic compounds. An infusion of broom, agrimony and dandelion root is excellent in remedying bladder, kidney and liver trouble. *Cytisus* should be used carefully as the sparteine has a strong effect on the heart and, depending upon dose, can cause weakness of the heart similar to that caused by hemlock (*Conium maculatum*). Death can occur in extreme cases if the respiratory organ's activity is impaired.

Administered as: fluid extract and infusion.

Chamomile *Anthemis nobilis. Common name*: Roman chamomile, double chamomile, manzanilla (Spanish), maythen (Saxon).

Occurrence: a low-growing plant found wild in the British Isles.

Parts used: the flowers and herb. The active principles therein are a volatile oil, anthemic acid, tannic acid and a glucoside.

Medicinal uses: tonic, stomachic, anodyne and antispasmodic. An infusion of chamomile tea was once thought to be a remedy for hysterical and nervous afflictions in women, as well as an emmenagogue. It has a powerful soothing and sedative effect that is harmless. A tincture is used to cure diarrhoea in children and it is used with purgatives to prevent griping, and as a tonic it helps dropsy. Externally, it can be applied alone or with other herbs as a poultice to relieve pain, swellings, inflammation and neuralgia. Its strong antiseptic properties make it invaluable for reducing swelling of the face due to abscess or injury. As a lotion, the flowers are good for resolving toothache and earache. The herb itself is an ingredient in herb beers. The use of chamomile can be dated back to ancient Egyptian times when they dedicated the plant to the sun because of its extensive healing properties.

Administered as: decoction, infusion, fluid extract and essential oil.

Clover, Red *Trifolium pratense. Common name*: Trefoil, purple clover.

Occurrence: widely distributed in Britain and Europe.

Parts used: the flowers.

Medicinal uses: alterative, sedative, antispasmodic. The fluid extract or infusion are excellent in treating bronchial and whooping coughs. External application of the herb in a poultice has been used on cancerous growths.

Administered as: fluid extract and infusion.

Coltsfoot *Tussilago farfara. Common name*: Coughwort, hallfoot, horsehoof, ass's foot, foalswort, fieldhove, bullsfoot, donnhove.

Occurrence: commonly found wild on waste ground and riverbanks in Great Britain.

Parts used: the leaves, flowers and root.

Medicinal uses: demulcent, expectorant and tonic. Coltsfoot is one of the most popular cough remedies and is generally taken in conjunction with horehound, marshmallow or ground ivy. It has been called 'Nature's best herb for the lungs' and it was recommended that the leaves be smoked to relieve a cough. Today, it forms the basis of British herb tobacco along with bogbean, eyebright, wood betony, rosemary, thyme, lavender and chamomile, which is said to relieve asthma, catarrh, bronchitis and lung troubles.

Administered as: syrup or smoked when dried.

Comfrey *Symphytum officinale. Common name*: Common comfrey, knitbone, knitback, bruisewort, slippery root, gum plant, consolida, ass ear, blackwort.

Occurrence: a native of Europe and temperate Asia but is common throughout England by rivers and ditches.

Parts used: the root and leaves. The roots contain a large quantity of mucilage, choline and allantoin.

Medicinal uses: demulcent, mildly astringent, expectorant and vulnerary. It is frequently used in pulmonary complaints, to soothe intestinal trouble and is a gentle remedy for diarrhoea and dysentery. A strong decoction or tea is administered in cases of internal haemorrhage whether it is the lungs, stomach, bowels or haemorrhoids. Externally, the leaves have been used as a poultice to promote healing of severe cuts, ulcers and abscesses and to reduce swelling, sprains and bruises. Allantoin is known to reduce swelling round damaged or fractured bones, thus allowing healing to occur faster and more thoroughly.

Administered as: a decoction, poultice and liquid extract.

Dandelion *Taraxacum officinale. Common name*: Priest's crown, swine's snout.

Occurrence: widely found across the northern temperate zone in pastures, meadows and waste ground.

Parts used: the root and leaves. The main constituents of the root are taraxacin, a bitter substance, and taraxacerin, an acid resin, along with the sugar inulin.

Medicinal uses: diuretic, tonic and slightly aperient. It acts as a general body stimulant, but chiefly acts on the liver and kidneys. Dandelion is used as a bitter tonic in atonic dyspepsia as a mild laxative and to promote increased appetite and digestion. The herb is best used in combination with other herbs and is used in many patent medicines. Roasted dandelion root is also used as a coffee substitute and helps ease dyspepsia, gout and rheumatism.

Administered as: fluid extract, decoction, infusion, tincture, solid extract and juice.

Elder *Sambucus nigra. Common name*: black elder, common elder, European elder, pipe tree, bore tree, bour tree.

Occurrence: frequently seen in Europe and Great Britain.

Parts used: the bark, leaves, flowers and berries.

Medicinal uses: the bark is a strong purgative and in large doses is emetic. It has been used successfully in epilepsy, and a tincture of the young bark relieves asthmatic symptoms and croup in children. A tea made from elder roots was highly effective against dropsy. The leaves are used both fresh and dried and contain the alkaloid sambucine, a glucoside called sambunigrin, as well as hydrogenic acid, cane sugar and potassium nitrate amongst other compounds. The leaves are used in preparation of green elder ointment, which is used domestically for bruises, haemorrhoids, sprains, chilblains and applied to wounds. Elder leaves have the same purgative effects as the bark (but produce more nausea) and have expectorant, diaphoretic and diuretic actions.

The elder flowers are either distilled into elderflower water or dried. The water is used in eye and skin lotions as it is mildly astringent and a gentle stimulant. When infused, the dried flowers make elderflower tea, which is gently laxative, aperient and diaphoretic. It is an old-fashioned remedy for colds and influenza when taken hot, before bed. The tea is also recommended to be drunk before breakfast as a blood purifier. Elder flowers would also be made into a lotion or poultice for use on inflamed areas and into an ointment that was good on wounds, scalds and burns. The ointment was used on the battlefields in World War I and at home for chapped hands and chilblains.

Administered as: an infusion, tincture, ointment, syrup, lotion, distilled water, poultice and dried powder.

Evening primrose *Oenothera biennis. Common name*: Tree primrose, sun drop.

Occurrence: native to North America but has been naturalized to British and European gardens.

Parts used: the bark and leaves.

Medicinal uses: astringent, sedative. The drug from this herb is not extensively used but has been of benefit in treating gastro-intestinal disorders, dyspepsia, liver torpor and in female problems in association with pelvic illness. It has also been successfully used in whooping cough and spasmodic asthma.

Administered as: liquid extract.

Fennel *Foeniculum vulgare. Common name*: Hinojo, fenkel, sweet fennel, wild fennel.
Occurrence: found wild in most areas of temperate Europe and generally considered indigenous to the shores of the Mediterranean. It is cultivated for medicinal benefit in France, Russia, India and Persia.
Parts used: the seeds, leaves and roots. The roots are rarely used in herbal medicine today. The essential oil is separated by distillation with water. Fennel oil varies in quality and composition dependent upon where, and under what conditions, the fennel was grown.
Medicinal uses: aromatic, stimulant, carminative and stomachic. The herb is principally used with purgatives to allay their tendency to griping, and the seeds form an ingredient of the compound liquorice powder. Fennel water also acts in a similar manner to dill water in correcting infant flatulence.
Administered as: fluid extract, distilled water, essential oil.

Foxglove *Digitalis purpurea. Common name*: Witch's gloves, dead men's bells, fairy's glove, gloves of Our Lady, bloody fingers, Virgin's glove, fairy caps, folk's glove, fairy thimbles, fair women's plant.
Occurrence: indigenous and widely distributed throughout Great Britain and Europe.
Parts used: the leaves, which contain four important glucosides—digitoxin, digitalin, digitalein and digitonin—of which the first three listed are cardiac stimulants.
Medicinal uses: cardiac tonic, sedative, diuretic. Administering digitalis increases the activity of all forms of muscle tissue, particularly the heart and arterioles. It causes a very high rise in blood pressure and the pulse is slowed and becomes regular. Digitalis causes the heart to contract in size, allowing increased blood flow and nutrient delivery to the organ. It also acts on the kidneys and is a good remedy for dropsy, particularly when it is connected with cardiac problems. The drug has benefits in treating internal haemorrhage, epilepsy, inflammatory diseases and delirium tremens. Digitalis has a cumulative action whereby it is liable to accumulate in the body and then have poisonous effects. It should only be used under medical advice. Digitalis is an excellent antidote in aconite poisoning when given as a hypodermic injection.
Administered as: tincture, infusion, powdered leaves, injection.

Golden rod *Solidago virgaurea. Common name*: Verge d'or, solidago, woundwort, Aaron's Rod.

Occurrence: this is a plant normally found wild in woods in Great Britain, Europe, Central Asia and North America but it is also a common garden plant.
Parts used: the leaves contain tannin, with some bitter and astringent chemicals that are unknown.
Medicinal uses: aromatic, stimulant, carminative. This herb is astringent and diuretic and is highly effective in curing gravel and urinary stones. It aids weak digestion, stops sickness and is very good against diphtheria. As a warm infusion it is a good diaphoretic drug and is used as such to help painful menstruation and amenorrhoea (absence or stopping of menstrual periods).
Administered as: fluid extract, infusion, spray.

Hemlock *Conium maculatum. Common name*: Herb bennet, spotted conebane, musquash root, beaver poison, poison hemlock, poison parsley, spotted hemlock, vex, vecksies.
Occurrence: common in hedges, meadows, waste ground and stream banks throughout Europe and is also found in temperate Asia and north Africa.
Parts used: the leaves, fruits and seeds. The most important constituent of hemlock leaves is the alkaloid coniine, which is poisonous, with a disagreeable odour. Other alkaloids in the plant include methyl-coniine, conhydrine, pseudoconhydrine, ethyl piperidine.
Medicinal uses: sedative, antispasmodic, anodyne. The drug acts on the centres of motion and causes paralysis and so it is used to remedy nervous motor excitability, e.g. teething, cramp and muscle spasms of the larynx and gullet. When inhaled, hemlock is said to be good in relieving coughs, bronchitis, whooping cough and asthma. The method of action of *Conium* means it is directly antagonistic to the effects of strychnine, from nux vomica (*Strychnos nux-vomica*), and it is used as an antidote to strychnine poisoning and similar poisons. Hemlock has to be administered with care as narcotic poisoning may result from internal application and overdoses induce paralysis, with loss of speech and depression of respiratory function leading to death. Antidotes to hemlock poisoning are tannic acid, stimulants, e.g. coffee, mustard and castor oil.
Administered as: powdered leaves, fluid extract, tincture, expressed juice of the leaves and solid extract.

Honeysuckle *Lonicera caprifolium. Common name*: Dutch honeysuckle, goat's leaf, perfoliate honeysuckle.
Occurrence: it grows freely in Europe, Great Britain and through the northern temperate zone.
Parts used: the dried flowers and leaves.

Medicinal uses: expectorant, laxative. A syrup made of the flowers is used for respiratory diseases and asthma. A decoction of the leaves is laxative and is also good against diseases of the liver and spleen, and in gargles.

Administered as: syrup, decoction.

Juniper *Juniperus communis*.

Occurrence: a common shrub native to Great Britain and widely distributed through many parts of the world.

Parts used: the berry and leaves.

Medicinal uses: the oil of juniper obtained from the ripe berries is stomachic, diuretic and carminative and is used to treat indigestion and flatulence as well as kidney and bladder diseases. The main use of juniper is in dropsy, and aiding other diuretic herbs to ease the disease.

Administered as: essential oil from berries, essential oil from wood, fluid extract, liquid extract, solid extract.

Larch *Pinus larix. Common name: Larix europaea, Abies larix, Larix decidua, Laricus cortex,* European larch, Venice turpentine.

Occurrence: indigenous to hilly regions of central Europe, but was introduced into Great Britain in 1639.

Parts used: the inner bark, which contains tannic acid, larixinic acid and turpentine.

Medicinal uses: stimulant, diuretic, astringent, balsamic and expectorant. It is very useful as an external application for eczema and psoriasis. However, it is mainly used as a stimulant expectorant in chronic bronchitisand for internal haemorrhage and cystitis. Larch turpentine has also been suggested as an antidote in cyanide or opium poisoning and has been used as a hospital disinfectant.

Administered as: fluid extract or syrup.

Liquorice *Glycyrrhiza glabra. Common name*: Licorice, lycorys, *Liquiriha officinalis*.

Occurrence: a shrub native to southeast Europe and southwest Asia and cultivated in the British Isles.

Parts used: the root. The chief compound in the root is glychrrhizin along with sugar, starch, gum, tannin and resin.

Medicinal uses: demulcent, pectoral, emollient. A very popular and well-known remedy for coughs, consumption and chest complaints. Liquorice extract is included in cough lozenges and pastilles, with sedatives and expectorants. An infusion of bruised root and flax (linseed) is good for irritable coughs, sore throats and laryngitis. Liquorice is used to a greater extent as a medicine in China and other eastern countries. The herb is used by brewers to give colour to porter and stout and is employed in the manufacture of chewing or smoking tobacco.

Administered as: powdered root, fluid extract, infusion, solid extract.

Meadowsweet *Spiraea ulmaria. Common name*: Meadsweet, dolloff, queen of the meadow, bridewort, lady of the meadow.

Occurrence: a common wild plant in the British Isles, found growing in meadows or woods.

Parts used: the herb.

Medicinal uses: aromatic, astringent, diuretic, alterative. This herb is good against diarrhoea, stomach complaints and blood disorders. It is highly recommended for children's diarrhoea and dropsy and was used as a decoction in wine to reduce fevers. Meadowsweet makes a pleasant everyday drink when infused and sweetened with honey. It is also included in many herb beers.

Administered as: infusion, decoction.

Nettle *Urtica dioica, Urtica urens. Common name*: Common nettle, stinging nettle.

Occurrence: widely distributed throughout temperate Europe and Asia, Japan, South Africa and Australia.

Parts used: the whole herb, which contains formic acid, mucilage, mineral salts, ammonia and carbonic acid.

Medicinal uses: astringent, stimulating, diuretic, tonic. The herb is anti-asthmatic and the juice of the nettle will relieve bronchial and asthmatic troubles, as will the dried leaves when burnt and inhaled. The seeds are taken as an infusion or in wine to ease consumption or ague. Nettles are used widely as a food source and are made into puddings, tea, beer, juice and used as a vegetable. A hair tonic or lotion can also be made from the herb. In the Highlands of Scotland, they were chopped, added to egg white and applied to the temples as a cure for insomnia.

Administered as: expressed juice, infusion, decoction, seeds, dried herb, dietary item.

Peppermint *Mentha piperita. Common name*: Brandy mint, curled mint, balm mint.

Occurrence: found across Europe, was introduced into Britain and grows widely in damp places and waste ground.

Parts used: the herb and distilled oil. The plant contains peppermint oil, which is composed of menthol, menthyl acetate and isovalerate, menthone, cineol, pinene and limonene. The medicinal qualities are found in the alcoholic chemicals.

Medicinal uses: stimulant, antispasmodic, carminative, stomachic, oil of peppermint is extensively used in both medicine and commerce. It is good in dyspepsia, flatulence, colic and abdominal cramps. The oil allays sickness and nausea, is used for chorea and diarrhoea but is normally used with other medicines to disguise unpalatable tastes and effects. Peppermint water is in most general use and is used to raise body temperature and induce perspiration. Peppermint tea can help ward off colds and influenza at an early stage, can calm heart palpitations and is used to reduce the appetite.

Administered as: infusion, distilled water, spirit, essential oil and fluid extract.

Primrose *Primula vulgaris*.
Occurrence: a common wild flower found in woods, hedgerows and pastures throughout Great Britain.
Parts used: the root and whole herb. Both parts of the plant contain a fragrant oil called primulin and the active principle saponin.
Medicinal uses: astringent, antispasmodic, vermifuge, emetic. It was formerly considered to be an important remedy in muscular rheumatism, paralysis and gout. A tincture of the whole plant has sedative effects and is used successfully in extreme sensitivity, restlessness and insomnia. Nervous headaches can be eased by treatment with an infusion of the root, while the powdered dry root serves as an emetic. An infusion of Primrose flowers is excellent in nervous headaches and an ointment can be made out of the leaves to heal and salve wounds and cuts.
Administered as: infusion, tincture, powdered root and ointment.

Ragwort *Senecio jacobaea*. *Common name*: St James's wort, stinking nanny, staggerwort, ragweed, dog standard, cankerwort, stammerwort, fireweed.
Occurrence: an abundant wild plant, widely distributed over Great Britain, Europe, Siberia and northwest India.
Parts used: the herb.
Medicinal uses: diaphoretic, detergent, emollient, cooling, astringent. The leaves were used as emollient poultices, while the expressed juice of the herb was utilized as a wash in burns, eye inflammation, sores and cancerous ulcers. It has been successful in relieving rheumatism, sciatica, gout and in reducing inflammation and swelling of joints when applied as a poultice. Ragwort makes a good gargle for ulcerated throats and mouths and a decoction of its root is said to help internal bruising and wounds. The herb was previously thought to be able to prevent infection. This plant is poisonous to cattle and should be removed from their pastures. The alkaloids in the ragwort have cumulative effects in the cattle and low doses of the chemical eaten over a period of time can built up to a critical level, where the cattle show obvious symptoms and then die. It is uncertain if sheep are also susceptible to this chemical.
Administered as: poultice, infusion and decoction.

Rosemary *Rosmarinus officinalis*. *Common name*: Polar plant, compass-weed, compass plant, romero, *Rosmarinus coronarium*.
Occurrence: native to the dry hills of the Mediterranean, from Spain westward to Turkey. A common garden plant in Britain, having been cultivated prior to the Norman Conquest.
Parts used: the herb and root. Oil of rosemary is distilled from the plant tops and used medicinally. Rosemary contains tannic acid, a bitter principle, resin and a volatile oil.
Medicinal uses: tonic, astringent, diaphoretic, stimulant. The essential oil is also stomachic, nervine and carminative and cures many types of headache. It is mainly applied externally as a hair lotion that is said to prevent baldness and the formation of dandruff. The oil is used externally as a rubefacient and is added to liniments for fragrance and stimulant properties. Rosemary tea can remove headache, colic, colds and nervous diseases and may also lift nervous depression.
Administered as: infusion, essential oil and lotion.

Sorrel *Rumex acetosa*. *Common name*: Garden sorrel, green sauce, sour grabs, sour suds, cuckoo sorrow, cuckoo's meate, gowke-meat.
Occurrence: indigenous to Britain and found in moist meadows throughout Europe.
Parts used: the leaves, dried and fresh.
Medicinal uses: refrigerant, diuretic, antiscorbutic. Sorrel is given as a cooling drink in all febrile conditions and can help correct scrofulous deposits. Its astringent qualities meant it was formerly used to stop haemorrhages and was applied as a poultice on cutaneous tumours. Sorrel juice and vinegar are said to cure ringworm, while a decoction was made to cure jaundice, ulcerated bowel, and gravel and stone in the kidneys.
Administered as: expressed juice, decoction, poultice and dried leaves.

Tansy *Tanacetum vulgare*. *Common name*: Buttons.
Occurrence: a hardy perennial plant, commonly seen on waste ground all over Europe and Great Britain.

Parts used: the herb. It contains the chemicals tanacetin, tannic acid, a volatile oil, thujone, sugar and a colouring matter among others.

Medicinal uses: anthelmintic, tonic, emmenagogue, stimulant. Tansy is largely used for expelling worms from children. The herb is also used for slight fevers, for allaying spasms and as a nervine drug. In large doses, the herb is violently irritant and induces venous congestion of the abdominal organs. In Scotland, an infusion was administered to cure gout. Tansy essential oil, when given in small doses, has helped in epilepsy and has also been used externally to help some eruptive diseases of the skin. Bruised fresh leaves can reduce swelling and relieve sprains, as can a hot infusion used as a poultice.

Administered as: essential oil, infusion, poultice, fresh leaves, solid extract.

Thyme *Thymus vulgaris. Common name*: Garden or common thyme, tomillo.

Occurrence: cultivated in temperate countries in northern Europe.

Parts used: the herb. Thyme gives rise to oil of thyme after distillation of the fresh leaves. This oil contains the phenols, thymol and carvacrol, as well as cymene, pinene and borneol.

Medicinal uses: antiseptic, antispasmodic, tonic, carminative. The fresh herb, in syrup, forms a safe cure for whooping cough, as is an infusion of the dried herb. The infusion or tea is beneficial for catarrh, sore throat, wind spasms, colic and in allaying fevers and colds. Thyme is generally used in conjunction with other remedies in herbal medicine.

Administered as: fluid extract, essential oil and infusion.

Valerian *Valeriana officinalis. Common name*: all-heal, great wild valerian, amantilla, setwall, sete-wale, capon's tail.

Occurrence: found throughout Europe and northern Asia. It is common in England in marshy thickets, riverbanks and ditches.

Parts used: the root, which contains a volatile oil, two alkaloids called chatarine and Valerianine as well as several unidentified compounds.

Medicinal uses: powerful nervine, stimulant, carminative anodyne and antispasmodic herb. It may be given in all cases of nervous debility and irritation as it is not narcotic. The expressed juice of the fresh root has been used as a narcotic in insomnia and as an anticonvulsant in epilepsy. The oil of valerian is of use against cholera and in strengthening the eyesight. A herbal compound containing valerian was given to civilians during the Second World War, to reduce the effects of stress caused by repeated air raids and to minimize damage to health.

Administered as: fluid extract, tincture, essential oil, expressed juice.

Witch hazel *Hamamelis virginiana. Common name*: Spotted alder, winterbloom, snapping hazelnut.

Occurrence: native to the United States of America and Canada. *Parts used*: the dried bark, both fresh and dried leaves. The leaves contain tannic and gallic acids, volatile oil and an unknown bitter principle. The bark contains tannin, gallic acid, a physterol, resin, fat and other bitter and odorous bodies.

Medicinal uses: astringent, tonic, sedative. Valuable in stopping internal and external haemorrhages and in treating piles. Mainly used for bruises, swelling, inflammation and tumours as a poultice. It may also be utilized for diarrhoea, dysentery and mucous discharges. A decoction is used against tuberculosis, gonorrhoea, menorrhagia and the debilitated state resulting from abortion. Tea made from the bark or leaves aids bleeding of the stomach, bowel complaints and may be given as an injection for bleeding piles. Witch hazel is used to treat varicose veins as a moist poultice, as an extract to ease burns, scalds and insect and mosquito bites, and to help inflammation of the eyelids.

Administered as: liquid extract, injection, tincture, lotion, ointment, suppositories, poultice, infusion and decoction.

Homeopathy

Introduction

The aim of homeopathy is to cure an illness or disorder by treating the whole person rather than merely concentrating on a set of symptoms. Hence, in homeopathy the approach is holistic, and the overall state of health of the patient, especially his or her emotional and psychological wellbeing, is regarded as being very significant. A homeopath notes the symptoms that the person wishes to have cured, but also takes time to discover other signs or indications of disorder that the patient may regard as being less important. The reasoning behind this is that illness is a sign of disorder or imbalance within the body. It is believed that the whole 'make-up' of a person determines, to a great extent, the type of disorders to which that individual is prone and the symptoms likely to occur. A homeopathic remedy must be suitable both for the symptoms and the characteristics and temperament of the patient. Hence, two patients with the same illness may be offered different remedies according to their individual natures. One remedy may also be used to treat different groups of symptoms or ailments.

Homoeopathic remedies are based on the concept that 'like cures like', an ancient philosophy that can be traced back to the 5th century BC when it was formulated by Hippocrates. In the early 1800s, this idea awakened the interest of a German doctor, Samuel Hahnemann, who believed that the medical practices at that time were too harsh and tended to hinder rather than aid healing. Hahnemann observed that a treatment for malaria, based on an extract of cinchona bark (quinine), actually produced symptoms of this disease when taken in a small dose by a healthy person. Further extensive studies convinced him that the production of symptoms was the body's way of combating illness. Hence, to give a minute dose of a substance that stimulated the symptoms of an illness in a healthy person, could be used to fight that illness in someone who was sick. Hahnemann conducted numerous trials (called 'provings') giving minute doses of substances to healthy people and recording the symptoms produced. Eventually, these very dilute remedies were given to people with illnesses, often with very encouraging results.

Modern homeopathy is based on the work of Hahnemann, and the medicines derived from plant, mineral and animal sources are used in extremely dilute amounts. Indeed it is believed that the curative properties are enhanced by each dilution because impurities that might cause unwanted side effects are lost. Substances used in homeopathy are first soaked in alcohol to extract their essential ingredients. This initial solution, called the 'mother tincture' is diluted successively either by factors of ten (called the 'decimal scale' and designated X), or 100 (the 'centesimal scale' and designated C). Each dilution is shaken vigorously before further ones are made and this is thought to make the properties more powerful by adding energy at each stage, while impurities are removed. The thorough shakings of each dilution are said to energize or 'potentiate' the medicine. The remedies are made into tablets or may be used in the form of ointment, solutions, powders, suppositories, etc. High potency (i.e. more dilute) remedies are used for severe symptoms and lower potency (less dilute) for milder ones.

The homeopathic view is that during the process of healing, symptoms are redirected from more important to less important body systems. It is also held that healing is from innermost to outermost parts of the body and that more recent symptoms disappear first, this being known as the 'law of direction of cure'. Occasionally, symptoms may worsen initially when a homeopathic remedy is taken, but this is usually short-lived and is known as a 'healing crisis.' It is taken to indicate a change and that improvement is likely to follow. Usually, with a homeopathic remedy, an improvement is noticed fairly quickly although this depends upon the nature of the ailment, health, age and wellbeing of the patient and potency of the remedy.

A first homeopathic consultation is likely to last about 1 hour so that the specialist can obtain a full picture of the patient's medical history and personal circumstances. On the basis of this information, the homeopathic doctor decides on an appropriate remedy and potency (which is usually 6C). Subsequent consultations are generally shorter and full advice is given on how to store and take the medicine. It is widely accepted that homeopathic remedies are very safe and non-addictive but they are covered by the legal requirements governing all medicines and should be obtained from a recognized source.

Potency table for homeopathic medicines

The centesimal scale

$1C = 1/100 \quad (1/100^{1)} \quad$ of mother tincture
$2C = 1/10\,000 \quad (1/100^{2}) \quad$ of mother tincture
$3C = 1/1\,000\,000 \quad (1/100^{3}) \quad$ of mother tincture
$6C = 1/1\,000\,000\,000\,000 \; (1/100^{6})$ of mother tincture

The decimal scale

$1X = 1/10 \;\; (1/10^{1})$ of mother tincture
$2X = 1/100 \;\; (1/10^{2})$ of mother tincture
$6X = 1/1\,000\,000 \;\; (1/10^{6})$ of mother tincture

The development of homeopathy

The Greek physician, Hippocrates, who lived several hundred years before the birth of Christ (460–370 BC), is regarded as the founding father of all medicine. The Hippocratic Oath taken by newly qualified doctors in orthodox medicine binds them to an ethical code of medical practice in honour of Hippocrates. Hippocrates believed that disease resulted from natural elements in the world in which people lived. This contrasted with the view that held sway for centuries that disease was some form of punishment from the gods or God. He believed that it was essential to observe and take account of the course and progress of a disease in each individual, and that any cure should encourage that person's own innate healing power. Hippocrates embraced the idea of 'like being able to cure like' and had many remedies that were based on this principle. Hence in his practice and study of medicine he laid the foundations of the homeopathic approach although this was not to be appreciated and developed for many centuries.

During the period of Roman civilization a greater knowledge and insight into the nature of the human body was developed. Many herbs and plants were used for healing by people throughout the world, and much knowledge was gained and handed down from generation to generation. However, the belief persisted that diseases were caused by supernatural or divine forces. It was not until the early 1500s that a Swiss doctor, Paracelsus (1493–1541) put forward the view that disease resulted from external environmental forces. He also believed that plants and natural substances held the key to healing and embraced the 'like can cure like' principle. One of his ideas, known as the Doctrine of Signatures, was that the appearance of a plant, or the substances it contained, gave an idea of the disorders it could cure.

In the succeeding centuries, increased knowledge was gained about the healing properties of plants and the way the human body worked. In spite of this, the methods of medical practice were extremely harsh and there is no doubt that many people suffered needlessly and died due to the treatment they received. It was against this background that Samuel Hahnemann, (1755–1843) the founding father of modern homeopathy, began his work as a doctor in the late 1700s. In his early writings, Hahnemann criticized the severe practices of medicine and advocated a healthy diet, clean living conditions and high standards of hygiene as a means of improving health and warding off disease. In 1790, he became interested in quinine, extracted from the bark of the cinchona tree, which was known to be an effective treatment for malaria. He tested the substance first on himself, and later on friends and close family members and recorded the results, and these early experiments were called 'provings'. The results led him to conduct many further investigations and provings of other natural substances, during the course of which he rediscovered and established the principle of like being able to cure like.

By 1812, the principle and practice of homeopathy, based on the work of Hahnemann, had become established and many other doctors adopted the homeopathic approach. Hahnemann himself become a teacher in homeopathy at the University of Leipzig and published many important writings—the results of his years of research. He continued to practice, teach and conduct research throughout his life, especially in producing more dilute remedies that were succussed or shaken at each stage and were found to be more potent. Although his work was not without its detractors, Hahnemann had attracted a considerable following by the 1830s. In 1831, there was a widespread cholera epidemic in central Europe for which Hahnemann recommended treatment with camphor. Many people were cured, including Dr Frederick Quin, (1799–1878), a medical practitioner at that time. He went on to establish the first homeopathic hospital in London in 1849. A later resurgence of cholera in Britain enabled the effectiveness of camphor to be established beyond doubt, as the numbers of people cured at the homeopathic hospital were far greater than those treated at other hospitals.

In the United States of America, homeopathy became firmly established in the early part of the 19th century and there were several eminent practitioners who further enhanced knowledge and practice. These included Dr Constantine Hering (1800–1880), who formulated the Laws of Cure, explaining how symptoms affect organ systems and move from one part of the body to another as a cure occurs. Dr James Tyler Kent (1849–1916) introduced the idea of constitutional types, which is now the basis of classical homeopathy, and advocated the use of high potency remedies.

In the later years of the 19th century, a fundamental split occurred in the practice of homeopathy, which was brought about by Dr Richard Hughes (1836–1902), who worked in London and Brighton. He insisted that physical symptoms and the nature of the disease itself were the important factors rather than the holistic approach, based on the make-up of the whole individual person. Hughes rejected the concept of constitutional types and advocated the use of low-potency remedies. Although he worked as a homeopath, his approach was to attempt to make homeopathy more scientific and to bring it closer to the practices of conventional medicine. Some other homeopathic doctors followed the approach of Hughes, and the split led to a collapse in faith in the whole practice of homeopathy during the early part of the century. However, as the century advanced, homeopathy regained its following and respect. Conventional medicine and homeopathy have continued to advance, and there is now a greater sympathy and understanding between the practitioners in both these important disciplines.

Among homeopathic remedies there are a small number of fundamental, regularly used compounds that are effective in treating many complaints. These are described below.

Basic remedies
Argenticum nitricum
Argent nit; silver nitrate, devil's stone, lunar caustic, hellstone.

Silver nitrate is obtained from the mineral acanthite, which is a natural ore of silver. White silver nitrate crystals are derived from a chemical solution of the mineral ore, and these are used to make the homeopathic remedy. Silver nitrate is poisonous in large doses and has antiseptic and caustic properties. In the past it was used to clean out wounds and prevent infection. In homeopathy, it is used to treat states of great anxiety, panic, fear or apprehension about a forthcoming event, e.g. taking an examination, having to perform a public role (speech-making, chairing a public meeting, acting, singing), going for an interview or any activity involving scrutiny and criticism by others. It was also used as a remedy for digestive complaints including indigestion, abdominal pain, wind, nausea and also for headache. Often, there is a longing for sweet 'comfort' or other types of food. Argent nit. may be given for laryngitis, sore throat and hoarseness, eye inflammation such as conjunctivitis and for period pains. Other types of pain, asthma and warts may benefit from argent nit.

Often, a person experiences symptoms mainly on the left side and these are worse for heat and at night. Also, they are made worse by anxiety and overwork, emotional tension and resting on the left side. Pains are made worse with talking and movement. Symptoms improve in cold or cool fresh air and are relieved by belching. Pains are helped by applying pressure to the painful part. People suitable for argent nit. are quick-witted and rapid in thought and action. They may appear outgoing and happy but are a prey to worry, anxiety and ungrounded fears that make them tense. All the emotions are quick to surface and argent nit. people are able to put on an impressive performance. They enjoy a wide variety of foods, particularly salty and sweet things, although these may upset the digestion. They have a fear of heights, crowds, of being burgled, of failure, and arriving late for an appointment. They also have a fear of serious illness, dying and madness. Argent nit. people are generally slim and full of restless energy and tension. They may have deeply etched features and lines on the skin that make them appear older than their actual age.

Arsenicum album
Arsen alb; white arsenic trioxide.

This is a widely used homeopathic remedy, the source being white arsenic trioxide derived from arsenopyrite, a metallic mineral ore of arsenic. Arsenic has been known for centuries as a poison and was once used as a treatment for syphilis. White arsenic trioxide used to be given to improve muscles and skin in animals such as horses. It is used to treat acute conditions of the digestive system and chest and mental symptoms of anxiety and fear. Hence it is a remedy for diarrhoea and vomiting caused by eating the wrong kinds of food, or food poisoning or over-indulgence in alcohol. Also, for dehydration in children following gastroenteritis or feverish illness. It is a remedy for asthma and breathing difficulty, mouth ulcers, carbuncle (a collection of boils), dry, cracked lips, burning skin, inflamed, watering stinging eyes and psoriasis. Also, for sciatica, shingles, sore throat and painful swallowing, candidiasis (fungal infection) of the mouth and motion sickness. There may be oedema (retention of fluid) showing as a puffiness around the ankles.

An ill person who benefits from arsen alb. experiences burning pains but also feels cold. The skin may be either hot or cold to the touch. The symptoms are worse for cold in any form, including cold food and drink, and between midnight and 3 a.m. They are worse on the right side and if the person is near the coast. Symptoms improve with warmth (including warm drinks), gentle movement and lying down with the head raised. People suitable for arsen alb. are precise, meticulous and ambitious and loathe any form of disorder. They are always immaculately dressed and everything in their life is neat and tidy. However, they tend to have great worries, especially about their financial security and their own health and that of their family. They fear illness and dying, loss of financial and personal status, being burgled, darkness and the supernatural. Arsen alb. people have strongly held views and do not readily tolerate contrary opinions or those with a more relaxed or disordered lifestyle. They enjoy a variety of different foods, coffee and alcoholic drinks. They are usually thin, with delicate, fine features and pale skin that may show worry lines. Their movements tend to be rapid and their manner serious and somewhat restless, although they are always polite.

Calcarea carbonica

Calc. carb; calcium carbonate.

This important homeopathic remedy is made from powdered mother-of-pearl, the beautiful, translucent inner layer of oyster shells. Calcium is an essential mineral in the body, being especially important for the healthy development of bones and teeth. The calc. carb. remedy is used to treat a number of different disorders especially those relating to bones and teeth, but also certain skin conditions and symptoms relating to the female reproductive system. It is a remedy for weak or slow growth of bones and teeth and fractures that take a long time to heal. Also, for teething problems in children, pains in bones, teeth and joints, headaches and eye inflammations affecting the right side, and ear infections with an unpleasant-smelling discharge. Premenstrual syndrome, heavy periods and

menopausal disorders are helped by calc. carb, and also chapped skin and eczema.

Calc. carb. may be used as a remedy for verruca (a type of wart) and thrush infections. People who benefit from calc. carb. are very sensitive to the cold, particularly in the hands and feet and tend to sweat profusely. They suffer from fatigue and anxiety, and body secretions (sweat and urine) smell unpleasant. Children who benefit from calc. carb. have recurrent ear, nose and throat infections, especially tonsillitis and glue ear. Symptoms are made worse by draughts and cold, damp weather and also at night. They are worse when the person first wakens in the morning and for physical exercise and sweating. In women, symptoms are worse premenstrually. They improve in warm, dry weather and are better later on in the morning and after the person has eaten breakfast. People suitable for calc. carb. are often overweight or even obese with a pale complexion. They are shy and very sensitive, quiet in company and always worried about what other people think of them. Calc. carb. people are hard-working, conscientious and reliable and easily upset by the suffering of others. They need constant reassurance from friends and family and tend to feel that they are a failure. Usually, calc. carb. people enjoy good health but have a tendency for skeletal weakness. They enjoy a wide variety of different foods and tend to overeat, but are upset by coffee and milk. They are afraid of dying and serious illness, the supernatural, madness, being a failure and becoming poor and they tend to be claustrophobic.

Graphites

Graphite; black pencil lead

Graphite is a form of carbon that is the basis of all life. It is found in older igneous or metamorphic rocks, such as granite and marble and is mined for its industrial uses, e.g. in batteries, motors, pencil leads, cleaning and lubricating fluids. It was investigated and proved by Hahnemann after he learned that it was being used by some factory workers to heal cold sores. The powder used in homeopathy is ground graphite and it is mainly used for skin disorders that may be caused by metabolic imbalances and stomach ulcers. It is a remedy for eczema, psoriasis, acne, rough, dry skin conditions with pustules or blisters, scarring and thickened cracked nails and cold sores. Also, for stomach ulcers due to a thinning or weakness in the lining of the stomach wall, problems caused by excessive catarrh, loss of hair and cramping pains or numbing of the feet and hands. In women it is used to treat some menstrual problems. The symptoms are worse in draughty, cold and damp conditions and for eating sweet meals or sea foods. Also, the use of steroids for skin complaints and, in women, during menstruation. Symptoms are often worse on the left side. They improve with warmth, as long as the air is fresh and it is not stuffy, when it is dark and with eating and sleep. People suitable for graphites are usually well built and may be overweight, often having dark hair. They like to eat well but lack physical fitness and sweat or flush with slight exertion. They are prone to dry, flaky skin conditions that may affect the scalp. Graphites people are usually lethargic and may be irritable, lacking in concentration for intellectual activities. They are prone to mood swings and subject to bouts of weeping, especially when listening to music. A graphites person feels that he or she is unlucky and is inclined to self-pity, often feeling fearful and timid.

Ignatia amara
Agnate; strychnos Ignatii, St Ignatius' bean
Ignatia amara is a large tree that is native to the Philippine Islands, China and the East Indies. The tree has many branches and twining stems and produces stalked white flowers. Later, seed pods are produced, each containing ten to twenty large, oval seeds, that are about one inch long and are embedded in pulp. The seeds are highly poisonous and contain strychnine, which affects the central nervous system. Similar active constituents and properties are found in *Nux vomica*. The tree is named after the founder of the Jesuits, Ignatius Loyola (1491–1556), and Spanish priests belonging to this order brought the seeds to Europe during the 1600s. The homeopathic remedy is made from the powdered seeds and is used especially for emotional symptoms. It is used for grief, bereavement, shock and loss, particularly when a person is having difficulty coming to terms with his or her feelings and is inclined to suppress the natural responses. Accompanying symptoms include sleeplessness, anger and hysteria. Similar emotional and psychological problems are helped by this remedy, including anxiety and fear especially of appearing too forward to others, a tendency to burst into fits of crying, self-doubt, pity, blame and depression. Nervous tension headaches and digestive upsets, feverish symptoms, chills and pains in the abdomen may be helped by *Ignatia*. Some problems associated with menstruation, especially sharp pains or absence of periods, are relieved by this remedy as are conditions with changeable symptoms. These are worse in cold weather or conditions, with

emotional trauma, being touched, for smoking and drinking coffee. They improve with warmth, moving about, eating, lying on the side or area that is painful and after passing urine.

The person for whom *Ignatia* is suitable is usually female and with a tendency towards harsh, self-criticism and blame; she is usually a creative, artistic person, highly sensitive but with a tendency to suppress the emotions. She is perceptive and intelligent but inclined to be hysterical and subject to erratic mood swings. Typically, the person expects a high standard in those she loves. The person enjoys dairy products, bread and sour foods but sweets, alcoholic drinks and fruit upset her system. She is afraid of crowds, tends to be claustrophobic, and fears being burgled. Also, she is afraid of being hurt emotionally, and is very sensitive to pain. The person is usually dark-haired and of slim build with a worried expression and prone to sighing, yawning and excessive blinking.

Lachesis
Trigonocephalus lachesis; lachesis muta, venom of the bushmaster or Surukuku snake
This South African snake produces a deadly venom that may prove instantly fatal due to its effects upon the heart. The venom causes the blood to thin and flow more freely, hence increasing the likelihood of haemorrhage. Even a slight bite bleeds copiously with a risk of blood poisoning or septicaemia. The snake is a ferocious hunter and its African name, Surukuku describes the sound it makes while in pursuit of prey. The properties of the venom were investigated in the 1800s by the eminent American homeopathic doctor, Constantine Hering , who tested and proved the remedy on himself. It is effective in treating a variety of disorders, particularly those relating to the blood circulation and where there is a risk of blood poisoning or septicaemia. It is used to treat varicose veins and problems of the circulation indicated by a bluish tinge to the skin. The remedy is useful for those suffering from a weak heart or angina, palpitations and an irregular, fast or weak pulse. There may be symptoms of chest pain and breathing difficulty. It is of great benefit in treating uterine problems, particularly premenstrual congestion and pain that is relieved once the period starts. Also, this is an excellent remedy for menopausal symptoms, especially hot flushes, and for infections of the bladder and rectum. It is used to treat conditions and infections where symptoms are mainly on the left side, such as headache or stroke when the left side is involved. Also, as a treatment for sore throats and

throat infections, tonsillitis, lung abscess, boils, ulcers, wounds that only heal slowly, vomiting due to appendicitis and digestive disorders, fevers with chills and shivering, nosebleeds and bleeding piles.

It is used to treat severe symptoms of measles and serious infections including scarlet fever and smallpox. Symptoms are made worse for touch and after sleep and by tight clothing. They are worse for hot drinks and baths, and exposure to hot sun or direct heat in any form. For women, symptoms are worse during the menopause. They improve with being out in the fresh air and drinking cold drinks and with release of normal bodily discharges. People suitable for *Lachesis* tend to be intelligent, creative, intense and ambitious. They have strong views about politics and world affairs and may be impatient of the views of others. They may be somewhat self-centred, possessive and jealous, which can cause problems in close relationships with others. They dislike being tied down and so may be reluctant to commit themselves to a relationship. *Lachesis* people have a liking for sour pickled foods, bread, rice and oysters and alcoholic drinks. They like coffee, but hot drinks and wheat-based food tends to upset them. They have a fear of water, people they do not know, being burgled and of dying or being suffocated. *Lachesis* people may be somewhat overweight and are sometimes red-haired and freckled. Alternatively, they may be thin and dark-haired, pale and with a lot of energy. Children tend to be somewhat jealous of others and possessive of their friends, which can lead to naughty or trying behaviour.

Lycopodium clavatum

Lycopodium; club moss, wolf's claw, vegetable sulphur, stagshorn moss, running pine
This plant is found throughout the northern hemisphere, in high moorlands, forests and mountains. The plant produces spore cases on the end of upright forked stalks, which contain the spores. These produce yellow dust or powder that is resistant to water and was once used as a coating on pills and tablets to keep them separate from one another. The powder was also used as a constituent of fireworks. It has been used medicinally for many centuries, as a remedy for digestive disorders and kidney stones in Arabian countries and in the treatment of gout. The powder and spores are collected by shaking the fresh, flowering stalks of the plant and its main use in homeopathy is for digestive and kidney disorders. It is used to treat indigestion, heartburn, the effects of eating a large meal late at night, sickness, nausea, wind,

bloatedness and constipation. Also, in men, for kidney stones, with the production of a red-coloured urine containing a sand-like sediment and enlarged prostate gland. It is used in the treatment of some problems of male impotence and bleeding haemorrhoids or piles. Symptoms that occur on the right side are helped by *Lycopodium*, and the patient additionally tends to crave sweet, comfort foods. Nettlerash, psoriasis affecting the hands, fatigue due to illness and ME (Myalgic encephalomyelitis), some types of headache, cough and sore throat are relieved by this remedy. It is used to relieve emotional states of anxiety, fear and apprehension caused by chronic insecurity, or relating to forthcoming events such as taking an examination or appearing in public (stage fright). Also, night terrors, sleeplessness, shouting or talking in the sleep and being frightened on first waking up can all benefit from this treatment.

The symptoms are worse between 4 p.m. and 8 p.m. and in warm, stuffy rooms and with wearing clothes that are too tight. They are also worse in the early morning between 4 a.m. and 8 a.m., for eating too much and during the Spring. They improve outside in cool fresh air, after a hot meal or drink and with loosening tight clothing, with light exercise and at night. People suitable for *Lycopodium* tend to be serious, hard-working and intelligent, often in professional positions. They seem to be self-possessed and confident but are, in reality, rather insecure with a low self-opinion. They are impatient of what they perceive as being weakness and are not tolerant or sympathetic of illness. *Lycopodium* people are sociable but may keep their distance and not get involved; they may be sexually promiscuous. They have a great liking for sweet foods of all kinds and enjoy hot meals and drinks. They are easily filled but may carry on eating regardless of this and usually complain of symptoms on the right side. *Lycopodium* people are afraid of being left on their own, of failure in life, of crowds, darkness and the supernatural and tend to be claustrophobic. They are often tall, thin and pale with receding hair or hair that turns grey early in life. They may be bald, with a forehead lined with worry lines and a serious appearance. They tend to have weak muscles and are easily tired after physical exercise. They may have a tendency to unconsciously twitch the muscles of the face and to flare the nostrils.

Mercurius solubilis

Merc sol; quicksilver
The mineral cinnabar, which is found in volcanic crystalline rocks, is an important ore of mercury and

is extracted for a variety of uses, including dental fillings and in thermometers. Mercury is toxic in large doses, and an affected person produces copious quantities of saliva and suffers repeated bouts of vomiting. Mercury has been used since ancient times and was once given as a remedy for syphilis. A powder of precipitate of mercury is obtained from dissolving liquid mercury in a dilute solution of nitric acid, and this is the source of the remedy used in homeopathy. It is used as a remedy for conditions that produce copious bodily secretions that often smell unpleasant, with accompanying symptoms of heat or burning and a great sensitivity to temperature. It is used as a remedy for fevers with profuse, unpleasant sweating, bad breath, inflammation of the gums, mouth ulcers, candidiasis (thrush) of the mouth, infected painful teeth and gums and excessive production of saliva. Also, for a sore infected throat, tonsillitis, mumps, discharging infected ear and a congested severe headache and pains in the joints. It is good for eye complaints including severe conjunctivitis, allergic conditions with a running nose, skin complaints that produce pus-filled pustules, spots and ulcers, including varicose ulcers. The symptoms are made worse by extremes of heat and cold and also for wet and rapidly changing weather. They are worse at night and for sweating and being too hot in bed.

Symptoms improve for rest and in comfortable temperatures where the person is neither too hot nor too cold. People suitable for merc. sol. tend to be very insecure although they have an outwardly calm appearance. They are cautious and reserved with other people and consider what they are about to say before speaking so that conversation may seem laboured. Merc. sol. types do not like criticism of any kind and may suddenly become angry if someone disagrees with their point of view. They tend to be introverted but their innermost thoughts may be in turmoil. They tend to be hungry and enjoy bread and butter, milk and other cold drinks but dislike alcohol with the exception of beer. They usually do not eat meat and do not have a sweet tooth. They dislike coffee and salt. Merc. sol. people often have fair hair with fine, unlined skin and an air of detachment. They are afraid of dying and of mental illness leading to insanity, and worry about the wellbeing of their family. They fear being burgled and are afraid or fearful during a thunderstorm.

Natrum muriaticum

Natrum mur; common salt, sodium chloride

Salt has long been prized for its seasoning and preservative qualities, and Roman soldiers were once paid in salt, such was its value. (Salary comes from the latin word *salarium*, which refers to this practice). Sodium and chlorine are essential chemicals in the body, being needed for many metabolic processes, particularly the functioning of nerve tissue. In fact, there is seldom a need to add salt to food as usually enough is present naturally in a healthy, well-balanced diet. (An exception is when people are working very hard physically in a hot climate and losing a lot of salt in sweat). However, people and many other mammals frequently have a great liking for salt. If the salt/water balance in the body is disturbed, a person soon becomes very ill and may even die.

In ancient times, salt was usually obtained by boiling sea water, but natural evaporation around the shallow edges of salt lakes results in deposits of rock salt being formed. Rock salt is the usual source of table salt and also of the remedy used in homeopathy. This remedy has an effect on the functioning of the kidneys and the salt/water balance of body fluids, and is used to treat both mental and physical symptoms. Emotional symptoms that benefit from natrum mur. include sensitivity and irritability, tearfulness and depression, suppressed grief and premenstrual tension. Physical ailments that respond to this remedy are often those in which there is a thin, watery discharge of mucus and in which symptoms are made worse by heat. Hence natrum mur. is used in the treatment of colds with a runny nose or other catarrhal problems. Also, for some menstrual and vaginal problems, headaches and migraines, cold sores, candidiasis (thrush) of the mouth, mouth ulcers, inflamed and infected gums and bad breath. Some skin disorders are helped by natrum mur. including verruca (a wart on the foot), warts, spots and boils and cracked, dry lips. It may be used in the treatment of fluid retention with puffiness around the face, eyelids and abdomen, etc, urine retention, constipation, anal fissure, indigestion, anaemia and thyroid disorders (goitre). When ill, people who benefit from this remedy feel cold and shivery but their symptoms are made worse, or even brought on, by heat. Heat, whether from hot sun and fire or a warm, stuffy room exacerbate the symptoms, which also are made worse in cold and thundery weather. They are worse on the coast from the sea breeze, and in the morning between 9 and 11 o'clock. Too much physical activity and the sympathy of others exacerbate the symptoms. They improve in the fresh, open air and for cold applications or a cold bath or swim. Also, sleeping on a hard bed and sweating and fasting make the symptoms better.

People suitable for natrum mur. are often women who are highly sensitive, serious-minded, intelligent and reliable. They have high ideals and feel things very deeply, being easily hurt and stung by slights and criticism. They need the company of other people but, being so sensitive, can actually shun them for fear of being hurt. They are afraid of mental illness leading to loss of self-control and insanity and of dying. Also, they fear the dark, failure in work, crowds, being burgled and have a tendency to be claustrophobic. They worry about being late and are fearful during a thunderstorm. Natrum. mur. people tend to become introverted and react badly to the criticism of others. They are highly sensitive to the influence of music, which easily moves them to tears. Natrum mur. people are usually of squat or solid build with dark or fairish hair. They are prone to reddened, watery eyes as though they have been crying, and a cracked lower lip. The face may appear puffy and shiny with an air of stoicism.

Nux vomica
Strychnos nux vomica; poison nut, Quaker buttons
The strychnos nux vomica tree is a native of India but also grows in Burma, Thailand, China and Australia. It produces small, greenish-white flowers and later, apple-sized fruits, containing small, flat, circular pale seeds covered in fine hair. The seeds, bark and leaves are highly poisonous, containing strychnine, and have been used in medicine for many centuries. In medieval times, the seeds were used as a treatment for the plague. Strychnine has severe effects upon the nervous system but in minute amounts can help increase urination and aid digestion. The seeds are cleaned and dried and used to produce the homeopathic remedy. Nux vomica is used in the treatment of a variety of digestive complaints including cramping, colicky abdominal pains, indigestion, nausea and vomiting, diarrhoea and constipation. Also, indigestion or stomach upset caused by over-indulgence in alcohol or rich food and piles that cause painful contractions of the rectum. Sometimes, these complaints are brought on by a tendency to keep emotions, particularly anger, suppressed and not allowing it to show or be expressed outwardly. Nux vomica is a remedy for irritability, headache and migraine, colds, coughs and influenza-like symptoms of fever, aching bones and muscles and chills and shivering. It is a useful remedy for women who experience heavy, painful periods that may cause fainting, morning sickness during pregnancy and pain in labour. It is also used to treat urinary frequency and cystitis.

The type of person who benefits from this remedy is frequently under stress and experiences a periodic flare-up of symptoms. The person may be prone to indigestion and heartburn, gastritis and stomach ulcer and piles or haemorrhoids. The person usually has a tendency to keep everything bottled up but has a passionate nature and is liable to outbursts of anger. Nux vomica people are very ambitious and competitive, demanding a high standard of themselves and others and intolerant of anything less than perfection. They enjoy challenges and using their wits to keep one step ahead. Often, they are to be found as managers, company directors, scientists, etc, at the cutting edge of their particular occupation. They are ungracious and irritable when ill and cannot abide the criticism of others. This type of person is afraid of being a failure at work and fears or dislikes crowded public places. He or she is afraid of dying. The person enjoys rich, fattening foods containing cholesterol and spicy meals, alcohol and coffee although these upset the digestive system. Symptoms are worse in cold, windy, dry weather and in winter and between 3 and 4 a.m. They are aggravated by certain noises, music, bright lights and touch, eating (especially spicy meals) and with overwork of mental faculties. Nux vomica people usually look serious, tense and are thin with a worried expression. They have sallow skin and tend to have dark shadows beneath the eyes.

Phosphorus
Phos; white phosphorus
Phosphorus is an essential mineral in the body, found in the genetical material (DNA), bones and teeth. White phosphorus is extremely flammable and poisonous and was once used in the manufacture of matches and fireworks. Due to the fact that it tends to catch fire spontaneously when exposed to air, it is stored under water. In the past it has been used to treat a number of disorders and infectious diseases such as measles. In homeopathy, the remedy is used to treat nervous tension caused by stress and worry, with symptoms of sleeplessness, exhaustion and digestive upset. Often there are pains of a burning nature in the chest or abdomen. It is a remedy for vomiting and nausea, heartburn, acid indigestion, stomach ulcer and gastroenteritis. It is also used to treat bleeding, e.g. from minor wounds, the gums, nosebleeds, gastric and profuse menstrual bleeding.

Severe coughs that may be accompanied by retching, vomiting and production of a blood-tinged phlegm are treated with phos. as well as some other severe respiratory complaints. These include pneumonia, bronchitis, asthma and laryngitis. Styes that tend to recur and poor circulation may also be helped by phos. Symptoms are worse in the evening and morning and before or during a thunderstorm. They are also made worse for too much physical activity, hot food and drink and lying on the left side. Symptoms improve in the fresh open air and with lying on the back or right side. They are better after sleep or when the person is touched or stroked. People who need phos. do not like to be alone when ill and improve for the sympathy and attention of others. They are warm, kind, affectionate people who are highly creative, imaginative and artistic. They enjoy the company of other people and need stimulation to give impetus to their ideas. Phos. people have an optimistic outlook, are full of enthusiasm but sometimes promise much and deliver little. They are very tactile and like to be touched or stroked and offered sympathy when unhappy or unwell. They enjoy a variety of different foods but tend to suffer from digestive upsets. Phos. people are usually tall, slim and may be dark or fair-haired, with an attractive, open appearance. They like to wear brightly coloured clothes, and are usually popular, having many friends. They have a fear of illness, especially cancer, and of dying and also of the dark and supernatural forces. They are apprehensive of water and fear being a failure in their work. Thunderstorms make them nervous.

Pulsatilla nigricans

Pulsatilla; *Anemone pratensis*, meadow anemone
This attractive plant closely resembles *Anemone pulsatilla*, the pasque flower, which is used in herbal medicine, but has smaller flowers. *Anemone pratensis* is a native of Germany, Denmark and Scandinavia and has been used medicinally for hundreds of years. The plant produces beautiful deep purple flowers with orange centres and both leaves and flowers are covered with fine, silky hairs. The whole fresh plant is gathered and made into a pulp and liquid is extracted to make the remedy used in homeopathy. It is used to treat a wide variety of disorders with both physical and mental symptoms. It is a useful remedy for ailments in which there is a greenish-yellowish discharge. Hence it is used for colds and coughs and sinusitis with the production of profuse catarrh or phlegm. Also, eye infections with discharge such as styes and conjunctivitis. Digestive disorders are helped by pulsatilla, particularly indigestion, heartburn, nausea and sickness caused by eating too much fatty or rich food. The remedy is helpful for female disorders in

which there are a variety of physical and emotional symptoms. These include premenstrual tension, menstrual problems, menopausal symptoms and cystitis, with accompanying symptoms of mood swings, depression and tearfulness. It is a remedy for headaches and migraine, swollen glands, inflammation and pain in the bones and joints as in rheumatic and arthritic disorders, nosebleeds, varicose veins, mumps, measles, toothache, acne, frequent urination and incontinence.

Symptoms are worse at night or when it is hot, and after eating heavy, rich food. Symptoms improve out in the cool fresh air and with gentle exercise such as walking. The person feels better after crying and being treated sympathetically by others. Pulsatilla people are usually women who have a mild, passive nature and are kind, gentle and loving. They are easily moved to tears by the plight of others and love animals and people alike. The person yields easily to the requests and demands of others and is a peacemaker who likes to avoid a scene. An outburst of anger is very much out of character and a pulsatilla person usually has many friends. The person likes rich and sweet foods, although these may upset the digestion, and dislikes spicy meals. Pulsatilla people may fear darkness, being left alone, dying and any illness leading to insanity. They are fearful of crowds, the supernatural and tend to be claustrophobic. Usually, they are fair and blue-eyed with clear, delicate skin that blushes readily. They are attractive and slightly overweight or plump.

Sepia officinalis

Sepia; ink of the cuttlefish
Cuttlefish ink has been used since ancient times, both for medicinal purposes and as a colour in artists' paint. The cuttlefish has the ability to change colour to blend in with its surroundings and squirts out the dark brown/black ink when threatened by predators. Sepia was known to Roman physicians who used it as a cure for baldness. In homeopathy it is mainly used as an excellent remedy for women experiencing menstrual and menopausal problems. It was investigated and proved by Hahnemann in 1834. It is used to treat premenstrual tension, menstrual pain and heavy bleeding, infrequent or suppressed periods, menopausal symptoms such as hot flushes and postnatal depression. Physical and emotional symptoms caused by an imbalance of hormones are helped by sepia. Also, conditions in which there is extreme fatigue or exhaustion with muscular aches and pains. Digestive complaints, including nausea and sickness, abdominal pain and

wind, caused by eating dairy products, and headaches with giddiness and nausea are relieved by sepia. Also, it is a remedy for incontinence, hot, sweaty feet and verruca (a wart on the foot). A woman often experiences pelvic, dragging pains frequently associated with prolapse of the womb. Disorders of the circulation, especially varicose veins and cold extremities benefit from sepia.

Symptoms are worse in cold weather and before a thunderstorm and in the late afternoon, evening and early in the morning. Also, before a period in women and if the person receives sympathy from others. The symptoms are better with heat and warmth, quick vigorous movements, having plenty to do and out in the fresh open air. People suitable for sepia are usually, but not exclusively, women. They tend to be tall, thin and with a yellowish complexion and are rather self-contained and indifferent to others. Sepia people may become easily cross, especially with family and close friends, and may harbour resentment. In company, they make a great effort to appear outgoing and love to dance. A woman may be either an externally hard, successful career person or someone who constantly feels unable to cope, especially with looking after the home and family. Sepia people have strongly held beliefs and cannot stand others taking a contrary opinion. When ill, they hate to be fussed over or have the sympathy of others. They like both sour and sweet foods and alcoholic drinks but are upset by milk products and fatty meals. They harbour deep insecurity and fear being left alone, illness resulting in madness and loss of their material possessions and wealth. One physical attribute is that they often have a brown mark in the shape of a saddle across the bridge of the nose.

Silicea terra
Silicea; silica.

Silica is one of the main rock-forming minerals and is also found in living things where its main function is to confer strength and resilience. In homeopathy, it is used to treat disorders of the skin, nails and bones and recurring inflammations and infections, especially those that occur because the person is somewhat run-down or has an inadequate diet. Also, some disorders of the nervous system are relieved by silicea. The homeopathic remedy used to be derived from ground flint or quartz but is now prepared by chemical reaction. The remedy is used for catarrhal infections such as colds, influenza, sinusitis, ear infections including glue ear. Also, for inflammations producing pus such as a boil, carbuncle, abscess, stye, whitlow (infection of the

finger nail) and peritonsillar abscess. It is beneficial in helping the natural expulsion of a foreign body such as a splinter in the skin. It is a remedy for a headache beginning at the back of the head and radiating forwards over the right eye and for stress-related conditions of over-work and sleeplessness.

Symptoms are worse for cold, wet weather, especially when clothing is inadequate, draughts, swimming and bathing, becoming chilled after removing clothes and in the morning. They are better for warmth and heat, summer weather, warm clothing, particularly a hat or head covering and not lying on the left side. People who are suitable for silicea tend to be thin with a fine build and pale skin. They often have thin, straight hair. They are prone to dry, cracked skin and nails and may suffer from skin infections. Silicea people are usually unassuming, and lacking in confidence and physical stamina. They are conscientious and hard-working to the point of working too hard once a task has been undertaken. However, they may hesitate to commit themselves through lack of confidence and fear of responsibility. Silicea people are tidy and obsessive about small details. They may feel 'put upon', but lack the courage to speak out, and may take this out on others who are not responsible for the situation. They fear failure and dislike exercise due to physical weakness, often feeling mentally and physically exhausted. They enjoy cold foods and drinks.

Sulphur
Sulphur; flowers of sulphur, brimstone.

Sulphur has a long history of use in medicine going back to very ancient times. Sulphur gives off sulphur dioxide when burnt, which smells unpleasant ('rotten eggs' odour) but acts as a disinfectant. This was used in medieval times to limit the spread of infectious diseases. Sulphur is deposited around the edges of hot springs and geysers and where there is volcanic activity. Flowers of sulphur, which is a bright yellow powder, is obtained from the natural mineral deposit and is used to make the homeopathic remedy. Sulphur is found naturally in all body tissues and, in both orthodox medicine and homeopathy, is used to treat skin disorders. It is a useful remedy for dermatitis, eczema, psoriasis and a dry, flaky, itchy skin or scalp. Some digestive disorders benefit from sulphur especially a tendency for food to rise back up to the mouth and indigestion caused by drinking milk. Sulphur is helpful in the treatment of haemorrhoids or piles, premenstrual and menopausal symptoms, eye inflammations such as conjunctivitis, pain in the lower part of the back, catarrhal colds and coughs, migraine headaches and feverish symptoms. Some mental symptoms are helped by this remedy particularly those brought about by stress or worry including depression, irritability, insomnia and lethargy. When ill, people who benefit from sulphur feel thirsty rather than hungry and are upset by unpleasant smells. The person soon becomes exhausted and usually sleeps poorly at night and is tired through the day. The symptoms are worse in cold, damp conditions, in the middle of the morning around 11 a.m. and in stuffy, hot, airless rooms. Also, for becoming too hot at night in bed and for wearing too many layers of clothes. Long periods of standing and sitting aggravate the symptoms and they are worse if the person drinks alcohol or has a wash. Symptoms improve in dry, clear, warm weather and for taking exercise. They are better if the person lies on the right side.

Sulphur people tend to look rather untidy and have dry, flaky skin and coarse, rough hair. They may be thin, round-shouldered and inclined to slouch or be overweight, round and red-faced. Sulphur people have lively, intelligent minds full of schemes and inventions, but are often useless on a practical level. They may be somewhat self-centred with a need to be praised, and fussy over small unimportant details. They enjoy intellectual discussion on subjects that they find interesting and may become quite heated although the anger soon subsides. Sulphur people are often warm and generous with their time and money. They enjoy a wide range of foods but are upset by milk and eggs. They have a fear of being a failure in their work, of heights and the supernatural.

Additional homeopathic medicines in common use

Aconitum nepalese (aconite, monkshood, wolfsbane, friar's cap, mousebane)

Actea racemosa (black snakeroot, rattleroot, bugbane, rattleweed, squaw root)

Allium (Spanish onion)

Apis mellifica (the honey bee)

Arnica montana (arnica; leopard's bane, sneezewort)

Atropa belladonna (belladonna; deadly nightshade, black cherry, devil's cherries, naughty man's cherries, devil's herb)

Aurum metallicum (aurum met; gold)

Bryonia alba (bryonia; European white bryony, black-berried white bryony, wild hops)

Calcarea fluorica (calc. fluor; fluorite, calcium fluoride, fluoride of lime)

Calcarea phosphorica (calc. phos; phosphate of lime, calcium phosphate)

Calendula officinalis (calendula; marigold, garden marigold)

Cantharis vesicatoria (cantharis; Spanish fly)

Carbo vegetablis (carbo veg; vegetable charcoal)

Chamomilla (chamomile; common chamomile, double chamomile)

China officinalis (cinchona succiruba; china, Peruvian bark, Jesuit's bark)

Citrullus colocynthus (colocynthis; bitter cucumber, bitter apple)

Cuprum metallicum (cuprum met; copper)

Daphne mezereum (daphne; spurge laurel, wild pepper, spurge olive, flowering spurge, dwarf bay)

Drosera rotundifolia (drosera; sundew, youthwort, red rot, moor grass)

Euphrasia officinalis (euphrasia; eyebright)

Ferrum phosphoricum (ferrum phos; phosphate of iron, iron phosphate)

Gelsemium sempervirens (gelsemium; yellow jasmine, false jasmine, Carolina jasmine, wild woodbine)

Guaiacum offinale (guaiac; resin of lignum vitae)

Hamamelis virginiana hamamelis (witch hazel; spotted alder, snapping hazelnut, winterbloom)

Hepar sulphuris calcareum (hepar sulph; sulphide of calcium)

Hypericum perforatum (hypericum, St John's wort)

Ipecacuanha (ipecac; cephalis ipecacuanha, psychotria ipeca-cuanha, the ipecac plant)

Kalium bichromicum (kali bich; potassium dichromate, potassium bichromate)

Kalium iodatum (kali iod; kali hydriodicum, potassium iodide)

Kalium phosphoricum (kali phos; potassium phosphate, phosphate of potash)

Ledum palustre (ledum; marsh tea, wild rosemary)

Rhus toxicodendron (rhus tox; rhus radicaris, American poison ivy, poison oak, poison vine)

Ruta graveolens (ruta grav; rue, garden rue, herbygrass, ave-grace, herb-of-grace, bitter herb)

Tarentula cubensis (tarentula cub; Cuban tarentula)

Thuja occidentalis (thuja; tree of life, yellow cedar, arbor vitae, false white cedar)

Urtica urens (urtica; stinging nettle)

Glossary of terms used in homeopathy

aggravations a term first used by Dr Samuel Hahnemann to describe an initial worsening of symptoms experienced by some patients, on first taking a homeopathic remedy, before the condition improved. In modern homeopathy this is known as a'healing crisis'. To prevent the occurrence of aggravations, Hahnemann experimented with further dilutions of remedies and, in particular, vigorous shaking (succussing) of preparations at each stage of the process.

allopathy a term first used by Dr Samuel Hahnemann meaning 'against disease'. It describes the approach of conventional medicine, which is to treat symptoms with a substance or drug with an opposite effect in order to suppress or eliminate them. This is called the Law of Contraries and is in direct contrast to the 'like can cure like,' the Law of Similars or *Similia Similibus Curentur* principle, which is central to the practice of homeopathy.

centesimal scale of dilution the scale of dilution used in homeopathy based on one part (or drop) of the remedy in 99 parts of the diluent liquid (a mixture of alcohol and water).

classical the practice of homeopathy based on the work of Dr Samuel Hahnemann and further developed and expanded by other practitioners, particularly Dr Constantine Hering and Dr James Tyler Kent.

constitutional prescribing and constitutional types the homeopathic concept, based on the work of Dr James Tyler Kent, that prescribing should be based on the complete make-up of a person, including physical and emotional characteristics, as well as on the symptoms of a disorder.

decimal scale of dilution the scale of dilution used in homeopathy based on one part (or drop) of the remedy in nine parts of the diluent liquid (a mixture of alcohol and water).

healing crisis the situation in which a group of symptoms first become worse after a person has taken a homeopathic remedy, before they improve and disappear. The occurrence of a healing crisis is taken to indicate a change and that improvement is likely to follow. It is usually short-lived, (*see also* aggravations).

homeopathy the system of healing based on the principle of 'like can cure like' and given its name by Samuel Hahnemann. The word is derived from the Greek *homeo* for similar and *pathos* for suffering, or 'like disease'.

laws of cure, law of direction of cure three concepts or 'laws' formulated by Dr Constantine Hering to explain the means by which symptoms of disease are eliminated from the body in homeopathy.

1. Symptoms move in a downwards direction.
2. Symptoms move from the inside of the body outwards.
3. Symptoms move from more important vital organs and tissues to those of less importance.

Herin g was also responsible for the view in homeopathy that more recent symptoms disappear first before ones that have been present for a longer time. Hence symptoms are eliminated in the reverse order of their appearance.

materia medica detailed information about homeopathic remedies, listed alphabetically and includes details of the symptoms that may respond to each remedy, based on previous research and experience. Details about the source of each remedy are also included. This information is used by a homeopathic doctor when deciding upon the best remedy for each particular patient and group of symptoms.

miasm a chronic constitutional weakness that is the aftereffect of an underlying suppressed disease that has been present in a previous generation or earlier in the life of an individual. The concept of miasm was formulated by Samuel Hahnemann who noted that some people were never truly healthy but always acquired new symptoms of illness. He believed that this was due to a constitutional weakness that he called a miasm, which may have been inherited and was caused by an illness in a previous generation. These theories were put forward in his research writings entitled *Chronic Diseases*. Three main miasms were identified, psora, sycosis and syphilis.

modalities a term applied to the responses of the patient, when he or she feels better or worse, depending upon factors in the internal and external environment. These are unique from one person to another depending upon the individual characteristics that apply at the time, although there are common features within each constitutional type. Modalities include responses, fears and preferences to temperature, weather, foods, emotional responses and relationships, etc, which all contribute to a person's total sense of wellbeing. Modalities are particularly important when a person has symptoms of an illness in prescribing the most beneficial remedy.

mother tincture (symbol O) the first solution obtained from dissolving a substance in a mixture of alcohol and water (usually in the ratio of $9/_{10}$ pure alcohol to $1/_{10}$ distilled water). The mother tincture is subjected to further dilutions and succussions (shakings) to produce the homeopathic remedies.

nosode a term used to describe a remedy prepared from samples of infected diseased tissue, often to treat or prevent a particular illness. They were first investigated by Wilhelm Lux, not without considerable controversy. Examples are *Medorrhinum and Tuberculinum*.

organon *The Organon of Rationale Medicine*. One of the most important works of Samuel Hahnemann, published in Leipzig in 1810, in which he set out the principles and philosophy of modern homeopathy. The *Organon* is considered to be a classic work and basic to the study of homeopathy.

polycrest a remedy suitable for a number of illnesses, disorders or symptoms.

potency the dilution or strength of a homeopathic remedy. Dr Samuel Hahnemann discovered that by further diluting and succussing (shaking) a remedy, it became more effective or potent in bringing about a cure. It is held that the process of diluting and shaking a remedy releases its innate energy or dynamism, even though none of the original molecules of the substance may remain. Hence the greater the dilution of a remedy, the stronger or more potent it becomes. Hahnemann called his new dilute solutions 'potentizations'.

potentiate the release or transfer of energy into a homeopathic solution by succussing or vigorous shaking of the mixture.

principle of vital force 'vital force' was the term given by Samuel Hahnemann to the inbuilt power or ability of the human body to maintain health and fitness and to fight off illness. Illness is believed to be the result of stresses that cause an imbalance in the vital force, and assail all people throughout life and include inherited, environmental and emotional factors. The symptom of this 'disorder' is illness, and this is held to be the physical indication of the struggle of the body's vital force to regain its balance. A person with a strong vital force will tend to remain in good health and to fight off illness. A person with a weak vital force is more likely to suffer from long-term, recurrent symptoms and illnesses. Homoeopathic remedies are believed to act upon the vital force, stimulating it to heal the body and restore the natural balance.

provings the term given by Samuel Hahnemann to experimental trials he carried out to test the reactions of healthy people to homeopathic substances. These trials were carried out under strictly controlled conditions (in advance of the modern scientific approach), and the symptoms produced were meticulously recorded. Quinine was the substance that Hahnemann first investigated in this way, testing it initially on himself and then on close friends and family members. He continued over the next few years to investigate and prove many other substances, building up a wealth of information on each one about the reactions and symptoms it produced. After conducting this research, Hahnemann went on carefully to prescribe the remedies to those who were sick. Provings are still carried out in modern homeopathy to test new

substances that may be of value as remedies. Usually, neither the prescribing physician nor those taking the substance—the 'provers'—know the identity of the material or whether they are taking a placebo.

psora one of three miasms identified by Samuel Hahnemann believed to be caused by suppression of scabies. Psora was believed to have an inherited element or to be caused by suppression of an earlier infection in a particular individual.

Schussler tissue salts Wilhelm Heinrich Schussler was a German homeopathic doctor who introduced the Biochemic Tissue Salt system in the late 1800s. Schussler believed that many symptoms and ailments resulted from the lack of a minute, but essential, quantity of a mineral or tissue salt. He identified twelve such tissue salts that he regarded as essential and believed that a cure could be obtained from replacing the deficient substance. Schussler's work was largely concentrated at the cell and tissue level rather than embracing the holistic view of homeopathy.

similia similibus curentur the founding principle of homeopathy that 'like can cure like' or 'let like be treated by like', which was first put forward by Hippocrates, a physician of ancient Greece. This principle excited the interest of Paracelsus in the Middle Ages, and was later restated and put into practice by Samuel Hahnemann with the development of homeopathy.

simillimum a homeopathic remedy that in its natural state is able to produce the same symptoms as those being exhibited by the patient.

succussion vigorous shaking of a homeopathic remedy at each stage of dilution, along with banging the container and holding it against a hard surface, therebycausing further release of energy.

sycosis one of the three major miasms identified by Samuel Hahnemann and believed to result from a suppressed gonorrhoeal infection. Sycosis was believed to have an inherited element or to be due to suppression of an earlier infection in a particular individual.

syphilis the third of the three major miasms identified by Samuel Hahnemann believed to result from a suppressed syphilis infection. Syphilis was believed to have an inherited element or to be due to suppression of an earlier infection in a particular individual.

trituration the process, devised by Samuel Hahnemann, of rendering naturally insoluble substances soluble so that they can be made available as homeopathic remedies. The process involves repeated grinding down of the substance with lactose powder until it becomes soluble. The substance usually becomes soluble at the third process of trituration. Each trituration is taken to be the equivalent of one dilution in the centesimal scale. Once the substance has been rendered soluble, dilution can proceed in the normal way.

Massage

As long ago as 3000 BC massage was used as a therapy in the Far East, making it one of the most ancient treatments used by the human race. In 5 BC in ancient Greece, Hippocrates recommended that to maintain health a massage using oils should be taken daily after a perfumed bath. The physicians there were well used to treating people who suffered from pain and stiffness in the joints.

Massage increased in popularity when, in the 19th century, Per Henrik Ling, a Swedish athlete, created the basis for what is now known as Swedish massage. Swedish massage is a combination of relaxing effects and exercises that work on the joints and muscles, but it is still based on the form that was practised in ancient times. More recently, a work was published by George Downing in the 1970s called *The Massage Book,* and this introduced a new concept in the overall technique of massage, that the whole person's state should be assessed by the therapist and not solely the physical side. The emotional and mental states should be part of the overall picture. Also combined in his form of massage were the methods used in reflexology and shiatsu, and this was known as therapeutic massage. The aim of this is to use relaxation, stimulation and invigoration to promote good health.

This massage is commonly used to induce general relaxation, so that any tension or strain experienced in the rush of daily life can be eased and eliminated. It is found to be very effective, working on the mind as well as the body. It can be used to treat people with hypertension (high blood pressure), sinusitis, headaches, insomnia and hyperactivity, including people who suffer from heart ailments or circulatory disorders. At the physical level, massage is intended to help the body make use of food and to eliminate the waste materials, as well as stimulating the nervous and muscular system and the circulation of blood. Neck and back pain are conditions from which many people suffer, particularly if they have not been sitting correctly, such as in a slightly stooped position with their shoulders rounded. People whose day-to-day work involves a great deal of physical activity, such as dancers and athletes, can also derive a great deal of benefit from the use of massage. Stiffness can be a problem that they have after training or working, and this is relieved by encouraging the toxins that gather in the muscles to disperse. Massage promotes a feeling of calmness and serenity, and this is particularly beneficial to people who frequently suffer from bouts of depression or anxiety. Once the worry and depression have been dispelled, people are able to deal with their problems much more effectively and, being able to do so, will boost their self-confidence.

In hospitals, massage has been used to ease pain and discomfort as well as being of benefit to people who are bedridden, since the flow of blood to the muscles is stimulated. It has also been used for those who have suffered a heart attack and has helped their recovery. A more recent development has been the use of massage for cancer patients who are suffering from the after-effects of treatment, such as chemotherapy, as well as the discomfort the disease itself causes. Indeed, there are few conditions when it is not recommended. However, it should not be used when people are suffering from inflammation of the veins (phlebitis), varicose veins, thrombosis (clots in the blood) or if they have a raised temperature such as occurs during a fever. It is then advisable to contact a doctor before using massage. Doctors may be able to recommend a qualified therapist, a health centre may be able to help or contact can be made with the relevant professional body.

It is quite usual nowadays for a masseur or masseuse to combine treatment with the use of other methods, such as aromatherapy, acupuncture or reflexology. Massage can be divided into four basic forms, and these are known as *percussion* (also known as drumming); *friction* (also called pressure); *effleurage* (also called stroking) and *petrissage* (also called kneading). These four methods can be practised alone or in combination for maximum benefit to the patient. Massage is a therapy in which both parties derive an overall feeling of wellbeing—the therapist by the skilful use of the hands to impart the relaxation, and the patient through the therapy being administered.

Percussion is also called tapotement, which is derived from *tapoter*, a French word that means 'to drum', as of the fingers on a surface. As would be expected from its name, percussion is generally done with the edge of the hand with a quick, chopping movement, although the strokes are not hard. This type of movement would be used on places like the buttocks, thighs, waist or shoulders where there is a wide expanse of flesh.

Friction is often used on dancers and athletes who experience problems with damaged ligaments or tendons. This is because the flow of blood is stimulated and the movement of joints is improved. Friction can be performed with the base of the hand, some fingers or the upper part of the thumb. It is not advisable to use this method on parts of the body that have been injured in some way, for example where there is bruising.

Effleurage is performed in a slow, controlled manner using both hands together with a small space between the thumbs. If the therapist wishes to use only light pressure he or she will use the palms of the hands or the tips of the fingers, whilst for increased pressure the knuckles or thumbs will be used.

Petrissage employs a kneading action on parts of a muscle. As the therapist works across each section, an area of flesh is grasped and squeezed, and this action stimulates the flow of blood and enables tensed muscles to relax. People such as athletes can have an accumulation of lactic acid in certain muscles, and this is why cramp occurs. Parts of the body on which this method is practised are along the stomach and around the waist.

A session may be undertaken in the patient's home, or he or she can attend the masseur or masseuse at a clinic. At each session the client will undress, leaving only pants or briefs on, and will lie on a firm, comfortable surface, such as a table that is designed especially for massage. The massage that follows normally lasts from 20 minutes to one hour. Women in labour have found that the pain experienced during childbirth can be eased if massage is performed on the buttocks and back. The massage eases the build-up of tension in the muscles, encouraging relaxation and easing of labour pains. It is said to be more effective on women who had previously experienced the benefits and reassurance of massage.

For anyone who is competent and wishes to provide some simple massage for a partner, there are some basic rules to follow. The room should be warm and peaceful. The surface on which the person lies is quite comfortable but firm. A futon (a quilted Japanese mattress) can be used, and to relieve the upper part of the body from any possible discomfort, a pillow should be placed underneath the torso. Any pressure that may be exerted on the feet can be dispelled by the use of a rolled-up towel or similar placed beneath the ankles. Both people should be relaxed, and to this end soft music can be played. All the movements of the hand should be of a continuous nature. It is suggested that the recipient always has one hand of the masseur or masseuse placed on him or her. Vegetable oil (about one teaspoonful) is suitable but should not be poured straight on to the person. It should be spread over the hands by rubbing, which will also warm it sufficiently for use. Should the masseur or masseuse get out of breath, he or she should stop for a rest, all the while retaining a hand on the person.

Massage of the head and face begins with the forehead, which should be massaged using the thumbs. This is done by stroking them outwards from the centre across the forehead. This can also be repeated for the cheeks. The jawline can then be squeezed along its full extent using the thumb and forefinger in a circular motion.

The head can be massaged by all the fingers using a circular motion. Whilst the person's head is being supported at the side, the muscles in the neck can be gently massaged, commencing at the top and moving downwards. To exercise the upper chest or pectoral muscles, move the base of the hands from the sternum (breastbone) outwards across these muscles. Both hands can be used to work upwards and also across the stomach area. Once the hands have moved across so that they are under the person's waist, raise the body slightly, thus stretching it. Another technique for the abdominal area is to glide the hands across but moving in opposite ways. The arm can be massaged by the fingers and thumb and then the fingers can be pressed and gently pulled, with the wrist being held at all times.

Effleurage (as described previously) can be used on the upper leg as far up as the hip on the outside of the leg. Once the person is lying face downwards (with support under the chest), continue to use effleurage movements on the back of the lower leg. Continue as before but work on the upper leg, avoiding the knee. The muscles in the buttocks can be worked upon with both hands to squeeze but making sure that the hands are moving in opposite ways. The foot will benefit from massage using the thumb in small circular movements. For a person suffering from stress or being 'on edge' at the end of a day's work, a back massage can help to ease these problems. With the hands in the position for using effleurage, start the movements at the lowest part of the back and work up and then sideways to the shoulders. The pressure used should be kept up, but as soon as the hands move downwards it should be released. This should be repeated so that all of the back is massaged. Next, using the palms of both hands, work on the top of the shoulder by moving the hands in opposite directions. If the right shoulder is being massaged, the person's head should be turned to the left. The area beside the spine can be massaged, although one should avoid the spinal column. Using both thumbs, one on each side of the spine itself, massage this area by pressing gently in a circle.

Massage has a wide range of uses for a variety of disorders. Its strengths lie in the easing of strain and tension and inducing relaxation and serenity, plus the physical contact of the therapist. Although doctors make use of this therapy in conjunction with orthodox medicine, it is not to be regarded as a cure for diseases in itself and serious problems could occur if this were the case.